Procedures

Chapter 2: The Professional Medical Assistant
Procedure 2-1: Locating and Defining a State's Legal Scope of Practice

Chapter 3: Ethics and Law for the Medical Office
Procedure 3-1: Separating Personal and Professional Ethics
Procedure 3-2: Incorporating the Patient's Bill of Rights
Procedure 3-3: Reporting Illegal Activities and Complying with Public Health Statutes

Chapter 4: Interacting with Patients
Procedure 4-1: Demonstrating Effective and Respectful Verbal and Nonverbal Communication
Procedure 4-2: Maintaining Boundaries and Demonstrating Respect for Boundaries in Communications

Chapter 17: Medical Asepsis and the OSHA Standard
Procedure 17-1: Handwashing
Procedure 17-2: Applying an Alcohol-Based Hand Rub
Procedure 17-3: Application and Removal of Clean Disposable Gloves

Chapter 18: Sterilization and Disinfection
Procedure 18-1: Sanitization of Instruments
Procedure 18-2: Wrapping Instruments Using Paper or Muslin
Procedure 18-3: Wrapping Instruments Using a Pouch
Procedure 18-4: Sterilizing Articles in the Autoclave

Chapter 19: Vital Signs
Procedure 19-1: Measuring Oral Body Temperature—Electronic Thermometer
Procedure 19-2: Measuring Axillary Body Temperature—Electronic Thermometer
Procedure 19-3: Measuring Rectal Body Temperature—Electronic Thermometer
Procedure 19-4: Measuring Aural Body Temperature—Tympanic Membrane Thermometer
Procedure 19-5: Measuring Temporal Artery Body Temperature
Procedure 19-6: Measuring Pulse and Respiration
Procedure 19-7: Measuring Apical Pulse
Procedure 19-8: Performing Pulse Oximetry
Procedure 19-9: Measuring Blood Pressure
Procedure 19-10: Determining Systolic Pressure by Palpation

Chapter 20: The Physical Examination
Procedure 20-1: Measuring Weight and Height
Procedure 20-2: Sitting Position
Procedure 20-3: Supine Position
Procedure 20-4: Prone Position
Procedure 20-5: Dorsal Recumbent Position
Procedure 20-6: Lithotomy Position
Procedure 20-7: Sims Position
Procedure 20-8: Knee-Chest Position
Procedure 20-9: Fowler Position
Procedure 20-10: Wheelchair Transfer
Procedure 20-11: Assisting with the Physical Examination

Chapter 21: Eye and Ear Assessment and Procedures
Procedure 21-1: Assessing Distance Visual Acuity—Snellen Chart
Procedure 21-2: Assessing Color Vision—Ishihara Test
Procedure 21-3: Performing an Eye Irrigation
Procedure 21-4: Performing an Eye Instillation
Procedure 21-5: Performing an Ear Irrigation
Procedure 21-6: Performing an Ear Instillation

Chapter 22: Physical Agents to Promote Tissue Healing
Procedure 22-1: Applying a Heating Pad
Procedure 22-2: Applying a Hot Soak
Procedure 22-3: Applying a Hot Compress
Procedure 22-4: Applying an Ice Bag
Procedure 22-5: Applying a Cold Compress
Procedure 22-6: Applying a Chemical Pack
Procedure 22-7: Measuring for Axillary Crutches
Procedure 22-8: Instructing a Patient in Crutch Gaits

Procedure 22-9: Instructing a Patient in the Use of a Cane
Procedure 22-10: Instructing a Patient in the Use of a Walker

Chapter 23: The Gynecologic Examination and Prenatal Care
Procedure 23-1: Breast Self-Examination Instructions
Procedure 23-2: Assisting with a Gynecologic Examination
Procedure 23-3: Assisting with a Return Prenatal Examination

Chapter 24: The Pediatric Examination
Procedure 24-1: Measuring the Weight and Length of an Infant
Procedure 24-2: Measuring Head and Chest Circumference of an Infant
Procedure 24-3: Calculating Growth Percentiles
Procedure 24-4: Applying a Pediatric Urine Collector

Chapter 25: Minor Office Surgery
Procedure 25-1: Applying and Removing Sterile Gloves
Procedure 25-2: Opening a Sterile Package
Procedure 25-3: Pouring a Sterile Solution
Procedure 25-4: Changing a Sterile Dressing
Procedure 25-5: Removing Sutures and Staples
Procedure 25-6: Applying and Removing Adhesive Skin Closures
Procedure 25-7: Assisting with Minor Office Surgery

Chapter 26: Administration of Medication and Intravenous Therapy
Procedure 26-1: Administering Oral Medication
Procedure 26-2: Preparing an Injection
Procedure 26-3: Reconstituting Powdered Drugs
Procedure 26-4: Administering a Subcutaneous Injection
Procedure 26-5: Administering an Intramuscular Injection
Procedure 26-6: Z-Track Intramuscular Injection Technique
Procedure 26-7: Administering an Intradermal Injection

Chapter 27: Cardiopulmonary Procedures
Procedure 27-1: Running a 12-Lead, Three-Channel Electrocardiogram
Procedure 27-2: Measuring Peak Flow Rate

Chapter 28: Specialty Examinations and Procedures: Colon Procedures, Male Reproductive Health, and Radiology and Diagnostic Imaging
Procedure 28-1: Fecal Occult Blood Testing: Guaiac Slide Test
Procedure 28-2: Developing the Hemoccult Slide Test

Chapter 30: Urinalysis
Procedure 30-1: Clean-Catch Midstream Specimen Collection Instructions
Procedure 30-2: Chemical Testing of Urine with the Multistix 10 SG Reagent Strip
Procedure 30-3: Prepare a Urine Specimen for Microscopic Examination: Kova Method
Procedure 30-4: Performing a Urine Pregnancy Test

Chapter 31: Phlebotomy
Procedure 31-1: Venipuncture—Vacuum Tube Method
Procedure 31-2: Venipuncture—Butterfly Method
Procedure 31-3: Skin Puncture—Disposable Semiautomatic Lancet Device

Chapter 32: Hematology
Procedure 32-1: Hematocrit
Procedure 32-2: Preparation of a Blood Smear for a Differential Cell Count

Chapter 33: Blood Chemistry and Immunology
Procedure 33-1: Blood Glucose Measurement Using the Accu-Chek Advantage Glucose Meter

Chapter 34: Medical Microbiology
Procedure 34-1: Using the Microscope
Procedure 34-2: Collecting a Throat Specimen

Chapter 36: Emergency Preparedness and Protective Practices
Procedure 36-1: Demonstrating Proper Use of a Fire Extinguisher
Procedure 36-2: Participating in a Mock Exposure Event

Chapter 38: The Medical Record
Procedure 38-1: Completion of a Procedure Consent Form
Procedure 38-2: Release of Medical Information

Procedure 38-3: Obtaining Patient History and Formulating Chief Complaint

Chapter 39: Patient Reception
Procedure 39-1: Opening the Medical Office
Procedure 39-2: Closing the Medical Office
Procedure 39-3: Obtaining New Patient Information
Procedure 39-4: Explaining Office Policies and Procedures

Chapter 41: Telephone Techniques
Procedure 41-1: Performing Telephone Screening
Procedure 41-2: Taking a Telephone Message
Procedure 41-3: Taking Requests for Medication or Prescription Refills
Procedure 41-4: Telephoning a Patient for Follow-Up

Chapter 42: Scheduling Appointments
Procedure 42-1: Setting up the Appointment Schedule
Procedure 42-2: Making an Appointment
Procedure 42-3: Managing the Appointment Schedule
Procedure 42-4: Scheduling Inpatient or Outpatient Diagnostic Tests or Procedures
Procedure 42-5: Scheduling Inpatient or Outpatient Admissions

Chapter 43: Medical Record Management
Procedure 43-1: Preparing a Medical Record
Procedure 43-2: Filing Patient Records: Alphabetic
Procedure 43-3: Filing Patient Records: Numeric
Procedure 43-4: Filing Reports

Chapter 44: Written Communications
Procedure 44-1: Composing a Business Letter
Procedure 44-2: Sending a Fax

Chapter 45: Mail
Procedure 45-1: Processing Incoming Mail
Procedure 45-2: Looking Up a ZIP code
Procedure 45-3: Preparing Envelopes for Mailing

Chapter 46: Managing Practice Finances
Procedure 46-1: Completing a Patient Charge Slip
Procedure 46-2: Posting Charges
Procedure 46-3: Posting Payments and/or Adjustments
Procedure 46-4: Writing a Check
Procedure 46-5: Preparing a Bank Deposit

Chapter 47: Medical Coding
Procedure 47-1: Performing CPT Coding
Procedure 47-2: Performing HCPCS Coding
Procedure 47-3: Performing ICD Coding

Chapter 48: Medical Insurance
Procedure 48-1: Interpreting Information on an Insurance Card
Procedure 48-2: Verifying Insurance Eligibility and Benefits
Procedure 48-3: Obtaining Insurance Preauthorization (Precertification)
Procedure 48-4: Completing and Reviewing an Insurance Claim Form
Procedure 48-5: Communicating Effectively Regarding Insurance and/or Managed Care

Chapter 49: Billing and Collections
Procedure 49-1: Processing Patient Statements
Procedure 49-2: Posting a Check Returned for Non-sufficient Funds (NSF)
Procedure 49-3: Processing a Credit Balance and Refund
Procedure 49-4: Creating and Examining an Accounts Receivable Aging Record
Procedure 49-5: Writing a Collection Letter

Chapter 50: The Medical Assistant as Office Manager
Procedure 50-1: Creating an Environmental Checklist and Performing a Safety Inspection
Procedure 50-2: Complying with Safety Signs, Symbols, and Labels
Procedure 50-3: Performing Routine Maintenance of Equipment
Procedure 50-4: Taking a Supply or Equipment Inventory
Procedure 50-5: Locating and Facilitating Referrals to Community Resources
Procedure 50-6: Completing an Incident Report

TODAY'S
MEDICAL
ASSISTANT

THIRD EDITION

THIRD EDITION

TODAY'S MEDICAL ASSISTANT

Clinical & Administrative Procedures

Kathy Bonewit-West, BS, MEd
Coordinator and Instructor
Medical Assistant Technology
Hocking College
Nelsonville, Ohio
Former Member, Curriculum Review
    Board of the American Association
    of Medical Assistants

Sue A. Hunt, MA, RN, CMA (AAMA)
Professor Emeritus
Medical Assisting Program
Middlesex Community College
Lowell, Massachusetts

Edith Applegate, MS
Professor of Biological Sciences
Kettering College of Medical Arts
Kettering, Ohio

ELSEVIER

ELSEVIER

3251 Riverport Lane
St. Louis, Missouri 63043

Notices

Knowledge and best practice in this field are constantly changing. As new research and experience broaden our understanding, changes in research methods, professional practices, or medical treatment may become necessary.

Practitioners and researchers must always rely on their own experience and knowledge in evaluating and using any information, methods, compounds, or experiments described herein. In using such information or methods they should be mindful of their own safety and the safety of others, including parties for whom they have a professional responsibility.

With respect to any drug or pharmaceutical products identified, readers are advised to check the most current information provided (i) on procedures featured or (ii) by the manufacturer of each product to be administered, to verify the recommended dose or formula, the method and duration of administration, and contraindications. It is the responsibility of practitioners, relying on their own experience and knowledge of their patients, to make diagnoses, to determine dosages and the best treatment for each individual patient, and to take all appropriate safety precautions.

To the fullest extent of the law, neither the Publisher nor the authors, contributors, or editors, assume any liability for any injury and/or damage to persons or property as a matter of products liability, negligence or otherwise, or from any use or operation of any methods, products, instructions, or ideas contained in the material herein.

Previous editions copyrighted 2013 and 2009.

International Standard Book Number: 978-0-323-31127-4

Executive Content Strategist: Jennifer Janson
Content Development Manager: Luke Held
Senior Content Development Specialist: Jennifer Bertucci
Publishing Services Manager: Julie Eddy
Book Production Specialist: Celeste Clingan
Design Direction: Maggie Reid

Printed in Canada

Last digit is the print number: 9 8 7 6 5

Working together
to grow libraries in
developing countries

www.elsevier.com • www.bookaid.org

For Marlene,
Thank you for being you. You gently reach out and touch the lives of many with grace and
compassion, making our world a better place. But above it all, I want to thank you for
the privilege of being able to call you my best friend.
KBW

For Melissa
Thank you for your support
SH

For Stan—my best friend and husband for over 55 years
You are the GPS in my life
EA

Reviewers

Karen Dennis, LVN, CMA (AAMA)
Medical Assistant Clinical
ABC Adult School
Cerritos, California

Linda Dente, BS, CMA (AAMA)
Program Director, Medical Assisting Program
Massasoit Community College
Canton, Massachusetts

Pat DeVoy, EdS, LPN, RHIT, CMA (AAMA)
Faculty
Davenport University
Warren, Michigan

Starra Herring, BSAH, BSHS, CMA (AAMA), AHI
Medical Assisting Program Director; Practicum
    Coordinator
Stanly Community College
Locusts, North Carolina

Jeanne Lawo, RN, MSN
Clinical Manager—SLUCare Practice
Saint Louis University
Saint Louis, Missouri

Nikki Marhefka, EdM, MT(ASCP), CMA (AAMA)
Medical Assisting Program Director
Central Penn College
Summerdale, Pennsylvania

Brigitte Niedzwiecki, RN, BSN
Medical Assisting Program Director
Chippewa Valley Technical College
Eau Claire, Wisconsin

Julie Pepper, CMA (AAMA)
Instructor, Medical Assisting Program
Chippewa Valley Technical College
Eau Claire, Wisconsin

Judith D. Symons, MA, Voc Ed Cert
Medical Assistant
Geisinger Medical Center
Danville, Pennsylvannia

Preface

Medical assistants, for many years an integral part of most physicians' staff, now fulfill an ever-expanding and varied role in the medical office, both clinically and administratively. With increased responsibilities, however, comes a greater need for professional knowledge and skills. This text has been designed to provide the basics of administrative and clinical competency combined with background knowledge of anatomy and physiology.

The underlying principle of this book is to provide a format for the achievement of professional competency in skills performed in the medical office, and the understanding of their application to real-life or on-the-job situations. When professional competency is achieved in the classroom, less of a gap should exist between the academic world and the real world, and thus the transition from student to practicing medical assistant is made more easily.

Although the book's usefulness to students in medical assisting educational programs has been emphasized, the practicing medical assistant will also find this text helpful as a learning and reference source. The organization of the text lends itself well to individualized instruction and convenient reference use.

FEATURES IN THIS TEXTBOOK

This third edition provides up-to-date information in both the administrative and clinical areas, and it incorporates current trends in technology.

IMPORTANT UPDATES INCLUDE THE FOLLOWING:

- Information about compliance to all aspects of HIPAA in the medical office
- Current information on the OSHA Bloodborne Pathogens Standard
- New pathology tables added to anatomy and physiology chapters
- Completely updated and revamped chapter on emergency procedures and protective practices
- Updated information on the new hazard communication standard
- Revised and updated information on the new safety data sheet
- Completely new chapter on nutrition
- Modernized and updated photography throughout
- Expanded information on the Electronic Medical Record (EMR)

- Fully updated chapter on the medical record
- Up-to-date information on ICD-10 coding
- Information on the updated claim form
- Completely modernized and updated throughout to comply with general curriculum updates and industry standards
- Maps and corresponds to the updated 2014 ABHES competencies and curriculum standards, as well as the most recent CAAHEP core curriculum, content areas, and competencies.

STANDARD PEDAGOGICAL FEATURES IN THIS TEXTBOOK

Other very important features include valuable learning aids:

- **On the Web Resources** allow students to access websites containing additional information relating to the chapter.

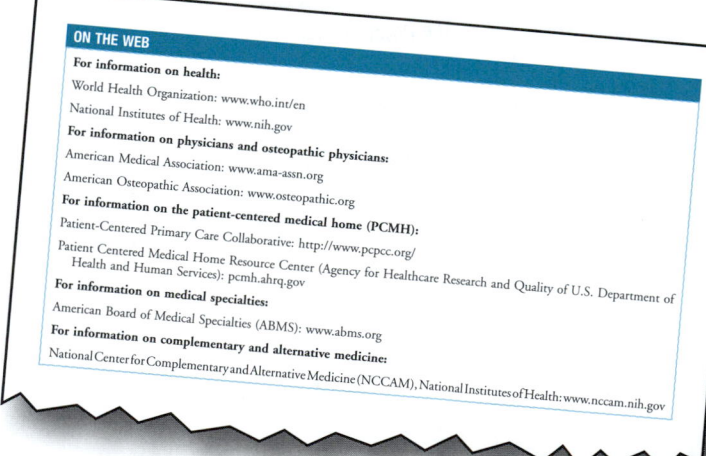

ON THE WEB

For information on health:
World Health Organization: www.who.int/en
National Institutes of Health: www.nih.gov

For information on physicians and osteopathic physicians:
American Medical Association: www.ama-assn.org
American Osteopathic Association: www.osteopathic.org

For information on the patient-centered medical home (PCMH):
Patient-Centered Primary Care Collaborative: http://www.pcpcc.org/
Patient Centered Medical Home Resource Center (Agency for Healthcare Research and Quality of U.S. Department of Health and Human Services): pcmh.ahrq.gov

For information on medical specialties:
American Board of Medical Specialties (ABMS): www.abms.org

For information on complementary and alternative medicine:
National Center for Complementary and Alternative Medicine (NCCAM), National Institutes of Health: www.nccam.nih.gov

- The organizational format of this textbook facilitates the learning process by providing students and educators with detailed objectives and an in-depth study of the most current and up-to-date administrative and clinical procedures performed in the medical office. Presented at the beginning of each chapter are **Learning Objectives** and related **Procedures,** a **Chapter Outline,** and **Key Terms.** The learning objectives address the cognitive knowledge required to perform the procedures. Procedures coincide with the objectives to delineate the task or skill to be mastered by the student. (In the student Study Guide, most procedures are expanded into detailed performance objectives, including outcomes, and conditions and standards of acceptable performance.) The chapter outline provides a quick reference of the cognitive knowledge included in that chapter. The Key Terms list designates the terms and definitions that should be mastered for each chapter.

- **Procedures** for each skill follow the theory section and are designed to help the student perform the skill with the level of competency required on the job. Each procedure is presented in an organized step-by-step format, with underlying principles and illustrations accompanying the techniques. A charting example follows each clinical procedure to provide the student with a guide for charting his or her own procedure. Where appropriate, examples of charting in the electronic medical record (EMR) are also included. Students should find it much easier to acquire competency in charting with these examples.

- The **knowledge** or **theory** that the student must acquire to perform each skill is presented in a clear and concise manner. **Numerous illustrations** accompany the theory section to aid the student in acquiring the knowledge relating to each skill.

- The unique and memorable medical assistant biographical profiles (**Memories from Practicum** and **Putting It All into Practice**) help students "connect" with their future beyond the classroom. The medical assistants featured are real people sharing their fears, likes, hopes, and aspirations, providing a "real-world" feel to the book and an inspiration for the student.

Putting It All Into Practice

My name is Sergio Martinez, and I am a Registered Medical Assistant. I work in a large clinic that is associated with a medical school. At present, I work in the family medicine department, but I also have worked in dermatology and internal medicine. Family medicine is the area I enjoy most because of the wide variety of tasks that are performed. There is rarely a dull moment.

I focus primarily on clinical medical assisting. Taking vital signs is a big part of my job responsibilities. It is routine at my clinic to take height, weight, TPR, and blood pressure on every patient seen at the clinic, no matter what the reason for his or her visit. I assist the physician with various procedures, examinations, and minor office surgery, and I administer injections, run electrocardiograms, and perform various laboratory tests.

Taking vital signs and length and weight on small children can be very challenging at times. Some children start to cry as soon as they are put on the scale. Taking a temperature on an uncooperative toddler can be very difficult. I try to calm the child as much as possible, and for good behavior, I give a lot of praise. Stickers also are a great reward for cooperative behavior. Usually when small children learn that they can trust you, they are not as frightened by the experience. It is rewarding when a child learns not to be afraid of being evaluated for routine vital signs. ■

Memories *from* Practicum

Sergio Martinez: One experience that stands out in my memory occurred during my practicum at a family practice medical office. I needed to take the blood pressure on an active 6-year-old boy. After I put the cuff on his arm, his eyes started filling up with tears. I stopped, removed the cuff, and asked him if something was wrong. He said he was afraid that when I started squeezing that thing around his arm, his hand would fall off. I sat down next to him, spent some time talking with him, and reassured him that his hand would be perfectly fine and would not fall off. I put the cuff on my own arm and pumped it up to show him that he would be safe. He then agreed to let me take his blood pressure. After I took his blood pressure, he wiggled his hand, gave me a big smile, and said that it didn't hurt at all. That situation made me realize that children may have a lot of fears about what might happen to them at the medical office. Since that experience, I always take the time to explain procedures to children before I perform them. ■

- **Patient Teaching** boxes emphasize this important aspect of the medical assistant's job and present it in context to make it more relevant, thereby making it more memorable.

PATIENT TEACHING   Acute Otitis Media

Answer questions that patients have about otitis media.

What is a middle ear infection?
An infection of the middle ear is medically referred to as *acute otitis media*. It is an inflammation of the middle ear caused by an infection and can occur in one or both ears. It is common in young children 3 months to 3 years old, but is unusual in adults. A middle ear infection is not serious if treated promptly and effectively. If not treated, however, middle ear infections can lead to serious complications, such as acute mastoiditis, meningitis, and permanent hearing loss.

What causes a middle ear infection?
A middle ear infection is often the result of an upper respiratory infection or allergy that causes the eustachian tube to swell and become blocked. The blockage causes fluid to build up in the middle ear. This fluid is an ideal place for bacteria to grow. If this occurs, the result is acute otitis media.

What are the symptoms of a middle ear infection?
The most common symptoms are intense pain, fever, and temporary hearing loss. Other symptoms may include dizziness, nausea and vomiting, and (if the eardrum ruptures) drainage from the ear.

How does the physician know whether a middle ear infection is present?
The physician examines the ears with an otoscope. If a middle ear infection is present, the eardrum is red and swollen (see illustration) as a result of irritation from the infection, and pus and mucus can be seen behind the eardrum.

How is the infection treated?
A middle ear infection is usually treated with an oral antibiotic for 10 to 14 days. It is important to take all of the antibiotic prescribed; otherwise, the ear infection may recur. The physician also may recommend a decongestant to help open the blocked eustachian tube. After the acute infection is over, fluid may remain trapped in the middle ear. This condition is known as *serous otitis media* (see illustration) and, if not treated, may last for days, weeks, months, or even a year. Although fluid in the middle ear is painless, it may result in a feeling of fullness or pressure in the ears and temporary hearing loss.

Serous otitis media. (From Swartz MH: *Textbook of physical diagnosis*, ed 5, Philadelphia, 2006, Saunders.)

- **Case Studies** are designed to assist the student in responding to "real-life" situations that occur in the medical office. A practitioner's response is given for each case study too, as a means of comparison for the student.

What Would You Do? What Would You *Not* Do? RESPONSES

Case Study 1
Page 1194

What Did Sandra Do?
☐ Explained to the patient that the original referral authorized treatment of only the lesion on the patient's neck, and the insurance carrier would not pay for other treatment without authorizing it.
☐ Explained that Sandra would contact the insurance carrier and primary care physician and take care of any required paperwork.
☐ Promised to minimize delay as much as possible.
☐ Told the patient that she would be responsible for the cost of removal if proper authorization was not obtained from her insurance carrier.

What Did Sandra Not Do?
☐ Did not assume that the referral covered additional lesions not specifically mentioned on the referral form.

☐ Did not assure the patient that her insurance would automatically cover the cost of removing the additional lesions.
☐ Did not schedule the removal of the additional lesions before she received insurance authorization or the patient promised to pay for the procedure.

Case Study 2
Page 1204

What Did Sandra Do?
☐ Explain...
covera...
that c...
☐ Asked...
birth d...
☐ Explain...
covere...
comes...

What Would You Do?   What Would You *Not* Do?

Case Study 1
Diane Bennett is a 35-year-old woman who has come to the office for treatment of a lesion on her neck. She has been referred from her primary care physician for up to three visits for consultation, diagnostic studies, and treatment. She is seen by one of the dermatologists in the practice, who recommends that the lesion be removed surgically in the office with a biopsy. During this visit the patient tells the physician that she has two other lesions she would like to have removed, one on her arm and one on her abdomen. The physician inspects the lesions and asks Sandra to contact the patient's managed care plan for authorization to treat the additional lesions. The patient says, "My physician gave me a referral to be treated by you. What's the problem? If these lesions need to be removed, I don't want any delay." ■

- **Key Terms** identified at the beginning of the chapter are defined at the end of the chapter in the **Terminology Review**, providing students with a valuable terminology overview for each chapter. The Terminology Review now contains a helpful "Word Parts" column for key terms that are easily broken down into meaningful word portions.

KEY TERMS

bacilli (bah-SILL-ie)
cocci (KOK-sie)
contagious (kon-TAE-jus)
culture
culture medium
false-negative result

incubate (IN-kyoo-bate)
incubation period
infectious disease
microbiology (mie-kroe-bie-OL-oe-jee)
mucous membrane (MYOO-kus MEM-brain)

normal flora
sequela (SEK-kwe-lah)
smear
specimen (SPESS-ih-men)
spirilla (spa-RILL-ah)

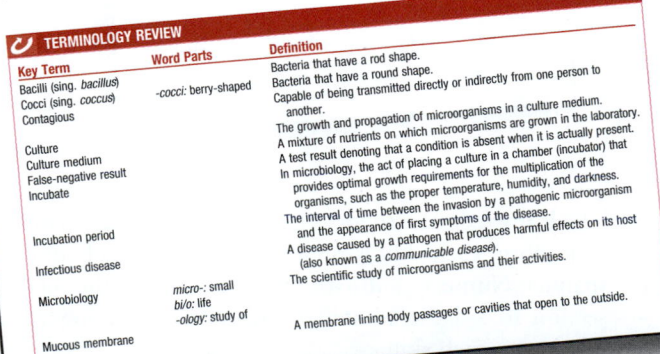

↻ TERMINOLOGY REVIEW

Key Term	Word Parts	Definition
Bacilli (sing. *bacillus*)		Bacteria that have a rod shape.
Cocci (sing. *coccus*)	-cocci: berry-shaped	Bacteria that have a round shape.
Contagious		Capable of being transmitted directly or indirectly from one person to another.
Culture		The growth and propagation of microorganisms in a culture medium.
Culture medium		A mixture of nutrients on which microorganisms are grown in the laboratory.
False-negative result		A test result denoting that a condition is absent when it is actually present.
Incubate		In microbiology, the act of placing a culture in a chamber (incubator) that provides optimal growth requirements for the multiplication of the organisms, such as the proper temperature, humidity, and darkness.
Incubation period		The interval of time between the invasion by a pathogenic microorganism and the appearance of first symptoms of the disease.
Infectious disease		A disease caused by a pathogen that produces harmful effects on its host (also known as a *communicable disease*).
Microbiology	micro-: small bi/o: life -ology: study of	The scientific study of microorganisms and their activities.
Mucous membrane		A membrane lining body passages or cavities that open to the outside.

Continuing education is of utmost importance in such a rapidly changing profession. New techniques and developments in the field of medicine have a direct influence on the medical assisting profession. Continuing education helps the medical assistant maintain and improve existing skills and learn new skills.

The authors hope that individuals who use this approach to medical assisting will view this text not as a stopping place but as a means of opening doors to new paths to be explored in the medical assisting profession.

EXTENSIVE SUPPLEMENTAL RESOURCES

PROCEDURAL VIDEOS

The most impressive feature of this textbook is the inclusion of clinical and administrative skills videos on the Evolve site, which present many of the skills outlined in the textbook. An icon ⓔ is placed within the procedural title bar of the procedures in this text that have accompanying procedural videos. Students will have the invaluable opportunity to watch these procedures at home or at school, using any computer and internet connection. This should greatly enhance the learning of these clinical and administrative skills and provide the medical assistant graduate with competence and confidence to perform clinical and administrative skills in the medical office.

EVOLVE RESOURCES

An Evolve site accompanies the textbook and is designed for students to apply the theory and skills learned throughout the textbook. Organized by chapter, the site includes Apply Your Knowledge questions (multiple-choice questions that give students an opportunity to "apply the knowledge" they learned in that particular chapter), **Procedure Videos, Video Evaluations** (True/False questions that quiz students on their knowledge of the procedures shown in the procedure videos), **Practicum Activities** for your practicum, and various games and interactive activities (i.e., "Quiz Show" and "Road to Recovery") that provide entertainment while learning important concepts related to selected chapters, matching exercises, labeling exercises, identification exercises, and other helpful activities for the student. New to this edition's Evolve site are SimChart® for the Medical Office activities and four medical assisting credentialing practice examinations (CMA, RMA, CMAA, and CCMA). An icon ⓔ is placed at the beginning of each chapter to prompt students to access the site and see what each chapter has to offer.

STUDY GUIDE

The student *Study Guide* that accompanies the textbook greatly enhances the learning value of the textbook. Full of practice, critical-thinking questions, and various other ways students can practice their content knowledge, the Study Guide is a valuable supplemental resource for any student who is looking to get the most out of his or her textbook. In addition, its outcome-based approach meets the criteria required for outcome-based program accreditation as stipulated by the Commission on Accreditation of Allied Health Educational Programs (CAAHEP) and the Curriculum Review Board of the American Association of Medical Assistants (AAMA), as well as meets all of the most recently updated ABHES and CAAHEP competencies and curriculum standards. Included are extensive exercises for each chapter, as well as performance checklists for all textbook procedures (and even a few extras not included in the textbook). The Study Guide also includes pretests and posttests, which help better prepare students for chapter tests, a student Study Guide assignment sheet for documenting completion of assignments and calculating points earned for each assignment, a laboratory assignment sheet to keep track of student procedure performance, and various ways for students to practice their content knowledge, through multiple-choice questions, true/false questions, critical-thinking exercises, and other stimulating practice activities.

Acknowledgments

The completion of the third edition of this text permits the opportunity to relay appreciation to the medical assisting educators who so eagerly and enthusiastically use and enjoy this text. To them, the authors are also indebted for their helpful assistance and suggestions for this new text.

The photographs in the textbook were taken by Brian Blauser and Jack Foley, professional photographers. We are indebted to them for their careful precision and patience in taking and editing the photographs, thus greatly enhancing the learning value of this text.

We would like to acknowledge Harvard Vanguard Medical Associates in Burlington, Massachusetts for allowing us to create new photographs for this edition in the administrative area of the practice.

We would like to gratefully acknowledge the following practicing medical assistants for contributing many hours to be photographed for demonstration of the clinical procedures in the text: Megan Baer, Dawn Bennett, Trudy Browning, Janet Canterbury, Theresa Cline, Marlyne Cooper, Hope Fauber, Dori Glover, Jennifer Hawk, Kevin Hickey, Cammie Lindner, Judy Markins, Korey McGrew, Natalie Morehead, Traci Powell, Linda Proffitt, Latisha Sharpe, Michelle Shockey, Kara Van Dyke, Michelle Villers, and Huang Ying.

We would also like to acknowledge the following individuals who portrayed patients and other individuals in the text: Brian Adevc, Travis Allman, Jessica Bennett, Kim Bingham, Pamela Bitting, Caitlin Brennan, David Brennan, Hollie Bonewit, Sarah Buckley, Phillip Carr, Chloe Cline, Angie Coffin, Brittany Cogar, Chad Cron, Dawn Decaminada, Elizabeth Feeny, Aja Fox, Markly Georges, Erika Giertz, Ciera Hart, Connie Hazlett, Gary Hazlett, Isabella Ipacs, Joey Ipacs, Susan Ipacs, Charles Larimer, Pam Larimer, Christopher Mace, Leah Moran, Deborah Murray, Delaney Murray, Michael Nkrumah, Heather Pike, Megan Powell, Quincy Sheets, Dawn Shingler, Jan Six, Megan Skidmore, Colton Smith, Janice Smith, Sydney Smith, Melissa Spencer, Clinton Swart, Faye Townsend, Tristen West, Devin White, Lynn Witkowski, and Judith Zappala.

We would like to extend our appreciation to the authors, publishers, and equipment companies who have granted us permission to use their illustrations.

The publication of this text was accomplished through the capable guidance of many talented individuals at Elsevier. First and foremost, this book could not have attained this level of excellence without the exceptional capabilities of Jennifer Bertucci, Senior Content Development Specialist. Also, many thanks to Celeste Clingan for her outstanding production work and to Bruce Siebert for his extensive multimedia knowledge and expertise. Maggie Reid created these beautiful interior and cover designs. And, finally, we want to relay a very special thank you to Jennifer Janson, Executive Content Strategist, for her dedication to quality medical assisting education and her encouragement in helping us achieve our very best in this edition.

With warm regard, we would like to recognize those very important individuals—the medical assisting students, graduates, and practicing medical assistants—who continually strive for excellence in meeting the demands and ever-increasing requirements of such a challenging profession. A quote by an unknown author really says it better: "Celebrate your talents, for they are what make you unique."

Kathy Bonewit-West, BS, MEd
Sue A. Hunt, MA, RN, CMA (AAMA)
Edith Applegate, MS

Clinical Procedure Icons

The OSHA Bloodborne Pathogens Standard must be followed when performing many of the clinical procedures presented in this text. To assist the student in following the OSHA Standard, icons have been incorporated into the procedures. An illustration of each icon along with its description is outlined below.

 HAND HYGIENE is an important medical aseptic practice and is crucial in preventing the transmission of pathogens in the medical office. The medical assistant should sanitize the hands frequently, using proper technique. When performing clinical procedures, the hands should always be sanitized before and after patient contact, before applying gloves and after removing gloves, and after contact with blood or other potentially infectious materials.

 CLEAN DISPOSABLE GLOVES should be worn when it is reasonably anticipated that you will have hand contact with the following: blood and other potentially infectious materials, mucous membranes, nonintact skin, and contaminated articles or surfaces.

 BIOHAZARD CONTAINERS are closable, leakproof, and suitably constructed to contain the contents during handling, storage, transport, or shipping. The containers must be labeled or color coded and closed before removal to prevent the contents from spilling.

 APPROPRIATE PROTECTIVE CLOTHING such as gowns, aprons, and laboratory coats should be worn when gross contamination can reasonably be anticipated during performance of a task or procedure.

 FACE SHIELDS OR MASKS IN COMBINATION WITH EYE-PROTECTION DEVICES must be worn whenever splashes, spray, spatter, or droplets of blood or other potentially infectious materials may be generated, posing a hazard through contact with your eyes, nose, or mouth.

Contents

SECTION 1
Introduction to Medical Assisting

1. **The Health Care System,** *1*
   Introduction to Health and the Health Care System, *2*
   Modern Trends in Health Care, *2*
   Health Insurance and Patient Care: Competing Forces Facing the
      Medical Office in the Twenty-First Century, *2*
   Ambulatory Care, *6*
   Parts of the Medical Office, *10*
   Medical Specialties, *12*
   Practice Types, *15*
   Complementary and Alternative Medicine, *16*

2. **The Professional Medical Assistant,** *19*
   Introduction to Professional Medical Assisting, *20*
   Educational Programs for Medical Assistants, *20*
   Characteristics of Medical Assistants, *21*
      *Procedure 2-1: Locating and Defining a State's Legal Scope
         of Practice, 24*
   Professionalism, *25*
   Certification for Medical Assistants, *26*
   Professional Organizations, *28*
   Role of the Medical Assistant, *28*
   Employment Opportunities, *31*

3. **Ethics and Law for the Medical Office,** *34*
   Introduction to Medical Ethics, *36*
   Reasons to Study Ethics, *36*
   Ethics and Health Care, *36*
      *Procedure 3-1: Separating Personal and Professional
         Ethics, 42*
   Introduction to Law, *43*
   Law and Professional Liability, *44*
      *Procedure 3-2: Incorporating the Patient's Bill
         of Rights, 48*
   Federal and State Laws Affecting the Medical
      Office, *52*
      *Procedure 3-3: Reporting Illegal Activities and Complying with
         Public Health Statutes, 56*

4. **Interacting with Patients,** *61*
   Introduction to Communication, *62*
   Communicating with Patients, *62*
   Understanding and Meeting the Needs of Patients, *69*
      *Procedure 4-1: Demonstrating Effective and Respectful Verbal and
         Nonverbal Communication, 71*
      *Procedure 4-2: Maintaining Boundaries and Demonstrating Respect
         for Boundaries in Communications, 73*

SECTION 2
Anatomy and Physiology

5. **Introduction to Anatomy and Physiology,** *80*
   A Brief Summary of Medical History, *81*
   The Human Body, *82*
   Cell Structure and Function, *89*
   Tissues and Membranes, *99*

6. **Integumentary System,** *111*
   Introduction to the Integumentary System, *111*
   Structure of the Skin, *112*
   Skin Color, *113*
   Epidermal Derivatives, *113*
   Functions of the Skin, *114*
   Aging of the Integumentary System, *115*

7. **Skeletal System,** *118*
   Introduction to the Skeletal System, *119*
   Overview of the Skeletal System, *119*
   Bones of the Axial Skeleton, *122*
   Bones of the Appendicular Skeleton, *127*
   Articulations, *131*
   Aging of the Skeletal System, *133*

8. **Muscular System,** *136*
   Introduction to the Muscular System, *137*
   Characteristics and Functions of the Muscular
      System, *137*
   Structure of Skeletal Muscle, *137*
   Contraction of Skeletal Muscle, *138*
   Skeletal Muscle Groups, *140*
   Aging of the Muscular System, *147*

9. **Nervous System,** *151*
   Introduction to the Nervous System, *152*
   Functions of the Nervous System, *152*
   Organization of the Nervous System, *152*
   Nerve Tissue, *153*
   Nerve Impulses, *155*
   Central Nervous System, *158*
   Peripheral Nervous System, *164*
   Aging of the Nervous System, *167*

10. **The Senses,** *173*
   Introduction to the Senses, *174*
   Receptors and Sensations, *174*
   General Senses, *174*
   Gustatory Sense, *175*
   Olfactory Sense, *176*

Visual Sense, *176*
Auditory Sense, *179*
Sense of Equilibrium, *181*
Aging of the Senses, *181*

11. Endocrine System, *186*

Introduction to the Endocrine System, *187*
Comparison of the Endocrine and Nervous Systems, *187*
Comparison of Exocrine and Endocrine Glands, *187*
Characteristics of Hormones, *187*
Endocrine Glands and their Hormones, *187*
Aging of the Endocrine System, *195*

12. Circulatory System, *196*

Introduction to the Circulatory System, *197*
Heart, *197*
Blood, *202*
Blood Vessels, *209*
Lymphatic System, *213*
Resistance to Disease, *214*
Aging of the Circulatory System, *216*

13. Respiratory System, *224*

Introduction to the Respiratory System, *225*
Functions and Overview of Respiration, *225*
Ventilation, *225*
Respiration, *228*
Regulation of Respiration, *229*
Aging of the Respiratory System, *230*

14. Digestive System, *235*

Introduction to the Digestive System, *236*
Functions of the Digestive System, *236*
General Structure of the Digestive Tract, *236*
Components of the Digestive Tract, *238*
Accessory Organs of Digestion, *245*
Chemical Digestion, *247*
Absorption, *248*
Aging of the Digestive System, *248*

15. Urinary System, *254*

Introduction to the Urinary System, *255*
Components of the Urinary System, *255*
Urine Formation, *262*
Aging of the Urinary System, *264*

16. Reproductive System, *266*

Introduction to the Reproductive System, *267*
Male Reproductive System, *267*
Female Reproductive System, *272*
Development, *279*
Aging of the Reproductive System, *282*

SECTION 3
Clinical Component

17. Medical Asepsis and the OSHA Standard, *290*

Introduction to Medical Asepsis and the OSHA
   Standard, *291*

Microorganisms and Medical Asepsis, *291*
   Procedure 17-1: *Handwashing, 296*
   Procedure 17-2: *Applying an Alcohol-Based Hand Rub, 298*
   Procedure 17-3: *Application and Removal of Clean Disposable Gloves, 300*
OSHA Bloodborne Pathogens Standard, *301*
Regulated Medical Waste, *309*
Bloodborne Diseases, *312*

18. Sterilization and Disinfection, *318*

Introduction to Sterilization and Disinfection, *319*
Definitions of Terms, *319*
Hazard Communication Standard, *319*
Sanitization, *326*
   Procedure 18-1: *Sanitization of Instruments, 329*
Disinfection, *333*
Sterilization, *334*
   Procedure 18-2: *Wrapping Instruments Using Paper or Muslin, 338*
   Procedure 18-3: *Wrapping Instruments Using a Pouch, 340*
   Procedure 18-4: *Sterilizing Articles in the Autoclave, 345*

19. Vital Signs, *350*

Introduction to Vital Signs, *352*
Temperature, *352*
   Procedure 19-1: *Measuring Oral Body Temperature—Electronic Thermometer, 359*
   Procedure 19-2: *Measuring Axillary Body Temperature—Electronic Thermometer, 362*
   Procedure 19-3: *Measuring Rectal Body Temperature—Electronic Thermometer, 363*
   Procedure 19-4: *Measuring Aural Body Temperature—Tympanic Membrane Thermometer, 365*
   Procedure 19-5: *Measuring Temporal Artery Body Temperature, 367*
Pulse, *370*
Respiration, *374*
Pulse Oximetry, *377*
   Procedure 19-6: *Measuring Pulse and Respiration, 381*
   Procedure 19-7: *Measuring Apical Pulse, 382*
   Procedure 19-8: *Performing Pulse Oximetry, 384*
Blood Pressure, *386*
   Procedure 19-9: *Measuring Blood Pressure, 396*
   Procedure 19-10: *Determining Systolic Pressure by Palpation, 400*

20. The Physical Examination, *405*

Introduction to the Physical Examination, *406*
Definition of Terms, *406*
Preparation of the Examining Room, *407*
Preparation of the Patient, *408*
Measuring Weight and Height, *409*
   Procedure 20-1: *Measuring Weight and Height, 415*
Body Mechanics, *418*
Positioning and Draping, *420*
   Procedure 20-2: *Sitting Position, 421*
   Procedure 20-3: *Supine Position, 422*
   Procedure 20-4: *Prone Position, 423*
   Procedure 20-5: *Dorsal Recumbent Position, 424*
   Procedure 20-6: *Lithotomy Position, 425*
   Procedure 20-7: *Sims Position, 426*
   Procedure 20-8: *Knee-Chest Position, 427*
   Procedure 20-9: *Fowler Position, 428*

Wheelchair Transfer, *429*
   Procedure 20-10: Wheelchair Transfer, 430
Assessment of the Patient, *434*
Assisting the Physician, *436*
   Procedure 20-11: Assisting with the Physical Examination, 436

21. Eye and Ear Assessment and Procedures, *441*

Introduction to the Eye, *442*
Visual Acuity, *442*
Assessment of Color Vision, *446*
   Procedure 21-1: Assessing Distance Visual Acuity—Snellen Chart, 447
   Procedure 21-2: Assessing Color Vision—Ishihara Test, 449
Eye Irrigation, *450*
Eye Instillation, *450*
   Procedure 21-3: Performing an Eye Irrigation, 451
   Procedure 21-4: Performing an Eye Instillation, 453
Introduction to the Ear, *455*
Assessment of Hearing Acuity, *455*
Ear Irrigation, *458*
Ear Instillation, *458*
   Procedure 21-5: Performing an Ear Irrigation, 460
   Procedure 21-6: Performing an Ear Instillation, 463

22. Physical Agents to Promote Tissue Healing, *467*

Introduction to Tissue Healing, *468*
Local Application of Heat and Cold, *468*
   Procedure 22-1: Applying a Heating Pad, 471
   Procedure 22-2: Applying a Hot Soak, 472
   Procedure 22-3: Applying a Hot Compress, 473
   Procedure 22-4: Applying an Ice Bag, 474
   Procedure 22-5: Applying a Cold Compress, 475
   Procedure 22-6: Applying a Chemical Pack, 476
Ambulatory Aids, *477*
   Procedure 22-7: Measuring for Axillary Crutches, 480
   Procedure 22-8: Instructing a Patient in Crutch Gaits, 481
   Procedure 22-9: Instructing a Patient in Use of a Cane, 484
   Procedure 22-10: Instructing a Patient in Use of a Walker, 484

23. The Gynecologic Examination and Prenatal Care, *487*

Introduction to the Gynecologic Examination and Prenatal Care, *488*
Gynecologic Examination, *488*
Gynecology, *488*
Breast Examination, *489*
Pelvic Examination, *490*
   Procedure 23-1: Breast Self-Examination Instructions, 498
   Procedure 23-2: Assisting with a Gynecologic Examination, 501
Vaginal Infections, *504*
Prenatal Care, *508*
Obstetrics, *508*
Prenatal Visits, *508*
   Procedure 23-3: Assisting with a Return Prenatal Examination, 522

24. The Pediatric Examination, *529*

Introduction to the Pediatric Examination, *530*
Pediatric Office Visits, *530*
Developing a Rapport, *531*
Carrying the Infant, *531*
Growth Measurements, *533*

   Procedure 24-1: Measuring the Weight and Length of an Infant, 536
   Procedure 24-2: Measuring Head and Chest Circumference of an Infant, 537
   Procedure 24-3: Calculating Growth Percentiles, 539
Pediatric Blood Pressure Measurement, *542*
Collection of a Urine Specimen, *543*
   Procedure 24-4: Applying a Pediatric Urine Collector, 544
Pediatric Injections, *546*
Immunizations, *548*
Newborn Screening Test, *555*

25. Minor Office Surgery, *560*

Introduction to Minor Office Surgery, *562*
Surgical Asepsis, *562*
Instruments Used in Minor Office Surgery, *563*
Commercially Prepared Sterile Packages, *568*
   Procedure 25-1: Applying and Removing Sterile Gloves, 569
   Procedure 25-2: Opening a Sterile Package, 571
   Procedure 25-3: Pouring a Sterile Solution, 573
Wounds, *573*
Sterile Dressing Change, *575*
   Procedure 25-4: Changing a Sterile Dressing, 576
Sutures, *578*
   Procedure 25-5: Removing Sutures and Staples, 583
   Procedure 25-6: Applying and Removing Adhesive Skin Closures, 586
Assisting with Minor Office Surgery, *590*
   Procedure 25-7: Assisting with Minor Office Surgery, 594
Medical Office Surgical Procedures, *598*
Bandaging, *607*

26. Administration of Medication and Intravenous Therapy, *613*

Introduction to the Administration of Medication, *615*
Administering, Prescribing, and Dispensing Medication, *615*
Legal Aspects, *615*
Routes of Administration, *615*
Drug References, *616*
Food and Drug Administration, *618*
Drug Nomenclature, *619*
Classification of Drugs Based on Preparation, *619*
Classification of Drugs Based on Action, *620*
Systems of Measurement for Medication, *632*
Converting Units of Measurement, *634*
Controlled Drugs, *635*
Prescription, *635*
Medication Record, *641*
Factors Affecting Drug Action, *644*
Guidelines for Preparation and Administration of Medication, *645*
Oral Administration, *645*
   Procedure 26-1: Administering Oral Medication, 646
Parenteral Administration, *647*
   Procedure 26-2: Preparing an Injection, 657
   Procedure 26-3: Reconstituting Powdered Drugs, 661
   Procedure 26-4: Administering a Subcutaneous Injection, 662
   Procedure 26-5: Administering an Intramuscular Injection, 664
   Procedure 26-6: Z-Track Intramuscular Injection Technique, 667
Tuberculin Skin Testing, *668*
Allergy Testing, *673*
   Procedure 26-7: Administering an Intradermal Injection, 678
Intravenous Therapy, *681*

27. Cardiopulmonary Procedures, 687

Introduction to Electrocardiography, 689
Cardiac Cycle, 689
Electrocardiograph Paper, 691
Standardization of the Electrocardiograph, 691
Electrocardiograph Leads, 692
Paper Speed, 696
Patient Preparation, 696
Maintenance of the Electrocardiograph, 696
Electrocardiographic Capabilities, 697
Artifacts, 699
    Procedure 27-1: Running a 12-Lead, Three-Channel Electrocardiogram, 701
Holter Monitor Electrocardiography, 704
Cardiac Dysrhythmias, 705
Pulmonary Function Tests, 706
Peak Flow Measurement, 706
    Procedure 27-2: Measuring Peak Flow Rate, 711
Home Oxygen Therapy, 713

28. Specialty Examinations and Procedures: Colon Procedures, Male Reproductive Health, and Radiology and Diagnostic Imaging, 719

Colon Procedures, 721
Introduction to Colon Procedures, 721
Blood in the Stool, 721
Fecal Occult Blood Test, 721
    Procedure 28-1: Fecal Occult Blood Testing: Guaiac Slide Test, 725
    Procedure 28-2: Developing the Hemoccult Slide Test, 728
Other Types of Stool Tests, 729
Sigmoidoscopy, 730
Colonoscopy, 733
Male Reproductive Health, 734
Introduction to Male Reproductive Health, 734
Prostate Cancer, 734
Prostate Cancer Screening, 735
Testicular Self-Examination, 736
Radiology and Diagnostic Imaging, 736
Introduction to Radiology, 736
Contrast Media, 737
Fluoroscopy, 738
Positioning the Patient, 738
Specific Radiographic Examinations, 738
Introduction to Diagnostic Imaging, 742
Ultrasonography, 742
Computed Tomography, 744
Magnetic Resonance Imaging, 744
Nuclear Medicine, 746
Digital Radiology, 747

29. Introduction to the Clinical Laboratory, 752

Introduction to the Clinical Laboratory, 753
Laboratory Tests, 754
Purpose of Laboratory Testing, 754
Types of Clinical Laboratories, 755
Laboratory Requests, 760
Laboratory Reports, 764
Laboratory Documents and the EMR, 767
Patient Preparation and Instructions, 767
Collecting, Handling, and Transporting Specimens, 770

Clinical Laboratory Improvement Amendments, 773
CLIA-Waived Laboratory Testing, 776
Quality Control, 778
Categories of Test Results, 782
Recording Test Results, 782
Laboratory Safety, 782

30. Urinalysis, 786

Composition of Urine, 787
Collection of Urine, 787
    Procedure 30-1: Clean-Catch Midstream Specimen Collection Instructions, 790
Analysis of Urine, 791
    Procedure 30-2: Chemical Testing of Urine with the Multistix 10 SG Reagent Strip, 797
    Procedure 30-3: Prepare a Urine Specimen for Microscopic Examination: Kova Method, 804
    Procedure 30-4: Performing a Urine Pregnancy Test, 809
Urine Pregnancy Testing, 807
Serum Pregnancy Test, 808

31. Phlebotomy, 814

Introduction to Phlebotomy, 815
Venipuncture, 815
General Guidelines for Venipuncture, 816
Vacuum Tube Method of Venipuncture, 824
    Procedure 31-1: Venipuncture—Vacuum Tube Method, 830
Butterfly Method of Venipuncture, 835
    Procedure 31-2: Venipuncture—Butterfly Method, 837
Problems Encountered with Venipuncture, 842
Obtaining a Serum Specimen, 845
Skin Puncture, 846
Puncture Sites, 846
Skin Puncture Devices, 846
    Procedure 31-3: Skin Puncture—Disposable Semiautomatic Lancet Device, 848
Microcollection Devices, 850
Guidelines for Performing a Finger Puncture, 850

32. Hematology, 854

Introduction to Hematology, 855
Hemoglobin Determination, 855
Hematocrit, 857
    Procedure 32-1: Hematocrit, 858
White Blood Cell Count, 861
Red Blood Cell Count, 861
Red Blood Cell Indices, 861
White Blood Cell Differential Count, 862
    Procedure 32-2: Preparation of a Blood Smear for a Differential Cell Count, 863
PT/INR, 866

33. Blood Chemistry and Immunology, 870

Introduction to Blood Chemistry and Immunology, 871
Blood Chemistry, 871
Collection of a Blood Chemistry Specimen, 871
Automated Blood Chemistry Analyzers, 872
Blood Glucose, 874
Tests for Management of Diabetes, 876
Glucose Meters, 880

Procedure 33-1: Blood Glucose Measurement Using the Accu-Chek Advantage Glucose Meter, 883
Cholesterol, 886
Triglycerides, 889
Blood Urea Nitrogen, 890
Immunology, 890
Immunologic Tests, 890
Rapid Mononucleosis Testing, 891

34. Medical Microbiology, 896

Introduction to Microbiology, 897
Normal Flora, 898
Infection, 898
Microorganisms and Disease, 899
Microscope, 901
  Procedure 34-1: Using the Microscope, 903
Microbiologic Specimen Collection, 906
  Procedure 34-2: Collecting a Throat Specimen, 908
Streptococcus Testing, 909
Sensitivity Testing, 909
Microscopic Examination of Microorganisms, 909
Prevention and Control of Infectious Diseases, 912

35. Nutrition, 915

Introduction to Nutrition, 916
Nutrients, 917
Dietary Supplements, 927
Nutrition Guides, 928
Food Labels, 929
Nutrition Therapy, 932
Weight Management, 932
Cardiovascular Disease, 935
Hypertension, 936
Diabetes, 937
Lactose Intolerance, 939
Gluten Intolerance, 940
Food Allergies, 941

36. Emergency Preparedness and Protective Practices, 944

Introduction to Disaster and Emergency Planning, 945
Categories of Disasters, 945
Psychological Effects of Emergencies, 946
Emergency Preparedness in the Medical Office, 949
Fire Safety in the Medical Office, 952
  Procedure 36-1: Demonstrating Proper Use of a Fire Extinguisher, 957
  Procedure 36-2: Participating in a Mock Exposure Event, 959
Employee Education and Training, 963
Emergency Practice Drills, 963
Medical Assistant's Role, 964

37. Emergency Medical Procedures and First Aid, 967

Introduction to Emergency Medical Procedures, 968
Office Crash Cart, 968
Emergency Medical Services System, 969
First Aid Kit, 969
OSHA Safety Precautions, 969
Guidelines for Providing Emergency Care, 970

SECTION 4
Administrative Component

38. The Medical Record, 991

Introduction to the Medical Record, 992
Types of Medical Records, 993
Medical Record Formats, 994
Administrative Section of the Medical Record, 996
  Procedure 38-1: Completion of a Procedure Consent Form, 1001
  Procedure 38-2: Release of Medical Information, 1001
Clinical Section of the Medical Record, 1002
Taking a Health History, 1007
Documentation in the Medical Record, 1011
  Procedure 38-3: Obtaining Patient History and Formulating Chief Complaint, 1017

39. Patient Reception, 1025

Introduction to Patient Reception, 1025
Preparing for Patients, 1026
  Procedure 39-1: Opening the Medical Office, 1027
  Procedure 39-2: Closing the Medical Office, 1028
Patient Check-In, 1029
  Procedure 39-3: Obtaining New Patient Information, 1035
Orienting Patients to the Medical Office, 1036
  Procedure 39-4: Explaining Office Policies and Procedures, 1037

40. Medical Office Computerization, 1040

Introduction to Medical Office Computerization, 1042
Computer Concepts, 1042
Data Processing Cycle, 1042
Components of the Computer System, 1043
Main Computer Unit, 1046
Computer Monitor, 1048
Input Devices, 1049
Printer, 1050
Storage Devices, 1052
Medical Office Computerization, 1053
Electronic Information Transfer, 1055
Medical Assistant's Use of the Electronic Medical Record, 1057
Physician's Use of the Electronic Medical Record, 1057
Computer Network Security, 1057
Backups, 1058
System Maintenance, 1058
Service Agreements, 1059

41. Telephone Techniques, 1063

Introduction to Telephone Techniques, 1064
Using the Telephone Effectively, 1064
Telephone Technology, 1065
Incoming Calls, 1067
  Procedure 41-1: Performing Telephone Screening, 1071
  Procedure 41-2: Taking a Telephone Message, 1072
  Procedure 41-3: Taking Requests for Medication or Prescription Refills, 1073
Outgoing Calls, 1074
  Procedure 41-4: Telephoning a Patient for Follow-Up, 1076

42. Scheduling Appointments, 1078

Introduction to Appointment Scheduling, 1079
Guidelines for Appointment Scheduling, 1079

Scheduling Appointments, *1080*
Daily Appointment Schedule, *1080*
Types of Scheduling, *1080*
Setting Up the Appointment Schedule, *1082*
  Procedure 42-1: Setting Up the Appointment Schedule, 1084
Guidelines for Scheduling, *1085*
  Procedure 42-2: Making an Appointment, 1088
Managing the Appointment Schedule, *1089*
  Procedure 42-3: Managing the Appointment Schedule, 1090
Scheduling Referral Appointments, Diagnostic Tests, Procedures, and Admissions, *1091*
  Procedure 42-4: Scheduling Inpatient or Outpatient Diagnostic Tests or Procedures, 1093
  Procedure 42-5: Scheduling Inpatient or Outpatient Admissions, 1094

43. Medical Records Management, *1098*
Introduction to Medical Records, *1099*
Paper-Based Medical Records, *1099*
Equipment and Supplies for Paper-Based Medical Records, *1099*
Preparing a Paper-Based Medical Record for a New Patient, *1102*
  Procedure 43-1: Preparing a Medical Record, 1102
Filing Systems, *1104*
  Procedure 43-2: Filing Patient Records: Alphabetic, 1107
  Procedure 43-3: Filing Patient Records: Numeric, 1108
Retrieving or Filing a Paper-Based Medical Record, *1108*
  Procedure 43-4: Filing Reports, 1110
Electronic Medical Record, *1110*
Storing Medical Records, *1111*

44. Written Communications, *1115*
Introduction to Written Communication, *1116*
Business Letters, *1116*
  Procedure 44-1: Composing a Business Letter, 1121
Preparing Memoranda, *1122*
Grammar and Punctuation, *1122*
Spelling and Proofreading, *1125*
Electronic Data Transmission, *1125*
  Procedure 44-2: Sending a Fax, 1127
Photocopying, *1128*

45. Mail, *1131*
Introduction to Mail and Shipping, *1132*
U.S. Postal System, *1132*
Other Package Delivery Services, *1136*
Processing Incoming Mail, *1136*
  Procedure 45-1: Processing Incoming Mail, 1137
Automated Mail Processing, *1138*
Postal Addressing Standards, *1139*
  Procedure 45-2: Looking Up a ZIP Code, 1141
Outgoing Mail, *1142*
  Procedure 45-3: Preparing Envelopes for Mailing, 1144

46. Managing Practice Finances, *1146*
Introduction to Daily Financial Activities, *1147*
Maintaining Patient Accounts, *1147*
Components of a Patient Account, *1148*
  Procedure 46-1: Completing a Patient Charge Slip, 1152
  Procedure 46-2: Posting Charges, 1155
  Procedure 46-3: Posting Payments and/or Adjustments, 1156
Other Financial Accounts, *1157*
Banking Activities, *1157*

  Procedure 46-4: Writing a Check, 1163
  Procedure 46-5: Preparing a Bank Deposit, 1165
Accounts Payable or Record of Cash Disbursements, *1165*
Petty Cash, *1165*

47. Medical Coding, *1168*
Introduction to Coding, *1169*
Procedure Coding, *1169*
Current Procedural Terminology (CPT) Codes, *1170*
  Procedure 47-1: Performing CPT Coding, 1175
Healthcare Common Procedure Coding System (HCPCS) Level II Codes, *1177*
  Procedure 47-2: Performing HCPCS Coding, 1178
Diagnosis Coding, *1179*
ICD-9-CM Manual, *1179*
ICD-10-CM Manual, *1181*
Improving Coding Accuracy, *1185*
  Procedure 47-3: Performing ICD Coding, 1185

48. Medical Insurance, *1189*
Introduction to Health Insurance, *1190*
History of Health Insurance, *1191*
Obtaining Health Insurance, *1191*
Paying for Health Insurance and Health Care, *1192*
Factors Affecting Insurance Reimbursement, *1192*
Types of Insurance, *1193*
Insurance and Managed Care Policies and Procedures, *1198*
  Procedure 48-1: Interpreting Information on an Insurance Card, 1200
  Procedure 48-2: Verifying Insurance Eligibility and Benefits, 1201
  Procedure 48-3: Obtaining Insurance Preauthorization (Precertification), 1201
Insurance Claim Forms, *1202*
Completing the Insurance Claim Form, *1204*
  Procedure 48-4: Completing and Reviewing an Insurance Claim Form, 1205
Submitting Insurance Claims, *1209*
Tracking Insurance Reimbursement, *1210*
Effective Communication Regarding Managed Care and/or Insurance, *1212*
  Procedure 48-5: Communicating Effectively Regarding Insurance and/or Managed Care, 1213

49. Billing and Collections, *1217*
Introduction to Billing, *1218*
Billing Cycle, *1218*
Billing Process, *1218*
  Procedure 49-1: Processing Patient Statements, 1220
Billing Problems, *1220*
  Procedure 49-2: Posting a Check Returned for Non-Sufficient Funds (NSF), 1221
  Procedure 49-3: Processing a Credit Balance and Refund, 1222
Account Aging, *1223*
  Procedure 49-4: Creating and Examining an Accounts Receivable Aging Record, 1225
Collection Activities, *1226*
  Procedure 49-5: Writing a Collection Letter, 1231

50. The Medical Assistant as Office Manager, *1233*
Introduction to Medical Office Management, *1234*
Maintaining the Office, *1234*
Routine Maintenance, *1236*
Patient and Employee Safety, *1237*

Procedure 50-1: Creating an Environmental Checklist and Performing a Safety Inspection, *1239*
Procedure 50-2: Complying with Safety Signs, Symbols, and Labels, *1240*
Maintaining Equipment, *1240*
Procedure 50-3: Performing Routine Maintenance of Equipment, *1242*
Supplies, *1242*
Procedure 50-4: Taking a Supply or Equipment Inventory, *1245*
Creating an Environment for Teamwork, *1245*
Preparing Payroll, *1246*
Managing Physician and Employee Schedules, *1247*
Providing Resources for Staff and Patients, *1248*
Procedure 50-5: Locating and Facilitating Referrals to Community Resources, *1249*

Risk Management, *1250*
Procedure 50-6: Completing an Incident Report, *1252*

51. Obtaining Employment, *1255*
Introduction to Obtaining Employment, *1256*
Successful Job Search, *1256*
Tools for a Job Search, *1256*
Getting the Job, *1263*
Lifelong Learning, *1266*
Planning for Job Advancement or Career Change, *1268*

Glossary, *1271*

Index, *1293*

The Health Care System

1

e Check out the Evolve site at http://evolve.elsevier.com/Bonewit/today/ to access additional interactive activities and exercises to help you study and prepare for success.

LEARNING OBJECTIVES

1. Describe the role of medical office care in the health care system.
2. Describe the historical development of managed care.
3. Identify the flow of activity in ambulatory care.
4. Identify the various types of health care professionals, and describe the job responsibilities of each professional.
5. State the educational requirements for physicians.
6. List and describe the parts of the medical office.
7. Identify and describe the various types of medical specialties.
8. Describe the philosophy of the patient-centered medical home (PCMH) as a means of delivering primary care.
9. Identify three medical practice types.
10. Compare and contrast various complementary and traditional medical treatments.

CHAPTER OUTLINE

INTRODUCTION TO HEALTH AND THE HEALTH CARE SYSTEM
MODERN TRENDS IN HEALTH CARE
HEALTH INSURANCE AND PATIENT CARE: COMPETING FORCES FACING THE MEDICAL OFFICE IN THE TWENTY-FIRST CENTURY
Fee-for-Service Insurance Plans
Government Insurance Plans
Managed Care
Health Care Reform
AMBULATORY CARE
Flow of Activity in Ambulatory Care
The Health Care Team
Members of the Health Care Team
Effective Teamwork

PARTS OF THE MEDICAL OFFICE
Reception Area and Waiting Room
Examination Rooms and Laboratory
Medical Records Storage and Business Office
Additional Areas Found in Many Offices
MEDICAL SPECIALTIES
Primary Care and the Patient-Centered Medical Home
Osteopathy
Podiatry
Chiropractic
PRACTICE TYPES
Solo Practice
Group Practice
Clinic
COMPLEMENTARY AND ALTERNATIVE MEDICINE

KEY TERMS

ambulatory (AM-byoo-la-toe-ree) care
capitation (cap-ih-TAY-shun)
curative (KYUR-a-tive) treatment
empirical (em-PEER-ih-cle)
fee-for-service

formulary (FORM-you-lay-ree)
health insurance
holistic (hole-IH-stick)
managed care
palliative (PAL-ee-a-tive) treatment

patient-centered medical home (PCMH)
residency (RES-ih-dense-ee)
symptomatic (simp-toe-MA-tick) treatment
utilization review

INTRODUCTION TO HEALTH AND THE HEALTH CARE SYSTEM

The World Health Organization (WHO) defines *health* as the absence of illness or disease and a state of being in which the individual feels well and is able to carry out the daily functions of life with no difficulties and no pain. In reality, no one reaches this optimum level of health. Everyone has aches and pains, psychological if not physical.

In our health care system, the physician's responsibility is to examine hundreds of people in the course of a week and to try to focus on medical problems that meet the following criteria: The problem is causing or can cause severe difficulties in carrying out the daily functions of life, and the problem can be treated either by reducing the effects of the symptoms or by eradicating the problem altogether.

Each individual the physician sees has a different group of presenting physical symptoms as well as a different set of social circumstances and emotional issues. The physician listens to the patient's description of his or her life, performs objective laboratory and diagnostic tests, identifies medical problems, and assesses the nature of each problem.

Physicians know that the vast majority of medical problems do not pose a long-term threat to health. Most medical conditions get better over time. Effective treatments are available to cure many conditions (**curative treatment**). In other cases the physician can reduce the symptoms even if the underlying medical condition is not significantly affected. This type of treatment is called **symptomatic treatment** (responding to symptoms) or **palliative treatment** (seeking to reduce the effects of a disease or condition without curing the underlying disease). For example, a patient with a urinary tract infection who is given a prescription for antibiotics receives curative treatment, whereas a patient who has diabetes mellitus receives palliative treatment. The patient is prescribed insulin, which alleviates the symptoms of the diabetes; however, the treatment does not cure the diabetes.

Most treatments are based on scientific study. In Western scientific medicine, as in no other medical tradition, approaches to diagnosis and treatment have been studied and tested over hundreds of years. As long ago as the fourth century BCE, a physician named Hippocrates in Greece believed that disease was not a punishment for transgressions against the gods, but rather the result of physiologic and environmental factors that could be studied. Since the time of Hippocrates, the practice of medicine has changed considerably in response to scientific discoveries.

MODERN TRENDS IN HEALTH CARE

Several trends running through modern medicine have a strong influence on the way in which health care is provided in ambulatory settings.

The first trend is the desire of those who pay the bills—employers, the federal and state governments, and insurance companies—to reduce the costs of health care, especially care for chronic diseases, and to make health care providers responsible for effective management of patients who require care over time without duplication of services and without medical errors. Medicare is encouraging several initiatives to encourage doctors and other health care providers to coordinate patient care; these initiatives include Accountable Care Organizations (ACOs), formed voluntarily by groups of physicians, hospitals, and other health care providers to give coordinated and high-quality care to Medicare patients.

A second trend is to encourage the general public to become more responsible for their own good health and management of chronic conditions. There are several public initiatives to improve dietary practices, especially for children, to prevent obesity. Within the health care system there is an increasing emphasis on coaching patients to manage their health and to initiate changes that will improve their health (including dietary changes, smoking cessation, and adherence to a healthy exercise program.)

The third trend is an increased understanding, through **empirical** evidence (information learned from experimental research), that people *feel better* the less they must be confined to a hospital or go to a hospital for treatment. Being able to be diagnosed and treated in an outpatient setting with follow-up at home allows people to feel more in control of their lives as medical patients. There is increasing development of remote medicine and telemedicine applications so that patients can be monitored and coached to health at any time.

This is especially important for people who have frequent contact with the medical system, such as the parents of infants and children, the elderly, and those with chronic illnesses. Many people who would have been hospitalized for long periods or possibly even institutionalized 50, 25, or even 10 years ago are currently living independently in the community.

Today the hospital's role is primarily to provide acute care and diagnostic services. For a patient to be hospitalized, his or her condition must be unstable or necessitate constant regulation of therapy. If the patient does not meet these strict criteria, he or she goes home to be followed as an outpatient; is transferred to a rehabilitation facility for intense, regular rehabilitative treatment; or is sent to a nursing home for long-term maintenance care.

HEALTH INSURANCE AND PATIENT CARE: COMPETING FORCES FACING THE MEDICAL OFFICE IN THE TWENTY-FIRST CENTURY

FEE-FOR-SERVICE INSURANCE PLANS

Traditionally, medical care in the United States was paid for on a **fee-for-service** basis. Each service was billed and paid for as a separate charge: so much for the office visit, so much for the electrocardiogram, so much for the urinalysis, and so on. Fee-for-service payments can be thought of as ordering food at a restaurant à la carte: so much for the main course, so much for a salad, so much for coffee.

During the first part of the twentieth century, health insurance (if the patient had any) paid only for hospitalization, and usually the patient completed most of the paperwork. **Health insurance** is a system by which a person or the person's employer pays an insurance company a yearly amount of money, and the insurance company pays some or most of the person's medical expenses for that year. The theory behind insurance is that although a few people will have large medical bills over the course of the year, most people will have small bills. By setting the fee for everyone at a level above the actual cost of care for most people, the insurance company can pay for the care of the well, the occasionally ill, and the often ill and still make a profit.

This system encouraged health care providers to provide a high level of care for everyone with health insurance because the insurance paid for every test and every procedure. Physicians' incomes soared between the end of World War II and the early 1980s. With the increasing costs of laboratory and diagnostic testing, hospital services, and office visits, the cost of medical care increased far more rapidly than the cost of other goods and services in the U.S. economy. (In economic terms, health care inflation increased much more rapidly than the general rate of inflation.)

During this time, ever-better health insurance became a standard employee benefit at many companies. The first kind of health insurance offered, in the 1950s and 1960s, was coverage for hospital care. Coverage for office visits became standard in the 1970s.

HIGHLIGHT on the History of Medical Treatment of Infectious Disease

Historians generally place the beginning of Western medicine with Hippocrates, an ancient Greek physician who saw medicine as an independent discipline based on clinical practice rather than prayer and ritual. For several centuries there were few treatment methods other than rest, exercise, diet, and a few medications derived from plants. The intensive study of the human body in the 1500s fostered a better understanding of physiologic processes. For example, the English scientist William Harvey, who rejected the traditional belief that blood was made up of "spirits" and that body fluids were "humors," developed a theory, later proved true, that blood flows from the heart to the lungs, throughout the body via arteries, and back to the heart via veins.

Physician in the Middle Ages taking a patient's pulse and holding a flask of urine. (Courtesy Blocker History of Medicine Collections, Moody Medical Library, University of Texas Medical Branch, Galveston, Tex.)

The first microscopic lens was invented in 1677 by Antony van Leeuwenhoek. Through his microscope van Leeuwenhoek saw yeasts, molds, and algae, adding evidence to the theory that diseases could be caused by particles too small to be seen with the eyes. He also identified red blood cells passing through capillaries.

Early microscope, about 1765. (Courtesy Blocker History of Medicine Collections, Moody Medical Library, University of Texas Medical Branch, Galveston, Tex.)

Throughout the nineteenth century, other scientists and physicians advanced the understanding of the cause of disease. Some found ways to combat disease without understanding the mechanism by which the disease acted; others determined the actual cause of a particular disease.

In the 1840s the Viennese obstetric assistant Ignaz Semmelweis discovered that the number of cases of puerperal fever, or so-called "childbed fever," a fatal illness of women who had just given birth, could be reduced if physicians washed their hands.

Continued

HIGHLIGHT on the History of Medical Treatment of Infectious Disease—cont'd

Semmelweis conducted what today would be called an *epidemiologic study.* He studied the records of women who had died and determined which physicians and medical students had attended which birth. His study of the records led him to conclude that most of the women who died had been attended to by physicians and medical students who had come into the birthing room directly from the anatomy laboratory, where they had worked with cadavers, without first washing their hands. Most of Semmelweis's colleagues dismissed his notion that simple handwashing could reduce childbirth deaths as nonsense, and during his lifetime Semmelweis was ridiculed. It was not until decades later that physicians regularly began washing their hands.

Extracting blood for a transfusion, eighteenth century. (Courtesy National Library of Medicine.)

The Scottish surgeon Joseph Lister worked on similar ideas to develop the first practice of antisepsis (cleaning areas where germs may be) and later asepsis (creating a germ-free environment). Lister started by pouring carbolic acid on the wounds of those who had just undergone surgery. Over time, he found milder substances. Lister found that far fewer patients who were treated with these substances died from gangrene that developed in the open wounds.

Semmelweis, Lister, and others worked empirically, which means they sought results through experiments that could be repeated with the same results. Although they were able to decrease infection rates, they never completely understood what caused infectious diseases. Other scientists sought to determine that bacteria caused specific diseases.

The German physician Robert Koch is called the "Father of Microbiology" because of his work with specific bacteria such as *Mycobacterium tuberculosis,* the bacterial agent that causes tuberculosis. Koch also isolated the bacterial agent that causes anthrax. Koch grew the anthrax bacillus in a number of different liquid media in his laboratory, used the microscope to identify it, injected the organism into a healthy animal, waited for the animal to become sick, and then recovered the same organism from the sick animal. This proved that one specific type of bacteria causes one specific disease. Today we know that it is possible to break the chain of illness by keeping those who are contagious away from those who are vulnerable to disease.

The work of Louis Pasteur and Koch, among others, helped set the stage for the understanding of infectious disease and for worldwide vaccination programs to eradicate smallpox and to try to eradicate the "childhood illnesses" of mumps, measles, and rubella (German measles).

The first vaccination actually had been performed a century earlier. Edward Jenner, an English physician in the farming country of Gloucestershire, used the pus from one person's cowpox lesion to vaccinate another individual against smallpox in 1796.

Edward Jenner vaccinating an infant. (Courtesy National Library of Medicine.)

Cowpox is a variant of smallpox. It is lethal to animals but relatively harmless to humans. For centuries, people had realized that people who had been infected with cowpox did not develop smallpox. Today, we understand what happened—their immune systems had developed antibodies to cowpox that also prevented smallpox infection by attacking the smallpox virus.

Jenner used "humanized cowpox" to establish immunity by taking pus from a lesion on a human infected with cowpox and rubbing it into an open wound on another human. A couple of weeks later, he inoculated the second person with smallpox. Not only did the individual not become ill, but he also was not contagious. A century later Pasteur would discover fully the mechanism by which vaccination works. Vaccines were discovered for many diseases. By the beginning of the twentieth century, vaccines had been developed for diphtheria and tetanus, and most children received these vaccines as infants by the middle of the twentieth century. New immunizations continue to be developed not only for infants but also for adolescents, adults, and the elderly.

Medications to kill bacteria were another important tool in the fight against infectious disease. Paul Ehrlich is credited with the development of the first medication to kill bacteria. In 1909 he developed a drug called *Salvarsan* (arsphenamine), which could be used to effectively treat syphilis. Unfortunately the medication itself was extremely toxic. The first of the sulfanilamide drugs, Prontosil, was developed in 1932 in Germany. It was effective against infections caused by streptococci and some other types of bacteria. The sulfanilamides became popular before and during World War II because they were the only antiinfective agents widely available. Penicillin, a mold that kills bacteria, had been discovered in 1922 by Alexander Fleming in London after it attacked bacteria that he was growing on agar plates. Initially the scientific community did not believe that it would be effective inside the body, and little follow-up research was done. During World War II, two medical researchers, Howard Florey and Ernst Chain, took up the research on penicillin and managed to prove that the medication was effective. The first human was treated in 1941, and within a few years mass production had been established and penicillin was in widespread use.

Discovery of the first virus is credited to Dimitri Ivanowski, a Russian botanist, in 1892. He discovered that a substance could pass through a ceramic filter that trapped all known bacteria and still cause a disease of tobacco called *mosaic tobacco disease.* We now know that the culprit is the tobacco mosaic virus. Yellow fever was the first viral disease of humans to be identified. During construction of the Panama Canal, workers were devastated by this disease. Research done by Walter Reed established that the disease was caused by a virus transmitted by mosquitoes and not direct contact. Controlling mosquitoes facilitated the work on the canal. The development of the electron microscope in 1930 allowed viruses to be seen, but progress to control viral diseases was slow. For most viruses the body has adequate defenses to overcome the infection, but there are some significant exceptions. The retroviruses, such as human immunodeficiency virus (HIV), are notable because they are able to overcome the body's immune system. In the 1970s the first deaths from acquired immunodeficiency syndrome (AIDS) were reported in the United States. Within the next 20 years, a worldwide epidemic occurred. By 1997 more than 6 million deaths worldwide had been caused by the AIDS virus. Treatments have been developed to slow the progression of the disease, but to date there is no effective immunization or cure for this disease. The ability of viruses to mutate rapidly has resulted in recent viral pandemics from diseases such as severe acute respiratory syndrome (SARS) in 2004 and H1N1 influenza in 2009. ∎

GOVERNMENT INSURANCE PLANS

Recognizing that there were large segments of the population without insurance because they were not employed, the federal government began to provide health insurance to large segments of the population starting in the 1960s. Medicaid began to provide health insurance for low-income children without parental support and later expanded to cover all the medically indigent. Medicare initiated health insurance for the elderly, the disabled, and those with end-stage kidney disease. The Civilian Health and Medical Program of the Uniformed Services (CHAMPUS; now called *TRICARE*) provided health insurance for dependents of active-duty military personnel. With these programs, the federal government has become the primary insurer for more than 50 million Americans. These plans, which included payments for office visits for illness, greatly increased the number of Americans who had medical insurance. There was little incentive for the consumer (the patient) to control costs because insurance was covering those costs, and care in most cases was "free" to the consumer.

Although most Americans who were insured did not feel that they were "paying" for their medical care, they were, indirectly. The huge increases in health care costs were one of the major sources of the generally high rates of inflation in the 1970s. Employers who paid for the insurance had to pay ever-rising premiums and offset these large premium increases with small increases in cash wages, which did not keep up with inflation. So American workers did, in fact, pay for health insurance and health care costs in lower purchasing power for the cash they received as salary.

MANAGED CARE

Health maintenance organizations (HMOs) were originally formed with a belief that consistent, routine care would help prevent later expensive care. Managed care was based on the belief that increasing prevention and promoting early detection and diagnosis of chronic and life-threatening medical conditions would reduce costs. At that time traditional health insurance only covered office visits for illness or injury and did not cover so-called "routine care" (well-child visits, immunizations, regular checkups, or physical examinations). The HMO movement, which gained acceptance in the 1970s, pushed traditional health insurance companies to begin providing coverage for routine care.

In the late 1970s, insurance companies began to respond to escalating health care costs by reviewing care to find out if it was medically necessary. This process, called **utilization review**, identifies patients who, according to the insurance companies, no longer need to be hospitalized. Originally, utilization review was used by Medicare and Medicaid and only for hospitalized patients. Other insurance companies soon realized that shortening hospital stays was an important way of reducing overall health care costs. The combination of HMO insurance plans and strict utilization review for hospitalized patients is the basis of what we call **managed care**. Utilization review is now used for both inpatients and outpatients to control healthcare costs.

The original HMO model had two components: insurance and services including diagnostic tests and pharmacy. HMO plans set up full-service medical clinics. Physicians were employees. The HMO established a contractual relationship with a hospital for inpatient services, and patients had to go to the specific hospital with which the HMO had a contract.

In the late 1980s HMO services began to separate from HMO insurance. A second type of HMO model based on networks of physicians who agreed to provide care for HMO patients came into being. Some of these networks operated under the old fee-for-service plans but agreed to discounted fees from the HMOs in exchange for access to the rapidly growing patient populations enrolled in HMOs. In an effort to reduce payments, HMOs tried to have physicians accept a flat monthly fee for each subscriber in their practice and agree to provide all necessary primary care for that fee. This type of payment is called **capitation**. This reduces the incentive to provide extra services because their cost will not be reimbursed separately.

The managed care movement in general, as well as the trend to decrease reimbursement for primary care in particular, put the burden on physicians to compete with one another to provide the most care for the least money. As a result, physicians often feel pressure to limit diagnostic tests, reduce hospitalizations and the number of days patients stay in the hospital, and use generic instead of brand-name drugs. (Generics are identical in chemical formulation to brand-name drugs and can be manufactured only after the brand-name drug's patent protection has expired.)

Managed care also puts pressure on physicians to see more patients, spend less time with each patient, and justify all services including diagnostic tests and referrals. The expense of handling sicker patients is expected to be balanced by those patients who use less than the average amount of medical services.

In addition, insurance plans have tried to reduce their costs for prescription medications by restricting drug coverage to lists of approved drugs. Such a list, called a **formulary**, usually includes one or two of the less expensive drugs for each possible medical condition. Exceptions are made if the physician can show that the less expensive drugs have been ineffective for his or her patient and that a more expensive drug is necessary. In some plans the patient can receive a more expensive medication by paying more of the cost.

HEALTH CARE REFORM

Despite these measures, however, beginning in the late 1990s, both insurance premiums and health care costs began to increase at more than double and even triple the underlying rate of inflation. There has also been an increase in the number of individuals and families who do not qualify for government insurance plans and also do not have health insurance through their employers. This may be because they work part-time or are self-employed. The Patient Protection and Affordable Care Act, which became law in March 2010, expanded insurance coverage to an estimated 32 million Americans who were previously uninsured. Among the provisions that went into effect in September 2010, insurance companies are no longer allowed to exclude children with preexisting health conditions or to drop customers after discovering technical mistakes on applications. As of 2014 this law required all individuals to purchase health insurance or pay an annual fine. Even though this law has been challenged in the courts, a strong belief persists that society has an obligation to make appropriate health care accessible to all citizens.

AMBULATORY CARE

There is no such thing as a "typical" medical office. The style of any particular medical office depends on the personality of the physician or physicians who practice there, as well as the general population of patients who come there. Regardless of the physician's personality and the patients' personal backgrounds, the same kinds of activities occur in any physician's office setting.

Today, the trend in medical care is toward an increasing amount of **ambulatory care**—defined as the patient coming to the care rather than the patient receiving care in a home or hospital setting (Figure 1-1). To take advantage of ambulatory care, the patient must be able to walk into the physician's office or at least be brought to the office in a wheelchair. In addition to private physicians' offices, offices of physicians who make up a staff model HMO, community health centers, multispecialty clinics, and hospitals are increasingly making more space available for outpatient care.

FLOW OF ACTIVITY IN AMBULATORY CARE

The flow of activities for each patient in an outpatient setting is similar. The patient will do the following:
- Enter the office.
- Approach the reception desk, identify the physician and time of appointment, provide the office staff with personal and payment information, and make a copayment (if necessary).

Figure 1-1 The patient check-in area in a clinic.

- Be seen by a physician (or by a nurse practitioner [NP] or physician assistant [PA] if the practice uses such personnel).
- Undergo diagnostic or laboratory tests in the office.
- Receive a diagnosis, treatment, or a referral to another health care provider.
- Receive instruction for follow-up care and any laboratory or diagnostic tests to be done elsewhere before leaving the medical office; if seriously ill, the patient may be admitted to the hospital.

Figure 1-2 is a flowchart of how a patient moves through the medical office.

Once a patient has been seen in the medical office, the office begins the process of obtaining payment for its services. The medical payment may come from a private insurance plan, a government-funded insurance program, and/or from the patient. The patient may be responsible for a percentage of the charges or the entire bill if he or she does not have insurance.

After the examination the patient receives instructions to prepare for a test or procedure to be performed or information about medication that has been prescribed. Patients who are seen regularly because of a chronic illness may spend time with a physician or medical assistant reviewing the patient's individual treatment plan. A follow-up appointment is made if necessary.

Most medical offices provide health education materials in print or online. These materials may consist of

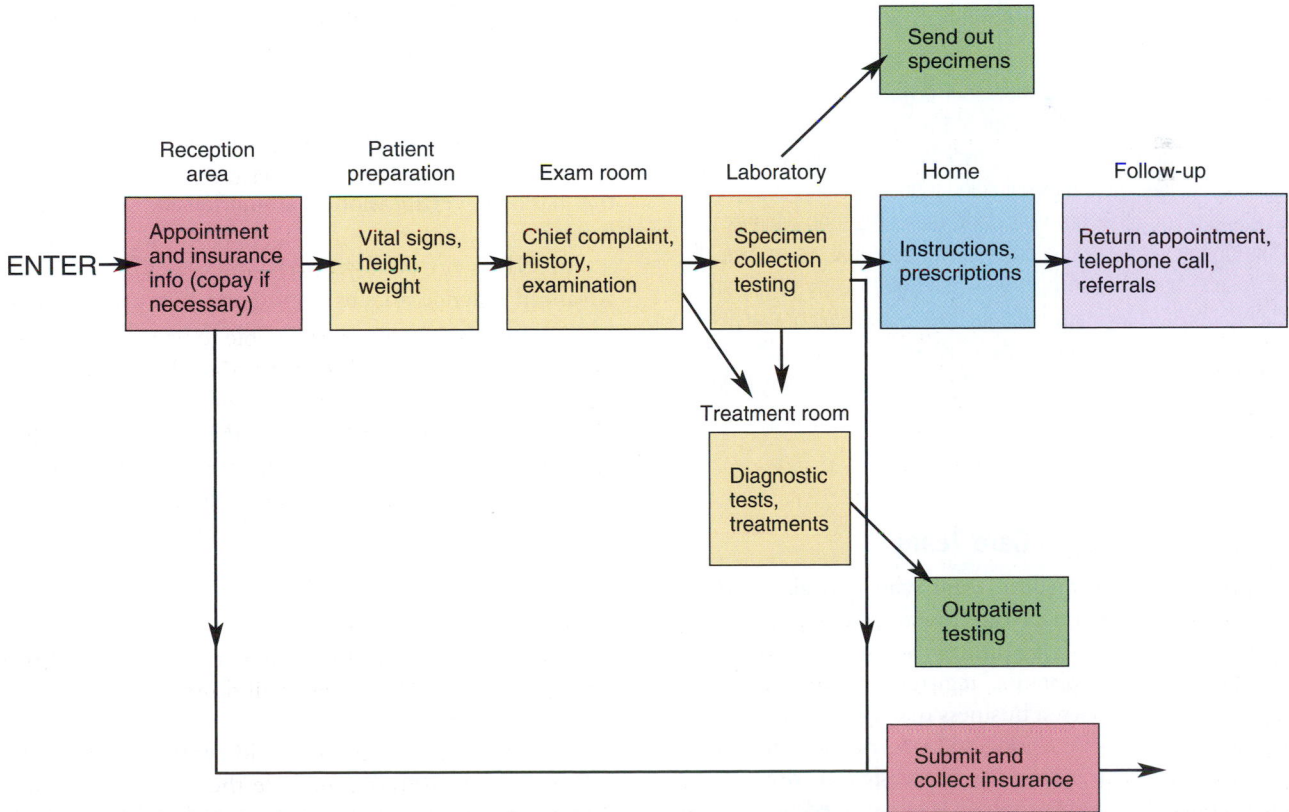

Figure 1-2 Patient progress through a medical office.

pamphlets, article reprints, health education videos, or health news reports specially prepared for viewing in the medical office.

THE HEALTH CARE TEAM

A medical assistant works as a member of a dedicated health care team. The physician or group of physicians expects each medical assistant to fill a slightly different role within the office team. This role will depend on the style of the practice, the region of the country where the practice is located, and what types of medical professionals make up the team.

As the operations of a medical practice become more complex, physicians may employ individuals with more specialized medical business and medical management experience to run the business side of the office. In these offices, medical assistants play more of a clinical role. In smaller offices, medical assistants usually perform both clinical and administrative activities.

Putting It All Into Practice

My name is Aida Reyes, and I am the Medical Assistant for a primary care physician. I have been working here for 12 years, and in that time it seems to get busier and busier. We used to see about 15 patients in a typical morning or afternoon, and now we are seeing an average of 20 to 25. When I first took the job, I thought it would be a fairly relaxed environment. How busy could it be with only one physician? Since I first began, our practice has merged with another practice and expanded, so that there are now four physicians and two nurse practitioners. We have hired a lot of front desk and billing staff, so that I primarily work with my physician, preparing patients for examination, keeping the examination rooms stocked, taking vital signs and doing other pre-visit work, then preparing patients for follow-up laboratory testing and making sure that we receive all test results back. I also help with referrals for my physician's patients because so many patients have some type of managed care insurance. We are fortunate to have a laboratory on the first floor of our building, but I still have to enter the laboratory orders into the computer as soon as possible after the patients are seen by the physician. ■

Members of the Health Care Team

The members of the medical team who typically work in ambulatory care, be it a private practice, a community or public health clinic, or a hospital clinic, include physicians, NPs, PAs, medical assistants, registered nurses (RNs) or licensed practical nurses, a business manager, a receptionist, a medical secretary, file clerks, and one or more insurance specialists. Medical transcription is occasionally done in the medical office, but increasingly it is outsourced or replaced by the electronic medical record or voice recognition software. If the office performs moderate- or high-complexity laboratory tests, a certified medical technologist may also be on the staff or serve as a consultant.

Hospital or community-based clinics will possibly also have a staff of social workers, outreach workers, and case managers to provide social services to patients. Practices specializing in women's health (obstetrics and gynecology) may also have certified nurse-midwives.

Table 1-1 lists various nurses and allied health professionals and describes their roles.

Physicians and Other Health Care Providers

Physicians have either an MD (medical doctor) or a DO (doctor of osteopathy) degree, either of which is awarded after 4 years of college, then 4 years of medical or osteopathic school. In addition, they complete a hospital-based, intensive postgraduate training period, traditionally called a **residency**, which lasts from 2 to 7 years, depending on the specialty. To receive a medical license from the state where he or she will practice, the physician must pass Parts I, II, and III of the U.S. Medical Licensing Examination (USMLE). The first two parts of the examination are taken during medical school, but Part III cannot be taken until the physician has completed at least 1 year of residency (sometimes called an *internship*).

If a physician wants to be "board certified" in a specialty, he or she must pass another examination, administered by the certification board of the particular specialty. The physician does not need to be board certified to obtain a state license to practice medicine.

A PA must have at least 2 years of college plus 2 years of PA school, although most PA programs award a master's degree. A PA usually specializes (e.g., in pediatrics, in adult medicine) and manages a group of patients receiving routine care. He or she must practice with a physician. All states have laws regulating PAs, and students must pass the national certification examination to obtain a state license.

An NP is an RN who has completed a program in advanced practice nursing, a program that usually grants a Master of Science in Nursing (MSN) or higher degree. NPs can specialize in pediatrics, family practice, gerontology, or other specialty areas. In primary care, NPs help with all aspects of patient care including physical examination, diagnosis, treatment, consultations, and patient education. They may serve as a patient's primary care provider. They are licensed as NPs by the state in which they practice.

The educational requirements and scope of an NP's ability to practice independently are determined by each state. In all states, NPs are allowed to carry a caseload and manage routine patient care. Most states allow NPs to write prescriptions; in other states a physician must cosign the order. In some states, NPs are allowed to practice independently, but in most they must practice in an office with supervision by a physician. In a few states, NPs are allowed to admit patients to hospitals.

Table 1-1 Nurses and Allied Health Professionals

Occupation	Credentials	Responsibilities
Certified Professional Coder Certified Coding Associate	CPC CCA	Assigns codes to patient charges and diagnoses for insurance billing. There are many coding certifications depending on knowledge and specialty.
Diagnostic Medical Sonographer	DMS	Performs ultrasound scans in hospitals and ambulatory care facilities. Ultrasound uses high-frequency sound waves to produce images. A sonographer may specialize in ultrasound of the heart (echocardiography).
Emergency Medical Technician Paramedic	EMT; paramedic	Provides emergency services and life support in the community. Several levels of emergency service personnel exist, depending on training and experience.
Health Information Specialist	RHIA; RHIT	Works with patient medical records; may provide assistance in planning, managing information, gathering data for medical research, and policy making.
Medical Assistant	CMA (AAMA); RMA	Performs administrative and clinical tasks in ambulatory care.
Medical (Clinical) Technologist	MT; MLT	Performs laboratory tests in the clinical laboratory and may supervise laboratory operations or provide consulting services.
Medical Secretary	CMS	Secretary who specializes in administrative procedures in a health care setting.
Nuclear Medicine Technologist	CNMT	Operates devices that detect and map absorption of radioactive substances given by injection to create diagnostic images.
Nurse, Practical	LPN; LVN	Performs direct patient care and clinical procedures. May work in hospitals, nursing homes, and ambulatory care settings.
Nurse Practitioner	NP	Specializes in a specific area such as internal medicine, pediatrics, and women's health and often manages routine patient care in ambulatory care settings.
Nurse, Registered	RN	Plans and provides nursing care in inpatient settings. Provides supervision for caregivers in both inpatient and outpatient settings.
Occupational Therapist Occupational Therapy Assistant	OT; OTA	Plans therapeutic activities for rehabilitation, especially for activities of daily living (ADLs). Implements treatment plans.
Physical Therapist Physical Therapy Assistant	PT; PTA	Plans exercises for large muscle groups for rehabilitation and implements treatment plans.
Physician Assistant	PA	Manages routine patient care under the supervision of a physician. Usually works in ambulatory care.
Radiologic Technologist	RT	Takes radiographs and assists with special radiographic examinations. After completing education, may specialize in computed tomography, mammography, or therapeutic radiation.
Registered Dietician	RD	Assists with nutrition of patients in hospitals and ambulatory care. Performs nutrition screening and counseling. Coordinates all aspects of food service in many settings.
Respiratory Therapist	RRT	Provides respiratory treatments and manages patients on ventilators.
Surgical Technologist	CST	Assists during surgery in hospital and day surgery centers by setting up operating rooms, preparing instruments and equipment, and passing instruments during surgery.

What Would You Do? What Would You *Not* Do?

Case Study 1

In the examination room, Alicia Darwin, a new patient, tells Aida that she has switched physicians because she had often been seen by a nurse practitioner in the medical office where she used to go. "I don't think a nurse practitioner has as much experience as a doctor," she says, "and besides, the nurse practitioner can't give me medication if I need it." She asks Aida to confirm that she will always be seen by the physician in this office. She adds, "I don't have anything against nurses like you; I just want to have a real doctor take care of me." ∎

Effective Teamwork

Working as an effective health care team does not just happen. To be effective, team members work together to provide appropriate care for each patient. The more people involved, the more crucial this teamwork is. Each member of the team must be committed to problem solving, communicating, and coordinating effective care.

Teamwork is reinforced at regular staff meetings, which can be directed by either the medical or the business director of the office, depending on the particular topics of the meeting. But the true test of teamwork occurs on a daily basis as health care is provided.

Each health care team member has certain responsibilities and restrictions on activities and areas about which he or she is allowed to make decisions. Sometimes this scope is defined by federal or state law. For example, medical assistants are allowed to administer injections in some states, but in others they cannot. The medical assistant must learn what areas fall within the proper scope of practice and decision-making responsibility in his or her state.

The specific education and role of the medical assistant is discussed in Chapter 2. The medical assistant plays an important role by keeping the work of the office flowing smoothly. He or she must communicate well with other health team members. Because a patient will not always repeat all information to the physician, the medical assistant must communicate anything related to the patient's health verbally or through the medical record. At the same time, the medical assistant must be careful to avoid using diagnostic terminology in the medical record or giving medical advice to the patient (unless following specific guidelines established by the physician).

Teamwork is enhanced when each team member helps and supports other members and avoids blaming or criticizing others. Because the number of employees in a medical office is often small, it is important for everyone to do his or her best to get along and deal with conflict. When a problem arises, it is important to try to find solutions to the problem rather than focusing on who caused the problem or whose fault it is. It is also helpful to maintain perspective and accept that things do go wrong, and most problems can be dealt with. In any conflict situation, it is important to listen to the point of view of others and validate their feelings. Effective communication techniques are discussed in more detail in Chapter 4.

PARTS OF THE MEDICAL OFFICE

A physician's office has a number of different physical spaces in it. Each space has a particular purpose. Every physician's office has three basic areas: a reception area and waiting room, examination and treatment rooms, and an area for other activities. This may include medical records storage, if the office uses paper medical records; storage for supplies; and staff offices or cubicles.

In most offices, physicians also have their own offices, separate from examination rooms, but some physicians have examination tables in their offices, combining the two spaces in one room.

Larger offices may have several additional areas such as an office laboratory; separate treatment rooms or special procedure rooms; a business office, which is separate from the front office (reception, telephones, appointments); and a lunch or break room for the staff.

All physicians' offices must meet a number of specifications laid out by regulatory agencies. These include the federal Occupational Safety and Health Administration (OSHA), which regulates workplace health and safety. Physicians' offices also must meet the specifications of the Americans with Disabilities Act, which requires that doorways be at least 3 feet wide and hallways at least 5 feet wide. Restroom facilities must be available for both patients and staff. Office laboratories are regulated by the Clinical Laboratory Improvement Amendments of 1988 (CLIA '88). Local boards of health also inspect and regulate hospitals and clinics.

Figure 1-3 shows the layout of a small medical office.

Figure 1-3 Layout of a small medical office.

RECEPTION AREA AND WAITING ROOM

The reception area and waiting room are the first place any new or prospective patient will see. First impressions are important. The waiting room should be clean and well lit. Furniture should be arranged and not haphazardly placed. Up-to-date, general-interest reading material should be available; many physicians also have patient education materials available in the waiting room. Waiting rooms in pediatric and family practice offices also have toys available for children. Large pediatric practices may have a separate waiting room for sick children or for adolescents.

The waiting room should have enough chairs for two people per patient visit, multiplied by the number of patients seen in 2 hours. It needs to present a calm atmosphere and look professional. Usually the waiting area is carpeted. It should have comfortable chairs, grouped in blocks if possible rather than just lined up around the walls. Colors should be muted, and music should be soft. Red, yellow, and orange are typically avoided; today, physician's office decor often uses shades of green, dusty pink, or salmon. Music is usually played from a CD or radio station of the "easy listening" variety.

The reception area adjoins the waiting room. The medical assistant at the reception desk should greet each patient as he or she enters the waiting room. Most reception areas have a counter so that the patient can fill out or sign forms, and many have a sliding window so that patients cannot hear the conversations occurring behind the receptionist.

Patients check in here when they enter the office. New patient forms are received here, and health insurance cards are copied. Copayments are taken from patients whose insurance is provided through HMOs. Appointments may be made by the receptionist or in a separate area of the office.

EXAMINATION ROOMS AND LABORATORY

Examination rooms are designed for the convenience of the physician and assisting personnel who will work there. However, they also need to be as comfortable and calming to the patient as possible. Reading material should be available in each examination room. Although good scheduling will ensure that patients will not wait too long in these rooms for a physician, most physicians do see patients in at least two examination rooms. Additional delays may occur if the physician has to respond to urgent telephone calls or office emergencies (Figure 1-4).

Many physicians perform treatments or diagnostic procedures in examination rooms, but complex procedures (such as suturing a laceration) are often performed in larger rooms with extra equipment and/or supplies. These are called *treatment rooms.*

If laboratory tests are performed in the medical office, there is a special room or area set aside for this. CLIA '88

Figure 1-4 Examination rooms are usually compact, but each should be large enough to accommodate a wheelchair. (From Proctor D, Adams A: *Kinn's the medical assistant*, ed 12, St Louis, 2014, Saunders.)

regulates laboratory testing. Medical assistants are trained to perform low-complexity tests (CLIA-waived tests) such as dipstick urinalysis, urine pregnancy tests, and rapid strep tests. They may also perform more complex texts with special training.

CLIA '88 specifies who can supervise laboratories and lays out the process for inspection and accreditation. It sets strict guidelines for quality control, quality assurance, handling of hazardous materials, documentation, and proficiency training. Offices that perform only CLIA-waived laboratory tests may perform laboratory testing in the patient preparation area. Ideally the bathroom is adjacent to this area, with an opening in the wall so that urine samples can be passed directly into the laboratory area.

MEDICAL RECORDS STORAGE AND BUSINESS OFFICE

If the office uses paper records, the medical records may be stored near the reception area, in the business areas, adjacent to the patient preparation area, or in a separate room. Charts of active patients—those who have been seen within the past 2 to 3 years—are kept in the records storage area in the office. Inactive charts are removed regularly and stored in a less accessible location such as the basement of the building or off-site in a facility that maintains records in storage. Charts needed for patients who will be coming in during a specified period—morning, afternoon, or an entire day—are removed from the storage area and prepared for use.

The majority of medical practices have moved away from paper records to computerized medical records. In this case, patient records are stored on a computer's hard disk and are simply pulled up from the database as needed. The process of placing old records into the computerized record is lengthy, and some offices that use an electronic health record store the former paper records of established patients in an accessible area for 1 to 2 years after the transition to the electronic health record.

Posting of patient charges, billing, and computer operations may be performed in an area behind the reception desk or in a separate business office. If the practice has one or more satellite locations, the billing and insurance tasks are usually done in the practice's main office for all locations. Some offices contract billing and insurance claim processing to an outside company, which may even be located in another state.

What Would You Do? What Would You *Not* Do?

Case Study 2

The physician complains to Aida that there are always dishes in the sink in the break room and crumbs and used paper coffee cups on the table. Even though the area is not seen by patients, the physician is concerned that an insect or rodent problem could develop. Aida knows that the part-time file clerk and the part-time receptionist have a tendency to leave dirty dishes and trash after their afternoon break. She herself is so busy that she rarely has time to either clean or sit down in the break room. ■

ADDITIONAL AREAS FOUND IN MANY OFFICES

Physicians' private offices are often a reflection of their personal tastes. This room is where a physician meets privately with patients, patients' families, and other visitors. He or she usually displays degrees and certificates of membership in professional organizations on the walls of the office. Even if the practice has a small library for the use of all staff, physicians will usually have at least a few important references in this office. Art and memorabilia that show the physician's personal taste also help to make the private office a pleasant place for the physician to do quiet work and hold meetings.

Recognizing the needs of staff for a quiet place to take their breaks and eat their lunch, newer offices often include a staff break or lunch room. This room may have a refrigerator and microwave for staff to prepare lunches they bring from home. There should be at least one table and chairs. The lunch or break room should not double as a storage area, and staff should avoid using the room for meetings that deprive others of use of the room.

Depending on the type of medical practice, particular rooms may be set aside for specific treatments or diagnostic procedures. Types of special rooms include the following:

- A pediatrics examination or treatment room in a family practice group's office
- A surgical procedure room in a general surgery group's office

- A room for more complex testing such as colposcopy and pelvic ultrasounds in a group practice specializing in obstetrics and gynecology
- A trauma room in a large clinic or community health center

Memories *from* Practicum

Aida Reyes: The clinic where I did my practicum was so large that at first I kept getting lost. Another thing that confused me was the doors that the staff used to get from one part of the clinic to another. It was arranged by department, but the layout of rooms in each department was different. I spent the majority of my time in internal medicine working with one medical assistant and one physician, but my preceptor arranged for me to spend time in other departments like medical records, billing, and pediatrics and with the referral coordinator. In addition to the full-time physicians, there were some specialists who came in once or twice a week, including a neurologist, an orthopedic surgeon, and an ophthalmologist. The clinic also employed a social worker and a dietician. In each department there was a nurse and there were at least two medical assistants in addition to the receptionist. The amazing thing was how quickly I adapted and became comfortable finding my way around. After only a few weeks, it felt like I belonged there. I was so proud when my preceptor said, "Aida, you have become one of the team. I don't know how we ever got along without you." ■

MEDICAL SPECIALTIES

Since the middle of the twentieth century, the practice of medicine has been broken down into fields of specialty and subspecialty. In 1950 most Americans received their medical care from a general practitioner, who took care of adults and children, often delivered babies, and performed many general surgical procedures.

Today, Americans may see two, three, or more physicians routinely. Box 1-1 describes the medical specialties recognized by the American Board of Medical Specialties. In many areas, there are several subspecialties. If the physician wants to work in a subspecialty, after the residency training he or she participates in additional training called a *fellowship* for 2 to 3 years. It is not possible to be board certified in any specialty or subspecialty without completing a residency.

PRIMARY CARE AND THE PATIENT-CENTERED MEDICAL HOME

Primary care physicians specialize in internal medicine (treatment of the internal organs of adults by other than surgical means), pediatrics (general medical care of children and adolescents), or family medicine (general medical care

BOX 1-1   Medical Specialties

Allergy and Immunology (Allergist, Immunologist): Treats adults and/or children with allergies and problems of the immune system. Many individuals experience allergies and/or asthma in the presence of allergens. The immune system can also malfunction either through inherited or acquired diseases. Allergists and immunologists diagnose, manage, and treat allergic diseases, immunodeficiency conditions, and autoimmune diseases.

Anesthesiology (Anesthesiologist): Provides anesthesia during surgery and other procedures, as well as medical care to patients before, during, and after surgery. The anesthesiologist also supervises other anesthesia personnel in the operating room such as nurse anesthetists and anesthesiology residents.

Colon and Rectal Surgery: Performs surgical treatment of the large intestine and rectum. These surgeons specialize in the diagnosis and treatment of diseases of the colon and rectum in addition to full training in general surgery. They perform diagnostic and screening procedures and perform surgery when necessary.

Dermatology (Dermatologist): Specializes in conditions of the skin. Dermatologists diagnose skin diseases and also perform surgery on the skin. Laser treatments are commonly used for skin conditions in addition to medication, cryotherapy, and surgery.

Emergency Medicine: Treats patients for emergency conditions, usually in the emergency department of a hospital. Emergency medicine focuses treatment of acute illnesses and injuries that require immediate care. The physician is often an employee of a hospital emergency department or other urgent care center.

Family Medicine (Family Practitioner): Treats adults and children for routine care and complaints; often the primary care physician for all family members. The family practitioner is concerned with the total health of the individual and the family.

Internal Medicine (Internist): Provides medical treatment for conditions of various body systems. The internist may be the primary care provider for adults. Within the discipline of internal medicine there are several subspecialties based on patient age groups, body system, or type of disease.

Medical Genetics: Provides diagnostic procedures and treatment for individuals with genetically linked diseases. Also provides genetic counseling and prenatal diagnosis.

Neurologic Surgery (Neurosurgeon): Performs prevention, diagnosis, surgical and nonsurgical treatment, and rehabilitation for conditions of the brain, spine, and nervous system. Also provides surgical and nonsurgical treatment of pain.

Neurology (Neurologist): Provides diagnosis and medical treatment of diseases of the peripheral and central nervous system. Neurologists are usually either generalists or have special qualifications in child neurology.

Nuclear Medicine: Specializes in diagnosis using radionuclides, atoms that give off electromagnetic radiation. Nuclear physicians are usually employed by a hospital or university (or both) and have little direct patient care. They are responsible for diagnosis and recommending treatment of abnormalities detected through the various imaging modalities used in the nuclear medicine department.

Obstetrics (Obstetrician) and Gynecology (Gynecologist): Specializes in care during pregnancy and delivery (obstetrician); specializes in other care and surgery of the female reproductive system (gynecologist). The gynecologist is responsible for screening procedures, diagnostic procedures, and both medical and surgical treatments. He or she also frequently uses hormone-modulating treatments.

Ophthalmology (Ophthalmologist): Specializes in the care of the eye. The ophthalmologist manages diseases and conditions of the eye with both medical and surgical treatment including laser treatments. May also manage errors of refraction and prescribe corrective lenses, although this is often delegated to an optometrist.

Orthopedic Surgery (Orthopedic Surgeon): Specializes in diagnosis and treatment of acute and traumatic injuries of the musculoskeletal system, as well as diseases of the muscular or skeletal system. Both surgical and nonsurgical treatments are used.

Otolaryngology (Otolaryngologist or ENT): Specializes in the care of the ear, nose, throat, head, and neck. The physician, often called an ENT (for ear, nose, and throat), is responsible for the diagnosis and surgical or nonsurgical treatment of a variety of disorders affecting the specified organs.

Pathology (Pathologist): Examines cells, tissues, and other specimens to determine whether their structure is normal or abnormal; attempts to determine the nature or cause of disease. Pathologists examine tissue biopsies and other specimens to identify abnormal cells. They also perform autopsies. They may be trained within two primary specialty areas: clinical pathology and/or anatomic pathology.

Pediatrics (Pediatrician): Specializes in the care of children from birth through adolescence. In the United States, pediatricians are considered to be primary care practitioners. However, many pediatricians specialize, and almost every specialty for adult medicine is represented as a pediatric subspecialty.

Physical Medicine and Rehabilitation (Physiatrist): Specializes in the treatment and rehabilitation of patients with disabling conditions such as spinal cord injury and stroke. A physiatrist sees patients across several age groups and specialty areas and focuses on restoring maximal function to patients. He or she may specialize in specific age groups or types of injury such as spinal cord injury.

Plastic Surgery: Specializes in surgical and nonsurgical treatment of physical defects of various areas of the body. The plastic surgeon performs procedures for cosmetic

Continued

BOX 1-1   Medical Specialties—cont'd

enhancement or reconstruction of various parts of the body. Cosmetic surgery has become popular in the past two decades. Reconstructive surgery includes craniofacial surgery, hand surgery, and maxillofacial surgery to repair congenital defects and problems that result from injury or disease.

Preventative Medicine: Includes aerospace medicine, occupational medicine, and public health. In this medical specialty, physicians practice in one of the specialty areas or one of the subspecialties (clinical informatics, medical toxicology, or undersea and hyperbaric medicine).

Psychiatry (Psychiatrist): Specializes in preventing, diagnosing, and treating mental illness. Psychiatrists have completed the same general training as any other physician, and they are able to prescribe medication for mental illness and monitor the effects of medication therapy. Like other mental health professionals, they usually also have training in psychotherapy, psychoanalysis, and/or cognitive behavioral therapy.

Radiology (Radiologist): Specializes in the use of x-ray and other ionizing radiation for diagnosis (diagnostic radiology),

treatment (radiation oncology), or medical physics. A diagnostic radiologist has the training to manage several types of diagnostic imaging including x-ray studies, computed tomography (CT) scans, and magnetic resonance imaging (MRI).

Surgery (General Surgeon): Performs general surgical procedures. A general surgeon performs primarily abdominal surgery using traditional methods or laparoscopic methods.

Thoracic Surgery (Thoracic Surgeon): Performs surgery of the chest including cardiac surgery, although thoracic surgeons usually specialize in surgery of the chest or cardiac surgery.

Urology (Urologist): Specializes in the care of the urinary system in males and females and the reproductive tract in males; also specializes in surgery of the urinary tract and male reproductive tract. The urologist may provide medical treatment as for infections or surgical repair for abnormal growths or correction of congenital malformations.

Vascular Surgery (Vascular Surgeon): Performs surgery of the arteries and veins (except for the blood vessels of the heart and brain).

---

of children, adolescents, and adults—today's equivalent of general practice).

Over the course of time, the activities of different types of physicians have shifted. For instance, fewer family practitioners deliver babies today than did general practitioners in the 1950s and 1960s, preferring to leave that task to obstetricians owing to the cost of malpractice insurance. Although some women continue to see a gynecologist for an annual pelvic examination and Pap test, the primary care provider performs these activities more often today than in the past.

Primary care has been greatly influenced in the past decade by the movement to establish a **patient-centered medical home (PCMH)** as the provider of a patient's primary care. The PCMH is a model of primary care that emphasizes patient-centered health care based on a personal relationship between a patient, a physician, and the patient's care team. The PCMH movement incorporates several elements:

- It is patient centered, and health care teams are jointly responsible for patient care and safety.
- It is comprehensive, including prevention, acute care, and chronic care.
- Care is coordinated across the entire health care system including specialty care, hospitals, home care, and community services.
- Patients receive high-quality care; both patients and families are encouraged to make informed decisions about their health.

Most states have adopted an initiative to support the PCMH movement and encourage primary care practices to

become recognized PCMHs. There is a strong relationship between PCMH practices and ACOs mandated by the Center for Medicare and Medicaid Services (CMS), which are intended to increase the quality of care of Medicare patients. Within the PCMH movement, medical assistants play an important role in enhancing access to care. They are often expected to undertake more advanced duties than were formerly assigned to them.

OSTEOPATHY

Osteopathy is a mix of traditional scientific medicine and **holistic** medicine, which focuses more on healing the entire person than a specific disease or condition. This branch of medical practice seeks to balance the structure and function of the body through manipulation of muscles and joints. Osteopathy was started in the late 1800s by Andrew Taylor Still (1828-1917). Osteopaths see disease as the result of dysfunction in the skeletal and muscular systems. Pain, "asymmetry" (the difference in anatomy or joint movement between one side of the body and the other), and tissue tenderness are used to gauge symptoms. Osteopaths, who hold DO degrees, today are given all the privileges of those with MD degrees. The majority of osteopaths practice as primary care doctors, where they believe their holistic and structural approach can be most effective.

PODIATRY

Podiatrists use traditional medical and surgical techniques but are limited in their practice to treatment of disorders of

Figure 1-5 Spinal adjustment with patient in prone position. (From Gatterman M: *Foundations of chiropractic: subluxation*, ed 2, St Louis, 2005, Mosby.)

the feet and ankles. Since the 1970s, podiatry has worked to enlarge its area of practice by focusing on surgery of the foot to alleviate such problems as bone spurs and bunions. Podiatrists work closely with primary care doctors in the management of diabetic patients and the elderly, who often require specialized foot care.

CHIROPRACTIC

Chiropractic is the technique of spinal manipulation. Chiropractors believe that vertebral subluxations (partially dislocated spinal joints) cause nerve blockages, which in turn lead to pain in the back, neck, shoulders, and legs. Begun in 1895 by Daniel David Palmer (1845-1913), chiropractic holds that the body has its own ability to heal and maintain balance. According to chiropractic theory, the nervous system is the center of all disease and healing. Some chiropractors believe that subluxation is the reason for all disease. Today's chiropractors, who are licensed by the state in which they practice, limit their treatment to discomfort clearly associated with the spine and integrate their practices into standard Western medical practice.

Figure 1-5 demonstrates a chiropractic adjustment.

PRACTICE TYPES

Fifty years ago most physicians who were not full-time members of hospital staffs worked by themselves in an office, either in their home or in an office building. They paid their office expenses, taxes, and liability insurance out of their income, and the difference was considered their "net income" from their practice. As their practice got busier, their income increased. Today many physicians work with other physicians. Some of them have an ownership position in the practice or facility in which they work, but others are employees and receive a salary from their employer. The following categories refer to the way the office is structured, not the business arrangement or ownership.

SOLO PRACTICE

It is still possible for a physician to work in a solo practice. But to do so, he or she must make a number of trade-offs. Solo practices are limited in their size by the number of patients one physician can manage. When a physician practices alone, the medical assistant is usually responsible for aspects of both administrative and clinical support.

Even if a solo practitioner employs an NP or a PA to see additional patients, the physician still must factor into his or her workday some time to oversee the work of these nonphysician professionals. In addition, the physician, as the employer, is usually responsible for paying the malpractice insurance premiums for all of the licensed professionals in his or her office. Physicians in solo practice are also completely responsible for their patients. Usually they make arrangements with other physicians to share after-hours and weekend call responsibilities and to cover for vacations.

GROUP PRACTICE

Many physicians today participate in a group practice. The most common type of group practice includes three or four physicians of the same medical specialty who band together to share resources such as office space and personnel. In these groups, medical assistants usually specialize in either clinical or administrative work, although they expect to help out in other areas.

Depending on the business form used, patients are the responsibility of either one physician or "the group." In either case, if a patient's regular physician is not available, another physician in the office can see the patient. In addition, physicians who work in group practices usually share after-hours and weekend call responsibilities. They usually split the cost of malpractice insurance, and the policy is written for the group rather than for each individual.

Large medical groups with physicians who provide primary care, as well as physicians with other medical specialties, are becoming increasingly common throughout the country. Their names often include the words "associates" or "medical associates." This organizational form allows a sharing of resources that, in turn, allows each physician in the group to provide a broader range of services. In the past, these groups were more common in particular regions and in rural areas where a single group of physicians has the responsibility of being both the physicians in town and the staff of a small, rural hospital. HMOs that provide all services in one building, so-called "closed-panel HMOs," also operate as multispecialty groups.

These practices often have separate administrative departments for billing, appointment scheduling, and referrals and separate clinical departments for phlebotomy, electrocardiography, laboratory work, and radiography. In such practices, medical assisting jobs can be limited in scope, and specific responsibilities depend on the department in which the medical assistant works.

CLINIC

Traditionally a clinic was connected to a hospital and provided ambulatory care, often to patients with limited financial resources. Patients were either seen at no charge or billed by the clinic, and physicians were paid a salary for their services and/or saw patients as part of their residency program. Today a *clinic* usually refers to a public or nonprofit facility that provides outpatient public health services, although private solo or group practices may use the word "clinic" in their name. Community health centers, established by the federal government in the late 1960s, operate as clinics and have physicians as well as NPs, PAs, and nurse-midwives all on salary.

COMPLEMENTARY AND ALTERNATIVE MEDICINE

Numerous other practices are used for the treatment of illness, some of which have a long tradition and some of which have developed more recently. Studies from the early 1990s found that Americans annually spend literally millions of dollars on therapies that are not part of their physician's standard approach. Patients often do not even tell their physicians about these other treatments. When practices have been used for extended periods in specific cultures, they may be called *traditional medicine.* The term *complementary medicine* is usually used for medical treatments that patients use in addition to standard medical treatments. The term *alternative medicine* refers to practices that are used instead of standard medical treatment. For many patients, these may overlap. Acupuncture, for example, has been a definitive method of treatment in traditional Chinese medicine for centuries (Figure 1-6). In the United States it has become a popular treatment method used in addition to standard treatment. It has become so popular that there are many schools to train practitioners, and the practice of acupuncture requires a license in most states.

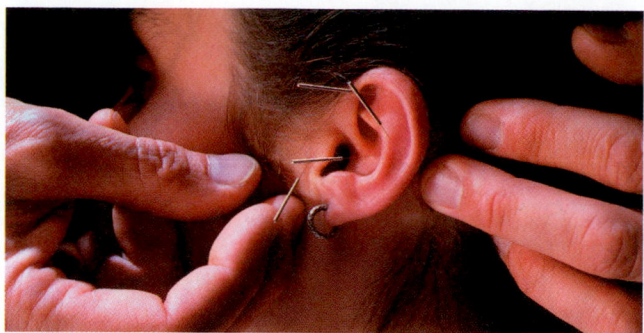

Figure 1-6 Acupuncture involves the placement of several extremely thin needles in various parts of the body.

Since the early 1990s, scholars of medicine have begun to take an interest in studying complementary and alternative practices scientifically. The federal government has since established the National Center for Complementary and Alternative Medicine within the National Institutes of Health. This agency coordinates and funds scientific research to study the effectiveness of these health practices. The most well respected medical journals such as the *New England Journal of Medicine* and *JAMA* have published a number of studies about the effectiveness of various nonstandard therapies, and numerous specialized journals have also been established to publish research about such therapies. When research demonstrates that a practice is effective, physicians trained in the classic Western medical tradition are more accepting and may even incorporate some of these practices or refer patients to practitioners.

What Would You Do?	What Would You *Not* Do?

Case Study 3
While Aida is taking John Carter's medical history, he mentions that he has been getting acupuncture and taking several herbal preparations that he buys at a health food store. He also says that he wears shoe insoles with magnets in them because he has had heel pain for several months. He says, "You should try them. They have really helped my heel pain." ∎

What Would You Do?	What Would You *Not* Do?	RESPONSES

Case Study 1
Page 9

What Did Aida Do?
❑ Accepted Alicia Darwin's reason for changing medical offices without making a judgment.
❑ Stated that she hopes Alicia will feel comfortable as a patient in their practice.
❑ Stated that she is a medical assistant, not a nurse, and explain the difference briefly.
❑ Clarified the legal position of a nurse practitioner in her state related to prescribing medications.

What Did Aida Not *Do?*
❑ Agreed verbally or by implication that she is a nurse.
❑ Asked for additional information about Alicia's previous physician or medical office.
❑ Made any critical remarks about nurse practitioners or Alicia's previous physician.
❑ Made any statement that could be interpreted as a guarantee that Alicia will like this physician better.

What Would You Do? What Would You *Not* Do? RESPONSES—cont'd

Case Study 2
Page 12

What Did Aida Do?
❑ Agreed that the condition of the break room could be improved.
❑ Promised to talk to all staff members about keeping the break room clean.
❑ Arranged time to speak to staff members either individually or as a group to discuss ways to keep the break room clean and make a plan.
❑ Encouraged all staff members to take an active part in developing a plan to keep the break room clean.
❑ Followed up to be sure that any plan made was implemented and was effective.

What Did Aida Not Do?
❑ Did not focus on identifying who was responsible when talking to either the physician or other staff members.
❑ Did not become defensive when talking to the physician or other staff members.
❑ Did not single out any staff member(s) as responsible for the problem.

❑ Did not complain about one staff member's behavior to any other staff member.

Case Study 3
Page 16

What Did Aida Do?
❑ Accepted John Carter's description of his complementary and alternative medical practices.
❑ Documented all practices in the medical record.
❑ Asked questions to explore the underlying problems such as heel pain or the reason for acupuncture.

What Did Aida Not Do?
❑ Did not tell John that he might be endangering his health because of his use of complementary or alternative medical practices.
❑ Did not tell John that acupuncture, magnets, or herbs will not help him.
❑ Did not ask John where to buy foot insoles with magnets.
❑ Did not dismiss John's practices as insignificant and fail to document them.

TERMINOLOGY REVIEW

Key Term	Word Parts	Definition
Ambulatory care	*ambulare:* to walk *-ory:* pertaining to	Medical care that is provided on an outpatient basis. The patient is able to come to the facility providing care and return home after having received services.
Capitation		A set payment provided by managed care insurance per patient per month regardless of the amount of service the patient receives.
Curative treatment		Treatment that cures disease.
Empirical	*empiricus:* experienced *-al:* pertaining to	Learned from observation or experiment.
Fee-for-service		A means of payment for health care in which the cost for each service provided is reimbursed in full or in part.
Formulary		A list of prescription drugs covered or preferred by a managed care insurance company.
Health insurance		Purchase of protection for covered services related to health care.
Holistic	*holos:* whole *-ic:* pertaining to	Considering the whole; in medicine, considering the entire person when providing health care.
Managed care		A system that manages the delivery of health care with the intention of controlling costs.
Palliative treatment		Therapy that reduces the effects of a disease or condition but does not remove the disease itself.
Patient-centered medical home (PCMH)		A model of primary care that emphasizes patient-centered health care based on a personal relationship among a patient, a physician, and the patient's care team.
Residency		A program to provide training in a medical specialty to a physician who has finished medical school.
Symptomatic treatment		Therapy for symptoms of a disease or condition that does not remove the disease itself.
Utilization review		Assessment of medical services to determine whether they are appropriate, necessary, and of high quality.

ON THE WEB

For information on health:

World Health Organization: www.who.int/en

National Institutes of Health: www.nih.gov

For information on physicians and osteopathic physicians:

American Medical Association: www.ama-assn.org

American Osteopathic Association: www.osteopathic.org

For information on the patient-centered medical home (PCMH):

Patient-Centered Primary Care Collaborative: http://www.pcpcc.org/

Patient Centered Medical Home Resource Center (Agency for Healthcare Research and Quality of U.S. Department of Health and Human Services): pcmh.ahrq.gov

For information on medical specialties:

American Board of Medical Specialties (ABMS): www.abms.org

For information on complementary and alternative medicine:

National Center for Complementary and Alternative Medicine (NCCAM), National Institutes of Health: www.nccam.nih.gov

The Professional Medical Assistant

LEARNING OBJECTIVES

1. Describe the history of the medical assisting profession.
2. Explain how a medical assisting educational program becomes accredited.
3. List character and personality traits of effective medical assistants.
4. Describe the appearance and behavior of a professional medical assistant.
5. Describe principles of effective time management.
6. Define *professionalism* for physicians and medical assistants.
7. Identify organizations and publications that guide professional behavior for physicians and medical assistants.
8. Differentiate between various national credentials for medical assistants.
9. Describe how professional organizations support the profession of medical assisting.
10. Identify the administrative tasks and clinical tasks performed by a medical assistant.
11. Discuss the medical assistant's role in the operation of the medical office and patient education.
12. List employment opportunities for medical assistants.

PROCEDURES

Locate and define the legal scope of practice in own state.

CHAPTER OUTLINE

INTRODUCTION TO PROFESSIONAL MEDICAL ASSISTING
EDUCATIONAL PROGRAMS FOR MEDICAL ASSISTANTS
CHARACTERISTICS OF MEDICAL ASSISTANTS
Character Traits
Personality Traits
Appearance
Initiative and Behavioral Skills
PROFESSIONALISM
Professionalism for Physicians
Professionalism for Medical Assistants
CERTIFICATION FOR MEDICAL ASSISTANTS
American Association of Medical Assistants
American Medical Technologists
California Certifying Board for Medical Assistants
National Healthcareer Association

National Center for Competency Testing
Obtaining Additional Credentials
PROFESSIONAL ORGANIZATIONS
Peer Support
Continuing Education
Legislative Advocacy
Publications, Newsletters, and Websites
ROLE OF THE MEDICAL ASSISTANT
Administrative Responsibilities
Clinical Responsibilities
Managing the Medical Office
Patient Education and Coaching
Patient Navigation
EMPLOYMENT OPPORTUNITIES

KEY TERMS

accreditation
continuing education unit (CEU)
fee splitting

health coaching
initiative
patient navigator

practicum
risk management
time management

INTRODUCTION TO PROFESSIONAL MEDICAL ASSISTING

Medical assisting came into existence as a career during the second half of the twentieth century. Around the middle of the 1900s, most physicians established their own practice when they completed their medical education and hospital training. A physician (almost always a man) usually saw patients and had no assistance, except possibly from his wife who answered the telephone and often did the billing.

The physician spent a large portion of each day making house calls. During a house call the physician would examine a patient with only the equipment he could carry in his medical bag. The physician's office was often located in a room in his house or the first floor of a building, with the physician living in an apartment above. Patients who went to the physician's office may or may not have had an appointment. They expected to wait to be seen.

In the first 20 years after World War II (before the increasing use of technology caused medical costs to skyrocket), a physician usually charged $2 to $5, possibly $10, for an office visit, a sum that seems small today. For some patients, however, even this small charge was more than a day's pay. For physicians the low fee was enough because the expenses of the practice were also low. In fact, physicians rarely pressed poor patients for full payment. They always had many patients who owed them money, and it was not uncommon for patients to pay small amounts on a weekly basis for many months or even years, especially the parents of young children. Sometimes physicians would even barter by exchanging medical care for goods or services provided by the patient. For example, a patient might pay for his medical care by bringing the physician fresh produce from his farm.

During the past 60 years, the practice of medicine has changed dramatically. This, in turn, has changed the way in which physicians operate their medical practices. With the advent of government insurance programs, not only were office visits covered by insurance, but the medical office was also expected to complete and submit the insurance forms to receive payment. Physicians soon discovered that the cost of employing a person to complete these forms was offset by improved collections and cash flow. Gradually almost all insurance billing shifted to the health care provider.

Advances in medical science made many more diagnostic tests, laboratory tests, and treatments available and even necessary for good medical care. It made sense to have an assistant in the office to perform these tests and allow the physician to concentrate on seeing patients.

Even as laboratory and diagnostic testing has increased in amount and in complexity, so too have the administrative equipment and technology used in a physician's office. Today there are computers, wireless electronic devices, printers, fax machines, photocopiers, intercoms, and voice-mail systems.

Physicians send claims to a number of different insurance companies. Many insurance plans require prior approval for certain medical procedures, referrals to specialists, or surgical procedures. Insurance companies and government programs prefer electronic claims filing and often make electronic payments directly into physicians' office accounts at banks. This creates a need not only for more staff, but also for more highly trained staff.

Physicians have also almost completely stopped making house calls. Because of this, physicians need more office space. In addition, patients with more complex needs are seen in physicians' offices rather than in the hospital emergency department or outpatient department. Sometimes a patient must occupy an examination or treatment room for an extended period of time, such as when an individual with asthma is receiving an inhalation treatment.

Another change that has had an impact on the medical practice involves the increase in medical litigation. Since the 1970s, physicians have practiced what has come to be called "defensive medicine." Because of the fear of a malpractice lawsuit and the high cost of malpractice insurance, physicians began to perform more laboratory and diagnostic tests to rule out even the most unlikely cause of an illness. Another factor stimulating the expanded use of laboratory tests in outpatient care is the increased number of Clinical Laboratory Improvement Amendments (CLIA)–waived tests that are available.

As services expanded, physicians employed nurses to help them in their offices. This helped ease their burden of performing procedures and caring for patients, but nurses were often unable and unwilling to assist with the administrative aspects of the practice. As a result, many physicians found a willing candidate and trained that person to assist first with administrative duties and then with both patient care and administrative duties. This evolved over time into what today is the medical assistant profession.

In 1956, medical assistants from 15 states organized to form the American Association of Medical Assistants (AAMA). In 1978 the profession was recognized by the U.S. Department of Education. The AAMA and other organizations, especially the American Medical Technologists (AMT), have worked to define professional training for the medical assistant and to provide certification for medical assistants through national examinations.

EDUCATIONAL PROGRAMS FOR MEDICAL ASSISTANTS

Initially, medical assistants received on-the-job training, but as the profession grew, formal educational programs were established. These programs vary in length from 6 months to 2 years. Medical assisting programs include theoretical and practical preparation in all aspects of the medical assisting profession. To maintain quality, many of these programs seek **accreditation,** credit, or recognition from a regional or national organization for maintaining certain standards. The two recognized accrediting agencies for medical assisting programs are the Commission on Accreditation of Allied Health Education Programs (CAAHEP) in collaboration with the AAMA and the Accrediting Bureau of Health Education Schools (ABHES).

A medical assisting program seeking accreditation from one of these agencies must prepare a written report showing how the educational standards of the agency are being met. After the report has been submitted, an accreditation visit is made to validate the information presented in the report. Once accreditation has been granted, graduates of the program are eligible to take either the certified medical assistant (CMA) (AAMA) or registered medical assistant (RMA) certification examination. Accredited programs must include at least 160 hours of practical work experience in a medical office or clinic, known as a **practicum** or practical experience (formerly called an *externship*).

CHARACTERISTICS OF MEDICAL ASSISTANTS

Medical assistants possess or develop a number of characteristics that make them effective in their work. Although a person's character and personality have been shaped by heredity and environment, a medical assisting student can work to enhance the traits that are important for health care delivery. Appearance and behavior are also an important means of projecting competence in the medical office (Figure 2-1).

CHARACTER TRAITS

The most important character traits of a competent medical assistant are dependability, honesty, and tolerance.

Figure 2-1 A professional appearance projects competence and increases the patient's confidence in the medical assistant.

Character is closely related to the moral and ethical values of an individual. It is often regarded as the true self and reveals itself through actions over time. As an integral part of the office practice, for example, medical assistants must arrive at work on time and not take days off except when ill or if a family emergency arises. Medical assistants who come to work promptly every day demonstrate that dependability is part of their character.

A medical assistant projects honesty by working within his or her "scope of practice"—that is, doing only what he or she is trained to do and being comfortable in saying "I don't know" or "I don't know how to" when appropriate. State laws regulating the scope of practice for medical assistants vary greatly, so it is important always to be aware of legal restrictions (Procedure 2-1). Medical assistants must always maintain confidentiality and behave ethically. They must recognize that a high level of trust is an important component of high-quality patient care. Tolerance or a willingness to accept the beliefs and practices of others is another important character trait. Tolerance allows medical assistants to work effectively with co-workers and patients from a variety of religious, ethnic, and cultural backgrounds. The patient-centered medical home in primary care emphasizes seeing each patient as a whole person and responding to needs throughout the life span.

Putting It All Into Practice

My name is Beth Ann Wilson, and I am a Certified Medical Assistant. I attended a medical assisting training program at the community college near my home. I was the first person in my family to go to college, and my family was very proud of me. After the first year (two semesters), I received a certificate in medical assisting, and I found a job in our town at a group practice specializing in obstetrics and gynecology. My instructor encouraged me to take the CMA (AAMA) examination, and I was glad when I found out that I had passed it. I continued to take night classes so that I could get my associate's degree. I also attend the state and local chapter meetings of the AAMA so that I can get the contact hours I need to renew my CMA (AAMA) certification.

When I started working, I spent most of my time at the front desk answering the telephone, checking patients in, and filing, but after about 8 months I began to escort patients back to the examination rooms, prepare them for examinations, perform laboratory tests, and assist during examinations. We do some specialized tests in our office, including colposcopy, and I was trained to set up for the test and assist the physicians. Janice, our office manager, who is also a CMA (AAMA), has asked me to be responsible for ordering all the supplies for the office and taking inventory. She has also encouraged me to take business courses and attend seminars related to changes in insurance billing. Not too long ago, Janice told me that she is planning to cut back her hours in the spring, and she hopes that I will be able to take over some of her duties in running the practice. That will be a big challenge, but I think I am ready for it. I have a few ideas of my own, and I will be glad for an opportunity to try them out. ■

PERSONALITY TRAITS

Certain personality traits are essential to being a successful medical assistant. Personality is closely related to character, but it refers more to the outward way that a person acts with others. Personality traits include being genuinely interested in helping people; being outgoing, warm, and caring; and having a sense of humor. The ability to remain calm in challenging or difficult situations is also important.

The practice of medicine is one of the "caring professions." Each professional in the medical office needs to have a serious interest in helping people and be able to communicate that when interacting with others. Although the medical assistant must know how to perform the necessary administrative activities effectively and efficiently, the first priority is the care of patients who visit the office.

The concepts of warmth and caring are discussed in more detail in Chapter 4 in the section on communication. For now, it is important to say that being able to interact in a caring manner is a valuable personality trait. Some aspects of caring can be learned and practiced. If an individual does not have a naturally caring personality, he or she will find it much harder to learn the communication skills needed to express caring.

The ability to put the needs of others first is important. The medical assistant must not allow personal circumstances to interfere with interactions with patients, colleagues, or physicians. Remaining objective and concentrating on the situation at hand are important. The patient's needs take precedence over the needs of the medical assistant.

The atmosphere in a medical office may change quickly from calm and orderly to rushed and somewhat disorganized. The medical assistant who can remain calm when things do not go as planned will be more successful than one who is thrown completely off balance by sudden changes in schedule or plans and who becomes emotionally unable to respond effectively.

What Would You Do? What Would You *Not* Do?

Case Study 1

It is a busy Monday and Beth Ann is getting ready to leave the office for her lunch break at 1:30 PM when a male physician steps out of an examination room and asks her to assist him with a Pap test and pelvic examination. Beth Ann knows that it is office policy to always have a female staff member in the examination room when a pelvic examination is done. She tells the physician that she is about to go for lunch, but she will find someone to assist him. She goes to the front and finds the receptionist at the desk checking in patients, but neither of the two other medical assistants working that day is in sight. ■

APPEARANCE

Personal appearance influences both the feelings and the behavior of the medical assistant. It also influences the way in which the patients respond to the medical assistant. Psychologists have long recognized the importance of physical appearance. Important judgments are made within seconds of meeting a stranger on the basis of appearance and body language.

When the medical assistant calls a patient to come from the waiting room to the examination or treatment room, the patient immediately forms an impression of the quality of care the medical assistant—and the physician—are going to provide (Figure 2-2). A medical assistant who is neat, clean, and well groomed projects a sense of professionalism, authority, and competence. When medical assistants are courteous, they project respect for a person's dignity. This is important because many patients feel awkward, especially when dressed in underwear and an examination gown. In the same way, anything that the patient experiences as negative can result in an instant feeling of doubt in the medical assistant's ability. This may be generalized to a general feeling of doubt about all office staff. Patients often react negatively to rumpled clothing, dirty or worn shoes, unpleasant body odor, strong scent from perfume or personal products, piercings, tattoos, or an appearance that seems too "dressed up" because of jewelry, false nails, heavy makeup, and/or elaborate hairstyle.

Most medical offices require that medical assistants wear a uniform when performing clinical tasks. The uniform worn by most medical assistants consists of scrub pants with a scrub top or short-sleeved shirt; clean, white, soft-soled shoes; and a laboratory coat or jacket as needed. The top and/or jacket may be patterned, especially in a pediatric practice. Both top and bottom should fit well without being too tight. Pants should be hemmed neatly so that they do not drag on the ground (Figure 2-3). In some practices all staff wear coordinated uniforms. When performing administrative tasks, the medical assistant wears scrubs or street clothes. If street clothes are worn, they should project a businesslike appearance (Figure 2-4). Jeans, for example, are always unacceptable attire in the medical office.

Neatness and good grooming are also important for health and safety reasons. Hair carries bacteria, even if regularly

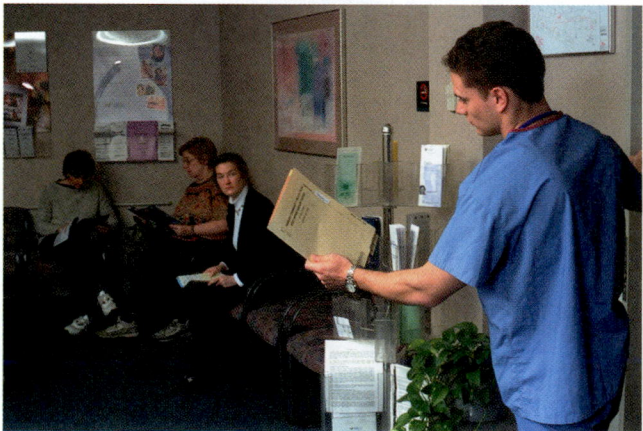

Figure 2-2 The patient judges the medical assistant's professionalism when called from the waiting room.

Figure 2-3 Scrub tops and pants should fit well and look professional.

Figure 2-4 Street clothes may be worn for administrative tasks in some offices.

washed. Medical assistants who perform clinical activities should pull their hair back and tie it, usually in a ponytail. A little bit of makeup can enhance a female medical assistant's professional image, but too much is not appropriate for a work environment. Both female and male medical assistants should always present a businesslike appearance.

Medical assistants should maintain scrupulous personal hygiene and avoid perfume or scented personal care products. Many patients have allergies or respiratory problems that can be aggravated by perfumes, colognes, and scented hairspray or deodorants.

Nails should be kept relatively short and should not be polished. Long nails are not functional for keyboard work, patient care, or laboratory procedures. The Centers for Disease Control and Prevention (CDC) recommends that artificial nails not be worn and fingernails be kept $\frac{1}{4}$ inch or shorter when one is caring for patients at high risk of acquiring infections.

Traditionally, health professionals were allowed to wear only "functional" jewelry—a wristwatch and a plain wedding band—because jewelry is not regularly washed and can become tangled in equipment. Today, most medical offices allow staff to wear small earrings that do not dangle below the earlobe and necklaces that can be tucked into the shirtfront. Wearing rings other than a wedding band is not a good idea. Rings can cut through protective gloves or scrape a patient. Also, they need to be taken off frequently for handwashing. Most medical offices do not allow visible piercings or implants, except for the ears. It may also be a policy of the medical office that visible tattoos and implants (microdermal or subdermal), must be covered. Those on the arms can be covered with a long-sleeved jersey worn under the scrub top or special sleeves designed specifically to cover tattoos or implants.

INITIATIVE AND BEHAVIORAL SKILLS

Initiative is the ability to begin or follow through on a plan without being supervised. Initiative is an important quality for a medical assistant. The willingness to take initiative and perform tasks that need to be done without being specifically instructed to do so improves the functioning of the office as a whole.

Initiative, however, does not mean taking over. The office is the physician's place of business, and the physician expects to run it. Initiative does not mean redecorating the waiting room without asking the physician. It does mean doing things that need to be done without being asked, keeping up with current issues in practice without being told, and identifying helpful educational opportunities and asking permission to attend. It also means finding useful things to do when the office is slow, such as restocking supplies, ordering supplies, and cleaning out cabinets and cupboards.

Office managers who supervise medical assisting students during externships relay that some medical assisting students do not take enough initiative. Taking appropriate initiative is an important skill to develop. While in school, students learn to wait for someone to tell them exactly what to do and how to do it. In the workplace the opposite quality is valued. A medical assistant is expected to figure out what needs to be done and how to help out—even during a practicum.

When a medical assistant begins a practicum or a new position, he or she must learn when to jump in and perform a task without being asked. The task that is most comfortable for the medical assistant to perform may not be the one that shows the most initiative. Medical assisting students can make an independent decision to restock examination rooms or make telephone calls to remind patients about appointments if they have no other pressing duties.

Initiative is a quality that employers look for in new medical assistants. An employer may even test a new employee's initiative by showing him or her how to do something, such as restocking an examination room at the end of the day, and then watching to see if the new medical assistant restocks the examination room without being told.

Managing activities, tasks, and schedules efficiently requires attention and effort first as a student and later as a professional medical assistant. This concept of **time management** goes beyond day-to-day use of time to include planning, setting goals, prioritizing, and analyzing the effectiveness of how time has been used.

Getting organized requires a method to keep track of personal, class, and/or work schedules. An effective schedule includes classes, work schedules, meetings, and/or other regular activities, but it can also be helpful to schedule time for specific tasks such as homework (for a student) or preparing an inventory (for a working medical assistant). There is a tendency to put off tasks that seem difficult or unappealing. Scheduling specific times to work on these types of tasks increases the likelihood of completing them so that they are done well and on time.

For class and work activities, it may be helpful to create and update a task list. In its simplest form, this is created daily as a list of tasks to be done; each task is checked off or crossed off when it is completed. Task lists do not have to be limited to a single day, and they can be prioritized with the tasks placed in order from most important to least important. In analyzing a schedule, some unimportant activities may stand out as items that can be eliminated or reduced in frequency. It may provide a psychological boost to limit the task list to tasks that can really be completed within the allotted time span.

To perform many tasks efficiently, it is important to have easy access to information including names, addresses, and telephone numbers of friends, classmates, or business contacts. Reference materials needed for the job or for schoolwork should also be easily accessible.

There are many tools to facilitate effective use of time, including a personal organizer, or personal planning book, or scheduling and information management software on a smartphone or computer. Address books and reference materials can also be in book or index card format or electronic format.

The willingness to adapt to change is important for medical assistants, as well as all health care workers. The pace of change within ambulatory care is fairly rapid, so it is unwise to become attached to one way of doing things. Changes in equipment, procedures, staff, and setting can occur quite frequently, but patient care needs to remain excellent. When the medical assistant approaches changes with tolerance and even enthusiasm, the office runs more smoothly. The medical assistant needs to adapt to the office setting rather than expecting the office to adapt to his or her preferences.

Finally, it is important for the medical assistant to work well with others and be a team player. Behavior that enhances patient care includes helping others, maintaining a positive attitude and not complaining, avoiding gossip, working within the established chain of command, and handling stress without losing emotional control or creating emotional scenes. Keeping perspective, accepting corrections or criticism without becoming defensive, and learning from mistakes are important. These behaviors facilitate working with others over the long term with a minimum of discord.

PROCEDURE 2-1   Locating and Defining a State's Legal Scope of Practice

Outcome

1. Locate and define the legal scope of practice of own state
2. Discuss delegation of procedures to the medical assistant

Equipment/Supplies

- Paper
- Pen
- Computer and printer
- Blank index cards

1. **Procedural Step.** Research the legal scope of practice for a medical assistant in your state.
2. Write a brief report summarizing what is included in the scope of practice for the medical assistant and what is not. Include a discussion of the consequences for medical assistants and patients if the medical assistant performs activities that are not included in the legal scope of practice. Describe what procedures can and cannot be delegated to the medical assistant by a physician, by a nurse (nurse practitioner or registered nurse) and by a physician assistant.
   Principle. It is important to know how each state defines (or is vague about) the scope of practice for a medical assistant if one is to practice professionally.
3. **Procedural Step.** Imagine two situations, one in which a medical assistant practices within the legal

scope of practice and one in which the medical assistant practices beyond the legal scope of practice. Summarize each on an index card. On the back of the card explain how the situation relates to the scope of practice for a medical assistant.

4. **Procedural Step.** Working in a small group, role-play the situations created by another classmate. When everyone in the group has finished the role-play, engage in a group discussion to identify the scenarios that do and do not fall within the legal scope of practice for a medical assistant.
   Principle. Discussion helps a person clarify and digest new information.
5. **Procedural Step.** Hand in your report and index cards to your instructor.

PROFESSIONALISM

Professionalism is behavior based on a body of knowledge and ethical standards to serve the public. The particular body of knowledge is different for each profession, but ethical standards for professionals are similar.

PROFESSIONALISM FOR PHYSICIANS

For physicians, *professionalism* means treating patients based on the body of scientific knowledge the physicians have accumulated, and continue to accumulate, over their working lifetime. In addition, physicians are bound by both ethical standards and legal regulations.

One source of guidance for physicians is the American Medical Association's (AMA's) *Principles of Medical Ethics.* The AMA code of ethics is reviewed and updated periodically by that organization.

Other sources of professional guidance for physicians include the following:

- State and federal regulations
- Regulations of the hospital(s) to which the physicians admit patients

- Any open-panel health maintenance organizations or preferred provider organizations in which the physicians participate
- The national medical board of their specialty or subspecialty

Physicians may have traditionally taken guidance from Hippocrates (c. 460-377 BCE). Hippocrates was an ancient Greek physician who wrote the Hippocratic Oath. The Hippocratic Oath served as a guide to good conduct for ancient physicians, and parts of it are still applicable today. Its philosophic underpinnings are still taught in medical school and adhered to by physicians, especially the key concept: "First, do no harm."

For more information on unprofessional activities of physicians, and by extension all office staff, see *Highlight on Unprofessional Conduct for a Physician.*

PROFESSIONALISM FOR MEDICAL ASSISTANTS

The AAMA maintains a code of ethics that is similar to the AMA principles for physicians. The AMT also maintains a set of standards that define professional practice. These codes of ethics can be viewed at the websites of each organization.

The medical assistant's ethical responsibilities are to admit mistakes, stay within his or her training and legal scope of practice, maintain confidentiality, stay current, and uphold the honor of the profession. This may mean having to confront a co-worker who is not adhering to such principles.

Dealing with a co-worker's inappropriate conduct is difficult, especially for a new employee or if the co-worker is higher in the organizational hierarchy. We live in a society that does not like "tattletales." On the other hand, unprofessional behavior in a medical office is disruptive to the concept of teamwork. Even if the unprofessional behavior does not pose an immediate threat to a patient, any behavior that results in people not working well together can lead

---

HIGHLIGHT on Unprofessional Conduct for a Physician

Even if they are not illegal, many activities are considered unprofessional for physicians, and by extension for their employees, including the following:

- Receiving payment for referrals to other physicians, laboratories, treatment centers, or pharmacies. Although physicians often make specific referrals, it is unethical for them to have arrangements to receive payments for those referrals, and especially to refuse to refer a patient unless a payment is made. This practice is sometimes called **fee splitting.** It is also unethical to charge a patient simply for being admitted to a hospital, without any other service being provided.

- Prescribing medication or diagnostic tests for financial gain rather than because of the patient's need for the test.
- Pressuring patients to use pharmacies or laboratories in which the physician has a financial interest. It is also unethical to prescribe medication, tests, or procedures that are not medically necessary. Billing an insurance company for unnecessary procedures is illegal.
- Accepting gifts from pharmaceutical companies or medical equipment manufacturers or suppliers in return for promoting the company's product or prescribing only the company's drug. Physicians may accept inexpensive or educational gifts

Continued

HIGHLIGHT on Unprofessional Conduct for a Physician—cont'd

if allowed by state law with the understanding that they have no obligation to promote the product.

- Allowing another physician or surgeon to perform surgery without informing the patient. The patient has the right to know who is performing a procedure.
- Failing to disclose the source of sperm used for artificial insemination (e.g., husband, sperm bank, paid donor). The physician may not substitute sperm without informing the patient.
- Failing to practice medicine appropriately.
- Practicing medicine under the influence of mind-altering drugs, alcohol, or any prescription medication that may impair mental function, alertness, or physical performance.
- Allowing an unlicensed person to practice medicine.
- Failing to order a consultation regarding any medical problem that is beyond a physician's personal experience and expertise. For example, a gynecologist should not treat a patient for renal failure.

- Withholding information about a patient's medical care from another medical facility just because the patient has an outstanding bill.
- Putting a patient at risk of human immunodeficiency virus (HIV) infection, or refusing to treat a patient who is HIV positive.
- Performing a procedure that might transmit the HIV virus to a patient if a physician or any other health care worker is HIV positive.
- Engaging in a sexual relationship with a patient. Something inherent in the relationship between two individuals in which one is perceived to be more influential than the other puts pressure on the "weaker" party to please the more powerful party. Because this makes it difficult to determine if consent is freely given, such a relationship should never be sexual in nature. Sexual relationships between professionals and the people they serve (e.g., physician-patient, attorney-client, teacher-student) are thus considered unethical and unprofessional. ■

to an uncomfortable or dangerous situation. The medical assistant should first discuss the situation with the co-worker by calmly and objectively describing the actions or behavior that he or she considers unprofessional. If the person does not correct the situation, it is appropriate to report the behavior to the office manager. If the behavior of a co-worker is illegal or threatens the health or safety of others, the medical assistant should report it as soon as possible to the individual's supervisor. Larger institutions often have a safety hotline where both patients and staff can report concerns anonymously. States maintain websites where complaints can be filed if health care professionals are believed to have performed illegal or unethical activities.

What Would You Do? What Would You *Not* Do?

Case Study 3

Before examining Ruth Mitchell, the physician asks Beth Ann to recheck Mrs. Mitchell's blood pressure. It is 190/100 in the right arm and 186/98 in the left arm. Beth Ann notices that the blood pressure had been taken that day by Diane, a medical assisting practicum student, who had recorded it as 130/80. Beth Ann asks Diane if she is confident about the blood pressure reading she obtained from Mrs. Mitchell. Diane says, "It was really faint, and I didn't hear it that well, so I wrote down the same blood pressure as she had the last time she was here. I didn't want to look incompetent. Besides, I was afraid it might affect my grade if you thought I was having trouble hearing the blood pressure." ■

CERTIFICATION FOR MEDICAL ASSISTANTS

Medical assistants usually graduate from an educational program that may vary in length from 6 months to 2 years. If the medical assistant graduates from a program accredited by CAAHEP or ABHES, he or she is automatically eligible to take a national certification examination. Certification is a process by which an organization, often a national body, validates the credentials of an individual or a program. Certification is important for health care professionals. Certification is also important for medical assistants, especially those who live in a state that does not regulate unlicensed health professionals. When an unbiased national organization validates knowledge and skills, the employer can be sure that the medical assistant has excellent qualifications.

Several organizations provide certification for medical assistants. Each has different requirements for eligibility, and some organizations offer more than one certification. In many areas, employers hire only medical assistants who have passed a certification examination. As medical assistants perform more specialized clinical tasks, employers have become increasingly concerned about validating skills and knowledge before hiring them.

AMERICAN ASSOCIATION OF MEDICAL ASSISTANTS

The AAMA administers the Certified Medical Assistant (AAMA) examination. To take the examination, an individual must have graduated from a medical assisting program accredited by CAAHEP or ABHES or be a CMA (AAMA) recertificant.

The examination is computer based and is administered online at testing centers. Most states have several testing locations.

Application materials can be obtained from the AAMA Certification Department, 20 North Wacker Dr., Suite 1565, Chicago, IL 60606-2903; from the director of accreditation at the medical assisting program attended; or from the AAMA website (www.aama-ntl.org).

Passing this examination allows a medical assistant to use the title CMA (AAMA) after his or her name on all official documents, including patient records and business cards.

AMERICAN MEDICAL TECHNOLOGISTS

The AMT is an organization that offers several certifications. Medical assistants may take an examination to be certified as an RMA, a certified medical administrative specialist (CMAS), and/or a registered phlebotomy technician (RPT). In addition, this organization certifies medical technologists and medical laboratory technicians.

To take the RMA examination, an individual must have (1) graduated from a medical assisting program accredited by CAAHEP or ABHES; (2) graduated from a medical assisting program that includes at least 720 hours of training in an institution that is accredited by an organization approved by the U.S. Department of Education; (3) graduated from a formal medical services program of the U.S. Armed Forces; or (4) been employed full-time in the profession of medical assisting for 5 years. The AMT may also grant the credential of RMA to an applicant who has passed another approved medical assisting certification examination.

Applications for the RMA examination can be obtained from the Registrar's Office, American Medical Technologists, 10700 W. Higgins, Suite 150, Rosemont, IL 60018, or the applicant can apply online. Information about the examination can be obtained from the AMT website (www.americanmedtech.org). The RMA examination may be given at a student's school, or an applicant may take the test online at testing centers located throughout the country.

Passing this examination entitles the medical assistant to use the initials RMA after his or her name on all official documents.

CALIFORNIA CERTIFYING BOARD FOR MEDICAL ASSISTANTS

The California Certifying Board for Medical Assistants (CCBMA) is one of the three organizations recognized by the Medical Board of California for certification of medical assistants (with the AAMA and the AMT). The CCBMA administers the California Certified Medical Assistant examination which is primarily taken by residents of

California. Information is available on the CCBMA website at www.ccbma.org.

NATIONAL HEALTHCAREER ASSOCIATION

The National Healthcareer Association (NHA) offers certifications for several allied health professions. Medical assistants may be interested in obtaining certification as a certified clinical medical assistant (CCMA), certified medical administrative assistant (CMAA), certified EKG technician (CET), and/or certified phlebotomy technician (CPT). The NHA also certifies other health professions. Information is available on the NHA website at www.nhanow.com.

NATIONAL CENTER FOR COMPETENCY TESTING

The National Center for Competency Testing (NCCT) offers testing for graduates of affiliated programs as well as medical assistants with experience or training through the military. It is possible to become certified as a medical assistant (NCMA), a medical office assistant (NCMOA), an ECG technician (NCET), and/or a phlebotomy technician (NCPT). The NCCT also certifies other health professions. Information is available on the NCCT website at www.ncctinc.com.

OBTAINING ADDITIONAL CREDENTIALS

A medical assistant may need to validate other skills as a condition of employment.

Training in cardiopulmonary resuscitation (CPR) is offered directly through the American Red Cross (ARC) and the American Heart Association (AHA) and by hospitals and other health care agencies. Like other health professionals, medical assistants recertify at the health care provider level every 2 years to be sure their skills are current as required by their professional organization and/or employer. Most health care facilities require current CPR credentials.

Medical assistants may also take courses in performing first aid, hearing tests, limited x-ray examinations, or other specialized tests, depending on state law and the needs of the medical practice. In many areas, medical assisting certification or registration is a valid qualification to perform phlebotomy, but some states and/or institutions require separate certification in phlebotomy. This can be obtained through organizations listed earlier as well as the American Society for Clinical Pathology (ASCP) or the American Society of Phlebotomy Technicians. The websites of these organizations are listed at the end of the chapter.

A medical assistant who obtains experience working for a podiatrist or an ophthalmologist may obtain certification as a podiatric medical assistant, certified (PMAC) or a certified ophthalmic assistant (COA).

If the medical assistant has specialized in the administrative area, additional credentials can be obtained as a medical administrative specialist. It is also possible to obtain one of the various certifications in medical coding with additional education, such as a certified professional coder (CPC) from the AAPC, an organization that specializes in coding training and certification. A medical assistant might also obtain certification as a certified coding associate (CCA), a certified coding specialist (CCS), or a certified coding specialist–physician-based (CCS-P) from the American Health Information Management Association (AHIMA).

PROFESSIONAL ORGANIZATIONS

The AAMA and the AMT are professional organizations for medical assistants. For an annual membership fee, many benefits are available. Medical assisting students can join either the AAMA or the AMT for a reduced annual rate and receive member services. Membership information is available at the website for each organization.

PEER SUPPORT

Through local and national meetings and workshops, medical assistants are able to enter a network of peers with whom they can share and from whom they can learn. They can also obtain insurance at reasonable cost, professional journals, and access to other sources of information important to the profession.

CONTINUING EDUCATION

With the constant change in the medical field, it is not merely important but necessary to keep skills up to date, attain new skills, and obtain new information about professional practices. Most health professions require a certain amount of continuing education for licensure or certification renewal. These are designed either as contact hours or continuing education units. A **continuing education unit (CEU)** is a unit of participation in professional continuing education.

Medical assisting contact hours and CEUs can be obtained from educational programs that have been approved by the particular certifying agency. The AAMA validates continuing education programs given through the state and national organization. Attending meetings of professional organizations is the best way to find educational programs specifically for the needs of professional medical assistants. Home study programs are also available to obtain continuing education credit.

An individual must be recertified as a CMA (AAMA) every 5 years. This can be accomplished by retaking the certification examination or by successfully completing the required continuing education programs. Sixty points must be accumulated during the 5-year period: 10 in the administrative area, 10 in the clinical area, and 10 in the general area, with 30 additional hours in any of the three categories. Of these, 30 points must be CEUs (1 contact hour each) from AAMA-approved programs.

If certified after January 2006, RMAs must accumulate 30 points of continuing education every 3 years. (One contact hour is equivalent to one point.) Those who were certified before this date are expected to keep up to date with current practice, but there are no specific continuing education requirements. Medical assistants who become certified through other organizations must that organization's requirements for recertification.

LEGISLATIVE ADVOCACY

One of the tasks of professional organizations is to monitor legislative initiatives at the state and national levels that may affect the profession. For example, the AAMA petitioned the CMS to designate medical assistants with a national certification as qualified for computerized physician order entry (CPOE) for Stage 2 of Meaningful Use of the electronic health record. This was allowed, and the wording of the CMS Stage 2 Final Rule was updated.

PUBLICATIONS, NEWSLETTERS, AND WEBSITES

Both the national and the state organizations provide a means for communication among professional medical assistants, including *CMA Today,* published by the AAMA, and the *Journal of Continuing Education Topics and Issues,* published by the AMT. The national organizations have state associations, often with several chapters within the state. The state organizations may produce newsletters and maintain websites. Conferences are held annually both nationally and at the state level to enhance communication and contact among members of the profession.

ROLE OF THE MEDICAL ASSISTANT
ADMINISTRATIVE RESPONSIBILITIES

Various administrative responsibilities must be performed on a daily basis in a medical office. We like to think of a physician's office as a place where patients receive medical treatment, but in reality much of the activity in a physician's office involves managing the logistics of scheduling patients, preparing to provide services, and receiving payment for services. The medical assistant may be responsible for a number of these activities, although larger offices may employ specialists to perform these tasks.

1. Scheduling appointments, both over the telephone and in person, is a primary responsibility of the medical

assistant. A patient may also need to have appointments made with other medical facilities; examples include a consultation with a specialist, a diagnostic procedure, outpatient surgery, continuing therapy or rehabilitation, and a hospital admission. Some patients may need to schedule multiple appointments with other facilities as the result of a single office visit. The medical assistant must learn the procedure for making and documenting each type of appointment.

2. Maintaining the medical record and filing records and reports has traditionally been one of the medical assistant's roles. With the increasing use of electronic medical records, there is less actual filing in many offices, but it still may be necessary to scan paper reports and keep track of laboratory and diagnostic test results. Each patient encounter with a clinician—physician, nurse practitioner (NP), or physician assistant (PA)—is followed by documentation of the patient's visit. Clinicians may enter information directly into an electronic medical record, or they may create handwritten or dictated patient notes. If the dictation method is used, it may be transcribed using voice recognition software or it may be sent to an outside service electronically. In this case the medical assistant prints the reports after they have been returned and files them after the physician has approved them. The medical assistant may prepare letters and other documents for the physician.

3. Every patient visit generates activities that are necessary for the physician to be paid for the services provided. The medical assistant must know how to accept and document payments, total and enter charges, code the procedures and/or diagnostic tests performed, and enter payments received. These charges and payments are entered into the office computer to keep track of money owed to and received by the practice. In turn, the charges are used to generate insurance claims and patient bills. In larger offices and clinics, a separate business office usually handles financial matters. Small offices often send billing information to an outside billing service. If billing is performed in the office, the medical assistant must be able to create patient bills and submit insurance claims.

4. On a regular basis, checks and cash need to be deposited into the office's bank account. Preparing bank deposits and recording the deposits in the office's checkbook are activities that medical assistants often perform.

5. Every business has bills to pay. These include rent (or mortgage, if the office is owned), electricity, lease payments on equipment, staff salaries, and a number of other regular payments, such as liability and malpractice insurance. Medical assistants, or business office personnel, usually pay these bills and maintain records of these and other bills owed by the office. (Some offices have an outside bookkeeping service perform these tasks. Even in offices that pay their own regular bills, salary may be managed by an outside payroll service.)

6. In the patient-centered medical home, the medical assistant may have additional administrative responsibilities

to enter health registry data into the medical record and to monitor patient progress by the use of disease-specific registries and tools. Pre-visit administrative tasks may be more extensive than in other types of medical practices.

CLINICAL RESPONSIBILITIES

Depending on the type of medical office, clinical activities may make up the bulk of the medical assistant's responsibilities. The medical assistant prepares patients for examination, performs diagnostic tests, performs treatments, and assists the physician with examination and treatment.

1. Medical assistants are often asked to collect and process specimens. Some specimens are tested in the office, and others are sent to an outside laboratory.

2. Medical assistants perform several diagnostic tests, such as electrocardiograms and respiratory testing.

3. Medical assistants prepare patients for examination, including taking medical histories, weighing the patient, measuring vital signs, and obtaining information about the chief complaint. Having this done by a medical assistant may allow the physician to see at least one extra patient per hour.

4. After each patient appointment, the medical assistant prepares the examination and/or treatment room for the next patient (Figure 2-5). This involves making sure that there is fresh paper on the table, the proper instruments and supplies are available for the next examination or procedure, and the necessary equipment is available and in working order.

5. Medical assistants help the physician with examinations and procedures. The medical assistant settles a patient into an examination room and positions and drapes the patient for portions of the examination. Another duty is to pass instruments and supplies to the physician during procedures. The medical assistant may also remove sutures and change sterile dressings. If minor surgery or sterile procedures are performed in the office, the medical

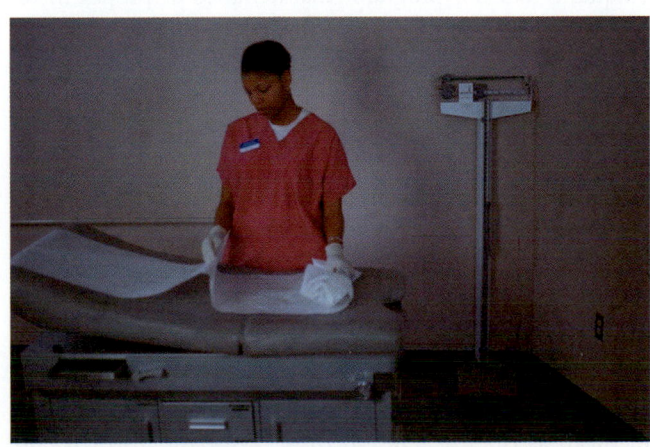

Figure 2-5 Medical assistant preparing an examination room.

assistant sets up the equipment and supplies and then assists the physician as needed.

6. Medical assistants perform treatments, including nebulizer treatments and application of hot and cold packs or compresses.

7. Medical assistants prepare and administer medications and immunizations depending on state law and office policy. The administration of medication requires concentration and precision. All medications must be documented according to office procedure.

8. Sometimes a medical assistant also has to perform emergency care and administer first aid or assist with an office emergency. This does not happen often, but every medical assistant must be prepared.

MANAGING THE MEDICAL OFFICE

The medical assistant may have many responsibilities to keep the medical office running smoothly.

1. Operational activities involve maintaining the inventory of supplies. This can include everything from purchasing tongue blades and gauze to contracting with a uniform service to launder the staff's laboratory coats or patient gowns. It may also involve evaluating and recommending changes in the supplies purchased and evaluating new equipment for potential purchase or lease.

2. A second group of activities involves personnel policy and procedures. Businesses are always reviewing their policies and procedures and updating and revising them as needed. As offices move from one or two physicians and a small staff to a larger organization, policies and procedures become more important to standardize the way all employees are dealt with.

3. **Risk management** is the development of policies and procedures that minimize the chances of the practice being sued by a patient or disciplined by a regulatory agency. Every physician's office needs to have one person responsible for risk management, which involves, among other areas, the promotion of health and safety for office personnel and patients, implementation of a quality control program, maintenance of proper infection control measures, fire prevention, and the proper disposal of hazardous waste and controlled substances.

4. Record keeping is an important activity for the individual who manages a medical office. In addition to patient records, many other kinds of records must be kept, including office insurance records, quality control records, maintenance contracts, personnel records, and financial records.

PATIENT EDUCATION AND COACHING

Instructing and coaching patients are important roles for medical assistants. The medical assistant instructs the patient in several types of situations.

1. The medical assistant is often responsible for educating the patient about office procedures, including giving information to a new patient who is making the first appointment, as well as instructing an established patient whose circumstances have changed.

2. The medical assistant may provide information about maintaining health to patients directly as directed by the physician or by making educational materials available in the office. These are always reviewed by the physician before being given to patients (Figure 2-6).

3. The medical assistant may teach a patient about ways to manage his or her disease or condition, especially if the patient is newly diagnosed. For example, a physician might ask a medical assistant to teach a patient how to take his or her own blood pressure using a sphygmomanometer and a stethoscope and keep a record of the results.

Maintaining the highest possible level of health requires more than knowledge. Patients must be motivated to make healthy choices to maintain their current level of health, as well as to prevent disease and comply with treatment plans prescribed by the physician. **Health coaching** is defined as a process that helps patients identify their values related to health, set health goals, and take steps to meet their personal goals. Coaching requires listening to patients, validating their concerns, and also encouraging them to make the changes that their own beliefs tell them are important. Medical assistants can work with patients to help them maintain health through proper diet, exercise and rest, and social interaction. They can also assist patients, especially those with risk factors, to take positive steps to prevent disease by identifying a specific target—for example, a lower cholesterol or low-density lipoprotein (LDL) level—setting goals to meet that target, and following up with the necessary behavior changes. Health coaching can also be an effective way to help a patient stick to a prescribed treatment plan. If the physician has prescribed a regimen of home glucose testing, insulin, and dietary modifications, a medical assistant might coach the patient to improve

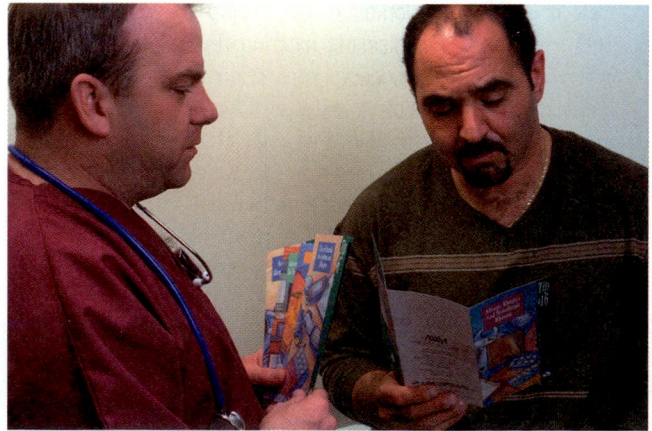

Figure 2-6 The medical assistant uses brochures to teach a patient.

compliance after initial teaching has been completed. If a patient needs services from the community, the medical assistant may provide brochures from community agencies or locate community resources for a patient—such as an exercise class given without cost at a center for senior citizens—but it might also be necessary to coach the patient to make specific plans to use those services. A patient might also require coaching to adapt to decreased balance or strength by avoiding behaviors that tend to cause falls.

PATIENT NAVIGATION

A **patient navigator** is a person whose role is to remove the obstacles patients face in accessing and receiving treatment. The concept was originally developed in relation to the treatment of cancer, which can involve a maze of doctors' offices, hospitals, outpatient centers, and patient-support organizations as well as numerous problems with insurance and payment systems. The patient-centered medical home model attempts to coordinate a patient's care through the office of the primary care provider; in this type of office or in any other type of medical office, the medical assistant may function as a patient navigator to help a patient with complex medical needs to access and receive appropriate referrals to community services or additional health care services.

EMPLOYMENT OPPORTUNITIES

According to the U.S. Department of Labor Bureau of Labor Statistics, medical assisting is projected to grow faster than the average for all occupations between 2012 and 2022. Federal legislation will expand the number of patients who have access to health insurance, increasing patient access to medical care. Certification may help to distinguish a medical assistant who meets recognized standards from an entry-level assistant.

The majority of medical assistants work in physicians' offices. Other common places of employment include hospitals and offices of other health practitioners, such as chiropractors, podiatrists, and optometrists. Medical assistants also work in outpatient care centers, schools or other educational facilities, medical laboratories, government agencies, insurance companies, employment services, and nursing care facilities.

The median annual income reported by medical assistants in May 2013 was $29,610 ($14.24 per hour), but salaries vary depending on geographic location, skill level, and type of facility in which the medical assistant is employed.

The most direct route for career advancement is probably to become an office, practice, or department manager. This may require additional education, especially in business administration, but often management skills can be learned mainly on the job. To become a medical assisting instructor, it is necessary to have an Associate in Science degree or a higher degree in a related field and to be either a CMA (AAMA) or an RMA (for an accredited medical assisting program). Clinical advancement usually requires additional training in a formal educational program preparing for a health career, such as dental hygiene, laboratory technology, nursing, radiologic technology, or respiratory therapy.

Memories *from* Practicum

Beth Ann Wilson: I couldn't believe how nervous I was before I went to my practicum the first day. I had worked at several jobs and even done filing at a medical office during the summer when I was in high school, but it felt totally different to know that I would be responsible to act like a "real" medical assistant. Fortunately, the staff members at my placement were wonderful. They let me shadow one of the medical assistants until I felt comfortable to work with patients on my own. They were also careful to expose me gradually to each part of the medical office, so it didn't get overwhelming. The person who helped me the most was Cheryl, the office manager. Every day she sought me out and asked how it was going. There was one time when a physician asked me to take out a patient's sutures, and I hadn't even seen someone perform that procedure. I didn't know what to say, but I told him I would find another medical assistant to help him. Then I went to Cheryl. She found someone else to perform the procedure and made sure that I had an opportunity to observe. I never could decide whether I liked checking patients in up front or assisting the physicians better, as long as I had a chance to interact with patients. It has always made me feel good to know that I am helping others. ■

What Would You Do? What Would You *Not* Do? RESPONSES

Case Study 1
Page 22

What Did Beth Ann Do?
- ❏ Looked in the back part of the office for an available staff member.
- ❏ Asked the receptionist if she knows where one of the other medical assistants is.
- ❏ Used the intercom to locate a medical assistant.
- ❏ Checked the examination rooms with open doors to see if a medical assistant might be almost finished checking in a patient.
- ❏ Assisted the physician if she was unable to find another medical assistant to do it.

What Did Beth Ann Not Do?
- ❏ Did not leave for lunch without finding someone to assist the physician.
- ❏ Did not tell the physician that she was sorry she could not assist him at this time.
- ❏ Did not knock on closed examination room doors.

Case Study 2
Page 25

What Did Beth Ann Do?
- ❏ Agreed to draw the blood without complaining.
- ❏ Tried to make the patient feel comfortable and confident.
- ❏ Explained to Diane later that some patients do not want students to perform certain procedures.
- ❏ Told Diane that she was glad Diane called her to help.

- ❏ Reinforced that even if Diane's pride was slightly hurt, Diane did the correct thing by not showing this to the patient.

What Did Beth Ann Not Do?
- ❏ Did not make the patient feel as if she were asking for special treatment.
- ❏ Did not tell Diane that she looked very young or unprofessional.
- ❏ Did not talk about the incident as a funny story in the break room to other staff.

Case Study 3
Page 26

What Did Beth Ann Do?
- ❏ Told the patient that the physician asked her to recheck the blood pressure because it sometimes changes when patients sit in a quiet examination room.
- ❏ Found a private place to speak to Diane and agreed with her that sometimes it is really hard to hear the blood pressure.
- ❏ Explained to Diane that it is important to take and record the blood pressure correctly even if she has to ask for assistance.
- ❏ Reminded Diane that the staff understands she is a student and will not be able to perform every procedure perfectly.
- ❏ Offered to work with Diane to improve her technique.

What Did Beth Ann Not Do?
- ❏ Did not talk down to Diane or try to make her feel bad.
- ❏ Did not tell others in the office not to rely on Diane's blood pressure measurements.
- ❏ Did not tell the patient that Diane had not been sure of her measurement.

↻ TERMINOLOGY REVIEW

Key Term	Word Parts	Definition
Accreditation		Credit or recognition from a regional or national organization for maintaining certain standards.
Continuing education unit (CEU)		A standard unit of measure of continuing education for professionals defined as 1 contact hour by the AAMA, but also commonly 10 contact hours of participation.
Fee splitting		The practice of sharing fees with colleagues, especially for making referrals.
Health coaching		A process that helps patients identify their values related to health, set health goals, and take steps to meet their personal goals.
Initiative		The ability to begin or carry through on a plan of action independently.
Patient navigator		A person whose role is to remove obstacles that patients face in accessing and receiving treatment.
Practicum		A supervised work experience that is required in an educational program and usually unpaid. Formerly called an *externship*.
Risk management		Processes to protect a health care facility from the risk of legal action.
Time management		Skills and techniques used to manage time to accomplish tasks and meet goals.

ON THE WEB

For information on professional organizations and certification:

Accrediting Bureau of Health Education Schools: www.abhes.org

American Association of Medical Assistants: www.aama-ntl.org

American Health Information Management Association: www.ahima.org

American Medical Association: www.ama-assn.org

American Medical Technologists: www.americanmedtech.org

American Society for Clinical Pathology: www.ascp.org

American Society of Phlebotomy Technicians: www.aspt.org

American Society of Podiatric Medical Assistants: www.aspma.org

California Certifying Board for Medical Assistants: www.ccbma.org

Commission on Accreditation of Allied Health Education Programs: www.caahep.org

Joint Commission on Allied Health Personnel in Ophthalmology: www.jcahpo.org

National Center for Competency Testing: www.ncctinc.com

National Healthcareer Association: www.nhanow.com

For information on occupational outlook for medical assistants:

U.S. Department of Labor Bureau of Labor Statistics: www.bls.gov

Ethics and Law for the Medical Office

Check out the Evolve site at http://evolve.elsevier.com/Bonewit/today/ to access additional interactive activities and exercises to help you study and prepare for success.

LEARNING OBJECTIVES	PROCEDURES

Ethics and Health Care

1. Identify key differences between law and ethics.
2. List reasons for medical assistants to study ethics.
3. Identify specific rights that patients have in relation to health care.
4. Correlate the concept of duties to the actions expected of health professionals.
5. Be a patient advocate.
6. Report illegal and/or unsafe activities and behaviors affecting patient care to proper authorities.
7. Describe how certain ethical issues generate ethical conflict in society.
8. Describe ways to separate and prioritize personal and professional ethics.   —   *Separate personal and professional ethics.*
9. Describe six steps that may be used to make ethical decisions.

Law and Professional Liability

10. Identify similarities and differences between public law and private law.
11. Identify the process through which laws are created at the federal and state level.
12. Differentiate among types of crimes, such as felonies and misdemeanors, as well as between violent and nonviolent crimes.
13. Differentiate between criminal law and civil law.
14. List and explain the elements of a valid contract.
15. State the rights and duties of each party in the physician-patient relationship.
16. Incorporate the Patient Bill of Rights into personal practice.   —   *Incorporate the Patient Bill of Rights.*
17. Define *standard of care,* and describe how this concept affects the behavior of health professionals.
18. Describe the medical assistant's role in obtaining informed consent.
19. Explain the principles of negligence and professional negligence as they apply to the behavior of health professionals.
20. Explain the purpose and need for professional liability insurance.
21. Describe the process of malpractice litigation.
22. List and explain specific defenses to intentional and unintentional torts.

Federal and State Laws Affecting the Medical Office

23. Describe and explain the laws regulating controlled substances and prescription medications.
24. List and explain several laws that protect employees of medical offices.
25. Describe how the provisions of the Health Insurance Portability and Accountability Act (HIPAA) affect the medical office.
26. List and explain the situations where mandatory reporting is required by the medical office.   —   *Report illegal activities and comply with public health statutes.*
27. Describe how states regulate the practice of medicine and health occupations.
28. Differentiate between licensing and voluntary accreditation for health care facilities.

CHAPTER OUTLINE

INTRODUCTION TO MEDICAL ETHICS
REASONS TO STUDY ETHICS
ETHICS AND HEALTH CARE
Ethical Concepts
Rights
Duties
Ethical Conflict
Reproductive Issues
Stem Cell Research
Genetic Engineering and Cloning
Refusing or Withholding Treatment and Physician-Assisted
    Suicide
Advance Directives
Personal, Professional, and Organizational Ethics
Process Used to Make Ethical Decisions
Gathering Information
Identifying Conflicting Values
Determining Relative Importance of Conflicting Claims
Exploring Alternatives
Choosing and Justifying One Alternative
Implementing the Decision
INTRODUCTION TO LAW
Difference Between Public Law and Private Law
Lawsuits
Specialized Areas of Law
Creation of Laws
Criminal Law
Nonviolent Crimes
Civil Law
LAW AND PROFESSIONAL LIABILITY
Physician-Patient Relationship
The Physician
The Patient
Terminating the Physician-Patient Relationship
Personal and Professional Liability
Standard of Care
Informed Consent
Professional Negligence
Professional Liability Insurance
Malpractice Litigation
Initiating a Lawsuit
Response to a Possible Lawsuit

Alternative Dispute Resolution
Tort Defenses
Privilege
Consent
Self-Defense or the Defense of Others
Expiration of the Statute of Limitations
Contributory or Comparative Negligence
Assumption of Risk
**FEDERAL AND STATE LAWS AFFECTING THE MEDICAL
    OFFICE**
Controlled Substances and Prescriptions
Controlled Substances
Prescriptions
Federal and State Laws Protecting Employees
Hiring and Firing
Preemployment Testing
The Americans with Disabilities Act and the Americans with
    Disabilities Act Amendments
Occupational Safety and Health Act of 1970
Family and Medical Leave Act
Sexual Harassment
Minimum Wage and Overtime
Employee Retirement Income Security Act
Genetic Information Nondiscrimination Act
**Health Insurance Portability and Accountability Act of
    1996**
Health Insurance Availability and Coverage
Privacy Rule
Transaction and Code Set Rule
Security Rule
Other Provisions
Patient Safety and Quality Improvement Act
**Health Information Technology for Economic and Clinical
    Health Act**
Patient Protection and Affordable Care Act
Mandatory Reporting
State Regulation of Health Occupations
Revoking or Suspending a Physician's License
Facility Licensing and Accreditation
State Requirements
Federal Requirements
Voluntary Accreditation

KEY TERMS

abandonment
act
advocate (ADD-va-kit)
arbitration
assumption of risk,
autonomy (ah-TAH-noe-mee)
beneficence (ben-IH-fih-sens)
bill
case law
civil law

cloning (KLOH-ning)
common law
comparative negligence (NEG-lih-jhens)
contingency (kon-TIN-jhen-see)
contributory negligence
controlled substance
crime
criminal law
defendant
deposition

do-not-resuscitate (DNR) orders
Drug Enforcement Administration (DEA)
duty
emancipated minor
embezzlement (em-BEZ-el-ment)
ethics
felony
fidelity
fraud
gene therapy

genetic engineering
health care proxy (PROX-ee)
informed consent
larceny
liability
license
licensure (LI-sen-sur)
litigation (lih-tih-GAY-shun)
living will
malfeasance (mal-FEE-suns)
malpractice
mature minor
mediation

medical durable power of attorney
misdemeanor (mis-de-MEAN-or)
misfeasance (mis-FEE-suns)
negligence (NEG-lih-jhens)
nonfeasance (non-FEE-suns)
nonmalfeasance (non-mal-FEE-suns)
plaintiff (PLANE-tiff)
prescription
privilege
prudent
reciprocity (re-sip-RAW-city)
res ipsa loquitur (ress-IHP-sah
    LOW-kwee-tour

respondeat superior (ray-SPON-day-at
    sue-PEER-ee-or)
right
standard of care
statute (STA-chewt) of limitations
statutory (STA-chew-toe-ree) law
stem cells
subpoena (su-PEE-na)
subpoena duces tecum (su-PEE-na
    DEW-chess TAY-come)
tort
veracity (ver-ASS-ih-tee)

INTRODUCTION TO MEDICAL ETHICS

Within a democracy, society tolerates a wide range of beliefs about *morals* (beliefs about what is right and wrong) and regulates public behavior using laws created by the democratic process. the democratic process to create rules and laws that regulate public behavior. This process allows for change and flexibility because laws are continually reviewed through the judiciary process.

It is important to remember that society's beliefs about right and wrong precede laws and also influence their interpretation. Currently the rapid pace of technologic innovation and changing beliefs places considerable stress on the social structure.

There is also a wide diversity of expectations about normal, acceptable behavior, sometimes called etiquette, or manners. Breaches of etiquette pose no true threat to the integrity of an individual or society. However, individuals may have just as strong an emotional reaction to what they see as bad manners as they would have to a true ethical breach.

In the context of the medical office, a patient may feel that being rushed by the physician and treated "as a number, not a name" by the front-office staff is being treated without dignity. The patient's emotional response to how he or she is treated may seem more important than the actual quality of care.

REASONS TO STUDY ETHICS

The branch of knowledge that deals with standards of behavior or beliefs is called **ethics**. Although it is an abstract discipline, medical assistants should study ethics for a number of reasons.

First, it is an important part of an individual's education to develop the intellectual skills to analyze complex problems and justify the choices made in particular situations. In the case of ethics, the choice is between alternative courses of action that have moral and social consequences.

Second, as society has become increasingly complex, average citizens are more aware that choices affect not only

people living now, but those who will live in the future. People hesitate to allow only elected and appointed officials to deal with these choices. Learning about ethics and social issues encourages ordinary people to have input into social beliefs and expectations. There is also a greater sense of interconnections involving the whole world, sometimes called *globalism*. Many individuals feel some level of responsibility for all human beings, and indeed for all living beings on the earth.

Third, in the specific realm of medicine and science, more sophisticated medical treatment and new technologies are constantly becoming available. However, society does not have unlimited resources to provide everything to everyone, even in the developed world. There is a need to make informed choices about what care will be provided to whom, and when, rather than simply responding to special interests.

Fourth, every year new biomedical research makes it possible to do more things with which the world has no previous experience. Society must have informed citizens who can analyze issues and guide the future. Within the health care system, health professionals, including medical assistants, need skills in considering ethical questions to improve health care for individuals and society.

ETHICS AND HEALTH CARE
ETHICAL CONCEPTS

Current thinking about biomedical ethics identifies several rights (very strong claims) for patients and duties (requirements) for the institutions and individuals who provide health care. Sources for these ideas include religious traditions, social belief systems, and political documents such as the Declaration of Independence and the U.S. Constitution and the Bill of Rights, as well as ethical theories developed by individual philosophers.

Rights

A **right** is a claim that is expected to be honored. It is stronger than a wish or a need.

The early leaders of the American government believed in natural rights and the duty of any government to preserve them. Natural rights were considered to exist through the natural order or to be granted by God. These include the following:

1. Right to life
2. Right to privacy
3. Right to autonomy
4. Right to the means to sustain life

Right to Life

One of the rights mentioned in the Declaration of Independence is the right to life.

Since the 1970s the term "right to life" has come to be associated with the movement against abortion. But in a broader context, it reflects the belief that human beings may not kill others. The belief in the right to life is found in all major religions and traditions.

The right to life has many implications for medicine. Historically, physicians and other health care workers may not harm patients because this may threaten their lives. They may not assist with suicide; this is expressly stated in the Hippocratic Oath. In the United States today, however, many individuals want some control over death, including the choice of suicide assisted by their physician.

Two important areas of conflict appeared in the middle of the twentieth century. First, advances in medical care made it possible to keep people alive who could not recover their health. Sometimes this sustaining of life came at the cost of prolonged suffering.

Second, the absolute right to life of an unborn fetus conflicts with the right of a woman to control her own reproductive capacity. Birth-control methods, artificial conception methods, and abortion, if necessary, are measures to control the size of a woman's family. Many women and their physicians have come to believe they have a right to make decisions related to reproduction, including use of available technology, as they see fit.

Right to Privacy

The Supreme Court has ruled that there is an implicit right to privacy in the Bill of Rights, specifically in the Fourth Amendment. A series of court decisions affirming a woman's right to use mechanical birth control and to an abortion hinged on justices' perceiving this right to privacy.

Patient confidentiality, which has been upheld by courts, is another manifestation of the right to privacy. Patient confidentiality is discussed in detail later in this chapter.

Right to Autonomy

Currently, medical ethics takes the position that an individual has the right to **autonomy,** which means the right to make independent decisions about his or her health care according to individual values and concerns, without constraint or coercion by others. This right is preserved even when the individual's decisions do not match the values of

the medical community or the individual physician. The right of autonomy is the basis for **informed consent.** Informed consent is consent based on understanding of a medical procedure and its possible outcomes. Health care professionals must provide complete information in order for patients to make informed decisions. The patient must have the mental capacity to reason and consider alternatives. Because of this, the law limits the autonomy of children or individuals with decreased mental capacity such as the mentally retarded or individuals whose mental capacity has been impaired by illness, those acting under the influence of drugs or alcohol, and those experiencing mental illness.

Respect for autonomy does not derive from the Hippocratic Oath. Rather, it comes from the thinking of European philosophers such as Immanuel Kant and John Locke.

Right to the Means to Sustain Life

Every society must grapple with the problem of equitable distribution of goods and services to its citizens and how to regulate that distribution over time.

This is not a problem when the supply is adequate, or when supply is greater than demand. For instance, in ordinary circumstances the supply of oxygen is more than adequate to meet the needs of the entire population.

It is when the amount of a particular resource is less than the desire for that resource that problems develop. In this case, resources are said to be *scarce,* and the society's government may take measures to determine who will have access to the scarce resources.

At a minimum, every individual should have access to what is necessary to sustain life and preserve human dignity. Consideration of justice in distribution and access is especially important in social and political movements. Any society must find ways to respond to need while also rewarding contribution and providing for stability within the social system.

Duties

A **duty** is a commitment to act in a certain way on the basis of religious beliefs, moral principles, or a particular professional code of conduct. Traditionally, five main duties of a health care professional have been identified.

Do No Harm

The concept of **nonmalfeasance** means, first of all, doing no harm in any treatment given. This duty is found in the Hippocratic Oath. It is not taken in a literal sense because many treatments can have adverse effects. Rather, it is taken to mean that medical benefits should outweigh adverse effects.

This concept applies especially to scientific research. Guidelines for ethical research not only require informed consent but also restrict research with possible harmful effects to those patients whose conditions are so serious that doing nothing is likely to be as dangerous as the treatment or procedure being studied.

Putting It All Into Practice

My name is Vicki Edmonds, and I have worked in a family practice for about 6 years. There are two physicians and two nurse practitioners in my practice, and I usually assist one of the physicians. Of course, if it is busy or one of the other medical assistants is ill, we all pitch in and help out. Neither of the physicians in my practice has ever been sued, and we all work together to be sure it stays that way. We do everything we can so that our patients not only receive great care but also are satisfied with their treatment. We also document everything carefully because our physicians are aware that you cannot prove that care was given if it isn't documented. Every once in a while we have a patient who constantly misses appointments or doesn't take his or her medication, and if the physician thinks that it is harmful to the patient's health, sometimes he will instruct the patient to find another practitioner to care for him or her. I remember one time when the patient lived far away, and she said that it was difficult for her to make the trip to our office. After she missed three appointments in a row, the physician had me write a letter suggesting that she find another physician nearer to her home. He explained that he couldn't be responsible for her if she was unable to keep appointments. In the letter he gave her a month to find another physician, and he offered to help her if she was having difficulty. We sent that letter by certified mail and obtained a return receipt. Then we documented everything in the patient's medical record. The patient sent a letter back saying that she was going to an office much closer to home, and she thought that would work out better for her. ■

Do the Best Possible

The concept of **beneficence,** doing the best possible, is seen in some systems of ethics as a separate duty, whereas in others it is considered an extension of doing no harm. It is often difficult to pinpoint exactly what harm and good are; they may vary with a particular individual's viewpoint.

Be Faithful to Reasonable Expectations

The concept of **fidelity,** being faithful, comes from the Latin term *fides,* which means "faith." In the case of medical practice, fidelity is usually interpreted as meaning being faithful to reasonable expectations. Although patient expectations vary, there is general agreement that a patient can reasonably expect to be treated with dignity, treated by individuals who honor their agreements, and treated by competent providers. Patients can also expect that they will be cared for by individuals who adhere to the ethical standards of their profession, to statutory law, and to accepted medical and scientific practice.

Be a Patient Advocate

The concept of fidelity includes the expectation that patient needs come first. An **advocate** is a person who intercedes on behalf of another person. A medical assistant functions as an advocate for patients by suggesting appropriate community referrals to the physician, by making sure that all insurance claims are complete, by following up to help patients receive insurance coverage if additional information will make that possible, and in general by working to protect patients' rights.

To protect patient safety, it may even be necessary for a medical assistant to report unsafe or illegal behavior to proper authorities. The first step is always to follow up within the organization by documenting and reporting to the supervisor any incident or situation that could cause potential harm. If no action is taken after a reasonable amount of time, the situation should be reported to the next person in the chain of command. If a medical assistant has followed up within the organization without resolution of an unsafe or illegal situation, he or she should report the incident to the appropriate government agency. Information about professionals whose licenses have been revoked or suspended is available online in many states.

Tell the Truth

The concept of **veracity** has increased in importance since the nineteenth century. Veracity is not found in the Hippocratic Oath. It has developed with the evolution of the scientific tradition. Today it is seen as a proactive duty—physicians and other health care professionals must provide truthful information without having to be asked. It is a tenet of modern science that scientific knowledge belongs to all. Results of experiments must be accurate and reviewed by other scientists to see if the results can be replicated, then published for the benefit of all.

Give Each Person a Fair Share

The concept of *justice* requires that each individual be given his or her due and implies that he or she deserves a fair share of resources. However, there is often an underlying belief that an individual must contribute or bear a portion of the burden before being allowed to get certain resources. Justice in the context of medical practice appears not only in terms of distribution of medical resources, but also in the belief in the right to compensation if a mistake is made.

Deciding what is "fair" is difficult because different situations may require different guidelines. In the United States,

What Would You Do? What Would You *Not* Do?

Case Study 1

Denise Fitzgerald is a 16-year-old girl who has come to the office with complaints of a sore throat and fever. While Vicki is taking vital signs, she notices a circular wound on Denise's arm that looks like a cigarette burn. It is red and has some crusted areas. When she asks Denise about it, the patient blushes and says in a low voice that her boyfriend burned her a few days ago to teach her a lesson. Then Denise says, "Please don't tell the doctor because he will tell my mother, and I'm afraid she will make me break up with my boyfriend." ■

the tendency is to believe in "first come, first served." But in an emergency department, serious conditions must take precedence.

ETHICAL CONFLICT

Many issues become controversial when there is a disagreement within society about the relative hierarchy of certain rights and duties.

Reproductive Issues

Conflict surrounds the issues of contraception, abortion, and other issues related to reproduction. With regard to pregnancy, some people feel that the duty to follow divine law or natural measures takes precedence over an individual's right to autonomy. This results in differing beliefs about how appropriate it is to use contraception and artificial measures to become pregnant. There has been controversy about the "morning-after pill" (marketed under the name *Plan B*). Because it has been found to be relatively safe, it was approved as an over-the-counter medication for women older than age 18 by the Food and Drug Administration (FDA) in 2006.

Another controversial issue is abortion. Some argue that the fetus's right to life outweighs the woman's right to privacy in determining—with her physician—the proper course of her medical care. Since the original U.S. Supreme Court decision in 1973 upholding a woman's right to obtain an abortion in any state *(Roe v Wade),* the Court has been called on to rule many times on various state laws that seek to limit this right. The Partial-Birth Abortion Ban Act of 2003, which prohibits a specific abortion procedure that can be done in the second trimester of pregnancy, is an example of a federal law that restricts a woman's right to abortion in some cases. It was upheld in the Supreme Court case of *Gonzales v Carhart* in 2007.

Stem Cell Research

A promising area of research for medical treatment involves the use of embryonic **stem cells.** These cells, taken from fetal tissue, are able to mature into different types of tissue. Embryonic cells may be found to be able to reduce, or possibly even reverse, the symptoms of Parkinson disease and other diseases.

The ethical conflict arises because the cells of live human embryos may be killed during research activities. In addition, a possible source of embryonic cell tissue is from aborted fetuses or fertilized ova not used for in vitro fertilization. Researchers who use fetal tissue stress that they use only tissue from spontaneous abortions (miscarriages). Antiabortion advocates argue that if there is an increased need for fetal tissue, a time may come when women might be influenced in their decision whether or not to have an abortion if they could sell their fetus's tissue for research and/or treatment. In 2001 the federal government introduced a policy that federal funding would be available only for research using the 64 then-existing stem cell lines. This

policy was reversed in 2009, and federal funding is now available for additional stem cell lines.

Genetic Engineering and Cloning

A number of ethical issues surround the practices of **genetic engineering** (making, altering, or repairing genetic material) and **cloning** (reproducing genetically identical cells or individuals).

One is the issue of genetically engineered crops and other food products. This encompasses practices as diverse as injecting milk cows with growth hormones to get them to produce more milk to incorporating material from bacteria into plant seeds. Opponents argue that we cannot predict all of the possible effects of manipulating genetic material and are likely to see unexpected and unwanted consequences to ourselves or other species.

Gene therapy is a term used for experimental treatments that attempt to treat or cure disease by giving patients new genes or parts of genes that may have been synthesized in the laboratory, taken from human tissue, or engineered from genetic material of animals or other species. Research efforts are overseen by the Recombinant DNA Advisory Committee of the National Institutes of Health (NIH). A clinical study of a gene therapy treatment for arthritis was suspended in July 2007 after the death of a patient.

Human cloning is prohibited by several states, but efforts to pass legislation on the federal level have not succeeded to date. Experiments in animal cloning continue, although critics claim that it results in unhealthy animals and needless suffering.

Refusing or Withholding Treatment and Physician-Assisted Suicide

The right to refuse treatment is well established for adults. The 1990 Patient Self-Determination Act establishes the duty of hospitals, nursing homes, and health maintenance organizations (HMOs) to inform patients or new subscribers of their right to express their wishes related to health care and to refuse treatment. The act also establishes the right of an individual to prepare an advance directive that specifies what treatments he or she would like to receive, and what ones he or she would not wish to receive, if the individual were to become incapable of making those decisions at a later time. Courts have held an individual's right to refuse treatment in such high regard that they have allowed mentally ill patients to refuse treatments for their mental illness.

When an individual requires resuscitation or life support to stay alive, there may come a point at which it seems that the treatment is resulting in more suffering (harm) than benefit. This is especially true if it is unlikely that the person can recover his or her health or normal function. If there is a written document expressing the person's wishes, life support may be removed or discontinued. In the absence of an advance directive, an individual's family may bring to court a petition to remove life support. Such a petition must be supported by witnesses other than those who file the petition, stating that the incompetent individual expressed a desire to avoid being kept alive by artificial means. Life support has been interpreted to include ventilators, antibiotics, and even tube feedings.

Physician-assisted suicide and euthanasia (literally, "good death"), sometimes called *mercy killing*, evoke fears that the power to take life will be abused—that it will be used more for the convenience of others than for the well-being of those who are dying. Advocates for the disabled have argued that allowing physician-assisted suicide or euthanasia could be the first step in society's determining that the severely disabled are too much of a financial and physical burden and having them euthanized.

Throughout the 1990s, an individual physician named Jack Kevorkian provided patients with degenerative, terminal illnesses a machine that delivered an injection of lethal drugs. He was sentenced to 10 to 25 years in prison in 1999 and was released after 8 years in 2007 after he promised not to assist in any additional deaths.

In 1997, Oregon became the first state to legalize physician-assisted suicide, allowing physicians to write a prescription for a patient of a lethal dose of pain killer or other medication. The physician is not allowed to administer the medication. The U.S. Supreme Court upheld a challenge to the Oregon law in 2006. The discussion about physician-assisted suicide occurs in every state, but to date only three other states allow physician-assisted suicide (Montana, Vermont, and Washington). Most other states have specific laws prohibiting assisted suicide, and a few states prohibit it by common law. Patients with a terminal illness and their families are often looking for a trusted advisor with whom they can discuss their fears and concerns. Even when a physician is not morally willing or legally able to provide a means for a patient to end his or her life, there is increasing recognition of the value of frank discussion and reassurance that patients will not be left to cope alone.

Advance Directives

On the basis of personal beliefs, patients can formalize their decisions about treatment in terminal or end-of-life situations in a number of ways. These include **do-not-resuscitate (DNR) orders,** living wills, health care proxies, and organ donor cards, all of which fall under the heading of "advance directives" (Box 3-1). An advance directive may specify care to be given or avoided and name a person to make medical decisions for the individual should he or she become incompetent. This is usually a spouse, child older than age 18, member of the clergy, or close friend. Medical advance directives should always name a single individual to make decisions, with an alternate if possible. This is often a difficult choice, especially for an elderly person with several children (Figure 3-1). In addition, the patient may want to provide for donation of any organs that are useful. Organ donation (or donation of one's entire body) and procedures for determining who may give permission if the patient has not left a directive are outlined in the Uniform

---

BOX 3-1   Advance Directives

Do-Not-Resuscitate (DNR) Order

Requested by either patient or health care agent. A written order from the physician in the patient's medical record that allows medical staff to not resuscitate in the event of cardiac or respiratory arrest.

Living Will

Executed by an individual before or during illness. Identifies the patient's wishes about which life-prolonging actions should or should not be taken. In states that accept it, it provides instructions to health professionals about treatment to be provided and may include instructions to a health care agent as to which treatments he or she should authorize. Provisions for organ donation, autopsy, or donation of remains to a medical school are also usually included in a living will.

Health Care Proxy

Executed by an individual before or during illness. Names a health care agent who has the ability to make decisions about care, including signing a DNR order. It may also outline the types of care that the individual does or does not wish to receive. It becomes effective only when the individual becomes incapable of making his or her own decisions.

Durable Power of Attorney

Provides a written authorization to act on the behalf of another that remains in effect, even if the grantor becomes incapacitated. An ordinary power of attorney, used in business affairs, expires when a person becomes incapacitated An authorization limited to health care decisions only is called a *durable power of attorney for health care decisions* or a **medical durable power of attorney**.

Organ Donation Status

Authorization to donate organs after death either by signing up with a website or including in a license application. Many states have done away with a separate organ donor card, preferring to place the organ-donor designation on an individual's driver's license or ID card. If a person has signed up using a state database exists, a separate card is not usually issued.

Anatomical Gift Act. The Patient Self-Determination Act (PSDA) of 1990 requires hospitals, nursing homes, health maintenance organizations (HMOs), and other facilities to provide information about advance directives to patients.

Signed originals rather than photocopies of the advance directives should be held by the named surrogate, and the patient should keep copies with his or her important papers. It should also be noted in the primary care physician's records with a copy if possible so that the surrogate can be contacted if necessary.

DNR orders should be in the medical record, and the staff should be informed of the patient's wishes. If the

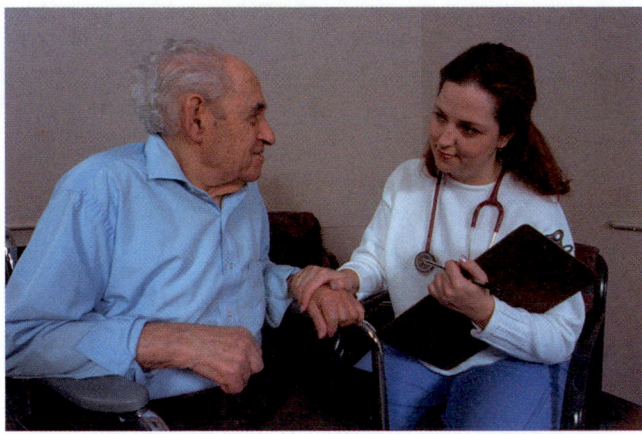

Figure 3-1 Elderly patients are grateful when office staff respond to their fears and concerns.

patient is at home, the family must have a copy of the DNR order to show emergency personnel, who otherwise will be legally obligated to resuscitate the patient.

Removal of life support means that no form of support, including mechanical breathing, feeding, or medications to prolong life, should be given. Pain medication and sedation are continued if necessary after removal of life support.

A **living will** is a document executed by an individual that gives medical professionals instructions about how that person wishes to be treated in the event he or she becomes incompetent. A living will may also give instructions regarding organ donation, autopsy, or donation of the remains to a medical school for anatomy dissection. Many states allow an individual's wishes to donate organs to be noted on his or her driver's license or on an organ donor card that can be carried in the wallet. In the event of a fatal auto accident, the police—who usually use the license or other documents to make identification—can notify ambulance personnel that the deceased is an organ donor.

A person usually names an agent to carry out his or her wishes if he or she is unable to do so. A **health care proxy** names the person who is charged with this responsibility and may also give specific instructions to the designated person concerning medical issues. Laws regulating living wills and health care proxies vary from state to state, and it is important for patients to use forms that will be valid where they live. This may require the assistance of an attorney.

PERSONAL, PROFESSIONAL, AND ORGANIZATIONAL ETHICS

It is important to distinguish between personal and professional ethics. In the work situation, professional ethics usually takes precedence over personal beliefs and morals. For example, a medical assistant may believe that a parent who is paying the medical bill should be given the results of laboratory tests done on his or her child. Legally, however, after age 18, information about a patient can be given only with the patient's consent. In this case, professional ethics requires that the medical assistant follow the law, no matter

what he or she believes personally, and maintain the patient's confidentiality.

Acting according to professional ethics means that the medical assistant cannot ethically withhold from the physician information given by the patient related to the medical condition. Even if the medical assistant does not agree with how the physician is managing a patient's care, the medical assistant cannot ethically (or legally) suggest another treatment plan for the patient.

It is important to clarify one's personal set of moral values and beliefs and identify areas where there may be potential conflict with professional ethics to avoid having to make a difficult decision on the spot. Using the process outlined in the following section, the medical assisting student should determine his or her own personal beliefs related to issues of potential ethical conflict. Then he or she should decide what professional ethics requires in those situations (Procedure 3-1).

An individual or medical practice can look to a professional organization for guidance related to ethical questions. Medical associations publish guidelines related to medical ethics. Professional associations for medical assistants can be a source of information and guidelines. For problems affecting the medical office, a discussion including all office staff may assist in decision making (Figure 3-2).

Organizational ethics includes the guidelines of an entire organization that influence the policies of the organization and conduct of employees in the workplace. An organization's mission statement is usually the best place to identify the specific principles and guidelines that are most important to it. The policy and procedure manual provides specific guidelines as well. In addition, there are several generally accepted principles for organizations. No organization should depend on unfair means to earn money. Employees should not manipulate or falsify information. Monetary transactions should be fair. Employees should not take or use office property for their own benefit. Employees should be treated fairly, and they should not be exploited. Employees should not be exposed to hazardous conditions without being provided with the means to protect their own safety.

PROCESS USED TO MAKE ETHICAL DECISIONS

Making ethical decisions involves measures to respond to conflict between different values and their relative importance. To decide on a course of action, it is helpful to clarify the conflict and make a thoughtful choice. A six-step process can be used to make these decisions. Actions should be well considered and in accordance with beliefs about what is right and wrong, rather than simply impulsive reactions.

Gathering Information

Information that needs to be gathered includes (1) background about the situation; (2) facts related to the specific problem; (3) information about the people involved, such as their knowledge of the situation or their mental capacity;

PROCEDURE **3-1**   Separating Personal and Professional Ethics

Outcome

1. Develop a plan for separation of personal and professional ethics
2. Examine the impact personal ethics and morals may have on the delivery of health care

Equipment/Supplies

- Paper
- Pen
- Computer and printer
- Blank index cards

1. Procedural Step. Research one of the following ethical issues: abortion, stem cell research, genetic engineering, cloning, refusing or withholding treatment, and physician-assisted suicide.

2. Procedural Step: Identify conflicting values related to the ethical issue you have chosen, and determine your own personal beliefs related to this ethical issue.
Principle. Analysis of ethical issues allows a person to identify personal values and beliefs.

3. Procedural Step: Write a summary of the ethical issue, your personal position on the issue, and the reasons for your position. Share this information with a group of your classmates.

4. Procedural Step: Imagine a possible situation involving a patient who has made a different choice from you related to this ethical issue, and describe the situation on an index card.
Principle. Different ethical values and beliefs must be respected to demonstrate sensitivity to patient rights.

5. Procedural Step. Role-play an interaction between yourself and the patient in which you maintain a professional demeanor.

6. Procedural Step: Participate in a group discussion in which you identify specific requirements for professionalism when there is a conflict between your personal beliefs and patient needs or rights.
Principle: Professional ethics places patient rights above personal ethical beliefs and values.

7. Procedural Step: Write a short description of the effect that personal ethics may have on professional behavior and the delivery of health care, and prepare a plan for how these can be separated.
Principle. Planning for the separation of personal and professional ethics increases a medical assistant's ability to respond in a professional way.

8. Procedural Step: Hand in your report to the instructor.

Figure 3-2 A staff meeting may be helpful to discuss problems affecting the medical office.

and (4) the laws or institutional policies that relate to the situation.

Identifying Conflicting Values

A conflict does not always involve lofty values. It may be as simple as one person's wish to not cause problems, to save time, or to avoid a hassle. However, this desire may conflict with professional duties or with another individual's right.

If a medical assistant is working in a facility where individual staff members do not always follow established procedures (e.g., do not always run controls for laboratory tests), the desire to go along with co-workers and avoid conflict may be strong; however, the duty to act with fidelity is not being met. The medical assistant may be personally performing the needed controls, but the knowledge that others are not doing so creates a conflict between personal reluctance to violate the autonomy of a co-worker and the professional duty of fidelity to patients.

Determining Relative Importance of Conflicting Claims

To determine the relative importance of conflicting claims, an individual needs to clarify his or her goals and weigh the conflicting values. It is important to remember that when values conflict, an individual or group makes a decision about importance that is valid within its own context but may not conform to the values of other individuals or groups.

For example, in the case of abortion, some people believe that the right of a fetus to life outweighs all other rights.

Others believe that a woman's right to autonomy in medical decisions about her body, and the consequences to a child of being unwanted, diminish or outweigh the absolute right to life in the early stages of a pregnancy.

Exploring Alternatives

Once it has been established which values are more important, it is important to consider the possible outcomes of possible actions. It is helpful to identify as many courses of action as possible, predict the consequences of each action, and project how different goals would be met or not met by following each possible course of action.

Choosing and Justifying One Alternative

Conflicting claims require choices. By analyzing hypothetic situations in detail, a person can construct some sort of personal framework for ethical decisions; once on the job, there is often little time to analyze each situation individually.

In the end, there are four ways to justify a decision:

1. By presenting logical arguments—deductions based on facts
2. By social justification—consideration of the larger consequences to society
3. By projection of consequences—imagining what might happen if a given alternative were chosen
4. By refuting alternative claims—stating explicitly why alternative choices have less merit than the one chosen

If it is impossible to select any alternative that seems comfortable, or "right," the choice to do nothing becomes a chosen alternative rather than simply the avoidance of a decision.

Implementing the Decision

The final step in this process is to put the ethical decision into action. This does not have to be a permanent solution. The decision can be reconsidered and another solution can be tried, or the question can be reconsidered at intervals to see if circumstances, beliefs, or knowledge has changed.

INTRODUCTION TO LAW

DIFFERENCE BETWEEN PUBLIC LAW AND PRIVATE LAW

The legal system in the United States is primarily divided into two parts, public law and private law. *Public law* refers to laws that define the relationship between the individual and society as a whole. The term **criminal law** is used to refer to the set of laws that protect society. Examples include laws against robbery, rape, and operating a motor vehicle while under the influence of alcohol or a controlled drug. Private law, also called **civil law,** is the set of laws that deal with relationships and disputes between individuals and/or groups of people. This may involve two individuals or groups of people; individuals and corporations, government, or other organizations; or one corporate, government, or organizational entity and another such entity. Contracts are considered a part of civil law, and disputes about contracts that go to court are tried as part of the civil court system.

LAWSUITS

Both civil and criminal action disputes can lead to lawsuits that are tried in the court system. In any court proceeding, there is a **plaintiff,** the person or entity that makes the complaint, and a **defendant,** the person or entity against whom a lawsuit is brought. In a criminal lawsuit, the plaintiff is the district or state's attorney, a representative of the government. In a civil lawsuit, the plaintiff is the injured party.

In criminal law the criminal activity itself is held to be harmful or potentially harmful to society or individual members of society. The act itself is punishable, regardless of whether anyone was actually harmed by the act. In civil law, an injury or damage that results because of someone's wrongful act results in **liability** (legal responsibility). The same misdeed can provoke both a criminal charge and a civil lawsuit. The criminal lawsuit will determine if the person is guilty of committing a crime punishable by an imprisonment or fine paid to the government. The civil lawsuit will determine what liability the person has to the injured party, if any.

A well-known example of this dual legal picture is the O. J. Simpson case. Simpson was found not guilty by a jury of the murder of his ex-wife, Nicole, and her friend, Ronald Goldman. However, her estate filed a civil suit against him on the grounds of "wrongful death." In the civil case, he was found liable for their deaths, and more than 30 million dollars was awarded in damages. In a criminal case the charge must be proven "beyond a reasonable doubt," but in a civil case the burden of proof is only to a level at which the supporting evidence is more convincing than the opposing evidence ("a preponderance of the evidence").

SPECIALIZED AREAS OF LAW

Specialized areas of law include constitutional law, international law, and administrative law. Constitutional law is the study of law of countries and other political organizations. International law concerns the relationships among countries and includes maritime law and regulations applying to ocean-going vessels. Administrative law arises from the actions of federal government agencies, such as the Social Security Administration and the Internal Revenue Service.

CREATION OF LAWS

Law was created by tradition through accepted social practices and decisions of the courts. This type of law is called **common law** or **case law.** Today most laws are created through a vote by a legislative body. The term for this is **statutory law.** Legislators are elected by popular vote to serve in either the state or the federal legislature. One of their important duties is to draft new legislation, which is called a **bill** while it is under consideration. Once passed by either the House of Representatives or the Senate, a bill that contains several parts becomes an **act.** Once passed by both houses, the act is signed into law by the President (for a federal law) or a state governor (for a law applicable to one state). Cities and towns can also enact laws, called *ordinances;* these usually have to do with local issues, such as smoking in public places, parking, leash laws for pets, and curfews at parks.

All employees of the medical office must be aware of the federal and state laws that regulate the provision of health care and insurance reimbursement, as well as those related to the operation of a business.

CRIMINAL LAW

The branch of law that describes offenses against the public welfare is called *criminal law.* A **crime** is an offense in violation of a law that prohibits or requires certain behavior. When a person is convicted of a crime (or pleads guilty to a crime), punishment is imposed. A **felony** is a serious crime, punishable by death or imprisonment in a state or federal penal institution for more than 1 year. A **misdemeanor** is a less serious crime, punishable by a fine or imprisonment for less than 1 year, often in a local or county penal institution. Another term sometimes used to describe a criminal act is **malfeasance**—a wrongdoing that is illegal or contrary to official obligation.

Nonviolent Crimes

Occasionally a physician is charged with manslaughter or criminal negligence if a patient dies or sustains serious injury as a result of incorrect or negligent treatment. This is usually in addition to a civil lawsuit brought by the patient or family for wrongful death (see the discussion of professional malpractice later in this chapter). Euthanasia and assisted suicide (except for physician-assisted suicide in states that allow it) are usually considered murder whether performed by a health professional or family member.

Two or more people who have joined together to commit an unlawful act may be accused of conspiracy; this may be applied to actions that are illegal in and of themselves, or actions to prevent detection of a prior crime.

Stealing another person's property (without violence) is called **larceny.** In the medical office, this may take the form of **embezzlement**—appropriation of funds from a client, customer, or employer.

A growing problem in the health care industry is **fraud**—deliberate deception carried out to secure unfair or unlawful gain. Billing for services not provided, billing for services provided to imaginary patients, performing unneeded services, and even deliberately using codes from a higher level of service than that provided are all forms of insurance fraud. Every instance of such a billing can be considered a separate act. If the fraud involves the use of mail (mail fraud) or electronic resources (wire fraud), it becomes a federal offense.

In the mind of an office employee, there may be a difference between billing an insurance company using a code for more complex service than was actually provided, "because they pay us so little anyway," and billing for procedures that were never performed. But from a legal perspective, both are considered fraud and, if proved, both carry serious penalties.

Insurance companies and agencies of the federal and state governments are victims of billions of dollars in fraudulent claims each year. They have increasing incentives to investigate health care facilities they suspect of fraudulent billing.

CIVIL LAW

The branch of law that regulates interactions among individuals, groups, organizations, and the government is civil law. Disputes arise when one individual or group believes that the actions of another individual or group have caused personal injury or damage to property. In medical offices these usually relate to the actual care received by the patient and/or the relationship between the patient and the physician or office staff. Two types of obligations that may give rise to civil lawsuits are contracts and torts.

Contracts involve agreements between two or more parties and are discussed in detail later. If a contract exists, failure to meet the terms of the contract by either party is called *breach of contract.* A **tort** is an injury or wrong against a person or property that does not involve breach of contract. If a person knows, or should know, the consequences of his or her action, the wrong is called an *intentional tort.* If the action is a mistake or has unintended consequences, it is called an *unintentional tort.* See Box 3-2 for a list of torts. Keep in mind that intentional torts may also be prosecuted as criminal acts if they are performed with specific intent to cause injury.

Two other terms may be used for acts that can result in civil lawsuits. The term **misfeasance** refers to a legal act performed in an improper way, especially if it causes injury or damage. The term **nonfeasance** means failing to perform an act that should have been performed to prevent injury or damage.

LAW AND PROFESSIONAL LIABILITY
PHYSICIAN-PATIENT RELATIONSHIP

The physician-patient relationship is a contractual relationship. Each party has certain rights and responsibilities under the relationship.

Several elements must be present for there to be a contract:

1. There must be a mutual agreement.
2. There must be intent to do (or not do) something that is legal.

BOX 3-2 Intentional and Unintentional Torts

Intentional Torts

Abandonment Failure to continue to provide medical care to a patient without proper notification.

Assault Threat to touch another person or his or her property without permission in a way that will cause pain, injury, or damage or is offensive.

Battery Touching of another person or his or her property without permission in a way that will cause pain, injury, or damage or is offensive.

Defamation Making a false claim that may harm a person's reputation, business, or group. If the claim is made verbally, it is called *slander*. If the claim is made in writing, it is called *libel*.

False imprisonment Confining a person without legal authority, such as using restraints without a proper physician order.

Invasion of privacy Public disclosure of private information, such as releasing medical information or photographs without consent of the patient.

Misrepresentation Providing information with knowledge that it is incorrect or reckless disregard for the truth.

Unintentional Torts

Negligence Failure to act with reasonable prudence in a situation. Negligence by a professional is also called *malpractice*.

Strict liability Responsibility for injury, even if there was no negligence. This is often applied when individuals are injured by products or equipment.

---

3. The action must occur in exchange for service (called *consideration*) or for payment.
4. The parties must be legally able to enter into a contract.

A contract does not have to be written or sometimes even discussed in detail. When clothes are left for dry cleaning, it is assumed that there will be an obligation to pay for the service. The same is true if a patient makes a visit to a medical office. Written contracts are used when there is a considerable amount of money at stake (such as a car loan or mortgage). In the medical office a patient may be asked to sign a statement confirming that payment will be made for any charges not covered by insurance.

Certain groups of people are not legally able to be a party to contracts, including most medical care contracts. These people are also not able to give informed consent. Such groups include the following:
1. Children younger than the age of 18
2. Mentally ill adults or adults with severe intellectual disabilities
3. Individuals who are temporarily mentally incapacitated (including those who have received narcotic analgesics or other mind-altering medications)

4. Individuals who are under threat or duress (fear of a threat)
5. Individuals who have been found incompetent to handle their affairs (as determined by a physician or court)

All consent forms should be signed and all implied contracts made with a competent party acting as a willing health care decision maker for the child or incompetent person. In some circumstances, adult rights, including the right to consent to medical treatment, are given to individuals younger than the age of 18. Such an individual is called an **emancipated minor.** In most states, an individual aged 14 to 18 years can obtain a court order from a judge to become free of control of a parent or guardian after proving the ability to be financially independent. If a minor is not emancipated, he or she may still be considered to have the maturity to choose or reject a particular health care treatment with or without parental consent. In this case the individual may be considered to be a **mature minor,** an individual younger than 18 with the maturity to provide informed consent for certain medical procedures. Depending on the jurisdiction, there may be specific laws or it may be a common law policy.

The Physician

Within the physician-patient relationship, the physician provides skillful care to the patient and continues to treat the patient unless the physician informs the patient that the relationship will be terminated. In this case the physician must give the patient time to make other arrangements for care. The physician arranges for someone else to treat the patient if the physician is unavailable (such as on nights, on weekends, and during vacations). The physician informs the patient about treatments or procedures and carries out only those treatments and procedures to which the patient consents. The physician informs the patient of test results, diagnoses, and medical conditions and gives the patient instructions for follow-up care and procedures to follow at home.

A physician has the following rights:
- To accept or decline to treat a patient
- To choose to limit the medical practice to a particular size or certain specialty
- To decide where to practice

Decisions not to treat particular patients must be based on general principles (such as limiting a practice to urology) rather than arbitrary decisions (based on a whim or subjective judgment).

The Patient

The patient agrees to keep appointments, give accurate information about his or her medical condition, provide an accurate medical history, follow directions, and pay for service.

The patient has the following rights:
- To refuse treatment
- To receive complete information about procedures
- To select a physician

- To expect continuity of care
- To expect confidentiality of verbal and written communication with the physician and the physician's agents
- To be treated with respect and dignity
- To receive complete information about the treatment suggested, alternatives, and possible consequences of alternatives or no treatment

Patients' rights may be legally defined by the state or an institution. The *Patient Bill of Rights* is a name that is often used to refer to the Consumer Bill of Rights and Responsibilities, which was adopted by the Presidential Advisory Commission on Consumer Protection and Quality in the Health Care Industry in 1998. This document was created to improve consumer trust in the health care system by defining the rights and responsibilities of consumers, health care professionals, health care institutions, and insurance plans. The Bipartisan Patient Protection Act (also known as the *McCain-Edwards-Kennedy Patients' Bill of Rights*) was an attempt to enact the findings of this commission into federal law. It failed in the U.S. House of Representatives in 2002. In the next decade, most individual states did pass legislation defining what was commonly called a "patient bill of rights," although the focus varies from state to state. Some concentrate primarily on rights of patients in residential facilities, whereas others have a broader scope (Figure 3-3). The medical assistant and all employees of the medical office must protect patients' rights (Procedure 3-2).

Terminating the Physician-Patient Relationship

To end a relationship with a patient, a physician must notify the patient in writing. It is recommended that such a letter be sent via certified mail with return receipt requested. The letter needs to be dated, must state the reasons for termination of care, and should describe how medical records will be made available. Copies of any correspondence regarding termination and receipts should be kept in the medical record. If the patient notifies the physician by telephone that he or she wishes to terminate the relationship, the physician should send a similar letter as documentation.

Common reasons for a physician terminating care of a patient include the following:

- The physician moves.
- The physician retires.
- The physician dies.
- The physician closes the practice for other reasons.
- The patient regularly and continually breaks appointments.
- The patient regularly and continually refuses to follow medical advice.

If a patient can convince a court that he or she was under the belief that a physician-patient relationship still existed and because of such belief did not seek out another practitioner, and sustained injury, a successful case can be made for **abandonment.** This is rare and should never happen if the physician keeps good written records about any termination notification.

PERSONAL AND PROFESSIONAL LIABILITY

A person is responsible for his or her actions and may be held liable if those actions injure another person. In daily life we are required to act as a reasonable person would act in the same circumstances. The failure to act—or to refrain from acting—as a reasonable person would act in similar circumstances is called **negligence.**

A common example of negligence relates to a wet floor. If someone washes the floor or spills water on the floor and does not wipe it up, the floor becomes slippery. When an unsuspecting person comes along and is not aware that the floor is wet, that person could slip and be injured. The person responsible for making the floor wet would be expected to know that the wet floor would be slippery and could cause someone to fall. A person who notices the spill would also be expected to know that the wet floor could cause a fall.

If a person falls, is injured, and files a lawsuit, the person who washed the floor, or another person with responsibility for public safety who noticed the spill, could be found to be negligent and be responsible (liable) to pay for the injured person's medical care, lost wages, and any other costs caused by the fall on the wet floor.

Standard of Care

A person without any special training is held only to the standard of a "reasonably prudent person." The term **prudent** means careful or using common sense. For instance, any reasonably prudent person is expected to realize that an infant or unconscious person will not be able to remove a heating pad that is too hot. If an infant or unconscious person is burned by a heating pad, the person who placed it will be considered liable and will be responsible for medical bills as well as compensation for pain and suffering.

In general, a medical assistant is held to a professional standard, especially when performing procedures that are often done by a licensed health professional. The medical assistant must be especially careful to avoid offering advice or making decisions that may be interpreted as diagnosing illness or prescribing treatment.

If the medical assistant administers medication, he or she must do so correctly and must follow proper procedures and precautions to protect the patient from injury. A physician must be on the premises (not necessarily in the room) any time medication is given by a medical assistant, because in most states the medical assistant can perform the procedure only under the authority and supervision of a physician. It is important for medical assistants to find out what they are legally allowed to do in the state where they work.

In emergency situations, when no qualified professional is available, health care practitioners are expected to give care for which they have been trained but at which they may not be proficient. For instance, any physician would

WALDEN-MARTIN
FAMILY MEDICAL CLINIC
1234 ANYSTREET ANYTOWN, ANYSTATE 12345
PHONE 123-123-1234   FAX 123-123-5678

Patient Bill of Rights

RIGHTS

1. **Medical Care and Dental Care.** The right to quality care consistent with available resources and accepted standards. The right to refuse treatment to the extent permitted by law and Government regulations, and to be informed of refusal consequences. When concerned about care received, the right to request review of care adequacy.

2. **Respectful Treatment.** The right to considerate and respectful care, with recognition of personal dignity.

3. **Privacy and Confidentiality.** The right, within law and military regulations, to privacy and confidentiality concerning medical care.

4. **Identity.** The right to know, at all times, the identity, professional status, and professional credentials of health care personnel, as well as the name of the health care provider primarily responsible for his or her care.

5. **Explanation of Care.** The right to an explanation concerning diagnosis, treatment, procedures, and prognosis of illness in terms the patient can understand. When it is not medically advisable to give such information to the patient, information should be provided to appropriate family members or, in their absence, another appropriate person.

6. **Informed Consent.** The right to be advised in non-clinical terms of information (significant complications, risks, benefits, and alternative treatments) needed to make knowledgeable decisions on treatment consent or refusal.

7. **Research Projects.** The right to be advised if the facility proposes to perform research associated with care. The right to refuse to participate in any research projects.

8. **Safe Environment.** The right to care and treatment in a safe environment.

9. **Medical Treatment Facility (MTF) or Dental Treatment Facility (DTF) Rules and Regulations.** The right to be informed of facility conduct rules and regulations. The patient should be informed about smoking rules and should expect compliance with those rules from other individuals. Patients are entitled to information about the MTF or DTF mechanism for the initiation, review and resolution of patient complaints.

RESPONSIBILITIES

1. **Providing Information.** The responsibility to provide, to the best of his or her knowledge, accurate and complete information about complaints, past illness, hospitalizations, medications, and other matters relating to his or her health. A patient has the responsibility to let his or her primary health care provider know whether he or she understands the treatment and what is expected of him or her.

2. **Respect and Consideration.** The responsibility for being considerate of the rights of other patients and MTF and DTF health care personnel and for assistance in the control of noise, smoking, and the number of visitors. The patient is responsible for being respectful of the property of other persons and of the facility.

3. **Compliance with Medical Care.** The responsibility for complying with medical and nursing treatment plans, including follow-up care, recommended by health care providers. This includes keeping appointments on time and notifying the MTF or DTF when appointments cannot be kept.

4. **Medical Records.** The responsibility for ensuring that medical records are promptly returned to the medical facility for appropriate filing and maintenance when records are transported by the patients for the purpose of medical appointment or consultation, etc.

5. **MTF and DTF Rules and Regulations.** The responsibility for following the MTF or DTF rules and regulations affecting patient care conduct. Regulations regarding smoking should be followed by all patients.

6. **Reporting of Patient Complaints.** The responsibility for helping the MTF or DTF commander provide the best possible care to all beneficiaries. Patients' recommendations, questions, or complaints should be reported to the patient contact representative.

Figure 3-3 The Patient Bill of Rights is found in the Forms Repository Section of SimChart for the Medical Office.

be expected to initiate emergency care for a patient who suddenly goes into cardiac arrest, even a specialist such as an ophthalmologist. Patients make an assumption that in a medical office they will receive medical treatment, even in the event of an emergency. All medical office personnel are expected to be able to give advice in an emergency or to activate the local emergency medical system if they cannot handle the situation.

Many, if not most, medical offices train all of their personnel in cardiopulmonary resuscitation (CPR) and first

PROCEDURE 3-2   Incorporating the Patient's Bill of Rights

Outcome Apply the Patient Bill of Rights and Health Insurance Portability and Accountability Act (HIPAA) Privacy Rule

Equipment/Supplies

- Paper
- Pen
- Computer and printer
- Role-play cards (from instructor)

1. **Procedural Step.** Make a list identifying policies or procedures a medical office should have in place to protect patient rights related to choice of treatment, consent for treatment, refusal of treatment, and privacy. Use Figure 3-3 (or print a copy of the Patient Bill of Rights from SimChart for the Medical Office) and identify a policy or procedure for each right and responsibility. Also include ways in which patient privacy should be protected.
   Principle. Patient rights are protected by moral obligation and sometimes also by federal and/or state law.

2. **Procedural Step.** Include specific examples of ways a medical assistant should behave to preserve patient rights related to choice of treatment, consent for treatment, and refusal of treatment. Describe how a medical assistant should respond if a patient refuses to undergo a diagnostic test or treatment. Give specific examples.

3. **Procedural Step.** Working with one or more classmates, role-play activities to identify how the Patient Bill of Rights can be applied to personal practice. During your role-play, demonstrate sensitivity to patient rights. Role-play at least one activity related to consent for or refusal of treatment.
   Principle. Medical assistants must apply legal and ethical principles to personal practice.

4. **Procedural Step.** Hand in your written list and descriptions to your instructor.

---

aid. If a medical assistant, secretary, or receptionist tells any patient that a problem is not serious, and it is, then he or she may be liable if there is injury to the patient caused by delay of treatment. Failure to respond correctly to an emergency can be considered a "breach of contract" because there is an implied contract between a patient and a medical office that any emergency will be handled by competent staff.

Health professionals are, in general, held to a high standard of care. For physicians and other health professionals, the term **standard of care** defines the level of appropriate care legally required of any other practitioner with the same education and training providing the same care in the same geographic region. In general, if a legal question arises, a medical assistant will be held to the standard of care of the professional who would normally perform the care in question.

For example, if a family practice physician prescribes blood pressure medication, he or she has to do it as competently as another family practice physician in the same area. If a nurse practitioner prescribes blood pressure medication, he or she has to meet the same standard as the family practice physician. If a patient sustains injury from taking the medication, in either case, the court would look at the appropriateness of the medication for the particular patient, the dose, and the follow-up to see whether either practitioner acted at an acceptable level.

Informed Consent

Consent can be implied by a patient's actions. If a medical assistant says, "Would you please roll up your sleeve so that I can give you an injection?" and the patient does so, the patient has given *implied* consent to the medical assistant to administer the injection. Even though the patient has not verbally agreed, the act of preparing for the injection suggests that the patient is willing to undergo the procedure.

Expressed consent can be verbal or written. We know, however, that simply expressing consent does not always represent understanding. Patients today have the legal right to completely understand what will be done to them or for them. For this reason, many medical offices now use written consent forms to obtain informed consent.

Written consent forms are now always used for surgery, for procedures involving entry into a sterile body cavity, for procedures that carry a risk to the patient's health, and for testing for human immunodeficiency virus (HIV), the virus that causes acquired immunodeficiency syndrome (AIDS). Written consent forms are increasingly being used as well for immunizations; treatment with birth control pills; transfusions of blood or blood products, such as plasma; and other treatments and procedures.

Legally it is not the form, but the understanding by the person on whom the treatment or procedure will be performed, that truly represents consent. It is the responsibility of the person performing the procedure, prescribing the medication, or performing the test or examination to provide the following information to the patient before consent is obtained:

1. The nature of the patient's condition
2. The nature and purpose of the recommended procedure
3. An explanation of risks involved with the procedure
4. Alternative treatments or procedures available
5. The likely outcome of the procedure (prognosis)
6. The risks of declining or delaying the procedure

The explanation must be given in terms the patient can understand, and the patient should be given an opportunity to ask questions regarding the information.

After the consent form has been personalized for the patient and the procedure has been explained, the medical assistant may be asked to obtain the signature. If the medical assistant believes that the patient does not fully understand what he or she is consenting to, the matter should be referred back to the physician. This is a good example of the medical assistant acting as a liaison between the patient and the physician and being an advocate for the patient. Depending on state law, there may be special consent forms for the release of information about HIV test results and/or treatment, drug and alcohol rehabilitation, services for mental health, or other health-related information.

A patient can rescind (withdraw) the authorization to release information at any time by notifying the medical office in writing.

What Would You Do? What Would You *Not* Do?

Case Study 2

Howard Morton is a 72-year-old patient who has come to the office because of severe back pain. After examining him, the physician referred him to an orthopedic surgeon for evaluation. While Vicki is preparing the referral form for Mr. Morton, he says, "If I see an orthopedic surgeon, he is probably going to want to do surgery. Do you think surgery is the best treatment for my kind of problem? What else could I try? Should I see a chiropractor? Or do you think acupuncture might help?" ■

Professional Negligence

Professional negligence is often called **malpractice.** To avoid lawsuits for malpractice, a health professional must be sure that he or she is acting within the limits of his or her profession and must act (or refrain from acting) in a given situation as a reasonable and prudent person of the same profession would. When the medical assistant performs procedures that are usually performed by other professionals, such as nurses, the medical assistant will be held to the same standard as the professional who usually performs the procedure. No one always does everything perfectly, and both negligence and malpractice are assumed to be mistakes and unintentional.

Requirements to Prove Professional Negligence

To prove that a professional is guilty of professional negligence and liable for the outcome, four things must be proved by a preponderance of the evidence. This means that they are more likely than not. Sometimes these things are called the *Four Ds of malpractice:*

1. The person who caused the injury has a *duty* to the person who was injured.
2. The person was *derelict* (neglectful) in performing that duty.
3. The failure to perform the duty was the *direct cause* of the injury and nothing could have intervened.
4. The failure to perform the duty caused *damage* or injury.

In some instances the plaintiff has no direct knowledge of the incident (e.g., if the plaintiff is under general anesthesia). In such a case a lawsuit may be allowed under the doctrine of **res ipsa loquitur,** whereby the court assumes that negligence must have occurred because of the type of injury. An example would be if the gallbladder was removed when the patient was scheduled for a hysterectomy.

A physician who gives casual medical advice at a party may not consider the person a patient he or she has a duty to take care of. But if the person fails to seek medical treatment on the basis of the physician's casual words, a court may have to decide if the physician owed a duty to the person.

If a professional does exactly what any other professional would have done and the patient has a poor outcome, the physician is not necessarily negligent. For example, even with the best sterile technique it is possible to get a wound infection. A person with a wound infection must show that proper technique was not used. If the injured person does not follow directions to keep the wound dry and the wound gets infected, the infection might have occurred because the patient did not follow directions.

If someone makes a mistake but there is no injury, the person who makes the mistake will not be liable and will not have to pay any damages. Many mistakes can be corrected if they are reported promptly.

Professional Liability Insurance

To protect against financial loss if the patient sues, physicians usually have professional liability insurance (also called *malpractice insurance*). This is for two reasons. One is to protect physicians for their own negligent actions. The second is to protect physicians if they are sued for the negligent actions of their employees while on the job.

If an injury occurs, the law allows the injured person to sue both the person responsible for causing the injury *and that person's employer,* provided that the incident occurred at work. This occurs under what is known as the doctrine of **respondeat superior.** The English translation of this Latin term is literally "let the master answer," meaning let the person at the head of the organization answer for the injuries caused by his or her employees.

This legal doctrine provides an incentive for employers to be sure that their employees are careful and gives the injured person a better chance of collecting damages for any injury. Even if the employee does not have insurance to cover such an incident or enough money to pay the amount received in judgment, the employer ought to have liability insurance. As the number of lawsuits for outpatient care increases, it is recommended that medical assistants carry their own malpractice insurance.

Laws that protect health professionals from being sued for giving emergency care at the scene of an accident are called *Good Samaritan Acts.* They vary from state to state and may cover physicians, nurses, emergency medical technicians, anyone certified to perform CPR, and other professionals.

MALPRACTICE LITIGATION

Litigation (the process of taking a lawsuit or criminal case through the courts) is complex. Having a general understanding of the process is important, even though less than 5% of all lawsuits brought against medical professionals or medical institutions ever reach the stage of going to trial.

Initiating a Lawsuit

A person who believes he or she has received inappropriate medical care consults an attorney, who obtains information from the patient and usually tries to obtain copies of the relevant medical records. A letter containing a patient's authorization to send a copy of medical records to a lawyer may be the first indication to the medical office that the patient is actively contemplating a lawsuit.

After having received written authorization from the patient, the medical office provides a copy of the record to a lawyer. Under the Health Insurance Portability and Accountability Act of 1996 (HIPAA), health care facilities, including physicians' offices, are allowed to charge a reasonable fee for copying paper records or preparing paper copies of electronic records sent to an attorney or requested by a patient.

At the time a lawsuit is actually filed, the patient signs a document releasing the physician from the requirements of patient confidentiality. This is necessary because information about the patient's medical record becomes part of the public record in the litigation process.

When he or she obtains the patient's medical records, the attorney has them reviewed by physicians or other health professionals uninvolved in the patient's treatment to determine if a case can clearly be made for malpractice. Appropriateness of care is clearly the major issue in a suit for malpractice. However, incomplete, illegible, or altered records decrease the medical record's credibility, even if the care actually given was appropriate.

Most malpractice suits are accepted by attorneys on a **contingency** basis. In such a case the individual filing the lawsuit pays for the attorney's time and effort only if he or she collects an award from the party being sued. This is usually a percentage of the settlement or judgment amount. Contingency payments to the attorney are usually from 20% to 40% of the amount collected.

Response to a Possible Lawsuit

The first thing a physician should do on receiving a request for patient records by an attorney or on being served with notice of a lawsuit is to inform the company that provides his or her professional liability insurance. If a suit is filed, the malpractice insurance provider will appoint an attorney to represent the physician as a policyholder. The physician may also wish to hire an independent attorney because the physician's interests are not always the same as the malpractice insurance carrier's. If other staff members are named in the lawsuit, it may be in their best interest to hire their own attorneys as well.

As the legal process continues, the attorneys usually negotiate a settlement to avoid the time and expense of going to court, as well as the possibility of a large damage award. Because juries are unpredictable, the attorneys appointed by the insurance provider will hesitate to risk a jury trial, even if there does not appear to be any negligence in the care provided to the plaintiff. If there is a trial, the court may issue a **subpoena,** a court order that requires an individual to be present to testify during some part of the trial process. A physician or nurse may provide a **deposition** before the actual trial, which is legal testimony given under oath to an officer of the court. To require that the original medical record be present, the court will issue a **subpoena duces tecum,** a court order requiring that documents (or other material evidence) be made available. An employee of the health care facility should bring the original paper medical record to court each day that it is required and be present wherever the medical record is at all times. Electronic health records (EHRs) contain more detailed patient information than paper medical records. Electronic tracking data and time stamps of clinical activity and the input of orders can be required by the court in most states. Electronic records contain an *audit trail* or *audit log,* a chronologic record that provides evidence of the sequence of activities that have occurred within the record. The printed version of the electronic record may not accurately reflect the screen seen at the time when information was entered. If a medical office is on notice of a credible probability that it will become involved in litigation, employees must be careful to preserve in the electronic record all information that may be relevant to the lawsuit.

Alternative Dispute Resolution

Instead of a trial, both parties may agree to have their dispute decided by a neutral third party. This process can reduce time, expense, and publicity of a dispute. Such a process may take the form of mediation or arbitration.

Mediation uses a facilitator to help two parties in conflict settle their differences. This can be done in different ways, and if no settlement is reached, either party may find recourse in the court system.

Arbitration is a process whereby a neutral party settles the dispute. The arbitration can be either binding or nonbinding.

In nonbinding arbitration, the parties do not have to accept the decision and one party can proceed with a court case. In binding arbitration, the parties agree at the beginning to be bound by the decision of the arbitrator(s).

Various organizations provide lists of arbitrators, and depending on the circumstances and applicable state law, the parties in arbitration either select a mutually acceptable arbitrator or are assigned one from a list prepared during the arbitration process.

Arbitration is not common in malpractice cases; it is far more common in commercial contract and labor contract disputes.

TORT DEFENSES

Privilege

Privilege is a special right or permission granted to a certain group of individuals. For example, a health care facility's policy and procedure manual may give physicians the power to order soft restraints or leather restraints for a patient in certain circumstances. With such an order, other health professionals may legally apply the restraints. A patient who is placed in restraints according to established procedures could not make a successful case for false imprisonment, an intentional tort.

Consent

Consent has been already discussed in detail. A patient may be asked to sign a consent form allowing photographs to be taken and published in a medical journal or textbook or used as a slide in a lecture (without personal identifying information) for the purpose of providing education. If informed consent was obtained, especially if it is in writing, the patient cannot make a case for invasion of privacy.

Self-Defense or the Defense of Others

Self-defense or the defense of others is another defense against intentional tort. When physical contact occurs, a person accused of assault and/or battery may assert that he or she was defending against contact initiated by another person.

Expiration of the Statute of Limitations

Several defenses can be used against a charge of negligence or malpractice. The **statute of limitations** is the law that limits the time period during which a person can sue. The period varies from 1 to 3 years, depending on the laws of the particular state and whether the suit is for negligence or malpractice (negligence usually has a shorter statute of limitations than malpractice).

Although state law can vary slightly, the statute of limitations usually begins at one of three points:
1. When the injury occurs
2. When the individual first realizes that an injury has occurred; for instance, if a hemostat is left in the body during surgery, the statute of limitations begins to run

when the instrument is discovered on a radiograph taken at a later date for another reason
3. When a minor reaches the age of majority or some other specific age (such as 21)

Contributory or Comparative Negligence

If the injured person has played a part in causing the injury, some states regard this as a complete defense (**contributory negligence**). Other states determine **comparative negligence**—how much of the negligence was caused by the professional and how much was caused by the injured individual. Judges and juries are asked to assess damages to the injured party depending on the percentage of the injury caused by the health care professional.

For example, after minor surgery a patient developed a wound infection that required additional surgery and resulted in an unsightly scar. The physician's attorney brought out that the patient had failed to seek medical attention for several days after noting swelling, drainage from the wound, and a fever of 102° F. Prompt medical attention, the attorney argued, would have prevented the second surgery and minimized scarring.

In a state using contributory negligence, establishing that the patient contributed to the injury would be a complete defense and the patient would not collect any damages. In a state using comparative negligence, the judge or jury would determine a percentage for the amount of negligence on the part of the physician and award the patient that percentage of the total damages established by the court.

Assumption of Risk

A patient who does not follow medical advice becomes responsible for any problems that occur as a result of his or her decision. This is called **assumption of risk.** This is easier to establish if the patient has signed a waiver, such as a form acknowledging that a patient is leaving the hospital against medical advice. In the medical office there is usually no form for the patient to sign, so a complete note should be written in the patient's medical record if he or she refuses to follow medical advice. This note should include the patient's exact words if possible, and the name of any staff or family member who was present during the discussion. If a patient frequently misses appointments, it is also an example of disregarding medical advice. By documenting all missed appointments, the medical assistant can provide evidence that the patient, not the physician, is responsible for any problem that may arise.

FEDERAL AND STATE LAWS AFFECTING THE MEDICAL OFFICE

CONTROLLED SUBSTANCES AND PRESCRIPTIONS

Controlled Substances

The **Drug Enforcement Administration (DEA)** enforces the Controlled Substances Act of 1970. A **controlled substance** is a drug that has a potential for addiction and/or abuse. Physicians who prescribe controlled substances must register with the DEA and renew their registration every year, but the physician's DEA number should not be preprinted on prescription forms. The DEA updates the five schedules of controlled substances annually. Schedule I controlled substances have the highest potential for abuse and currently have no accepted medical use in the United States, whereas Schedule V controlled substances have the lowest potential for abuse. The specific medications are discussed in more detail in Chapter 26.

Federal law requires that controlled substances be stored away from other medications, in a sturdy, locked cabinet. It is recommended to use a double-locked box or drawer—a box or drawer with an outer lock or key and an inner compartment that also has a lock or key. A physician may not legally obtain Schedule I controlled substances unless participating in an authorized experiment. Schedule II controlled substances are ordered from a manufacturer or a distributor with federal triplicate order form DEA Form 222. Schedule III through V controlled substances do not require the special triplicate form; however, they do require that invoices and packing slips be kept for 2 years.

If controlled substances are kept in a medical office, an inventory sheet must be maintained. The controlled substance stock should be counted daily and verified by a second person. The two people must sign the inventory sheet. Every 2 years, a record of daily inventory of controlled substances must be submitted to the DEA. If controlled substances need to be wasted or destroyed, two witnesses must sign the inventory sheet. If any controlled substances are stolen, local police must be alerted immediately.

Prescribing, dispensing, and/or administering controlled substances also requires documentation. States vary on what paperwork is necessary; some require a special narcotic prescription form for Schedule II prescriptions. Any physician copies of controlled substance prescription forms should be kept in a secure, fireproof safe or other storage. If controlled substances are administered or dispensed only rarely, records can be kept in the patients' records and made available to DEA investigators.

A medical assistant must know the legal requirements regarding controlled substances that have been set by the DEA and the state in which he or she works. A medical assistant will often be responsible for flagging the physician's DEA registration renewal date, as well as for providing security and inventory record keeping for all controlled substances. A medical assistant may also be responsible for properly disposing of expired controlled substances and keeping records. In some states medical assistants are not permitted to administer controlled substances, even if they are allowed to administer other medications.

Prescriptions

Federal law also identifies drugs that require a prescription. A **prescription** is an order from a physician or other licensed health care provider to a pharmacist to dispense a supply of medication. Individual states have different regulations within a set of federal guidelines. The medical assistant must know the laws of the state in which he or she works.

To prevent theft or alteration of written prescriptions, it is recommended that physicians adhere to the following recommendations related to written prescriptions:

1. Store all prescription blanks in a safe place where they cannot be stolen, and keep the number of prescription pads in use to a minimum.
2. Write out the actual amount prescribed in words in addition to the number. This makes it more difficult to alter the amount.
3. Use prescription blanks only for writing prescriptions and not for notes.
4. Do not sign prescription blanks in advance.
5. Use tamper-resistant prescription pads.

The physician may also write on the prescription whether a generic substitute may be provided. Different states have different laws regarding substitution of a generic preparation for a brand-name drug.

Electronic prescriptions are sent directly by the physician or other authorized provider to a pharmacy or mail-order pharmacy through a prescription program or the EHR. Usually the prescription function is limited to individuals with prescribing privileges. In most states it is now allowed to prescribe controlled substances electronically in addition to ordinary prescriptions. Both provider and pharmacy must follow state guidelines to avoid prescription drug misuse, abuse, and diversion.

FEDERAL AND STATE LAWS PROTECTING EMPLOYEES

Hiring and Firing

A person who works for an organization that has more than 15 employees is protected by federal Equal Opportunity Employment laws (Title VII of the Civil Rights Act of 1964) and the federal Age Discrimination in Employment Act of 1967. These laws make it illegal for a company to discriminate in hiring practices on the basis of race, sex, religion, national origin, or age. Some states also have legislation making it illegal to discriminate on the basis of sexual orientation. Complaints about discrimination in hiring are submitted to the federal Equal Employment Opportunity Commission (EEOC).

Employment policies must treat employees equally and cannot discriminate against any category of employees by paying one group (such as men) more than another group for the same duties. During an interview for employment, the interviewer may not ask questions related to race, sex, religion, national origin, or age (unless it relates to legal age for employment or serving alcoholic beverages).

Preemployment Testing

Preemployment testing is allowed only to determine if the potential employee has the skills and abilities to perform a specific job. If keyboarding is included in the job description, the employer may administer a keyboarding test to test a candidate's qualifications for the position. This also applies to any testing done before an individual with a disability is hired.

Preemployment drug tests have been ruled legal for any position. However, random drug tests while on the job are usually legal only if the demands of public safety outweigh the employee's right to privacy. Some health care facilities perform drug tests on all new employees.

Memories *from* Practicum

Vicki Edmonds: When I was at my practicum at a clinic affiliated with a community hospital, the employees were implementing a plan for the physicians to discuss advance directives with all patients. They hoped to have each patient prepare a written health care proxy and provide the office with a copy. When we pulled each patient's medical record for the visit, we checked the record to see if there was already a completed form. If not, we placed a blank health care proxy form loosely in the front of the folder for the physician to give to the patient. Then when patients checked out, we would remind them to return the completed form. At first I found this embarrassing because it seemed like such a private thing. Then one of our elderly patients told me that she was so grateful that her husband had signed a health care proxy before he had a stroke, which left him completely paralyzed and unable to speak. She said that the discussions they had had when he was preparing the form had helped her understand exactly what his wishes were. On the basis of those discussions, she had asked the hospital staff not to resuscitate him if he stopped breathing or his heart stopped. She told me that before they talked about it, she would not have been comfortable making that decision. I was impressed by this patient's ability to talk frankly about her family's preparations to face serious illness, and I was grateful because it helped me become more comfortable with the subject. ■

The Americans with Disabilities Act and the Americans with Disabilities Act Amendments

The Americans with Disabilities Act (ADA) discusses the need for employers to make "reasonable accommodations"

for any individual with a physical or mental disability who is otherwise qualified to perform the tasks necessary in the job. The law also deals with the necessity of making public accommodations accessible to disabled individuals. The EEOC also hears complaints about possible failure to comply with the workplace portions of the ADA.

The Americans with Disability Act Amendments (ADAA) were enacted in 2008 to make it easier for an individual to establish that he or she has a disability within the meaning of the law. Any substantial limitation in performing a major life activity (and this is intended to be interpreted broadly) would make it possible for an individual to require a reasonable accommodation. Previously it was required that an individual be severely or significantly restricted.

Occupational Safety and Health Act of 1970

The Occupational Safety and Health Administration (OSHA) was created in 1970 to be the federal agency responsible for the physical protection of employees in the workplace. OSHA regulates all workplace environments but has two specific functions related to the medical office. The Bloodborne Pathogens Standard relates to preventing exposure to pathogens that cause disease. This standard is discussed in detail in Chapter 17. OSHA also regulates the exposure of employees to hazardous chemicals in the workplace and requires employers to inform employees of the hazards of any chemicals used. See Chapter 18 for a discussion of the newest Hazard Communication Standard information. The 1988 Clinical Laboratory Improvement Amendments, which regulate office laboratories, are discussed in detail in Chapter 29.

Family and Medical Leave Act

The Family and Medical Leave Act of 1993 (FMLA) applies to employers with 50 or more employees. Under FMLA, employees are entitled to up to 12 weeks of unpaid leave annually to accommodate a serious health crisis of any family member or the birth or adoption of a child. The employee must notify the employer before the beginning of the leave how much of the leave he or she intends to take. After the employee returns, he or she must be given former job and seniority status.

Sexual Harassment

Sexual harassment is defined as any unwanted physical or verbal sexual attention from anyone an individual interacts with on the job that causes that individual to fear reprisal if the attention is refused. Sexual harassment is not flirting. Flirting occurs when both parties engage in actions or verbal exchanges intended to attract or compliment the other. Harassment occurs when one party (most often but not necessarily, a man) engages another party in unwanted comments or physical contact of a sexual nature. If a comment or attention is unwanted, it should be clearly stated to the offending party. Sometimes individuals hesitate to "hurt the other person's feelings" or are uncomfortable speaking out, and communication is unclear.

Minimum Wage and Overtime

The federal Fair Labor Standards Act regulates the minimum wage, although some states have a higher minimum wage than that set under federal law. The Fair Labor Standards Act also requires overtime pay of one-and-one-half times the employee's regular rate of pay for time worked beyond 40 hours in 1 week. Professional and supervisory employees are exempt from the law. Registered nurses and office managers are considered professional employees, but medical assistants are not and are covered by the overtime rules.

Employee Retirement Income Security Act

The Employee Retirement Income Security Act of 1974 (ERISA) regulates employee benefit plans, including managed care health plans, pension plans, and other employee benefits. ERISA sets minimum standards for pension plans to prevent unfair denial of pension rights. Under ERISA, employee health plans cannot use health status or medical condition to deny certain employees the right to insurance.

Genetic Information Nondiscrimination Act

The Genetic Information Nondiscrimination Act of 2008 prohibits the use of genetic information in health insurance and employment. Employers may not use an individual's genetic information to make hiring, firing, job placement, or promotion decisions. In addition, health insurers are prohibited from denying coverage to a healthy individual or charging higher premiums based on a genetic predisposition to develop a disease in the future.

HEALTH INSURANCE PORTABILITY AND ACCOUNTABILITY ACT OF 1996

HIPAA provides legislation related to several aspects of health insurance, privacy of patient information, and standards for filing health insurance claims electronically. This act has several sections.

Health Insurance Availability and Coverage

The first part deals with health insurance availability and coverage. It provides specific regulations for group health insurance plans to prevent eligibility rules that exclude patients with certain diagnoses or genetic conditions or require such patients to pay higher premiums.

Privacy Rule

The HIPAA Privacy Rule (one part of the law) went into effect in 2003. This rule provides patients with control over the use and disclosure of their health information. The Privacy Rule contains provisions that describe how personal health information may be used, stored, maintained, or transmitted electronically. In addition, it describes how patients must be informed of their right to control their health information.

1. The medical office must inform patients in writing how their protected health information (PHI) will be used by the medical office. This document is called a *Notice of Privacy Practices* (NPP). PHI includes written, oral, and electronic health information that contains data through which the patient can be identified, such as the Social Security number, name, and telephone number. Patients must sign to indicate that they have received a notice regarding privacy protection.
2. A patient's written consent is not required for the use or disclosure of PHI if the purpose of disclosure is medical treatment, payment, or health care operations. Therefore individuals who are involved in caring for the patient (including medical assistants and medical assisting students) may have access to PHI.
3. Patients have the right to access their medical records and to request changes to the records if they believe they are inaccurate.
4. The medical office must have procedures in place to prevent unnecessary or inappropriate access to PHI, including request forms for information; procedures to prevent unauthorized individuals from viewing records, appointment books, computer screens, or other material that might contain PHI; and procedures for storing and destroying records containing PHI so that no unauthorized access occurs.
5. Patients have a right to request an accounting of the transfer of their information for purposes other than treatment, payment, or health care operations.
6. The medical office must have written agreements with each outside agency that handles PHI, such as medical laboratories, transcription services, law and accounting firms, software and hardware consultants, and billing services, to ensure that these other agencies handle PHI in accordance with the HIPAA Privacy Rule.
7. All employees must be trained in privacy and security of PHI.

Transaction and Code Set Rule

The Transaction and Code Set Rule prescribes electronic data interchange standards for structuring information that must be used for Medicare and Medicaid insurance claims. Providers that file Medicare claims electronically must adhere to these electronic data interchange standards.

Security Rule

The Security Rule complements the Privacy Rule by setting standards to maintain security of personal health information that is transmitted electronically. It identifies administrative, physical, and technical security safeguards for electronic protected health information (EPHI). The final compliance date was April 21, 2006.

Other Provisions

The Unique Identifiers Rule established a new provider identification number called the *National Provider Identifier* (NPI), a 10-digit identification number issued to each provider by the Centers for Medicare and Medicaid Services (CMS). The NPI replaced other physician insurance identification numbers but not the DEA number or state physician license number.

The final part of HIPAA is the Enforcement Rule, which describes penalties for violating HIPAA rules.

PATIENT SAFETY AND QUALITY IMPROVEMENT ACT

The Patient Safety and Quality Improvement Act of 2005 (PSQIA) was passed to encourage reporting of adverse events, near misses, and unsafe conditions and decrease the number of preventable medical errors. It went into effect in January 2009. In addition to setting up Patient Safety Organizations (PSOs), the act also defined requirements for reporting events that threaten patient safety and patient safety work products (e.g., data, reports, and records assembled to report to a PSO) and the confidentiality protections for patients related to the patient safety evaluation system. Common formats for reporting various types of events have been developed for hospitals and will be developed in the future for ambulatory settings. Many states have passed specific laws defining mandated reports.

HEALTH INFORMATION TECHNOLOGY FOR ECONOMIC AND CLINICAL HEALTH ACT

The Health Information Technology for Economic and Clinical Health (HITECH) Act, part of the American Recovery and Reinvestment Act of 2009, includes incentives to encourage adoption of electronic health records by physicians and health care facilities and to create a national health care infrastructure. This act also includes a 1% reduction in the Medicare fee schedule if an electronic health record has not been adopted by 2015.

To continue to protect the individual's right to privacy in the face of increased sharing of health care data, this act also increases the security provisions of HIPAA and adds increased financial penalties for privacy violations. It requires notification of patients for unauthorized use and unencrypted disclosure of PHI; breaches involving more than 500 patients must be reported to federal agencies and sometimes local media. Privacy requirements are imposed directly on business associates, whereas formerly, health care providers were required to have contracts with business associates. Business associates also become liable for financial penalties for privacy violation.

PATIENT PROTECTION AND AFFORDABLE CARE ACT

One goal of the Patient Protection and Affordable Care Act of 2010 (commonly called the Affordable Care Act or "Obamacare") was to reform health insurance practices so that more Americans have access to affordable, high-quality

health insurance. A second goal was to reduce the growth in health care spending. Although provisions of the act, which have been implemented every year, have made some progress toward the first goal, opponents argue that instead of controlling costs, the law has increased health care costs—for example, as a result of the expansion of Medicaid coverage. The Supreme Court upheld a challenge to the law in June 2012. Provisions of the law will continue to roll out until 2022. Those that took effect in 2014 included prohibition against denying insurance coverage for medical conditions, expanded requirements for employers to offer health insurance, and creation of health insurance "exchanges" so that individuals and small businesses can buy insurance coverage at a reasonable cost.

MANDATORY REPORTING

For public health reasons and the good of society as a whole, physicians are required to make certain reports, usually to a state or local agency. Some are required by law and cannot be refused because the patient does not want the information released.

1. Records of births, stillbirths, and deaths.
2. Reports must be made to the medical examiner or coroner (the name depends on the state) for certain types of deaths that may indicate suspicious circumstances or may be a result of a crime. The medical examiner then decides whether to investigate.
3. Infectious disease cases have to be reported to the local board of health. Each state has a list of reportable diseases, which include diseases that pose a public health risk, such as rabies, measles, and AIDS. Dog bites and human bites must usually also be reported.
4. Injuries that may have occurred as a result of violence must be reported to the police. Sometimes a patient asks that the report not be made. Even if the injured person does not intend to press charges, the injury still must be reported. If there is a likely need for evidence to be collected from the injured person (e.g., in the case of a rape), the person should be directed to an emergency department, which has personnel trained in the procedure.
5. Possible abuse or neglect must be reported to the police or a particular state agency, depending on state law. Suspicion does not have to be backed up with evidence. Certain professions are mandated (legally required) to report, especially child abuse or elder abuse. Physicians and nurses are always required to make such reports, and in some states medical assistants, as allied health care professionals, are also included in the list of those required to make reports.
6. Crimes that occur in the office such as burglary, theft (especially theft of narcotics), and criminal assault must be reported to the police.
7. Various other reports are mandated by the states. Some states require reports of seizures (a symptom of epilepsy) to the department of motor vehicles, and some states

PROCEDURE **3-3**   Reporting Illegal Activities and Complying with Public Health Statutes

Outcome

1. Perform compliance reporting based on public health statutes
2. Report illegal activities in the health care setting

Equipment/Supplies

- Paper
- Computer with Internet capability
- Printer

1. Procedural Step. Do research using the Internet and make a written list of federal, state, and/or local agencies to report each of the following:
  a. Theft or diversion of controlled substances
  b. Wounds or injuries that might be the result of criminal activity or reportable abuse
  c. Public health threats (e.g., communicable diseases, animal bites)
2. Procedural Step. Print at least one report form from a government agency.
3. Procedural Step. Make a table with two columns identifying specific reportable conditions or actions

and the agency (or agencies) to which they must be reported.
4. Procedural Step. Discuss in writing the rights of a patient when a legal report is mandated.
Principle: Patients have a right to know how and why information about them is reported to a public agency.
5. Procedural Step: Role-play making a verbal report of an illegal activity and a public health threat.
6. Procedural Step: Hand in your list, table, and sample report form to your instructor.

---

require that all cancer cases treated by health professionals be reported to a state cancer registry.

Failure to make a mandated report is a crime. When a report is required by law, the patient should be informed why the report is required and to whom the report will be made (Procedure 3-3).

STATE REGULATION OF HEALTH OCCUPATIONS

The laws that regulate the practice of medicine are called *medical practice acts,* and in general they contain the following two elements:
- Definition of the practice of medicine.
- Limitation to qualified practitioners by **licensure**—the process by which the state examines a person's qualifications and issues a **license** to practice medicine. All states require a license to practice medicine, although a physician may practice in certain federal facilities and agencies with a license from a different state than the one in which the facility is located. Practicing medicine without a license is a criminal act.

Physicians can also be licensed in most states if they have held a medical license in another state for more than 5 to 10 years. This is called **reciprocity** or *reciprocal licensing.* Usually this is simply a matter of requesting a license if a physician is moving from one state to another. In states with many physicians, reciprocal licensing is more difficult to obtain. Florida severely limits reciprocal licensing in an effort to keep older physicians from "retiring" to Florida

and then opening practices or taking hospital or clinic jobs. The physician licensing board approves the original application for a license then renews the license yearly or biannually (every 2 years).

A physician who works as a *locum tenens* (temporary physician; from the Latin "place holder") must have a license for the state where she or he is assigned as well as hospital privileges (if the assignment is in a hospital). Temporary physician placements are often handled by an agency that also obtains necessary state and hospital physicians.

Revoking or Suspending a Physician's License

A physician licensing board can revoke or suspend a physician's license for conviction of a crime, unprofessional activity, and physical or mental incapacity, including alcoholism, drug abuse, and senility. If the physician is convicted of a crime, the seriousness and nature of the crime will influence the physician licensing board's decision about the length of time the person's license may be suspended.

Similar laws govern the licensure and revocation of licenses for such professionals as registered nurses, nurse practitioners, and physician assistants. These laws clarify what the member of the profession can and cannot do.

FACILITY LICENSING AND ACCREDITATION

State Requirements

Each state requires certain types of health care facilities to obtain a license. This gives the state oversight into the

| BOX 3-3 | List of Health Care Facilities That May be Licensed by the State |

BOX 3-3   List of Health Care Facilities That May be Licensed by the State

- Ambulatory surgical centers
- Blood banks
- Clinics or community clinics
- Commercial independent laboratories
- Substance abuse treatment facilities
- End-stage renal disease centers
- Health departments
- Home health agencies
- Hospices
- Hospitals
- Intermediate care facilities
- Nursing homes
- Physician office laboratories
- Pregnancy counseling centers

Federal Requirements

In addition to state licensure, health care facilities that bill Medicare and Medicaid for services fall under CMS oversight and are responsible for meeting all regulatory standards.

The CMS also participates with state and private agencies to regulate clinical laboratories and determine compliance with regulations for quality assurance. This is discussed in more detail in Chapter 29.

Voluntary Accreditation

Many health care facilities, including hospitals, ambulatory surgical centers, clinical laboratories, health clinics, and physician offices, seek accreditation by independent accrediting agencies as a means to improve health care and maintain high standards. Accreditation may also be a means to comply with regulations for state licensure and regulations of the CMS.

The Joint Commission (formerly the Joint Commission on Accreditation of Healthcare Organizations [JCAHO]) was originally established in 1951 to accredit hospitals, rehabilitation centers, and nursing homes. In recent years it has expanded its activities to accredit almost all kinds of health care facilities, including clinics and physician offices. To become accredited, the health care facility must prepare a report demonstrating compliance with all standards of the Joint Commission. This is followed by a survey visit with follow-up to improve in any areas of weakness that might be found during that visit.

The Accreditation Association for Ambulatory Health Care (AAAHC) performs a similar type of accreditation for most types of ambulatory health care facilities.

activities of the facility and allows for on-site surveys to maintain quality standards. A list of these types of facilities can be found in Box 3-3. Physician offices are usually not included, but if laboratory testing is done in the office, it may be necessary to get a license or certificate of waiver for the laboratory depending on the type of testing being done. Health insurance companies and HMOs are also licensed by the state, which sets certain requirements for their business operations.

What Would You Do? | What Would You *Not* Do? | RESPONSES

Case Study 1
Page 38

What Did Vicki Do?
- ❑ Told Denise that she would have to point out the burn to the physician because he needed to be sure it was healing properly.
- ❑ Told Denise that she would have to tell the physician what Denise had said about the burn.
- ❑ Explained that burning someone with a cigarette is not acceptable behavior and encouraged Denise to discuss the incident with the physician or another adult.
- ❑ Asked Denise if her boyfriend had hurt her any other time.

What Did Vicki Not Do?
- ❑ Did not tell Denise that she needs to break up with her boyfriend immediately.
- ❑ Did not agree to hide the information about the burn from the physician.

- ❑ Did not promise that the physician would not tell her parents.
- ❑ Did not discuss Denise's burn or explanation for it with anyone other than the physician.

Case Study 2
Page 49

What Did Vicki Do?
- ❑ Told Mr. Morton that the orthopedic surgeon specializes in musculoskeletal conditions and does not always recommend surgery.
- ❑ Asked Mr. Morton if he questioned the physician about other kinds of treatments.
- ❑ Asked Mr. Morton if he wanted her to complete the referral and make the appointment.
- ❑ Reported to the physician if Mr. Morton refused the referral.
- ❑ Asked Mr. Morton if he needs more time to speak to the physician.

Continued

What Did Vicki* Not *Do?

❑ Did not make recommendations about other types of treatment for back pain.

❑ Did not give an opinion about the benefits of one type of procedure compared with another.

❑ Did not promise that the orthopedic surgeon will not want to do surgery.

❑ Did not tell Mr. Morton that the physician should have done a better job explaining possible treatments.

Case Study 3

Page 51

What Did Vicki Do?

❑ Told the physician politely that she had to finish cleaning up the spill in the hall because someone might slip and fall.

❑ Worked as quickly as possible to dry the floor of the hall and then call the next patient.

❑ Asked the physician if he wants to talk to the next patient before she takes the vital signs.

❑ Obtained the electrocardiogram (ECG) for the patient in room 4 after calling and preparing the physician's next patient.

What Did Vicki* Not *Do?

❑ Did not leave the spilled water on the floor while she calls the next patient and takes the ECG.

❑ Did not ask if the physician thinks she can do two things at once.

❑ Did not go around the office later trying to find out who spilled water without cleaning it up.

TERMINOLOGY REVIEW

Key Term	Word Parts	Definition
Abandonment		Failure to continue to provide medical care to a patient without proper notification.
Act		A bill or measure that has become law. Often refers to legislation with several parts.
Advocate		A person who intercedes on another person's behalf.
Arbitration		A formal process whereby the parties to a dispute agree to submit to the decision of a neutral party.
Assumption of risk		A defense to a lawsuit that establishes that the plaintiff assumed the risk of whatever caused the injury.
Autonomy		Ability to make independent decisions without constraint or coercion by others.
Beneficence		Acting in the best possible way; performing good deeds.
Bill		A law proposed by a legislative body.
Case law		Law established by decisions of previous court cases.
Civil law		Law that regulates relationships and interactions between individuals and groups.
Cloning		Producing genetically identical cells or individuals artificially.
Common law		Unwritten body of law based on general custom.
Comparative negligence		A defense to a lawsuit that establishes a percentage of responsibility for injury on the part of the plaintiff.
Contingency		A condition that must be met before a contract is binding.
Contributory negligence		A defense to a lawsuit that establishes any responsibility for injury on the part of the plaintiff.
Controlled substance		A drug that has the potential for addiction or abuse.
Crime		An offense in violation of a law that prohibits or requires certain behavior.
Criminal law		Law that regulates offenses against the public welfare.
Defendant		The person or group against which an action is brought in a court of law.
Deposition		Testimony given under oath to an officer of the court before a trial.
Do-not-resuscitate (DNR) order		A medical order signed by a physician that relieves health care personnel from the obligation to resuscitate a patient who stops breathing or whose heart stops.
Drug Enforcement Administration (DEA)		The federal agency that enforces the Controlled Substances Act of 1970.
Duty		Commitment to act in a certain way.
Emancipated minor		A person younger than the age of 18 with the rights of an adult including the ability to consent to medical care.
Embezzlement		Fraudulent appropriation of funds or property of an employer or client.
Ethics		The branch of knowledge that deals with standards of behavior or beliefs.
Felony		A serious crime punishable by death or imprisonment.

TERMINOLOGY REVIEW—cont'd

Key Term	Word Parts	Definition
Fidelity		Faithfulness.
Fraud		Intentional deception resulting in injury or loss.
Gene therapy		Giving patients new genes or parts of genes to treat a disease or condition.
Genetic engineering		Making, altering, or repairing genetic material.
Health care proxy		A legal document that names an agent to make decisions about a person's medical care if he or she becomes unable to make wishes known.
Informed consent		Agreement to a medical procedure based on understanding of the procedure and its possible consequences and effects.
Larceny		Stealing another person's property or money without violence.
Liability		Legal responsibility.
License		Official permission to perform an activity or practice a profession.
Licensure		The process by which the state examines qualifications and gives permission to an individual or organization to engage in a profession or business.
Litigation		The process of taking a lawsuit through the courts.
Living will		A legal document that specifies the kind of medical treatment a patient wants or does not want if he or she becomes incapacitated.
Malfeasance		A crime or wrongdoing that is illegal or contrary to official obligation.
Malpractice		Negligence by a professional.
Mature minor		An individual younger than 18 with the maturity to provide informed consent for certain medical procedures.
Mediation		Negotiation by a third party to help two parties resolve a dispute.
Medical durable power of attorney		A written authorization to make health care decisions for a specified individual that is in effect if the individual becomes incapacitated.
Misdemeanor		A less serious crime, punishable by a fine or imprisonment for less than 1 year.
Misfeasance		Performing a legal act in an improper way.
Negligence		Failure to act (or to refrain from acting) as a reasonably prudent person would in similar circumstances.
Nonfeasance		Failing to perform an act that should have been performed, resulting in injury.
Nonmalfeasance		Ethical concept requiring that an action do no harm, or do less harm than good.
Plaintiff		The person or group that makes the complaint in a lawsuit.
Prescription		An order to a pharmacist to dispense a supply of a medication.
Privilege		A special immunity that protects against legal liability.
Prudent		Using care or common sense.
Reciprocity		Automatic issuing of a license in one state to the holder of a license in another state.
Res ipsa loquitur		A legal doctrine that assumes negligence because of the type of injury
Respondeat superior		A legal doctrine making an employer liable for the negligent acts of employees.
Right		A claim that is expected to be honored.
Standard of care		Level of appropriate care required of a health professional.
Statute of limitations		A law limiting the time period for beginning a lawsuit.
Statutory law		Law enacted by a legislative body.
Stem cells		Cells that have the capacity to develop into various types of body tissue.
Subpoena		A court order for a witness to appear and give testimony.
Subpoena *duces tecum*		A court order to produce documents or records.
Tort		An injury or wrong against a person or property that does not involve breach of contract.
Veracity		Truthfulness.

ON THE WEB

For information on accreditation of ambulatory care facilities:

Accreditation Association for Ambulatory Health Care (AAAHC): www.aaahc.org

The Joint Commission: www.jointcommission.org

For information on federal supervision of laboratories:

U.S. Department of Health and Human Services, Centers for Medicare and Medicaid Services: www.cms.gov/clia

For information on genetic engineering:

Office of Biotechnology Activities, National Institutes of Health: http://oba.od.nih.gov

For information on organ and tissue donation:

U.S. Department of Health and Human Services, Information on Organ and Tissue Donation and Transplantation: www.organdonor.gov

For information on National Provider Identifier (NPI) numbers:

NPI Registry Search: https://nppes.cms.hhs.gov/NPPES/NPIRegistryHome.do

For information on the Patient Bill of Rights:

Executive Summary of the Consumer Bill of Rights and Responsibilities from the *Report of the President's Advisory Commission on Consumer Protection and Quality in the Health Care Industry*: www.hcqualitycommission.gov

For information on the Patient Protection and Affordable Care Act:

Healthcare.gov website: https://www.healthcare.gov/

Medicaid.gov website: http://www.medicaid.gov/AffordableCareAct/Affordable-Care-Act.html

U.S. Department of Health and Human Services: http://www.hhs.gov/healthcare/rights/

Interacting with Patients

4

(e) Check out the Evolve site at http://evolve.elsevier.com/Bonewit/today/ to access additional interactive activities and exercises to help you study and prepare for success.

LEARNING OBJECTIVES

Communicating with Patients
1. Describe the steps in the communication process.
2. Differentiate between verbal and nonverbal communication.
3. List several types of nonverbal communication.
4. Identify and describe factors that can interfere with effective communication.
5. Explain the elements of active listening.
6. Describe how eye contact can have different meanings based on cultural background.
7. Give examples of techniques that encourage a patient to continue speaking.
8. Explain how to overcome sensory and language barriers to communication.
9. Describe ways to evaluate if communication has been effective.

Establishing Relationships to Meet Patient Needs
10. List factors that affect patient expectations of health care.
11. Explain the levels of Maslow's hierarchy of needs.
12. Correlate the existence of unmet needs to types of patient behavior in the health care setting.
13. List several ways to establish caring relationships with patients.
14. Describe the importance of maintaining appropriate self-boundaries.
15. Explain the role of empathy in the relationship between the medical assistant and patients.
16. Describe how the medical assistant can handle common emotional responses to illness.
17. Clarify how empathy helps improve the relationship between the medical assistant and the patient.
18. Describe ways to support the terminally ill patient in all stages of the grieving process.
19. Demonstrate respect for cultural and ethnic diversity in approaching patients and families.

PROCEDURES

Demonstrate effective and respectful verbal and nonverbal communication.

Maintain boundaries and demonstrate respect for boundaries in communication.

CHAPTER OUTLINE

INTRODUCTION TO COMMUNICATION
COMMUNICATING WITH PATIENTS
Verbal and Nonverbal Communication
Interference with Communication
Listening Skills
Nonverbal Measures to Facilitate Communication
Interviewing Techniques
Closed Questions
Open Questions

Keeping the Conversation Going
Drawing Patients Out
Styles of Communication
Avoiding Responses That Inhibit Communication
Barriers to Effective Communication
Impaired Level of Understanding
Sight Impaired
Hearing Impaired
Language Barriers

UNDERSTANDING AND MEETING THE NEEDS OF PATIENTS
Patient Expectations of Health Care
How Basic Needs Affect the Behavior of Patients
Maslow's Hierarchy of Needs
Effects of Unmet Needs During Illness
Developmental Stages
Establishing Caring Relationships
Empathy
Expression of Caring
Value of Effective Relationships with Patients
Self-Boundaries

Emotional Responses to Illness
Guilt
Loss of Control
Anxiety
Anger
The Grieving Process
Cultural Influences Affecting Health Care
Causes of Illness
Treatments and Traditional Practices
Behavioral Requirements

KEY TERMS

active listening	hierarchy (HIGH-er-ark-ee)	projection
anxiety	hospice (HOSS-piss)	reflecting
body language	judgmental	self-actualization
chronic	nonverbal	summarizing
closed questions	open questions	sympathy
denial	oral	terminal phase
ego defense mechanism	paraphrasing	verbal
empathy	physiologic	webcam

INTRODUCTION TO COMMUNICATION

To respond to a patient effectively, the medical assistant must be able to communicate effectively. Major components of health care include reducing a patient's fear and anxiety and helping the patient understand how to promote health and manage illness. To assess a patient's perception of his or her health status, the medical assistant must be effective at both sending and receiving messages.

COMMUNICATING WITH PATIENTS

Figure 4-1 outlines the basic model of communication. A sender sends a message to a receiver. The message can be **verbal,** meaning that spoken or written words are used to send the message. It can also be **nonverbal,** meaning that the message is expressed without words through body language, facial expression, and other means. Most messages are sent using a combination of verbal and nonverbal communication. The *feedback* from the receiver to the sender, also verbal or nonverbal, helps the sender decide whether to initiate a new message, expand on the original message, or clarify the message.

VERBAL AND NONVERBAL COMMUNICATION

Verbal communication is either **oral** (spoken) or written. Written communication has traditionally been thought of as more formal than oral conversation—a letter rather than a phone call. Today, however, with the increasing use of e-mail, written communication may be as informal as oral communication.

Nonverbal communication refers to information that is received from body language. **Body language** is the way a person's body signals feelings or emotions. For example, hands folded across the chest and a rigid posture may signal anger. Nonverbal communication also includes the secondary communication that occurs during oral conversation. Secondary communication consists of tone of voice, voice pitch, voice volume, and voice quality. Nonverbal communication often provides more information than the words themselves (Figure 4-2).

The response to a simple question such as "How are you feeling today, Mr. Jackson?" may consist only of the words "All right." The quality of the voice—pinched, pained, flat, excited, spoken with a deep sigh—gives more information than the words about Mr. Jackson's physical condition and his state of mind.

Other types of nonverbal communication include facial expression, body position, and gestures used while speaking. These are known as *nonverbal cues.*

INTERFERENCE WITH COMMUNICATION

Numerous elements can interfere with communication between the sender and receiver. An analogy for interference is listening to the radio. The radio station can be thought of as the sender of a message. The message is sent through radio signals. Any number of outside elements can interfere with the radio station's signal to the receiver, such as a storm that causes electrical interference in the atmosphere, air traffic controllers switching to a radio frequency that interferes with the broadcast frequency, or the receiver driving through a tunnel or over a bridge with steel suspension. In addition, interference can be caused by elements inside the receiver, such as having strong emotions, thinking about something else, or needing to concentrate on driving carefully.

Similarly, in communicating with a patient, interference can come from the outside or inside. Examples of outside

interference include a distracting environment, noise, and lack of privacy during communication. Examples of inside interference include fatigue, fear, anxiety, anger, or being preoccupied with something else. All of these factors can cause the message to be diluted, changed, or not completely understood by the receiver. Other barriers arise because understanding or senses are impaired.

The ability to identify a patient's strong emotions or feelings from the nonverbal cues exhibited by the patient may cross cultural boundaries. For example, infants and children from all cultures cry when they receive immunizations. The ability of the medical assistant or a patient to interpret subtle feelings or gestures, however, does not typically cross cultural boundaries. For example, shaking the head from side to side does not always mean "no." In some cultures it may mean "yes," or it may be used to express other meanings such as an acknowledgement that the listener has heard what was said.

Individuals who come from different cultures also have a different idea of personal space and may interpret physical touch in a different way. Cultural sensitivity is especially important if communication is to be effective. Nonverbal communication that is accepted in the sender's culture, such as smiling, looking straight into the speaker's eyes, or lightly touching someone's shoulder to show concern, may create interference if the gesture has a different significance in the listener's culture. The medical assistant should learn as much as possible about cultural or ethnic differences, especially for those groups that are frequent patients of the medical practice where the medical assistant works.

First impressions based on personal appearance may influence the way an individual is addressed. For example, it is easy to assume that an individual who looks homeless, who is dressed in dirty clothing, or who has a strong body odor is also uneducated. In the same way, individuals who are dressed in expensive suits often are treated with great respect. It is important to be aware of this tendency and respond to each patient as an individual.

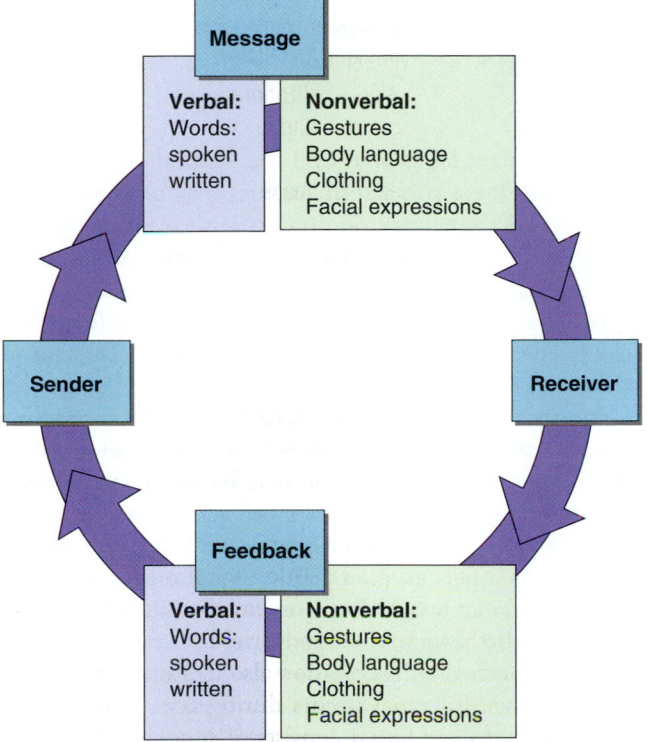

Figure 4-1 Model of communication.

Figure 4-2 Most adults can easily identify the people in these photographs as expressing **A,** pleasure; **B,** uncertainty or lack of confidence; **C,** confusion.

LISTENING SKILLS

Good listening skills are major components of good communication. Some health professionals are naturally better listeners than others, but listening skills can be learned and practiced.

The most important listening skill is known as *active listening*. **Active listening** means being "in the moment" and paying close attention to what is being said without thinking about anything else. Focusing all the attention on the sender of the message is important. To receive a message clearly, the listener cannot allow emotions or thoughts to interfere with the sender's message.

What a sender says will naturally trigger a response. Letting go of the urge to respond verbally, take over the conversation, and air one's own views is important. By focusing on the sender, the medical assistant will not be tempted to let his or her own mental responses become spoken responses. It will also prevent the medical assistant from focusing on his or her mental responses, thereby preventing messages from the sender from being received clearly.

Additional guidelines for the medical assistant to demonstrate good listening techniques include the following:

1. Checking to make sure the patient's interpretation of a message is correct. This may involve asking the patient to repeat what has been said by rephrasing a question.
2. Listening for feelings. Medical assistants should be alert for key words or themes the patient uses frequently to describe his or her medical condition. These can be important clues to the patient's emotional state. The medical assistant should also be aware of changes in his or her own feelings. The medical assistant's emotions may mirror the emotions of patients. For example, if the medical assistant begins to get impatient or aggravated with a patient, it may be a clue that the patient is upset or angry.
3. Being observant while listening. The patient's facial expressions, body language, tone of voice, and other nonverbal cues can tell a lot about what the patient is feeling.
4. Being patient and listening completely. Patients should be allowed to "tell their story" in their own time and in their own way. Interruption interferes with this process. Although there are questions that need to be asked, the medical assistant should introduce questions in a way that interferes as little as possible with the patient's natural storytelling flow.

Nonverbal Measures to Facilitate Communication

In the United States, eye contact is important (Figure 4-3). Maintaining eye contact is a sign of interest and involvement. However, being aware that in many cultures it is not respectful to look directly at older people is important. This is especially true in Asian and Native American cultures. Many Latinos also do not look directly at a person they respect, such as a teacher or a physician.

Figure 4-3 Photograph showing a comfortable talking distance and eye contact that is typical for the United States.

If the patient looks away and the medical assistant continues to seek eye contact, the patient may perceive this as aggression. Maintaining eye contact with someone who is culturally uncomfortable with that nonverbal communication creates a barrier between the two individuals.

For the most part, control of body language is unconscious. Therefore it is important for the medical assistant to be aware of the patient's nonverbal messages. Being alert to the patient's body language allows the medical assistant to notice when a patient feels uncomfortable or anxious. When a patient's words and body language do not match, the body language is usually a more genuine reflection of the patient's feelings.

Touching a person, even gently, can also be interpreted in many different ways. Moving closer can indicate interest, but it may also be viewed as aggressive. Many adults do not like to be touched by people they do not know well.

Cultural sensitivity is extremely important. For example, some Asians do not like to have their heads or their children's heads touched. This may present a problem when the medical assistant must measure the head circumference of an Asian infant. If this occurs, the medical assistant should stress to the infant's parent in a reassuring tone of voice that measuring head circumference is an important health assessment procedure and that there is no disrespect intended in the action.

A gentle pat on the shoulder can be reassuring to a patient, but it is important to notice if the patient becomes tense or appears uncomfortable when touched. If the medical assistant steps back, the patient will usually relax. In the United States, people normally maintain a distance of about 3 to 4 feet for conversation with others, but in other cultures this comfort zone varies. If a patient is standing too close for comfort, before responding the medical assistant should consider the patient's cultural or ethnic background. This allows a choice between a response that sets limits for the patient and a response that gives information about typical conversational distance in the United States.

If the medical assistant must penetrate the patient's personal comfort zone for a procedure, it may help to make a statement that prepares the patient for movement into the patient's personal space. For example, when applying a sterile dressing to a wound, the medical assistant might say, "I'm going to have to move in now so I have a better view of the area."

What Would You Do? | What Would You *Not* Do?

Case Study 1
Nancy Walker, CMA (AAMA), has called Jennifer Boland, a 32-year-old married mother of three, from the waiting room. Nancy notices that Jennifer is not looking at her, but the patient cooperates with getting her weight and vital signs. When Nancy asks the reason for today's visit, it seems to take Jennifer a long time to answer. She picks at the sleeve of her jersey and finally says in a low voice that she is afraid she might be pregnant. Her voice cracks a little, and then she wipes one of her eyes. ■

INTERVIEWING TECHNIQUES

Closed Questions

Two types of questions can be used in conducting a patient interview. These include closed questions and open questions. **Closed questions** are questions that can be answered with one word (e.g., yes or no) or a short answer (e.g., I was born on January 16, 1985). Closed questions are especially effective when the medical assistant needs to obtain specific information.

Examples of closed questions include the following:
- What is your date of birth?
- Who referred you to our office?
- Have you taken any medication for your pain?
- What medications are you currently taking?

Open Questions

Open questions consist of questions that encourage the patient to open up and talk. Examples of open questions include the following:
- What brings you to see the doctor today?
- What is your pain like?
- What has been going on with you since you were last here?
- How has your appetite changed over the past few months?
  Open questions help the patient do the following:
- Identify what is important
- Express feelings
- Relay perceptions

Open questions are particularly effective in allowing the patient to describe a problem in his or her own words and explain how the patient feels about the problem. Because of this, open questions should be used to obtain a patient's chief complaint and conduct a patient interview. In using open questions, it is important for the medical assistant to employ active listening techniques.

If the medical assistant asks primarily closed questions, the patient may fail to give important details or mention other problems. If the medical assistant asks directly if the patient has been following a special diet or taking prescribed medication, the patient may feel pressure to agree, even if this has not always been the case. When a patient is encouraged to talk freely, a more realistic picture may emerge.

Keeping the Conversation Going

On occasion the medical assistant will need to employ techniques to keep a conversation going with a patient. For example, the medical assistant may need additional information from a patient, but the patient stops talking. When this occurs, the medical assistant should employ techniques that encourage the patient to continue speaking without steering the conversation in a particular direction. A useful technique in such a situation is to ask the patient an open question; however, "why" questions should not be used. Examples of "why" questions include the following:
- Why aren't you taking your medication?
- Why aren't you following your diet?

"Why" questions tend to make people defensive. Rather than having the patient justify his or her actions, it is important to identify the underlying reasons as to why the patient did not take the medication or stay on the diet. Effective questions that keep the conversation flowing without making a patient defensive include the following:
- How do you set up your meals and snacks?
- What problems are you having taking your medication?
- What do you think about having to take medication at school?

In answering these questions, the patient may provide clues as to the underlying reasons for not staying with the prescribed treatment plan.

Drawing Patients Out

Active listening includes techniques to draw a patient out and/or clarify what a patient is saying. This is especially important when the patient is trying to cope with strong feelings about his or her medical problems. Refer to Table 4-1 for a full listing of communication techniques that demonstrate active listening.

Styles of Communication

Communication is most effective when all contributors are clear, direct, and respectful in their communication. For a variety of reasons, individuals may hold back and not participate completely, or be too active and disregard the feelings of others when communicating. Passive communication occurs when an individual avoids expressing feelings even in response to hurtful or anger-inducing situations. Passive communicators do not stand up for themselves and tend to try to keep the peace at all costs. The opposite type of communicators is aggressive in interactions with others. Aggressive communicators express their feelings and opinions as if they were more important than those of other speakers. They may not give others a chance to speak, and they may

Table 4-1 Communication Techniques That Demonstrate Active Listening

Technique	Description	Example
Using open questions	Asking questions that do not expect a particular answer, especially a yes or no answer.	"What's been going on lately?" "How would you describe your stomach pain?"
Repeating or rephrasing	Saying the same thing as the patient, either as a statement or a question, to encourage agreement, disagreement, or clarification.	*Patient:* "It feels like someone is stabbing me in the side." *Medical assistant:* "Like a knife in your side…"
Translating a nonverbal message into words	Translating the patient's nonverbal expression of emotion into a verbal expression.	*Patient:* "All the doctor visits, the medication, the pain—it's really too much." *Medical assistant:* "You sound like you feel overwhelmed."
Reflecting	**Reflecting** is turning a question or statement around to reflect back to the patient; this gives the patient confidence to continue.	*Patient:* "Would you have this surgery if you were me?" *Medical assistant:* "What do you think about having the surgery?"
Paraphrasing and summarizing	**Paraphrasing** puts the patient's statement into the medical assistant's own words; **summarizing** restates the meaning but may leave out some of the details. The purposes are to validate that the medical assistant has understood and to encourage clarification.	*Medical assistant:* "So for the past week the pain has been getting steadily more intense and more frequent, and since this morning it hasn't let up at all."
Providing silence	Simply waiting for the patient to continue; allows the patient to choose whether to continue or choose a new topic.	(Silence)
Verbalizing the implied	Saying what the patient seems to mean but has not expressed.	*Patient:* "Usually I don't mind coming to see Dr. Hughes." *Medical assistant:* "But you didn't want to come today…"
Asking for clarification	Asking for more detail or a clearer statement; lets the patient know that the medical assistant has not understood and may show the patient how to make the message clearer.	*Medical assistant:* "It's not clear to me how often you have been taking this medication. Do you take it before every meal, or just when you are at home?"

interrupt and criticize others. They tend to blame others instead of taking responsibility for their own behavior. Some individuals have characteristics of both types of communication. Passive-aggressive communication is a style in which a person appears passive on the surface but acts in an unfriendly way later or is sarcastic and exhibits facial expressions that do not match the underlying feelings of anger. The most respected style of communication is assertive communication, by which individuals clearly state their opinions and feelings and advocate for their rights without violating the rights of others. To be assertive, an individual must own his or her feelings and behavior but maintain self-control. Assertive communicators listen without interrupting, but state their needs clearly and respectfully.

Avoiding Responses That Inhibit Communication

The medical assistant should avoid communication techniques that exhibit disapproval or blame as well as statements that are challenging or not genuine. If a patient feels that the medical assistant is not really listening, does not understand his or her point of view, or does not validate emotions, the patient may become defensive or stop speaking altogether. The medical assistant's ability to demonstrate acceptance of strong emotions experienced by the patient is especially important.

When a patient expresses concerns, it is tempting to try to reassure the patient. For example, a patient might express anxiety about the results of a diagnostic test. If the medical assistant reassures the patient that the results will probably be normal, the fact that the patient is worried is not validated and the reassurance implies that the patient's worry is unreasonable or unacceptable. If the medical assistant confirms that it is difficult to wait for test results, the patient is more likely to feel that his or her feelings have been accepted.

Because the medical assistant's job is to make the person feel comfortable, it is important to avoid being too casual or familiar with a patient. If a subject is sensitive, but it is important to ask about it, the medical assistant can do so in a somewhat tentative way to make it easier for the patient to reply. The medical assistant can identify what the patient might be feeling, but the patient will not always agree. Many people are not always aware of their feelings and may deny feelings that they are communicating nonverbally. This should be respected. Others are only too glad to have their feelings recognized.

Medical assistants should express themselves honestly, without being **judgmental,** which means critical or negative. They can disagree with what a patient is saying, especially if that disagreement will get the patient to elaborate on what is being said. But they should not argue because arguing sets up a competitive situation. Because the medical assistant represents medical authority, the patient can easily feel threatened and unworthy.

Table 4-2 Responses That Inhibit Communication

Technique	Description	Example
Offering false reassurance	Telling the patient that everything will be all right; implies that the patient should not feel anxiety or concern. Especially inappropriate when the medical assistant does not know what will happen.	"Don't worry; your husband will come through this with flying colors."
Disapproving, blaming	Making a negative value judgment about the patient's thinking or behavior; by implying or stating that a patient is responsible for his or her health problem, the medical assistant encourages the patient to defend against attack rather than establishing trust.	"You shouldn't be smoking, you know. No wonder you have trouble breathing."
Challenging	Insisting that the patient prove a statement or belief.	"Just show me something in writing that says people should never take a bath."
Defending	Protecting oneself or someone else from criticism, (implies that the patient does not have the right to have a different opinion).	"Dr. Lawler's patients never have to wait very long."
Asking for explanations of feelings or behavior	Because patients often don't know why they feel or act as they do, asking why may be frustrating and cause them to become defensive.	"Why don't you stick to your diet?" "Why are you angry?"
Belittling or negating feelings	Acting as if feelings are less intense than they are or not even present; this implies that the patient's feelings are not real or not justified	"You're really making a big deal out of a little cut."

The responses that should be avoided are summarized in Table 4-2.

BARRIERS TO EFFECTIVE COMMUNICATION

Impaired Level of Understanding

Occasionally a patient with an impaired level of understanding visits the medical office. When this occurs, the medical assistant needs to simplify his or her method of speaking. The medical assistant should use short sentences and simple words. Speaking slowly in a normal speaking tone is important. Raising one's voice does not help in this situation. The tone of voice should express concern and empathy without being condescending or implying that the patient is not intelligent. Strong and constant eye contact also helps the patient to focus.

It may be necessary to say the same thing more than once, either by repeating it or by saying the same thing in a different way. In addition, gestures and demonstration help to reinforce the information.

Those with limited understanding of medical information need constant reassurance. This includes children, the elderly (especially those with some degree of dementia), and those who are mentally disabled. Giving a direct and complete explanation at the patient's level of understanding is important. Even young children need to be informed about what is going to be done to them. For instance, if the medical assistant is going to draw blood, it is not enough to say, "I'm going to draw your blood. It's going to hurt for just a moment."

It may be necessary to say something like, "I'm going to use this needle to take some blood from your arm. I'm going to put it through the skin, into where your blood is. It will feel kind of like someone is pinching you, but only for a second. Then I'll put a Band-Aid on it, and it will stop bleeding."

After an explanation to an individual with impaired understanding, the medical assistant should ask the patient to repeat the explanation back in his or her own words. If the patient simply repeats a small part of the explanation, communication may have been ineffective. If the medical assistant explains a procedure such as a colonoscopy, for example, he or she should then ask the patient, "Can you tell me what a colonoscopy is?" An answer that may indicate lack of understanding is, "It's when they do a colonoscopy." The medical assistant can then make another attempt to provide a simple explanation.

A young child or an individual with an impaired level of understanding cannot give informed consent. This must be obtained from an individual who can legally give informed consent for the impaired patient before the medical assistant can proceed.

Sight Impaired

Many degrees of vision loss exist. Total blindness is the complete inability to perceive light and form. *Legally blind* is a term used to describe individuals whose vision cannot be corrected beyond 20/200 in the better eye. This means that with glasses, at 20 feet the person sees the same as or less than a person with normal vision sees at 200 feet. A person may be called *sight impaired* if his or her vision is better than 20/200 but he or she still has low vision or a decreased field of vision.

It is important for the medical assistant to be verbally descriptive when working with a patient with impaired vision. The medical assistant should use touch and guidance when escorting patients who cannot see to walk safely from the waiting room to the examination room and also when helping them around the examination room. Patients with impaired vision usually prefer to take the medical assistant's arm and follow his or her movements rather than vice versa. To explain exactly where things are, a clock image sometimes helps. Saying that the examination table is at three o'clock tells a blind patient that the examination table is on the right directly to the side.

Hearing Impaired

The term *deaf* is usually used when individuals cannot hear well enough to use the sense of hearing to process information. However, there are many more individuals whose hearing is impaired than those who are deaf, especially in certain tone ranges or when sound is not loud enough.

Special techniques should be used with patients who are hearing impaired. The medical assistant should speak clearly, slowly, and in short sentences. The medical assistant's voice should be slightly louder than normal but not so loud that it loses clarity or sounds like shouting. Eye contact is also important when communicating with a hearing-impaired patient. Even if the hearing-impaired patient does not lip-read, most people who lose their hearing learn how to associate facial expression and mouth shape with words they know and recognize.

When beginning a conversation with a hearing-impaired patient, it may be necessary to touch the person gently to get his or her attention. If the patient is wearing a hearing aid, it may be helpful to ask if the hearing aid has been working well for him or her.

Sign language is often used to communicate with the deaf. Hand and finger positions represent letters or words. Several different systems exist, but American Sign Language is the recognized language in the United States.

Because each sign can represent an entire word, a person who uses sign language may be able to communicate as fast as, or faster than, a person who is speaking. Sign language has its own structure and grammar system, so it takes considerable practice to become fluent. A patient who uses sign language to communicate is usually accompanied by an interpreter. If the patient does not have an interpreter, the law requires the office to provide one. Sign language interpretation can be provided by an interpreter. It can also be provided by setting up a video relay service account. Video service links the deaf patient with a sign language interpreter. When a sign language interpreter's services are being used, it is important that the medical assistant maintain eye contact with the patient. Hearing-impaired and deaf patients are able to obtain information from facial expressions and body language. They may also be able to read lips.

Language Barriers

A language barrier interferes with communication when two people speak different languages. Depending on the patient's facility with English, this interference may vary from slight to severe.

The best way to work around language barriers is with translation assistance. It is preferred to use trained medical interpreters or translators whenever possible. When scheduling an appointment for a patient with a language barrier, the medical assistant should arrange translation assistance at the same time. Sometimes a patient with a language barrier brings a child to translate. The medical assistant

should be aware that children are the least reliable interpreters because they have a tendency to skip over medical words they do not understand or cannot translate without realizing that important information may be lost. It may also be embarrassing for a patient to discuss certain medical problems if a child is translating for him or her. Some facilities require a trained or certified medical interpreter for the health care provider, even if a family member is also present and translating for the patient.

When conversing with a patient through an interpreter, the medical assistant should speak to the patient and not to the interpreter. The medical assistant should allow the interpreter to translate a sentence before going on to the next sentence. The medical assistant should speak slowly and carefully, using simple terms and short sentences. Many people who do not feel comfortable speaking English can still understand much of what is said to them in English.

At times the medical assistant may need to improvise when working with a patient with a language barrier. This may be required during the following circumstances: the office does not have translation services, the interpreter is busy, or the patient's family member is translating but the patient wants to converse with the medical assistant in private. In these situations the medical assistant should use gestures and pantomime to convey his or her ideas.

Translation assistance is required before a patient with a language barrier gives written consent to an invasive procedure or minor office surgery. The law states that a patient must be fully informed as to the nature of his or her surgery or procedure. Consent forms are usually written in English, but the verbal explanation of the procedure needs to be in a language the patient understands well. If a practice has a large number of non–English-speaking patients, it is a good idea to have routine consent forms and instructional materials translated and available.

Telephone and video translation services can be purchased from several companies. Telephone translation assistance allows the patient, medical assistant, and/or physician to speak to the interpreter via a speakerphone. A video translation service requires a computer, a **webcam** (small video camera attached to the computer), and a speakerphone and allows all parties to see one another during the conversation.

What Would You Do? What Would You *Not* Do?

Case Study 2

When Nancy calls Harold Underwood, a 67-year-old man, from the waiting room, he does not answer until she has repeated his name three times. Because he is a new patient, Nancy introduces herself. He says that he has moved into senior housing nearby so that he can be close to his daughter. Nancy finds that she has to repeat all instructions, and she notices that Harold is wearing a hearing aid in his left ear. When she asks him if he needs help to step up to sit on the examination table, he looks at her blankly. ■

UNDERSTANDING AND MEETING THE NEEDS OF PATIENTS

PATIENT EXPECTATIONS OF HEALTH CARE

Patient expectations depend on many factors including unmet needs and experiences the person has had in the past. Previous interactions with health care facilities also shape a patient's expectations. For example, if there is a long waiting time, a patient who has always had to spend 30 to 40 minutes in the waiting room will be less upset than a patient who is used to being seen within 10 minutes.

Patients usually want to be seen by a physician within a reasonable amount of time, and they hope that the physician will "fix" whatever is wrong. Patients do not expect to have long-term problems. They want to be treated as if they were cars and physicians were mechanics—"fix what's broken and get me back on the road of life!"

In addition, people expect physicians to take care of them when they are really sick and not fuss too much over them when they are, in general, well. People certainly do not want physicians to nag them about changing their lifestyle to improve their health. But physicians are much more likely today to bring up lifestyle issues, such as eating healthy foods in reasonable portions, not smoking, reducing alcohol intake, exercising, and using seat belts. Physicians are well aware that a healthy lifestyle can reduce the amount and intensity of medical care a person needs in the future.

Patients are sometimes so wrapped up in their primary concern—to get relief from pain or other symptoms—that they have difficulty accepting that physicians are often looking for the cause of their illness, not just to alleviate symptoms. This can cause a lot of frustration for patients, especially if no significant relief can be given or if the physician does not seem to think that alleviating the symptoms would be appropriate.

A common example of this is a viral illness such as the common cold. A patient may have a fever, muscle aches, weakness, vomiting, and diarrhea. Once the physician establishes that the patient does not have a more serious condition, the physician may recommend only rest, fluids, and over-the-counter medications (e.g., acetaminophen or ibuprofen for fever reduction and relief of soreness). This plan of treatment can be frustrating for a patient who wants to feel better and have a speedy recovery.

HOW BASIC NEEDS AFFECT THE BEHAVIOR OF PATIENTS

Maslow's Hierarchy of Needs

Abraham Maslow was an American psychiatrist. In his book *Motivation and Personality,* he defined what has come to be known as "Maslow's hierarchy of needs." A **hierarchy** is an arrangement in order of importance. Maslow describes human needs as a hierarchy with the most important needs at the lowest level. The image of a pyramid is often used to

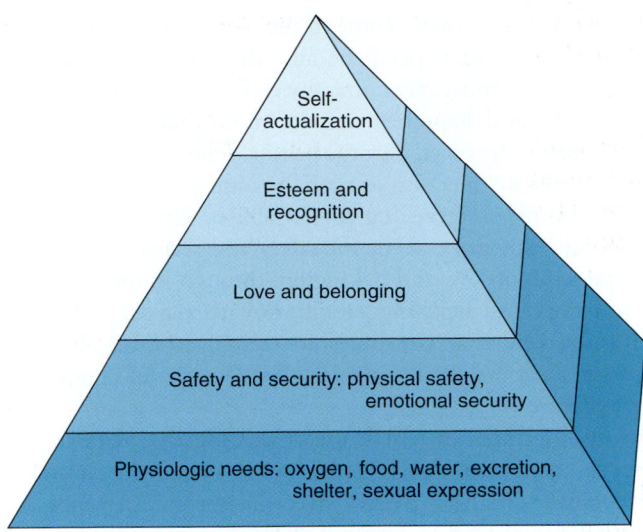

Figure 4-4 Maslow's hierarchy of needs.

depict this visually, as shown in Figure 4-4. On the bottom of the pyramid (Level 1) are the **physiologic** needs. These are the basic biologic needs for survival, which include oxygen, water, food, excretion, sleep, shelter, and sexual expression.

On the next level of the pyramid (Level 2) are the needs for safety and security. Level 2 needs include avoiding harm, attaining physical safety, and the emotional security that comes with freedom from fear and anxiety.

On the middle level of the pyramid (Level 3) are the needs for love and belonging. Level 3 needs include both receiving and giving personal affection, companionship with another individual, and identification with a group.

On the fourth level of the pyramid (Level 4) are the needs for esteem and recognition. Level 4 needs include self-esteem, the respect of others in one's peer group, success in work, and prestige in the community.

Finally, at the pyramid's pinnacle (Level 5) is the need for **self-actualization.** This is the fulfillment of each individual's potential.

Effects of Unmet Needs during Illness

Understanding that an individual cannot step up to the next level on Maslow's pyramid until his or her needs have been fully met at the current level is important. An individual's current level may shift several times, even in the course of a day, as different needs are experienced. An individual moves up or down the pyramid depending on what needs are currently unmet. Only when lower-level needs are met will the person be able to devote a significant amount of energy or concern to needs that are higher on the pyramid. In fact, a person has all the needs (outlined on the pyramid) all the time but becomes aware of higher-level needs only once the lower-level needs have been met.

This has a number of implications for how patients relate to the medical care they receive.

Many patients who come to the medical office are struggling to meet basic needs because they are ill. Health care professionals must recognize any difficulties in that area.

Health and happiness require more than just meeting basic needs, however. Part of the role of health professionals is to foster the meeting of needs beyond physiologic needs. For example, intervening for an abused child or battered woman helps meet needs for safety and security, as well as some sense of love and belonging, through knowledge that someone cares. Teaching patients how to manage a **chronic** disease—one that continues to exist over time—helps a person's self-esteem by making the person feel competent in self-care.

Another area in which understanding the hierarchy of needs helps in the health care setting includes learning to recognize situations when attention-getting behavior by patients might be an attempt to satisfy needs for love and belonging, or for esteem and recognition. When people are ill, their usual means for meeting their attention needs (both for love and belonging, as well as esteem and recognition) may be interrupted.

Medical assistants must be able to recognize that they cannot meet all of a patient's needs. For example, the medical assistant is not a close friend and should not attempt to be one, but by recognizing when a patient feels a loss in this area, the medical assistant helps the person to identify his or her feelings and to cope with whatever need is not being met.

DEVELOPMENTAL STAGES

A patient's developmental level also affects his or her relationships with health care providers. The sociologist Erik Erikson identified eight stages of psychosocial developmental through the life cycle with a challenge for the individual at each stage. Mastery of the challenge would strengthen the individual's development and prepare him or her to meet the challenges of each subsequent state. Although individuals do not all pass through the stages at the same rate, they are helpful for understanding the challenges and pitfalls of the life cycle (Table 4-3).

The task of infancy is to develop a sense of trust that the infant's needs will be met and a hope for the future. The task of a toddler is to develop a sense of self with a certain amount of self-control.

Skills that reflect this are toilet training and the ability to tolerate frustration for short periods. The task of a preschool-age child is to develop the ability to explore and act independently. During the grade-school years, children develop self-confidence and the ability to devote themselves to school or sports. In adolescence, social relationships develop along with greater tolerance for differences among people. As a young adult, a person becomes more aware of the requirements for successful intimate relationships and develops closer friendships and/or romantic relationships. In the adult years, people find satisfaction in work or family responsibilities and anxiety about meeting responsibilities may result when they are diagnosed with serious illness. The challenge in the final stage of life is to remain engaged and feel satisfied with one's life, even in the face of physical and mental decline.

ESTABLISHING CARING RELATIONSHIPS

A patient who visits the medical office is often fragile, emotionally as well as physically. Illness interrupts an individual's daily routine and threatens self-concept and self-esteem. A patient who is ill often has a difficult time meeting his or her physiologic needs. One of the primary roles of a medical assistant is to create and maintain a caring relationship with the patient. The medical assistant is often the patient's earliest, most frequent, and most consistent point of contact with the medical office.

Empathy

To meet a patient's needs, the medical assistant must first be able to identify the patient's feelings. In addition, the medical assistant must be able to understand those feelings, not in an intellectual way but in an emotional way. This understanding is called *empathy*. **Empathy** is the capacity to make an emotional connection with another person's feelings without allowing the emotional connection to become overpowering. Empathy is often contrasted with sympathy. **Sympathy** is defined as experiencing the same emotions as another. Sympathy is often accompanied by a feeling of pity.

Table 4-3 Erickson's Stages of Psychosocial Development			
Developmental Stage	**Approximate Age**	**Developmental Task**	**Examples**
Infancy	0-2 years	Trust versus mistrust	Crying, being comforted
Toddlerhood	2-4 years	Autonomy versus shame and doubt	Toilet training, getting dressed
Preschool Age	4-5 years	Initiative versus guilt	Exploring, using tools
School Age	6-12 years	Industry versus inferiority	School, sports
Adolescence	13-19 years	Identity versus role confusion	Social relationships
Young Adult	20-25 years	Intimacy versus isolation	Romantic relationships
Adulthood	26-64 years	Generativity versus stagnation	Job or profession, family
Old Age	65 and older	Integrity versus despair	Reflection on life

PROCEDURE 4-1 Demonstrating Effective and Respectful Verbal and Nonverbal Communication

Outcomes

1. Responds to nonverbal communication
2. Demonstrates nonverbal communication, empathy, and active listening when communicating with patients, family and staff

Equipment/Supplies

- Index cards with situations
- Paper
- Pen
- Computer and printer

1. **Procedural Step.** Working in groups of three, role-play three situations in which one person plays a medical assistant, one person plays a patient with a terminal illness, and one person plays a family member. The medical assistant should demonstrate empathy and active listening toward the patient and family member.
2. **Procedural Step.** After each role-play, describe the nonverbal communication of the "patient" and the "medical assistant," and evaluate the effectiveness of communication.
   Principle: Nonverbal communication is an important part of every interaction.
3. **Procedural Step.** Role-play an additional situation in which a "medical assistant" and "another staff person" disagree, and discuss how each displayed active listening and empathy toward the other.

Principle: The ability to listen closely to and identify with the feelings of another person (empathy) enhances communication, even if the two people disagree strongly.

4. **Procedural Step.** Write a short description of the nonverbal communication that occurred during the role-play situations, and discuss the messages communicated nonverbally. Include ways that empathy is communicated both verbally and nonverbally. Include examples of active listening. Explain how important it is to communicate nonverbally in an effective way. If there were places where nonverbal communication was not effective in the role-play situations, describe them.
5. **Procedural Step.** Hand in the description of the role-play and discussion to your instructor.

Empathy is more objective than sympathy. Experiencing empathy requires a person to retain perspective and have confidence that strong emotions are not dangerous. The medical assistant must be sensitive to the feelings patients have when they go through the medical office routine. It is important for the medical assistant to be constantly aware that strong emotions may arise when individuals experience a threat such as an illness. By showing empathy to patients, a medical assistant can support them more effectively (Procedure 4-1).

Expression of Caring

Caring can be expressed through words and body language. The medical assistant expresses caring through words, by drawing patients out and letting them tell their story in their own way, in their own time. This was described earlier in this chapter in the section on interviewing techniques. The medical assistant should accept and validate a patient's feelings. Patients benefit by being acknowledged and having someone else accept them.

Caring can also be expressed nonverbally through body language and through the way a medical assistant positions himself or herself during conversations with patients (Figure 4-5). The medical assistant should be positioned at the

Figure 4-5 Allowing a preschool child to handle and use the blood pressure cuff may prevent anxiety by giving the child a sense of control.

patient's eye level and at a distance of no more than 3 to 4 feet. If the medical assistant stands while the patient sits at a lower level, the patient may feel intimidated or inferior. Typically, the patient sits on the examining table while the medical assistant stands, which has both at almost equal height. If the patient is more comfortable sitting in the examining room chair, the medical assistant can sit on the

Putting It All into Practice

My name is Nancy Walker, and I have been working for an oncologist for the past 5 years. Our patients have many different types of cancer and are at many different stages of their diseases. One thing that they all have in common is that they need a lot of emotional support. We provide this primarily by keeping the lines of communication open. We try to create an atmosphere where patients feel able to discuss whatever is on their minds. Some patients never say the word "cancer," and they talk about future plans as if they will be in the peak of health. Other patients are amazingly open and frank, even if they have not responded well to treatment. One patient told me that this is the only place she can talk about dying because her husband and her daughter become so emotional that she feels she has to spare them. We do not push patients to talk about anything they are uncomfortable with, but we do make time if patients want to talk about their feelings. The physicians also refer our patients to support groups or counselors because they believe that it is equally important to manage a patient's emotions and physical symptoms. ∎

physician's stool, which again puts both at about equal height. This is much more friendly than if the medical assistant stands while the patient sits in the chair.

Maintaining eye contact and lightly touching the patient, if it seems appropriate, also communicate interest and caring.

Value of Effective Relationships with Patients

The medical assistant is often the patient's most frequent, and long-term, point of contact with the medical office. A medical assistant who gets to know a patient well can be of invaluable assistance to both the patient and the physician, through trust established over time.

The experience of being understood and cared for is one of the most important steps in beginning to heal or cope effectively with illness, especially if the patient has a chronic illness. Ideally, each professional with whom the patient comes in contact at the office will convey this sense, but it is most important for those who are performing procedures. If the patient feels understood, he or she will also develop trust and be able to relax during procedures. This makes the procedure easier and less painful for the patient. It also makes it easier for the medical assistant to perform the procedure.

SELF-BOUNDARIES

Self-boundaries or personal boundaries include physical, mental, and spiritual guidelines or limits that a person uses to define how close other people can come without posing a threat to personal integrity. Self-boundaries indicate a sense of being separate from others instead of defined and controlled by others. The medical assistant and other health professionals allow others to maintain the personal physical space that is necessary for them to feel comfortable, and they do not allow others to intrude into their own physical space. They should also have a clear sense of their own responsibility and right to decide how to behave based on clear moral and ethical principles without intruding into the personal space of others.

It is not uncommon to encounter individuals with mental boundaries that are too weak or too strong. A person who is very unsure about his or her boundaries goes along with his or her companions and is easily manipulated. The opposite type of person maintains rigid control, refuses to be influenced, and usually keeps others at a distance so that no one can get close. Either of these types of individuals may be totally self-absorbed, seeing themselves as the center of the universe and treating others as if their only function is to meet the individuals' needs.

When interacting with an individual who does not respect physical or emotional boundaries, it is important for the medical assistant to recognize what is happening and take appropriate steps to maintain self boundaries. If possible, this should be done in a straightforward way without acting upset or angry. For example, a patient may act as if he or she is a good friend of the medical assistant or flirt with the medical assistant and ask for a cell phone number or a date. Initially most medical assistants would offer excuses not to comply. If the patient continues to ask for a telephone number, for example, the medical assistant may state calmly that he or she does not give his or her cell phone number to patients (Procedure 4-2). To maintain a professional relationship, the medical assistant should always avoid sharing too much personal information, spending time with patients outside the professional relationship, performing or accepting personal favors, or abusing the relationship in any other way.

EMOTIONAL RESPONSES TO ILLNESS
Guilt

Patients may feel guilt about their illness. The amount of guilt they feel varies from one patient to another. The amount of guilt that a patient is willing to express, as opposed to the amount that is repressed, varies from one patient to the next.

Some individuals engage in behaviors that are known to be risky to health, such as cigarette smoking, drinking, and drug abuse. These patients sometimes feel guilty about a respiratory disease, but others may display a devil-may-care attitude about their disease. People often know intellectually that their high-calorie, high-fat diet or sedentary lifestyle predisposes them to certain illnesses or conditions. Smokers, for example, have been bombarded with scientifically valid information for almost 40 years about the link between smoking and heart disease, lung cancer, and chronic obstructive pulmonary disease. Yet many of these individuals continue established habits without an outward sense of guilt. It seems as though they have convinced

---

PROCEDURE 4-2   **Maintaining Boundaries and Demonstrating Respect for Boundaries in Communications**

Outcomes

1. Demonstrates the principles of self-boundaries
2. Demonstrates respect for individual diversity, including: a. gender, b. race, c. religion, d. age, e. economic status, f. appearance

Equipment/Supplies

- Paper
- Pen
- Computer and printer

1. **Procedural Step.** Create three situations in which a medical assistant is taking vital signs for each of the following patients:
   a. An indigent person with strong body odor and an undiagnosed skin condition
   b. An 80-year-old Hispanic woman who is hard of hearing and speaks poor English
   c. A woman from Ethiopia who does not look at the medical assistant and whose husband speaks for her and says she will not undress
2. **Procedural Step.** Write dialog including actions of all individuals for a short scene for each situation.
3. **Procedural Step.** Write an analysis of each situation explaining how the appearance of the patient, self-boundaries, and/or personal bias with respect to gender, race, religion, age, appearance, and economic status may influence the interaction. Identify your own biases as honestly as possible.
4. **Procedural Step.** Explain how a medical assistant should protect his or her own and patients' self-boundaries and demonstrate respect for individual diversity in each of the situations described.
   Principle. Patients are entitled to considerate and respectful care according to the Patient Bill of Rights.
5. **Procedural Step.** Role-play each scene with a classmate, and demonstrate respect for individual diversity with respect to gender, race, religion, age, economic status, and appearance.
6. **Procedural Step.** Hand in your situations and discussion to your instructor.

---

themselves that their risky behavior is not the cause of their disease or that they are somehow immune to the consequences of their behavior.

On the other hand, patients with conditions totally out of their control may experience guilt. For example, someone with pancreatic cancer might say that he could have avoided the disease if he had taken better care of himself, eaten a healthy diet, or gotten more exercise.

As with other emotions, the medical assistant should accept and validate a patient's description of his or her feelings. If the patient's previous behavior is partially responsible for current medical problems, the patient requires support and acceptance. If it is unlikely that previous behavior is related to the medical problem, the medical assistant can encourage the patient to discuss the causes of his or her condition with the physician.

Loss of Control

When people are ill, they often have a feeling of a loss of control. This is especially true if they have sought medical care for their condition. In addition to physiologic changes that may be unwelcome, they feel unable to control their schedule and/or environment. Some decisions are made for them. They have to take off their clothes. People get physically close to them and sometimes even touch them. People tell them to do things they do not want to do. They are anxious and become defensive. The medical assistant should respond to the patient's irritation with patience and kindness. It is important to give the patient choices and make every effort to accommodate the patient's wishes.

Anxiety

Anxiety is a response to a perceived threat. A person who is moderately to severely anxious is not able to converse coherently and will not pick up nonverbal cues that he or she would normally notice. When working with a patient who is anxious, the medical assistant must first get the person's attention, slow down the conversation, and then help the person to focus on the conversation. It is important to validate the patient's concern, which reduces his or her anxiety level. This allows the patient's energy to be channeled in a more productive way. When patients are anxious, they may not remember what they are told. The medical assistant can help the patient by creating memory aids. For example, the medical assistant can prompt the patient to record a follow-up appointment in his or her appointment calendar. It is also a good idea to write the instructions down or provide the patient with a preprinted instruction sheet.

Severe anxiety can be medically problematic. Physical symptoms occur with a full-blown anxiety attack, often termed a *panic attack.* An overly anxious person hyperventilates, has an extremely rapid heart rate, and becomes unresponsive. Some people experience numbness in their fingers and toes; others feel a sensation of fullness in their ears. Some people become intensely fearful and have an overpowering sense of dread.

An anxiety attack must be dealt with as a medical issue first. Helping the patient acknowledge the anxiety is important. Acknowledging the anxiety helps a person gain control. In addition, having strong emotions accepted by another person decreases the sense of fear that many people have about their emotions.

If the patient is breathing rapidly, the medical assistant should encourage the patient to take slow, deep breaths. Experts no longer recommend having a patient breathe into a brown paper bag because this may cause blood oxygen levels to fall dangerously low.

If possible, the medical assistant should encourage the patient to validate that anxiety is present without minimizing its significance. If the patient has not experienced severe anxiety before, he or she may not realize the effects it can

cause. The medical assistant can explain that any physical symptoms are the result of anxiety and stay with the patient until the symptoms begin to subside. With most patients, the symptoms begin to diminish after 1 or 2 minutes. After the person has returned to a level of relative calm, it may be possible to discuss how the person handles anxiety. The physician may also refer the patient to a counselor to work on strategies to manage it.

Anger

Anger is a natural response to a perceived threat. Anger is often a subconscious response, which means that the patient is unaware of its cause, its intensity, or even its presence. A patient may express anger at a target that did not actually cause the angry feeling. Anger can also escalate quickly if it triggers an angry response from another individual. When dealing with an angry patient, the medical assistant needs to identify the emotion without feeling attacked. If possible, the medical assistant should help the angry person identify the true source of the anger.

Anger is one of the more difficult of the incapacitating emotions to deal with. Anger tests a medical assistant's empathy and ability to put aside private issues to help patients. The first instinct is to defend oneself against a perceived attack by the angry patient, but this is counterproductive. It is more effective to respond with calmness and control using a quiet voice. Accepting that a patient is angry is not the same as allowing the patient to threaten office staff or other patients. It is perfectly acceptable to set personal boundaries by telling the patient that he or she is acting inappropriately, that he or she is making it difficult for other patients, or that shouting will not be tolerated. To protect the confidentiality of the patient who is temporarily out of control, the medical assistant should escort the patient to a private area. It is also appropriate for the medical assistant to request assistance from the office manager in dealing with an angry patient. Sometimes anger, like electricity, loses intensity when the connection is broken.

What Would You Do? What Would You *Not* Do?

Case Study 3

Julie Ann Reynolds is a 20-year-old patient who comes to the office and describes four or five recent episodes of shortness of breath, palpitations, faintness, sweating, and nausea. She states that she has just started taking classes at a local university after transferring from a community college. The episodes have occurred mainly in the car on the way to school or shortly after arrival. She says that on one occasion her heart was beating so fast that she had to pull her car over and wait for about 10 minutes before she felt well enough to drive. She says that she has never had a heart problem, but now she is afraid that there is something wrong with her heart. She also says that her mother is worried about her and has suggested that she get an electrocardiogram and other tests because she might have a serious medical condition. ■

HIGHLIGHT on Ego Defense Mechanisms

An **ego defense mechanism** is an unconscious mental process that offers psychological protection. Everyone uses defense mechanisms at some time or another to protect against being overwhelmed by painful feelings. Although people are sometimes aware of using these mechanisms, usually they operate on an unconscious level—that is, people are not aware that they are disguising or blocking emotions or impulses.

Everyone tends to use defense mechanisms that have been effective in the past to reduce stress or anxiety. When a person first encounters a situation that would provoke strong feelings, such as a diagnosis of serious illness, a defense mechanism such as denial helps him or her avoid feeling overwhelmed and unable to cope. (**Denial** is unconsciously refusing to acknowledge something that is difficult to accept.) People say things like, "It doesn't seem real to me" or "This must be a mistake."

Denial allows the truth to penetrate gradually so the person has a chance to get used to the threat, to seek privacy to experience intense emotion, and to avoid total disorientation. However, if a person continues to use denial without attempting to accept the situation, negative consequences may occur.

The person may not take appropriate actions to respond to illness. Friends and family may respond negatively to the person's perceived lack of responsibility. And the person may miss the opportunity to grow and strengthen his or her sense of self-worth and ability to cope with adversity.

If a medical assistant can identify a patient's defense mechanisms and coping patterns, he or she can gain a better understanding of the patient's underlying fears and concerns. The medical assistant can try to respond to these concerns but should not directly challenge the defenses or label them.

HIGHLIGHT on Ego Defense Mechanisms—cont'd

When defense mechanisms are attacked, it takes more energy to defend against threatening emotions. On the other hand, accepting defenses tends to promote a feeling of being understood and may decrease the need for rigidity in the defenses.

Example

Mr. Sykes has had to wait for about 45 minutes past his appointment time to see Dr. Lopez. When Kathy, the medical assistant, takes him back to the examination room, he says, "I think you should know that some of the people in the waiting room are really upset about how long they have been waiting."

Kathy may suspect that this is an example of **projection**— unconsciously identifying thoughts or feelings as originating in someone else when they really are one's own thoughts and feelings. She can be helpful to Mr. Sykes by responding in a way that reassures him that it is understandable for a person to be upset when there is an unusually long wait. Responses that are not helpful (because they reinforce Mr. Sykes's fear that it would be dangerous to express a negative emotion directly) are as follows:

1. Making it seem as though Mr. Sykes is overreacting and should not feel upset ("Oh, it hasn't been that long.")
2. Labeling or challenging the defense mechanism ("Do you always project your own feelings on people around you?")
3. Defending the physician or office staff ("Dr. Lopez has been very busy with several sick patients.")
4. Talking negatively about the patients in the waiting room ("Some people are never happy, no matter how quickly they are seen.")

In the accompanying box is a list of several other ego defense mechanisms, with examples that might occur in a medical office. Remember that using defense mechanisms usually helps people adapt to stressful situations. ■

Other Ego Defense Mechanisms

Selective inattention	Failing to hear or pay attention to information that may provoke anxiety	A patient says he was told that his cancer will definitely be cured if he has the primary tumor removed.
Regression	Returning to the emotional adjustment of an earlier stage of growth and development	An ill person who could be independent asks for assistance with personal hygiene.
Depersonalization	Removing feeling from something that is perceived as stressful	A medical assistant who is assisting with a lumbar puncture on a young child experiences the child as looking like a toy or doll.
Rationalization	Assigning logical reasons or excuses for actions that may have been motivated by self-interest or other emotions the person does not wish to acknowledge	A patient might justify not telling the physician that he smokes by saying to himself, "The doctor isn't interested because he didn't ask about it."
Repression	Unconsciously excluding unacceptable ideas, impulses, or emotions from awareness	A diabetic patient who hates finger sticks often forgets to test her blood sugar.
Suppression	Deciding to put uncomfortable or painful thoughts out of awareness	A patient says, "I don't want to think about my surgery until the day before."
Displacement	Shifting an emotion or behavior from the original object to a more acceptable substitute	A medical assistant who has just been given a poor evaluation is extremely rude to the next person she talks to on the telephone.
Undoing	An attempt to make amends for a feeling or behavior that makes a person feel guilty	A patient notices that she hates the medical assistant's hairstyle and hair color. Immediately she tells the medical assistant that she has beautiful eyes.
Compensation	Attempting to overcome a real or perceived handicap by developing some other ability or trait	A person who thinks that she isn't very intelligent in school always offers to help the teacher.

THE GRIEVING PROCESS

Any time a disease causes actual or potential loss including loss of function as well as loss of life, both the patient and family go through a fairly predictable sequence of stages called the *grieving process*. This process was described in detail by the spiritual author Elisabeth Kübler-Ross in relation to individuals with a terminal illness. The **terminal phase** is defined as when the patient is not expected to live longer than 6 months. People go through this sequence over varying lengths of time and may move from one stage to another out of the order presented here. Although the process is individual, it is important to know that even a dying person can come to a type of acceptance, and after death has occurred there is a time when the grieving relatives and friends will again be able to engage in loving and fulfilling relationships.

The following five steps are those described by Kübler-Ross for the patient with a terminal illness:

1. *Denial.* This is the initial response to knowledge that one has a terminal illness. It is a state of shock and disbelief. Most people simply deny the idea. Denial can be useful; it can provide a period of time to find a way to deal with death or disability. If a patient is using denial, the medical assistant should remember that this is a defense against unmanageable anxiety.

   The medical assistant should listen to the patient actively, without confronting unrealistic statements. Acceptance of the patient's need to deny reality provides support for a patient to accept at his or her own pace. The patient and family will start to accept reality when they are ready to handle the strong emotions.

2. *Anger.* Frustration and anger usually follow denial. The patient is in the "Why me?" mode. The illness seems unfair, and the patient may respond by being belligerent, uncooperative, and critical of those around him or her. Health care providers may become targets of this anger and criticism. The medical assistant must keep in mind that any such display of anger is not directed at him or her personally but toward the situation and circumstances over which the patient has no control.

3. *Bargaining.* In this stage, which usually follows anger closely, the patient may try to give something up to gain more time. Most bargaining is done between the patient and his or her personal concept of God. If bargaining is verbalized, the medical assistant should be accepting of the patient's wish to make a bargain that will reverse his or her condition or prolong his or her life.

4. *Depression.* The patient recognizes the facts that cannot be denied and becomes depressed. Most people become silent at this stage and prefer to be alone. The patient who is withdrawn is more difficult to deal with than the person who is openly angry. In this situation, a medical assistant needs to be available and present with the patient for companionship and to provide a nonjudgmental listening ear. The medical assistant should always strive to maintain communication with a patient in the depression stage. Counseling and support groups may be appropriate referrals for both patients and family members in this stage.

5. *Acceptance.* Some people find a degree of peace within themselves when they accept their imminent death. They willingly stop resisting death and rest quietly. This is seldom seen by professionals who work in medical offices, because those who reach this stage may be in a hospital, in a hospice center, or at home. The dying person may want loved ones present at death and may not interact with others at all. Most people fear dying alone and want the comfort of having someone, preferably a loved one, present in the final moments.

A dying person has a number of fears, such as fear of the unknown, fear of pain, and fear of helplessness. It is a challenge for all health care professionals to accept the difficult feelings of fear.

Listening closely to the patient allows the medical assistant to help the patient respond to all hints of deterioration, as well as actual problems, as soon as they become apparent. The patient may need to be seen by several health care professionals while receiving additional care at home. The medical assistant can be helpful by being aware of community resources and by communicating the needs of the patient and his or her family to the doctor. This requires knowledge of insurance benefits and of the types of insurance the office accepts, as well as other sources of funding assistance the patient may be able to obtain.

A patient whose condition has stabilized or whose active treatment has ended but who still requires pain relief, nursing care, and/or comfort measures must receive them at home, in a nursing home, in a rehabilitation center, or in a hospice center. A **hospice** is an organization that provides comfort, pain relief, and personal care for dying patients.

Most hospices provide nursing care, nursing assistants, and volunteers to visit terminal patients in their homes, working with the families to increase the individual's comfort once active treatment is no longer effective or desired. There are also some hospice centers, which provide centralized care. In some areas a patient can receive similar services from home health care agencies and visiting nurse associations.

The medical assistant may serve as a patient navigator or liaison to obtain appropriate referrals from the doctor and assist the patient and/or family to locate providers of needed services. Communication on this level must be two-way; if a patient is being seen by visiting nurses, hospice, or other health professionals, the medical assistant may be the person who facilitates communication between the doctor and these other parties.

CULTURAL INFLUENCES AFFECTING HEALTH CARE

Patients often come from cultures that have some level of distrust of Western scientific medicine and/or strong belief in their own medical traditions. In addition to seeking care from a physician, these patients may complement their care by visiting traditional practitioners. In many traditional practices, religion and medicine are tightly interwoven. Both patients and practitioners hope to affect health by influencing spirits or gods in the unseen world. People from many cultures believe in the effectiveness of sacred words, tattoos, or amulets (objects worn to prevent injury or evil), as well as specific rituals that may involve chanting, fire, or even animal sacrifice.

Causes of Illness

Many cultures distinguish between illness caused by bad spirits or evil people and illness with physiologic origins. It is important to not ridicule these theories if patients believe them. When patients feel that health professionals do not respect their beliefs, they may not follow recommendations

Memories *from* Practicum

Nancy Walker: I did my practicum in the adult medicine area of a clinic in a large metropolitan area. We had several African patients who came to our area as refugees from Somalia. If they were recent immigrants, we had to explain many things about our clinic to them because they were not familiar with preventative care from their own country. The female patients were modest; they did not shake hands with male physicians and avoided undressing for examinations. We tried to assign them to female practitioners, if possible, and everyone in the office learned to adapt procedures by having the patient remove the minimum possible amount of clothing. For example, the physicians usually listened to a female patient's heart and respirations just by placing the stethoscope under her clothing. One of these patients told me that some offices were not as accepting of their customs as we were. She said that it is considered immodest for a woman to remove clothing in front of any male, even a physician. She told me that if she had to do it, she would just stay sick. ■

or return for follow-up care. An open attitude and the willingness to listen to the patient's beliefs are required to establish a relationship of trust with the patient.

Fundamentals of scientific medical practice—such as frequent handwashing to remove invisible organisms, taking medicine when one does not feel ill, and causing pain to healthy children by giving them immunizations—may be foreign to certain traditional practices.

Treatments and Traditional Practices

When patients have beliefs that do not correspond to those of the health care team, it is important to keep the lines of communication open. Patients need to be able to discuss other treatments that are being used. They also need to understand the importance of the treatments being offered by scientific medicine so that they can comply with standard medical treatment regimens in addition to their traditional practices.

As a general rule, the health care team should accept any traditional practice that is not dangerous. For example, some patients from Cambodia and other parts of Southeast Asia believe that rubbing the skin with the side of a coin dipped in a camphor preparation is a treatment for colds and headaches. This treatment leaves bruises on the skin but does not cause breaks in the skin. A child with bruises from this type of treatment is not a victim of child abuse, but the bruises might look like abuse. The medical assistant should learn about traditional treatments used by patients in the practice where he or she works.

One area in which family and cultural traditions may be strong relates to diet and herbal preparations. In many traditions, certain diseases and conditions are considered "hot" and others are considered "cold." The patient may be advised to either eat or avoid certain foods or to take certain herbal preparations to restore balance. If the patient can describe traditional treatments, it will be easier for the physician to identify any practices that might be harmful or that might interfere with prescribed medical treatments.

Behavioral Requirements

In some cultures there are specific behavioral requirements for women and men. There may be cultural norms requiring women to have a male escort when they leave their homes. In some cultures the oldest male in the family must make important decisions. For some individuals there are also cultural requirements prohibiting the removal of clothing, jewelry, and head coverings, even for medical examinations. Medical assistants must learn about cultural norms and respond with acceptance and sensitivity. If necessary, adaptations must be made so that the patient is not forced to violate personal standards.

What Would You Do? What Would You *Not* Do? RESPONSES

Case Study 1
Page 65

What Did Nancy Do?
❏ Maintained a warm and accepting posture and a friendly tone of voice.
❏ Used an open response to encourage Jennifer to say more about how she feels about possibly being pregnant.
❏ Identified verbally that Jennifer seemed a little upset.

What Did Nancy *Not* Do?
❏ Did not immediately congratulate Jennifer or respond as if this was good news.
❏ Did not immediately assume a businesslike tone of voice and ask closed questions to obtain information.

❏ Did not act as if the patient has nothing on her mind.
❏ Did not appear to be in a hurry to finish the interview.

Case Study 2
Page 68

What Did Nancy Do?
❏ Made sure that Harold was looking at her when she spoke to him.
❏ Spoke clearly and a little more slowly than usual, using a strong voice.
❏ Asked Harold if his hearing aid was working well for him.
❏ Used gestures to reinforce her directions.
❏ Used short sentences.
❏ Repeated instructions or questions as needed.

Continued

What Would You Do? | What Would You *Not* Do? RESPONSES—cont'd

What Did Nancy **Not** *Do?*
- ❑ Did not shout.
- ❑ Did not express impatience in her tone of voice or body language.
- ❑ Did not speak in long, complicated sentences.
- ❑ Did not turn away from the patient and keep talking.
- ❑ Did not drop her voice at the end of sentences.

Case Study 3
Page 74

What Did Nancy Do?
- ❑ Expressed to Julie Ann that these symptoms are upsetting.
- ❑ Agreed that it is a good decision to see the doctor.

- ❑ Asked Julie Ann to describe the emotions she was experiencing during these episodes.
- ❑ Maintained an open, friendly, and calm demeanor during the interview.

What Did Nancy **Not** *Do?*
- ❑ Did not try to identify the cause of the episodes for Julie Ann.
- ❑ Did not rush through the interview so that the patient would be ready for the physician quickly.
- ❑ Did not say, "It's probably just anxiety."
- ❑ Did not say that there was probably nothing seriously the matter with Julie Ann.

↻ TERMINOLOGY REVIEW

Key Term	Word Parts	Definition
Active listening		Paying close attention to a speaker without thinking of anything else.
Anxiety		A vague, unpleasant emotion of fear or dread often accompanied by restlessness or nervousness.
Body language		Communication that is expressed through facial expressions, body position, muscle activity, and other nonverbal means.
Chronic		Existing over a long period of time.
Closed questions		Questions that anticipate a yes or no or a short answer.
Denial		Failure to acknowledge the reality of a situation.
Ego defense mechanism		Unconscious mental process that offers psychological protection.
Empathy		Objective awareness and sensitivity to the feelings and emotions of others.
Hierarchy		Classified according to rank or importance.
Hospice		An organization that manages care for dying patients including comfort, pain relief, and personal care.
Judgmental		Critical or negative; making judgments about what is good or bad based on personal opinion.
Nonverbal	*non-:* not *verbum:* word *-al:* pertaining to	Communication that occurs without words, such as through body posture or facial expression.
Open questions		Questions that could have a variety of answers and encourage a personal response.
Oral	*os* (gen. *oris*): mouth *-al:* pertaining to	Spoken; pertaining to the mouth.
Paraphrasing		A restatement of the words of another, often to clarify meaning.
Physiologic	*physis:* nature *logia:* study *-ic:* pertaining to	Pertaining to body processes.
Projection		Experiencing one's own emotions as those of another.
Reflecting		Expressing the meaning and emotion of another's words back to the person.
Self-actualization		The fulfillment of each individual's potential.
Summarizing		Expressing the most important points of a conversation or written document.
Sympathy		Feeling the same emotions as another.
Terminal phase		The last stage of illness, usually used when death is expected to occur within 6 months.
Verbal	*verbum:* word *-al:* pertaining to	Using words to communicate.
Webcam		Small video camera attached to a computer that allows video to be transmitted on the Internet.

ON THE WEB

For information on multicultural resources:

U.S. National Library of Medicine—Multi-Cultural Resources for Health Information: sis.nlm.nih.gov/outreach/multi-cultural.html

For information on hearing impairment:

National Association of the Deaf: www.nad.org

For information on limited English proficiency:

Department of Health and Human Services Office for Civil Rights: Limited English Proficiency (LEP): www.hhs.gov/ocr/civilrights/resources/specialtopics/lep

For information on psychology:

American Psychological Association: www.apa.org

Social Psychology Network: www.socialpsychology.org

For information on vision impairment:

American Foundation for the Blind: www.afb.org

The Blind Reader's Page: blindreaders.info

Introduction to Anatomy and Physiology

e Check out the Evolve site at http://evolve.elsevier.com/Bonewit/today/ to access additional interactive activities and exercises to help you study and prepare for success.

LEARNING OBJECTIVES

1. Explain why it is important for the medical assistant to be knowledgeable about anatomy and physiology.
2. Explain the relationship between anatomy and physiology.
3. State the six levels of organization within the human body.
4. List the 11 organ systems of the body, and describe the function of each.
5. Describe homeostasis and its importance to the human body.
6. Explain how the body maintains homeostasis through use of a negative feedback system.
7. List the four criteria used to describe the anatomic position.
8. Identify body planes, body regions, and relative positions using anatomic terms.
9. Distinguish between the dorsal body cavity and the ventral body cavity, and list the subdivisions of each cavity.
10. Describe the cell membrane.
11. Describe the composition of the cytoplasm.
12. Describe the components of the nucleus, and state the function of each component.
13. Identify and describe each of the cytoplasmic organelles, and state the function of each organelle.
14. Explain how the cell membrane regulates the composition of the cytoplasm.
15. Describe the various mechanisms that result in the transport of substances across the cell membrane.
16. List the phases of a cell cycle, and describe the events that occur in each phase.
17. Explain the difference between mitosis and meiosis.
18. List the four main types of tissues found in the body.
19. Describe the various types of epithelial tissues in terms of structure, location, and function.
20. Describe the general characteristics of connective tissue.
21. List three types of connective tissue cells, and state the function of each.
22. Describe the features and location of the various types of connective tissue.
23. Explain the differences among skeletal muscle, smooth muscle, and cardiac muscle in terms of structure, location, and control.
24. State the two categories of cells in nerve tissue, and explain their function.

CHAPTER OUTLINE

A BRIEF SUMMARY OF MEDICAL HISTORY
THE HUMAN BODY
Anatomy and Physiology
Levels of Organization
Chemical Level
Cells
Tissues
Organs
Body Systems
Total Organism
Organ Systems
Integumentary System
Skeletal System
Muscular System

Nervous System
Endocrine System
Cardiovascular System
Lymphatic System
Digestive System
Respiratory System
Urinary System
Reproductive System
Homeostasis
Negative and Positive Feedback
Anatomic Terms
Anatomic Position
Directions in the Body
Planes and Sections of the Body

Body Cavities
Regions of the Body
CELL STRUCTURE AND FUNCTION
Structure of the Generalized Cell
Plasma Membrane
Cytoplasm
Nucleus
Cytoplasmic Organelles
Filamentous Protein Organelles
Cell Functions
Movement of Substances Across the Cell Membrane
Cell Division
DNA Replication and Protein Synthesis

TISSUES AND MEMBRANES
Body Tissues
Epithelial Tissue
Connective Tissue
Muscle Tissue
Body Membranes
Mucous Membranes
Serous Membranes
Synovial Membranes
Meninges

KEY TERMS

active transport (AK-tiv TRANS-port)
anatomic position (an-ah-TOM-ik poh-ZIH-shun)
axon (AKS-on)
chondrocytes (KON-droh-sytes)
collagenous fibers (koh-LAJ-eh-nuss FYE-burs)
cutaneous membrane (kyoo-TAY-nee-us MEM-brayn)
cytokinesis (sye-toh-kih-NEE-sis)
dendrites (DEN-drytes)
diffusion (dif-YOO-zhun)
elastic fibers (ee-LAS-tick FYE-burs)
erythrocytes (ee-RITH-roh-sytes)
fibroblasts (FYE-broh-blasts)

histology (hiss-TAHL-oh-jee)
homeostasis (hoh-mee-oh-STAY-sis)
human anatomy (ah-NAT-o-mee)
human physiology (fiz-ee-AHL-oh-jee)
leukocytes (LOO-koh-sytes)
macrophages (MAK-roh-fay-esj)
mast cell (MAST SELL)
meiosis (mye-OH-sis)
meninges (meh-NIN-jeez)
mitosis (mye-TOH-sis)
mucous membranes (MYOO-cus MEM-brayns)
negative feedback (NEG-ah-tiv FEED-bak)
neuroglia (noo-ROG-lee-ah)

neurons (NOO-rons)
osmosis (os-MOH-sis)
osteocytes (AH-stee-oh-sytes)
passive transport (PASS-iv TRANS-port)
pericardium (pair-ih-KAR-dee-um)
peritoneum (pair-ih-toe-NEE-um)
phagocytosis (fag-oh-sye-TOH-sis)
pinocytosis (pin-oh-sye-TOH-sis)
pleura (PLOO-rah)
serous membranes (SEER-us MEM-brayns)
synovial membranes (sih-NOH-vee-al MEM-brayns)
thrombocyte (THROM-boh-syte)
tissue (TISH-yoo)

A BRIEF SUMMARY OF MEDICAL HISTORY

Studies of illness and aging of the human body are major components in the field of medicine. The study of "modern" medicine began in the fifth century BCE.

Hippocrates, who was born in approximately 460 BCE on the Greek island of Cos, is recognized as the "Father of Medicine." After his death, all the existing writings on medicine were gathered into a work called the *Hippocratic Collection* and attributed to him whether he wrote them or not. The Hippocratic Oath, which is still in use today, is from the *Collection*. Hippocrates concluded that illness had rational explanations instead of being caused by evil spirits or disfavor of the gods. This freed medicine from superstition and allowed for scientific study.

Leonardo da Vinci advanced the understanding of human anatomy by carefully dissecting corpses and making detailed anatomic drawings during the fifteenth century. William Harvey published *An Anatomical Essay on the Motion of the Heart and Blood in Animals* in 1628, detailing how blood was pumped from the heart throughout the body and then returned to the heart and recirculated. Shortly after this, Robert Hooke invented a primitive microscope. A Dutch cloth merchant, Antony van Leeuwenhoek, by grinding his own glass lenses, greatly improved the microscope's design and magnification. Using his new and improved microscope, van Leeuwenhoek discovered blood cells in 1670. He also observed bacteria, yeast cells, spermatozoa, and protozoa. The microscope allowed capillaries to be observed, thus showing the link between arteries and veins and confirming Harvey's theory of blood circulation.

Edward Jenner, an English microbiologist, is known as the "Father of Immunology." He observed that people who had contracted cowpox seemed immune to the deadly smallpox. He theorized that deliberately infecting people with cowpox would protect them from smallpox. He tested his theory on a young boy in 1796 and then demonstrated that the lad was indeed immune to smallpox.

William Beaumont, while serving as an army post surgeon, treated a patient who had been blasted by a musket at close range. The resulting large wound affected part of his lung, two ribs, and his stomach. Beaumont treated the wounds but was unable to get the hole in the stomach to completely close; repeated bandaging was required to prevent food and drink from coming out. Recognizing this as an opportunity to study the digestion process, he tied small pieces of food with silk string and dangled them through the hole in the patient's stomach, then removed the items at 1-hour intervals. He published his observations in 1833.

Medicine truly came of age during the second half of the nineteenth century. Louis Pasteur and Robert Koch established the germ theory of disease. Florence Nightingale showed the importance of hygiene and sanitation in reducing hospital infections. Sir Humphry Davy discovered the anesthetic properties of nitrous oxide, and Joseph Lister pioneered the use of carbolic acid as an antiseptic to clean wounds and surgical instruments. His antiseptic technique reduced deaths from infection after surgery from about 60% to under 4%. Then in 1895 a German scientist named Wilhelm Roentgen discovered x-rays. Medicine has never been the same since.

The twentieth century continued to build on all these discoveries. The pharmaceutical industry mushroomed with the development of thousands of new medicines. Vaccines were developed to prevent polio, measles, mumps, and many other diseases. Cardiac pacemakers and defibrillators were invented. Medical imaging advanced with the development of computed tomography (CT), magnetic resonance imaging (MRI), positron emission tomography (PET), ultrasound, and many other techniques. Numerous advances occurred in surgery, including open-heart surgery and organ transplants. Radiation therapy and chemotherapy for the treatment of cancer were developed. Kidney dialysis machines were invented, and hospital intensive care units (ICUs) were established to better treat very ill patients. In the latter part of the twentieth century, a Swedish neurosurgeon, Lars Leksell, developed the Gamma Knife. This is a radiologic technique used to treat tumors in the brain that are not amenable to conventional surgery.

The beginning of the twenty-first century brought the development of the da Vinci Surgical System, a robotic system that uses a minimally invasive approach. The da Vinci System translates the surgeon's movements into micro-movements of the instruments through small incisions. The result is a minimally invasive procedure with less pain, less blood loss, shorter hospital stays, and quicker recovery than with other surgical methods. The list of medical advances goes on and on and is added to every year.

THE HUMAN BODY

The human body is an awesome masterpiece. Imagine billions of microscopic parts, each with its own identity, working together in an organized manner for the benefit of the total being. The human body is more complex than the greatest computer, yet it is personal. The study of the human

body is as old as history itself because people have always had an interest in how the body is put together, how it works, why it becomes defective (illness), and why it wears out (aging).

The study of the human body is essential for those planning a career in health sciences, just as knowledge about automobiles is necessary for those planning to repair them. How can you fix an automobile if you do not know how it is put together or how it works? How can you help fix a human body if you do not know how it is put together or how it works?

ANATOMY AND PHYSIOLOGY

Human anatomy is the study of the shape and structure of the human body and its parts. It encompasses a wide range of topics, including the development and microscopic organization of structures, the relationship between structures, and the interrelationship between structure and function. Gross human anatomy deals with the large structures of the human body that can be seen through normal dissection. Microscopic anatomy deals with the smaller structures and fine detail that can be seen only with the aid of a microscope.

Human physiology is the scientific study of the functions or processes of the human body. It answers how, what, and why anatomic parts work. Anatomy and physiology are interrelated because structure and function are always closely associated. The function of an organ, or how it works, depends on how it is put together. Conversely, the anatomy or structure provides clues to understanding how it works. The structure of the hand, with its long, jointed fingers, is related to its function of grasping things. The heart is designed as a muscular pump that can contract to force blood into the blood vessels. By contrast, lungs are made of a thin tissue and function to exchange oxygen and carbon dioxide between the outside environment and the blood. Imagine what would happen if the heart were made of thin tissue and the lungs were made of thick muscle. Structure and function are always related.

LEVELS OF ORGANIZATION

Among the most outstanding features of the complex human body are its order and organization—how all the parts, from tiny cells to visible organs, work together to make a functioning whole. The organizational scheme of the body has six levels (Figure 5-1).

Starting with the simplest and proceeding to the most complex, the six levels of organization are chemical, cellular, tissue, organ, body system, and total organism. The structural and functional characteristics of all organisms are determined by their chemical makeup.

Chemical Level

The *chemical level* deals with the interactions of atoms, such as hydrogen and oxygen, and their combinations into

Figure 5-1 Organizational scheme of the body. From simple to complex, the levels are chemical, cellular, tissue, organ, body system, and total organism. (From Applegate E: *The anatomy and physiology learning system,* ed 4, St Louis, 2011, Saunders.)

molecules, such as water. Molecules contribute to the makeup of a cell, which is the basic unit of life.

Cells

Cells, discussed later in this chapter, are the basic living units of all organisms. Estimates indicate that there are about 75 trillion dynamic, living cells in the human body. These cells represent a variety of sizes, shapes, and structures and provide a vast array of functions.

Tissues

Cells with similar structure and function are grouped together as *tissues.* All of the tissues of the body are grouped into four main types: epithelial, connective, muscle, and nervous. The tissue level of organization is discussed later in this chapter.

Organs

Two or more tissue types that form a more complex structure and work together to perform one or more functions make up *organs,* the next higher level of organization.

Examples of organs include the skin, heart, ear, stomach, and liver.

Body Systems

A *body system* consists of several organs that work together to accomplish a set of functions. Some examples of body systems include the nervous system, the digestive system, and the respiratory system.

Total Organism

Finally, the most complex of all the levels is the *total organism,* which is made up of several systems that work together to maintain life.

ORGAN SYSTEMS

The human body has 11 major organ systems, each with specific functions, yet all are interrelated and work together to sustain life. Each system is described briefly here and then in more detail in later chapters. The organ systems are illustrated and summarized in Table 5-1.

Table 5-1 Organ Systems of the Body

Integumentary System

Components: Skin, hair, nails, sweat, sebaceous glands

Functions: Covers and protects body; regulates temperature

Skeletal System

Components: Bones, cartilage, ligaments

Functions: Provides body framework and support; protects; attaches muscles to bones; provides calcium storage

Muscular System

Components: Muscles

Functions: Produces movement; maintains posture; provides heat

Nervous System

Components: Brain, spinal cord, nerves, sense receptors

Functions: Coordinates body activities; receives and transmits stimuli

Endocrine System

Components: Pituitary, adrenal, thyroid, other ductless glands

Functions: Regulates metabolic activities and body chemistry

Cardiovascular System

Components: Heart, blood vessels, blood

Functions: Transports material from one part of the body to another; defends against disease

Table 5-1 Organ Systems of the Body—cont'd

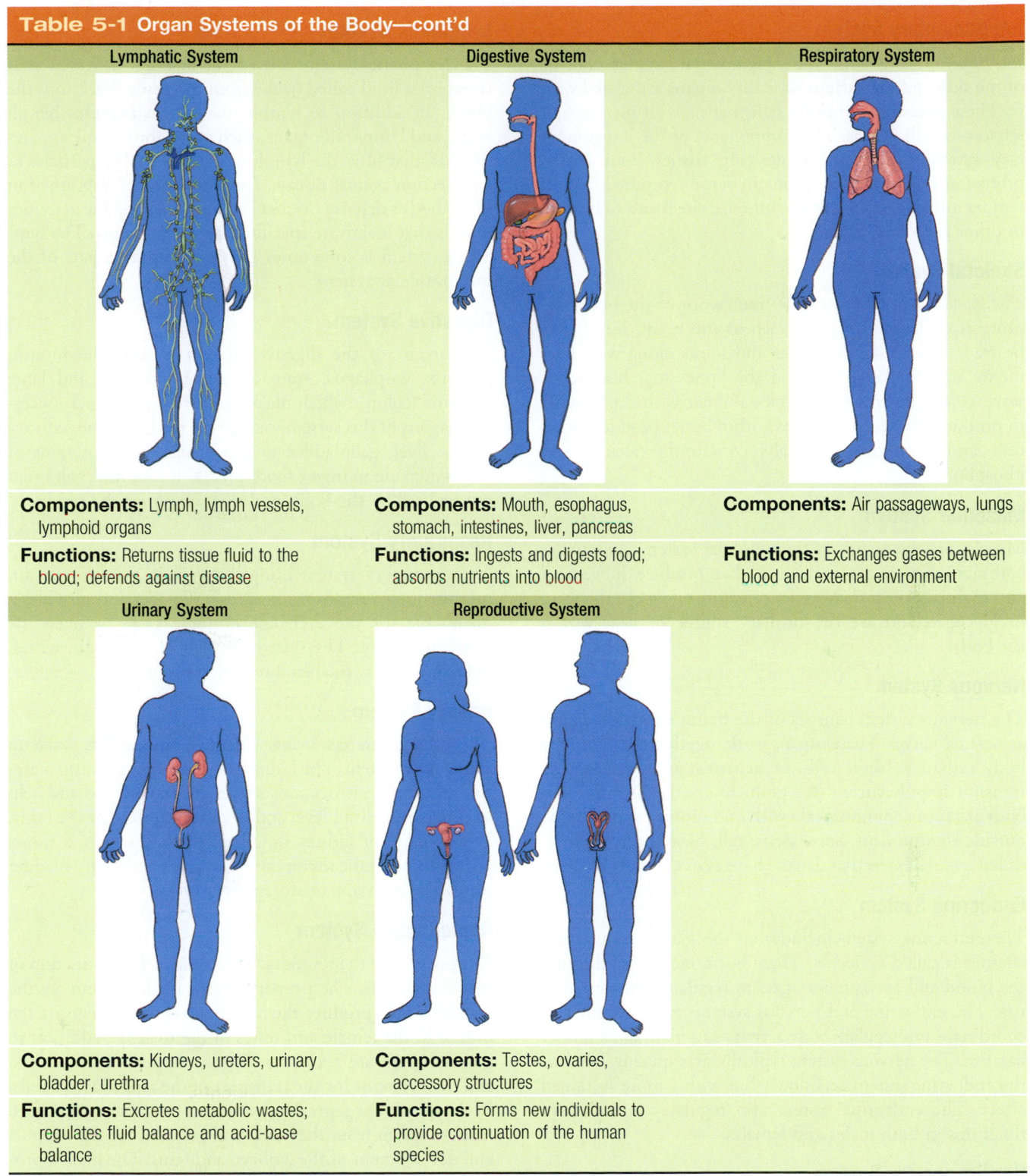

Lymphatic System	Digestive System	Respiratory System
Components: Lymph, lymph vessels, lymphoid organs	**Components:** Mouth, esophagus, stomach, intestines, liver, pancreas	**Components:** Air passageways, lungs
Functions: Returns tissue fluid to the blood; defends against disease	**Functions:** Ingests and digests food; absorbs nutrients into blood	**Functions:** Exchanges gases between blood and external environment

Urinary System	Reproductive System
Components: Kidneys, ureters, urinary bladder, urethra	**Components:** Testes, ovaries, accessory structures
Functions: Excretes metabolic wastes; regulates fluid balance and acid-base balance	**Functions:** Forms new individuals to provide continuation of the human species

From Applegate E: *The anatomy and physiology learning system,* ed 4, St Louis, 2011, Saunders.

Integumentary System

Integument means skin. The integumentary system consists of the skin and the various accessory organs associated with it. These accessories include hair, nails, sweat glands, and sebaceous (oil) glands. The components of the integumentary system protect the underlying tissues from injury, protect against water loss, contain sense receptors, help in temperature regulation, and synthesize chemicals to be used in other parts of the body.

Skeletal System

The skeletal system forms the framework of the body and protects underlying organs, such as the brain, lungs, and heart. It consists of the bones and joints along with ligaments and cartilage that bind the bones together. Bones serve as attachments for muscles and act with the muscles to produce movement. Tissues within bones produce blood cells and store inorganic salts containing calcium and phosphorus.

Muscular System

Muscles are the organs of the muscular system. As muscles contract, they create the forces that produce movement and maintain posture. Muscles can store energy in the form of glycogen and are the primary source of heat within the body.

Nervous System

The nervous system consists of the brain, spinal cord, and associated nerves. These organs work together to coordinate body activities. Nerve cells, or **neurons,** are specialized to transmit impulses from one point to another. In this way, body parts can communicate with one another and with the outside environment. Some nerve cells have special endings called *sense receptors* that detect changes in the environment.

Endocrine System

The endocrine system includes all the glands that secrete chemicals called *hormones.* These hormones travel through the blood and act as messengers to regulate cellular activities. The endocrine and nervous systems work together to coordinate and regulate body activities to maintain a proper balance. The nervous system typically acts quickly, whereas the endocrine system acts slowly but with a more sustained effect. The endocrine system also regulates reproductive functions in both males and females.

Cardiovascular System

The cardiovascular system consists of the blood, heart, and blood vessels. The blood transports nutrients, hormones, and oxygen to tissue cells and removes waste products such as carbon dioxide. Certain cells within the blood known as *white blood cells* defend the body against disease. The heart acts as a pump to create the forces necessary to maintain blood pressure and to circulate the blood. The blood vessels serve as pipes or conduits for the flow of blood.

Lymphatic System

The lymphatic system consists of a series of vessels that transport a fluid called *lymph* from the tissues back into the blood. In addition to lymph, the system includes lymph nodes and lymphoid organs, such as the tonsils, spleen, and thymus, that filter the lymph to remove foreign particles as a protection against disease. Lymphoid organs also function in the body's defense mechanism by enhancing the activities of cells that inactivate specific pathogenic agents. The lymphatic system is sometimes considered to be a part of the cardiovascular system.

Digestive System

The organs of the digestive system include the mouth, pharynx, esophagus, stomach, small intestine, and large intestine (colon), which make up the digestive tract. Accessory organs of this system include the teeth, tongue, salivary glands, liver, gallbladder, and pancreas. The functions of this system are to ingest food, process it into molecules that can be used by the body, and then eliminate the residue.

Respiratory System

The respiratory system brings oxygen, in the form of air, into the lungs; removes the carbon dioxide; and provides a membrane for the exchange of these gases between the blood and lungs. The system consists of the nasal cavities, pharynx, larynx, trachea, bronchi, and lungs.

Urinary System

The kidneys, ureters, urinary bladder, and urethra make up the urinary system. The kidneys remove various waste materials, especially nitrogenous wastes, from the blood and help to regulate the fluid level and chemical content of the body. The product of kidney function is urine, which is transported through the ureters and urethra. The urinary bladder serves as a reservoir or storage area for the urine.

Reproductive System

The purpose of the reproductive system is the production of new individuals. The primary organs of the system are the gonads, which produce the reproductive cells. These are the ovaries in the female and testes in the male. In addition to gonads, there are accessory glands, supporting structures, and duct systems for the transport of the reproductive cells. In the female the reproductive system produces ova or eggs, receives sperm from the male, and provides for the support and development of the embryo and fetus. The male reproductive system is concerned with the production and maintenance of sperm and the transfer of these cells to the female.

HOMEOSTASIS

Homeostasis refers to the constant internal environment that must be maintained for the cells of the body. The word is derived from two Greek words: *homeo,* which means "alike" or "the same," and *stasis,* which means "always" or "staying." Putting these together, the word *homeostasis* means "staying the same." When the body is healthy, the internal environment always stays the same. It remains stable within a limited normal range.

Everyone is familiar with aspects of the external environment—whether it is cold or hot, humid or dry, smoggy or clear. The internal environment is not quite as obvious. It involves the tissue fluid that surrounds and bathes every cell of the body. Normal functional activities of the cell depend on the internal environment being maintained within a limited normal range. The chemical content, volume, temperature, and pressure of the fluid must stay the same, regardless of external conditions, so that the cell can function properly. If the conditions in the tissue fluid deviate from normal, mechanisms respond that try to restore conditions to normal. If the mechanisms are unsuccessful, the cell malfunctions and dies. This leads to illness and disease. Ultimately the goal of medical treatment is to restore homeostasis.

Negative and Positive Feedback

Any condition or stimulus that disrupts the homeostatic balance in the body is a *stressor*. When a stressor causes internal conditions to deviate from normal, all the body systems work to bring conditions back to the normal range. This is usually accomplished by a **negative feedback** mechanism in which a stimulus initiates reactions that reduce the stimulus. This mechanism works similarly to a thermostat connected to a furnace and an air conditioner. When the temperature in the room decreases (stressor) below the thermostat setting (normal), the sensing device in the thermostat detects the change and causes the furnace to add heat to the room. When the room becomes too warm, the furnace stops and the air conditioner begins to cool the room. Negative feedback mechanisms do not prevent variation, but they keep variation within a normal range.

An example of a physiologic negative feedback mechanism in the human body involves blood pressure. When blood pressure decreases below normal, body sensors detect the deviation and initiate changes that bring the pressure back within the normal range. When the pressure increases above normal, changes occur to decrease the pressure to normal. Variations in blood pressure occur, but homeostatic mechanisms keep them within the limits of a normal range.

The nervous and endocrine systems work together to control homeostasis, but all the organ systems in the body help maintain the normal conditions of the internal environment. The brain contains centers that monitor temperature, pressure, volume, and the chemical conditions of body fluids. Endocrine glands secrete hormones in response to deviations from normal conditions, and these hormones affect other organs. The changes required to bring conditions back to the normal range are mediated by various organ systems. Good health depends on homeostasis. Illness results when the negative feedback mechanisms that maintain homeostasis are disrupted. Medical therapy attempts to assist the negative feedback process to restore balance, or homeostasis.

ANATOMIC TERMS

Certain basic terms need to be understood if one is to communicate effectively in the health care profession. In other words, you have to speak the language. This section explains some basic terms that relate to the anatomy of the body. They are used to describe directions and regions of the body.

Anatomic Position

If directional terms are to be meaningful, there must be some knowledge of the beginning position. If you give a person directions to go somewhere, you must have a starting reference point. When using directions in anatomy and physiology, it is assumed that the body is in **anatomic position.** In this position, the body is standing erect, the face is forward, and the arms are at the sides with the palms and toes directed forward. Figure 5-2 illustrates the body in anatomic position. It is important for medical assistants to understand anatomic positioning because all patient documentation is done as if the patient were in anatomic position.

Directions in the Body

Directional terms are used to describe the relative position of one part to another. Note that in the following list of

Face forward

Arms at sides

Palms directed forward

Standing erect

Toes directed forward

Figure 5-2 The body in anatomic position. (From Applegate E: *The anatomy and physiology learning system,* ed 4, St Louis, 2011, Saunders.)

directional terms, the two items in each pair of terms are opposites.

Superior means that a part is above another part, or closer to the head. The nose is superior to the mouth. *Inferior* means that a part is below another part, or closer to the feet. The heart is inferior to the neck.

Anterior (or ventral) means toward the front surface. The heart is anterior to the vertebral column. *Posterior* means that a part is toward the back. The heart is posterior to the sternum.

Medial means toward, or nearer, the midline of the body. The nose is medial to the ears. *Lateral* means toward, or nearer, the side, away from the midline. The ears are lateral to the eyes.

Proximal means that a part is closer to a point of attachment, or closer to the trunk of the body, than another part. The elbow is proximal to the wrist. The opposite of proximal is *distal,* which means that a part is farther away from a point of attachment than is another part. The fingers are distal to the wrist.

Superficial means that a part is located on or near the surface. The superficial (or outermost) layer of the skin is the epidermis. The opposite of superficial is *deep,* which means that a part is away from the surface. Muscles are deep to the skin.

Visceral pertains to internal organs or the covering of the organs. The visceral pericardium covers the heart. *Parietal* refers to the wall of a body cavity. The parietal peritoneum lines the wall of the abdominal cavity.

Planes and Sections of the Body

To aid in visualizing the spatial relationships of internal body parts, anatomists use three imaginary planes, each of which is cut through the body in a different direction. Figure 5-3 illustrates these three planes. These planes are often used to describe surgical incisions and x-ray positions.

The *sagittal* plane refers to a lengthwise cut that divides the body into right and left portions. This is sometimes called a *longitudinal section.* If the cut passes through the midline of the body, it is called a *midsagittal plane,* and it divides the body into right and left halves.

The *transverse plane* or horizontal plane is perpendicular to the sagittal plane and cuts across the body horizontally to divide it into superior and inferior portions. Sections cut this way are sometimes called *cross sections.*

The *frontal plane* divides the body into anterior and posterior portions. It is perpendicular to both the sagittal plane and the transverse plane. This is sometimes called a *coronal plane.*

Body Cavities

Spaces within the body that contain the internal organs or viscera are called *body cavities.* The two main cavities are the

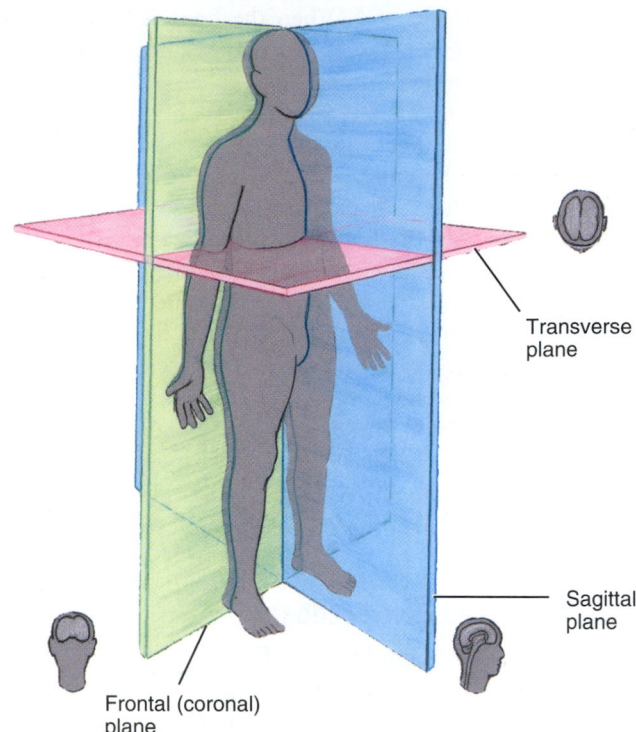

Figure 5-3 Transverse, sagittal, and frontal planes of the body. (From Applegate E: *The anatomy and physiology learning system,* ed 4, St Louis, 2011, Saunders.)

dorsal cavity and the larger *ventral cavity,* which are illustrated in Figure 5-4. The dorsal cavity is divided into the *cranial cavity,* which contains the brain, and the *spinal cavity,* which contains the spinal cord. The cranial and spinal cavities join with each other to form a continuous space.

The ventral cavity is much larger than the dorsal cavity and is subdivided into the *thoracic cavity* and the *abdominopelvic cavity.* The thoracic cavity is superior to the abdominopelvic cavity and contains the heart, lungs, esophagus, and trachea. It is separated from the abdominopelvic cavity by the muscular diaphragm. Although there is no clear-cut partition to divide it, the abdominopelvic cavity is separated into the superior *abdominal cavity* and the inferior *pelvic cavity.* The stomach, liver, gallbladder, spleen, and most of the intestines are in the abdominal cavity. The pelvic cavity contains portions of the small and large intestines, the rectum, the urinary bladder, and the internal reproductive organs.

To help describe the location of body organs or pain, health care professionals frequently divide the abdominopelvic cavity into regions using imaginary lines. One such method uses the midsagittal plane and a transverse plane that passes through the umbilicus. This divides the abdominopelvic area into four quadrants, illustrated in Figure 5-5. Another system uses two sagittal planes and two transverse planes to divide the abdominopelvic area into the nine regions illustrated in Figure 5-6. The three central regions are, from superior to inferior, the *epigastric, umbilical,* and

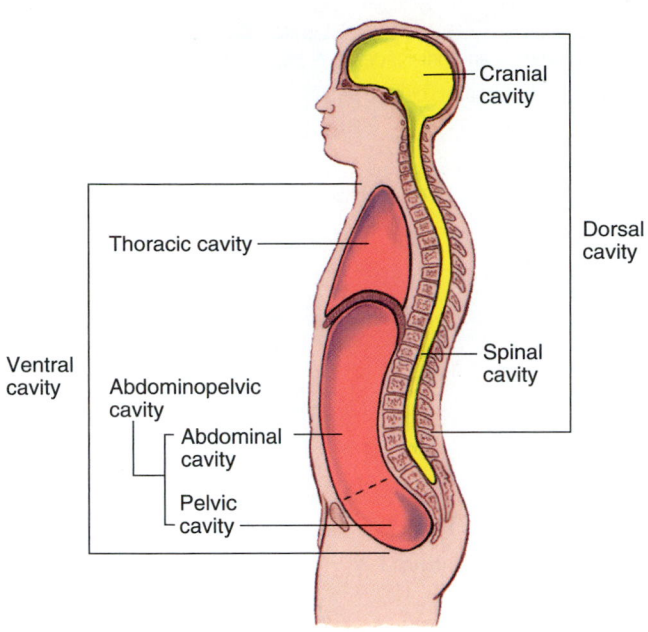

Figure 5-4 The two major cavities in the body and their subdivisions. (From Applegate E: *The anatomy and physiology learning system,* ed 4, St Louis, 2011, Saunders.)

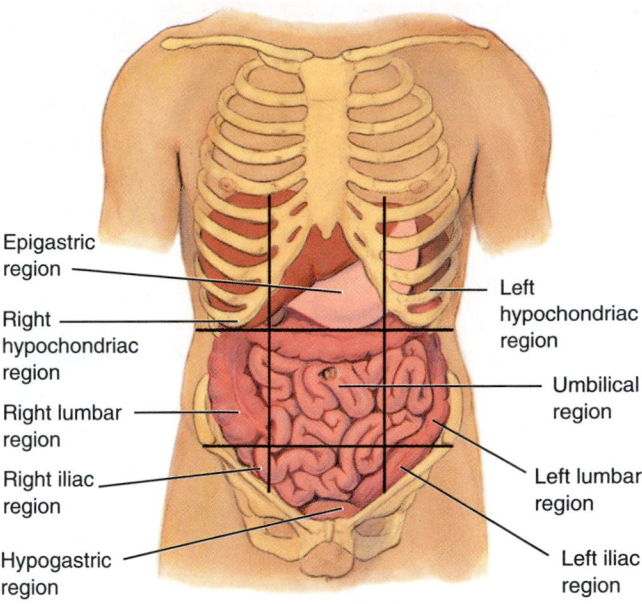

Figure 5-6 Nine abdominopelvic regions formed by two sagittal planes and two transverse planes. (From Applegate E: *The anatomy and physiology learning system,* ed 4, St Louis, 2011, Saunders.)

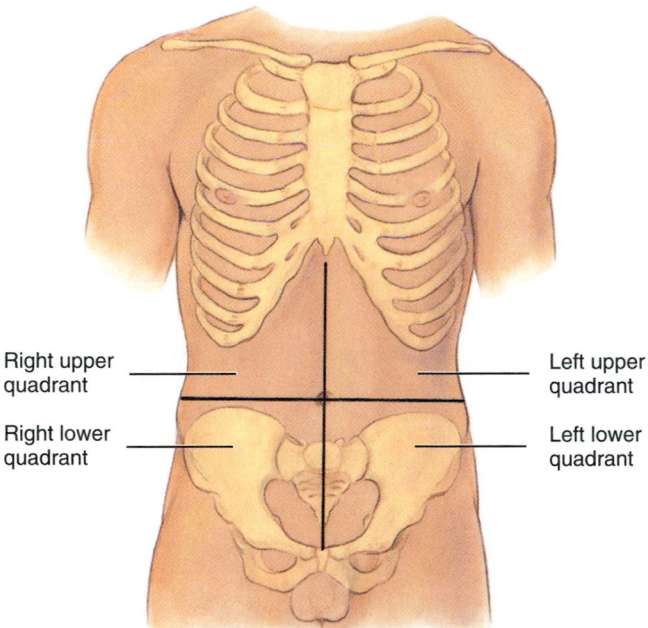

Figure 5-5 Abdominopelvic quadrants that are formed by a midsagittal plane and a transverse plane through the umbilicus. (From Applegate E: *The anatomy and physiology learning system,* ed 4, St Louis, 2011, Saunders.)

hypogastric regions. Lateral to these, from superior to inferior, are the right and left *hypochondriac,* right and left *lumbar,* and right and left *iliac* or *inguinal* regions.

Regions of the Body

The body may be divided into the *axial* portion, which consists of the head, neck, and trunk, and the *appendicular* portion, which consists of the limbs. The trunk, or *torso,* includes the thorax, abdomen, and pelvis. In addition to these terms and the nine abdominopelvic regions identified in the previous section, numerous other terms are applied to specific body areas. Some of these are listed in Table 5-2 and are identified in Figure 5-7.

CELL STRUCTURE AND FUNCTION

STRUCTURE OF THE GENERALIZED CELL

Every individual begins life as a single cell, a fertilized egg. This single cell divides into two cells, then four, eight, 16, and on and on, until the adult human body has an estimated 75 trillion cells. Cells are the structural and functional units of the human body. Homeostasis depends on the interaction between the cell and its environment.

During development, cells become specialized in size, shape, characteristics, and function, resulting in a large variety of cells in the body. For descriptive purposes it is convenient to imagine a typical, generalized cell that contains the components of all the different cell types. Not all the components of a "generalized" cell are present in every

Table 5-2 Body Area Terms

Abdominal (ab-DAHM-ih-nal)	Portion of the trunk between the thorax and pelvis; celiac region
Antebrachial (an-te-BRAY-kee-al)	Region between the elbow and wrist; forearm; cubital region
Antecubital (an-te-KYOO-bih-tal)	Space in front of elbow
Axillary (AK-sih-lair-ee)	Armpit area
Brachial (BRAY-kee-al)	Arm; proximal portion of upper limb
Buccal (BUK-al)	Region of cheek
Buttock (BUT-tuck)	Posterior aspect of lower trunk; gluteal region
Carpal (KAR-pal)	Wrist
Celiac (SEE-lee-ak)	Abdomen
Cephalic (seh-FAL-ik)	Head
Cervical (SER-vih-kal)	Neck region
Costal (KAHS-tal)	Ribs
Cranial (KRAY-nee-al)	Skull
Crural (KROO-rahl)	Portion of lower extremity between knee and foot; leg
Cubital (KYOO-bih-tal)	Forearm; region between elbow and wrist; antebrachial
Cutaneous (kyoo-TAY-nee-us)	Skin
Femoral (FEM-or-al)	Thigh; part of lower extremity between hip and knee
Frontal (FRUN-tal)	Forehead
Gluteal (GLOO-tee-al)	Buttock region
Groin (GROYN)	Depressed region between abdomen and thigh; inguinal
Inguinal (IN-gwih-nal)	Depressed region between abdomen and thigh; groin
Leg (LEG)	Portion of lower extremity between knee and foot; also called *crural region*
Lumbar (LUM-bar)	Region of lower back and side between lowest rib and pelvis
Mammary (MAM-ah-ree)	Pertaining to the breast
Navel (NAY-vel)	Middle region of abdomen; umbilical region
Occipital (ahk-SIP-ih-tal)	Lower portion of the back of the head
Ophthalmic (off-THAL-mik)	Pertaining to the eyes
Oral (OH-ral) or (AW-ral)	Pertaining to the mouth
Otic (OH-tik)	Ears
Palmar (PAWL-mar)	Palm of hand
Pectoral (PEK-toh-ral)	Chest region
Pedal (PED-al)	Foot
Pelvic (PEL-vik)	Inferior region of abdominopelvic cavity
Perineal (pair-ih-NEE-al)	Region between anus and pubic symphysis; includes region of external reproductive organs
Plantar (PLAN-tar)	Sole of foot
Popliteal (pop-LIT-ee-al or pop-lih-TEE-al)	Area behind knee
Sacral (SAY-kral)	Posterior region between hip bones
Sternal (STIR-nal)	Anterior midline of the thorax
Tarsal (TAHR-sal)	Ankle and instep of foot
Thigh (THIGH)	Part of lower extremity between hip and knee; femoral region
Thoracic (tho-RAS-ik)	Chest; part of trunk inferior to neck and superior to diaphragm
Umbilical (um-BIL-ih-kal)	Navel; middle region of abdomen
Vertebral (ver-TEE-bral or VER-teh-bral)	Pertaining to spinal column; backbone

From Applegate E: *The anatomy and physiology learning system,* ed 4, St Louis, 2011, Saunders.

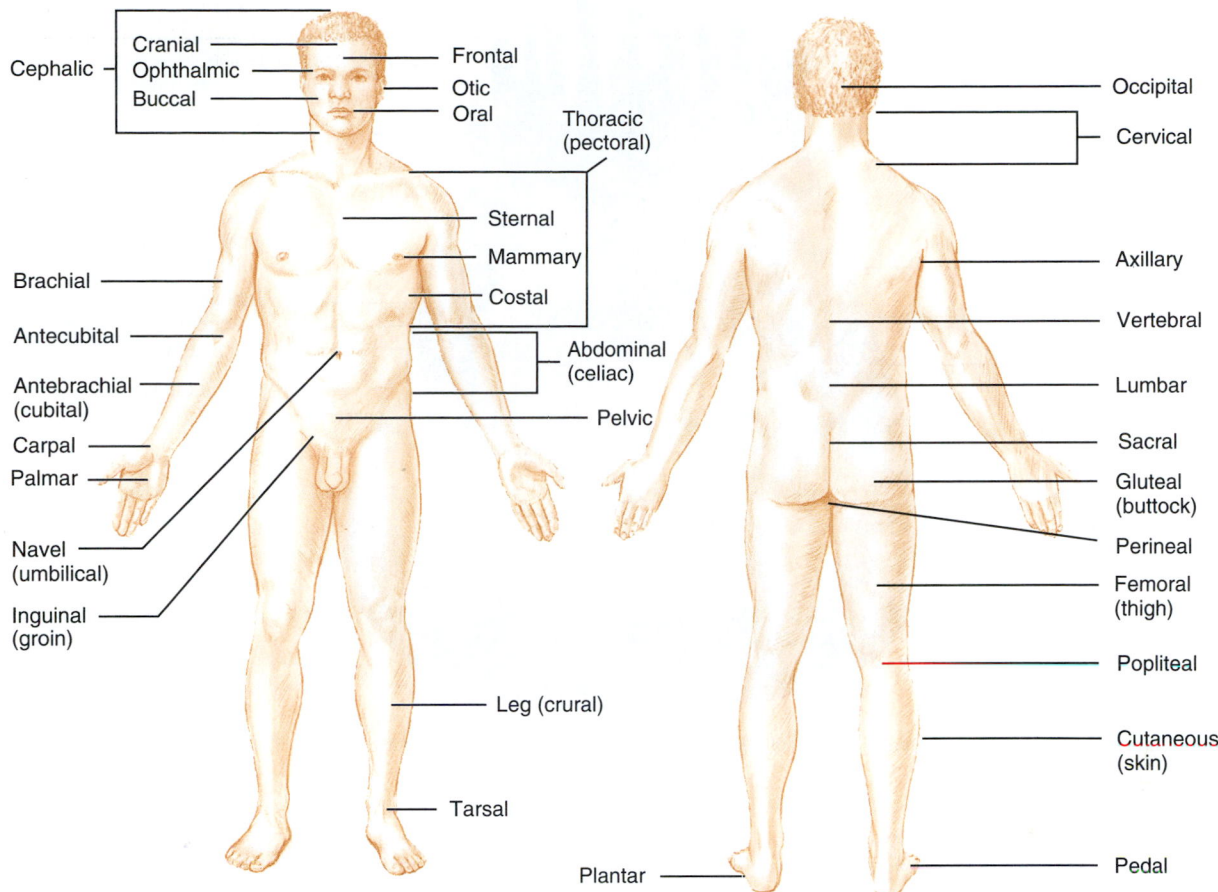

Figure 5-7 Terms for selected regions of the body. (From Applegate E: *The anatomy and physiology learning system,* ed 4, St Louis, 2011, Saunders.)

cell type, but each component is present in some cells and has its particular function to maintain life. A generalized cell is illustrated in Figure 5-8, and the structure and functions of the cellular components are summarized in Table 5-3.

Plasma Membrane

Every cell in the body is enclosed by a *plasma (cell) membrane.* The plasma membrane separates the material outside the cell (extracellular) from the material inside the cell (intracellular). If the membrane breaks, the cell dies. The plasma membrane determines what can go into or out of the cell. It is *selectively permeable,* which means that some substances can pass through the membrane but others cannot. The main structural components of the plasma membrane are *phospholipids* and *proteins.*

Cytoplasm

The *cytoplasm* is the gel-like fluid inside the cell. The cytoplasm has numerous small structures, called *organelles,* suspended in it. These organelles, or "little organs," are the functional machinery of the cell, and each organelle type has a specific role in the metabolic reactions that take place in the cytoplasm.

The cytoplasm is primarily water known as the *intracellular fluid.* About two thirds of the water in the body is in the cytoplasm of cells. The intracellular fluid contains dissolved electrolytes, metabolic waste products, and nutrients such as amino acids and simple sugars.

Nucleus

The *nucleus* is the control center that directs the activities of the cell. All cells have at least one nucleus at some time during their existence; some, however, such as red blood cells, lose their nucleus as they mature. Other cells, such as skeletal muscle cells, have multiple nuclei.

The nucleus is a relatively large, spherical body that is usually located near the center of the cell (see Figure 5-8). It is enclosed by a double-layered *nuclear membrane* that separates the cytoplasm of the cell from the *nucleoplasm,* the fluid portion inside the nucleus.

The nucleus contains the genetic material of the cell. In the nondividing cell, the genetic material, deoxyribonucleic acid (DNA), is present as long, slender, filamentous threads called *chromatin* (see Figure 5-8). When the cell starts to divide or replicate, the chromatin condenses and becomes tightly coiled to form short, rodlike *chromosomes.* Each chromosome, composed of DNA with some protein,

Mitochondrion
Secretory vesicle
Nuclear membrane
Nucleolus
Centrioles
Cytoplasm
Cell membrane

Cilia
Rough endoplasmic reticulum
Ribosomes
Lysosome
Chromatin
Microtubules
Nucleus
Golgi apparatus
Smooth endoplasmic reticulum

Figure 5-8 Generalized cell. (From Applegate E: *The anatomy and physiology learning system,* ed 4, St Louis, 2011, Saunders.)

Table 5-3 Structure and Function of Cellular Components

Component	Structure	Function
Plasma membrane	Bilayer of phospholipid and protein molecules	Maintains integrity of cell; controls passage of materials into and out of cell
Cytoplasm	Water; dissolved ions and nutrients; suspended colloids	Medium for chemical reactions; suspending medium for organelles
Nucleus	Spheric body near center of cell; enclosed in a membrane	Contains genetic material; regulates activities of cell
Nuclear membrane	Double-layered membrane around nucleus; has pores	Separates cytoplasm from nucleoplasm; pores allow passage of material as needed
Chromatin	Strands of DNA in nucleus	Genetic material of cell; becomes chromosomes during cell division
Nucleolus	Dense, nonmembranous body in nucleus; composed of RNA and protein molecules	Forms ribosomes
Mitochondria	Rod-shaped bodies enclosed by a double-layered membrane in cytoplasm; folds of inner membrane form cristae	Major site of adenosine triphosphate synthesis; convert energy from nutrients into a form that is usable by the body
Ribosomes	Granules of RNA in cytoplasm	Protein synthesis
Endoplasmic reticulum	Interconnected membranous channels and sacs in cytoplasm	Transports material through cytoplasm; rough endoplasmic reticulum aids in synthesis of protein; smooth endoplasmic reticulum involved in lipid synthesis
Golgi apparatus	Group of flattened membranous sacs usually near nucleus	Packages products for secretion; forms lysosomes
Lysosomes	Membranous sacs of digestive enzymes in cytoplasm	Digest material taken into cell, debris from damaged cells, worn-out cell components
Cytoskeleton	Protein microfilaments and microtubules in cytoplasm	Provides support for cytoplasm; helps in movement of organelles
Centrioles	Pair of rod-shaped bodies composed of microtubules; located near nucleus at right angles to each other	Distribute chromosomes to daughter cells during cell division
Cilia	Membrane-enclosed bundles of microtubules that extend outward from cell membrane; short and numerous	Move substances across surface of cell
Flagella	Similar to cilia, except usually long and single	Cell locomotion

From Applegate E: *The anatomy and physiology learning system,* ed 4, St Louis, 2011, Saunders.

contains several hundred genes arranged in a specific linear order. Human cells have 23 pairs of chromosomes that together contain all the information necessary to direct the synthesis of more than 100,000 different proteins.

The *nucleolus* ("little nucleus") appears as a dark-staining, discrete, dense body within the nucleus (see Figure 5-1). It has no enclosing membrane, and the number of nucleoli may vary from one to four in any given cell. The function of the nucleolus is to produce ribonucleic acid (RNA) and combine it with protein to form ribosomes. Ribosomes function in protein synthesis, as described later in this section. In growing cells and other cells that are making large amounts of protein, the nucleoli are large and distinct.

Cytoplasmic Organelles

Cytoplasmic organelles are "little organs" that are suspended in the cytoplasm of the cell. Each type of organelle has a definite structure and a specific role in the function of the cell.

Mitochondria

Mitochondria are elongated, oval, fluid-filled sacs in the cytoplasm that contain their own DNA and can reproduce themselves (see Figure 5-8). Enzymes necessary for the production of adenosine triphosphate (ATP) are located inside the mitochondria. ATP is a chemical that stores chemical energy within the cell and provides energy for use by the body cells. Mitochondria could be called the "power plant" of the cell because they convert energy from nutrients into ATP.

Ribosomes

Ribosomes consist of small granules of RNA located in the cytoplasm. The RNA in the ribosomes is from the nucleolus; when fully assembled, ribosomes function in protein synthesis. Some ribosomes are found free in the cytoplasm. These ribosomes function in the synthesis of proteins for use within that same cell. Other ribosomes are attached to the membranes of the endoplasmic reticulum (ER) and function in the synthesis of proteins that are exported from the cell and used elsewhere.

Endoplasmic Reticulum

The *endoplasmic reticulum* (ER) is a complex series of membranous channels extending throughout the cytoplasm. The interconnected membranes form fluid-filled flattened sacs and tubular canals. The membranes are connected to the outer layer of the nuclear membrane, to the inner layer of the cell membrane, and to certain other organelles. The ER provides a path to transport materials from one part of the cell to another.

Some of the membranes of the ER have granular ribosomes attached to the outer surface (see Figure 5-8). This is called *rough endoplasmic reticulum* (RER) and, because of the ribosomes, it functions in the synthesis and transport of protein molecules. Other portions of the ER lack the

ribosomes and appear smooth. This is the *smooth endoplasmic reticulum* (SER), which functions in the synthesis of certain lipid molecules, such as steroids.

Golgi Apparatus

The *Golgi apparatus* is a series of four to six flattened membranous sacs, usually located near the nucleus, and is connected to the ER (see Figure 5-8). It is the "packaging and shipping plant" of the cell.

Proteins and lipids are carried through the channels of the ER to the Golgi apparatus. Within the Golgi apparatus, the proteins become surrounded by a piece of the Golgi membrane. Then they are pinched off the end of the apparatus to become a *secretory vesicle,* a temporary inclusion in the cytoplasm. The secretory vesicles move to the cell membrane and release their contents to the exterior of the cell.

The Golgi apparatus is especially abundant and well developed in glandular cells that secrete a product, but it also functions in nonsecretory cells. In these cells it appears to package intracellular enzymes in the form of lysosomes. Because of the vesicles pinching off the ends of the flattened membranous sacs, the Golgi apparatus is sometimes described as looking like a stack of pancakes with syrup dripping off the edge.

Lysosomes

Lysosomes are membrane-enclosed sacs of various enzymes that have been packaged by the Golgi apparatus. When cells are damaged, these enzymes destroy the cellular debris. They also function in the destruction of worn-out cell parts. The enzymes break down particles, such as bacteria, that have been taken into the cell. When a white blood cell engulfs bacteria, the enzymes from the lysosomes destroy the bacteria. Lysosomal activity also seems to be responsible for decreasing the size of some body organs at certain periods. Atrophy of muscle because of lack of use, reduction in breast size after breastfeeding, and decrease in the size of the uterus after parturition all seem to be caused by lysosomal function.

Filamentous Protein Organelles

Several types of protein filaments are considered to be cellular organelles. The cytoskeleton and centrioles are in the cytoplasm, but the cilia and flagella project outward, away from the cell surface.

Cytoskeleton

The *cytoskeleton* helps to maintain the shape of the cell. At times it anchors certain organelles in position, but it may also move organelles from one position to another. Some parts of the cytoskeleton may move a portion of the cell membrane, whereas others may move the entire cell. The cytoskeleton also plays a role in muscle contraction.

The cytoskeleton is made up of protein *microfilaments* and *microtubules*. Microfilaments are long, slender rods of protein that support small projections of the cell membrane called *microvilli*. Microtubules are thin hollow cylinders. They are found in centrioles, cilia, and flagella.

Centrioles

A dense area called the *centrosome* is located near the nucleus and contains a pair of *centrioles* (see Figure 5-8). Each centriole is a nonmembranous rod-shaped structure composed of microtubules. Centrioles function in cell reproduction by aiding in the distribution of chromosomes to the new daughter cells.

Cilia

Cilia are short, cylindric, hairlike processes that project outward from the cell membrane. Each cilium consists of specialized microtubules surrounded by a membrane and anchored under the cell membrane. Cilia create a wavelike motion to move substances across the surface of the cell. They are found in large quantities on the surfaces of cells that line the respiratory tract. Their motion moves mucus, in which particles of dust are embedded, upward and away from the lungs.

Flagella

Similar in structure to cilia, *flagella* are much longer and fewer. In contrast to cilia, which move substances across the surface of the cell, flagella beat with a whiplike motion to move the cell itself. In the human, the tail of the spermatozoon, or sperm cell, is a single flagellum that causes the swimming motion of the cell.

CELL FUNCTIONS

The structural and functional characteristics of different types of cells are determined by the nature of the proteins present. Cells of various types have different functions because cell structure and function are closely related. A very thin cell is not well suited for a protective function. Bone cells do not have an appropriate structure for nerve impulse conduction. Just as there are many cell types, there are varied cell functions. The specific functions of cells will become more apparent as the tissues, organs, and systems are studied. This section deals with the more generalized cell functions—the functions that relate to the sustained viability and continuation of the cell itself. These functions include movement of substances across the cell membrane, cell division to make new cells, and protein synthesis.

Movement of Substances Across the Cell Membrane

The cell membrane provides a surface through which substances enter and leave the cell. The cell membrane controls the composition of the cell's cytoplasm by regulating the passage of substances through the membrane. If the membrane breaks, this control is removed and the cell dies. The survival of the cell depends on maintaining the difference between extracellular and intracellular material. Mechanisms of movement across the cell membrane include

Table 5-4 Summary of Membrane Transport Mechanisms

Mechanism	Description
Passive	
Simple diffusion	Molecular movement down a concentration gradient
Osmosis	Movement of solvent toward high solute (low solvent) concentration; requires membrane
Filtration	Movement of solvent using hydrostatic pressure; requires membrane filter
Active	
Active transport	Movement of ions or molecules against a concentration gradient; requires carrier molecule and adenosine triphosphate (ATP)
Phagocytosis	Ingestion of solid particles by creation of vesicles; requires ATP
Pinocytosis	Ingestion of fluid by creation of vesicles; requires ATP
Exocytosis	Secretion of cellular products by creation of vesicles, then liberation of contents to outside of cell; requires ATP

From Applegate E: *The anatomy and physiology learning system,* ed 4, St Louis, 2011, Saunders.

diffusion, osmosis, filtration, active transport, endocytosis, and exocytosis. These are summarized in Table 5-4.

Diffusion

Diffusion is the movement of substances from a region of high concentration to a region of low concentration. Odors permeate a room because the aromatic molecules diffuse through the air. A crystal of dye will color a whole beaker of water because the dye particles diffuse from the region of high concentration in the dye crystal to regions of low concentration in the water (Figure 5-9).

In the examples of diffusion cited, there has been no membrane involved. Diffusion can also occur across a membrane as long as the membrane is permeable to the substances involved. For example, oxygen and carbon dioxide are able to diffuse through the cell membrane. When carbon dioxide builds up in the capillaries to a concentration that is higher than in the lungs, the carbon dioxide diffuses into the lungs to be exhaled. Similarly, when the level of oxygen in the capillaries is lower than the level of oxygen in the lungs, oxygen diffuses into the capillaries for distribution to the body cells. In this way, the gases are exchanged between the air and the blood in the lungs, and between the blood and the cells of the various tissues (Figure 5-10).

Osmosis

Osmosis involves the movement of *solvent* (water) molecules through a *selectively permeable* membrane from a region of higher concentration of water molecules (where the *solute* concentration is lower) to a region of

Figure 5-9 Simple diffusion. Molecules of solute diffuse throughout the solvent until equilibrium exists. (From Applegate E: *The anatomy and physiology learning system,* ed 4, St Louis, 2011, Saunders.)

Figure 5-10 Diffusion of oxygen and carbon dioxide in the lungs. Oxygen moves from the higher concentration in the lung into the lower concentration in the capillary. Carbon dioxide moves in the opposite direction. (From Applegate E: *The anatomy and physiology learning system,* ed 4, St Louis, 2011, Saunders.)

lower concentration of water molecules (where the solute concentration is higher). Figure 5-11 illustrates osmosis. When equilibrium is reached, the solutions on both sides of the membrane have the same concentration, but the solution that was more concentrated at the start will now have a greater volume. Water molecules continue to pass through the membrane after equilibrium, but because they move in both directions at the same rate there is no change in concentration or volume.

If a red blood cell, which contains 5% glucose, is placed in a container of 5% glucose solution, water will move in both directions at the same rate because the glucose concentrations inside and outside the cell are the same. Solutions that have the same solute concentration are *isotonic* (Figure 5-12, *A*).

When a red blood cell is placed in a 10% glucose solution, water will leave the cell (where there are more water molecules) and enter the surrounding fluid (where there are fewer water molecules). When fluid leaves the cells, they will shrink or *crenate*. The 10% glucose solution has a greater solute concentration than the cell. It is *hypertonic* to the cell (Figure 5-12, *B*).

When a red blood cell is placed in distilled water, water will enter the cell because there are more water molecules outside the cell than inside. The distilled water has a lower solute concentration than the cell. It is *hypotonic* to the cell. As water enters the cell, it will swell because of the increased volume. If enough water goes into the cell, it may rupture. This is called *lysis*. When this happens to a red blood cell, it is called *hemolysis* (Figure 5-12, *C*).

The terms *isotonic, hypotonic,* and *hypertonic* are relative. They are used to compare two solutions. A 5% glucose solution is hypertonic to distilled water but hypotonic to a 10% glucose solution.

Filtration

In diffusion and osmosis, particles (whether solute, solvent, or both) pass through a membrane by virtue of their own random movement, which is directed by a difference in concentration. In *filtration,* however, pressure pushes the particles through a membrane. Drip coffee makers, for example, use this principle. Water first drips through the coffee, and then the water and small particles pass through a filter. The large granules of coffee are too big to go through

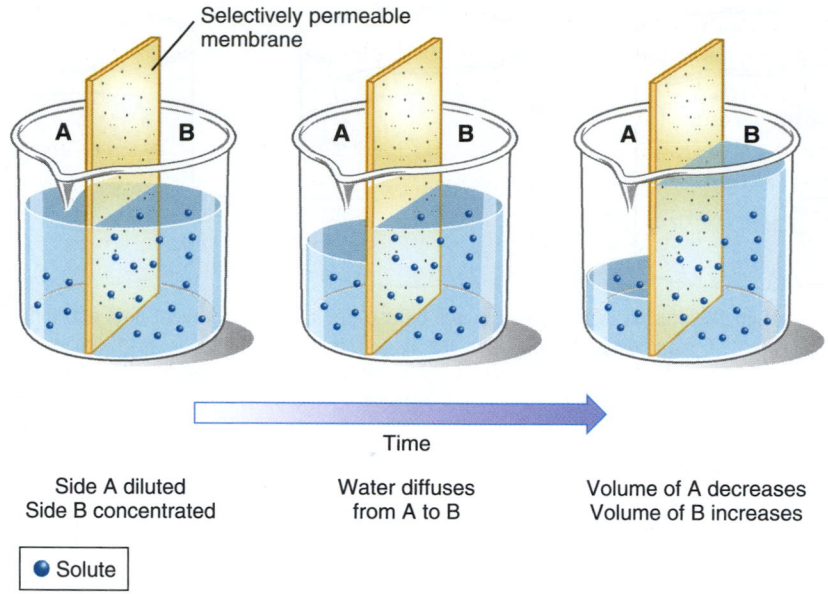

Side A diluted
Side B concentrated

Water diffuses
from A to B

Volume of A decreases
Volume of B increases

● Solute

Figure 5-11 Osmosis. Solvent molecules move across the membrane but solute molecules do not because the membrane is selectively permeable. (From Applegate E: *The anatomy and physiology learning system,* ed 4, St Louis, 2011, Saunders.)

Figure 5-12 **A,** Isotonic solution. The extracellular concentration equals the intracellular concentration and there is no net movement of solvent. **B,** Hypertonic solution. The extracellular concentration is greater than the intracellular concentration, and fluid moves from the cell into the surrounding fluid. The cell shrinks (crenates). **C,** Hypotonic solution. The extracellular concentration is less than the intracellular concentration, and the solvent moves into the cell. The cell expands. (From Applegate E: *The anatomy and physiology learning system,* ed 4, St Louis, 2011, Saunders.)

the pores in the filter. The size of the pores determines the size of the particles that can pass through the filter. The pressure is created by the weight of the water on the paper filter.

Contraction of the heart creates pressure in the blood. This fluid pressure or *hydrostatic pressure,* which is greater inside the blood vessels, pushes fluid, dissolved nutrients, and small ions through the capillary walls to form tissue fluid. The large protein molecules and blood cells are unable to pass through the pores in the capillary membrane. Blood is filtered through specialized membranes in the kidney as the initial step in urine formation. Water and small molecules and ions pass through the filtration membrane

while blood cells and protein molecules remain in the blood.

Active Transport

In the transport mechanisms discussed thus far, no cellular energy has been involved and the molecules and/or ions have moved from a region of high concentration to one of low concentration. **Active transport** differs from these processes in that it moves molecules and ions "uphill" from an area of lower concentration to an area of higher concentration. To accomplish this, cellular energy is required in the form of ATP. If ATP is not available, active transport ceases immediately. Active transport also uses a carrier molecule.

As a result of active transport, some substances are present in significantly higher concentrations on one side of the cell membrane than on the other. For example, sodium ions are more concentrated outside the plasma membrane than inside the cell. Potassium is just the opposite; its concentration is higher inside the cell. Active transport maintains concentration gradients. Normal **passive transport,** such as diffusion and osmosis, tends to equalize the concentrations on the two sides of the membrane.

Endocytosis

Endocytosis refers to the formation of vesicles to transfer particles and droplets from outside to inside the cell. In this case the material is too large to enter the cell by diffusion or active transport. The process requires energy in the form of ATP. **Phagocytosis,** which means "cell eating," is a form of endocytosis that involves solid material. The cell membrane engulfs a particle to form a vesicle in the cytoplasm. Lysosomes fuse with the vesicle, and the enzymes digest the particle. Certain white blood cells are called *phagocytes* because they engulf and destroy bacteria in this manner. Another form of endocytosis is **pinocytosis** or "cell drinking." It differs from phagocytosis in that the vesicles that are formed are much smaller and their contents are fluids. Pinocytosis is important in cells that function in absorption.

Exocytosis

In certain cells, secretory products are packaged into vesicles by the Golgi apparatus and are then released from the cell by a process called *exocytosis.* The secretory vesicle moves to the cell membrane, where the vesicle membrane fuses with the cell membrane, and the contents are discharged to the outside of the cell. Secretion of digestive enzymes from the pancreas and secretion of milk from the mammary glands are examples of exocytosis. Exocytosis and endocytosis are similar except for working in opposite directions. They are both active processes that require cellular energy (ATP). Exocytosis releases substances to the outside of the cell, and endocytosis transports substances to the inside of the cell.

Cell Division

Cell division is the process by which new cells are formed for growth, repair, and replacement in the body. This process includes division of the nuclear material and division of the cytoplasm. Periods of growth and repair are special periods in the life of an individual when it is obvious that new cells are needed either to increase the number of cells or to repair tissues after an injury. General maintenance and replacement needs of the body may not be quite as obvious. More than 2 million red blood cells are worn out and replaced in the body every second of every day. Skin cells are continually sloughed off the body's surface and must be replaced. The lining of the stomach is replaced every few days. All cells in the body (somatic cells), except those that give rise to the eggs and sperm (gametes), reproduce by *mitosis.* Egg and sperm cells are produced by a special type of nuclear division called *meiosis,* in which the

number of chromosomes is halved. Division of the cytoplasm is called **cytokinesis**.

Mitosis

All somatic cells reproduce by **mitosis,** in which a single cell divides to form two new "daughter cells," each identical to the parent cell. Humans have 23 pairs of chromosomes (or 46 chromosomes) in their cells. Each new cell that forms must also have that same number. For this to occur, events must proceed in an organized manner, chromosome material must replicate exactly, and then the chromosomes must separate precisely so that each new cell receives a set of chromosomes that is a carbon copy of the parent cells. For descriptive purposes, it is convenient to divide the events of mitosis into stages, as illustrated in Figure 5-13. It is important to remember that the process is a continual one and that there are no starting and stopping points along the way.

Except for size, the two newly formed daughter cells are exact copies of the parent cell. The two daughter cells carry out designated cellular functions and undergo mitosis as needed.

Normally, body cells divide at a rate required to replace the dying ones. Normal cells are subject to control mechanisms that prevent overpopulation and competition for nutrients and space. Occasionally a series of events occurs that alters some cells, so they lack the control mechanisms that tell them when to stop dividing. When the cells do not stop their mitotic activity, they form an abnormal growth called a *tumor* or neoplasm.

Meiosis

Meiosis is a special type of cell division that occurs in the production of the gametes, or eggs and sperm. These cells have only 23 chromosomes, one half the number found in somatic cells, so that when fertilization takes place the resulting cell will again have 46 chromosomes, 23 from the egg and 23 from the sperm. Meiosis consists of two cell divisions, but the DNA is replicated only once. The result is four cells, but each one has only 23 chromosomes. Figure 5-14 compares mitosis and meiosis.

DNA Replication and Protein Synthesis

Proteins that are synthesized in the cytoplasm function as structural materials, enzymes that regulate chemical reactions, hormones, and other vital substances. Because DNA in the nucleus directs the synthesis of the proteins in the cytoplasm, it ultimately determines the structural and functional characteristics of an individual. Whether a person has blue or brown eyes, brown or blond hair, or light or dark skin is determined by the types of proteins synthesized in response to the genetic information contained in the DNA in the nucleus. The portion of a DNA molecule that contains the genetic information for making one particular protein molecule is called a *gene.* If a cell produced for replacement or repair is to function exactly as its predecessor, then it must have the same genes, a carbon copy of the DNA. This is the purpose of DNA replication in cell division.

Figure 5-13 Mitosis. **A,** Interphase is the period between active cell divisions. During this time the DNA, mitochondria, and centrioles replicate. It is the longest period of the cell cycle. **B,** Prophase is the first stage in mitosis. The chromatin shortens and thickens to form chromosomes, each with two chromatids connected by a centromere. Spindle fibers form and the nucleolus and nuclear membrane disintegrate. **C,** Metaphase shows the chromosomes aligned along the center of the cell. **D,** Anaphase shows the spindle fibers pulling each chromatid of a chromosome to opposite ends of the cell. **E,** Telophase shows the chromosomes reaching the centrioles at the ends of the cell. A new nuclear membrane and nucleolus form. Cytokinesis occurs. **F,** Daughter cells are two new interphase cells exactly like the parent cell. (From Applegate E: *The anatomy and physiology learning system,* ed 4, St Louis, 2011, Saunders.)

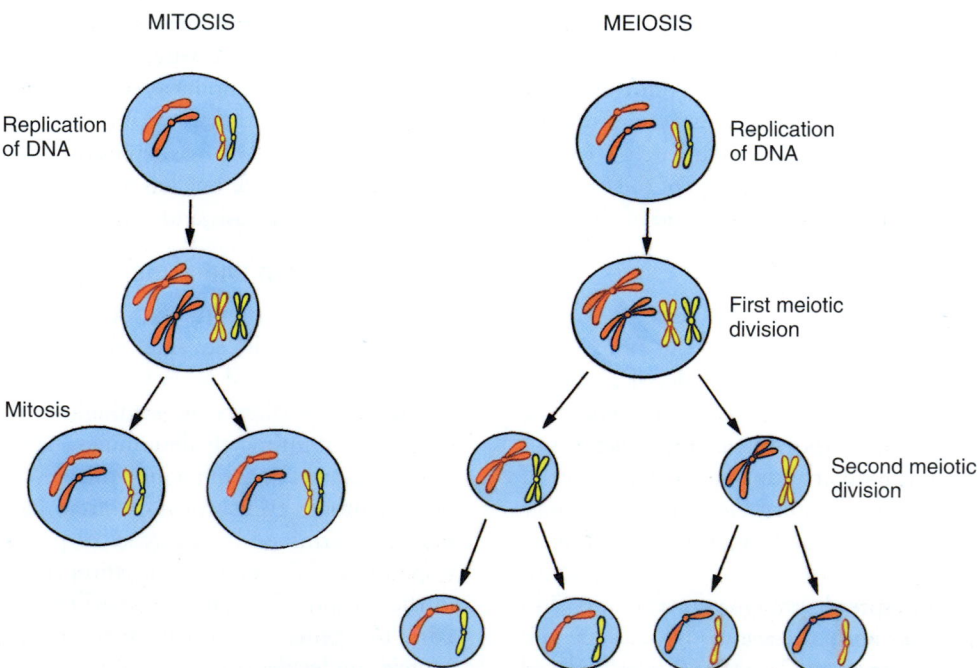

Figure 5-14 Comparison of mitosis and meiosis. The result of mitosis in humans is two cells, each with 46 chromosomes (23 pairs). Meiosis results in four cells, each with 23 chromosomes. (From Applegate E: *The anatomy and physiology learning system,* ed 4, St Louis, 2011, Saunders.)

HIGHLIGHT on Cells and Tissues

Congenital Abnormalities

Often, congenital anatomic abnormalities must be surgically repaired so that disruptions in physiology are corrected. For example, a cleft palate (anatomy) is repaired so that food will enter (physiology) the pharynx instead of the nasal cavity. Broken bones (anatomy) are reset so that function (physiology) is restored.

Kidney Dialysis

Normally functioning kidneys remove waste products from the blood. When the kidneys do not function properly, waste molecules can be removed from the blood artificially by a process called *dialysis.* Dialysis is a form of diffusion in which the size of the pores in a selectively permeable membrane separates smaller solute particles from larger solutes. In kidney dialysis, small waste molecules pass through the membrane and are removed from the blood. The protein molecules, which are needed in the blood, are too large to pass through the pores and thus are retained.

Neoplasms

A benign neoplasm consists of highly organized cells that closely resemble normal tissue. In contrast, a malignant neoplasm, or cancer, consists of unorganized and immature cells that are incapable of normal function. These cells may detach from the tumor site and travel in the blood or lymph to another site and establish a new tumor. This is called *metastasis* and is probably the most devastating property of malignant cells. Tumors are named according to the tissue from which they are derived. For example, a

benign tumor of glandular epithelial cells is called an *adenoma.* A *lipoma* is derived from fat cells, a *myoma* is formed from muscle tissue, and a *papilloma* may occur on any epithelial surface or lining. Carcinomas are solid cancerous tumors that are derived from epithelial tissue. An adenocarcinoma is a cancerous tumor arising from glandular cells. S*arcomas* are malignant growths derived from connective tissue cells. Approximately 85% of all malignant neoplasms are carcinomas. These account for approximately 10% of all malignant neoplasms.

Genetic Disorders

Genetic disorders are pathologic conditions caused by mistakes, or mutations, in a cell's genetic code. Mutations may occur naturally, or they may be induced by mutagens, such as radiation and certain chemicals. If the mutations occur in the gametes, the faulty code is passed from one generation to the next. Errors in the genes (DNA) cause the production of abnormal proteins, which result in abnormal cellular function. For example, in sickle cell anemia, a genetic blood disorder, red blood cells have abnormal hemoglobin because there is an "error" in the gene that directs hemoglobin synthesis.

Peritonitis

An inflammation of the serous membranes in the abdominal cavity is called *peritonitis.* This is sometimes a serious complication of an infected appendix. ∎

TISSUES AND MEMBRANES

A **tissue** is a group of cells that have similar structure and that function together as a unit. The microscopic study of tissues is called **histology.** A nonliving material called the *intercellular matrix* fills the spaces between cells. This may be abundant in some tissues and scarce in others. The intercellular matrix may contain special substances, such as salts and fibers, that are unique to a specific tissue and give the tissue distinctive characteristics.

BODY TISSUES

Four main tissue types are found in the body: epithelial, connective, muscle, and nervous. Each is designed for specific functions.

Epithelial Tissue

Epithelial tissues are widespread throughout the body. They form the covering of all body surfaces, line body cavities and hollow organs, and are the major tissue in glands. They perform a variety of functions that include protection, secretion, absorption, excretion, filtration, diffusion, and sensory reception.

The cells in epithelial tissue are tightly packed with little intercellular matrix. Because the tissues form coverings and linings, the cells have one free surface that is not in contact with other cells. Opposite the free surface, the cells are attached to underlying connective tissue by a noncellular *basement membrane.* Because epithelial tissues are typically *avascular* (without blood vessels), they must receive their nutrients and oxygen supply by diffusion from the blood vessels in the underlying tissues. Another characteristic of epithelial tissues is that they regenerate, or reproduce, quickly. For example, the cells of the skin and stomach are continually damaged and replaced, and skin abrasions heal quite rapidly.

Epithelia are classified according to cell shape and the number of layers in the tissue. Classified according to shape, the cells are squamous, cuboidal, or columnar, and the shape of the nucleus corresponds to the cell shape. *Squamous* cells are flat and the nuclei are usually broad and thin. *Cuboidal* cells are cubelike, as tall as they are wide, and the nuclei are spherical and centrally located. *Columnar* cells are tall and narrow, resembling columns, and the nuclei are usually in the lower portion of the cell near the basement membrane. According to the number of layers, epithelia are *simple* if they have only one layer of cells and *stratified* if they have multiple layers. Stratified epithelia are named

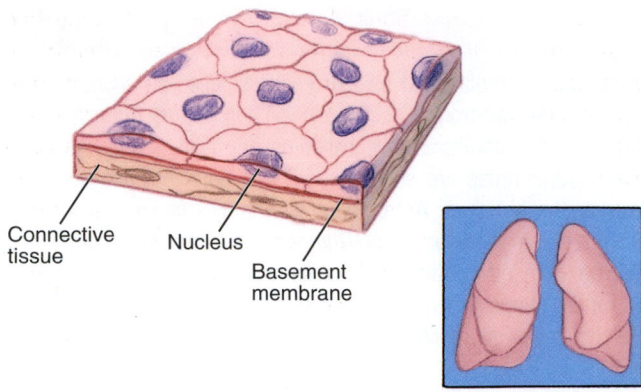

Figure 5-15 Simple squamous epithelium in the alveoli of the lungs. It is also found in capillary walls and in renal corpuscles of the kidney. (From Applegate E: *The anatomy and physiology learning system,* ed 4, St Louis, 2011, Saunders.)

Figure 5-16 Simple cuboidal epithelium in the kidney tubules. It is also found in many glands and as a covering of the ovary. (From Applegate E: *The anatomy and physiology learning system,* ed 4, St Louis, 2011, Saunders.)

according to the type of cells at the free surface of the tissue.

Simple Squamous Epithelium

Simple squamous epithelium (Figure 5-15) consists of a single layer of thin, flat cells that fit closely together with little intercellular matrix. Because it is so thin, simple squamous epithelium is well suited for areas in which diffusion and filtration take place. The alveoli or air sacs of the lungs, where diffusion of oxygen and carbon dioxide gases occurs, are made of simple squamous epithelium. This tissue is also found in the kidney, where the blood is filtered. Capillary walls, where oxygen and carbon dioxide diffuse between the blood and tissues, are made of simple squamous epithelium. Because it is so thin and delicate, this tissue is damaged easily and offers little protective function.

Simple Cuboidal Epithelium

Simple cuboidal epithelium (Figure 5-16) consists of a single layer of cube-shaped cells. These cells have more volume than squamous cells and also have more organelles. Simple cuboidal epithelium is found as a covering of the ovary, as a lining of kidney tubules, and in many glands, such as the thyroid, pancreas, and salivary glands. In the kidney tubules, the tissue functions in absorption and secretion. In glands, simple cuboidal cells form the secretory portions and the ducts that deliver the products to their destination.

Simple Columnar Epithelium

A single layer of cells that are taller than they are wide makes up *simple columnar epithelium* (Figure 5-17). The nuclei are in the bottom portion of the cell near the basement membrane. Simple columnar epithelium is found lining the stomach and intestines, where it secretes digestive enzymes and absorbs nutrients. Because the cells are taller (or thicker) than either squamous or cuboidal cells, this tissue offers some protection to underlying tissues.

In regions where absorption is of primary importance, such as in parts of the digestive tract, the cell membrane on

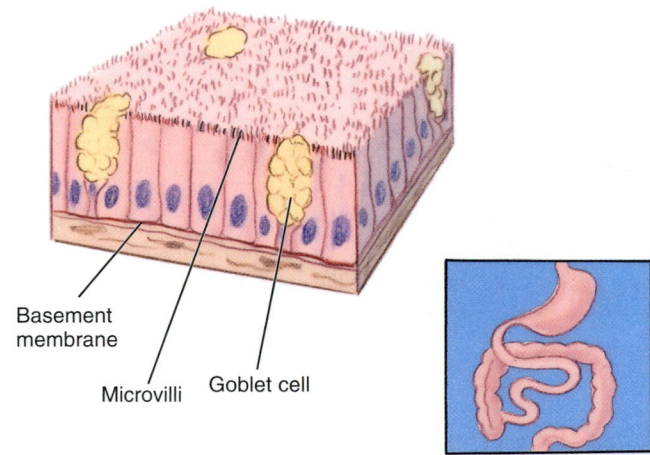

Figure 5-17 Simple columnar epithelium in the lining of the stomach and intestines. (From Applegate E: *The anatomy and physiology learning system,* ed 4, St Louis, 2011, Saunders.)

the free surface has numerous small projections called *microvilli.* Microvilli increase the surface area that is available for absorption of nutrients. *Goblet cells* are frequently interspersed among the simple columnar cells. Goblet cells are flask- or goblet-shaped cells that secrete mucus onto the free surface of the tissue. Cilia may be present to move secretions along the surface.

Pseudostratified Columnar Epithelium

Pseudostratified columnar epithelium (Figure 5-18) appears to have multiple layers (stratified), but it really does not. This is because the cells are not all the same height. Some cells are short and some are tall, and the nuclei are at different levels. Close examination reveals that all the cells are attached to the basement membrane but that not all cells reach the free surface of the tissue. Cilia and goblet cells are often associated with pseudostratified columnar epithelium. This tissue lines portions of the respiratory tract in which

Figure 5-18 Pseudostratified columnar epithelium in the respiratory tract. It also lines some parts of the male reproductive system. (From Applegate E: *The anatomy and physiology learning system,* ed 4, St Louis, 2011, Saunders.)

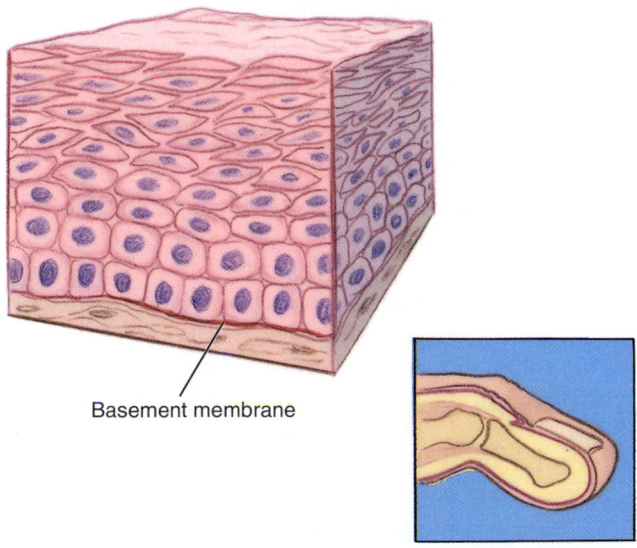

Figure 5-19 Stratified squamous epithelium from the outer layer of the skin. Note the numerous cell layers and the flattened cells at the surface. (From Applegate E: *The anatomy and physiology learning system,* ed 4, St Louis, 2011, Saunders.)

the mucus, produced by the goblet cells, traps dust particles and is then moved upward by the cilia. Pseudostratified columnar epithelium also lines some of the tubes of the male reproductive system. Here the cilia help propel the sperm from one region to another.

Stratified Squamous Epithelium

Stratified squamous epithelium, the most widespread stratified epithelium, is thick because it consists of many layers of cells (Figure 5-19). The cells on the bottom layer, next to the basement membrane, are usually cuboidal or columnar, and these are the cells that undergo mitosis. As the cells are pushed toward the surface, they become thinner, so the

surface cells are squamous. As the cells are pushed farther away from the basement membrane, it is more difficult for them to receive oxygen and nutrients from underlying connective tissue, and the cells die. As cells on the surface are damaged and die, they are sloughed off and replaced by cells from the deeper layers. Because this tissue is thick, it is found in areas in which protection is a primary function. Stratified squamous epithelium forms the outer layer of the skin and extends a short distance into every body opening that is continuous with the skin.

Transitional Epithelium

Transitional epithelium is a specialized type of tissue that has several layers but can be stretched in response to tension. The lining of the urinary bladder is a good example of this type of tissue. When the bladder is empty and contracted, the epithelial lining has several layers of cuboidal cells. As the bladder fills and is distended or stretched, the cells become thinner and the number of layers decreases.

Glandular Epithelium

Glandular epithelium consists of cells that are specialized to produce and secrete substances. Glandular epithelium normally lies deep to the epithelia that cover and line parts of the body. If the gland secretes its product onto a free surface via a duct, it is called an *exocrine gland.* Examples of exocrine glands include sebaceous glands, mammary glands, and salivary glands. If the gland secretes its product directly into the blood, it is a ductless gland, or *endocrine gland.* Endocrine glands are discussed in Chapter 11.

Connective Tissue

Connective tissues bind structures together, form a framework and support for organs and the body as a whole, store fat, transport substances, protect against disease, and help repair tissue damage. They occur throughout the body. Connective tissues are characterized by an abundance of intercellular matrix with relatively few cells. Connective tissue cells are able to reproduce but not as rapidly as epithelial cells. Most connective tissues have a good blood supply, but some do not. Examples of connective tissue include adipose tissue, cartilage, and bone.

The intercellular matrix in connective tissue has a gel-like base of water, nonfibrous protein, and other molecules. Various mineral salts in the matrix of some connective tissues, such as bone, make them hard. Two types of fibers, collagenous and elastic, are frequently embedded in the matrix. **Collagenous fibers,** composed of the protein collagen, are strong and flexible but are only slightly elastic. They are able to withstand considerable pulling force and are found in areas in which this is important, such as in tendons and ligaments. When collagenous fibers are grouped together in parallel bundles, the tissue appears white, so they are sometimes called *white fibers.* **Elastic fibers,** composed of the protein elastin, are not very strong, but they are elastic. They can be stretched and will return to their original shape and length when released. Elastic fibers, also called *yellow fibers,* are located where structures are stretched and released, such as the vocal cords.

Numerous cell types are found in connective tissue. Three of the most common are the *fibroblast, macrophage,* and *mast cell.* As the name implies, **fibroblasts** produce the fibers that are in the intercellular matrix. **Macrophages** are large phagocytic cells that are able to move about and clean up cellular debris and foreign particles from the tissues. **Mast cells** contain heparin, an anticoagulant, and histamine, a substance that promotes inflammation and that is active in allergies.

Loose Connective Tissue

Loose connective tissue, also called *areolar connective tissue,* is one of the most widely distributed tissues in the body. It is the packing material in the body. It attaches the skin to the underlying tissues and fills the spaces between muscles. Most epithelial tissue is anchored to this tissue by the basement membrane, and the blood vessels in the loose connective tissue supply nutrients to the epithelium above. The matrix is characterized by a loose network of collagenous and elastic fibers. The predominant cell is the fibroblast, but other connective tissue cells are also present (Figure 5-20).

Adipose Tissue

Commonly called *fat, adipose tissue* is really a specialized form of loose connective tissue in which there is little intercellular matrix. Some of the cells accumulate liquid triglyceride, or fat, droplets. When this happens, the cytoplasm and nucleus are pushed off to one side, and the cells swell and become closely packed together. Fat cells have the ability to take up fat and then release it at a later time. Adipose tissue forms a protective cushion around the kidneys, heart, eyeballs, and various joints. It also accumulates under the skin, where it provides insulation for heat. Adipose tissue is an efficient energy storage material for excess calories.

Dense Fibrous Connective Tissue

Dense fibrous connective tissue is characterized by closely packed parallel bundles of collagenous fibers in the intercellular matrix. There are relatively few cells, and the ones that are present are fibroblasts to produce the collagenous fibers. This is the tissue that makes up *tendons,* which connect muscles to bones, and *ligaments,* which connect bones to bones. Dense fibrous connective tissue has a poor blood supply, and this, along with the relatively few cells, accounts for the slow healing of this tissue.

Elastic Connective Tissue

Elastic connective tissue has closely packed elastic fibers in the intercellular matrix. This type of tissue yields easily to a pulling force and then returns to its original length as soon as the force is released. The vocal cords and the ligaments that connect adjacent vertebrae are composed of elastic connective tissue.

Cartilage

Cartilage has an abundant matrix that is solid, yet flexible, with fibers embedded in it. The matrix contains the protein *chondrin.* Cartilage cells, or **chondrocytes**, are located in spaces called *lacunae* that are scattered throughout the matrix. Typically, cartilage is surrounded by a dense fibrous connective tissue covering called the *perichondrium.* The perichondrium has blood vessels, but they do not penetrate the cartilage itself, and the cells obtain their nutrients by diffusion through the solid matrix. Cartilage heals slowly because there is no direct blood supply, and this also contributes to slow cellular reproduction. Cartilage protects underlying tissues, supports other structures, and provides a framework for attachments.

Hyaline cartilage (Figure 5-21) is the most common type of cartilage. It has fine collagenous fibers in the matrix and a shiny, white, opaque appearance. It is found at the ends of long bones, in the costal cartilage that connects the ribs to the sternum, and in the supporting rings of the trachea. Most of the fetal skeleton is formed of hyaline cartilage before it is replaced by bone.

Fibrocartilage has an abundance of strong collagenous fibers embedded in the matrix. This allows it to withstand compression, act as a shock absorber, and resist pulling forces. It is found in the intervertebral discs, or pads between the vertebrae; in the symphysis pubis, or pad between the two pubic bones; and between the bones in the knee joint.

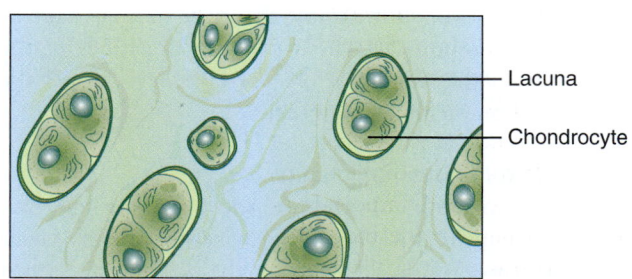

Figure 5-20 Loose (areolar) connective tissue. Note the fibroblasts and the two types of fibers embedded in a gel-like matrix. (From Applegate E: *The anatomy and physiology learning system,* ed 4, St Louis, 2011, Saunders.)

Figure 5-21 Hyaline cartilage. Note the chondrocytes within the lacunae. (From Applegate E: *The anatomy and physiology learning system,* ed 4, St Louis, 2011, Saunders.)

Figure 5-22 Compact bone (osseous tissue). Note the osteons with a central haversian canal and concentric lamellae of matrix. Canaliculi extend from the osteocytes, which are located within lacunae. (From Applegate E: *The anatomy and physiology learning system,* ed 4, St Louis, 2011, Saunders.)

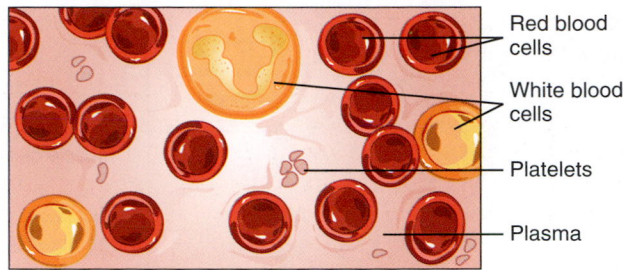

Figure 5-23 Blood. Note the blood cells and platelets, which are suspended in a liquid plasma. (From Applegate E: *The anatomy and physiology learning system,* ed 4, St Louis, 2011, Saunders.)

Figure 5-24 Skeletal muscle. Note the long cylindric fibers with striations. (From Applegate E: *The anatomy and physiology learning system,* ed 4, St Louis, 2011, Saunders.)

Elastic cartilage has numerous yellow elastic fibers embedded in the matrix, which makes it more flexible than hyaline cartilage or fibrocartilage. It is found in the framework of the external ear, the epiglottis, and the auditory tubes.

Bone

Osseous tissue or *bone* is the most rigid of all the connective tissues. Collagenous fibers in the matrix give strength to bone, and its hardness is derived from the mineral salts, particularly calcium, that are deposited around the fibers. Bones form the framework for the body and help protect underlying tissues. They serve as attachments for muscles and act as mechanical levers in producing movement. Bone also contributes to the formation of blood cells and functions as a storage area for mineral salts.

Cylindric structural units, called *osteons* or *haversian systems,* are packed together to form the substance of compact bone (Figure 5-22). The center or hub of the osteon is a tubular *osteonic* or *haversian canal* that contains a blood vessel. The matrix is deposited in concentric rings called *lamellae* around the canal. **Osteocytes,** or bone cells, are located in lacunae between the lamellae, so they are also arranged in concentric rings. Slender processes from the bone cells extend through tiny tubes in the matrix called *canaliculi* to other cells or to the osteonic canals. This provides a readily available blood supply for the bone cells, which allows a faster repair process for bone than for cartilage.

Blood

Blood is a unique connective tissue because it is the only one that has a liquid matrix. It is a vehicle for transport of substances throughout the body. **Erythrocytes**, or red blood cells, and **leukocytes**, or white blood cells, are suspended in a liquid matrix called *plasma* (Figure 5-23). The red blood cells transport oxygen from the lungs to the tissues. White blood cells are important in fighting disease. Another formed element in the blood is the *platelet,* or **thrombocyte,** which is not actually a cell but a fragment of a giant cell in the bone marrow. Platelets are important in initiating the blood clotting process. Blood is discussed in more detail in Chapter 12.

Muscle Tissue

Muscle tissue is composed of cells that have the special ability to shorten or contract to produce movement of body parts. The tissue is highly cellular and is well supplied with blood vessels. The cells are long and slender, so they are sometimes called *muscle fibers,* and these are usually arranged in bundles or layers that are surrounded by connective tissue. Muscle tissue is of three types: skeletal muscle, smooth muscle, and cardiac muscle.

Skeletal Muscle

Skeletal muscle tissue (Figure 5-24) is what is commonly thought of as "muscle." It is the meat of animals, and it constitutes about 40% of an individual's body weight. Skeletal muscle cells (fibers) are long and cylindric with many nuclei (multinucleated) peripherally located next to the cell membrane. The cells have alternating light and dark bands that are perpendicular to the long axis of the cell. These bands are a result of the organized arrangement of the contractile proteins in the cytoplasm and give the cell a *striated* appearance. Skeletal muscle fibers are collected into bundles and wrapped in connective tissue to form the muscles, which are attached to the skeleton and which cause body movements when they contract in response to nerve stimulation. Skeletal muscle action is under conscious or voluntary control. Chapter 8 describes skeletal muscles in more detail.

Smooth Muscle

Smooth muscle tissue (Figure 5-25) is found in the walls of hollow body organs, such as the stomach, intestines, urinary

Figure 5-25 Smooth muscle. Note the spindle-shaped cells with tapered ends. (From Applegate E: *The anatomy and physiology learning system,* ed 4, St Louis, 2011, Saunders.)

Figure 5-26 Cardiac muscle. Note the branching striated cells and intercalated disks. (From Applegate E: *The anatomy and physiology learning system,* ed 4, St Louis, 2011, Saunders.)

Figure 5-27 Neuron (nervous tissue). Note the dendrites, axon, and cell body. (From Applegate E: *The anatomy and physiology learning system,* ed 4, St Louis, 2011, Saunders.)

bladder, uterus, and blood vessels. It normally acts to propel substances through the organ by contracting and relaxing. It is called *smooth muscle* because it lacks the striations evident in skeletal muscle. Because it is found in the viscera or body organs, it is sometimes called *visceral muscle.* Smooth muscle cells are shorter than skeletal muscle cells, are spindle-shaped and tapered at the ends, and have a single, centrally located nucleus. Smooth muscle usually cannot be stimulated to contract by conscious or voluntary effort, so it is called *involuntary muscle.*

Cardiac Muscle

Cardiac muscle tissue (Figure 5-26) is found only in the wall of the heart. The cardiac muscle cells are cylindric and appear striated, similar to skeletal muscle cells. Cardiac muscle cells are shorter than skeletal muscle cells and have only one nucleus per cell. The cells branch and interconnect to form complex networks. At the point where one cell attaches to another, there is a specialized intercellular connection called an *intercalated disc.* Cardiac muscle appears striated like skeletal muscle, but its contraction is involuntary. It is responsible for pumping the blood through the heart and into the blood vessels.

Nervous Tissue

Nervous tissue is found in the brain, spinal cord, and nerves. It is responsible for coordinating and controlling many body activities. It stimulates muscle contraction, creates an awareness of the environment, and plays a major role in emotions, memory, and reasoning. To do all of these things,

cells in nervous tissue need to be able to communicate with one another by way of electrical nerve impulses.

The cells in nervous tissue that generate and conduct impulses are called *neurons* or *nerve cells.* These cells have three principal parts: the dendrites, the cell body, and one axon (Figure 5-27). The main part of the cell, the part that carries on the general functions, is the *neuron cell body.* **Dendrites** are extensions, or processes, of the cytoplasm that carry impulses to the cell body. An extension or process called an **axon** carries impulses away from the cell body.

Nervous tissue also includes cells that do not transmit impulses but instead support the activities of the neurons. These are the *glial cells,* together termed the **neuroglia.** Supporting, or glial, cells bind neurons together and insulate the neurons. Some are phagocytic and protect against bacterial invasion, whereas others provide nutrients by binding blood vessels to the neurons. Further detail on nerve tissue is presented in Chapter 9.

BODY MEMBRANES

Body membranes are thin sheets of tissue that cover the body, line body cavities, cover organs within the cavities, and line the cavities in hollow organs. By this definition, the skin is a membrane because it covers the body, and indeed, the skin, or integument, is sometimes called the **cutaneous membrane.** This membrane is discussed in Chapter 6. This section examines two epithelial membranes and two connective tissue membranes. Epithelial membranes consist of epithelial tissue and the connective tissue to which it is attached. The two main types of epithelial membranes are the mucous membranes and serous membranes. Connective tissue membranes contain only connective tissue. Synovial membranes and meninges belong to this category.

Mucous Membranes

Mucous membranes are epithelial membranes that consist of epithelial tissue attached to underlying loose connective tissue. These membranes (sometimes called *mucosae*) line the body cavities that open to the outside. The entire digestive tract is lined with mucous membranes. Other examples include the respiratory, urinary, and reproductive tracts. The type of epithelium varies depending on its function. In the mouth the epithelium is of the stratified squamous type for its protection function, but the stomach and intestines are lined with simple columnar epithelium for absorption and secretion. The mucosa of the urinary bladder is transitional epithelium so that it can expand. Mucous membranes get their name from the fact that the epithelial cells secrete mucus for lubrication and protection.

Serous Membranes

Serous membranes line body cavities that do not open directly to the outside, and they cover the organs located in those cavities. A serous membrane, or *serosa*, consists of a thin layer of loose connective tissue covered by a layer of simple squamous epithelium called *mesothelium.* These membranes always have two parts. The part that lines a cavity wall is the *parietal* layer, and the part that covers the organs in the cavity is the *visceral* layer (Figure 5-28). Serous membranes are covered by a thin layer of *serous fluid* that is secreted by the epithelium. Serous fluid lubricates the membrane and reduces friction and abrasion when organs in the thoracic or abdominopelvic cavity move against one another or the cavity wall.

Serous membranes have special names according to their location. The serous membrane that lines the thoracic cavity and covers the lungs is the **pleura,** with the parietal pleura lining the cavity and the visceral pleura covering the lungs. The **pericardium** lines the pericardial cavity and covers the heart. The serous membrane in the abdominopelvic cavity is the **peritoneum.**

Synovial Membranes

Synovial membranes are connective tissue membranes that line the cavities of the freely movable joints such as the shoulder, elbow, and knee. Similar to serous membranes, they line cavities that do not open to the outside. Unlike serous membranes, they do not have a layer of epithelium. Synovial membranes secrete *synovial fluid* into the joint cavity, and this lubricates the cartilage on the ends of the bones so that they can move freely and without friction. In certain types of arthritis, these membranes become inflamed and the fluid becomes viscous. This reduces lubrication and

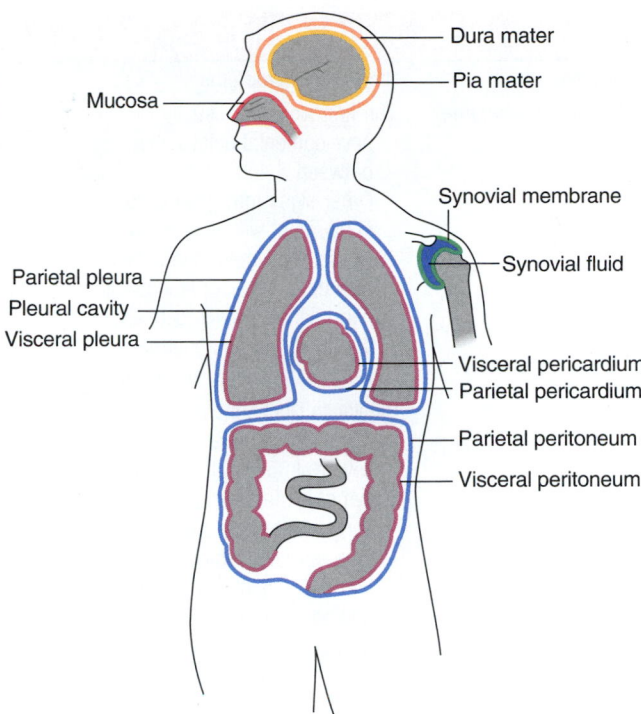

Figure 5-28 Body membranes. (From Applegate E: *The anatomy and physiology learning system,* ed 4, St Louis, 2011, Saunders.)

increases friction, and movement becomes difficult and painful.

Meninges

The connective tissue coverings around the brain and spinal cord, within the dorsal cavity, are called **meninges.** They provide protection for these vital structures. Inflammation of the meninges is *meningitis.* Further discussion of the meninges appears in Chapter 9.

HIGHLIGHT on Conditions Affecting Tissues

Adhesion: Abnormal joining of tissues by fibrous scar tissue
Carcinoma: A malignant growth derived from epithelial cells
Lipoma: Benign tumor derived from fat (adipose) cells
Myoma: Benign tumor formed of muscle tissue
Papilloma: Benign epithelial tumor; may occur on any epithelial surface or lining
Sarcoma: A malignant growth derived from connective tissue cells
Scurvy: A condition caused by a deficiency of vitamin C in the diet, which results in abnormal collagen synthesis ▪

Genetic Diseases and Disorders

Disease	Signs and Symptoms	Etiology	Diagnosis and Treatment
Angelman syndrome (AS)	The first signs are usually developmental delays observed between 6 and 12 month of age. Other signs may include speech impairment with little or no use of words, movement and balance disorders, frequent laughter and hand flapping, microcephaly, seizures, and an abnormal electroencephalogram (EEG).	The syndrome is most often caused by deletion or inactivation of genes on the maternally inherited chromosome 15.	Confirmation of the diagnosis requires genetic studies of a blood sample from the child. There is no cure for AS. Treatment focuses on managing the signs and symptoms and may include antiseizure medication, physical therapy, speech therapy, and behavioral therapy.
Becker muscular dystrophy (BMD)	Similar to Duchenne muscular dystrophy but later onset and less severe. In general, signs and symptoms appear in the teens or early 20s to mid-20s and include frequent falls, difficulty in running or jumping, waddling gait, difficulty getting up from a lying or sitting position, and large calf muscles.	A mutation in a specific gene on the X chromosome disrupts the synthesis of dystrophin, a protein that helps keep muscle cells intact. In BMD the protein is only partially functional, causing muscles to weaken and degenerate.	Diagnosis involves enzyme tests, electromyography, muscle biopsy, and genetic testing. There is no cure. Treatment focuses on managing the symptoms. Gene therapy may eventually provide a treatment protocol to slow the progression of the disease.
Cystic fibrosis (CF)	Secretions such as mucus, sweat, and pancreatic juice are salty and thick. Thick mucus in the lungs leads to impaired breathing and increased infections. The pancreatic ducts become plugged, which stops the flow of digestive enzymes. Signs and symptoms vary greatly depending on the severity of the disorder.	Caused by mutations in a gene that produces a protein called CFTR that controls the flow of salt and water in and out of the cells. This results in secretions that are thick and salty.	Every state in the United States now routinely screens newborns for cystic fibrosis by testing a blood sample. Older children and adults are diagnosed through a sweat test and genetic testing using DNA. The goals of treatment include preventing and controlling lung infections, loosening and removing mucus from the lungs, preventing and treating intestinal blockage, and providing adequate nutrition.
Down syndrome (DS)	Signs and symptoms include physical growth delays, characteristic facial patterns, and intellectual impairment.	This is the most common chromosomal disorder. It is a genetic disorder caused by the presence of all or part of a third copy of chromosome 21 (trisomy 21).	Screening tests offered as a routine part of prenatal care can indicate likelihood of a Down syndrome baby. Diagnostic tests during pregnancy include amniocentesis and chorionic villus sampling. Diagnosis for newborns depends on chromosomal karyotype. There is no cure. Treatment and medical care are aimed at providing resources for the individual to develop skills as fully as possible.
Duchenne muscular dystrophy (DMD)	Similar to Becker muscular dystrophy but earlier onset and more severe. Signs and symptoms appear when the child begins to walk and include frequent falls, difficulty in running or jumping, waddling gait, difficulty getting up from a lying or sitting position, and large calf muscles. As the disease progresses, the heart and respiratory muscles may weaken, leading to cardiac and respiratory difficulties.	DMD is a severe form of muscular dystrophy that is caused by a total absence of the protein dystrophin, a protein that helps keep muscle cells intact. It is the result of a mutation on the X chromosome. It most commonly occurs in young boys and is characterized by muscle degeneration and weakness.	Diagnosis involves enzyme tests, electromyography, muscle biopsy, and genetic testing. There is no cure. Treatment focuses on managing the symptoms. Gene therapy may eventually provide a treatment protocol to slow the progression of the disease.

Genetic Diseases and Disorders—cont'd

Disease	Signs and Symptoms	Etiology	Diagnosis and Treatment
Fragile X syndrome (FXS)	The variety and degree of the signs and symptoms depend on the extent of the mutation in the gene, but may include impaired intellectual functioning, distinctive physical features such as large ears and long face, social anxiety, aggressive behavior, language difficulties, and autism-like behavior.	Caused by a mutation in a specific gene on the X chromosome. The mutated gene is unable to direct the synthesis of a protein needed for normal brain development. This is the most common known genetic cause of autism spectrum disorder.	Diagnosis is determined by direct analysis of the specific gene site on the X chromosome. Prenatal testing includes amniocentesis and chorionic villus sampling. There is no cure. Early intervention is key to realizing the child's full potential through appropriate education accompanied by behavioral and/or physical therapy as needed.
Huntington disease (HD)	Usually develops in midlife and may include involuntary movements, impairment of voluntary motor skills, cognitive impairment, and psychiatric disorders such as depression, social withdrawal, and bipolar disorder.	An inherited disorder caused by a defect in a single gene that results in the progressive degeneration of brain cells; an autosomal dominant disorder.	Diagnosis is based on medical history, physical examination, evaluation of motor and sensory functions, neurologic testing, psychiatric evaluation, and genetic testing. No treatments can cure or alter the course of the disorder. Medical management is likely to evolve as the condition progresses and may include medications and physical, speech, and/or occupational therapy.
Klinefelter syndrome	Occurs only in males and may not be noticeable until puberty or adulthood. The signs and symptoms are associated with low testosterone levels: less body and facial hair, broad hips, gynecomastia, hypogonadism, and hypospermia.	A condition in which a male has an extra X chromosome (XXY instead of XY). It is caused by an error during meiosis so that the zygote receives an extra X.	Diagnosis can be confirmed by hormone testing and chromosome analysis. Treatment may include testosterone replacement therapy, surgical removal of breast tissue, and fertility treatments.
Noonan syndrome	Unusual facial characteristics, heart defects, short stature, and abnormal bruising or bleeding.	An autosomal dominant congenital disorder that affects both males and females equally. The mutation may be inherited from a parent or occur as a result of a new mutation.	Diagnosis is confirmed by molecular genetic testing. There is no cure. Treatment focuses on controlling the symptoms and complications.
Phenylketonuria (PKU)	Seizures, microcephaly, progressive impairment of cerebral function, hyperactivity, severe learning disabilities, a "musty" odor to sweat and urine.	An autosomal recessive genetic disorder that inhibits the metabolism of the amino acid phenylalanine. As phenylalanine accumulates, it hinders the development of the brain. In PKU, phenylalanine is converted to phenylketones that appear in the urine.	Babies born in the United States and many other countries are screened for PKU soon after birth. Treatment involves controlling phenylalanine through diet. The U.S. Food and Drug Administration (FDA) has approved the drug sapropterin for treatment of PKU. It increases tolerance to phenylalanine in some people.

Continued

Genetic Diseases and Disorders—cont'd

Disease	Signs and Symptoms	Etiology	Diagnosis and Treatment
Sickle cell anemia (SCA)	Major features include fatigue and anemia, dactylitis, bacterial infections, pooling of blood in the spleen, liver congestion, and lung and heart injury. Signs and symptoms are the direct result of lack of oxygen to the organs with impaired circulation.	SCA is a hereditary blood disorder characterized by red blood cells that are rigid and sickle-shaped. The sickling occurs because of a mutation in the gene that codes for hemoglobin. The abnormal red blood cells clump together and block blood flow through the vessels.	Diagnosis can be made by microscopic observation of the abnormally shaped sickle cells and can be confirmed by using hemoglobin electrophoresis. Prenatal diagnosis is possible with use of amniocentesis or chorionic villus sampling. In general, treatment is directed at management and prevention of acute manifestations of the disease and therapies to prevent cells from sticking together. There is no remedy to reverse the condition.
Tay-Sachs disease (TSD)	In the most common form, infantile onset TSD, a baby about 6 months old will begin to show signs of the disorder. The child's body loses function, leading to blindness, deafness, paralysis, and death, usually by age 4.	Rare genetic autosomal recessive disorder passed from parents to child. A fatty substance in the brain accumulates to toxic levels and damages the nerve cells.	Initial testing involves an enzyme assay to determine the activity of hexosaminidase, which is reduced in TSD. This may be followed by molecular analysis. All patients with infantile onset TSD have a "cherry red" macula in the retina. There is no cure. Gene therapy research may eventually lead to a cure or treatment protocol.
Thalassemias	Disruption in normal hemoglobin synthesis causes low hemoglobin levels and a high rate of red blood cell destruction. The result is anemia with fatigue, weakness, jaundice, abdominal swelling, and dark urine.	Caused by hereditary mutations in the DNA of cells that make hemoglobin. There are numerous forms of thalassemia determined by the number of mutations and the part of the hemoglobin molecule that is affected.	Diagnosis is by blood tests that evaluate the quantity and quality of red blood cells and hemoglobin. DNA analysis is also useful. Prenatal testing can be done using amniocentesis or chorionic villus sampling. Treatment depends on the specific type of thalassemia; mild cases may need no treatment, and severe forms may need blood transfusions or a stem cell transplant.
Turner syndrome	Lymphedema, short stature, reproductive sterility, amenorrhea, webbed neck, heart problems, horseshoe kidney, defective vision and hearing.	Chromosomal abnormality in females in which all or part of one of the sex chromosomes is missing. In most cases of Turner syndrome, the functional X chromosome comes from the mother. The missing or abnormal chromosome is the result of an error in meiosis in the father.	Prenatal diagnosis is by amniocentesis or chorionic villus sampling. Postnatally, it is often diagnosed subsequent to heart problems associated with the disease. It may go undetected until the changes normally associated with puberty do not occur. Chromosome analysis is the diagnostic test of choice. There is no cure. Treatment is focused on minimizing the symptoms and may include growth hormone and estrogen replacement therapy.

TERMINOLOGY REVIEW

Key Term	Word Parts	Definition
Active transport	*trans-*: across, through	Process that moves substances across or through a membrane and requires cellular energy.
Anatomic position		Standard reference position for the body.
Axon		Efferent process of a neuron.
Chondrocyte	*chondr/o*: cartilage *-cyte*: cell	Cartilage cell.
Collagenous fibers	*-ous*: pertaining to	Strong and flexible connective tissue fibers that contain the protein collagen.
Cutaneous membrane	*cutane/o*: skin *-ous*: pertaining to	A type of epithelial membrane; skin.
Cytokinesis	*cyt/o*: cell *-kinesis*: movement	Division of the cell at the end of mitosis to form two separate daughter cells.
Dendrites	*dendr-*: tree	Treelike processes of a neuron; efferent processes.
Diffusion		Movement of substances from a region of high concentration to a region of low concentration.
Elastic fibers		Yellow connective tissue fibers that are not particularly strong but can be stretched and will return to their normal shape when released.
Erythrocytes	*erythr/o*: red *cyte*: cell	Red blood cell.
Fibroblast	*fibr/o*: fiber *-blast*: to form, immature cell	Connective tissue cell that produces fibers.
Histology	*-hist/o*: tissues *-logy*: study	Branch of microscopic anatomy that studies tissues.
Homeostasis	*home/o*: sameness, unchanging, constant *-stasis*: to stop, control, place	A normal stable condition in which the body's internal environment remains the same; constant internal environment.
Human anatomy	*anatomy*: structure	Study of human body shape and structure and the relationships of its parts.
Human physiology	*physi/o*: nature, function *-logy*: study	Study of the functions of humans and their separate parts.
Leukocytes	*leuk/o*: white *cyte*: cell	White blood cells.
Macrophage	*macro-*: large *-phage*: eat, swallow	Large phagocytic connective tissue cell that functions in the immune response.
Mast cell		A connective tissue cell that produces heparin and histamine.
Meiosis		Type of nuclear division in which the number of chromosomes is reduced to one half the number found in a body cell; results in the formation of egg or sperm.
Meninges	*Mening/o*: membrane	Connective tissue membranes that cover the brain and spinal cord.
Mitosis		Process by which the nucleus of a body cell divides to form two new cells, each identical to the parent cell.
Mucous membrane		Epithelial membrane that lines body cavities that open directly to the exterior; secretes mucus.
Negative feedback		A mechanism of response in which a stimulus initiates reactions that reduce the stimulus.
Neuroglia	*neur/o*: nerve *-glia*: glue	Supporting cells of nervous tissue; cells in nervous tissue that do not conduct impulses; nerve "glue."
Neuron	*neur/o*: nerve	Nerve cell, including its processes; conducting cell of nervous tissue.
Osmosis		Diffusion of water through a selectively permeable membrane.

Continued

↻ TERMINOLOGY REVIEW—cont'd

Key Term	Word Parts	Definition
Osteocyte	*oste/o:* bone *-cyte:* cell	Mature bone cell.
Passive transport	*trans-:*	Process that moves substances across or through a membrane and does not require cellular energy.
Pericardium	*peri:* around, surrounding *cardi/o:* heart	Membrane that surrounds the heart.
Peritoneum	*periton:* peritoneum	Serous membrane associated with the abdominopelvic cavity
Phagocytosis	*phag/o:* eat, swallow *-cyt-:* cell *-osis:* condition	Condition of cell eating; a form of endocytosis in which solid particles are taken into the cell.
Pinocytosis	*pin/o:* to drink *-cyt-:* cell *-osis:* condition	Condition of cell drinking; a form of endocytosis in which fluid droplets are taken into the cell.
Pleura	*pleur/o:* pleura	Serous membrane that surrounds the lungs.
Serous membrane	*ser/o:* serous, serum	Epithelial membrane that lines closed body cavities.
Synovial membrane	*synov/o:* synovia	Membrane that lines the cavities of freely movable joints.
Thrombocyte	*thromb/o:* blood clot *cyt/o:* cell	A formed element of the blood that functions in blood clotting; platelet.
Tissue		Group of similar cells specialized to perform a certain function.

ON THE WEB

For information on the human body:

American Medical Association: www.ama-assn.org

Cell Biology: www.cytochemistry.net/cell-biology

Cells Alive: www.cellsalive.com

Healthfinder: www.healthfinder.gov

Inner Body: Human Anatomy Online: www.innerbody.com

Loyola University Medical Education Network: www.lumen.luc.edu/lumen/meded/histo/frames/histo_frames.html

MadSci Network: www.madsci.org

MedlinePlus Tutorials: www.nlm.nih.gov/medlineplus/tutorials

Medscape: www.medscape.com

Medtropolis: The Virtual Body: www.medtropolis.com

The Virtual Cell Web Page: www.ibiblio.org/virtualcell

The Visible Human Project: www.nlm.nih.gov/research/visible

University of Utah Health Sciences Center: library.med.utah.edu

Integumentary System

6

Check out the Evolve site at http://evolve.elsevier.com/Bonewit/today/ to access additional interactive activities and exercises to help you study and prepare for success.

LEARNING OBJECTIVES

1. Describe the structure of the two layers of the skin.
2. State three names for the layer of tissue that anchors the skin to underlying organs, and describe the structure of this layer.
3. List three factors that influence skin color.
4. Describe the structure of hair and nails and their relationship to the skin.
5. Discuss the characteristics and functions of the various glands associated with the skin.
6. List and describe four functions of the integumentary system.
7. Describe ways in which the aging of an individual affects the integumentary system.
8. Identify pathology related to the integumentary system.

CHAPTER OUTLINE

INTRODUCTION TO THE INTEGUMENTARY SYSTEM
STRUCTURE OF THE SKIN
Epidermis
Dermis
Subcutaneous Layer
SKIN COLOR
EPIDERMAL DERIVATIVES
Hair and Hair Follicles
Nails
Glands

Sebaceous Glands
Sweat (Sudoriferous) Glands
Ceruminous Glands
FUNCTIONS OF THE SKIN
Protection
Sensory Reception
Regulation of Body Temperature
Synthesis of Vitamin D
AGING OF THE INTEGUMENTARY SYSTEM

KEY TERMS

arrector pili (ah-REK-tor PY-lee)
ceruminous glands (see-ROOM-in-us GLANDS)
cutaneous membrane (kyoo-TAY-nee-us MEM-brayn)
dermis (DER-mis)
epidermis (ep-ih-DER-mis)
hypodermis (hye-poh-DER-miss)

keratinization (ker-ah-tin-ih-ZAY-shun)
melanin (MEL-ah-nin)
melanocytes (meh-LAN-oh-sytes)
sebaceous glands (see-BAY-shus GLANDS)
sebum (SEE-bum)
stratum corium (STRAY-tum KOR-ee-um)

stratum corneum (STRAY-tum KOR-nee-um)
subcutaneous layer (sub-kyoo-TAY-nee-us LAY-ER)
sudoriferous glands (soo-door-IF-er-us GLANDS)
sweat glands (SWET GLANDS)

INTRODUCTION TO THE INTEGUMENTARY SYSTEM

The skin and the glands, hair, nails, and other structures that are derived from it make up the *integumentary system*.

Because it is on the outside of the body, this organ system is our contact with the external environment and is subjected to continual abuse from the environment. However, the skin is resilient and versatile. In general, it quickly repairs itself and continues to perform its many functions year after year.

111

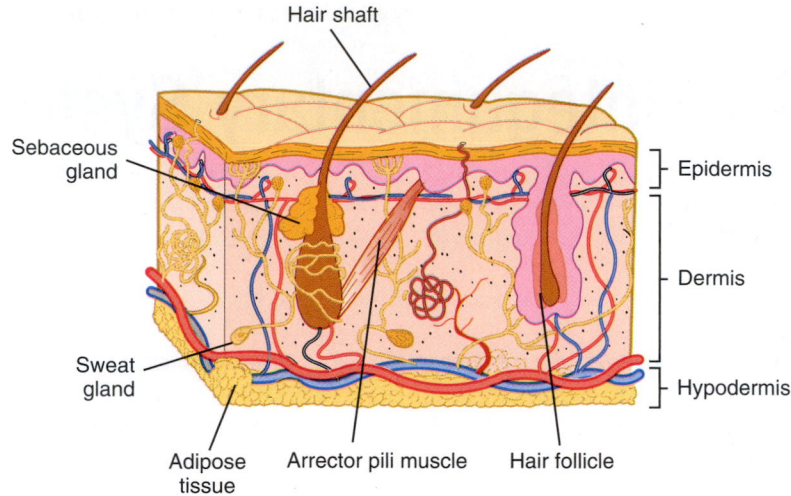

Figure 6-1 Structure of the skin. Note the epidermis, dermis, and hypodermis. (From Applegate E: *The anatomy and physiology learning system*, ed 4, St Louis, 2011, Saunders.)

STRUCTURE OF THE SKIN

The skin (sometimes called the **cutaneous membrane**) consists of two distinct layers of tissues. The outer layer is the *epidermis,* and the inner layer is the *dermis.* These are anchored to underlying structures by a third layer, the *hypodermis* or *subcutaneous tissue.*

The structure of the skin is illustrated in Figure 6-1.

EPIDERMIS

The outer layer of the skin is the **epidermis.** This layer consists of stratified squamous epithelium (see Figure 6-1). There are no blood vessels present in the epidermis, and the cells receive their nutrients by diffusion from vessels in the underlying tissue. The bottom row of cells in the epidermis is called the *stratum basale.* It consists of actively dividing (mitotic) columnar cells and **melanocytes.** This is the layer next to the basement membrane and closest to the blood supply. As older cells are pushed upward toward the surface by the growing cells next to the basement membrane, they receive fewer nutrients. They also undergo a process called **keratinization.** During keratinization, a protein called *keratin* is deposited in the cell. This causes the chemical composition of the cell to change, and the cell changes shape. By the time the cells reach the surface, they are flat or squamous. They are also dead from lack of nutrients and are sloughed off. They are replaced by other cells that are pushed upward from the stratum basale. About one fourth of the cells in the stratum basale are melanocytes. *Melanocytes* are specialized epithelial cells that produce a dark pigment called **melanin,** which is primarily responsible for skin color.

The outermost or surface region of the epidermis is the **stratum corneum.** It makes up about three fourths of the epidermal thickness and consists of 20 to 30 layers of flattened, dead, completely keratinized cells. The cells in the stratum corneum are continually shed and replaced. About 5 weeks after a cell has been produced in the stratum basale, it is sloughed off the surface of the stratum corneum. The keratin that is present is a tough, water-repellent protein, and its inclusion in the stratum corneum provides protection against water loss from the body.

DERMIS

The **dermis,** or **stratum corium,** is dense connective tissue that is deeper and usually thicker than the epidermis (see Figure 6-1). Hair, nails, and certain glands (although derived from the stratum basale of the epidermis) are embedded in the dermis. The dermis contains both collagenous and elastic fibers to give it strength and elasticity. If the skin is overstretched, the dermis may be damaged, leaving white scars called *striae,* commonly called "stretch marks." Fibers also form a framework for the numerous blood vessels and nerves that are present in the dermis but generally absent in the epidermis. Many of the nerves in the dermis have specialized endings called *sensory receptors* that detect changes in the environment, such as heat, cold, pain, pressure, and touch. Because there are no nerves in the epidermis, these receptors are the body's contact with the environment.

The upper region of the dermis has numerous *papillae,* or projections, that extend into the epidermis. Blood vessels, nerve endings, and sensory receptors extend into the papillae to bring them into closer proximity to the epidermis and the surface. On the palms, the fingertips, and the soles of the feet, the papillae form distinct patterns or ridges that provide friction for grasping objects. The patterns are genetically determined and are unique for each individual. These are the basis of fingerprints and footprints.

SUBCUTANEOUS LAYER

The **subcutaneous layer** (see Figure 6-1) is not actually a part of the skin, but it loosely anchors the skin to underlying organs. Because it is beneath the dermis, it is sometimes called the **hypodermis.** It is also referred to as *superficial fascia.* The subcutaneous layer consists largely of loose connective tissue and adipose tissue. The fibers in the loose connective tissue are continuous with those in the dermis, and as a result there is no distinct boundary between the dermis and the subcutaneous tissue.

The adipose tissue in the subcutaneous layer cushions the underlying organs from mechanical shock and acts as a heat insulator in temperature regulation. Fat in the adipose tissue can be mobilized and used for energy when necessary. The distribution of subcutaneous adipose tissue is largely responsible for the differences in body contours between men and women.

SKIN COLOR

Skin color is a result of many factors: some genetic, some physiologic, and some environmental. Basic skin color is caused by the dark pigment *melanin* produced by the melanocytes in the stratum basale of the epidermis. Everyone has about the same number of melanocytes. The activity of the melanocytes, however, is genetically controlled. Although many genes are responsible for skin color, a single mutation can result in an inability to produce melanin. This results in a condition called *albinism* in which

individuals have light skin, white hair, and unpigmented irises in the eyes.

Some people have the yellowish pigment *carotene* in addition to melanin. This gives a yellow tint to the skin. A pinkish tint in the skin is attributable to the blood vessels in the dermis. Ultraviolet light increases melanocyte activity so that more melanin is produced and the skin becomes darker or tanned.

EPIDERMAL DERIVATIVES

Accessory structures of the skin include hair, nails, sweat glands, and sebaceous glands. They are derived from the stratum basale of the epidermis and are embedded in the dermis. Figure 6-1 illustrates some of the accessory structures associated with the skin.

HAIR AND HAIR FOLLICLES

Hair is found on nearly all body surfaces, but it is absent on the palms of the hands and the soles of the feet. All hair has essentially the same structure. It consists of a shaft and a root that are composed of dead, keratinized epithelial cells. The root is enclosed in a hair follicle that extends through the epidermis and is embedded in the dermis.

The *shaft* of a hair is that portion that extends beyond the surface of the epidermis. It is the part that you can see. Because it contains no nerves, it can be cut with no sensation of pain. The *root* is the portion of the hair that is below the surface of the skin. It is surrounded by a hair follicle.

HIGHLIGHT on the Integumentary System

Skin
For an "average" person, the skin weighs about 5 kg (11 lb), has a surface area of approximately 2 m² (21 ft²), and varies in thickness from 0.05 to 0.4 cm (0.02 to 0.16 inch).

Acne
Acne is a problem that plagues many teenagers. Increased hormone activity at puberty causes an increase in sebaceous gland activity. Sebum and dead cells may block the hair follicle and form blackheads. Bacteria infect the blocked follicle, and the sebum–dead cell mixture accumulates until the follicle ruptures. This initiates an inflammatory response that soon appears on the surface as a pus-filled pimple.

Adipose Tissue
People who lose weight rapidly may feel cold because they have reduced their adipose insulation.

Blister
A blister is a fluid-filled pocket between the dermis and the epidermis. When the skin is burned or irritated, some plasma escapes

from the blood vessels in the dermis and accumulates between the two layers, where it forms the blister.

Dermal Blood Vessels
In people with light skin, when dermal blood vessels dilate and blood flow increases (e.g., during blushing and increased temperature), the skin may be quite red. If the vessels constrict and blood flow decreases, the individual is pale or "white as a sheet."

Dermis
The dermis is the portion of an animal's skin that is used to make leather because the collagen in the dermis becomes tough when treated with tannic acid.

Hair Type
The shape of the hair shaft determines whether hair is straight or curly. If the shaft is round, the hair is straight. If it is oval, the hair is wavy. If it is flat, the hair is curly or kinky. To make their hair curly, individuals often get a "permanent," which flattens the hair. ■

The shaft and root are continuous and together make up the hair, which is produced by the hair follicle. The outermost covering on a hair is a single layer of overlapping, keratinized cells called the *cuticle.* On the shaft of the hair, the cuticle is exposed to the environment and subjected to abrasion. It tends to wear away at the tip of the shaft. When this happens, the inner portion projects from the tip of the shaft, resulting in "split ends."

The root of a hair is enclosed in a tubular *hair follicle* that is embedded in the dermis. Blood vessels in the dermis provide the blood supply for the epithelial cells of the hair follicle. Stratum basale cells, like those in the skin, provide the mitotic cells that divide and undergo keratinization to produce the hair.

Hair color is determined by the type of melanin produced by the melanocytes in the stratum basale. The shaft of the hair without melanin is clear and transparent. Yellow, brown, and black pigments are present in varying proportions to produce different hair colors. With age, the melanocytes become less active and the hair appears to have less color.

A bundle of smooth muscle cells, called the **arrector pili** muscle, is associated with each hair follicle. Most hair follicles are at a slight angle to the surface of the skin. The arrector pili muscles are attached to the hair follicles in such a way that contraction pulls the hair follicles into an upright position or causes the hair to "stand on end." Contraction of the arrector pili muscles also causes raised areas on the skin, or "goose bumps." Action of the arrector pili muscles is controlled by the nervous system in response to cold and fright.

NAILS

Nails are thin plates of dead stratum corneum that contain a very hard type of keratin and cover the dorsal surfaces of the distal ends of the fingers and toes. Each nail has a *free edge;* a *nail body,* which is the visible portion; and a *nail root,* which is covered with skin. The *eponychium* or *cuticle* is a fold of stratum corneum that grows onto the proximal portion of the nail body. Stratum basale from the epidermis grows under the nail body and is responsible for nail growth. The portion of the body over the growth area appears as a whitish, crescent-shaped area called the *lunula.* Nails appear pink because of the rich supply of blood vessels in the underlying dermis.

GLANDS

The two major glands associated with the skin are the *sebaceous glands* and the *sweat glands* (also called *sudoriferous glands*). A third type, the *ceruminous glands,* are modified sweat glands.

Sebaceous Glands

In general, **sebaceous glands** are associated with hair follicles and are found in all areas of the body that have hair (see Figure 6-1). Those not associated with hair follicles open directly onto the surface of the skin. The oily secretion, called **sebum,** is transported by a duct into a hair follicle, and from there it reaches the surface of the skin. Sebum functions to keep hair and skin soft and pliable. It also inhibits growth of bacteria on the skin and helps to prevent water loss. Secretory activity of the sebaceous glands is stimulated by sex hormones; consequently, the glands are relatively inactive in childhood, become highly active during puberty, and decrease in activity during old age. Decreased sebum, in part, accounts for the dry skin and brittle hair that are common in older people.

Sweat (Sudoriferous) Glands

Sweat glands (also called **sudoriferous glands**) are widely distributed over the body. They are most numerous in the palms and soles. The glandular portion of a sweat gland is a coiled tube that is embedded in the dermis of the skin, and the duct opens onto the surface of the skin through a *sweat pore* (see Figure 6-1). The secretion of these glands is primarily water with a few salts. When the body's temperature increases, the glands are stimulated to produce sweat, which evaporates and has a cooling effect. Sweat, or *perspiration,* is also produced in response to nerve stimulation as a result of emotional stress.

Ceruminous Glands

Ceruminous glands are modified sweat glands that are found in the external auditory (ear) canal. They secrete an oily, sticky substance called *cerumen,* or earwax, that is thought to repel insects and trap foreign material.

FUNCTIONS OF THE SKIN
PROTECTION

The skin forms a protective covering over the entire body. The keratin in the cells waterproofs the cells and helps prevent fluid loss from the body. This waterproofing also prevents too much water from entering the body during swimming and bathing. Unbroken skin forms the first line of defense against bacteria and other invading organisms. The oily secretions of the sebaceous glands are acidic and inhibit bacterial growth on the skin. Melanin pigment absorbs light and helps protect underlying tissues from the damaging effects of ultraviolet light. Skin also protects underlying tissues from mechanical, chemical, and thermal injury.

SENSORY RECEPTION

The dermis contains numerous sensory receptors for heat, cold, pain, touch, and pressure. Even though hair itself has no sensory receptors, the movement of hair can be detected by receptors clustered around a hair follicle. The sensory receptors in the dermis relay information about the environment to the brain so that changes can be made to prevent or minimize injury. The sensory receptors are also a means of communication between individuals.

REGULATION OF BODY TEMPERATURE

Normally, body temperature is maintained at 37°C (98.6°F). It is important that body temperature be regulated because changes in temperature alter the speed of chemical reactions in the body. The skin helps to regulate body temperature in two ways: by dilation and constriction of blood vessels, and by activity or inactivity of the sweat glands. Both of these mechanisms are examples of negative feedback in maintaining homeostasis. Blood vessels dilate and sweat glands become active in response to an increase in body temperature. Both mechanisms tend to remove heat from the body. In response to cold, blood vessels constrict and sweat glands are inactive to conserve body heat. The adipose tissue in the subcutaneous layer also helps by acting as an insulator.

SYNTHESIS OF VITAMIN D

Vitamin D is required for calcium and phosphorus absorption in the small intestine. The calcium and phosphorus are essential for normal bone metabolism and muscle function. Skin cells contain a precursor molecule that is converted to vitamin D when the precursor is exposed to ultraviolet rays in sunlight. It takes only a small amount of ultraviolet light to stimulate vitamin D production, so this should not be used as an excuse to expose the skin to sun unnecessarily and to risk the damage that may result.

AGING OF THE INTEGUMENTARY SYSTEM

As the skin ages, the number of elastic fibers decreases and adipose tissue is lost from the dermis and subcutaneous layer. This causes the skin to wrinkle and sag. Loss of collagen fibers in the dermis makes the skin more fragile and makes it heal more slowly. Mitotic activity in the stratum basale slows so that the skin becomes thinner and appears more transparent. Reduced sebaceous gland activity causes dry, itchy skin. Loss of adipose tissue in the subcutaneous layer and reduced sweat gland activity lead to an intolerance to cold and susceptibility to heat. The ability of the skin to regulate temperature is reduced. There is a general reduction in melanocyte activity, which decreases protection from ultraviolet light, resulting in increased susceptibility to sunburn and skin cancer. Some melanocytes, however, may increase melanin production, resulting in "age spots."

Despite all the creams and "miracle" lotions, there is no known way to prevent skin from aging. Good nutrition and cleanliness may slow the aging process. Because skin that is exposed to sunlight ages more rapidly than unexposed skin, one of the best ways to slow the aging process is to avoid exposure by wearing protective clothing and by using sunblock whenever possible.

Common Pathology of the Integumentary System

Disease	Signs and Symptoms	Etiology	Diagnosis and Treatment
Alopecia	Absence of hair from skin areas where it normally grows.	May be caused by chemotherapy, injury, or disease. Baldness may be hereditary.	Diagnosis is evident by lack of hair. Medications may help prevent further hair loss. Hair transplants are sometimes indicated.
Cellulitis	Affected area appears swollen and red and feels hot.	Infection of connective tissue with severe inflammation of the dermis and subcutaneous layers of the skin. Caused by bacteria, usually *Streptococcus* or *Staphylococcus*, entering the skin by way of a cut or abrasion.	Diagnosis is by physical examination. Blood tests and a wound culture may be useful. Treatment includes resting the affected area. Cutting away dead tissue may be necessary. Oral antibiotics are usually prescribed.
Dermatitis	Affected area exhibits a red, itchy rash. In some forms, blisters may develop; in others, oily scales may appear.	Inflammation of a region of the skin; commonly an allergic reaction to a specific allergen such as poison ivy.	Diagnosis is by examination. Treatment is typically with moisturizers and steroid creams.
Eczema	Skin shows red, itching, vesicular lesions that may crust over.	Inflammatory skin disease believed to be the result of a combination of hereditary and environmental factors.	Diagnosis is by examination of the skin. Treatment aims to heal the affected skin and to prevent recurrence of the symptoms; may include mild soap and moisturizers, hydrocortisone, and antihistamines. Good skin care is the key for controlling eczema.

Continued

Common Pathology of the Integumentary System—cont'd

Disease	Signs and Symptoms	Etiology	Diagnosis and Treatment
Impetigo	Superficial skin infection characterized by vesicles, pustules, and crusted-over lesions, usually on the face.	Highly contagious skin disorder caused by staphylococcal or streptococcal bacteria. Most common in children.	Diagnosis is by examination of the distinctive sores. Antibiotics are usually prescribed. Mild cases may be treated with bactericidal ointment.
Tinea	Red scaly patches on the skin.	A fungal infection of the skin; Caused by dermatophytes, a type of fungus. Growths on the dead keratinized cells of the skin multiply in warm, damp environments on the body and can be transmitted by touch. Common forms are ringworm, athlete's foot, and jock itch.	Diagnosis is by examination. Treatment includes thoroughly washing and drying the affected area and applying antifungal creams, powders, or sprays.
Urticaria	Skin rash notable for pale red, raised, itchy bumps; commonly called *hives*.	Many different substances in the environment may cause urticaria, including medications, food and physical agents.	Diagnosis is by examination. Treatment includes avoiding the triggers that cause the outbreaks. Acute episodes may be relieved by antihistamines and hydrocortisone. There are no guaranteed means of controlling attacks.
Warts	The appearance of small, rough skin growths resembling cauliflower.	Caused by human papilloma virus infection of the squamous epithelium.	Diagnosis is by examination. Treatments and procedures associated with wart removal include the use of salicylic acid and cryosurgery.
Decubitus ulcers	Localized open sores on the skin.	Caused by pressure being applied to soft tissue resulting in completely or partially obstructed blood flow. Typically occurs over a bony prominence; commonly called *bedsores.*	Diagnosis is by examination. Treatment involves removing the pressure from the affected areas. Patients with pressure ulcers should not lie or sit on them. In most cases, necrotic tissue should be removed.
Psoriasis	Skin disease characterized by red, scaly patches that usually itch.	In general, considered a genetic disease thought to be triggered or influenced by environmental factors.	Diagnosis is by examination. Treatment includes topical agents for mild disease, phototherapy for moderate disease, and prescribed systemic agents for severe disease.
Skin cancer, basal cell	Typically appears as a waxy bump or a skin sore that does not heal within 2 months while increasing in size.	Damage to the DNA of basal cells is a result of ultraviolet B (UVB) exposure from sunlight or tanning beds.	Early diagnosis by examination and a biopsy by a trained medical professional are vital. Treatments include surgical excision, liquid nitrogen freezing, electrodessication, and curettage.
Skin cancer, melanoma	A skin mole with the following characteristics: *Asymmetry*—irregular shape *Border*—rough, irregular *Color*—nonuniform *Diameter*—more than $\frac{1}{4}$ inch	Probably caused by excessive exposure to UVB rays from sunlight or tanning beds.	Early diagnosis by examination and a biopsy by a trained medical professional are vital. Treatments include surgery and radiation therapy.
Skin cancer, squamous cell	A firm lump on the skin with a rough, scaly or crusty surface.	Typically caused by excessive exposure to UVB rays from sunlight or tanning beds.	Early diagnosis by examination and a biopsy by a trained medical professional are vital. Treatments include Mohs surgery, radiation therapy, excision, and cryosurgery.

⟳ TERMINOLOGY REVIEW

Key Term	Word Parts	Definition
Arrector pili	*pil/o:* hair	Muscle associated with hair follicles.
Ceruminous glands	*cerumin/o:* cerumen	Glands in the ear canal that produce cerumen or ear wax.
Cutaneous membrane	*cutane/o:* skin	Another name for the skin.
Dermis	*derm/o:* skin	Inner layer of the skin that contains the blood vessels, nerves, glands, and hair follicles.
Epidermis	*epi-:* above, upon *-derma:* skin	Outermost layer of the skin.
Hypodermis	*hypo:* below, under *-derma:* skin	Below the skin; a sheet of areolar connective tissue and adipose beneath the dermis of the skin.
Keratinization	*kerat/o:* hard, horny tissue *-ation:* process, condition	Process by which the cells of the epidermis become filled with keratin and move to the surface where they are sloughed off.
Melanin	*melan/o:* black	A dark brown or black pigment found in parts of the body, especially skin and hair.
Melanocytes	*melan/o:* black *cyte:* cell	Cells that produces the dark or black pigment melanin.
Sebaceous glands	*seb/o:* sebum *-ous:* pertaining to	Oil glands of the skin that produce sebum or body oil.
Sebum	*seb/o:* oil	Oily secretion from sebaceous glands.
Stratum corium	*strat:* layer	Another name for the dermis, a layer of the skin.
Stratum corneum	*strat:* layer *corne/:* dead, flattened, scaly	Outermost layer of the epidermis; consists of flattened, dead, keratinized cells.
Subcutaneous layer	*sub-:* under, below *cutane/o:* skin *-ous:* pertaining to	A sheet of areolar connective tissue and adipose tissue beneath the dermis of the skin; also called *hypodermis* or *superficial fascia.*
Sudoriferous glands	*sud-:* sweat *-ous:* pertaining to	Glands in the skin that produce perspiration; also called *sweat glands.*
Sweat glands		Glands in the skin that produce perspiration; also called *sudoriferous glands.*

ON THE WEB

For information on the integumentary system:

British Medical Journal: Dermatology: www.bmj.com/cgi/collection/dermatology

Loyola University Medication Education Network: Dermatology Atlas: www.meddean.luc.edu/lumen/MedEd/medicine/dermatology/melton/title.htm

Merck Manual—Dermatologic Disorders: www.merck.com/mmpe *(Click on "Dermatologic Disorders")*

Skin Cancer Risk Analyzer: www.telemedicine.org/melanoma.htm

University of Delaware—Integumentary System: www.udel.edu/biology/Wags/histopage/colorpage/cin/cin.htm

7 Skeletal System

LEARNING OBJECTIVES

1. List and describe five functions of the skeletal system.
2. Explain the difference between compact and spongy bone.
3. Classify bones according to size and shape.
4. Identify the general features of a long bone.
5. Explain the process by which long bones grow in length.
6. Explain the difference between the axial and appendicular skeletons.
7. Identify the bones of the skull.
8. Identify the structural features of vertebrae.
9. List and describe the divisions of the vertebral column.
10. Describe the structural features of the sternum and ribs.
11. Identify the parts of the pectoral girdle.
12. Identify the bones of the upper extremities.
13. Identify the parts of the pelvic girdle.
14. Identify the bones of the lower extremities.
15. List and describe the different types of joints.
16. Describe ways in which the aging of an individual affects the skeletal system.
17. Identify pathology related to the skeletal system.

CHAPTER OUTLINE

INTRODUCTION TO THE SKELETAL SYSTEM
OVERVIEW OF THE SKELETAL SYSTEM
Functions of the Skeletal System
Support
Protection
Movement
Storage
Blood Cell Formation
Structure of Bone Tissue
Compact Bone
Spongy (Cancellous) Bone
Classification of Bones
General Features of a Long Bone
Bone Development and Growth
Bone Growth in Length
Divisions of the Skeleton
BONES OF THE AXIAL SKELETON
Skull
Cranium
Facial Bones
Auditory Ossicles
Hyoid Bone
Vertebral Column

General Structure of Vertebrae
Composition of the Vertebral Column
Thoracic Cage
Sternum
Ribs
BONES OF THE APPENDICULAR SKELETON
Pectoral Girdle
Upper Extremity
Arm
Forearm
Hand
Pelvic Girdle
Lower Extremity
Thigh
Leg
Foot
Patella
ARTICULATIONS
Synarthroses
Amphiarthroses
Diarthroses
AGING OF THE SKELETAL SYSTEM

KEY TERMS

amphiarthroses (am-fee-ahr-THROH-sseez)

appendicular skeleton (ap-pen-DIK-yoo-lar SKEL-eh-ton)

appositional growth (ap-poh-ZISH-un-al GROWTH)

articular cartilage (ahr-TIK-yoo-lar KAR-tih-layj)

articulation (ahr-TIK-yoo-lay-shun)

axial skeleton (AK-see-al SKEL-eh-ton)

diaphysis (dye-AF-ih-sis)

diarthroses (dye-ahr-THROH-seez)

endosteum (end-AH-stee-um)

epiphyseal line (ep-ih-FIZ-ee-al LINE)

epiphyseal plate (ep-ih-FIZ-ee-al PLATE)

epiphysis (ee-PIF-ih-sis)

hematopoiesis (hee-mat-oh-poy-EE-sis)

osteoblasts (AH-stee-oh-blasts)

osteoclasts (AH-stee-oh-clasts)

osteocytes (AH-stee-oh-sytes)

osteogenesis (AH-stee-oh-jen-eh-sis)

osteon (AH-stee-ahn)

pectoral girdle (PEK-toh-ral GIR-dull)

pelvic girdle (PEL-vik GIR-dull)

periosteum (pair-ee-AH-stee-um)

sutures (SOO-chers)

synarthroses (sin-ahr-THROH-seez)

INTRODUCTION TO THE SKELETAL SYSTEM

The skeletal system consists of the bones and the cartilage, ligaments, and tendons associated with the bones. It accounts for about 20% of the body weight. Bones are rigid structures that form the framework for the body. People often think of bones as dead, dry, inert pipes and plates because that is how they are seen in the laboratory. In reality, the living bones in our bodies contain active tissues that consume nutrients, require a blood supply, use oxygen and discharge waste products in metabolism, and change shape or remodel in response to variations in mechanical stress. The skeletal system is strong but lightweight. It is well adapted for the functions it must perform. It is a masterpiece of design.

OVERVIEW OF THE SKELETAL SYSTEM

FUNCTIONS OF THE SKELETAL SYSTEM

The skeletal system gives form and shape to the body. Without the skeletal components, we would appear as big "blobs" inefficiently "oozing" around on the ground. In addition to contributing to shape and form, our bones perform several other functions and play an important role in homeostasis.

Support

Bones provide a rigid framework that supports the soft organs of the body. Bones support the body against the pull of gravity, and the large bones of the lower limbs support the trunk when standing.

Protection

The skeleton protects the soft body parts. The fused bones of the cranium surround the brain to make it less vulnerable to injury. The vertebrae surround and protect the spinal cord. The bones of the rib cage help protect the heart and lungs in the thorax.

Movement

Bones provide sites for muscle attachment. Bones and muscles work together as simple mechanical lever systems to produce body movement.

Storage

The intercellular matrix of bone contains large amounts of calcium salts, the most important being calcium phosphate. Calcium is necessary for vital metabolic processes. When blood calcium levels decrease below normal, calcium is released from the bones so that there will be an adequate supply for metabolic needs. When blood calcium levels are increased, the excess calcium is stored in the bone matrix. Storage and release are dynamic processes that go on almost continually.

Blood Cell Formation

Blood cell formation, called **hematopoiesis,** takes place mostly in the red marrow of bones. Red marrow is found in the cavities of most bones in an infant. With age, it is largely replaced by yellow marrow for fat storage. In the adult, red marrow is limited to the spongy bone in the skull, ribs, sternum, clavicles, vertebrae, and pelvis. Red marrow functions in the formation of red blood cells, white blood cells, and blood platelets.

STRUCTURE OF BONE TISSUE

There are two types of bone tissue: compact and spongy. As the names imply, the two types differ in density, or how tightly the tissue is packed together. Three types of cells contribute to bone homeostasis: **osteoblasts, osteoclasts, and osteocytes.** Osteoblasts are bone-forming cells, osteoclasts resorb or break down bone, and osteocytes are mature bone cells. An equilibrium between osteoblasts and osteoclasts maintains bone tissue.

Compact Bone

The microscopic unit of compact bone is known as the **osteon** (haversian system). The osteon consists of a central canal called the *osteonic* (haversian) *canal,* which is surrounded by concentric rings (lamellae) of hard, calcified matrix. Between the rings of matrix, the bone cells (osteocytes) are located in spaces called *lacunae.* Small channels (canaliculi) radiate from the lacunae to the osteonic (haversian) canal to provide passageways through the hard matrix. In compact bone the haversian systems are packed tightly together to form what appears to be a solid mass. The osteonic canals contain blood vessels that are parallel to the long axis of the bone. These blood vessels interconnect, by way of perforating (Volkmann) canals, with vessels on the surface of the bone. The microscopic structure of compact bone is illustrated in Figure 7-1.

Spongy (Cancellous) Bone

Spongy (cancellous) bone is lighter and less dense than compact bone (see Figure 7-1). Spongy bone consists of plates and bars of bone adjacent to small, irregular cavities that contain red bone marrow. The plates of bone are called *trabeculae.* The canaliculi, instead of connecting to a central haversian canal, connect to the adjacent cavities to receive their blood supply. It may appear that the trabeculae are arranged in a haphazard manner, but they are organized to provide maximum strength in the same way that braces are used to support a building. The trabeculae of spongy bone follow the lines of stress and can realign if the direction of stress changes.

CLASSIFICATION OF BONES

Bones come in a variety of sizes and shapes. Bones that are longer than they are wide are called *long bones.* They consist of a long shaft with two bulky ends or extremities. They are primarily compact bone but may have a large amount of spongy bone at the ends. Examples of long bones are those in the thigh, leg, arm, and forearm.

Short bones are roughly cube-shaped with vertical and horizontal dimensions approximately equal. They consist primarily of spongy bone, which is covered by a thin layer of compact bone. Examples of short bones include the bones of the wrist and ankle.

Flat bones are thin, flattened, and often curved. They are usually arranged like a sandwich with a middle layer of spongy bone called the *diploë.* The diploë is covered on each side by a layer of compact bone; these layers are called the *inner* and *outer tables.* Most of the bones of the cranium are flat bones.

Bones that are not in any of the previously mentioned three categories are classified as *irregular bones.* They are

Figure 7-1 Structure of compact and spongy bone. Note the osteons packed together for compact bone and trabeculae of spongy bone. (From Applegate E: *The anatomy and physiology learning system,* ed 4, St Louis, 2011, Saunders.)

primarily spongy bone that is covered with a thin layer of compact bone. The vertebrae and some of the bones in the skull are irregular bones.

GENERAL FEATURES OF A LONG BONE

Most long bones have the same general features, which are illustrated in Figure 7-2.

Diaphysis: The shaft of a long bone is called the **diaphysis.** It is formed from relatively thick compact bone that surrounds a hollow space called the *medullary cavity.*

Medullary cavity: In adults the medullary cavity contains yellow bone marrow, so it is sometimes called the *yellow marrow cavity.*

Epiphysis: At each end of the diaphysis, there is an expanded portion called the **epiphysis.** The epiphysis is spongy bone covered by a thin layer of compact bone. The end of the epiphysis, where it meets another bone, is covered by hyaline cartilage, called the **articular cartilage.** This provides smooth surfaces for movement in the joints. In growing bones, there is an **epiphyseal plate** of hyaline cartilage between the diaphysis and epiphysis. Bones grow in length at the epiphyseal plate. Growth ceases when the cartilaginous epiphyseal plate is replaced by a bony epiphyseal line.

Periosteum: Except in the region of the articular cartilage, the outer surface of long bones is covered by a tough, fibrous connective tissue called the **periosteum.** The periosteum is richly supplied with nerve fibers, lymphatic vessels, blood vessels, and osteoblasts.

Nutrient foramina: Blood vessels enter the diaphysis of the bone through small openings called *nutrient foramina.*

Endosteum: The surface of the medullary cavity is lined with a thinner connective tissue membrane, the **endosteum,** which contains osteoclasts.

In addition to the general features that are present in most long bones, all bones have surface markings and characteristics that make a specific bone unique. Bones have holes, depressions, smooth facets, lines, projections, and other markings. These usually represent passageways for vessels and nerves, points of articulation with other bones, or points of attachment for tendons and ligaments.

BONE DEVELOPMENT AND GROWTH

The terms **osteogenesis** and *ossification* are often used synonymously to indicate the process of bone formation. Parts of the skeleton form during the first few weeks after conception. By the end of the eighth week after conception, the skeletal pattern is formed in cartilage and connective tissue membranes and ossification begins. Bone development continues throughout adulthood. Even after adult stature has been attained, bone development continues for repair of fractures and for remodeling to meet changing lifestyles. Three types of cells are involved in the development, growth, and remodeling of bones. *Osteoblasts* are bone-forming cells; *osteocytes* are mature bone cells; and *osteoclasts* break down and reabsorb bone.

BONE GROWTH IN LENGTH

Bones grow in length at the *epiphyseal plate* located between the diaphysis and epiphysis of a long bone. The hyaline cartilage in the region of the epiphyseal plate next to the epiphysis continues to grow by mitosis. The chondrocytes in the region next to the diaphysis age and degenerate. Osteoblasts move in and ossify the matrix to form bone. This process continues throughout childhood and adolescence until the cartilage growth slows and finally stops. When cartilage growth ceases, usually in the early 20s, the epiphyseal plate completely ossifies so that only a thin **epiphyseal line** remains and the bones can no longer grow in length. Bone growth occurs under the influence of growth hormone from the anterior pituitary gland and sex hormones from the ovaries and testes.

Even though bones stop growing in length in early adulthood, they can continue to increase in thickness or diameter

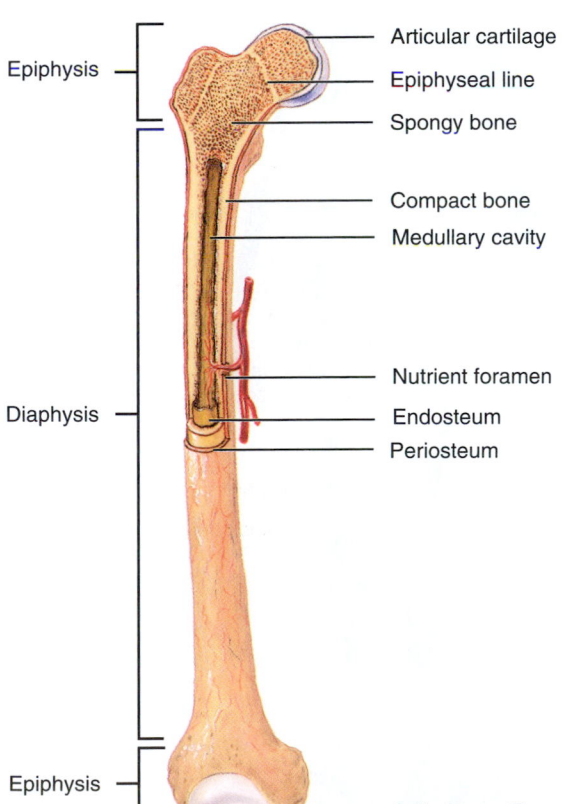

Epiphysis

Articular cartilage
Epiphyseal line
Spongy bone

Compact bone
Medullary cavity

Diaphysis

Nutrient foramen
Endosteum
Periosteum

Epiphysis

Articular cartilage

Figure 7-2 General features of long bones. (From Applegate E: *The anatomy and physiology learning system,* ed 4, St Louis, 2011, Saunders.)

throughout life in response to stress from increased muscle activity or to weight gain. The increase in diameter is called **appositional growth.** Osteoblasts in the periosteum form compact bone around the external bone surface. At the same time, osteoclasts in the endosteum break down bone on the internal bone surface, around the medullary cavity. These two processes together increase the diameter of the bone and at the same time keep the bone from becoming excessively heavy and bulky.

DIVISIONS OF THE SKELETON

The typical adult human skeleton consists of 206 named bones. For convenience, the bones of the skeleton are grouped in two divisions, as illustrated in Figure 7-3. The 80 bones of the **axial skeleton** form the vertical axis of the body. They include the bones of the head, vertebral column, ribs, and breastbone or sternum. The **appendicular skeleton** consists of 126 bones and includes the free appendages and their attachments to the axial skeleton. The free appendages are the upper and lower extremities, or limbs, and their

attachments are called *girdles.* Table 7-1 lists the named bones of the body by category.

BONES OF THE AXIAL SKELETON

The axial skeleton, with 80 bones, is divided into the skull, hyoid, vertebral column, and rib cage.

SKULL

The skull has 28 bones, as illustrated in Figures 7-4 and 7-5. The eight bones of the *cranium* are interlocked to enclose the brain. The anterior aspect of the skull, the *face,* consists of 14 bones. The remaining six bones are the *auditory ossicles,* tiny bones in the middle ear cavity. With the exception of the lower jaw, or mandible, and the auditory ossicles, the bones in the skull are tightly interlocked along irregular lines called **sutures.** Some of the bones in the skull contain *sinuses,* which are air-filled cavities lined with mucous membranes. The sinuses help to reduce the weight

Figure 7-3 Divisions of the skeleton with major bones identified. *Yellow,* axial skeleton. *Blue,* appendicular skeleton. (From Applegate E: *The anatomy and physiology learning system,* ed 4, St Louis, 2011, Saunders.)

HIGHLIGHT on the Skeletal System

Epiphyseal plate: The epiphyseal plates of specific long bones ossify at predictable times. Radiologists frequently can determine a young person's age by examining the epiphyseal plates to see whether they have ossified. A difference between bone age and chronologic age may indicate some type of metabolic dysfunction.

Sinus problems: The bones with paranasal sinuses are the frontal, the sphenoid, the ethmoid, and the two maxillae. The sinuses are lined with mucous membranes that are continuous with the nasal cavity. Allergies and infections cause inflammation of the membranes, which results in sinusitis. The swollen membranes may reduce drainage from the sinuses so that pressure within the cavities increases, resulting in sinus headaches.

Soft spots: The bones in the skull of a newborn are not completely joined together but are separated by fibrous membranes. The six large areas of membranes are called *fontanels,* or soft spots. The anterior fontanel is on the top of the head, at the junction of the frontal and parietal bones. The posterior fontanel is at the junction of the occipital and parietal bones. On each side of the head there is a mastoid (posterolateral) fontanel near the mastoid region of the temporal bone and a sphenoid (anterolateral) fontanel just superior to the sphenoid bone.

Abnormal spinal curvatures: An abnormally exaggerated lumbar curvature is called lordosis, or swayback. This is often seen in pregnant women as they adjust to their changing center of gravity. An increased roundness of the thoracic curvature is kyphosis, or hunchback. This is frequently seen in elderly people. Abnormal side-to-side curvature is scoliosis. Abnormal curvatures may interfere with breathing and other vital functions.

Yes and no: The atlas holds up the skull and permits you to nod "yes." The axis allows you to rotate your head from side to side to indicate "no."

Marrow biopsy: The sternum is frequently used for a red marrow biopsy because it is accessible. The sample for biopsy is obtained by performing a sternal puncture, in which a large needle is inserted into the sternum to remove a sample of red bone marrow.

Fractured clavicle: The clavicle is the most frequently fractured bone in the body because it transmits forces from the arm to the trunk. The force from falling on the shoulder or outstretched arm is often sufficient to fracture the clavicle.

Pelvic outlet and childbirth: The female pelvis is shaped to accommodate childbearing. Because the fetus must pass through the pelvic outlet, the physician carefully measures this opening to make sure there is enough room. The distance between the two ischial spines is a good indication of the size of the pelvic outlet. If the opening is too small, a cesarean delivery is indicated.

Broken hip: Elderly people, particularly those with osteoporosis, are susceptible to "breaking a hip." The femur is a weight-bearing bone, and when it is weakened, it cannot support the weight of the body and the neck of the femur fractures under the stress. Instead of saying, "Grandma fell and broke her hip," often it is more appropriate to say, "Grandma broke her hip, then fell." ∎

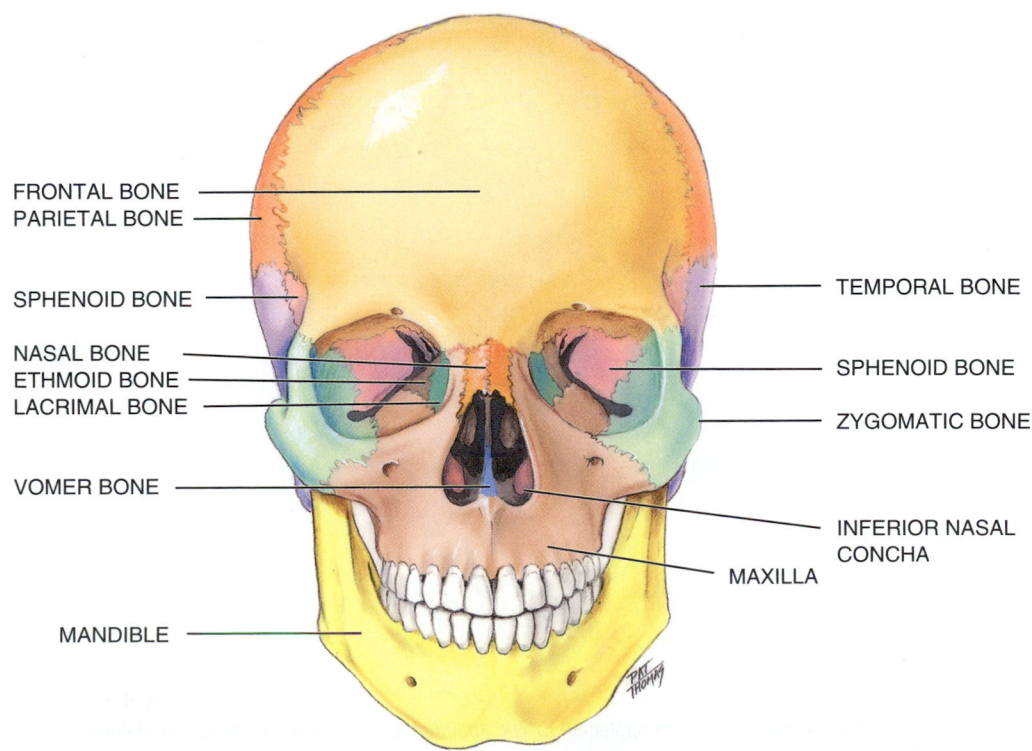

Figure 7-4 Skull, anterior view. (From Applegate E: *The anatomy and physiology learning system,* ed 4, St Louis, 2011, Saunders.)

Table 7-1 Names of Bones of the Body Listed by Category

Bones	Number	Bones	Number
Axial Skeleton (80 Bones)		Thoracic cage	25
Skull (28 bones)		Sternum (1)	
Cranial bones	8	Ribs (24)	
Parietal (2)			
Temporal (2)		**Appendicular Skeleton (126 Bones)**	
Frontal (1)		Pectoral girdles	4
Occipital (1)		Clavicle (2)	
Ethmoid (1)		Scapula (2)	
Sphenoid (1)		Upper extremity	60
Facial bones	14	Humerus (2)	
Maxilla (2)		Radius (2)	
Zygomatic (2)		Ulna (2)	
Mandible (1)		Carpals (16)	
Nasal (2)		Metacarpals (10)	
Palatine (2)		Phalanges (28)	
Inferior nasal concha (2)		Pelvic girdle	2
Lacrimal (2)		Coxal, innominate, or hip bones (2)	
Vomer (1)		Lower extremity	60
Auditory ossicles	6	Femur (2)	
Malleus (2)		Tibia (2)	
Incus (2)		Fibula (2)	
Stapes (2)		Patella (2)	
Hyoid	1	Tarsals (14)	
Vertebral column	26	Metatarsals (10)	
Cervical vertebrae (7)		Phalanges (28)	
Thoracic vertebrae (12)			
Lumbar vertebrae (5)			
Sacrum (1)			
Coccyx (1)			

From Applegate E: *The anatomy and physiology learning system,* ed 4, St Louis, 2011, Saunders.

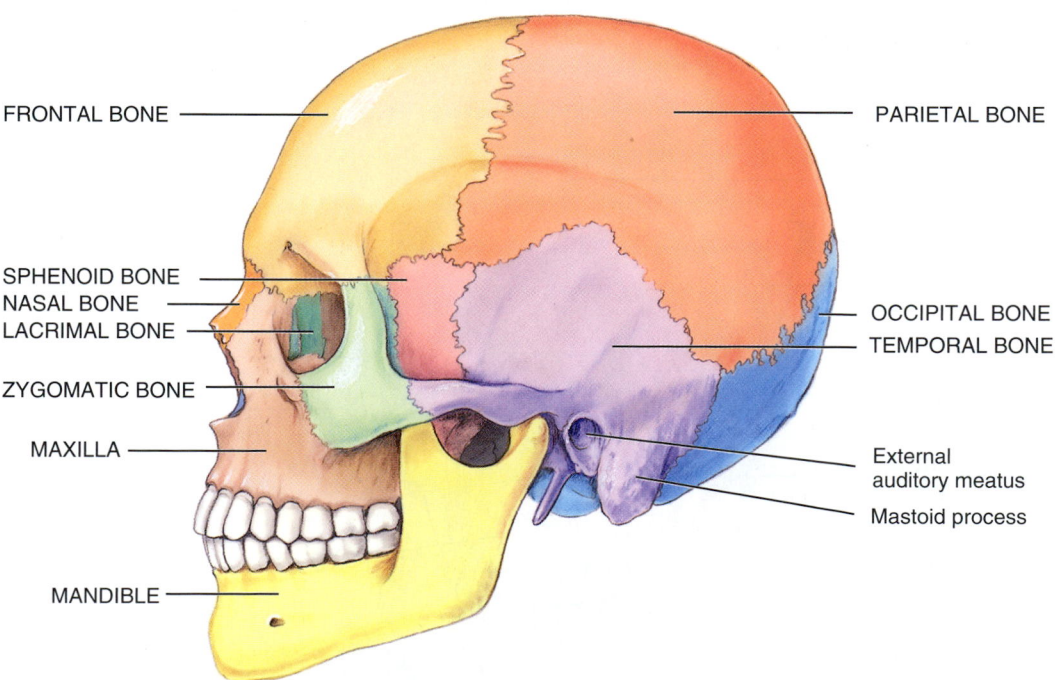

Figure 7-5 Skull, lateral view. (From Applegate E: *The anatomy and physiology learning system,* ed 4, St Louis, 2011, Saunders.)

of the skull. The paranasal sinuses are arranged around the nasal cavity and drain into it.

Cranium

Frontal Bone

The frontal bone forms the anterior portion of the skull above the eyes (forehead). The paranasal *frontal sinuses* are cavities in the frontal bone.

Parietal Bones

The two parietal bones form most of the superolateral aspect of the skull.

Occipital Bone

The single occipital bone forms most of the posterior part of the skull. The *foramen magnum* is a large opening on the lower surface of the occipital bone. The spinal cord passes through this opening. *Occipital condyles* are rounded processes on each side of the foramen magnum. They articulate with the first cervical vertebra.

Temporal Bones

The two temporal bones, one on each side of the head, form parts of the sides and base of the cranium. Near the inferior margin of the temporal bone, there is an opening, the *external auditory meatus,* which is a canal that leads to the middle ear. Just anterior to the external auditory meatus, the temporal bone articulates with the mandible to form the *temporomandibular joint* (TMJ). Posterior and inferior to each external auditory meatus, there is a rough protuberance, the *mastoid process.* The mastoid process contains air cells that drain into the middle ear cavity.

Sphenoid Bone

The sphenoid bone is an irregularly shaped bone that spans the entire width of the cranial floor. It is wedged between other bones in the anterior portion of the cranium. The sphenoid bone contains paranasal *sphenoid sinuses.*

Ethmoid Bone

The ethmoid bone is located anterior to the sphenoid bone and forms most of the bony area between the nasal cavity and the orbits. The ethmoid bone contains many small, paranasal *ethmoidal sinuses.*

Facial Bones

The 14 facial bones form the basic framework and shape of the face. They also provide attachments for the muscles that control facial expression and move the jaw for chewing. All facial bones except the vomer and mandible are paired. Facial bones are illustrated in Figures 7-4 and 7-5.

Maxillary Bones

The maxillary bones, or *maxillae,* form the upper jaw and the anterior part of the hard palate or roof of the mouth. Each maxilla has a large paranasal *maxillary sinus.* These are the largest of all the paranasal sinuses.

Palatine Bones

The palatine bones are behind, or posterior to, the maxillae and form the posterior portion of the hard palate.

Nasal Bones

The two nasal bones are small rectangular bones that form the bridge of the nose.

Lacrimal Bones

The small, thin lacrimal bones are located in the medial walls of the orbits, between the ethmoid bone and the maxilla. Each one has a small *lacrimal groove* that is a pathway for a tube that carries tears from the eyes to the nasal cavity.

Zygomatic Bones

The zygomatic bones, also called *malar* bones, form the prominences of the cheeks.

Inferior Nasal Conchae

The inferior nasal conchae are thin, curved bones that are attached to the lateral walls of the nasal cavity and project into the nasal cavity.

Vomer

The thin, flat vomer is in the inferior portion of the midline in the nasal cavity. It forms part of the *nasal septum.*

Mandible

The mandible is the lower jaw. It articulates with the temporal bone to form the *temporomandibular joint.*

Auditory Ossicles

Three tiny bones form a chain in each middle ear cavity in the temporal bone. These are the *malleus, incus,* and *stapes.* These bones transmit sound waves from the tympanic membrane, or eardrum, to the inner ear, where the sound receptors are located.

HYOID BONE

The hyoid bone is not really part of the skull, so it is listed separately. It is a U-shaped bone in the neck, suspended under the mandible. It is unique because it is the only bone in the body that does not articulate directly with another bone. It functions as a base for the tongue and as an attachment for several muscles associated with swallowing.

VERTEBRAL COLUMN

The vertebral column extends from the skull to the pelvis and contains 26 bones called *vertebrae* (singular, *vertebra*). The bones are separated by pads of fibrocartilage called *intervertebral discs.* The discs act as shock absorbers and allow the column to bend. Normally there are four curvatures, illustrated in Figure 7-6, that increase the strength and resilience of the column. They are named according to

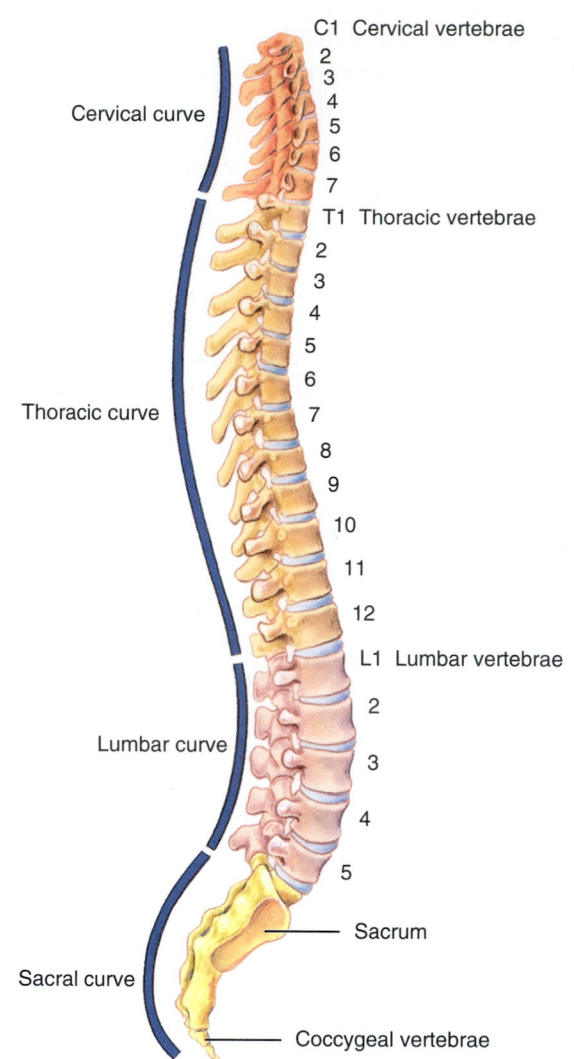

C1 Cervical vertebrae
2
3
4
Cervical curve
5
6
7
T1 Thoracic vertebrae
2
3
4
5
6
Thoracic curve
7
8
9
10
11
12
L1 Lumbar vertebrae
2
Lumbar curve
3
4
5
Sacrum
Sacral curve
Coccygeal vertebrae

Figure 7-6 Curvatures of the vertebral column. The thoracic and sacral curvatures are concave anteriorly, and the cervical and lumbar curvatures are convex anteriorly. (From Applegate E: *The anatomy and physiology learning system,* ed 4, St Louis, 2011, Saunders.)

the region in which they are located. The *thoracic* and *sacral curvatures* are concave anteriorly and are present at birth. The *cervical curvature* develops when an infant begins to hold his or her head erect. The *lumbar curvature* develops when an infant begins to stand and walk. Both the cervical and lumbar curvatures are convex anteriorly.

General Structure of Vertebrae

All vertebrae have a common structural pattern, illustrated in Figure 7-7, although there are variations among them. The thick anterior, weight-bearing portion is the *body* or *centrum.* The posterior curved portion is the *vertebral arch.* The vertebral arch and body surround a central large opening, the *vertebral foramen.* When all the vertebrae are stacked together in a column, the vertebral foramina make a canal that contains the spinal cord. *Transverse processes* project laterally from the vertebral arch, and in the posterior midline there is a *spinous process.* These processes are places

Body (centrum)
Vertebral foramen
Transverse process
Vertebral arch
Spinous process

Figure 7-7 General features of vertebrae, viewed from above. (From Applegate E: *The anatomy and physiology learning system,* ed 4, St Louis, 2011, Saunders.)

for muscle attachment. The spinous processes can be felt as bony projections along the midline of the back.

Composition of the Vertebral Column

The seven *cervical vertebrae* are designated C1 through C7. The 12 *thoracic vertebrae* are designated T1 through T12. Five *lumbar vertebrae,* designated L1 through L5, make up the part of the vertebral column in the small of the back. The lumbar vertebrae have large, heavy bodies because they support most of the body weight and have many back muscles attached to them.

The *sacrum* is a triangular bone just below the lumbar vertebrae. In the child there are five separate bones, but these fuse to form a single bone in the adult. The sacrum articulates with the pelvic girdle laterally, at the *sacroiliac joint,* and forms the posterior wall of the pelvic cavity.

The *coccyx,* or tailbone, is the last part of the vertebral column (Figure 7-8). A child has four (the number varies from three to five) separate small bones, but these fuse to form a single bone in the adult.

THORACIC CAGE

The thoracic cage, or bony thorax, protects the heart, lungs, and great vessels. It also supports the bones of the shoulder girdle and plays a role in breathing. The components of the thoracic cage are the thoracic vertebrae dorsally, the ribs laterally, and the sternum and costal cartilage anteriorly.

Sternum

The *sternum,* or breastbone, is in the anterior midline (see Figure 7-8). An important anatomic landmark, the *jugular (suprasternal) notch* is an easily palpable, central indentation in the superior margin of the sternum. The superior portion of the sternum articulates with the clavicles and the first two pairs of ribs. The body of the sternum has notches along the sides where it attaches to the cartilage of the third through seventh ribs.

Ribs

Twelve pairs of *ribs,* illustrated in Figure 7-8, form the curved, lateral margins of the thoracic cage. One pair is attached to each of the 12 thoracic vertebrae. The upper

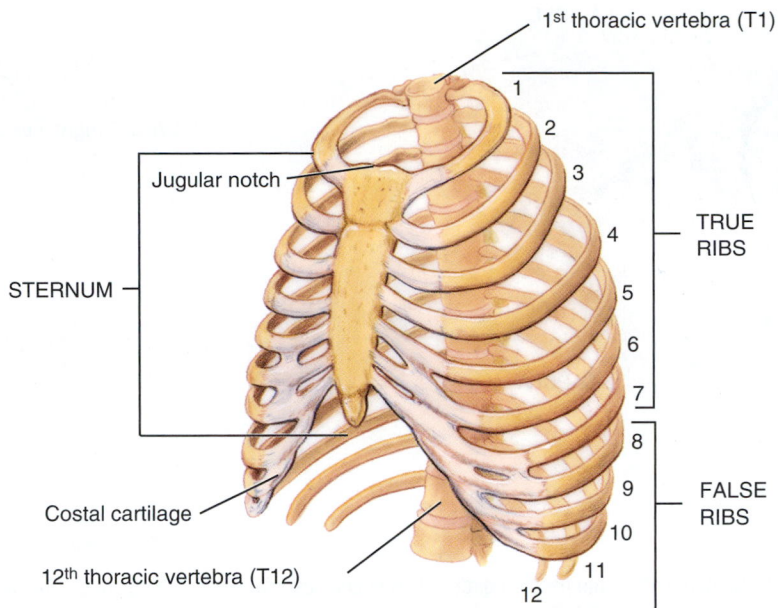

1st thoracic vertebra (T1)

Jugular notch

STERNUM

Costal cartilage

12th thoracic vertebra (T12)

1
2
3
4
5
6
7
8
9
10
11
12

TRUE
RIBS

FALSE
RIBS

Figure 7-8 Thoracic cage. (From Applegate E: *The anatomy and physiology learning system,* ed 4, St Louis, 2011, Saunders.)

seven pairs of ribs are called *true,* or *vertebrosternal, ribs* because they attach to the sternum directly by their individual *costal cartilage.* The lower five pairs of ribs are called *false ribs* because their costal cartilage does not reach the sternum directly. The first three pairs of false ribs reach the sternum indirectly by joining with the cartilage of the ribs above. These are called *vertebrochondral ribs.* The bottom two rib pairs have no anterior attachment and are called *vertebral ribs* or *floating ribs.*

BONES OF THE APPENDICULAR SKELETON

The 126 bones of the appendicular skeleton are suspended from two yokes or girdles that are anchored to the axial skeleton. They are additions or appendages to the axis of the body. The appendicular skeleton is designed for movement. If a portion of the appendicular skeleton is immobilized for a period of time, movement can be awkward.

PECTORAL GIRDLE

Each half of the **pectoral girdle,** or *shoulder girdle,* consists of two bones: an anterior *clavicle* and a posterior *scapula.* The bones of the pectoral girdle, illustrated in Figure 7-9, form the connection between the upper extremities and the axial skeleton. The clavicles and scapulae, with their associated muscles, also form the shoulder.

The *clavicle* is commonly called the *collarbone.* It is an elongated, S-shaped bone that articulates proximally with the manubrium of the sternum. The distal end articulates with the scapula.

The *scapula,* commonly called the *shoulder blade,* is a thin, flat triangular bone on the posterior surface of the thoracic wall. It articulates with the clavicle and the humerus. The *acromion process* of the scapula forms the point of the shoulder. On the lateral margin of the scapula there is a shallow depression, the *glenoid cavity* (fossa), where the head of the humerus connects to the scapula. The clavicle and scapula provide attachments for numerous muscles.

UPPER EXTREMITY

The upper extremity (limb) consists of the bones of the arm, forearm, and hand.

Arm

The arm, or *brachium,* is the region between the shoulder and the elbow. It contains a single long bone, the *humerus,* illustrated in Figure 7-10. The *head* is the large, smooth, rounded end that fits into the scapula. The deltoid muscle attaches to the humerus along the shaft of the humerus. At the distal end, on the posterior surface, there is a depression, the *olecranon fossa,* where the ulna fits with the humerus to form the hinged elbow joint. Two smooth, rounded projections are evident on the distal end of the humerus. The capitulum is on the lateral side and articulates with the radius of the forearm. The trochlea is on the medial side and articulates with the ulna of the forearm.

Forearm

The forearm, or *antebrachium,* is the region between the elbow and wrist. It is formed by the *radius* on the lateral side and the *ulna* on the medial side when the forearm is in anatomic position. When the hand is turned so that the

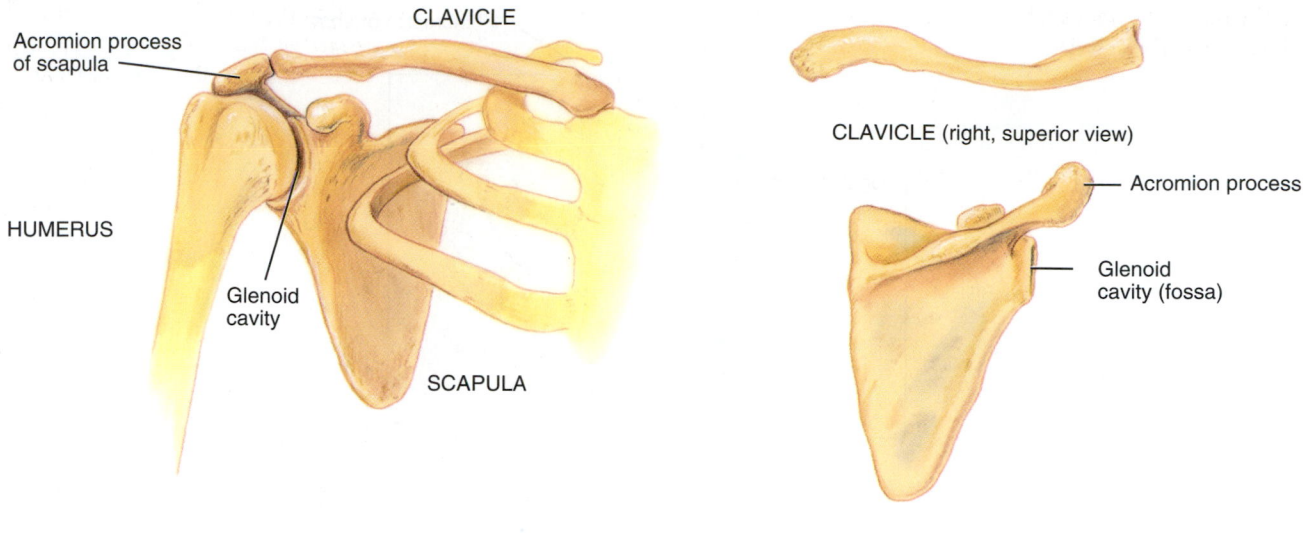

Figure 7-9 Components of the pectoral girdle: clavicle and scapula. (From Applegate E: *The anatomy and physiology learning system,* ed 4, St Louis, 2011, Saunders.)

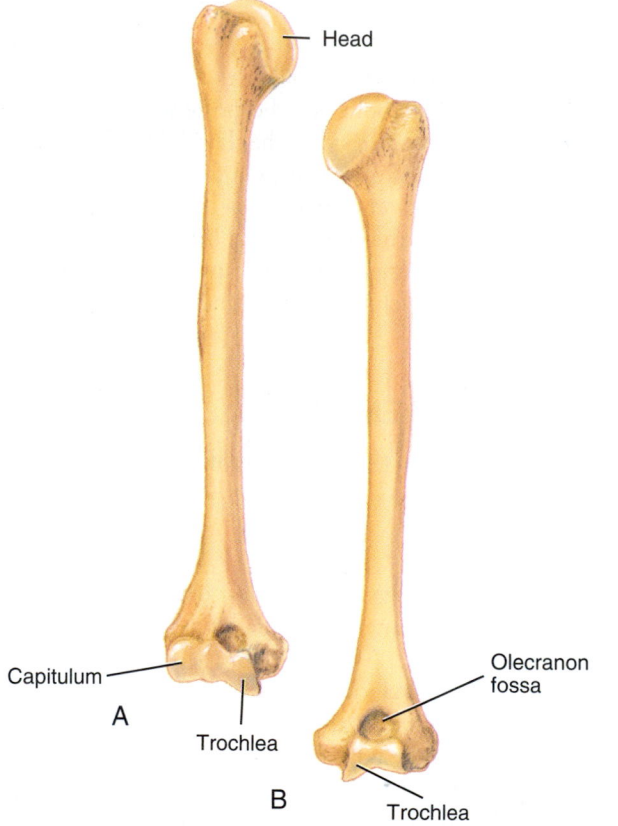

Figure 7-10 Humerus. **A,** Anterior view. **B,** Posterior view. (From Applegate E: *The anatomy and physiology learning system,* ed 4, St Louis, 2011, Saunders.)

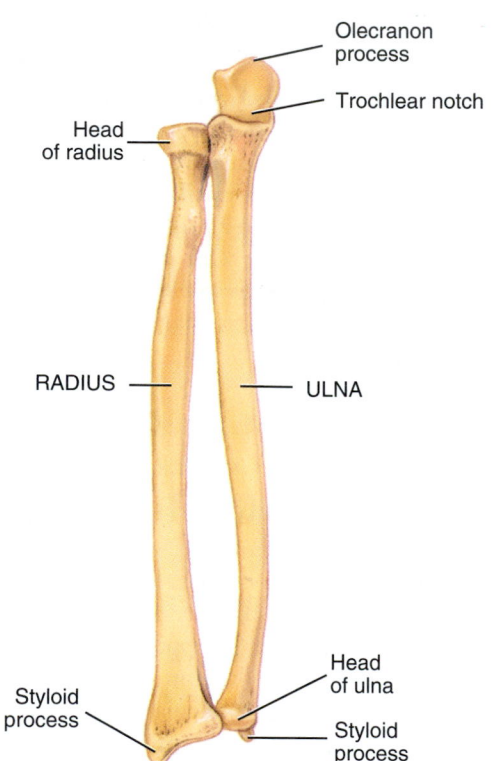

Figure 7-11 Radius and ulna, anterior view. The radius is on the lateral side, and the ulna is the medial bone. (From Applegate E: *The anatomy and physiology learning system,* ed 4, St Louis, 2011, Saunders.)

palm faces backward, the radius crosses over the ulna. The radius and ulna are illustrated in Figure 7-11.

The radius has a circular, disclike *head* on the proximal end. This articulates with the capitulum of the humerus. On the distal end, the prominent marking is the *styloid process,* a pointed projection on the lateral side.

The proximal end of the ulna has a wrenchlike shape, with the opening of the wrench being the *trochlear notch,* or semilunar notch. The projection at the upper end of the notch is the *olecranon process,* which fits into the olecranon fossa of the humerus and forms the bony point of the elbow. The *head* is at the distal end, and on the medial side of the head the pointed *styloid process* serves as an attachment point for ligaments of the wrist.

Hand

The hand, illustrated in Figure 7-12, is composed of the wrist, palm, and five fingers. The wrist, or *carpus,* contains eight small *carpal bones,* tightly bound by ligaments. The palm of the hand, or *metacarpus,* contains five *metacarpal bones,* one in line with each finger. These bones are not named but are numbered one through five starting on the thumb side. The 14 bones of the fingers are called *phalanges.* Some people refer to these as *digits.* Three phalanges are in each finger (a proximal, middle, and distal phalanx) except the thumb, or *pollex,* which has two. The thumb lacks a middle phalanx. The proximal phalanges articulate with the metacarpals.

PELVIC GIRDLE

The **pelvic girdle,** or *hip girdle,* attaches the lower extremities to the axial skeleton and provides a strong support for the weight of the body. It also provides support and protection for the urinary bladder, a portion of the large intestine, and the internal reproductive organs, which are located in the pelvic cavity.

The pelvic girdle consists of two *coxal* (hip) *bones,* illustrated in Figure 7-13. The coxal bones are also called the *ossa coxae,* or *innominate bones.* Anteriorly, the two bones articulate with each other at the *symphysis pubis;* posteriorly, they articulate with the sacrum at the *iliosacral joints.* During childhood, each coxal bone consists of three separate parts: the *ilium, ischium,* and *pubis.* In the adult, these bones are firmly fused to form a single bone. Where the three bones meet, there is a large depression, the *acetabulum,* which holds the head of the femur. The *obturator foramen* is a large opening between the pubis and ischium that functions as a passageway for blood vessels, nerves, and muscle tendons.

Together, the sacrum, coccyx, and pelvic girdle form the basin-shaped pelvis. The *false pelvis* (greater pelvis) is

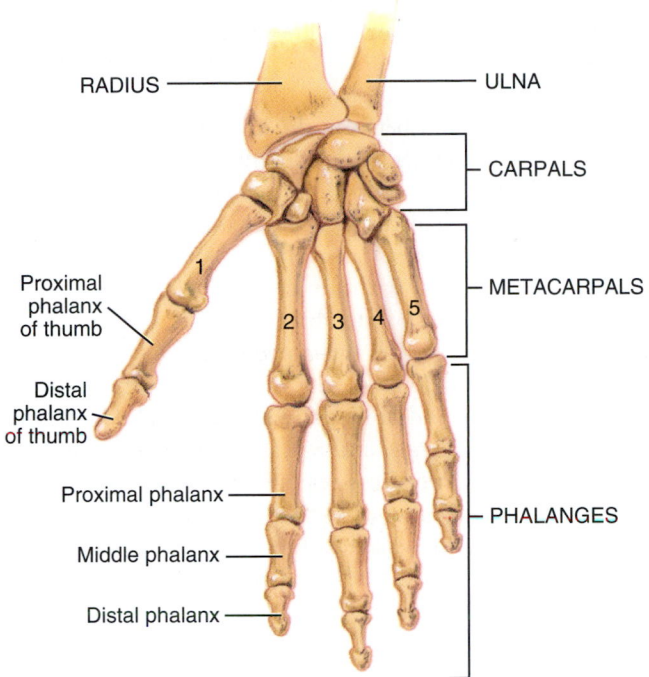

Hand (right, palmar aspect)

Figure 7-12 Hand. The carpals form the wrist, the metacarpals form the palm, and the phalanges form the fingers. (From Applegate E: *The anatomy and physiology learning system,* ed 4, St Louis, 2011, Saunders.)

PELVIC GIRDLE (anterior view)   OS COXAE (right, lateral view)

Figure 7-13 Bones of the pelvic girdle. The right and left ossa coxae form the pelvic girdle. Posteriorly, the two bones are separated by the sacrum. Anteriorly, they meet at the symphysis pubis. (From Applegate E: *The anatomy and physiology learning system,* ed 4, St Louis, 2011, Saunders.)

surrounded by the flared portions of the ilium bones and the lumbar vertebrae. The *true pelvis* (lesser pelvis) is smaller and inferior to the false pelvis. It is the region below the *pelvic brim,* or *pelvic inlet,* and it is encircled by bone. The large opening at the bottom of this region is the *pelvic outlet.* The dimensions of the true pelvis are especially important in childbirth.

LOWER EXTREMITY

The lower extremity (limb) consists of the bones of the thigh, leg, foot, and patella, or kneecap. The lower extremities support the entire weight of the body when we are erect, and they are exposed to tremendous forces when we walk, run, and jump. With this in mind, it is not surprising that the bones of the lower extremity are larger and stronger than those in the upper extremity.

Thigh

The *thigh* is the region from the hip to the knee. It contains a single long bone, the *femur,* illustrated in Figure 7-14. It is the largest, longest, and strongest bone in the body.

The large, smooth, ball-like *head* of the femur has a small depression called the *fovea capitis.* A ligament attaches here.

Prominent projections at the proximal end, the *greater* and *lesser trochanters,* are major sites for muscle attachment. The *neck* is between the head and the trochanters. The distal end is marked by two large, rounded surfaces, the *lateral* and *medial condyles.* These form joints with the bones of the leg. The *intercondylar notch* is a depression between the condyles that contains ligaments associated with the knee joint. On the anterior surface, between the condyles, a smooth *patellar surface* marks the area for the kneecap.

Leg

The *leg* is the region between the knee and the ankle. It is formed by the slender *fibula* on the lateral side and the larger, weight-bearing *tibia,* or shin bone, on the medial side. The tibia articulates with the femur to form the knee joint and with the *talus* (one of the foot bones) to allow flexion and extension at the ankle.

The proximal end of the fibula is the *head,* and the projection at the distal end is the *lateral malleolus,* which forms the lateral bulge of the ankle. The superior surface of the tibia is flattened and smooth, with two slightly concave regions called the *lateral* and *medial condyles.* The condyles of the femur fit into these regions. The *anterior crest* is a sharp ridge on the anterior surface and forms the shin. On the medial side of the distal end, the *medial malleolus* forms the medial bulge of the ankle. Figure 7-15 illustrates the tibia and fibula.

FEMUR and PATELLA (right)

Figure 7-14 Femur and patella *(right).* **A,** Anterior view. **B,** Posterior view. (From Applegate E: *The anatomy and physiology learning system,* ed 4, St Louis, 2011, Saunders.)

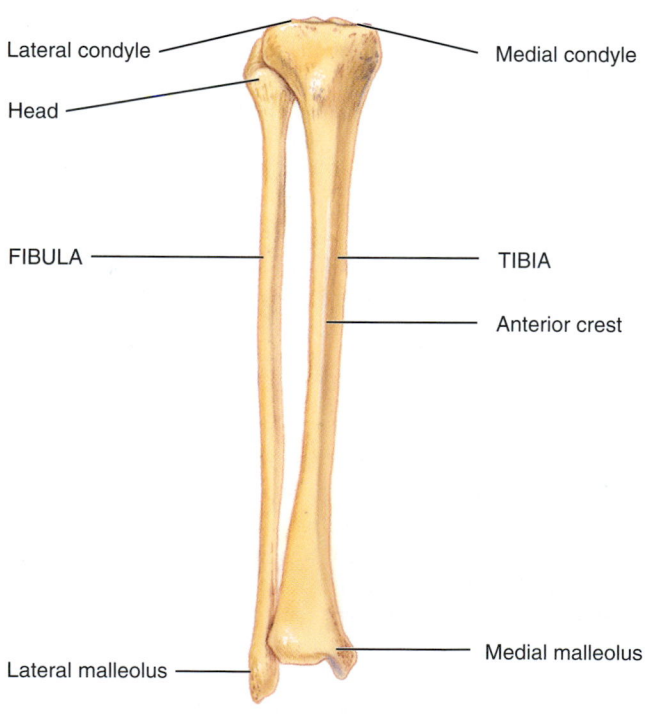

Anterior view (right)

Figure 7-15 Tibia and fibula, anterior view *(right).* The fibula is on the lateral side of the leg, and the tibia is on the medial side. (From Applegate E: *The anatomy and physiology learning system,* ed 4, St Louis, 2011, Saunders.)

Figure 7-16 Bones of the foot. **A,** Superior view. **B,** Lateral view. (From Applegate E: *The anatomy and physiology learning system,* ed 4, St Louis, 2011, Saunders.)

Foot

The *foot,* illustrated in Figure 7-16, is composed of the ankle, instep, and five toes. The ankle, or *tarsus,* contains seven *tarsal bones.* These correspond to the carpals in the wrist. The largest tarsal bone is the *calcaneus,* or heel bone. The *talus,* another tarsal bone, rests on top of the calcaneus and articulates with the tibia. The instep of the foot, or *metatarsus,* contains five *metatarsal bones,* one in line with each toe. The distal ends of these bones form the ball of the foot. These bones are not named but are numbered one through five starting on the medial side. The tarsals and metatarsals, together with strong tendons and ligaments, form the arches of the foot. The 14 bones of the toes are called *phalanges.* Three phalanges are in each toe (a proximal, middle, and distal phalanx), except in the great (or big) toe, or *hallux,* which has only two. The great toe lacks a middle phalanx. The proximal phalanges articulate with the metatarsals.

Patella

The *patella,* or *kneecap,* is a flat, triangular bone enclosed within the major tendon that anchors the anterior thigh muscle to the tibia. It provides a smooth surface for the tendon as it turns the corner between the thigh and leg when the knee is flexed. It also protects the knee joint anteriorly.

ARTICULATIONS

An **articulation,** or joint, is where two bones come together. In terms of the amount of movement that articulations allow, there are three types of joints: immovable, slightly movable, and freely movable.

SYNARTHROSES

Synarthroses are immovable joints. The singular form is *synarthrosis.* In these joints, the bones come in close contact and are separated by only a thin layer of fibrous connective tissue. The *sutures* in the skull are examples of immovable joints.

AMPHIARTHROSES

Slightly movable joints are called **amphiarthroses.** The singular form is *amphiarthrosis.* In this type of joint, the bones are connected by hyaline cartilage or fibrocartilage. The ribs connected to the sternum by costal cartilage are slightly movable joints connected by hyaline cartilage. The symphysis pubis is a slightly movable joint in which there is a fibrocartilage pad between the two bones. The joints between the vertebrae, the intervertebral discs, are also of this type.

DIARTHROSES

Most joints in the adult body are **diarthroses** or freely movable joints. The singular form is *diarthrosis.* In this type of joint, the ends of the opposing bones are covered with hyaline cartilage, the **articular cartilage**, and they are separated by a space called the *joint cavity.* The components of the joints are enclosed in a dense fibrous *joint capsule* (Figure 7-17).

The outer layer of the capsule consists of the ligaments that hold the bones together. The inner layer is the *synovial membrane,* which secretes *synovial fluid* into the joint cavity for lubrication. Because all of these joints have a synovial membrane, they are sometimes called *synovial joints.*

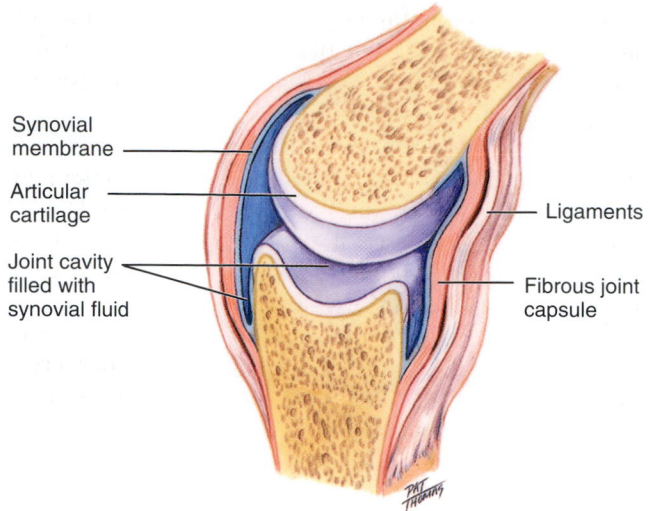

Figure 7-17 Generalized structure of a synovial joint. (From Applegate E: *The anatomy and physiology learning system*, ed 4, St Louis, 2011, Saunders.)

Some diarthroses have pads and cushions associated with them. The knee has fibrocartilaginous pads, called *semilunar cartilages* or the *lateral meniscus* and *medial meniscus,* which rest on the lateral and medial condyles of the tibia. The pads help stabilize the joint and act as shock absorbers. *Bursae* are fluid-filled sacs that act as cushions and help reduce friction. Bursae are lined with a synovial membrane that secretes synovial fluid into the sac. They are commonly located between the skin and underlying bone or between tendons and ligaments. Inflammation of a bursa is called *bursitis.*

There are six types of diarthrotic or freely movable joints based on the shapes of their parts and the types of movement they allow. These are described and illustrated in Figure 7-18.

Figure 7-18 Types of freely movable joints. (From Applegate E: *The anatomy and physiology learning system,* ed 4, St Louis, 2011, Saunders.)

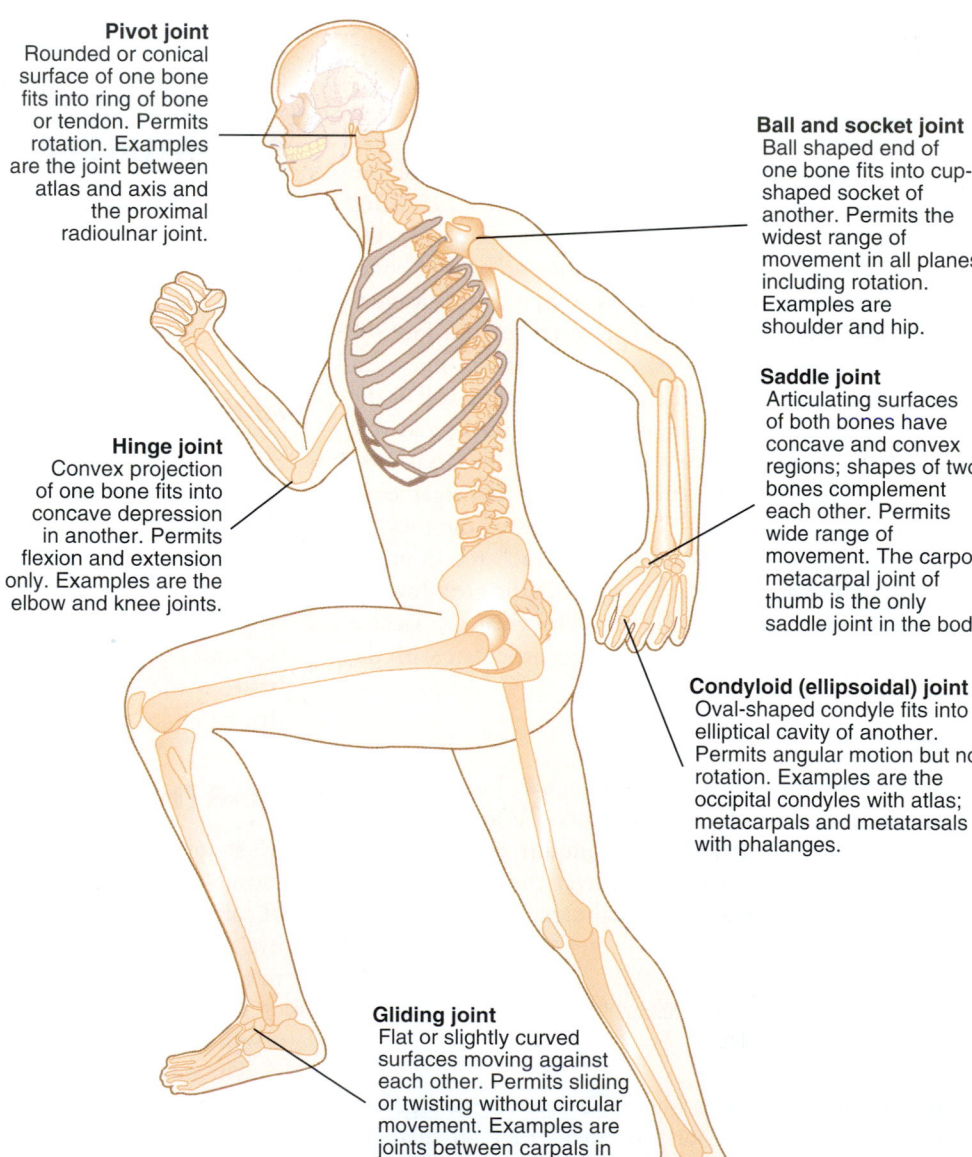

Pivot joint
Rounded or conical surface of one bone fits into ring of bone or tendon. Permits rotation. Examples are the joint between atlas and axis and the proximal radioulnar joint.

Ball and socket joint
Ball shaped end of one bone fits into cup-shaped socket of another. Permits the widest range of movement in all planes, including rotation. Examples are shoulder and hip.

Saddle joint
Articulating surfaces of both bones have concave and convex regions; shapes of two bones complement each other. Permits wide range of movement. The carpometacarpal joint of thumb is the only saddle joint in the body.

Hinge joint
Convex projection of one bone fits into concave depression in another. Permits flexion and extension only. Examples are the elbow and knee joints.

Condyloid (ellipsoidal) joint
Oval-shaped condyle fits into elliptical cavity of another. Permits angular motion but not rotation. Examples are the occipital condyles with atlas; metacarpals and metatarsals with phalanges.

Gliding joint
Flat or slightly curved surfaces moving against each other. Permits sliding or twisting without circular movement. Examples are joints between carpals in wrist and between tarsals in ankle.

Synovial membrane

Articular cartilage

Joint cavity filled with synovial fluid

Ligaments

Fibrous joint capsule

AGING OF THE SKELETAL SYSTEM

The major age-related change in the skeletal system is the loss of calcium from the bones. Calcium loss occurs in both men and women, but it starts at an earlier age and is more severe in women. The exact reasons for the loss are unknown and possibly involve a combination of several factors. These may include an imbalance between osteoblast and osteoclast activity, imbalance between calcitonin and parathormone levels, reduced absorption of calcium and/or vitamin D from the digestive tract, poor diet, and lack of exercise. Whatever the cause, there is no sure way of preventing the loss, but adequate calcium and vitamin D in the diet may help reduce the effects.

Another change with age is a decrease in the rate of collagen synthesis. This means that the bones have less strength and are more brittle. Bones fracture more readily in elderly individuals, and the healing process may be slow or incomplete. Tendons and ligaments become less flexible because of the changes in collagen.

The articular cartilage at the ends of bones tends to become thinner and deteriorates with age. This causes joint disorders that are commonly found in older individuals. People also appear to get shorter as they get older. This is caused partially by loss of bone mass and partially by compression of the intervertebral discs.

Age-related changes in the skeletal system cannot be prevented. An active and healthy lifestyle with appropriate exercise and an adequate diet help reduce the effect of the changes in the skeletal system.

Common Pathology of the Skeletal System

Disease	Signs and Symptoms	Etiology	Diagnosis and Treatment
Sprain	Painful swelling and/or bruising of a joint area with decreased movement ability.	Joint ligament damage caused by the joint being taken beyond its functional range of motion.	Diagnosis is by examination and imaging modalities. Treatment is RICE: *Rest* the sprain. *Ice* should be applied. *Compress* with wraps, immobilize. *Elevate* to minimize swelling.
Strain	Localized stiffness, discoloration, and bruising in the muscle area.	The muscle fibers associated with a joint tear as a result of overstretching.	Diagnosis is by examination and imaging modalities. Treatment is RICE: *Rest* the strain *Ice* should be applied *Compress* with wraps, immobilize *Elevate* to minimize swelling
Spina bifida	A baby is born with an opening in the back through which the meninges and spinal cord may protrude.	There may be a genetic basis for the condition. It most likely results from the interaction of multiple genes and environmental factors.	Prenatal testing for spina bifida includes blood tests, ultrasound, and amniocentesis. Mild forms may require no treatment. More severe forms require surgery to close the opening. There is no known cure for nerve damage caused by spina bifida.
Osteosarcoma	Recurring limb pain that may be worse at night. If the tumor is large it can appear as a swelling. The affected bone may fracture easily.	Osteoblasts multiply without control and form large tumors in bones.	Diagnosis is by x-ray examination followed by other scan modalities. Current standard treatment uses chemotherapy followed by surgical resection.
Osteoporosis	There are no symptoms. As bone loss becomes more severe, there may be back pain, and bone fractures occur more frequently.	Immobilization and lack of exercise can cause bone loss. Endocrine disorders also may be involved, along with malnutrition and inadequate calcium intake and/or adsorption.	Diagnosis can be made by measuring the bone mineral density. Medications can be used to reduce further bone loss.
Tennis elbow	Pain and swelling at the elbow joint.	Repeated contraction of muscles that control hand and wrist movements cause their proximal attachments on the humerus to become irritated, inflamed, and painful.	Diagnosis is made by clinical signs and symptoms. Minor cases may be treated by simply relaxing the affected arm. Eccentric exercise using a rubber bar may be effective at reducing pain and increasing strength.

Continued

Common Pathology of the Skeletal System—cont'd

Disease	Signs and Symptoms	Etiology	Diagnosis and Treatment
Arthritis	Painful inflammation of one or more joints, often accompanied by swelling.	The inflammation is a result of damage to the joint from disease, daily wear and tear on the joint, and/or muscle strains.	Diagnosis is made by clinical examination by an appropriate health professional and may be supported by other tests such as radiology and blood tests. Treatment focuses on relieving pain and reducing swelling.
Osteoarthritis	Pain during movement, stiffness in the morning or after periods of inactivity, and loss of flexibility.	Characterized by the degeneration of articular cartilage and changes in the synovial membrane.	Diagnosis is based on history, physical examination, and imaging tests. Treatment is aimed at relieving the symptoms.
Rheumatoid arthritis	Tends to first affect the smaller joints such as fingers and toes and then progresses to the knees and hips.	Caused by changes that occur in the connective tissues of the body, especially the joints. It may be an autoimmune disease.	Diagnosis is based on physical examination, blood tests, and imaging modalities. Medications are used to relieve pain, and physical therapy can help maintain flexibility of the joints.
Osteomalacia	Early stages present no symptoms. As the condition progresses, there may be a dull, aching bone pain and muscle weakness. Bones bend easily under stress and become deformed; in childhood this is called *rickets*.	The bones soften because of inadequate amounts of calcium and phosphorus as a result of a lack of vitamin D in the diet. Vitamin D is necessary for the body to absorb the minerals necessary for healthy bones.	Diagnostic techniques include blood and urine tests for levels of calcium, phosphorus, and vitamin D combined with imaging modalities and a biopsy. Treatment may require vitamin D and calcium or phosphate supplements in the diet. For severe cases injection of large doses of vitamin D may be required.
Osteomyelitis	Tenderness and swelling around the affected bone with fever, fatigue and nausea. If located in the vertebrae, severe back pain is present, especially at night.	Caused by an inflammation of the bone marrow as a result of bacterial infection. The bacteria may enter via the bloodstream, from penetrating trauma, or after internal fixation of fractures.	Diagnosis is based on radiologic results showing a lytic center with a ring of sclerosis. Culture of material taken from a bone biopsy is needed to identify the specific pathogen. Treatment requires prolonged antibiotic therapy.
Dislocation	Difficulty in moving a joint, accompanied by intense pain, joint instability, and deformity of the joint area.	A bone has been dislodged from its joint or socket with the tearing of ligaments, tendons, and the articular capsule.	Diagnosis is by physical examination and imaging modalities. A dislocated joint usually can be successfully returned to its normal position by a trained medical professional.
Gout	A red, tender, hot, swollen joint. The metatarsal-phalangeal joint at the base of the big toe is affected most often.	Caused by an excessive accumulation of uric acid that forms needle-like crystals within the joint.	The disorder is diagnosed by aspiring joint fluid and observing the crystals under the microscope. It can be effectively treated with antiinflammatory drugs and dietary adjustments.
Ankylosing spondylitis	Sacroiliitis is typically the first manifestation, accompanied by a chronic dull pain, felt deep in the lower lumbar or gluteal region, and morning stiffness.	An inflammation causes some of the vertebrae to fuse together. Genetic factors may be involved.	Diagnosis involves imaging tests to observe the changes in the bones and joints. Antiinflammatory drugs are prescribed to relieve pain. Physical therapy may help in maintaining flexibility in the joints.

TERMINOLOGY REVIEW

Key Term	Word Parts	Definition
Amphiarthroses	*arthr/o:* joint *-osis:* condition of	Slightly movable joints; singular, *amphiarthrosis.*
Appendicular skeleton	*appendicul-:* little attachment	Bones that are attached to the body; upper and lower extremities.
Appositional growth		Growth resulting from material being deposited on the surface, such as the growth in diameter of long bones.
Articular cartilage	*artic-:* joint	Thin layer of hyaline cartilage that covers the ends of long bones in joints.
Articulation	*artic-:* joint	A joint; area of contact between two bones.
Axial skeleton		Bones of the head, neck, and trunk.
Diaphysis	*dia-:* through	The long straight shaft of a long bone.
Diarthroses	*arthr/o:* joint *-osis:* condition of	Freely movable joints characterized by a joint cavity; also called a *synovial joint;* singular, *diarthrosis.*
Endosteum	*end/o:* within, inward *oste/o:* bone	Membranous lining of a cavity within a bone.
Epiphyseal line	*epi-:* above, upon, on *-phys:* to grow	The remnant of the epiphyseal plate after the cartilage calcifies and growth ceases.
Epiphyseal plate	*epi-:* above, upon, on *-phys:* to grow	The cartilaginous plate between the epiphysis and diaphysis of a bone; responsible for the lengthwise growth of a long bone.
Epiphysis	*epi-:* above, upon, on	The end of a long bone.
Hematopoiesis	*hem/o:* blood *poie-:* making	Production of blood or its cells.
Osteoblasts	*oste/o:* bone *-blast:* immature cell	Bone-forming cells; immature bone cells.
Osteoclasts	*oste/o:* bone *-clast:* to break	Cells that destroy, break down, or resorb bone tissue.
Osteocytes	*oste/o:* bone *-cyte:* cell	Mature bone cells.
Osteogenesis	*oste/o:* bone *-genesis:* production	Formation of bone; also called *ossification.*
Osteon	*oste/o:* bone	Structural unit of bone; haversian system.
Pectoral girdle	*pect/o:* chest	Attachment for the upper extremities in the chest region; clavicle and scapula.
Pelvic girdle	*pelv:* basin	Attachment for the lower extremities; bones collectively shaped like a basin; ilium, ischium, pubis.
Periosteum	*peri:* around *oste/o:* bone	Tough white outer membrane that covers a bone.
Sutures		Immovable fibrous joints between the flat bones of the skull
Synarthroses	*syn-:* together *arthr-:* joint *-osis:* condition of	Immovable joinst; singular, *synarthrosis.*

ON THE WEB

For information on the skeletal system:

Loyola University Medical Education Network: Pick a Bone: www.meddean.luc.edu/lumen/MedEd/GrossAnatomy/learnem/bones/main_bone.htm

Merck Manual—Bone, Joint, and Muscle Disorders: www.merck.com/mmhe *(Click on "Bone, Joint, and Muscle Disorders")*

National Osteoporosis Foundation: www.nof.org

8

Muscular System

e Check out the Evolve site at http://evolve.elsevier.com/Bonewit/today/ to access additional interactive activities and exercises to help you study and prepare for success.

LEARNING OBJECTIVES

1. State the characteristics and functions of muscle tissue.
2. Describe the structure of a skeletal muscle.
3. List and describe the sequence of events involved in the contraction of a skeletal muscle fiber.
4. Explain how energy is provided for a muscle contraction.
5. Describe oxygen debt.
6. Describe and illustrate the movements accomplished by the contraction of skeletal muscle.
7. Identify and describe the major muscles making up the axial skeleton.
8. Identify and describe the major muscles making up the appendicular skeleton.
9. Describe ways in which the aging of an individual affects the muscular system.
10. Identify pathology related to the muscular system.

CHAPTER OUTLINE

INTRODUCTION TO THE MUSCULAR SYSTEM
CHARACTERISTICS AND FUNCTIONS OF THE MUSCULAR SYSTEM
STRUCTURE OF SKELETAL MUSCLE
Whole Skeletal Muscle
Skeletal Muscle Fibers
Nerve and Blood Supply
Skeletal Muscle Attachments
CONTRACTION OF SKELETAL MUSCLE
Stimulus for Contraction
Energy Sources and Oxygen Debt
Movements
SKELETAL MUSCLE GROUPS
Naming Muscles
Muscles of the Head and Neck
Muscles of Facial Expression

Muscles of Mastication
Neck Muscles
Muscles of the Trunk
Vertebral Column Muscles
Thoracic Wall Muscles
Abdominal Wall Muscles
Pelvic Floor Muscles
Muscles of the Upper Extremity
Muscles That Move the Shoulder and Arm
Muscles That Move the Forearm and Hand
Muscles of the Lower Extremity
Muscles That Move the Thigh
Muscles That Move the Leg
Muscles That Move the Ankle and Foot
AGING OF THE MUSCULAR SYSTEM

KEY TERMS

acetylcholine (ah-see-till-KOH-leen)
acetylcholinesterase
   (ah-see-till-koh-lin-ES-ter-ase)
antagonists (an-TAG-oh-nists)
aponeurosis (ah-pah-noo-ROE-sis)
contractility (kon-track-TILL-ih-tee)
elasticity (ee-lass-TISS-ih-tee)

epimysium (ep-ih-MYE-see-um)
excitability (eks-eye-tah-BILL-ih-tee)
extensibility (eks-ten-sih-BILL-ih-tee)
insertion (in-SIR-shun)
motor unit (MOH-toar YOO-nit)
neuromuscular junction (noo-roe-MUSK-
   yoo-lar JUNK-shun)

neurotransmitter
   (noo-roh-TRANS-mit-ter)
origin (OR-ih-jin)
prime mover (PRYM MOO-ver)
sarcolemma (sar-koh-LEM-mah)
sarcoplasm (sar-koh-plazm)
synergists (SIN-er-gists)

INTRODUCTION TO THE MUSCULAR SYSTEM

As described in Chapter 5, there are three types of muscle tissue: skeletal, visceral, and cardiac. These are reviewed in Table 8-1. This chapter takes a closer look at skeletal muscle, which makes up about 40% of an individual's body weight. It forms more than 600 muscles that are attached to the bones of the skeleton. Skeletal muscles are under conscious control, and when they contract they move the bones. Skeletal muscles also allow us to smile, frown, pout, show surprise, and exhibit other forms of facial expression.

CHARACTERISTICS AND FUNCTIONS OF THE MUSCULAR SYSTEM

Skeletal muscle has four primary characteristics that relate to its functions:
- **Excitability**: Excitability is the ability to receive and respond to a stimulus. To function properly, muscles have to respond to a stimulus from the nervous system.
- **Contractility**: Contractility is the ability to shorten or contract. When a muscle responds to a stimulus, it shortens to produce movement.
- **Extensibility**: Extensibility means that a muscle can be stretched or extended. Skeletal muscles are often arranged in opposing pairs. When one muscle contracts, the other muscle is relaxed and stretched.
- **Elasticity**: Elasticity is the capacity to recoil or return to the original shape and length after contraction or extension.

Table 8-1 Summary of Muscle Tissue

Feature	Skeletal	Visceral	Cardiac
Location	Attached to bones	Walls of internal organs and blood vessels	Heart
Function	Produce body movement	Contraction of viscera and blood vessels	Pump blood through heart and blood vessels
Cell shape	Cylindric	Spindle-shaped; tapered ends	Cylindric, branching
Number of nuclei	Many	One	One
Striations	Present	Absent	Present
Type of control	Voluntary	Involuntary	Involuntary

From Applegate E: *The anatomy and physiology learning system*, ed 4, St Louis, 2011, Saunders.

Muscle contraction fulfills four important functions in the body:
- Movement
- Posture
- Joint stability
- Heat production

Nearly all movement in the body is the result of muscle contraction. Some exceptions to this are the action of cilia, the motility of the flagella on sperm cells, and the ameboid movement of some white blood cells. The integrated action of joints, bones, and skeletal muscles produces obvious movements such as walking and running. Skeletal muscles also produce more subtle movements that result in various facial expressions, eye movements, and respiration. Posture, such as sitting and standing, is maintained as a result of muscle contraction. The skeletal muscles are continually making fine adjustments that hold the body in stationary positions. Skeletal muscles contribute to joint stability. The tendons of many muscles extend over joints and in this way contribute to joint stability. This is particularly evident in the knee and shoulder joints, where muscle tendons are a major factor in stabilizing the joint. Heat production, to maintain body temperature, is an important by-product of muscle metabolism. Nearly 85% of the heat produced in the body is the result of muscle contraction.

STRUCTURE OF SKELETAL MUSCLE

A whole skeletal muscle is considered an organ of the muscular system. For example, the biceps brachii muscle is an organ of the muscular system. Each organ or muscle consists of skeletal muscle tissue, connective tissue, nerve tissue, and blood or vascular tissue.

WHOLE SKELETAL MUSCLE

An individual skeletal muscle such as the biceps muscle may consist of hundreds, or even thousands, of muscle cells (fibers) bundled together and wrapped in a connective tissue covering. Each muscle is surrounded by a connective tissue sheath called the **epimysium**. Fascia consists of connective tissue located outside the epimysium. Fascia surrounds and separates the muscles. Skeletal muscle cells (fibers), like other body cells, are soft and fragile. The connective tissue coverings furnish support and protection for the delicate cells and allow them to withstand the forces of contraction. The coverings also provide pathways for the passage of blood vessels and nerves.

SKELETAL MUSCLE FIBERS

Each individual skeletal muscle fiber consists of a single cylindric muscle cell. The cell membrane is called the **sarcolemma**, and the cytoplasm is the **sarcoplasm**. Multiple nuclei are next to the sarcolemma at the periphery of the cell. There are numerous mitochondria to provide the initial

Rigor mortis: The term *rigor mortis* means the "stiffness of death." Within a short time of death, the adenosine triphosphate in muscles breaks down. This causes the myofilaments to remain locked in a contracted position and the body becomes rigid. A day or so later, muscle proteins begin to deteriorate and the rigor mortis disappears.

Tetanus: The word *tetanus* is often confusing because it means different things to different people. In reference to muscle contraction, the term denotes a steady contraction of a muscle fiber, without a relaxation phase. The word also refers to a disease, commonly called "lockjaw," that is caused by the bacterium *Clostridium tetani*. The toxin from the bacteria causes nerves to be highly excitable, which in turn causes uncontrollable muscle contractions, or spasms. A third use of the word is to denote a condition caused by a deficiency of calcium ions in the extracellular fluid. The lack of calcium increases nerve excitability with resulting muscle spasms, particularly of the extremities. The word *tetany* is also sometimes used to mean tetanus.

Wryneck: Injury to one of the sternocleidomastoid muscles may result in torticollis, or wryneck. This is characterized by a twisting of the neck and an unnatural position of the head.

Diaphragm: Voluntary forceful contractions of the diaphragm increase intraabdominal pressure to assist in urination, defecation, and childbirth.

Electrical shock: The muscles that flex the fingers and hand are stronger than the extensor muscles. In a normal relaxed position the fingers are slightly flexed because the normal muscle tone is greater in the flexors. Persons who receive a high-voltage electrical shock through the arms flex their hands tightly and "can't let go." All of the flexors and extensors receive the electrical stimulus, but because the flexor muscles are stronger, they contract more forcefully.

Intramuscular injections: The gluteus medius is a common site for intramuscular injections. In general, the injection is given in the center of the upper outer quadrant of the buttock, or gluteal, area. The gluteus medius, rather than the gluteus maximus, is used to avoid damaging the sciatic nerve.

Horseback riding: The adductor muscles in the medial compartment are the horse rider's muscles. These muscles adduct, or press, the thighs together to keep a person on a horse.

Quads: The quadriceps femoris group is a powerful knee extensor that is used in climbing, running, and rising from a chair. ∎

energy for contraction. The cells also contain systematically arranged threadlike organelles called *myofilaments* that slide across one another during contraction.

NERVE AND BLOOD SUPPLY

Skeletal muscles have an abundant supply of blood vessels and nerves. This is directly related to the primary function of skeletal muscle contraction. Before a skeletal muscle fiber can contract, it must receive an impulse from a nerve cell. Muscle contraction requires adenosine triphosphate (ATP), and blood vessels deliver the necessary nutrients and oxygen to produce it. Blood vessels also remove the waste products that are produced as a result of muscle contraction.

In general, an artery and at least one vein accompany each nerve that penetrates the epimysium of a skeletal muscle. Branches of the nerve and blood vessels follow the connective tissue components of the muscle so that each muscle fiber is in contact with a branch of a nerve cell and with one or more minute blood vessels called *capillaries*.

SKELETAL MUSCLE ATTACHMENTS

In some instances, fibers of the epimysium fuse directly with the periosteum of a bone to form a *direct* attachment. The fleshy part of the muscle is known as the *belly* or *gaster*. More commonly, the connective tissue coverings extend beyond the belly of the muscle to form a thick, ropelike

tendon or a broad, flat, sheetlike **aponeurosis**. The tendons and aponeuroses form *indirect* attachments from muscles to the periosteum of bones or to the connective tissue of other muscles. Typically, a muscle spans a joint and is attached to bones by tendons at both ends. One of the bones remains relatively fixed or stable, whereas the other end moves as a result of muscle contraction. The fixed or stable end is called the **origin** of the muscle, and the more movable attachment is called the **insertion**.

CONTRACTION OF SKELETAL MUSCLE

Skeletal muscle contraction is the result of a complex series of events based on chemical reactions at the cellular (muscle fiber) level. This chain of reactions begins with stimulation by a nerve cell and ends when the muscle fiber is again relaxed. Contraction of a whole muscle is the result of the simultaneous contraction of many muscle fibers.

STIMULUS FOR CONTRACTION

Skeletal muscles are stimulated to contract by special nerve cells called *motor neurons*. As the axon of the motor neuron penetrates the muscle, the axon branches, so there is an axon terminal for each muscle fiber. A single motor neuron and all the muscle fibers it stimulates make up a **motor unit**. Some motor units include several hundred individual fibers; others contain fewer than 10. Because all the muscle fibers

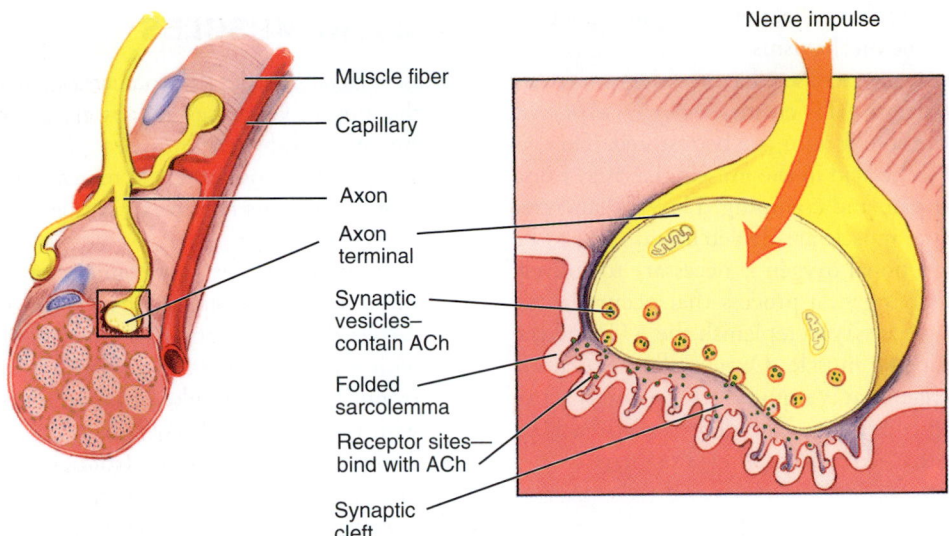

Nerve impulse

Muscle fiber

Capillary

Axon

Axon terminal

Synaptic vesicles— contain ACh

Folded sarcolemma

Receptor sites— bind with ACh

Synaptic cleft

Figure 8-1 Neuromuscular junction. The axon terminal fits into a depression on the sarcolemma. A nerve impulse travels down the axon to the axon terminal. The impulse causes the synaptic vesicles to release acetylcholine, which diffuses across the synaptic cleft and binds with receptors on the sarcolemma. (From Applegate E: *The anatomy and physiology learning system*, ed 4, St Louis, 2011, Saunders.)

in a motor unit receive a nerve impulse at the same time, all the fibers contract at the same time.

The region in which an axon terminal meets a muscle fiber is called a **neuromuscular junction** or myoneural junction, which is illustrated in Figure 8-1. The axon terminal does not actually touch the sarcolemma of the muscle cell but fits into a shallow depression in the cell membrane. The fluid-filled space between the axon terminal and sarcolemma is called a *synaptic cleft* (gap). **Acetylcholine** (ACh), a **neurotransmitter**, is contained within synaptic vesicles in the axon terminal. Receptor sites for the ACh are located on the sarcolemma.

When a nerve impulse reaches the axon terminal, ACh is released. The ACh diffuses across the synaptic cleft and binds with the receptor sites on the sarcolemma. This reaction is the stimulus that causes the myofilaments to slide across one another, resulting in contraction. This is called the *sliding filament theory of contraction.*

The ACh is rapidly inactivated by the enzyme **acetylcholinesterase**. This ensures that one nerve impulse will result in only one contraction of the muscle fiber. Anything that interferes with the production, release, or inactivation of ACh, or its ability to bind with the receptor sites on the sarcolemma, will have an effect on muscle contraction. Muscle relaxant drugs work in this manner.

ENERGY SOURCES AND OXYGEN DEBT

The immediate or initial source of energy for muscle contraction is ATP. Surprisingly, muscles have limited storage facilities for ATP. In working muscles the stored ATP is depleted in about 6 seconds, and new ATP must be regenerated if muscle contraction is to continue.

Creatine phosphate is a unique high-energy compound that is stored in muscles. This compound provides almost instantaneous regeneration of ATP.

This reaction is so effective that there is little change in ATP levels during the initial stages of muscle contraction. Muscles store enough creatine phosphate to regenerate sufficient ATP to sustain contraction for about 10 seconds.

When muscles are actively contracting for extended periods of time, *fatty acids* and *glucose* become the primary energy sources. As ATP and creatine phosphate stores are being used, more ATP is produced from the metabolism of glucose and fatty acids.

If adequate oxygen is available, fatty acids and glucose are broken down in the mitochondria by a process called *aerobic respiration.* The products are carbon dioxide, water, and large amounts of ATP.

When muscles are contracting vigorously for long periods of time, the circulatory system is unable to deliver oxygen fast enough to maintain the aerobic pathways. Processes that do not require oxygen are necessary. Under these conditions, glucose is the primary energy source. If adequate oxygen is not available, glucose is broken down by a process called *anaerobic respiration.* The products of the anaerobic pathway are lactic acid and a small amount of ATP.

Some of the lactic acid accumulates in the muscle and causes a burning sensation. Most of it diffuses out of the muscle and into the bloodstream, which takes it to the liver. Later, when sufficient oxygen is available, the liver converts the lactic acid back to glycogen, the storage form of glucose.

The aerobic pathway produces about 20 times more ATP than the anaerobic pathway. However, the anaerobic pathway provides ATP about two and one-half times faster than the aerobic pathway. Most of the energy for vigorous activity over a moderate period of time comes from anaerobic respiration. Prolonged activities requiring endurance depend on aerobic mechanisms.

Periods of strenuous exercise that require anaerobic mechanisms to regenerate ATP create an *oxygen debt* that must be repaid before equilibrium can be restored. There is an accumulation of lactic acid in the muscle that may cause temporary muscular pain and cramping. The ATP and creatine phosphate in the muscle are depleted and need to be replenished. This additional oxygen is necessary to convert the lactic acid into glycogen, a process that occurs in the liver. Oxygen is also necessary to replenish the ATP and the creatine phosphate in the muscle. Oxygen debt is defined as the additional oxygen that is required after physical activity to restore resting conditions. The debt is paid back by labored breathing that continues after the activity has stopped.

MOVEMENTS

Most intact skeletal muscles are attached to bones by tendons that span joints. When the muscle contracts, one bone (the insertion) moves relative to the other bone (the origin). Frequently muscles work in groups to perform a particular movement. If one muscle has a primary role in providing a movement, it is called a **prime mover**. Muscles that work with, or assist, the prime mover to cause a movement are called **synergists**. Often muscles span more than one joint, and a synergist will stabilize one joint while the prime mover acts on the other joint. For example, the fingers can be flexed to make a fist without bending the wrist because certain muscles fix the wrist in a stabilized position. **Antagonists** are muscles that oppose, or reverse, a particular movement. The biceps brachii muscle on the anterior arm flexes the forearm at the elbow. The triceps brachii muscle on the posterior arm extends the forearm at the elbow. The two muscles are on opposite sides of the humerus and have opposite functions. They are antagonists.

Bones and muscles work together to perform different types of movement at the various joints. Describing muscular action or movement at joints requires a frame of reference and descriptive terminology with definite meaning. Some terms that are commonly used to describe particular movements are defined and illustrated in Figure 8-2.

SKELETAL MUSCLE GROUPS

The body is composed of more than 600 skeletal muscles. A discussion of each muscle is certainly beyond the scope of this book. Only the more significant and obvious muscles are identified and described here. These are arranged in groups according to location and/or function. If you identify and learn the muscles as group associations, it will make them easier to remember. If you can locate a muscle on your own body, you will be able to contract the muscle and describe its action. Learning anatomy in this manner makes it more meaningful.

NAMING MUSCLES

Most skeletal muscles have names that describe some feature of the muscle. Often several criteria are combined into one name. Associating the muscles' characteristics with their names will help you learn and remember them. The following are some terms relating to muscle features that are used in naming muscles:

- *Size:* vastus (huge); maximus (large); longus (long); minimus (small); brevis (short)
- *Shape:* deltoid (triangular); rhomboid (like a rhombus with equal and parallel sides); latissimus (wide); teres (round); trapezius (like a trapezoid, a four-sided figure with two sides parallel)
- *Direction of fibers:* rectus (straight); transverse (across); oblique (diagonal); orbicularis (circular)
- *Location:* pectoralis (chest); gluteus (buttock or rump); brachii (arm); supra- (above); infra- (below); sub- (under or beneath); lateralis (lateral)
- *Number of origins:* biceps (two heads); triceps (three heads); quadriceps (four heads)
- *Origin and insertion:* sternocleidomastoid (origin on the sternum and clavicle, insertion on the mastoid process); brachioradialis (origin on the brachium or arm, insertion on the radius)
- *Action:* abductor (to abduct a structure); adductor (to adduct a structure); flexor (to flex a structure); extensor (to extend a structure); levator (to lift or elevate a structure); masseter (to chew)

MUSCLES OF THE HEAD AND NECK
Muscles of Facial Expression

Humans have well developed muscles in the face that permit a large variety of facial expressions. Because these muscles are used to show surprise, disgust, anger, fear, and other emotions, they are an important means of nonverbal communication. The following are some of the muscles used to produce facial expressions.

The *frontalis* lies over the frontal bone of the forehead. It is attached to the soft tissue of the eyebrow; when it contracts, it raises the eyebrows and wrinkles the forehead. The *orbicularis oris* is a sphincter that encircles the mouth. This muscle is used to close the mouth, to form words, and to pucker the lips as in kissing. The *orbicularis oculi* is another sphincter but lies around the eye (oculus). The actions of winking, blinking, and squinting use this muscle. The *buccinator* is the principal muscle in the cheek area and is used to compress the cheek when whistling, sucking, or blowing air out. It is sometimes called the *trumpeter's muscle*. The *zygomaticus* extends from the zygomatic arch to the corners of the mouth. It contracts to raise the corner of the mouth when we smile.

Muscles of Mastication

Four pairs of muscles are responsible for chewing movements or mastication. All of these muscles insert on the mandible, and they are some of the strongest muscles in the body. Two of the muscles, the *temporalis* and *masseter*, are superficial and are identified in Figure 8-3. The others, the lateral and medial pterygoids, are deep to the mandible and are not shown in the figure. The *temporalis* is the largest of the mastication muscles. As the name implies, it has its origin on the temporal bone. The *masseter* is located along the ramus of the mandible and is a synergist of the temporalis.

Neck Muscles

Only two of the more obvious and superficial neck muscles are considered here. Numerous muscles are associated with

Flexion (FLEK-shun)
Means to bend. Flexion usually brings two bones closer together and decreases the angle between them. Example: bending the elbow or the knee.

Dorsiflexion (dor-sih-FLEK-shun)
Flexion of the ankle in which the dorsum or top of the foot is lifted upward, decreasing the angle between the foot and leg. Example: standing on your heels.

Extension (ek-STEN-shun)
Means to straighten. Extension is the opposite of flexion. It increases the angle between two bones. Example: straightening the elbow or the knee after it has been flexed.

Plantar flexion (PLAN-tar FLEK-shun)
Plantar flexion is movement at the ankle that increases the angle between the foot and leg. Example: standing on your toes.

Hyperextension (hye-perk-ek-STEN-shun)
Hyperextension occurs when a part of the body is extended beyond the anatomical position. The joint angle becomes greater than 180°. Example: moving the head backward.

Abduction (ab-DUCK-shun)
Means to take away. Abduction moves a bone or limb away from the midline or axis of the body. Examples: the outward movement of the legs in "jumping jacks," moving the arms away from the body, or spreading the fingers apart.

Figure 8-2 Types of body movements. (From Applegate E: *The anatomy and physiology learning system,* ed 4, St Louis, 2011, Saunders.)

Continued

Adduction (ad-DUCK-shun)
Means to bring together. Adduction is the opposite of abduction. It moves a bone or limb toward the midline of the body. Examples: bringing the arms back to the sides of the body after they have been abducted or moving the legs back to anatomical position after abduction.

Circumduction (sir-kum-DUCK-shun)
Circumduction is the conelike, circular movement of a body segment. The proximal end of the segment remains relatively stationary while the distal end outlines a large circle. Example: the movement of the arm at the shoulder joint, with the elbow extended, so that the tips of the fingers move in a large circle.

Rotation (roh-TAY-shun)
Rotation is the movement of a bone around its own axis in a pivot joint. Example: shaking your head "no".

Inversion (in-VER-zhun)
Inversion is the movement of the sole of the foot inward or medially.

Supination (soo-pih-NAY-shun)
Supination is a specialized rotation of the forearm that turns the palm of the hand forward or anteriorly. If the elbow is flexed, supination turns the palm of the hand upward or superiorly.

Eversion (ee-VER-zhun)
Eversion is the opposite of inversion. It is the movement of the sole of the foot outward or laterally.

Pronation (proh-NAY-shun)
Pronation is the opposite of supination. It is a specialized rotation of the forearm that turns the palm of the hand backward or posteriorly. If the elbow is flexed, pronation turns the palm of the hand downward or inferiorly.

Figure 8-2, cont'd

Figure 8-3 Muscles of the head and neck. (From Applegate E: *The anatomy and physiology learning system*, ed 4, St Louis, 2011, Saunders.)

the throat, hyoid bone, and vertebral column, a discussion of which is beyond the scope of this text.

The *sternocleidomastoid* muscles ascend obliquely across the anterior neck from the sternum and clavicle to the mastoid process. When both of these muscles contract together, the neck is flexed and the head is bent toward the chest. When one of the muscles contracts, the head turns toward the direction opposite the side that is contracting. When the left muscle contracts, the head turns to the right. A portion of the *trapezius* muscle is in the neck region and moves the head. Each trapezius muscle extends from the occipital bone at the base of the skull to the end of the thoracic vertebrae and also inserts on the scapula laterally. A portion of this muscle extends the head and is antagonistic to the sternocleidomastoid.

MUSCLES OF THE TRUNK

The muscles of the trunk include those that move the vertebral column, the muscles that form the thoracic and abdominal walls, and those that cover the pelvic outlet.

Vertebral Column Muscles

The *erector spinae* group of muscles on each side of the vertebral column is a large muscle mass that extends from the sacrum to the skull. These muscles are primarily responsible for extending the vertebral column to maintain erect posture. Muscle contraction on only one side bends the vertebral column to that side.

Thoracic Wall Muscles

The muscles of the thoracic wall are involved primarily in the process of breathing. The intercostal muscles are located in spaces between the ribs. The *external intercostal muscles* contract to elevate the ribs during the inspiration phase of breathing. The *internal intercostals* contract during forced expiration.

The *diaphragm* is a dome-shaped muscle that forms a partition between the thorax and the abdomen. It has three openings in it for structures that have to pass from the thorax to the abdomen. The diaphragm is responsible for the major movement in the thoracic cavity during quiet, relaxed breathing. When the diaphragm contracts, the dome is flattened. This increases the volume of the thoracic cavity and results in inspiration. When the muscle relaxes, it again resumes its dome shape and decreases the volume of the thoracic cavity, which forces air out during expiration.

Abdominal Wall Muscles

The abdomen, unlike the thorax and pelvis, has no bony reinforcements or protection. The wall consists entirely of four muscle pairs, arranged in layers, and the fascia that envelops them (Figure 8-4). The aponeuroses of the muscles on opposite sides meet in the anterior midline to form the *linea alba* ("white line"), a band of connective tissue that extends from the sternum to the pubic symphysis. The outer muscle layer is the *external oblique*. The *internal oblique* lies just underneath it, and the deepest layer of muscle is the *transversus abdominis*. The arrangement of the muscle layers with the fibers in each layer going in different directions is similar to the type of construction found in plywood and adds strength to the anterolateral abdominal wall. The fascia of these muscles extends anteriorly to form a broad aponeurosis along much of the anterior aspect of the abdomen. The fascia also envelops the *rectus abdominis* muscle, which runs vertically from the pubic bones to the ribs and the sternum on each side of the midline. All of these muscles compress the abdominal wall and increase intraabdominal pressure. The rectus abdominis also flexes the vertebral column.

Pelvic Floor Muscles

The *pelvic diaphragm* forms the floor of the pelvic cavity. Most of the pelvic diaphragm is formed by the two *levator ani* muscles, which support the pelvic viscera. They resist increased pressure in the abdominopelvic cavity and thus play a role in the control of the urinary bladder and rectum.

MUSCLES OF THE UPPER EXTREMITY

The muscles of the upper extremity include those that attach the scapula to the thorax and in general move the scapula, those that attach the humerus to the scapula and in general move the arm, and those that are located in the arm or forearm and move the forearm, wrist, and hand. Figure 8-5 illustrates the anterior view of body musculature, and Figure 8-6 illustrates the posterior view.

Muscles That Move the Shoulder and Arm

The *trapezius* attaches the scapula to the axial skeleton. It is a large superficial triangular muscle of the back. When the trapezius contracts, it adducts and elevates the scapula, as in shrugging the shoulders.

Figure 8-4 Abdominal wall muscles. (From Applegate E: *The anatomy and physiology learning system*, ed 4, St Louis, 2011, Saunders.)

Both the *pectoralis major* and the *latissimus dorsi* muscles attach the humerus to the axial skeleton. The pectoralis major is a superficial muscle on the anterior chest. It has a broad origin on the sternum, costal cartilages, and clavicle, but then the fibers converge to insert on the humerus by way of a short tendon. The primary function of the pectoralis major is to adduct and rotate the arm medially across the chest. The latissimus dorsi is a large, superficial muscle located in the lower back region. It has an extensive origin from the spines of the thoracic vertebrae, ilium, and ribs and then extends upward to insert on the humerus. The latissimus dorsi adducts and rotates the arm medially and lowers the shoulder. It is an important muscle in swimming and rowing motions.

The *deltoid* is a large, fleshy muscle that covers the shoulder and attaches the humerus to the scapula. This muscle abducts the arm to a horizontal position. It is a common site for administering intramuscular injections. Another group of muscles, called the *rotator cuff muscles*, attaches the humerus to the scapula and moves the humerus in various ways . These muscles form a cuff or cap over the proximal humerus. A rotator cuff injury involves damage to one or more of these muscles or their tendons.

Muscles That Move the Forearm and Hand

The muscles that move the forearm are located along the humerus and are divided into anterior and posterior muscle compartments. The *triceps brachii*, the primary extensor of the forearm, is the only muscle in the posterior compartment. As the name implies, it has three heads of origin. The anterior muscle compartment contains the *biceps brachii*, a primary flexor of the forearm.

The 20 or more muscles that cause most wrist, hand, and finger movements are located along the forearm. These muscles are divided into anterior and posterior compartments. Most of the anterior compartment muscles flex the wrist and fingers, whereas the posterior muscles cause extension.

MUSCLES OF THE LOWER EXTREMITY

The muscles of the lower extremity include those that are located in the hip region and in general move the thigh, those that are located in the thigh and move the leg, and those that are located in the leg and move the ankle and foot. See Figures 8-5 and 8-6 to visualize these muscles.

Muscles That Move the Thigh

The muscles that move the thigh have their origins on some part of the pelvic girdle and their insertions on the femur. The largest muscle mass belongs to the posterior group, the gluteal muscles. The *gluteus maximus* forms the area of the buttocks. The *gluteus medius*, a common site for intramuscular injections, is superior and deep to the gluteus maximus. The *gluteus minimus* is the smallest and deepest of the gluteal muscles and is not illustrated. These muscles abduct the thigh—that is, they raise the thigh sideways to a horizontal position. The gluteus maximus also extends or straightens the thigh at the hip for walking or climbing stairs.

The anterior muscle that moves the thigh is the *iliopsoas*. This muscle is formed from the iliacus, which originates on the iliac fossa, and the psoas, which originates on the lumbar vertebrae. The fibers converge into the iliopsoas and insert on the femur. The iliopsoas flexes the thigh, making it antagonistic to the gluteus maximus.

The medial muscles adduct the thigh—that is, they press the thighs together. This group includes the *adductor longus*,

Deltoid

Biceps
brachii

Trapezius

Pectoralis major

Brachialis

Linea alba

External
abdominal
oblique

Iliopsoas

Adductor
longus

Adductor
magnus

Gracilis

Sartorius

Vastus medialis

Rectus femoris

Vastus lateralis

Gastrocnemius

Tibialis anterior

Soleus

Figure 8-5 General overview of body musculature. Anterior view. (From Applegate E: *The anatomy and physiology learning system*, ed 4, St Louis, 2011, Saunders.)

Cut edge of
trapezius

Deltoid

Trapezius

Latissimus
dorsi

Triceps brachii

Gluteus
medius

Gluteus
maximus

Adductor
magnus

Gracilis

Semitendinosus

Semimembranosus

Biceps femoris

Gastrocnemius

Soleus

Calcaneal
tendon

Peroneus longus

Figure 8-6 General overview of body musculature. Posterior view. (From Applegate E: *The anatomy and physiology learning system*, ed 4, St Louis, 2011, Saunders.)

adductor brevis, *adductor magnus*, and *gracilis* muscles. These muscles are often called the *horse rider's muscles* because their action keeps the rider on the horse.

Muscles That Move the Leg

Muscles that move the leg are located in the thigh region. The *quadriceps femoris* includes four muscles that are on the anterior and lateral sides of the thigh, namely the *vastus lateralis*, *vastus intermedius*, *vastus medialis*, and *rectus femoris*. As a group, these muscles are the primary extensors of the leg, straightening the leg at the knee. The other muscle on the anterior surface of the thigh is the long, straplike *sartorius*, which passes obliquely over the quadriceps group. The sartorius, the longest muscle in the body, flexes and medially rotates the leg when one sits cross-legged.

The posterior thigh muscles are called the *hamstrings*, and they are used to flex the leg at the knee. All have origins on the ischium and insert on the tibia. Because these muscles extend over the hip joint, as well as over the knee joint, they also extend the thigh. The strong tendons of these muscles can be felt behind the knee. These same tendons are present in hogs, and butchers used them to hang the hams for smoking and curing, so they were called "ham strings." The hamstring muscles are the *biceps femoris*, *semimembranosus*, and *semitendinosus*. A "pulled hamstring" is a tear in one or more of these muscles or their tendons.

Muscles That Move the Ankle and Foot

The muscles located in the leg move the ankle and foot and are divided into anterior, posterior, and lateral compartments. The *tibialis anterior* is the primary muscle in the anterior group, and its contraction causes dorsiflexion of the foot. The *peroneus* muscles occupy the lateral compartment of the leg. Contraction of these muscles everts the foot and also helps in plantar flexion. The *gastrocnemius* and *soleus* are the major muscles in the posterior compartment. These two muscles form the fleshy mass in the calf of the leg. They have a common tendon called the *calcaneal tendon* or *Achilles tendon*. These muscles are strong plantar flexors of the foot. They are sometimes called the *toe dancer's muscles* because they allow one to stand on tiptoe. Numerous other deep muscles in the leg cause flexion and extension of the toes.

AGING OF THE MUSCULAR SYSTEM

One of the most obvious age-related changes in skeletal muscles is the loss of muscle mass. This involves a decrease in both the number of muscle fibers and the diameter of the remaining fibers. Because muscle fibers are amitotic, once they are lost they cannot be replaced by new ones. Instead, they are replaced by connective tissue, primarily adipose. The number of muscle cells lost depends on several factors, including the amount of physical activity, the nutritional state of the individual, heredity, and the condition of the motor neurons that supply the muscle tissue. There is an age-related loss of motor neurons to skeletal muscle cells, and this is considered an important cause of muscle atrophy. It is probable that exercise enhances the ability of nerves to stimulate muscle fibers and to reduce atrophy.

As muscle mass decreases, there is a corresponding reduction in muscle strength. The amount of strength loss differs, depending to a large extent on the amount of physical activity. There is evidence that the mitochondria function less effectively in nonexercised muscle cells than in exercised cells. When mitochondria are inefficient, lactic acid accumulates, which contributes to muscle weakness.

There is a tendency for the skeletal muscles of older people to be less responsive, or to respond more slowly, than those of younger people. This is because the latent, contraction, and relaxation phases of muscle action all increase in duration. The increase in response time is less in muscles that are used regularly. Continued physical activity and good nutrition are probably the best deterrents to loss of muscle mass and muscle strength and to increased muscle response time.

Common Pathology of the Muscular System			
Disease	Signs and Symptoms	Etiology	Diagnosis and Treatment
Myopathy	Muscle weakness with cramps, stiffness, spasms, and tetany.	Myopathy results from several different disease processes. It may result from endocrine, inflammatory, infectious, drug- and toxin-induced, metabolic, and other systemic disorders.	Diagnosis of myopathy is based on symptoms; however, it is important to discover and treat the underlying cause. Treatments for myopathy range from management of the symptoms to very specific cause-targeting treatments. Physical therapy, drug therapy, support bracing, surgery, and massage are all current treatments for this wide variety of conditions.

Continued

Common Pathology of the Muscular System—cont'd

Disease	Signs and Symptoms	Etiology	Diagnosis and Treatment
Myalgia	Muscle pain.	Myalgia without a traumatic history is often the result of a viral infection. It is a symptom of many diseases and disorders. A common cause is the overuse or overstretching of a muscle or group of muscles. It can also be caused by medications or occur as a response to a vaccination.	Diagnosis is based on symptoms; however, it is important to discover and treat the underlying cause. The treatment or management of myalgia differs depending on the underlying causes. Mild cases may be treated with massage, a warm bath, or hot and cold packs. Pain-relieving medications may be required. Muscle relaxants are sometimes helpful.
Myositis	Muscle weakness, swelling, and pain are the common myositis symptoms. Myositis sometimes occurs as part of a systemic infection.	*Myositis* is a general term for inflammation of the muscles. Many such conditions are considered likely to be caused by autoimmune conditions, rather than directly by infection.	Diagnosis is based on symptoms and blood tests. There are two approaches to the treatment of myositis: medical and lifestyle changes. Nonsteroidal antiinflammatory drugs may be used for pain relief. Corticosteroids and other drugs that suppress the immune system may slow down the attack on healthy tissue.
Repetitive stress disorder (RSD)	The symptoms of RSD are pain, tingling, numbness, swelling, redness, loss of flexibility, and muscle weakness.	Conditions associated with RSD include repetitive tasks, forceful exertions, vibrations, mechanical compression, and/or sustained awkward positions.	Usually diagnosed by history and examination. Imaging modalities may be used to rule out other possible causes of the pain. The most-often prescribed treatments for early-stage RSD include drug therapies such as antiinflammatory medications combined with passive forms of physical therapy such as rest, splinting, and massage. Some patients may require more aggressive intervention including surgery.
Shin splint	Pain along the tibia (shinbone) and mild swelling in the lower leg.	Shin splints are caused by repeated stress of the tibia and the connective tissues that attach muscles to it, especially flexor muscles of the toes.	Usually diagnosed by history and examination. Imaging modalities may be used to rule out other possible causes of the pain. Initial treatment includes rest, ice, and pain medications, which allow the tibia to recover from high levels of stress and reduce the inflammation and pain. Surgery may be performed in more severe cases when more conservative options have been unsuccessful.
Contusion	Typically a moderately large area of the skin that has been darkened as the result of a hit or impact. Commonly called a *bruise*.	A contusion is a hematoma of tissue in which capillaries and sometimes venules are damaged by trauma, allowing blood to enter the surrounding interstitial tissues.	Diagnosis is by examination. Treatment for light bruises is minimal and may include *RICE* (rest, ice, compression, elevation), painkillers, and, later in recovery, light stretching exercises. In most cases hematomas spontaneously resolve, but in cases of large hematomas, the physician may optionally perform a puncture of the hematoma to allow the blood to exit.
Muscular dystrophy	A chronic and progressive weakening of the muscles. There are many forms of the condition ranging from mild to severe.	Caused by a mutation in one of the genes involved in directing the synthesis of proteins that protect muscle fibers from damage. The mutations may be inherited or occur spontaneously.	Diagnosis depends on patient history, physical examination, muscle enzyme tests, electromyography, muscle biopsy, and genetic testing. At present there is no cure. Treatment is aimed at alleviating the symptoms and complications.
Myasthenia gravis	Notable weakness and rapid fatigue of the skeletal muscles. The first signs occur in the face and throat, such as drooping eyelids and double vision.	Myasthenia gravis occurs when the immune system produces antibodies that block the acetylcholine receptors at the neuromuscular junction.	Diagnosis includes patient history and physical examination, reflex testing, muscle strength, coordination, and balance. Blood analysis may reveal the presence of the antibodies. At present there is no cure. Treatment is aimed at alleviating the symptoms.

Common Pathology of the Muscular System—cont'd

Disease	Signs and Symptoms	Etiology	Diagnosis and Treatment
Poliomyelitis	Flulike symptoms that progress to muscle paralysis. Although approximately 90% of polio infections cause no symptoms at all, affected individuals can exhibit a range of symptoms if the virus enters the bloodstream and affects the nerves. Advanced stages of the disease exhibit muscle weakness and acute flaccid paralysis. Different types of paralysis may occur, depending on the nerves involved.	Poliomyelitis is caused by a contagious enterovirus called the polio virus (PV) that forms colonies in the oropharynx and intestine. Polio is now extremely rare in the Western world because of very effective vaccination programs.	Paralytic poliomyelitis is suspected in individuals experiencing acute onset of flaccid paralysis in one or more limbs with decreased tendon reflexes. Recovery of the virus from a stool sample or throat swab confirms the diagnosis. There is no cure for polio. The focus of modern treatment has been on providing relief of symptoms, speeding recovery, and preventing complications.

TERMINOLOGY REVIEW

Key Term	Word Parts	Definition
Acetylcholine		A neurotransmitter at the neuromuscular junction.
Acetylcholinesterase	-ase: enzyme	An enzyme that inactivates acetylcholine.
Antagonists	anti-: against	Muscles that have an action opposite to that of the prime mover.
Aponeurosis		A broad flat sheet of connective tissue that connects one muscle to another
Contractility		The ability of muscle cells to shorten to produce movement.
Elasticity		The ability of tissue to return to its original shape after contraction or extension.
Epimysium	epi: above, around mys: muscle	Fibrous connective tissue that surrounds a whole muscle.
Excitability		The ability of muscle and nerve tissue to receive and respond to stimuli; also called irritability.
Extensibility		The ability of muscle tissue to stretch when pulled.
Insertion		The end of a muscle that is attached to a relatively movable part; the end opposite the origin.
Motor unit		A single neuron and all the muscle fibers it stimulates.
Neuromuscular junction	neur/o: nerve	The area of communication between the axon terminal of a motor neuron and the sarcolemma of a muscle fiber; also called a myoneural junction.
Neurotransmitter	neur/o: nerve trans-: across	A chemical substance that is released at the axon terminals to stimulate a muscle fiber contraction or an impulse in another neuron.
Origin		The end of a muscle that is attached to a relatively immovable part; the end opposite the insertion.
Prime mover		The muscle that is mainly responsible for a particular body movement; also called an agonist.
Sarcolemma	sarc/o: flesh, muscle lemm-: peel, rind	Covering of a muscle cell; the muscle cell membrane.
Sarcoplasm	sarc/o: flesh, muscle	Cytoplasm of a muscle cell.
Synergist	syn-: together erg/o: work	Muscles that assist a prime mover but are not capable of producing the movement by themselves; two or more muscles work together to produce a movement.

ON THE WEB

For information on muscles and joints:

Gateway Community College: Muscles Tutorial: www.gwc.maricopa.edu/class/bio201/muscle/mustut.htm

Loyola University Medical Education Network: Master Muscle List: www.meddean.luc.edu/lumen/meded/grossanatomy/dissector/mml/index.htm

Merck Manual—Musculoskeletal Disorders: www.merck.com/mmpe/sec04.html *(Click on "Musculoskeletal Disorders")*

San Diego State University College of Sciences: Actin Myosin Crossbridges: www.sci.sdsu.edu/movies/actin_myosin_gif.html

Science Animations: science.nhmccd.edu/biol/animatio.htm

Skeletal Muscles of the Human Body: ptcentral.com/muscles

Skeleton: The Joints: www.zoology.ubc.ca/%7Ebiomania/tutorial/bonejt/outline.htm

University of Washington: Lower Extremity Muscle Atlas: www.rad.washington.edu/atlas2

University of Washington: Upper Extremity Muscle Atlas: www.rad.washington.edu/atlas

University of Wisconsin Medical School: Anatomy Dissections: www.anatomy.wisc.edu/courses/gross/index.html

Nervous System

Check out the Evolve site at http://evolve.elsevier.com/Bonewit/today/ to access additional interactive activities and exercises to help you study and prepare for success.

LEARNING OBJECTIVES

1. Describe the organization and functions of the nervous system.
2. Describe the structure and functions of neurons and neuroglia.
3. Explain how an impulse is conducted along the length of a neuron.
4. List and describe the three layers of meninges around the central nervous system.
5. Describe the location, components, and functional areas of the cerebrum, diencephalon, brain stem, and cerebellum.
6. Compare the composition of gray matter and white matter.
7. Explain the function of cerebrospinal fluid.
8. Describe the structure and functions of the spinal cord.
9. Explain the difference in composition of sensory, motor, and mixed nerves.
10. List the 12 cranial nerves, and state the function of each.
11. Identify the region of the body that is innervated by each of the following spinal nerve plexuses: cervical, brachial, lumbosacral.
12. Explain the difference between the sympathetic and parasympathetic divisions of the autonomic nervous system.
13. Describe ways in which the aging of an individual affects the nervous system.
14. Identify pathology related to the nervous system.

CHAPTER OUTLINE

INTRODUCTION TO THE NERVOUS SYSTEM
FUNCTIONS OF THE NERVOUS SYSTEM
ORGANIZATION OF THE NERVOUS SYSTEM
Central Nervous System
Peripheral Nervous System
NERVE TISSUE
Neurons
Neuroglia
NERVE IMPULSES
Resting Membrane
Stimulation of a Neuron
Conduction Along a Neuron
Conduction Across a Synapse

Neuronal Pools
Reflex Arcs
CENTRAL NERVOUS SYSTEM
Meninges
Brain
Ventricles and Cerebrospinal Fluid
Spinal Cord
PERIPHERAL NERVOUS SYSTEM
Structure of a Nerve
Cranial Nerves
Spinal Nerves
Autonomic Nervous System
AGING OF THE NERVOUS SYSTEM

KEY TERMS

action potential (ACK-shun po-TEN-shall)
axons (AKS-ons)
basal ganglia (BAY-sal GANG-lee-ah)
brain stem (BRAYN STEM)
central sulcus (SEN-tral SULL-kus)
cerebellum (sair-eh-BELL-um)

cerebrospinal fluid (she-ree-broh-SPY-null FLOO-id)
cerebrum (se-REE-brum)
dendrites (DEN-drytes)
decussation (dee-kuh-SAY-shun)
diencephalon (dye-en-SEF-ah-lon)
myelin (MY-eh-lin)

neurilemma (noo-rih-LEM-mah)
neuroglia (noo-ROG-lee-ah)
neuron (NOO-ron)
neurotransmitters (nee-roh-TRANS-mit-ers)
nodes of Ranvier (nodes of ron-vee-AY)

refractory period (ree-FRAK-toar-ee
   PEE-ree-od)
saltatory conduction (SAL-tah-toar-ee
   kon-DUCK-shun)

somatomotor cortex (soh-mat-oh-MOH-
   ter KOR-tex)
somatosensory cortex (soh-mat-oh-
   SEN-soar-ee KOR-tex)

synapse (SIN-aps)
threshold stimulus (THRESH-hold
   STIM-yoo-lus)

INTRODUCTION TO THE NERVOUS SYSTEM

The nervous system is the major controlling, regulatory, and communicating system in the body. It is the center of all mental activity, including thought, learning, and memory. Together with the endocrine system, the nervous system is responsible for regulating and maintaining homeostasis. Through its receptors, the nervous system keeps us in touch with our environment, both external and internal.

Like other systems in the body, the nervous system is composed of organs, principally the brain, spinal cord, nerves, and ganglia. These, in turn, consist of various tissues, including nerve, blood, and connective tissues. Together these carry out the complex activities of the nervous system.

FUNCTIONS OF THE NERVOUS SYSTEM

The various activities of the nervous system can be grouped together as three general functions:
• Sensory functions
• Integrative functions
• Motor functions

Together these functions keep us in touch with our environments, maintain homeostasis, and account for thought, learning, and memory.

Millions of sensory receptors detect changes, called *stimuli,* that occur inside and outside the body. They monitor such things as temperature, light, and sound from the external environment. Inside the body, the internal environment, receptors detect variations in pressure, pH, carbon dioxide concentration, and the levels of various electrolytes. All of this gathered information is called *sensory input.*

Sensory input is converted into electrical signals called *nerve impulses* that are transmitted to the brain. In the brain the signals are brought together to create sensations, produce thoughts, or add to memory. Decisions are made each moment on the basis of sensory input. This is called *integration.*

Based on the sensory input and integration, the nervous system responds by sending signals to muscles, causing them to contract, or to glands, causing them to produce secretions. Muscles and glands are called *effectors* because they cause an effect in response to directions from the nervous system. This is the *motor output* or *motor function.*

ORGANIZATION OF THE NERVOUS SYSTEM

There is really only one nervous system in the body, although terminology seems to indicate otherwise. Although each subdivision of the system is also called a "nervous system," all of these smaller systems belong to the single, highly integrated nervous system. Each subdivision has structural and functional characteristics that distinguish it from the others. The nervous system as a whole is divided into two subdivisions: the *central nervous system* (CNS) and the *peripheral nervous system* (PNS) (Figure 9-1).

CENTRAL NERVOUS SYSTEM

The *brain* and *spinal cord* are the organs of the CNS. Because they are so vitally important, the brain and spinal cord, located in the dorsal body cavity, are encased in bone for protection. The brain is in the cranial vault, and the spinal cord is in the vertebral canal of the vertebral column. Although considered to be two separate organs, the brain and spinal cord are continuous at the foramen magnum.

PERIPHERAL NERVOUS SYSTEM

The organs of the PNS are the *nerves* and *ganglia.* Nerves are bundles of nerve fibers, much as muscles are bundles of muscle fibers. Cranial nerves (12 pairs) and spinal nerves (31 pairs) extend from the CNS to peripheral organs, such as muscles and glands. Ganglia are collections, or small knots, of nerve cell bodies outside the CNS.

The PNS is further subdivided into an *afferent (sensory) division* and an *efferent (motor) division.* The afferent or sensory division transmits impulses from peripheral organs to the CNS. The efferent or motor division transmits impulses from the CNS out to the peripheral organs to cause an effect or action.

Finally, the efferent or motor division is again subdivided into the *somatic nervous system* and the *autonomic nervous system* (ANS). The somatic nervous system, also called the *somatomotor* or *somatic efferent* nervous system, supplies motor impulses to the skeletal muscles. Because these nerves

Figure 9-1 Organization of the nervous system. (From Applegate E: *The anatomy and physiology learning system,* ed 4, St Louis, 2011, Saunders.)

permit conscious control of the skeletal muscles, the somatic nervous system is sometimes called the *voluntary nervous system.* The ANS, also called the *visceral efferent* nervous system, supplies motor impulses to cardiac muscle, smooth muscle, and glandular epithelium. It is further subdivided into *sympathetic* and *parasympathetic* divisions. Because the ANS regulates involuntary or automatic functions, it is sometimes called the *involuntary nervous system.*

NERVE TISSUE

Although the nervous system is complex, there are only two main types of cells in nerve tissue. The actual nerve cell is the **neuron.** It is the "conducting" cell that transmits impulses. It is the structural unit of the nervous system. The other type of cell is the *neuroglia* or *glial cell.* The word **neuroglia** means "nerve glue." These cells are

nonconductive and provide a support system for the neurons. They are a special type of "connective tissue" for the nervous system.

NEURONS

Neurons, or nerve cells, carry out the functions of the nervous system by conducting nerve impulses. They are highly specialized and amitotic. This means that if a neuron is destroyed, it cannot be replaced because neurons do not undergo mitosis.

Each neuron has three basic parts:
- Cell body
- One or more dendrites
- A single axon

Figure 9-2 illustrates a typical neuron. The main part of the neuron is the *cell body* or *soma.* In many ways the cell body is similar to other types of cells. It has a nucleus with

Figure 9-2 Structure of a typical neuron. (From Applegate E: *The anatomy and physiology learning system,* ed 4, St Louis, 2011, Saunders.)

at least one nucleolus and contains many of the typical cytoplasmic organelles. It lacks centrioles, however. Because centrioles function in cell division, the fact that neurons lack these organelles is consistent with the amitotic nature of the cell.

Dendrites and **axons** are cytoplasmic extensions, or processes, that project from the cell body. They are sometimes referred to as *fibers.* Dendrites are usually, but not always, short and branching, which increases their surface area to receive signals from other neurons. The number of dendrites on a neuron varies. They are called *afferent processes* because they transmit impulses to the neuron cell body. Only one axon projects from each cell body. It is usually elongated, and because it carries impulses away from the cell body, it is called an *efferent process.*

An axon may have infrequent branches called *axon collaterals.* Axons and axon collaterals terminate in many short branches or *telodendria.* The distal ends of the telodendria are slightly enlarged to form *synaptic bulbs.* Many axons are surrounded by a segmented, white, fatty substance called **myelin** or the *myelin sheath.* Myelinated fibers make up the white matter in the CNS, whereas cell bodies and unmyelinated fibers make up the gray matter. The unmyelinated regions between the myelin segments are called the **nodes of Ranvier.** In the PNS the myelin is produced by Schwann cells. The cytoplasm, nucleus, and outer cell membrane of the Schwann cell form a tight covering around the myelin and around the axon itself at the nodes of Ranvier. This covering is the **neurilemma,** which plays an important role in the regeneration of nerve fibers. In the CNS, *oligodendrocytes* produce myelin, but there is no neurilemma, which is why fibers within the CNS do not regenerate. The structure of an axon and its coverings is illustrated in Figure 9-2.

Functionally, neurons are classified as afferent, efferent, or interneurons (association neurons) according to the direction in which they transmit impulses relative to the CNS (Table 9-1). *Afferent,* or *sensory, neurons* carry impulses from peripheral sense receptors to the CNS. They usually

have long dendrites and relatively short axons. *Efferent,* or *motor, neurons* transmit impulses from the CNS to effector organs, such as muscles and glands. Efferent neurons usually have short dendrites and long axons. *Interneurons,* or *association neurons,* are located entirely within the CNS, where they form the connecting link between the afferent and efferent neurons. They have short dendrites and may have either a short or a long axon.

NEUROGLIA

Neuroglial cells do not conduct nerve impulses; instead, they support, nourish, and protect the neurons. They are far more numerous than neurons and, unlike neurons, are capable of mitosis.

Table 9-1 Types of Neurons Classified According to Function

Type of Neuron	Structure	Function
Afferent (sensory)	Long dendrites and short axon; cell body located in ganglia in PNS; dendrites in PNS; axon extends into CNS	Transmits impulses from peripheral sense receptors to CNS
Efferent (motor)	Short dendrites and long axon; dendrites and cell body located within CNS; axons extend to PNS	Transmits impulses from CNS to effectors, such as muscles and glands in periphery
Association (interneurons)	Short dendrites; axon may be short or long; located entirely within CNS	Transmits impulses from afferent neurons to efferent neurons

CNS, Central nervous system; *PNS,* peripheral nervous system.
From Applegate E: *The anatomy and physiology learning system,* ed 4, St Louis, 2011, Saunders.

HIGHLIGHT on the Nervous System

Brain tumors: Because neurons are not capable of mitosis, primary malignant tumors of the brain are tumors of the glial cells rather than of the neurons themselves. These tumors, called *gliomas,* have extensive roots, making them extremely difficult to remove.

Blood-brain barrier: Neuroglia, particularly astrocytes, form a wall around the outside of the blood vessels in the nervous system. This astrocyte wall plus the blood vessel wall form the blood-brain barrier. Water, oxygen, carbon dioxide, alcohol, and a few other substances are able to pass through this barrier and move between the blood and brain tissue. Other substances, such as toxins, pathogens, and certain drugs, cannot pass through this barrier. This is a protective mechanism to keep harmful substances out of the brain. It has clinical significance because drugs such as penicillin that may be used to treat disorders in other parts of the body have no effect on the brain because they do not cross the blood-brain barrier.

Anesthetics: Some anesthetics produce their effects by inhibiting the diffusion of sodium through the cell membrane and thus blocking the initiation and conduction of nerve impulses.

Meningitis: Meningitis is an acute inflammation of the pia mater and the arachnoid. It is most commonly caused by bacteria. However, viral infections, fungal infections, and tumors may also cause inflammation of the meninges. Depending on the primary cause, meningitis may be mild or it may progress to a severe and life-threatening condition.

Left and right brain: In most people (approximately 90%), the left cerebral hemisphere dominates for language and mathematic abilities. It is the reasoning and analytic side of the brain. The right cerebral hemisphere is involved with motor skills, intuition, emotion, art, and music appreciation. It is the poetic and creative side of the brain. In about 10% of people these sides are reversed. In some individuals, neither hemisphere dominates. This may result in "confusion" and learning disabilities.

Emotions: The *limbic system* consists of scattered but interconnected regions of gray matter in the cerebral hemispheres and diencephalon. The limbic system is involved in memory and in emotions such as sadness, happiness, anger, and fear. It is our emotional brain.

Hydrocephalus: In hydrocephalus, an obstruction in the normal flow of cerebrospinal fluid (CSF) causes the fluid to accumulate in the ventricles. The obstruction may be a congenital defect or an acquired lesion such as a tumor. As the fluid accumulates, it causes the ventricles to enlarge and CSF pressure to increase. When this happens in an infant, before the cranial bones ossify, the cranium enlarges. In an older child or adult the pressure damages the soft brain tissue.

Lumbar puncture: A lumbar puncture is the withdrawal of some CSF from the subarachnoid space in the lumbar region of the spinal cord. The extension of the meninges beyond the end of the cord makes it possible to do this without injury to the spinal cord. The needle is usually inserted just above or just below the fourth lumbar vertebra, and the spinal cord ends at the first lumbar vertebra. The CSF that is removed can be tested for abnormal characteristics that may indicate an injury or infection.

Carpal tunnel syndrome: Carpal tunnel syndrome is a common occupational injury to the hand and wrist that is associated with repetitive hand motions. It is also associated with several diseases, including arthritis, diabetes, and gout. Symptoms, which include tingling of the thumb and fingers, result from the compression of the median nerve because of inflammation and swelling of the tendons within the carpal tunnel. ∎

NERVE IMPULSES

The functional characteristics of neurons are *excitability* and *conductivity.* Excitability is the ability to respond to a stimulus; conductivity is the ability to transmit an impulse from one point to another. All the functions associated with the nervous system, including thought, learning, and memory, are based on these two characteristics. These functional characteristics are the result of structural features of the cell membrane.

RESTING MEMBRANE

A *resting membrane* is the cell membrane of a nonconducting, or resting, neuron. The membrane is impermeable to the passive diffusion of sodium (Na^+) and potassium (K^+) ions. Sodium ions are concentrated in the extracellular fluid, whereas potassium ions are inside the cell. Electrical measurements show the resting membrane to be polarized with the inside of the membrane more negative than the outside. This is called the resting *membrane potential* and measures about −70 mv.

STIMULATION OF A NEURON

A stimulus is a physical, chemical, or electrical event that alters the permeability of the neuron cell membrane. This allows sodium ions to move inside the cell, then potassium ions move to the outside. This ionic movement briefly changes the polarization of the membrane.

This response to a stimulus is called the **action potential.** Electrical measurements show the action potential to peak at approximately +30 mV (Figure 9-3). At the conclusion of the action potential, the sodium-potassium pump actively transports sodium ions out of the cell and potassium ions into the cell to completely restore resting conditions.

Figure 9-3 Recording of an action potential. The resting potential is −70 mV and the peak action potential is +30 mV. (From Applegate E: *The anatomy and physiology learning system,* ed 4, St Louis, 2011, Saunders.)

The minimum stimulus necessary to initiate an action potential is called a **threshold stimulus** or *liminal stimulus.* A weaker stimulus, called a *subthreshold (subliminal) stimulus,* does not cause sufficient depolarization to elicit an action potential.

CONDUCTION ALONG A NEURON

Once a threshold stimulus has been applied and an action potential generated, it must be conducted along the total length of the neuron either to an effector or to another neuron.

The threshold stimulus causes a localized action potential on the membrane. The rest of the membrane is in the resting condition. The action potential stimulates the next point. This continues point by point, in domino fashion, along the entire length of the neuron, creating a *propagated action potential,* or *nerve impulse.*

Saltatory Conduction

The conduction described in the previous paragraph is representative of an unmyelinated axon. Because myelin is an insulating substance, it inhibits the flow of current from one point to another. In myelinated fibers, an action potential occurs only at the places where there is no myelin, at the nodes of Ranvier. The action potential "jumps" from node to node. This "jumping" is **saltatory conduction,** which is faster than conduction in unmyelinated fibers.

Refractory Period

The period of time during which a point on the cell membrane is "recovering" from an action potential is called the **refractory period.** That point on the cell membrane cannot respond to a second stimulus, no matter how strong the stimulus.

All-or-None Principle

Nerve fibers obey the *all-or-none principle.* If a threshold stimulus is applied, an action potential is generated and propagated along the entire length of the neuron at maximum strength and speed for the existing conditions. A stronger stimulus does not increase the strength of the action potential or change the rate of conduction. A weaker stimulus is subthreshold and does not evoke an action potential. If a stimulus is at threshold level or greater, an impulse is conducted. If the stimulus is subthreshold, there is no conduction.

CONDUCTION ACROSS A SYNAPSE

A nerve impulse travels along a nerve fiber until it reaches the end of the axon; then it must be transmitted to the next neuron. The region of communication between two neurons is called a **synapse.** This is similar to the neuromuscular junction described in Chapter 8. A synapse has three parts (Figure 9-4):
• Synaptic knob
• Synaptic cleft
• Postsynaptic membrane

The first neuron, the one preceding the synapse, is called the *presynaptic neuron;* the second neuron, the one following the synapse, is called the *postsynaptic neuron.* Synaptic knobs are tiny bulges at the end of the telodendria on the presynaptic neuron. Small sacs within the synaptic knobs, called *synaptic vesicles,* contain chemicals known as **neurotransmitters.**

When a nerve impulse reaches the synaptic knob, a series of reactions releases neurotransmitters into the synaptic cleft. The neurotransmitters diffuse across the synaptic cleft and react with receptors on the postsynaptic cell membrane. This is synaptic transmission. To prevent prolonged reactions with the postsynaptic receptors, the transmitters are quickly inactivated by enzymes. One of the best known neurotransmitters is *acetylcholine,* which is inactivated by the enzyme *cholinesterase.* Table 9-2 lists some of the common neurotransmitters.

In *excitatory transmission,* the neurotransmitter-receptor reaction on the postsynaptic membrane depolarizes the membrane and initiates an action potential. This is excitation or stimulation. Acetylcholine is typically an excitatory neurotransmitter. Some neurotransmitters result in *inhibitory transmission.* In this case, the reaction between the neurotransmitter and the receptor makes it more difficult to generate an action potential. This is inhibition. Gamma-aminobutyric acid (GABA) is an inhibitory neurotransmitter in the CNS.

NEURONAL POOLS

The billions of neurons in the CNS are organized into functional groups called *neuronal pools.* The neuronal pools receive information, process and integrate that information,

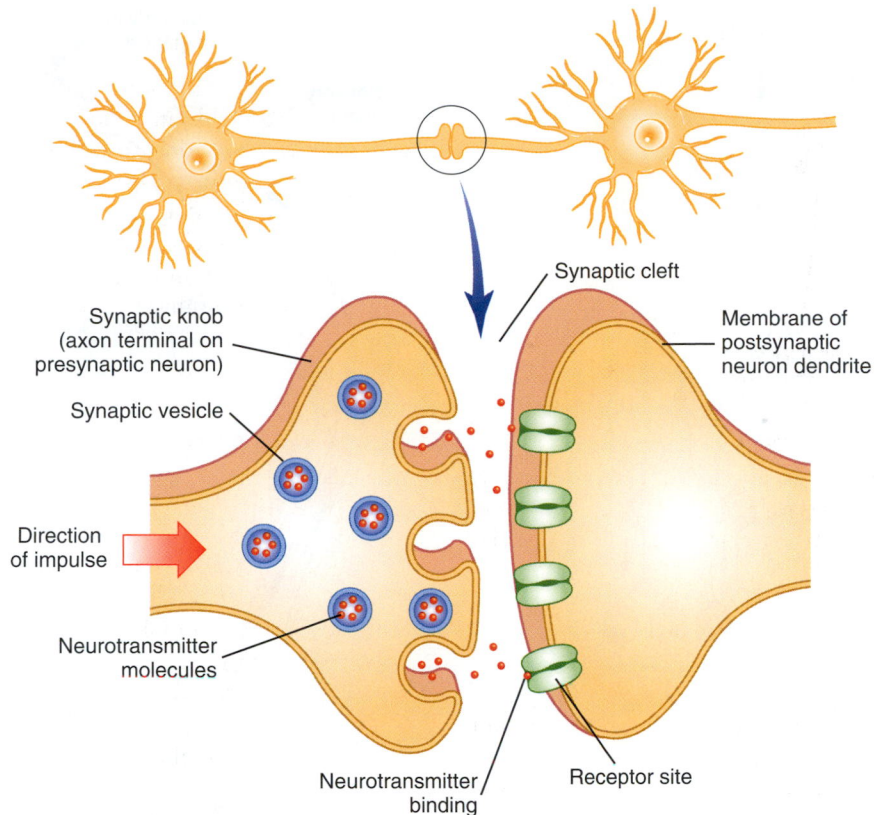

Figure 9-4 Components of a synapse. The impulse travels from the presynaptic neuron to the postsynaptic neuron. (From Applegate E: *The anatomy and physiology learning system,* ed 4, St Louis, 2011, Saunders.)

Table 9-2 Some Common Neurotransmitters			
Neurotransmitter	Location	Function	Comments
Acetylcholine	CNS and PNS	Generally excitatory but inhibitory to some visceral effectors	Found in skeletal neuromuscular junctions and in many ANS synapses
Norepinephrine	CNS and PNS	May be excitatory or inhibitory depending on receptors	Found in visceral and cardiac muscle neuromuscular junctions; cocaine and amphetamines exaggerate effects
Epinephrine	CNS and PNS	May be excitatory or inhibitory depending on receptors	Found in pathways concerned with behavior and mood
Dopamine	CNS and PNS	Generally excitatory	Found in pathways that regulate emotional responses; decreased levels in Parkinson disease
Serotonin	CNS	Generally inhibitory	Found in pathways that regulate temperature, sensory perception, mood, onset of sleep
Gamma-aminobutyric acid (GABA)	CNS	Generally inhibitory	Inhibits excessive discharge of neurons
Endorphins and enkephalins	CNS	Generally inhibitory	Inhibit release of sensory pain neurotransmitters; opiates mimic effects of these peptides

ANS, Autonomic nervous system; *CNS,* central nervous system; *PNS,* peripheral nervous system.
From Applegate E: *The anatomy and physiology learning system,* ed 4, St Louis, 2011, Saunders.

and then transmit it to some other destination. Neuronal pools are arranged in pathways, or circuits, over which the nerve impulses are transmitted. The simplest pathway is the *simple series circuit* (Figure 9-5, A) in which a single neuron synapses with another neuron, which in turn synapses with another, and so on. Most pathways are more complex. In a *divergence circuit* (Figure 9-5, B), a single neuron synapses with multiple neurons within the pool. This permits the same information to diverge or go along different pathways at the same time. This type of pathway is important in muscle contraction when many muscle fibers, or even several muscles, must contract at the same time. Another type of pathway is the *convergence circuit* (Figure 9-5, C). In this case, several presynaptic neurons synapse with a

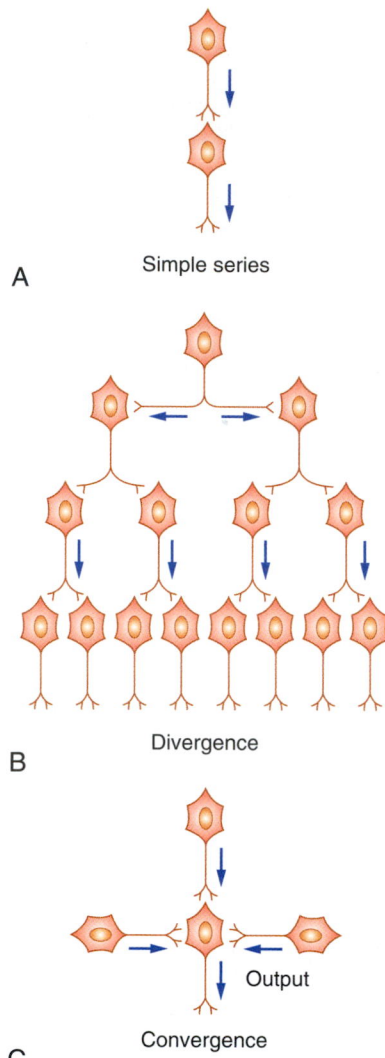

A   Simple series

B   Divergence

C   Convergence   Output

Figure 9-5 Neuronal pools. **A,** Simple series circuit: one neuron synapses with another. **B,** Divergence circuit: a single neuron synapses with multiple neurons. **C,** Convergence circuit: several neurons synapse with a single postsynaptic neuron. (From Applegate E: *The anatomy and physiology learning system,* ed 4, St Louis, 2011, Saunders.)

single postsynaptic neuron. This accounts for the fact that many different stimuli may have the same ultimate effect. For example, thinking about food, smelling food, and seeing food all have the same effect—the flow of saliva.

REFLEX ARCS

The neuron is the structural unit of the nervous system; the *reflex arc* is the functional unit. The reflex arc is a type of conduction pathway. It is similar to a one-way street because it allows impulses to travel in only one direction. The simplest reflex arc consists of two neurons, but most have three or more neurons in the conduction pathway. Figure 9-6 illustrates a three-neuron reflex arc. There are five basic components in a reflex arc (Table 9-3):

- Receptor
- Sensory neuron

Figure 9-6 Components of a generalized reflex arc. Note the five components of a reflex arc. (From Applegate E: *The anatomy and physiology learning system,* ed 4, St Louis, 2011, Saunders.)

- Integration center
- Motor neuron
- Effector

A *reflex* is an automatic, involuntary response to some change, either inside or outside the body. Reflexes are important in maintaining homeostasis by making adjustments to heart rate, breathing rate, and blood pressure. Reflexes are also involved in coughing, sneezing, and reactions to painful stimuli. Everyone is familiar with the withdrawal reflex. When you step on a tack or touch a hot iron, you immediately, without conscious thought, withdraw the injured foot or hand from the source of the irritation. Clinicians frequently test an individual's reflexes to determine if the nervous system is functioning properly.

CENTRAL NERVOUS SYSTEM

The CNS consists of the brain and spinal cord, which are located in the dorsal body cavity. These are vital to our well-being and are enclosed in bone for protection. The brain is surrounded by the cranium, and the spinal cord is protected by the vertebrae. The brain is continuous with the spinal cord at the foramen magnum in the occipital bone. In addition to bone, the CNS is surrounded by connective tissue membranes, called *meninges,* and by *cerebrospinal fluid* (CSF).

Table 9-3 Components of a Reflex Arc

Component	Description	Function
Receptor	Site of stimulus action; receptor end of dendrite or special cell in receptor organ	Responds to some change in internal or external environment
Sensory neuron	Afferent neuron; cell body is in ganglion outside CNS; axon extends into CNS	Transmits nerve impulses from receptor to CNS
Integration center	Always within CNS; in simplest reflexes, it consists of synapse between sensory and motor neurons; more commonly one or more interneurons are involved	Processing center; region in CNS where incoming sensory impulses generate appropriate outgoing motor impulses
Motor neuron	Efferent neuron; dendrites and cell body are in CNS; axon extends to periphery	Transmits nerve impulses from integration center in CNS to effector organ
Effector	Muscle or gland outside CNS	Responds to impulses from motor neuron to produce an action, such as contraction or secretion

CNS, Central nervous system.
From Applegate E: *The anatomy and physiology learning system,* ed 4, St Louis, 2011, Saunders.

Figure 9-7 Meninges of the central nervous system. (From Applegate E: *The anatomy and physiology learning system,* ed 4, St Louis, 2011, Saunders.)

MENINGES

Three layers of meninges surround the brain and spinal cord (Figure 9-7). The outer layer, the *dura mater,* is tough, white fibrous connective tissue. It is just inside the cranial bones and lines the vertebral canal. The dura mater contains channels, called *dural sinuses,* that collect venous blood to return it to the cardiovascular system.

The middle layer of meninges is the *arachnoid.* The arachnoid, which resembles a cobweb in appearance, is a thin layer with numerous threadlike strands that attach it to the innermost layer. The space under the arachnoid, the *subarachnoid space,* is filled with CSF and contains blood vessels.

The *pia mater* is the innermost layer of meninges. This thin, delicate membrane is tightly bound to the surface of the brain and spinal cord and cannot be dissected away without damaging the surface. It closely follows all surface contours.

BRAIN

The brain is divided into the cerebrum, diencephalon, brain stem, and cerebellum.

Cerebrum

The largest and most obvious portion of the brain is the **cerebrum,** which is divided by a deep *longitudinal fissure* into two *cerebral hemispheres.* The two hemispheres are two separate entities but are connected by an arching band of white fibers, called the *corpus callosum,* that provides a communication pathway between the two halves. The surface of the cerebrum is marked by convolutions, or *gyri,* that are separated by grooves, or *sulci.* The pia mater closely follows the convolutions and goes deep into the sulci and then up and over the gyri.

Each cerebral hemisphere is divided into five lobes, as illustrated in Figure 9-8. Four of the lobes have the same name as the bone over them. The *frontal lobe,* under the frontal bone, is the most anterior portion of each hemisphere. The posterior boundary of the frontal lobe is the **central sulcus.** The *parietal lobe* is immediately posterior to the central sulcus, under the parietal bone. The *occipital lobe,* under the occipital bone, is the most posterior portion of the cerebral hemisphere. Laterally, the *temporal lobe* is inferior to the frontal and parietal lobes. The *lateral sulcus* (fissure) separates the temporal lobe from the two lobes that are superior to it. A fifth lobe, the *insula* or *island of Reil,* lies deep within the lateral sulcus. It is covered by parts of the frontal, parietal, and temporal lobes.

The cerebral hemispheres consist of gray matter and white matter. A thin layer of *gray matter,* the *cerebral cortex,* forms the outermost portion of the cerebrum. Gray matter consists of neuron cell bodies and unmyelinated fibers. The *white matter,* which makes up the bulk of the cerebrum, is just beneath the cerebral cortex. White matter is myelinated nerve fibers that form communication pathways in the cerebrum.

Figure 9-8 Lobes and landmarks of the cerebrum. (From Applegate E: *The anatomy and physiology learning system,* ed 4, St Louis, 2011, Saunders.)

The cerebral cortex is the neural basis of what makes us "human." It is the center for sensory and motor functions. It is concerned with memory, language, reasoning, intelligence, personality, and all the other factors that we associate with human life. Even though the two cerebral hemispheres are nearly symmetric in structure, they are not always equal in function; instead, there are areas of specialization. However, there is considerable overlap in these regions and no area really works alone; all the areas are dependent on one another for mental "consciousness"—those abilities that involve higher mental processing, such as memory, reasoning, logic, and judgment.

It is possible to identify regions of the cerebral cortex that have specific functions. *Sensory areas* receive information from the various sense organs and receptors throughout the body. The primary sensory area, the **somatosensory cortex,** is located in the *postcentral gyrus* of the parietal lobe, immediately posterior to the central sulcus. This region receives sensory input from sensory receptors in the skin and skeletal muscles. The right side of the somatosensory cortex receives input from the left side of the body and vice versa. *Motor areas* responsible for muscle contraction are located in the frontal lobe. The primary motor area, the **somatomotor cortex,** is in the *precentral gyrus,* immediately anterior to the central sulcus. Neurons in this area allow us to consciously control our skeletal muscles. The right primary motor gyrus controls muscles on the left side of the body and vice versa. The primary motor cortex is also highly organized in a manner similar to the primary sensory cortex,

with neurons in a specific region responsible for controlling movement in a specific part of the body.

Association areas of the cerebral cortex are involved in the process of recognition. They analyze and interpret sensory information, and based on previous experiences they integrate appropriate responses through the motor areas. Table 9-4 describes some of the specific functional areas of the cerebral cortex.

The **basal ganglia** are functionally related regions of gray matter that are scattered throughout the white matter of the cerebral hemispheres. These regions function as relay stations, or areas of synapse, in pathways going to and from the cortex. The major effects of the basal ganglia are to decrease muscle tone and inhibit muscular activity. Because of these effects, they play an important role in posture and coordinating motor movements. Also, nearly all the inhibitory neurotransmitter dopamine is produced in the basal ganglia.

Diencephalon

The **diencephalon** is centrally located and is nearly surrounded by the cerebral hemispheres. Regions of the diencephalon are illustrated in Figure 9-9.

The *thalamus,* about 80% of the diencephalon, consists of two oval masses of gray matter that serve as relay stations for sensory impulses, except for the sense of smell, going to the cerebral cortex. The thalamus channels the impulses to the appropriate region of the cortex for discrimination, localization, and interpretation.

Table 9-4 Functional Regions of the Cerebral Cortex

Functional Region	Location	Description	Comments
Primary sensory cortex (somatosensory cortex)	Postcentral gyrus in parietal lobe	Receives sensory input from receptors in skin and skeletal muscles	Functions in sensations of temperature, touch, pressure, pain
Primary visual cortex	Posterior region of occipital lobe	Receives sensory input from retina of eye	Perceives current visual image
Auditory cortex	Superior margin of temporal lobe, along lateral sulcus	Receives auditory impulses related to pitch, rhythm, and loudness from inner ear	Allows the hearing of "sounds"
Olfactory cortex	Medial aspect of temporal lobe	Receives input from olfactory (smell) receptors in nasal cavity	Permits perception of different odors
Gustatory cortex	Parietal lobe where it is overlapped by temporal lobe	Receives input from taste buds on tongue	Permits perception of different tastes
Primary motor cortex (somatomotor cortex)	Precentral gyrus in frontal lobe	Initiates efferent action potentials that control voluntary movements	Permits skeletal muscle contraction
Premotor cortex	Anterior to primary motor cortex in frontal lobe	Controls learned motor skills that involve skeletal muscles, either simultaneously or sequentially	Examples of learned motor skills are playing piano, typing, writing
Broca area (motor speech area)	Inferior portion of frontal lobe in one hemisphere, usually the left	Programs and coordinates muscular movements necessary to articulate words	Person with injury in this area is able to understand words but is unable to speak because of inability to coordinate muscles necessary to form words
Prefrontal cortex	Anterior portion of frontal lobes	Involved with thought, reasoning, intelligence, judgment, planning, conscience	This area is well developed only in humans
Gnostic area (general interpretation area)	Region where parietal, temporal, and occipital lobes meet; found in one hemisphere (usually the left)	Integrates sensory interpretations from adjacent association areas to form thoughts; then transmits signals for appropriate responses	Stores complex memory patterns; allows person to recognize words and arrange them appropriately to express thoughts or to read and understand written ideas

From Applegate E: *The anatomy and physiology learning system,* ed 4, St Louis, 2011, Saunders.

Figure 9-9 Midsagittal section of the brain showing the major portions of the diencephalon, brain stem, and cerebellum. (From Applegate E: *The anatomy and physiology learning system,* ed 4, St Louis, 2011, Saunders.)

The *hypothalamus* is a small region below the thalamus. It plays a key role in maintaining homeostasis because it regulates many visceral activities. The hypothalamus also serves as a link between the nervous and endocrine systems because it regulates secretion of hormones from the pituitary gland. A slender stalk, the *infundibulum,* extends from the floor of the hypothalamus to the pituitary gland and acts as a connector between the two structures. Functions of the hypothalamus include the following:

- Regulates and integrates the ANS
- Regulates emotional responses and behavior
- Regulates body temperature
- Regulates food intake
- Regulates water balance and thirst
- Regulates endocrine system activity

The *epithalamus* is the most superior portion of the diencephalon. The *pineal gland,* or *body,* extends from its posterior margin. This small gland is involved with the onset of puberty and rhythmic cycles in the body. It is similar to a biologic clock.

Brain Stem

The **brain stem** is the region between the diencephalon and the spinal cord. It consists of three regions:

- Midbrain
- Pons
- Medulla oblongata

Regions of the brain stem are illustrated in Figure 9-9.

The *midbrain* is the most superior portion of the brain stem, the region next to the diencephalon. It consists of bundles of myelinated fibers that contain the voluntary motor tracts descending from the cerebral cortex. The *pons* is the bulging middle portion of the brain stem. This region primarily consists of nerve fibers that form conduction tracts between the higher brain centers and the spinal cord. Four cranial nerves originate in the pons. It also contains the *pneumotaxic* and *apneustic areas,* which help regulate breathing movements.

The *medulla oblongata,* or simply *medulla,* extends inferiorly from the pons. It is continuous with the spinal cord at the foramen magnum. All the ascending (sensory) and descending (motor) nerve fibers connecting the brain and spinal cord pass through the medulla. Most of the descending fibers cross over from one side to the other. In other words, fibers descending on the left side cross over to the right and vice versa. This is called **decussation.** Because the fibers decussate, or cross over, the brain controls motor functions on the opposite side of the body. The medulla contains three vital centers that control visceral activities. The *cardiac center* adjusts the heart rate and contraction strength to meet body needs. The *vasomotor center* regulates blood pressure by effecting changes in blood vessel diameter. The *respiratory center* acts with the centers in the pons to regulate the rate, rhythm, and depth of breathing. Other centers are involved in coughing, sneezing, swallowing, and vomiting.

Cerebellum

The **cerebellum,** the second largest portion of the brain, is located below the occipital lobes of the cerebrum. It consists of two *cerebellar hemispheres* connected in the middle by a structure called the *vermis.*

Like the cerebrum, the cerebellum consists of white matter surrounded by a thin layer of gray matter, the *cerebellar cortex.* Because the surface convolutions are less prominent in the cerebellum than in the cerebrum, the cerebellum has proportionately less gray matter.

Bundles of myelinated nerve fibers form communication pathways between the cerebellum and other parts of the CNS.

The cerebellum functions as a motor area of the brain that mediates subconscious contractions of skeletal muscles necessary for *coordination, posture,* and *balance.* The cerebellum coordinates skeletal muscles to produce smooth muscle movement rather than jerky, trembling motion. When the cerebellum is damaged, movements such as running, walking, and writing become uncoordinated. Posture is dependent on muscle tone, which is mediated by the cerebellum. Impulses from the inner ear concerning position and equilibrium are directed to the cerebellum, which uses that information to maintain balance.

VENTRICLES AND CEREBROSPINAL FLUID

A series of interconnected, fluid-filled cavities is found within the brain. These cavities are the *ventricles* of the brain, and the fluid is **cerebrospinal fluid.** The *lateral ventricles* in the cerebrum are the largest of these cavities. One lateral ventricle exists in each cerebral hemisphere. The CSF is a clear fluid that forms as a filtrate from the blood in specialized capillary networks, the *choroid plexus,* within the ventricles of the brain. It circulates through the ventricles and the central canal of the spinal cord and surrounds the brain in the subarachnoid space. From the subarachnoid space, CSF carrying waste products is returned to the blood. In addition to providing support and protection for the CNS, the CSF helps to nourish the brain and maintain constant ionic conditions for the brain and spinal cord and provides a pathway for removal of waste products.

SPINAL CORD

The *spinal cord,* illustrated in Figure 9-10, extends from the foramen magnum at the base of the skull to the level of the first lumbar vertebra, a distance of about 43 to 46 cm (approximately 17 to 18 inches). The cord is continuous with the medulla oblongata at the foramen magnum. Distally, it terminates in the *conus medullaris.* Like the brain, the spinal cord is surrounded by bone, meninges, and CSF. The spinal dura is separated from the vertebral bones by an *epidural space.* The meninges extend beyond the end of the spinal cord, down to the upper part of the sacrum. From there, a fibrous cord of pia mater, the *filum terminale*, extends down to the coccyx, where it is anchored.

The spinal cord is divided into 31 segments, with each segment giving rise to a pair of spinal nerves. At the distal end of the cord, many spinal nerves extend beyond the conus medullaris to form a collection that resembles a horse's tail. This is the *cauda equina*. There are two enlargements in the cord, one in the cervical region and one in the lumbar region. The *cervical enlargement* gives rise to the nerves that supply the upper extremity. Nerves from the *lumbar enlargement* supply the lower extremity.

In cross section, the spinal cord appears oval (Figure 9-11). Peripheral white matter surrounds a core of gray matter that resembles a butterfly or the letter *H*. The gray matter contains the terminal portions of sensory neuron axons, entire interneurons, and the dendrites and cell bodies of motor neurons. The central connecting bar between the two large areas of gray matter is the *gray commissure*. This surrounds the *central canal,* which contains CSF. The white matter that surrounds the gray matter contains longitudinal bundles of myelinated nerve fibers, called *nerve tracts.*

The spinal cord has two main functions. It is a conduction pathway for impulses going to and from the brain, and it serves as a reflex center. The conduction pathways that carry sensory impulses from body parts to the brain are called *ascending tracts.* Pathways that carry motor impulses from the brain to muscles and glands are *descending tracts.*

In addition to serving as a conduction pathway, the spinal cord functions as a center for spinal reflexes. The reflex arc, described earlier in this chapter and illustrated in

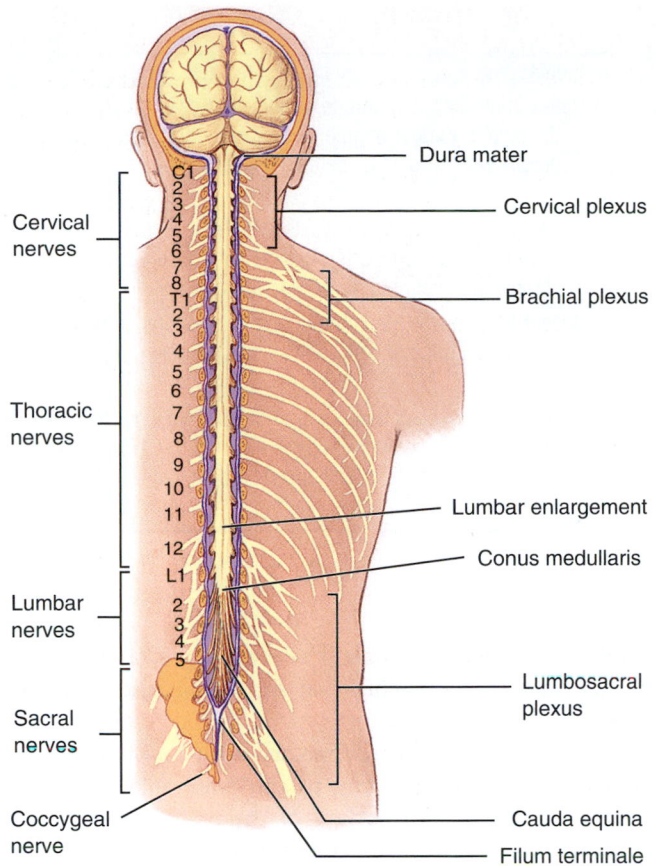

Figure 9-10 Gross anatomy of the spinal cord. (From Applegate E: *The anatomy and physiology learning system,* ed 4, St Louis, 2011, Saunders.)

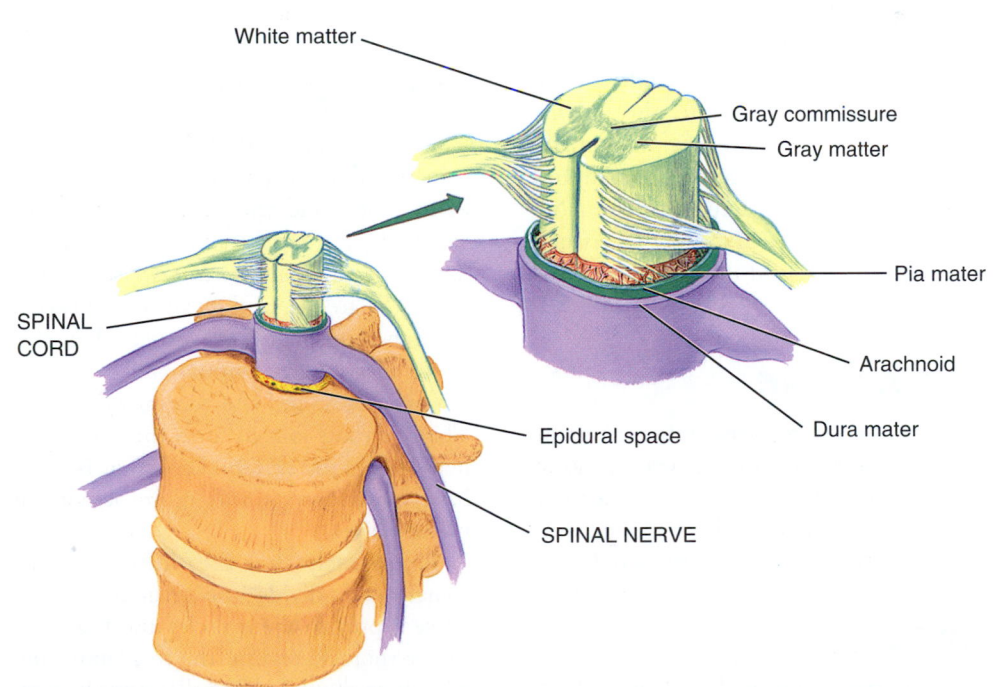

Figure 9-11 Cross section of the spinal cord. (From Applegate E: *The anatomy and physiology learning system,* ed 4, St Louis, 2011, Saunders.)

Table 9-5 Some Clinically Significant Reflexes

Reflex	Description	Indications
Patellar (knee-jerk reflex)	Stretch reflex; two-neuron path; reflex hammer strikes patellar tendon just below knee; receptors in quadriceps femoris muscle are stretched; reflex results in immediate "kick"	Reflex is blocked by damage to nerves involved and by damage to lumbar segments of spinal cord; also absent in people with chronic diabetes mellitus and neurosyphilis
Achilles tendon (ankle-jerk reflex)	Stretch reflex; two-neuron path; reflex hammer strikes Achilles tendon just above heel; gastrocnemius and soleus muscles contract to plantarflex foot	Weak or no reflex action indicates damage to nerves involved or to L5 to S2 segments of spinal cord; also absent in chronic diabetes, neurosyphilis, and alcoholism
Abdominal	Stroking lateral abdominal wall produces reflex action that compresses abdominal wall and moves umbilicus toward stimulus	Absent in lesions of peripheral nerves, in lesions in thoracic segments of spinal cord, and in multiple sclerosis
Babinski	Lateral sole of foot is stroked from heel to toe; positive sign results in dorsiflexion of big toe and spreading of other toes; negative sign results in toes curling under with a light inversion of foot	Positive Babinski sign is normal in children younger than 18 months of age; negative sign is normal after 18 months of age; if motor tracts in spinal cord are damaged, positive Babinski sign reappears

From Applegate E: *The anatomy and physiology learning system,* ed 4, St Louis, 2011, Saunders.

Figure 9-6, is the functional unit of the nervous system. Reflexes are responses to stimuli that do not require conscious thought, and consequently they occur more quickly than reactions that require thought processes. For example, with the withdrawal reflex, the reflex action withdraws the affected part before one is aware of the pain. Many reflexes are mediated in the spinal cord without going to the higher brain centers. Table 9-5 describes some clinically significant reflexes.

PERIPHERAL NERVOUS SYSTEM

The PNS consists of the nerves that branch out from the brain and spinal cord. These nerves form the communication network between the CNS and the remainder of the body. The PNS is further subdivided into the *somatic nervous system* and the *autonomic nervous system.* The somatic nervous system consists of nerves that go to the skin and muscles and is involved in conscious activities. The ANS consists of nerves that connect the CNS to the visceral organs such as the heart, stomach, and intestines. It mediates unconscious activities.

STRUCTURE OF A NERVE

A nerve contains bundles of nerve fibers, either axons or dendrites, surrounded by connective tissue. *Sensory nerves* contain only afferent fibers—long dendrites of sensory neurons. *Motor nerves* have only efferent fibers—long axons of motor neurons. *Mixed nerves* contain both types of fibers.

CRANIAL NERVES

Twelve pairs of cranial nerves, illustrated in Figure 9-12, emerge from the inferior surface of the brain. All of these nerves except the vagus nerve innervate structures in the head, neck, and facial region. The vagus nerve, cranial nerve X, has numerous branches that supply the viscera in the body.

The cranial nerves are designated both by name and by Roman numerals, according to the order in which they appear on the inferior surface of the brain. Most of the nerves have both sensory and motor components. Three of the nerves (I, II, VIII) are associated with the special senses of smell, vision, hearing, and equilibrium and have only sensory fibers. Five other nerves (III, IV, VI, XI, XII) are primarily motor in function but do have some sensory fibers for proprioception. The remaining four nerves (V, VII, IX, X) consist of significant amounts of both sensory and motor fibers. Table 9-6 itemizes the cranial nerves.

SPINAL NERVES

Thirty-one pairs of spinal nerves emerge laterally from the spinal cord. Each pair of nerves corresponds to a segment of the cord, and the nerves are named accordingly. This means there are *eight cervical nerves* (C1 to C8), *12 thoracic nerves* (T1 to T12), *five lumbar nerves* (L1 to L5), *five sacral nerves* (S1 to S5), and *one coccygeal nerve* (Co).

Each spinal nerve is connected to the spinal cord by a *dorsal root* and a *ventral root.* The dorsal root has only sensory fibers, and the ventral root has only motor fibers. The two roots join to form the spinal nerve just before the nerve leaves the vertebral column. Because all spinal nerves have both sensory and motor components, they are all mixed nerves.

Immediately after they leave the vertebral column, the spinal nerves divide into several branches that provide the nerve supply to the muscles and the skin of the body wall. In the thoracic region, the main portions of the nerves go directly to the thoracic wall, where they are called *intercostal nerves.* In other regions, the main portions of the nerves form complex networks called *plexuses* (see Figure 9-10). In

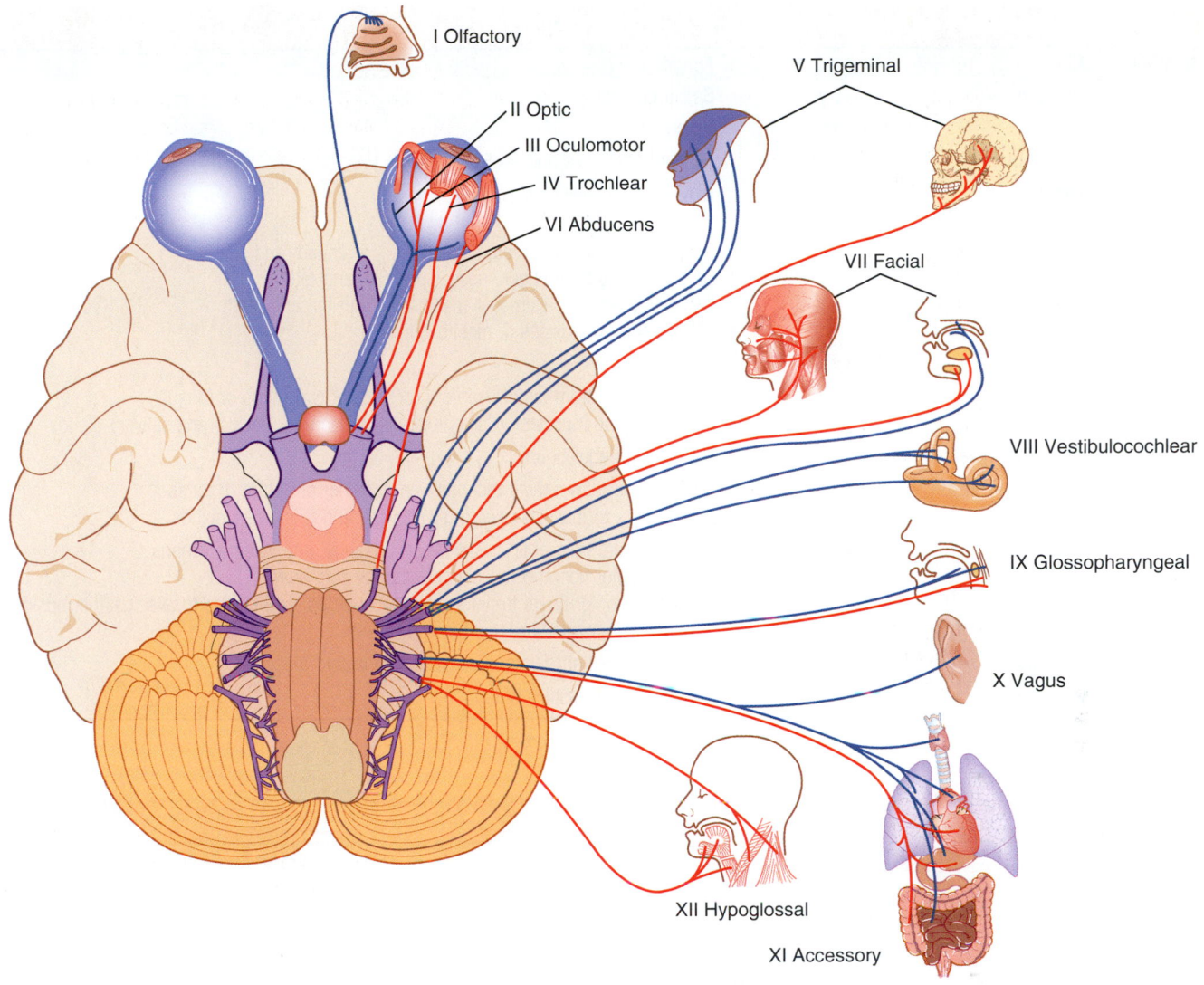

I Olfactory

V Trigeminal

II Optic

III Oculomotor

IV Trochlear

VII Facial

VI Abducens

VIII Vestibulocochlear

IX Glossopharyngeal

X Vagus

XII Hypoglossal

XI Accessory

Figure 9-12 Cranial nerves. The red lines indicate motor function, and the blue lines indicate sensory function. (From Applegate E: *The anatomy and physiology learning system,* ed 4, St Louis, 2011, Saunders.)

the plexus the fibers are sorted and recombined so that the fibers associated with a particular body part are together even though they may originate from different regions of the cord. The *cervical plexus* is located in the neck and sends nerves to the skin and muscles of the neck, shoulder, and diaphragm. The *brachial plexus* is deep to the clavicle and innervates the skin and muscles of the upper extremities. The *lumbosacral plexus* is in the lumbar region of the back. Nerves from this plexus go to the skin and muscles of the lower abdominal wall, the lower extremities, the buttocks, and the external genitalia.

AUTONOMIC NERVOUS SYSTEM

General Features

The ANS is a visceral efferent system, which means it sends motor impulses to the visceral organs. It functions automatically and continuously, without conscious effort, to innervate smooth muscle, cardiac muscle, and glands. It is

concerned with heart rate, breathing rate, blood pressure, body temperature, and other visceral activities that work together to maintain homeostasis.

The ANS has two parts: the *sympathetic division* and the *parasympathetic division* (Table 9-7). Many visceral organs are supplied with fibers from both divisions *(dual innervation).* In this case, one stimulates and the other inhibits. This antagonistic functional relationship serves as a balance to help maintain homeostasis.

Sympathetic Division

The sympathetic division, illustrated in Figure 9-13, is concerned primarily with preparing the body for stressful or emergency situations. Sometimes called the *fight-or-flight system,* it is an energy-expending system. It stimulates the responses that are necessary to meet the emergency and inhibits the visceral activities that can be delayed momentarily. For example, during an emergency the sympathetic system increases breathing rate, heart rate, and blood flow

Table 9-6 Summary of Cranial Nerves

Number	Name	Type	Function
I	Olfactory	Sensory	Sense of smell
II	Optic	Sensory	Vision
III	Oculomotor	Primarily motor	Movement of eyes and eyelids
IV	Trochlear	Primarily motor	Movement of eyes
V	Trigeminal Ophthalmic branch Maxillary branch Mandibular branch	Mixed	 Sensory fibers from cornea, skin of nose, forehead, and scalp Sensory fibers from cheek, nose, upper lip, and teeth Sensory fibers from skin over mandible, lower lip, and teeth Motor fibers to muscles of mastication
VI	Abducens	Primarily motor	Eye movement
VII	Facial	Mixed	Sensory fibers from taste receptors on anterior two thirds of tongue Motor fibers to muscles of facial expression, lacrimal glands, and salivary glands
VIII	Vestibulocochlear	Sensory	Hearing and equilibrium
IX	Glossopharyngeal	Mixed	Sensory fibers from taste receptors on posterior one third of tongue Motor fibers to muscles used in swallowing and to salivary glands
X	Vagus	Mixed	Sensory fibers from pharynx, larynx, esophagus, and visceral organs Somatic motor fibers to muscles of pharynx and larynx Autonomic motor fibers to heart, smooth muscles, and glands to alter gastric motility, heart rate, respiration, and blood pressure
XI	Accessory	Primarily motor	Contraction of trapezius and sternocleidomastoid muscles
XII	Hypoglossal	Primarily motor	Contraction of muscles of tongue

From Applegate E: *The anatomy and physiology learning system,* ed 4, St Louis, 2011, Saunders.

Table 9-7 Comparison of Sympathetic and Parasympathetic Actions on Selected Visceral Effectors

Visceral Effectors	Sympathetic Action	Parasympathetic Action
Pupil of eye	Dilates	Constricts
Lens of eye	Lens flattens for distance vision	Lens bulges for near vision
Sweat glands	Stimulates	No innervation
Arrector pili muscles of hair	Stimulates contraction; goose bumps	No innervation
Heart	Increases heart rate	Decreases heart rate
Bronchi	Dilates	Constricts
Digestive glands	Decreases secretion of digestive enzymes	Increases secretion of digestive enzymes
Digestive tract	Decreases peristalsis	Increases peristalsis
Digestive tract sphincters	Stimulates—closes sphincters	Inhibits—opens sphincters
Blood vessels to digestive organs	Constricts	No innervation
Blood vessels to skeletal muscles	Dilates	No innervation
Blood vessels to skin	Constricts	No innervation
Adrenal medulla	Stimulates secretion of epinephrine	No innervation
Liver	Increases release of glucose	No innervation
Urinary bladder	Relaxes bladder and closes sphincter	Contracts bladder and opens sphincter

From Applegate E: *The anatomy and physiology learning system,* ed 4, St Louis, 2011, Saunders.

to skeletal muscles. At the same time, it decreases activity in the digestive tract because that is not necessary to meet the emergency.

The sympathetic preganglionic fibers arise from the thoracic and lumbar regions of the spinal cord; thus the sympathetic division is sometimes called the *thoracolumbar division.*

Parasympathetic Division

The parasympathetic division is most active under ordinary, relaxed conditions (see Figure 9-13). It also brings the body's systems back to a normal state after an emergency by slowing the heart rate and breathing rate, decreasing blood pressure, decreasing blood flow to skeletal muscles,

Figure 9-13 Structure and function of autonomic nervous system. The red lines indicate the sympathetic division, and the blue lines indicate parasympathetic innervations. Note the location of the ganglia for each division. (From Applegate E: *The anatomy and physiology learning system,* ed 4, St Louis, 2011, Saunders.)

Legend in figure:
- Parasympathetic
- Sympathetic

Labels: Terminal ganglia, Constrict pupil, Increase saliva, Dilate pupil, Decrease saliva, Dilate bronchioles / Increase heart rate, Constrict bronchioles, Slow heart rate, Empty gallbladder / Increase digestion, Release glucose in liver / Decrease digestion, Increase intestinal activity, Decrease intestinal activity, Open sphincters of bladder and colon, Close sphincters of bladder and colon, Collateral ganglia, Sympathetic chain ganglia

and increasing digestive tract activity. Sometimes called the *rest-and-repose system,* it is an energy-conserving system.

The parasympathetic preganglionic fibers arise from the brain stem and sacral region of the spinal cord; thus the parasympathetic division is sometimes called the *craniosacral division.*

AGING OF THE NERVOUS SYSTEM

Aging of the nervous system is of major importance because changes in this system affect organs in other systems and can cause disturbances of many bodily functions. For example, changes in nerves decrease stimulation of skeletal muscle, which contributes to muscle atrophy with age. Because of its widespread consequences, aging of the nervous system is one of the most distressing aspects of growing old.

Like other cells, nerve cells are lost as a person ages, even in the absence of disease processes. Because neurons are amitotic, those that are lost are not replaced. Loss of neurons is largely responsible for the decrease in brain mass that occurs with aging. Fortunately, the brain has a large reserve supply of neurons, many more than are necessary to carry out its functions, so the decrease in neuron number alone is not devastating. The loss of neurons is not constant in all areas of the brain. For example, about 25% of the specialized cells in the cerebellum, which are responsible for coordinated movements, are lost during aging. This may affect balance and cause difficulty in coordinating fine movements. In other areas of the brain, the number of neurons remains essentially constant throughout life.

It is generally accepted that there is a decline in intelligence with aging, and this is thought to be associated with the loss of neurons. However, it is important to remember that there are wide variations in individuals regarding changes in intellect with age. Because a person is old does not mean that person is "dumb." Many elderly people retain a keen intellect until death. Along with the decline in intelligence, there may be a general decline in memory. Again, this varies from person to person. In general, short-term memory seems to be affected more than long-term memory. Intellect and memory appear to be retained better in people who remain mentally and physically active.

Another change observed in older people is a decrease in the rate of impulse conduction along an axon and across a synapse. A reduction in the amount of myelin around the axon probably accounts for the diminished conduction rate along the axon. Decreases in the quantity of neurotransmitter and in the number of receptor sites cause slower conduction across the synapses. These factors contribute to the slower reflexes and the longer time required to process information that are observed in many elderly people.

Common Pathology of the Nervous System

Disease	Signs and Symptoms	Etiology	Diagnosis and Treatment
Hydrocephalus	Signs and symptoms vary with age of onset. Infants: unusually large head and bulging fontanels. Toddlers: headache, blurred vision, poor coordination. Adults: distorted vision, poor coordination and balance, memory loss.	Caused by an accumulation of CSF in the brain as a result of overproduction, reduced absorption into the blood, or blockage in the pathway of flow. The accumulation of CSF increases pressure on the brain and destroys brain tissue.	Diagnosis is based on physical examination, neurologic examination, and brain imaging techniques. The most common treatment is the surgical insertion of a shunt system to increase the drainage of CSF.
Carpal tunnel syndrome	Tingling or numbness in the fingers and hand; weakness in the wrist and hand.	The condition is caused by compression of the median nerve as it passes through the carpal tunnel in the wrist.	Diagnosis is based on history, physical examinations, x-ray studies, EMG, and nerve conduction studies. Treatment begins with rest and ice for the affected wrist; wrist splinting and drugs to reduce inflammation and swelling may be beneficial. In severe cases, surgery may be necessary to relieve the pressure on the median nerve.
Dementia	A widespread group of disorders characterized by damage to nerve cells in the brain resulting in memory loss, impaired judgment or language, inability to perform daily activities, easily becoming disoriented, inability to reason, paranoia, and agitation. Some forms are progressive.	There are numerous causes including accumulation of toxic substances in the brain and reduced blood supply to the brain; it may also be secondary to other conditions.	Diagnosis is difficult. The health care professional may use a combination of medical history, physical examination, cognitive and neuropsychological tests, brain scans, and laboratory tests. Most types of dementia cannot be cured. Treatment protocols focus on managing the symptoms.
Alzheimer disease	The most common form of progressive dementia. Signs and symptoms include memory loss, impaired judgment or language, inability to perform daily activities, easily becoming disoriented, inability to reason, paranoia, and agitation.	Caused by a progressive destruction of brain cells. Hallmark abnormalities in the brain include plaques of protein fragments called *beta-amyloid*, tangles of protein fragments called *tau*, and a loss of connections among brain cells.	Diagnosis is difficult. The health care professional may use a combination of medical history, physical examination, cognitive and neuropsychological tests, brain scans, and laboratory tests. Treatment protocols focus on managing the symptoms and keeping the individual comfortable and physically healthy.
Epilepsy	Seizures of epilepsy can produce symptoms such as temporary confusion, staring spells, uncontrollable jerking movements of the arms and legs, loss of consciousness or awareness, and psychic symptoms. Focal seizures originate in one area of the brain; generalized seizures involve all areas of the brain.	Epilepsy is a CNS disorder in which the nerve cell activity in the brain is disturbed. In about half of the cases, there is no identifiable cause. In the other half, there may be genetic factors, head trauma, brain tumor or stroke, infectious diseases, prenatal injury, or developmental disorders.	Diagnosis is based on medical history, neurologic examination, blood tests, EEG, and a variety of imaging modalities. Many patients can be treated with antiseizure medications. Others may require surgery.
Bell palsy	Paralysis of the muscles on one side of the face with sagging of the mouth on the affected side; difficulty making facial expressions.	Caused by neuropathy of cranial nerve VII; cause of the neuropathy unknown; may be result of a viral infection.	No specific diagnostic test for Bell palsy; health professional may order EMG or an imaging scan. Many cases resolve spontaneously. Treatment options include corticosteroids, antiviral drugs, and physical therapy to restore muscle function.

Common Pathology of the Nervous System—cont'd

Disease	Signs and Symptoms	Etiology	Diagnosis and Treatment
Cerebral concussion	Symptoms range from mild to severe and may include fuzzy or blurry vision, headache, dizziness, nausea and vomiting, sensitivity to light or noise, sleep disturbances, and inability to concentrate.	Caused by a traumatic blow to the head that causes the brain to impact against the skull.	Diagnosis is based on physical and neurological findings. Initial treatment consists of observation to make sure the condition does not become more serious. Physical and cognitive rest usually allows the condition to resolve within 7 to 10 days.
Sciatica	Pain that radiates from the lumbar spine to the buttocks and down the back of the leg to the foot; varies from a mild ache to a sharp, burning type of pain.	Occurs when the sciatic nerve becomes pinched or compressed from a herniated disc, bone spur, or tumor.	For a diagnosis, the health professional will test muscle strength and reflexes. If the pain is severe and persists, imaging scans may be used. Treatment, if necessary, may include muscle relaxants, antiinflammatory drugs, and physical therapy. In some cases, injections of corticosteroids may be recommended.
Neuralgia	Sharp, shocking pain that follows the path of a nerve; increased sensitivity to the skin along the path of the nerve; weakness or paralysis of the muscles supplied by the nerve; nerve pain.	Causes include chemical irritation, renal insufficiency, infections, trauma, and pressure on a nerve; in many cases the cause is unknown.	No specific tests for neuralgia. Diagnosis depends on history and physical examination; blood tests, EMG, MRI may help locate the underlying cause of the pain. Pain relievers may help reduce the pain. Treatment should attempt to reverse or control the underlying cause of the pain.
Cerebral palsy	Signs and symptoms usually appear during infancy or early childhood and may include exaggerated reflexes, abnormalities in muscle tone, abnormal posture, tremors or involuntary movements, unsteadiness in walking, and stiff muscles.	Caused by an abnormality or disruption in brain development, usually in utero. The trigger for the disruption is unknown but may include mutations, fetal stroke, infant infections, lack of oxygen during a difficult delivery, or traumatic head injury.	The child is usually referred to a pediatric neurologist for diagnosis. A combination of medical history, physical examination, brain scans, and EEG is used. A cerebral palsy patient requires long-term care by a team of health professionals including physical therapists, occupational therapists, and speech therapists. Medications may lessen the muscle rigidity. Severe contractures may require surgery.
Cerebrovascular accident (CVA)	Symptoms depend on the area of the brain affected. A convenient system is FAST: *F*acial muscle weakness, *A*rm droop, *S*peech abnormalities, *T*ime to rush to the emergency room.	Most common brain disorder; may be caused either by a decreased blood supply to the brain (ischemic) or rupture of a blood vessel in the brain (hemorrhagic). Risk factors include hypertension, elevated blood lipids, and diabetes mellitus. Commonly called a *stroke*.	Diagnosis involves a neurologic examination, CT and/or MRI scans, Doppler ultrasound, and arteriography. Treatment options depend on the type and severity of the CVA. For the ischemic type, intervention restores blood flow; for the hemorrhagic type it may be necessary to reduce the pressure on the brain. Long-term stroke rehabilitation attempts to help patients return to normal life as much as possible.
Tic douloureux (trigeminal neuralgia)	Characterized by unilateral, intense, sharp, stabbing pain most commonly felt in the cheek, nose, upper lip, and upper teeth. A muscle spasm accompanies the pain.	Pain is caused by irritation of the trigeminal nerve (V), possibly by a blood vessel pressing on the nerve or other injury.	Diagnosis is based on symptoms, physical and neurologic examinations, and possibly CT and/or MRI scans. There is no specific test to confirm a diagnosis. Treatment options include medications that decrease the ability of the trigeminal nerve to fire off the impulses that cause the pain, muscle relaxants, and narcotic pain relievers. If medications are not effective, surgical procedures on the trigeminal nerve may be necessary.

Continued

Common Pathology of the Nervous System—cont'd

Disease	Signs and Symptoms	Etiology	Diagnosis and Treatment
Reye syndrome (RS)	Disorientation, lethargy, weakness or paralysis in arms and legs, and personality changes; may progress to a coma. Occurs primarily in children.	Exact cause is unknown. Seems to be triggered by use of aspirin to treat a viral illness, particularly influenza and chickenpox, especially in children with an underlying disorder in fatty acid metabolism. Exposure to toxins such as insecticides, herbicides, and paint thinner may be a contributing factor.	There is no specific test for RS. Screening for RS usually begins with blood and urine tests and tests for disorders in fatty acid oxidation. Treatment includes intravenous fluids, diuretics, antiseizure medications, and medications to prevent bleeding.
Transient ischemic attack (TIA)	Temporary cerebral dysfunction of sudden onset and short duration; like a stroke but with no permanent damage. Symptoms include weakness of facial and arm muscles, altered speech, blurred vision, and dizziness or loss of balance or coordination.	Common causes are blood clots and atherosclerosis that disrupt blood flow to the brain.	Because TIA is of short duration, diagnosis is based on medical history. Physician will use blood tests and imaging tests to determine underlying cause. Treatment is aimed at correcting the abnormality that caused the TIA and preventing a stroke. Antiplatelet drugs (aspirin) and anticoagulants may suffice. Other options are angioplasty and carotid endarterectomy.
Shingles	Blisters and pain spread over the skin in a bandlike pattern that follows the path of affected nerves.	Caused by the varicella-zoster (herpes zoster) virus, the same virus that causes chickenpox. After causing chickenpox, the virus lies dormant for years, only to reappear as shingles. The cause for reappearance is unknown but may be a result of lowered immunity.	Diagnosis is based on history, location of pain, and pattern of rash or blisters. There is no cure. Antiviral medications speed healing and reduce complications. Pain relievers help alleviate the pain.
Multiple sclerosis	Signs and symptoms include numbness or weakness in the extremities, double vision or total loss of vision, slurred speech, fatigue, dizziness, tremors, and a lack of coordination. There is progressive loss of function with periods of remission.	Progressive destruction of the myelin sheaths of the neurons in the CNS. Cause of destruction is unknown but evidence suggests the disease may be an autoimmune disorder. Destruction of myelin interferes with the neuron's ability to conduct impulses.	Diagnosis is based on medical history, physical examination. Blood tests, CSF analysis, and imaging scans may be used to rule out other conditions. There is no cure. Treatment focuses on managing the symptoms and slowing the progression of the disorder. Corticosteroids reduce the inflammation during attacks; immunosuppressants slow the progress; physical therapy and muscle relaxants reduce muscle stiffness.
Parkinson disease	Signs and symptoms include tremors, altered speech patterns, lack of facial expression, cognitive impairment, dysphagia, and emotional disorders. Occurs more frequently in men than in women. Signs and symptoms become more pronounced as disease progresses.	Neurons in the basal ganglia do not produce enough of the inhibitory transmitter dopamine, allowing excess excitatory signals to certain voluntary muscles. The reason for the lack of dopamine is unknown.	No specific test for Parkinson disease. Neurologist relies on the signs and symptoms, medical history, and physical examination. Other tests may be used to eliminate other conditions. There is no known cure, but levodopa and dopamine agonists may help control symptoms.

Common Pathology of the Nervous System—cont'd

Disease	Signs and Symptoms	Etiology	Diagnosis and Treatment
Amyotrophic lateral sclerosis (ALS) (Lou Gehrig disease)	Characterized by progressive muscular weakness and atrophy with spasticity and exaggerated reflexes. Early signs are muscle twitching in arms and legs; slurred speech. Eventually, there is inability to control muscles needed to move, speak, eat, and breathe.	Results from a degeneration of motor neurons in the CNS. The cause is unknown. Suggested causes are gene mutation, a chemical imbalance in the system that is toxic to neurons, and an autoimmune response.	No specific test that will confirm a diagnosis. Neurologist relies on a combination of signs and symptoms, medical history, physical examination, EMG, and nerve conduction studies. Treatment focuses on slowing the progress of the disease and managing complications. Medications may provide relief from symptoms, physical therapy addresses the mobility problems, breathing exercises may help when the respiratory muscles are involved. There is no known cure, and the disease eventually leads to death.

CSF, Cerebrospinal fluid; *CNS,* central nervous system; *CT,* computed tomography; *EEG,* electroencephalography; *EMG,* electromyography; *MRI,* magnetic resonance imaging.

TERMINOLOGY REVIEW

Key Term	Word Parts	Definition
Action potential	*act-:* motion	A nerve impulse; a rapid change in membrane potential that involves depolarization and repolarization.
Axons		The efferent processes of neurons that carry impulses away from the cell bodies
Basal ganglia	*gangli-:* knot	Paired regions of gray matter located within the white matter of the cerebrum.
Brain stem		The portion of the brain, between the diencephalon and spinal cord, that contains the midbrain, pons, and medulla oblongata.
Central sulcus	*sulc-:* furrow, ditch	The groove or furrow between the frontal and parietal lobes of the cerebrum; also called the *fissure of Rolando.*
Cerebellum	*cerebell/o:* cerebellum	Second largest part of the human brain, located posterior to the pons and medulla oblongata and involved in the coordination of muscular movements.
Cerebrospinal fluid	*cerebr/o:* cerebrum	A fluid, similar to plasma, that fills the subarachnoid space around the brain and spinal cord and is in the ventricles of the brain.
Cerebrum	*cerebr/o:* cerebrum	The largest and uppermost part of the human brain; concerned with consciousness, learning, memory, sensations, and voluntary movements.
Dendrites	*dendr-:* tree	The branching (treelike) afferent processes of a neuron that receive impulses from other neurons and transmit them to the cell body.
Decussation		A crossing over; usually refers to motor fibers that cross over to the opposite side in the medulla oblongata.
Diencephalon	*cephal/o:* head	Part of the brain between the cerebral hemispheres and the midbrain; includes the thalamus and hypothalamus.
Myelin		White, fatty substance that surrounds many nerve fibers.
Neurilemma	*neur/o:* nerve *-lemma:* sheath, covering	The layer of cells that surrounds a nerve fiber in the peripheral nervous system and in some cases produces myelin; also called *Schwann sheath.*
Neuroglia	*neur/o:* nerve *gli/a:* glue	Supporting cells of nervous tissue; cells in nervous tissue that do not conduct impulses.
Neuron	*neur/o:* nerve	Nerve cell including its processes; conducting cell of nervous tissue.
Neurotransmitters	*neur/o:* nerve	A chemical substance that is released from axon terminals to stimulate muscle fiber contraction or an impulse in another neuron.
Nodes of Ranvier		Short spaces between segments of myelin in a myelinated nerve fiber.
Refractory period		Time during which an excitable cell cannot respond to a stimulus that is usually adequate to initiate an action potential.

Continued

↻ TERMINOLOGY REVIEW—cont'd

Key Term	Word Parts	Definition
Saltatory conduction	*-tion:* process of	Process in which a nerve impulse travels along a myelinated nerve fiber by jumping from one node of Ranvier to the next.
Somatomotor cortex	*somat/o:* body	The primary motor area of the brain; located in the precentral gyrus; transmits motor impulses to the body.
Somatosensory cortex	*somat/o:* body	The primary sensory area of the brain; located in the postcentral gyrus; receives sensory impulses from the body.
Synapse	*syn-:* together, with	The region of communication between two neurons.
Threshold stimulus		Minimum level of stimulation that is required to start a nerve impulse or muscle contraction; also called *liminal stimulus.*

ON THE WEB

For information on the nervous system:

Inner Body: www.innerbody.com/html/body.html

Interactive Brain Atlases: www9.biostr.washington.edu/da.html

Martindale's Virtual Medical Center Brain and Neuro Center: www.martindalecenter.com/MedicalBrain.html

Neuroanatomy and Neuropathology: www.neuropat.dote.hu

Spinal Cord Injury Tracts: www.rexdonald.com/facts.htm

The Washington School of Medicine, Neuroscience Tutorial: http://thalamus.wustl.edu/course

University of Washington: Nervous System: faculty.washington.edu/chudler/ehc.html

The Senses 10

⬯ Check out the Evolve site at http://evolve.elsevier.com/Bonewit/today/ to access additional interactive activities and exercises to help you study and prepare for success.

LEARNING OBJECTIVES

1. Explain the difference between general senses and special senses, and state examples of each.
2. List and describe the five groups of sense receptors.
3. Identify the sense receptors for touch, pressure, proprioception, temperature, and pain.
4. List and identify the location of the four different taste sensations.
5. Locate the sense receptors for smell, and trace the impulse pathway to the cerebral cortex.
6. Describe the structure of the eye, and explain the function of each structure.
7. Explain how light is focused on the retina.
8. Explain the function of the following photoreceptor cells in the retina: rods and cones.
9. Explain how nerve impulses for sight are initiated in response to light.
10. Describe the structure of the ear, and explain the function of each structure.
11. Explain how nerve impulses for hearing are initiated in response to sound waves.
12. Explain the difference between static equilibrium and dynamic equilibrium.
13. Explain how impulses for static equilibrium and dynamic equilibrium are initiated.
14. Describe ways in which the aging of an individual affects the senses.
15. Identify pathology related to the senses.

CHAPTER OUTLINE

INTRODUCTION TO THE SENSES
RECEPTORS AND SENSATIONS
GENERAL SENSES
Touch and Pressure
Proprioception
Temperature
Pain
GUSTATORY SENSE
OLFACTORY SENSE
VISUAL SENSE
Protective Features and Accessory Structures of the Eye

Structure of the Eyeball
Pathway of Light and Refraction
Photoreceptors
Visual Pathway
AUDITORY SENSE
Structure of the Ear
Physiology of Hearing
SENSE OF EQUILIBRIUM
Static Equilibrium
Dynamic Equilibrium
AGING OF THE SENSES

KEY TERMS

accommodation (ah-kahm-
   oh-DAY-shun)
bulbus oculi (BUL-bus AHK-yoo-lye)
chemoreceptor (kee-moh-ree-SEP-tor)
cochlea (KOK-lee-ah)
crista ampullaris (KRIS-tah
   amp-yoo-LAIR-is)
general senses (JEN-er-uhl SEN-sez)
gustatory sense (GUS-tah-toar-ee SENS)

lacrimal apparatus (LACK-rih-mal
   ap-pah-RAT-us)
macula lutea (MACK-yoo-lah
   LOO-tee-aj)
mechanoreceptors
   (mek-ah-noh-ree-SEP-tors)
nociceptors (noh-see-SEP-tors)
olfaction (ohl-FAK-shun)
otoliths (OH-toe-liths)

photoreceptors (foh-toh-ree-SEP-tors)
proprioception (proh-pree-oh-SEP-shun)
refraction (ree-FRAK-shun)
rhodopsin (roe-DOP-sin)
sensory adaptation (SEN-soh-ree
   add-dap-TAY-shun)
special senses (SPESH-uhl SEN-sez)
thermoreceptors (ther-moh-
   ree-SEP-tors)

INTRODUCTION TO THE SENSES

Sensory perception depends on receptors that respond to various stimuli. When a stimulus triggers an impulse in a receptor, the action potentials travel to the cerebral cortex, where they are processed and interpreted. Only after this has occurred is a particular sensation perceived. Some senses, such as pain, touch, pressure, and proprioception, are widely distributed in the body. These are called **general senses.** Other senses, such as taste, smell, hearing, and sight, are called **special senses** because their receptors are localized in a particular area.

RECEPTORS AND SENSATIONS

Although there are many different kinds of sense receptors, they can be grouped into five types. The basis for these receptor types is the kind of stimulus to which they are sensitive or have a low threshold. The five types of receptors are chemoreceptors, mechanoreceptors, nociceptors, thermoreceptors, and photoreceptors (Table 10-1).

Perceived sensation occurs only after impulses have been interpreted by the brain. Steps involved in sensory perception include the following:

1. There must be a *stimulus.*
2. A *receptor* must detect the stimulus and create an action potential.
3. The action potential (impulse) must be *conducted* to the central nervous system (CNS).
4. Within the CNS, the impulse must be *translated* into information.
5. Information must be *interpreted* in the CNS into an awareness or perception of the stimulus.

The impulses from all the receptors are alike. The difference in perception is where they are interpreted in the brain. For example, all impulses going to one particular region are interpreted as sound, whereas those going to another region are interpreted as taste. As the brain interprets a sensation, it projects that sense back to its original source so that the "feeling" seems to come from the receptors that are stimulated. This projection allows us to locate the source of the stimulus.

Some sense receptors, when they are continually stimulated, undergo **sensory adaptation.** They have a decreased sensitivity to a continued stimulus and trigger impulses only if the strength of the stimulus is increased.

GENERAL SENSES

General senses, or *somatic senses,* are those that are found throughout the body. They are associated with the visceral organs, as well as the skin, muscles, and joints, and include touch, pressure, proprioception, temperature, and pain.

TOUCH AND PRESSURE

As a group, the receptors for touch and pressure are **mechanoreceptors** that are sensitive to forces that deform or displace tissues. They are widely distributed in the skin. Three of the mechanoreceptors involved in touch and pressure are free nerve endings, Meissner corpuscles, and pacinian corpuscles.

Free nerve endings are the dendritic ends of sensory neurons that are interspersed among the cells in epithelial tissue. They do not have a connective tissue covering. They are important in sensing objects, such as clothing, that are in continuous contact with the skin. *Meissner corpuscles* consist of the ends of sensory nerve fibers surrounded by connective tissue and are specific in localizing tactile sensations. They are located in the dermal papillae, just beneath the epidermis, where they are important in sensing light-discriminative touch stimuli. *Pacinian corpuscles* are called *lamellated corpuscles* because several layers of connective tissue surround the nerve endings. These are common in deeper dermis and subcutaneous tissues, tendons, and ligaments. They are stimulated by heavy pressure.

PROPRIOCEPTION

Proprioception is the sense of position or orientation. It allows us to sense the location and rate of movement of one body part relative to another. *Golgi tendon organs,* found at the junction of a tendon with a muscle, and *muscle spindles,* located in skeletal muscles, are important mechanoreceptors for proprioception.

TEMPERATURE

Thermoreceptors are located immediately under the skin and are widely distributed throughout the body. They are

Table 10-1 Types of Sense Receptors		
Receptor	**Stimulus**	**Example**
Chemoreceptors	Changes in chemical concentration of substances	Taste and smell
Mechanoreceptors	Changes in pressure or movement in fluids	Proprioceptors in joints, receptors for hearing and equilibrium
Nociceptors	Tissue damage	Pain receptors
Thermoreceptors	Changes in temperature	Heat and cold
Photoreceptors	Light energy	Vision

From Applegate E: *The anatomy and physiology learning system,* ed 4, St Louis, 2011, Saunders.

most numerous on the lips and are least numerous on some of the broad surfaces of the trunk. Thermoreceptors include at least two types of free nerve endings that are sensitive to temperature changes. In general, there are up to 10 times more *cold receptors* in a given area than *heat receptors.* Extremes in temperature stimulate pain receptors. A person determines gradations in temperatures by the degree of stimulation of each type of receptor. Extreme cold and extreme heat feel almost the same—both are painful— because the pain receptors are being stimulated. Thermoreceptors are strongly stimulated by abrupt changes in temperature and then fade after a few seconds or minutes. In other words, thermoreceptors show rapid **sensory adaptation.**

PAIN

The sense of pain is initiated by **nociceptors,** which are free nerve endings that are stimulated by tissue damage. They are widely distributed throughout the skin and in the tissues of the internal organs. The nervous tissue of the brain has no pain receptors; however, other tissues in the head, including the meninges and blood vessels, have an abundant supply. Pain receptors have a protective function because pain is usually perceived as unpleasant and is a signal to locate and remove the source of the tissue damage. Nociceptors usually do not adapt and may continue to send signals after the stimulus has been removed.

GUSTATORY SENSE

The **gustatory sense,** or *taste,* is one of the special senses. As previously explained, the senses of taste, smell, hearing, and sight are called *special senses* because their receptors are localized in a particular area.

The organs of taste, the *taste buds,* are localized in the mouth region, primarily on the surface of the tongue, where they lie along the walls of projections called *papillae* (Figure 10-1).

The receptors belong to the **chemoreceptor** category because they are sensitive to chemicals in the food we eat. For these chemicals to be detected by a chemoreceptor, they must be dissolved in water.

Within the taste bud, specialized epithelial cells called *gustatory cells* or *taste cells* are interspersed with supporting cells and nerve fibers (see Figure 10-1). The entire taste bud opens to the surface through a *taste pore.* Tiny *taste hairs* (microvilli) project from the taste cells through the taste pore, and it is these hairs on the taste cells that function as the receptors.

Although all the taste receptors appear to be alike, there are at least four different types, each one sensitive to a particular kind of stimulus. Consequently, there are four different taste sensations: salty, sweet, sour, and bitter.

When the microvilli, or taste hairs, are stimulated, an impulse is triggered on a nearby nerve fiber. Impulses from

---

HIGHLIGHT on the Senses

Odors: Nearly everyone is familiar with sensory adaptation in the sense of smell. A particular odor becomes unnoticed after a short time, even though the odor molecules are still present in the air, because the system quickly adapts to the continued stimulation. Odors have the quality of being interpreted as pleasant or unpleasant. Because of this, the sense of smell is as important as taste in the selection of food. For example, a person who has became sick after eating a certain type of food is often nauseated by the smell of that same food on a later occasion.

Cold adaptation: When a person first enters a cool swimming pool on a hot day, there is an abrupt change in temperature; therefore the cold receptors are strongly stimulated and there is a feeling of discomfort. After a brief time, the receptors adapt, the stimulation fades, and the cool water feels comfortable.

Headache: If there are no pain receptors in the nervous tissue of the brain, what are headaches? Headaches are a type of referred pain, pain that is referred to the surface of the head from deeper structures. The pain stimuli may originate in the meninges or blood vessels within the cranium. Other pain stimuli may originate outside the cranium from muscular spasms, the nasal sinuses, or the eyes.

Bitter taste: The taste receptors with the highest degree of sensitivity are those that are stimulated by bitter substances, and a highly intense bitter taste usually causes a person to reject that substance. This is probably an important protective mechanism because many of the deadly toxins found in poisonous plants have an intensely bitter taste.

Blinking: The eye blinks 6 to 30 times a minute. Blinking stimulates the lacrimal glands to secrete a sterile fluid, or "tears," and helps move the fluid across the eyes.

Corneal transplant: The cornea was one of the first organs transplanted. Surgical removal of deteriorating corneas and replacement with donor corneas is a common medical procedure for several reasons. The cornea is readily accessible and relatively easy to remove. The tissue is avascular, so there is no bleeding problem or difficulty in establishing circulatory pathways. Corneas are less active than other tissues immunologically and are less likely to be rejected. Long-term success after corneal implant surgery is excellent.

Pupil size: In addition to regulating the amount of light that enters the eye, pupillary reflexes may also reflect interest or emotional state. For example, frequently the pupils dilate during problem solving or when the subject is appealing. If the subject is boring or repulsive, the pupils constrict. ◼

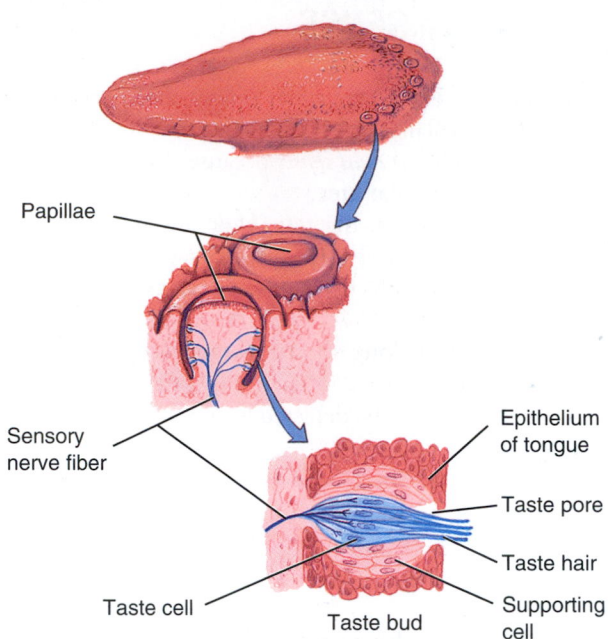

Figure 10-1 Taste buds on the papillae of the tongue. The taste hairs on taste (gustatory) cells are the receptors for taste. (From Applegate E: *The anatomy and physiology learning system,* ed 4, St Louis, 2011, Saunders.)

the anterior two thirds of the tongue travel along the *facial nerve,* and those from the posterior one third travel along the *glossopharyngeal nerve.* The impulses are interpreted in the sensory cortex on the parietal lobe of the cerebrum, near the lateral sulcus.

OLFACTORY SENSE

The receptors for **olfaction** (sense of smell) are neurons in the *olfactory epithelium* of the nasal cavity. The *olfactory neurons* are concentrated in the superior region of the cavity. These neurons have long cilia that extend to the surface and project into the nasal cavity. The cilia are believed to be the sensitive receptors of the neuron.

Like those for taste, the olfactory receptors are **chemoreceptors.** They are stimulated by chemicals dissolved in liquids. In this case, airborne molecules responsible for odors dissolve in the fluid on the surface of the olfactory epithelium and then bind to the receptors and trigger impulses. Axons from the olfactory neurons pass through foramina in the ethmoid bone and enter the olfactory bulb of the olfactory nerve (cranial nerve I). Here they synapse with association neurons that conduct the impulses to the olfactory cortex in the temporal lobe, where they are interpreted.

The senses of taste and smell are closely related and complement each other. They often have a combined effect when they are interpreted in the cerebral cortex. This implies that part of what we "taste" is really smell. Also, part of what we "smell" is taste because some airborne molecules move from the nose down to the mouth and stimulate taste buds.

VISUAL SENSE

Most of us consider vision to be one of the most important senses we have. The eyes, which contain the **photoreceptors,** are the organs of vision. They are protected by a bony socket and are assisted in their function of vision by accessory structures that protect and move them.

PROTECTIVE FEATURES AND ACCESSORY STRUCTURES OF THE EYE

Only a small portion of the eye is visible from the exterior. Most of it is surrounded by a protective bony orbit, or socket, that is formed by portions of seven cranial bones: frontal, lacrimal, ethmoid, maxilla, zygomatic, sphenoid, and palatine. It also contains fat, various connective tissues, blood vessels, and nerves.

Eyebrows help to keep perspiration, which can be an irritant, out of the eyes. Eyelids function to open and close the eye and to keep foreign objects from entering the eye. The muscles associated with the eyelids are the orbicularis oculi, which is a sphincter that closes the eye, and the levator palpebrae superioris, which elevates the eyelid to open the eye. The conjunctiva, a thin mucous membrane, lines the eyelid and then folds back to cover the anterior portion of the eyeball, except for the central portion, which is the cornea. Mucus from the conjunctiva helps keep the eye from drying out. Eyelashes line the margin of the eyelid and help trap foreign particles. Sebaceous glands associated with the eyelashes secrete an oily fluid that helps lubricate the region. Inflammation of the sebaceous glands is called a *stye.*

The **lacrimal apparatus,** shown in Figure 10-2, consists of the lacrimal gland and various ducts. The lacrimal gland is located in the superior and lateral region of the orbit. Tears produced by the lacrimal gland flow through lacrimal ducts and across the surface of the eye to the medial side, where they drain into two small lacrimal canals (canaliculi). From the lacrimal canals, the tears flow into the lacrimal sac, and then into the nasolacrimal duct, which opens into the nasal cavity. Tears moisten, lubricate, and cleanse the anterior surface of the eye. Tears also contain an enzyme (lysozyme) that helps destroy bacteria and prevent infections.

STRUCTURE OF THE EYEBALL

The eyeball, or **bulbus oculi,** is somewhat spherical, is 2 to 3 cm in diameter, and has an anterior bulge. It is surrounded by orbital fat within the orbital cavity. Figure 10-3 illustrates the structure of the bulbus oculi.

The wall of the eyeball is made up of three concentric layers or coats called *tunics.* The outermost layer is the *fibrous tunic.* It consists of the white, opaque *sclera* and the transparent *cornea.* The sclera, the white part of the eye, covers the posterior five sixths of the eyeball, and the muscles that move the eye are attached to it. The transparent cornea, which covers the anterior one sixth of the eyeball, is the "window" of the eye. It helps focus light rays entering the eye.

The middle layer of the eyeball is the *vascular tunic.* It consists of the *choroid, ciliary body,* and *iris.* The *choroid* is a highly vascular, brown-pigmented layer located between the sclera and the retina in the posterior portion of the eye. It is the largest part of the middle tunic and lines most of the sclera, although it is only loosely connected to the

fibrous coat and can be stripped away easily. The choroid is, however, firmly attached to the retina. The brown pigment in the choroid absorbs excess light rays that might interfere with vision. The blood vessels nourish the interior of the eye. Anteriorly, the choroid is continuous with the *ciliary body.* Numerous finger-like ciliary processes within the ciliary body secrete aqueous humor, a fluid in the anterior portion of the eye. The ciliary body also contains the ciliary muscle. Suspensory ligaments connect the ciliary body to the transparent, biconvex lens of the eye. When the ciliary muscle contracts, the suspensory ligaments relax and the lens bulges to allow focusing for close vision. The iris is the conspicuous, colored portion of the eye. It is a doughnut-shaped diaphragm with a central aperture, called the *pupil.* The iris contains two groups of smooth muscles, a radial group and a circular group. When the radial muscles contract, the pupil dilates; when the circular group contracts, the pupil gets smaller. These muscles of the iris continually contract and relax to change the size of the pupil, which regulates the amount of light entering the eye.

The innermost coat of the eyeball is the *nervous tunic,* or retina, which is found only in the posterior portion of the eye. It ends at the posterior margin of the ciliary body. The retina contains several layers. The outer layer is deeply pigmented and firmly attached to the choroid. The layer next to the pigmented layer contains the *rods and cones,* which are the photoreceptor cells. Other layers consist of bipolar neurons and ganglion cells. The axons of the ganglion cells converge to form the optic nerve, which penetrates the tunics at the optic disk and passes through the apex of the orbital cavity to reach the brain. Because there are no photoreceptor cells in the optic disk it is commonly

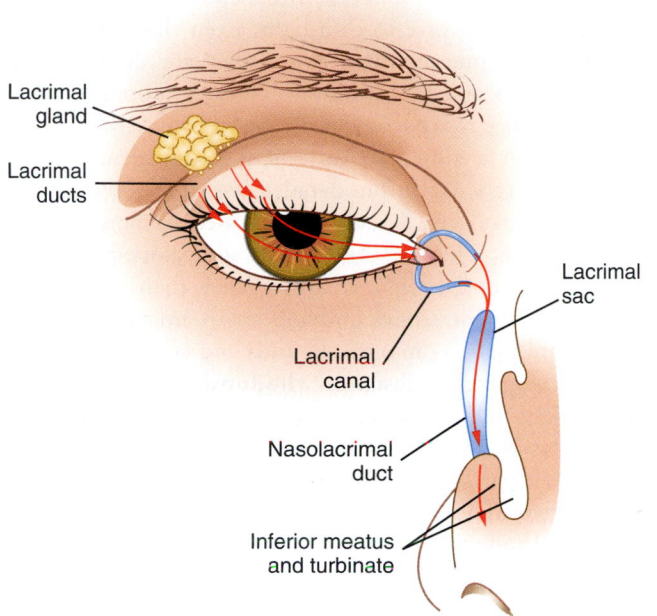

Lacrimal gland
Lacrimal ducts
Lacrimal sac
Lacrimal canal
Nasolacrimal duct
Inferior meatus and turbinate

Figure 10-2 Lacrimal apparatus of the eye. (From Applegate E: *The anatomy and physiology learning system,* ed 4, St Louis, 2011, Saunders.)

Ciliary body
Suspensory ligament
Cornea
Lens
Pupil
Anterior cavity filled with aqueous humor
Iris
Posterior cavity with vitreous humor
Conjunctiva
Sclera
Choroid
Retina
Optic disk
Optic nerve
Fovea centralis

Figure 10-3 Anatomy of bulbus oculi or eyeball. (From Applegate E: *The anatomy and physiology learning system,* ed 4, St Louis, 2011, Saunders.)

referred to as the "blind spot" of the eye. Just lateral to the optic disk near the center of the retina, there is a yellow spot called the **macula lutea**. The region of the retina that produces the sharpest image is a depression, the *fovea centralis*, in the center of the macula lutea.

The lens, suspensory ligaments, and ciliary body form a partition that divides the interior of the eyeball into two cavities. The space anterior to the lens, between the cornea and the lens, is the anterior cavity and is filled with *aqueous humor* secreted by the ciliary body. Aqueous humor helps maintain the shape of the anterior part of the eye and nourishes the structures in that region. It is largely responsible for the internal pressure of the eye. The aqueous humor circulates through the anterior cavity and then is reabsorbed into blood vessels at the junction of the sclera and cornea. The posterior cavity, between the lens and the retina, is filled with a colorless, transparent, gel-like *vitreous humor*. The vitreous humor presses the retina firmly against the wall of the eye, supports the internal parts of the eye, and helps maintain the eye's shape.

PATHWAY OF LIGHT AND REFRACTION

Vision depends on light rays. When a person sees an object, light rays from the object enter the eye. Light rays have two important properties—they travel in a straight line, and they can be bent. When light rays travel from one substance to another that has a different optical density, the rays bend. The bending of light rays is called **refraction.** When light rays hit a concave surface, they scatter or diverge. When the rays meet a convex surface, they get closer together or converge. The eyes have four refractive surfaces and media. In a normal eye, the cornea, aqueous humor, lens, and vitreous humor bend the light rays so that they focus on the retina. The image that forms on the retina is upside down and backward (Figure 10-4), but the brain turns it around and interprets the image in the correct position.

When an object is at least 20 feet away, the normal relaxed eye is able to focus the image on the retina. When the object is closer than 20 feet, the eye must make adjustments to focus the image. The primary adjustment for close vision is changing the shape of the lens. For distance vision, the ciliary muscle is relaxed, the suspensory ligaments are taut, and the lens is flat. When the eyes adapt for close vision, illustrated in Figure 10-5, the ciliary muscle

contracts, the suspensory ligaments become loose or relaxed, and the lens bulges or becomes more convex. The closer the object, the more the light rays have to bend to focus and the greater the curvature of the lens. These adjustments are called **accommodation.**

PHOTORECEPTORS

The retina contains two kinds of photoreceptor cells: rods and cones. *Rods* are thin cells with slender, rodlike projections and are sensitive to dim light. Even though rods are much more numerous than cones, they are absent in the fovea centralis and their number increases proportionately to the distance away from the fovea centralis. Many rods synapse with a single sensory fiber (convergence); thus vision with rods lacks fine detail. *Cones,* the receptors for color vision and visual acuity, are located primarily in the fovea centralis. They are thicker cells with short, blunt projections. Cones exhibit less convergence than rods, so in addition to color, cones provide sharp images and fine detail. Table 10-2 compares the rods and cones.

Rods contain a substance, **rhodopsin** (visual purple), that is very light sensitive. When even small amounts of light focus on the rods, rhodopsin breaks down into its component parts—opsin (a protein) and retinal (retinene), a derivative of vitamin A. This reaction triggers a nerve impulse. Rhodopsin is resynthesized from opsin and retinal to prepare the rods for receiving subsequent stimuli. The more rhodopsin there is in the rods, the greater the sensitivity to light. In bright light, nearly all the rhodopsin in the rods is decomposed. After entering a dimly lit area, it takes some time for the eyes to adapt to the dim light. During this period, rhodopsin is regenerated in the rods so that they become more sensitive.

Cones function similarly to rods. Light-sensitive pigments break down into component parts, and the reaction triggers nerve impulses. Three different types of cones exist, each with a different visual pigment. All the pigments contain retinal, but the protein portion is different. One type responds best to green light, another responds best to blue light, and a third type responds best to red light. The perceived color of an object depends on the quantity and combination of cones that are stimulated. If all the pigments are stimulated, the person senses white. If none are stimulated, the person senses black.

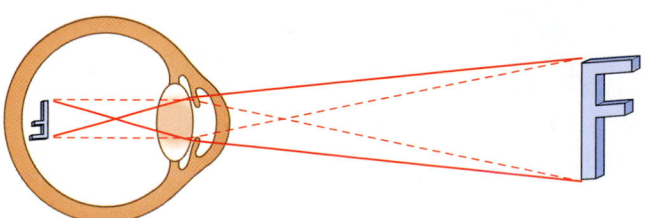

Figure 10-4 Formation of images on the retina. The image on the retina is upside down and backward. (From Applegate E: *The anatomy and physiology learning system,* ed 4, St Louis, 2011, Saunders.)

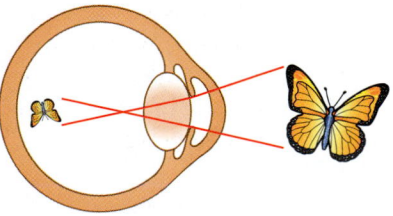

Figure 10-5 Accommodation for close vision. The ciliary muscles contract, the suspensory ligaments relax, and the lens becomes more convex. (From Applegate E: *The anatomy and physiology learning system,* ed 4, St Louis, 2011, Saunders.)

Table 10-2 Comparison of Rods and Cones

Feature	Rods	Cones
Shape	Long, slender projections	Short, thick projections
Location	None in fovea centralis; increase in density away from fovea centralis	Concentrated in fovea centralis; decrease in density away from fovea centralis
Quantity	More numerous than cones	Less numerous than rods
Convergence	High degree of convergence	Less convergence
Pigments	Single pigment, rhodopsin	Three pigments, one each for red, green, blue
Functions	Black and white vision; dim light; night vision; vision lacks detail	Color vision; bright light; precise vision with fine detail

From Applegate E: *The anatomy and physiology learning system,* ed 4, St Louis, 2011, Saunders.

VISUAL PATHWAY

Visual impulses generated in the rods and cones of the retina leave the eyes in the axons that form the optic nerves. Just anterior to the pituitary gland, these nerves form an X-shaped structure, the *optic chiasma.* Within the optic chiasma, the axons from the medial portion of each retina cross over to enter the *optic tract* on the opposite side (Figure 10-6). The right optic tract contains the fibers from the lateral portion of the right eye and the medial portion of the left eye. The left optic tract contains the fibers from the lateral portion of the left eye and the medial portion of the right eye. The optic tracts lead to the *thalamus,* where they synapse with neurons that carry the impulses in the *optic radiations* to the visual cortex of the occipital lobes. Because some of the fibers cross over to the other side in the optic chiasma, each occipital lobe receives an image of the entire object from each eye but from slightly different perspectives. This enables vision in three dimensions.

AUDITORY SENSE

The ear is the organ of hearing (auditory or acoustic organ). It is also the organ for the sense of equilibrium, which is covered later in this chapter. The receptors for hearing, located within the ear, are mechanoreceptors. Physical forces, in the form of sound vibrations, are responsible for initiating impulses that are interpreted as sound.

STRUCTURE OF THE EAR

The "ears" on the sides of the head are only a portion of the actual organ of hearing. A large part of the organ, actually the most important part, lies hidden from view and protected

Figure 10-6 Visual pathway. The optic nerves converge at the optic chiasma, where some axons cross to the opposite side. Impulses then travel to the thalamus, then to the visual cortex of the occipital lobe, where they are interpreted. (From Applegate E: *The anatomy and physiology learning system,* ed 4, St Louis, 2011, Saunders.)

in the temporal bone. Anatomically, the organ of hearing is divided into the external ear, middle ear, and inner ear. The anatomy of the ear is illustrated in Figure 10-7.

External Ear

The *external ear* consists of an auricle, or pinna, and the external auditory canal. The auricle, or pinna, is the fleshy part of the external ear that is visible on the side of the head and surrounds the opening into the external auditory meatus. The auricle collects sound waves and directs them toward the auditory canal.

The *external auditory canal* is an S-shaped tube, about 2.5 cm long, that extends from the auricle to the *tympanic membrane.* The skin that lines the external auditory canal has numerous hairs and *ceruminous glands,* which secrete a waxy substance called cerumen. The hairs and cerumen help prevent foreign objects from reaching the eardrum. The external ear ends at the tympanic membrane.

Middle Ear

The *middle ear* is an air-filled cavity, called the *tympanic cavity,* in the temporal bone. It begins at the tympanic

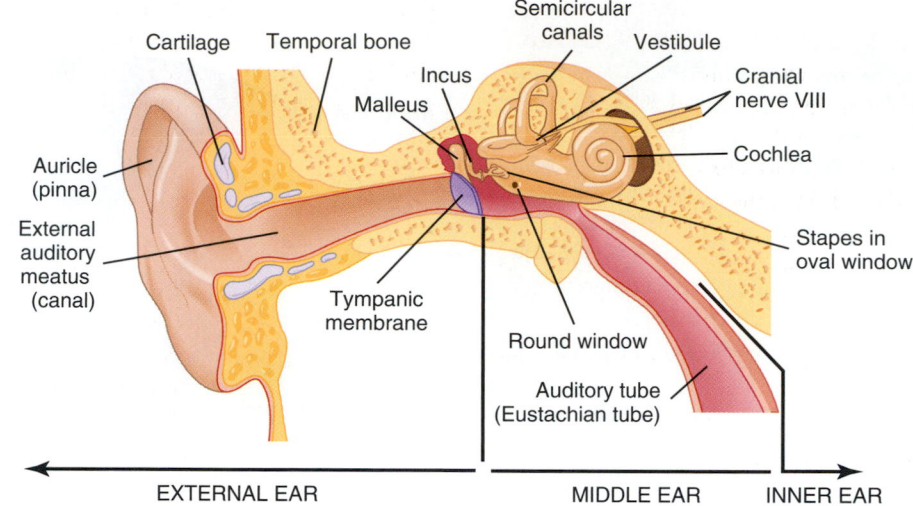

Figure 10-7 Anatomy of the ear. (From Applegate E: *The anatomy and physiology learning system,* ed 4, St Louis, 2011, Saunders.)

membrane, contains the auditory ossicles, and has an opening into the eustachian tube. The *oval window* and the *round window* in the medial wall of the middle ear connect the middle ear with the inner ear. The oval window is closed by the stapes, one of the bones in the middle ear. The round window is closed by a membrane.

The *tympanic membrane,* or eardrum, is a thin membrane that separates the external ear from the middle ear. Sound waves cause the tympanic membrane to vibrate.

An *auditory tube* (eustachian tube) connects each middle ear with the throat. Its purpose is to equalize the pressure between the outside air and the middle ear cavity, a condition necessary for normal hearing. Throat infections may spread to the middle ear through the auditory tube.

The *auditory ossicles* are three tiny bones: the malleus (hammer), incus (anvil), and stapes (stirrup). These bones are linked together by tiny ligaments and form a bridge across the space of the tympanic cavity. The malleus is attached to the tympanic membrane, and the stapes is attached to the oval window between the middle ear and the inner ear. The incus is between the malleus and stapes. When the tympanic membrane vibrates, the ossicles transmit the vibrations across the cavity to the oval window, which transfers the motion to the fluids in the inner ear. This fluid motion excites the receptors for hearing.

Inner Ear

The *inner ear* consists of a series of interconnecting chambers in the temporal bone. It is divided into the vestibule, semicircular canals, and cochlea. The vestibule and semicircular canals function in the sense of equilibrium. The cochlea functions in the sense of hearing.

The **cochlea** is the coiled portion of the inner ear. It encloses the *organ of Corti,* which contains the receptors for sound. The organ of Corti consists of supporting cells and hair cells (Figure 10-8). The hair cells are specialized sensory

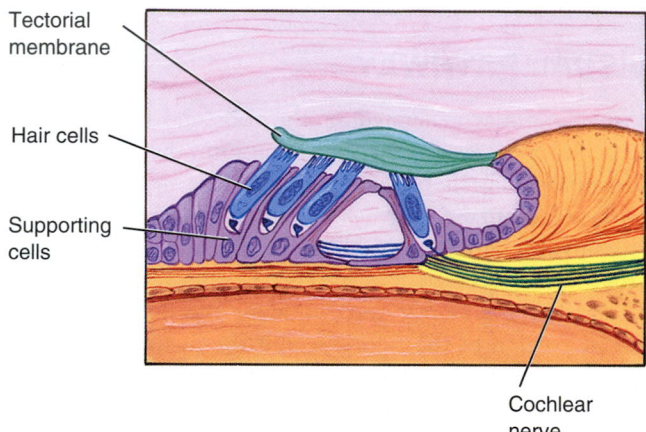

Figure 10-8 Organ of Corti enlarged to show the hair cells and tectorial membrane. (From Applegate E: *The anatomy and physiology learning system,* ed 4, St Louis, 2011, Saunders.)

cells that have hairlike projections (microvilli) extending from their free surface. The tips of the projections contact a gelatinous *tectorial membrane* that extends over them. Hair cells have no axons, but they are surrounded by sensory nerve fibers that form the *cochlear branch* of the *vestibulocochlear nerve* (cranial nerve VIII).

PHYSIOLOGY OF HEARING

Sound travels through the atmosphere in waves of alternating compressions and decompressions of molecules. Low-pitched tones create low-frequency sound waves; high-pitched tones create high-frequency sound waves. An individual with normal hearing should be able to hear the frequencies of normal speech, which range from 300 to 4000 vibrations per second. Hearing is most acute with frequencies between 2000 and 3000 vibrations per second.

Initiation of Impulses

The process of hearing begins when sound waves enter the external auditory canal. As the waves travel through the external ear, they hit the tympanic membrane and cause it to vibrate. Because the malleus is attached to the membrane, the vibrations are transferred from the tympanic membrane to the malleus, then to the incus, and then to the stapes, which creates vibrations in the membrane of the oval window. Movement of the oval window passes the vibrations to the inner ear.

The vibrations cause the organ of Corti to move and the hairs on the hair cells rub against the tectorial membrane. As the hairs contact the membrane, they bend, and this mechanical deformation initiates the nerve impulses that result in hearing. The following list summarizes the sequence of events in the initiation of auditory impulses:

1. The tympanic membrane vibrates in response to sound waves.
2. The malleus, incus, and stapes transfer vibrations to the oval window membrane.
3. Movement from the oval window starts oscillations within the cochlea.
4. As the cochlea moves, the hairs on the hair cells in the organ of Corti rub against the tectorial membrane and bend.
5. Bending of the hairs on the hair cells stimulates the formation of impulses.
6. Impulses are transmitted to the auditory cortex of the temporal lobe by the cochlear branch of cranial nerve VIII, the vestibulocochlear nerve.

Pitch and Loudness

Hair cells in the organ of Corti have varying sensitivities to different frequencies. Pitch is detected by the portion of the organ of Corti that vibrates in response to the sound and the sensitivity of the hair cells.

Loudness is determined by the intensity of the sound waves. Loud sounds create a greater magnitude of oscillation than low-level sounds. This means that more hair cells are stimulated and more impulses travel to the auditory cortex.

SENSE OF EQUILIBRIUM

The sense of equilibrium is a combination of two different senses: the sense of *static equilibrium* and the sense of *dynamic equilibrium.* Static equilibrium is involved in evaluating the position of the head relative to gravity. It occurs when the head is motionless or moving in a straight line. Dynamic equilibrium occurs when the head is moving in a rotational or angular direction.

STATIC EQUILIBRIUM

The organs of static equilibrium are located in the *vestibule* portion of the inner ear. The vestibule is divided into two portions, the *utricle* and the *saccule.* Each of these contains a small structure called a *macula,* which is the organ of static equilibrium. The macula consists of sensory hair cells, similar to those in the organ of Corti, and supporting cells. The projections, or hairs, of the hair cells are embedded in a gelatinous mass that covers the macula. Grains of calcium carbonate, called **otoliths,** are embedded on the surface of the gelatinous mass.

When the head is in an upright position, the hairs are straight. When the head tilts or bends forward, the otoliths and the gelatinous mass move in response to gravity. As the gelatinous mass moves, it bends some of the hairs on the receptor cells. This action initiates an impulse that travels to the CNS by way of the vestibular branch of the vestibulocochlear nerve. The CNS interprets the information and sends motor impulses out to appropriate muscles to maintain balance.

DYNAMIC EQUILIBRIUM

The sense organs for dynamic equilibrium, the equilibrium of rotational or angular movements, are located in the *semicircular canals.* Three semicircular canals, positioned at right angles to one another, exist in three different planes (see Figure 10-7). At the base of each canal, near where it attaches to the utricle, there is a swelling called the *ampulla.* The sensory organs of the semicircular canals are located within the ampullae. Each of these organs, called a **crista ampullaris,** contains sensory hair cells and supporting cells. The crista ampullaris is covered by a dome-shaped gelatinous mass called the *cupula.* The hairs of the hair cells are embedded in the cupula.

When the head turns rapidly, the semicircular canals move with the head but the cupula tilts to one side. As the cupula tilts, it bends some of the hairs on the hair cells, which triggers a sensory impulse. Because the three canals are in different planes, their cristae are stimulated differently by the same motion. This creates a mosaic of impulses that are transmitted to the CNS on the vestibular branch of the vestibulocochlear nerve. The CNS interprets the information and initiates appropriate responses to maintain balance. The cerebellum is particularly important in mediating the sense of balance and equilibrium.

AGING OF THE SENSES

As the body ages, a general decline in all of the special senses occurs. The most significant changes in the eye occur in the lens. It tends to become thicker and less elastic, which makes it less able to change shape to accommodate for near vision. This condition, called *presbyopia* or farsightedness of aging, probably is the most common age-related dysfunction of the eye. The lens also tends to become cloudy or opaque, forming cataracts. About 90% of people older than age 70 have some degree of cataract formation; however, it is not always significant enough to affect vision. The cornea tends to become more translucent and less spherical, which contributes to an increase in astigmatism in older people. Older people require more light to see well because atrophy of the muscles in the iris reduces the ability of the pupil to dilate and decreases the amount of light that reaches the retina. The chemical processes that rebuild the visual pigment, rhodopsin, are slower in older people, so dark adaptation takes longer and is not as complete as in young people. These changes in the eye may make it more difficult for older people to read and fill out forms correctly, especially if the forms are printed in small type and the individual is reading in dim light.

Most age-related changes in the external ear and middle ear have little effect on hearing. A buildup of cerumen, or earwax, in the external ear may contribute to hearing loss in the low-frequency range. The joints between the auditory ossicles in the middle ear may become less movable, which interferes with the transmission of sound waves to the inner ear, but in general it is not clinically significant. Most of the gradual loss of hearing that usually begins by the age of 40 is a result of degeneration of the receptor cells in the spiral organ of Corti in the inner ear. Another factor is the decrease in the number of nerve fibers in the vestibulocochlear nerve. The reduction in fibers in the cochlear branch contributes to hearing loss. A decrease in vestibular fibers affects balance and equilibrium. Age-related changes in the ear may make it more difficult for individuals to hear verbal instructions and other communication correctly, especially if there is background noise.

Taste and smell, both chemical senses, show a decline with age; however, the mechanism is unclear. Diminished perception may be caused by degeneration of the receptor cells, by changes in the way the impulses are processed in the brain, or by other factors. It is likely that decreases in sensory perception result from a combination of several factors. Whatever the cause, deterioration in the sense of taste may make food unappetizing. Loss in the sense of smell may lead to an inability to detect harmful odors such as smoke and gas.

Common Pathology of the Senses

Disease	Signs and Symptoms	Etiology	Diagnosis and Treatment
Nyctalopia	Difficulty seeing in low light; commonly known as *night blindness*.	Night blindness may exist from birth or may develop later because of injury or malnutrition. The most common cause is retinitis pigmentosa, a disorder in which the rod cells in the retina gradually lose their ability to respond to the light.	Treatment depends on the cause of the nyctalopia and may be a simple as increasing vitamin A in the diet. If the cause is cataracts, cataract surgery is indicated. There is no cure for retinitis pigmentosa.
Presbycusis	Progressive difficulty hearing sounds as a person ages. Over time, the detection of high-pitched sounds becomes more difficult, and speech perception is affected.	There are four pathologic types of presbycusis: sensory, characterized by degeneration of organ of Corti; neural, characterized by degeneration of cells of spiral ganglion; strial or metabolic, characterized by atrophy of stria vascularis in the cochlea; and cochlear conductive, caused by stiffening of the basilar membrane.	Diagnosis is based on medical history and a physical examination of the ear canal and eardrum along with audiometry tests. Devices such as hearing aids and cochlear implants may help improve the hearing of some elderly patients.
Presbyopia	Progressive difficulty in focusing on close objects as a person ages.	Thought to be caused by a loss of elasticity in the lens and/or weakness in the ciliary muscles of the eye.	Corrective lenses provide vision correction, often with varifocal or bifocal lenses to eliminate the need for a separate pair of reading glasses.
Myopia	Distant objects appear very blurry and out of focus, but close objects may be in focus; commonly called *nearsightedness*.	Myopia is a condition of the eye in which the light rays do not directly focus on the retina but tend to focus in front of it. Caused by too much curvature in the cornea and/or lens.	Diagnosis is determined with an eye examination performed by an eye specialist. The condition is normally treated through the use of corrective lenses, such as glasses or contact lenses. It may also be corrected by refractive surgery.
Hyperopia	Distant objects may be in focus, but close objects are blurry and out of focus; commonly called *farsightedness*.	Hyperopia is a condition of the eye in which the light that comes in does not directly focus on the retina but tends to focus behind it. Caused by too little curvature in the cornea and/or lens for accommodation.	Diagnosis is determined with an eye examination performed by an eye specialist. The condition is normally treated through the use of corrective lenses, such as glasses or contact lenses. It may also be corrected by refractive surgery.

Common Pathology of the Senses—cont'd

Disease	Signs and Symptoms	Etiology	Diagnosis and Treatment
Conjunctivitis	Red eye, swelling of the conjunctiva, and watering of the eyes are symptoms common to all forms of conjunctivitis; commonly called *pink eye*.	Conjunctivitis, when caused by an infection, is most commonly caused by a viral infection. Bacterial infections, allergies, other irritants and dryness are also common causes. Both bacterial and viral infections are contagious and passed from person to person, but can also spread through contaminated objects or water.	Differential diagnosis is necessary to determine the underlying cause of the conjunctivitis. Conjunctivitis often resolves without treatment. Antibiotics may be prescribed. Conjunctivitis caused by chemicals is treated by irrigation with Ringer's lactate or saline solution.
Strabismus	Fuzzy or unclear vision and headaches from eyestrain.	Strabismus is a disorder in which the two eyes do not work together. It may be classified based on the time of onset: congenital, acquired, or secondary to another pathologic process. It may be unilateral if one eye consistently deviates, or alternating if either of the eyes can be seen to deviate. To avoid double vision, the brain may adapt by ignoring one eye.	Tests are performed to determine how much the eyes are out of alignment. Strabismus is usually treated with a combination of eyeglasses, vision therapy, and surgery, depending on the underlying reason for the misalignment.
Sensorineural deafness	Inability to hear normal sounds or to comprehend what is being said.	Sensorineural deafness is a type of hearing loss in which the root cause lies in the vestibulocochlear nerve, the inner ear, or central processing centers of the brain. It can be mild, moderate, or severe, including total deafness. The great majority of cases are caused by abnormalities in the hair cells of the organ of Corti in the cochlea.	A differential diagnosis is required to determine if the condition is acquired or congenital. Sensorineural hearing loss can be treated with hearing aids or cochlear implants, which stimulate cochlear nerves directly.
Tinnitus	A ringing or buzzing sound in the ears when no sound is present.	Tinnitus is not a disease, but a condition that can result from a wide range of underlying causes. The most common cause is noise-induced hearing loss. Other causes include neurologic damage, physical and emotional stress, foreign objects in the ear, nasal allergies that prevent fluid drainage, and wax buildup.	Specialized tests are performed to diagnose tinnitus. Some of these tests measure the specific features of the tinnitus itself. These tests may include x-ray examination, audiograms, tinnitus pitch or loudness match, and residual inhibition. At present there are no medications that are effective for tinnitus.
Vertigo	A feeling of dizziness, loss of balance, and lightheadedness.	Vertigo is caused by problems with the inner ear or vestibular system. Any cause of inflammation such as common cold, influenza, and bacterial infections may cause transient vertigo if it involves the inner ear.	Vertigo is classified as either peripheral or central depending on the location of the dysfunction of the vestibular pathway. It can also be caused by psychological factors. Definitive treatment depends on the underlying cause of vertigo; there are many treatment modalities.
Macular degeneration	Loss of central vision and eventual blindness.	The exact cause of macular degeneration is unknown, but smoking, obesity, unhealthy diet, cardiovascular disease, and elevated cholesterol appear to be risk factors. It usually affects older adults and causes a loss of vision in the center of the visual field because of damage to the macula. Macular degeneration by itself will not lead to total blindness. There are two types, wet and dry. Dry is more common.	It is important to have periodic eye examinations in which an ophthalmologist examines the retina. A special type of angiogram may be used to observe the blood vessels in back of the eye to see if they are leaking fluid. At present there is no cure for macular degeneration. Medications may be prescribed to manage the condition, and vision assist devices are available to help an individual with visual tasks.
Glaucoma	A gradual and progressive visual field loss ending in blindness.	Glaucoma is one of the leading causes of blindness in the United States. It is a group of eye conditions that are characterized by increased intraocular pressure resulting in a loss of peripheral vision.	Diagnosis is based on an increase in intraocular pressure, tests for optic nerve damage, and visual field tests to detect peripheral vision loss. The focus of treatment is to lower the intraocular pressure, typically with eye drops.

Continued

Common Pathology of the Senses—cont'd

Disease	Signs and Symptoms	Etiology	Diagnosis and Treatment
Detached retina	The disorder is accompanied by peripheral flashes of light, an increase in the number of floaters, and a feeling of heaviness in the eye followed by a dense shadow that slowly progresses toward the central vision. Straight lines suddenly appear curved.	The sensory portion of the retina breaks away the underlying pigmented layer and the cells lose their oxygen supply. Detachment occurs when fluid accumulates beneath the retina, usually through small holes and tears.	Diagnosis is based on a visual examination of the retina with an ophthalmoscope and ultrasonography to create an image of the retina. Surgery is used to repair the holes and tears in the retina and to reattach it. The appearance of sudden flashes of light or a shower of floaters is a medical emergency.
Meniere disease	Spontaneous episodes of dizziness, ringing in the ear, fluctuating hearing loss, and a feeling of pressure in the ear.	Meniere disease is a chronic disorder of the inner ear caused by an abnormal volume or composition of the endolymph in the inner ear.	Diagnosis is based on physical examination and medical history, hearing assessment, and tests for balance. There is no known cure. The symptoms may be managed with motion sickness medications, diuretics, and hearing aids.
Otitis media	Patient experiences ear pain, often accompanied by fever and an upper respiratory tract infection.	*Otitis media* is the medical term for a middle ear infection. The common cause is blockage of the Eustachian tube. Because of the Eustachian tube blockage, the air volume in the middle ear is trapped and parts of it are slowly absorbed by the surrounding tissues, leading to a mild vacuum in the middle ear.	As its typical symptoms overlap with other conditions, clinical history alone is not sufficient to predict whether acute otitis media is present; it has to be complemented by visualization of the tympanic membrane. Oral and topical painkillers are effective to treat the pain caused by otitis media.

↻ TERMINOLOGY REVIEW

Key Term	Word Parts	Definition
Accommodation		Mechanism that allows the eye to focus at various distances, primarily achieved by changing the curvature of the lens.
Bulbus oculi	*ocul/o:* eye	The eyeball.
Chemoreceptor	*chem/o:* chemical	A sensory receptor that detects the presence of chemicals; responsible for taste, smell, and monitoring of the concentration of certain chemicals in body fluids.
Cochlea	*coch-:* snail	Spiral or snail-shaped portion of the inner ear.
Crista ampullaris		Receptor organ located within the ampulla of the semicircular canals; functions in dynamic equilibrium.
General senses		Senses that are located throughout the body; somatic senses.
Gustatory sense	*gust-:* taste	Sense of taste.
Lacrimal apparatus	*lacr-:* tears	The structures that produce and convey tears.
Macula lutea	*macul-:* spot, depression *lute-:* yellow	Yellowish depression on the retina.
Mechanoreceptors	*mechan/o:* mechanical	Sensory receptors that respond to a bending or deformation of the cell; examples include receptors for touch, pressure, hearing, and equilibrium.
Nociceptors	*noci:* causing harm or damage *-ceptor:* receptor	Sensory receptors that respond to tissue damage; pain receptors.
Olfaction	*olfact/o:* smell	Sense of smell.
Otoliths	*ot/o:* ear *lith:* stone	Little stones of calcium carbonate in the macula of the inner ear.
Photoreceptors	*phot/o:* light	Sensory receptors that detect light; located in the retina of the eye.
Proprioception	*propri/o:* one's own *-ceptor:* receptor	The sense of body position and movements; responds to stimuli originating within an organism or muscle.

TERMINOLOGY REVIEW—cont'd

Key Term	Word Parts	Definition
Refraction		The bending of light as it passes from one medium to another.
Rhodopsin	*rhod/o:* red	Photosensitive pigment in the rods; also called *visual purple.*
Sensory adaptation		Phenomenon in which some receptors respond when a stimulus is first applied but decrease their response if the stimulus is maintained; receptor sensitivity decreases with prolonged stimulation.
Special senses		Senses with receptors localized in a particular area; taste, smell, vision, hearing, and equilibrium
Thermoreceptors	*therm/o:* heat	Sensory receptors that detect changes in temperature.

ON THE WEB

For information on the senses:

Ear, Nose, and Throat: www.entusa.com

National Eye Institute: www.nei.nih.gov

National Institute on Deafness: www.nidcd.nih.gov

The Inner Ear: oto.wustl.edu/cochlea

The Joy of Visual Perception: A Web Book: www.yorku.ca/eye

Vestibular Disorders Association: www.vestibular.org

11 Endocrine System

ⓔ Check out the Evolve site at http://evolve.elsevier.com/Bonewit/today/ to access additional interactive activities and exercises to help you study and prepare for success.

LEARNING OBJECTIVES

1. Compare the actions of the nervous system and the endocrine system.
2. Compare the major chemical classes of hormones.
3. Discuss the general mechanisms of hormone action.
4. Identify the major endocrine glands—pituitary gland, thyroid gland, parathyroid glands, adrenal glands, pancreas, gonads, pineal gland, thymus—and discuss their hormones and function.
5. Describe ways in which the aging of an individual affects the endocrine system.
6. Identify pathology related to the endocrine system.

CHAPTER OUTLINE

INTRODUCTION TO THE ENDOCRINE SYSTEM
COMPARISON OF THE ENDOCRINE AND NERVOUS SYSTEMS
COMPARISON OF EXOCRINE AND ENDOCRINE GLANDS
CHARACTERISTICS OF HORMONES
Chemical Nature of Hormones
Mechanism of Hormone Action
ENDOCRINE GLANDS AND THEIR HORMONES
Pituitary Gland
Hormones of the Anterior Lobe (Adenohypophysis)
Hormones of the Posterior Lobe (Neurohypophysis)
Thyroid Gland
Thyroxine and Triiodothyronine

Calcitonin
Parathyroid Glands
Adrenal (Suprarenal) Glands
Hormones of the Adrenal Cortex
Hormones of the Adrenal Medulla
Pancreas—Islets of Langerhans
Gonads (Testes and Ovaries)
Testes
Ovaries
Pineal Gland
Thymus Gland
AGING OF THE ENDOCRINE SYSTEM

KEY TERMS

adenohypophysis (add-eh-noe-hye-PAH-fih-sis)
androgens (AN-droh-jenz)
circadian rhythms (sir-KAY-dee-an RIH-thimz)
endocrine gland (EN-doh-krin GLAND)
endocrinology (en-doh-krih-NOLL-oh-jee)

estrogens (ESS-troh-jenz)
exocrine gland (EKS-oh-krin GLAND)
glucocorticoids (gloo-koh-KOR-tih-koyds)
gonadocorticoids (go-nad-oh-KOR-tih-koyds)
hormones (HOAR-mohnz)

mineralocorticoids (min-er-al-oh-KOR-tih-koyds)
neurohypophysis (noo-roh-hye-PAH-fih-sis)
pinealocytes (PIE-nee-al-oh-cytes)
progesterone (proh-JESS-ter-ohn)
target tissue (TAR-get TISH-yoo)

INTRODUCTION TO THE ENDOCRINE SYSTEM

The endocrine system is composed of the endocrine glands, which secrete hormones into the blood. Unlike the organs in other systems, endocrine glands are scattered throughout the body. In addition, they are small and unimpressive; however, as you study this chapter, you will discover that they are extremely important. The study of endocrine glands and hormones is called **endocrinology**.

COMPARISON OF THE ENDOCRINE AND NERVOUS SYSTEMS

The endocrine system, along with the nervous system, functions in the regulation of body activities. The nervous system acts through electrical impulses and neurotransmitters to cause muscle contraction and glandular secretion. The effect is of short duration, measured in seconds, and localized. The endocrine system acts through chemical messengers called **hormones** that influence growth, development, and metabolic activities. The action of the endocrine system is measured in minutes, hours, or weeks and is more generalized than the action of the nervous system.

COMPARISON OF EXOCRINE AND ENDOCRINE GLANDS

The two major categories of glands in the body are exocrine and endocrine. **Exocrine glands** have ducts that carry their secretory product to a surface. These have a variety of functions and include the sweat, sebaceous, and mammary glands and the glands that secrete digestive enzymes. The **endocrine glands** do not have ducts to carry their product to a surface. They are called *ductless glands*. The word *endocrine* is derived from the Greek terms *endo*, meaning "within," and *krine*, meaning "to separate or secrete." The secretory products of endocrine glands are called **hormones** and are secreted directly into the blood and then carried throughout the body where they influence only those cells that have receptor sites for that hormone. Other cells are not affected. Endocrine glands have an extensive network of blood vessels, and organs with the richest blood supply include some of the endocrine glands, such as the thyroid and adrenal glands.

CHARACTERISTICS OF HORMONES

Each hormone produced in the body is unique. Each one is different in its chemical composition, structure, and action. In spite of the differences, there are similarities in these molecules.

CHEMICAL NATURE OF HORMONES

Chemically, hormones may be classified as either *proteins* or *steroids*. All of the hormones in the human body, except the sex hormones and those from the adrenal cortex, are proteins or protein derivatives. This means that their fundamental building blocks are amino acids. Protein hormones are difficult to administer orally because they are quickly inactivated by the acid and pepsin in the stomach. These hormones are usually administered by injection. Sex hormones and those from the adrenal cortex are steroids, which are lipid derivatives. These lipid-soluble hormones may be taken orally.

MECHANISM OF HORMONE ACTION

Hormones are potent substances. This means that small amounts of a hormone may have profound effects on metabolic processes. Hormones are carried by the blood throughout the entire body, yet they affect only certain cells. The specific cells that respond to a given hormone have receptor sites for that hormone. This is sort of a lock-and-key mechanism. If the key fits the lock, the door will open. If a hormone fits the receptor site, there will be an effect (Figure 11-1). If a hormone and a receptor site do not match, then there is no reaction. All the cells that have receptor sites for a given hormone make up the **target tissue** for that hormone. In some cases the target tissue is localized in a single gland or organ. In other cases the target tissue is diffuse and scattered throughout the body so that many areas are affected. Hormones bring about their characteristic effects on target cells by modifying cellular activity.

ENDOCRINE GLANDS AND THEIR HORMONES

The organs of the endocrine system are the glands that secrete hormones. Figure 11-2 illustrates that the eight major endocrine glands are scattered throughout the body; however, they are still considered to be one system because they have similar functions, similar mechanisms of influence, and many important interrelationships.

Some glands also have nonendocrine regions that have functions other than hormone secretion. The pancreas is one of these glands. It has a major exocrine portion that secretes digestive enzymes and an endocrine portion that secretes hormones. The ovaries and testes secrete hormones and also produce the ova and sperm. Some organs, such as the stomach, intestines, and heart, produce hormones, but their primary function is not hormone secretion. These organs are discussed in more detail in the chapters dealing with their predominant function. Table 11-1 summarizes the major endocrine glands and their hormones.

A cell producing protein hormones

A cell producing steroid hormones

Blood vessels

Protein hormone

Steroid hormone

Target cells

Receptor site

Receptor site

Second messenger

Unmatched hormone and receptor site

No effect

Effect

Effect

Figure 11-1 Hormone-receptor action. There must be a match between hormone and receptor. Receptors for protein hormones are on the cell surface. Receptors for steroid hormones are inside the cell. (From Applegate E: *The anatomy and physiology learning system*, ed 4, St Louis, 2011, Saunders.)

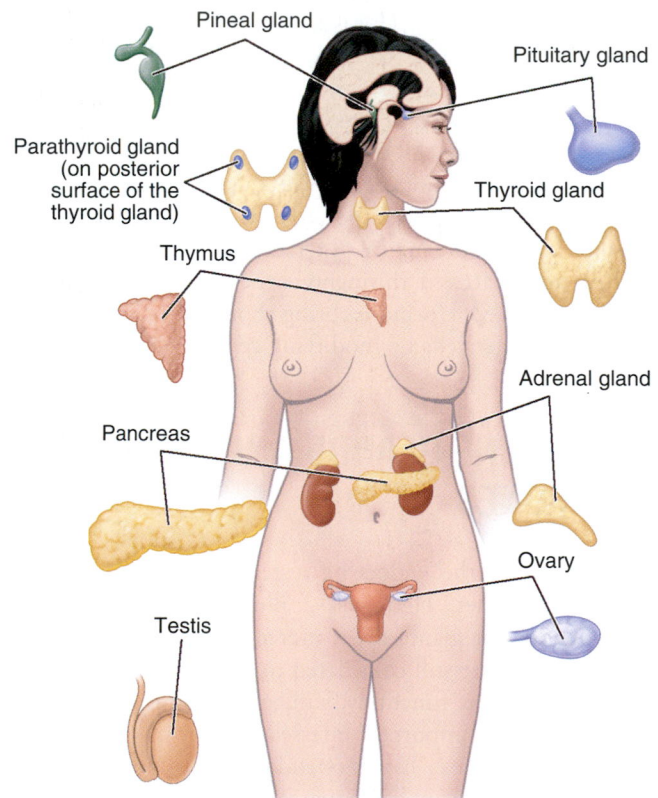

Pineal gland

Pituitary gland

Parathyroid gland (on posterior surface of the thyroid gland)

Thyroid gland

Thymus

Adrenal gland

Pancreas

Ovary

Testis

Figure 11-2 Major endocrine glands. (From Applegate E: *The anatomy and physiology learning system*, ed 4, St Louis, 2011, Saunders.)

PITUITARY GLAND

The *pituitary gland* or *hypophysis* is a small gland about 1 cm in diameter, or about the size of a pea. The gland is connected to the hypothalamus of the brain by a slender stalk called the *infundibulum*. The gland has two distinct regions.

The anterior portion is called the **adenohypophysis**. The posterior region is called the **neurohypophysis**. Table 11-1 and Figure 11-3 summarize the hormones from the pituitary gland.

Hormones of the Anterior Lobe (Adenohypophysis)

Growth Hormone

Growth hormone (GH) stimulates the growth of bones, muscles, and other organs by promoting protein synthesis. This hormone dramatically affects the appearance of an individual because it influences height. If there is too little of the hormone in a child, that person may become a pituitary dwarf of normal proportions but small stature. An excess of the hormone in a child results in exaggerated bone growth, and the individual becomes exceptionally tall or a giant. After ossification is complete and an increase in bone length is no longer possible, excess GH causes an enlargement in the diameter of the bones. The result is a condition called *acromegaly* in which the bones of the hands and face become abnormally large.

Thyroid-Stimulating Hormone

Thyroid-stimulating hormone (TSH), or thyrotropin, causes the glandular cells of the thyroid to secrete thyroid hormone. When there is a hypersecretion of TSH, the thyroid gland enlarges and secretes too much thyroid hormone. Hyposecretion of TSH results in atrophy of the thyroid gland and too little hormone.

Adrenocorticotropic Hormone

Adrenocorticotropic hormone (ACTH) reacts with receptor sites in the cortex of the adrenal gland to stimulate the secretion of cortical hormones, particularly cortisol. ACTH also affects the melanocytes in the skin and increases

Table 11-1 Principal Endocrine Glands and Their Hormones

Gland	Hormone	Target Tissue	Principal Actions
Anterior lobe of pituitary	Growth hormone (GH)	Most tissues in body	Stimulates growth by promoting protein synthesis
	Thyroid-stimulating hormone (TSH)	Thyroid gland	Increases secretion of thyroid hormone; increases size of thyroid gland
	Adrenocorticotropic hormone (ACTH)	Adrenal cortex	Increases secretion of adrenocortical hormones, especially glucocorticoids, such as cortisol
	Follicle-stimulating hormone (FSH)	Ovarian follicles in females; seminiferous tubules of testis in males	Follicle maturation and estrogen secretion in females; spermatogenesis in males
	Luteinizing hormone (LH); also called *interstitial cell–stimulating hormone* (ICSH) in males	Ovary in females, testis in males	Ovulation; progesterone production in females; testosterone production in males
	Prolactin	Mammary gland	Stimulates milk production
Posterior lobe of pituitary	Antidiuretic hormone (ADH)	Kidney	Increases water reabsorption (decreases water lost in urine)
	Oxytocin	Uterus; mammary gland	Increases uterine contractions; stimulates ejection of milk from mammary gland
Thyroid gland	Thyroxine and triiodothyronine	Most body cells	Increases metabolic rate; essential for normal growth and development
	Calcitonin	Primarily bone	Decreases blood calcium by inhibiting bone breakdown and release of calcium; antagonistic to parathyroid hormone (PTH)
Parathyroid gland	PTH or parathormone	Bone, kidney, digestive tract	Increases blood calcium by stimulating bone breakdown and release of calcium; increases calcium absorption in digestive tract; decreases calcium lost in urine
Adrenal cortex	Mineralocorticoids (aldosterone)	Kidney	Increases sodium reabsorption and potassium excretion in kidney tubules; secondarily increases water retention
	Glucocorticoids (cortisol)	Most body tissues	Increases blood glucose levels; inhibits inflammation and immune response
	Androgens and estrogens	Most body tissues	Secreted in small amounts so that effect is generally masked by hormones from ovaries and testes
Adrenal medulla	Epinephrine, norepinephrine	Heart, blood vessels, liver, adipose	Helps cope with stress; increases heart rate and blood pressure; increases blood flow to skeletal muscle; increases blood glucose level
Pancreas (islets of Langerhans)	Glucagon	Liver	Increases breakdown of glycogen to increase blood glucose levels
	Insulin	General, but especially liver, skeletal muscle, adipose	Decreases blood glucose levels by facilitating uptake and use of glucose by cells; stimulates glucose storage as glycogen and production of adipose
Testes	Testosterone	Most body cells	Maturation and maintenance of male reproductive organs and secondary sex characteristics
Ovaries	Estrogens	Most body cells	Maturation and maintenance of female reproductive organs and secondary sex characteristics; menstrual cycle
	Progesterone	Uterus and breast	Prepares uterus for pregnancy; stimulates development of mammary gland; menstrual cycle
Pineal gland	Melatonin	Hypothalamus	Inhibits gonadotropin-releasing hormone, which consequently inhibits reproductive functions; regulates daily rhythms, such as sleep and wakefulness

From Applegate E: *The anatomy and physiology learning system,* ed 4, St Louis, 2011, Saunders.

HIGHLIGHT on the Endocrine System

Antidiuretic hormone (ADH): Ingestion of alcoholic beverages inhibits ADH secretion and results in increased urine output. Certain drugs, called *diuretics*, counteract the effects of ADH and result in fluid loss. These drugs are sometimes prescribed for patients with high blood pressure or those with edema caused by congestive heart failure because the drugs have the effect of removing fluid from the body.

Thyroid function: When thyroxine and triiodothyronine, with their incorporated iodine, are released into the blood, more than 99% combines with plasma proteins. This iodine is called *protein-bound iodine* (PBI). The amount of PBI can be measured by a laboratory procedure and is widely used as a test of thyroid function.

Cortisone: Persons with inflamed joints often receive injections of a pharmaceutic glucocorticoid, cortisone, to relieve the pain and inflammation. Over-the-counter creams and ointments containing hydrocortisone are available to relieve the itching and inflammation of rashes.

Gonadocorticoids: Tumors that result in hypersecretion of gonadocorticoids may have dramatic effects in prepubertal boys and girls. There is a rapid onset of puberty and sex drive in males. Females develop the masculine distribution of body hair, including a beard, and the clitoris enlarges to become more like a penis.

Hypoglycemia: Hyperinsulinism is usually caused by an overdose of insulin. The result is hypoglycemia, or a low blood sugar level. The low blood sugar stimulates the secretion of glucagon, epinephrine, and growth hormone (GH), which causes anxiety, nervousness, tremors, and a feeling of weakness. Insufficient glucose levels in the brain lead to disorientation, convulsions, and unconsciousness. Death can occur quickly unless the blood glucose level is raised. The early symptoms can be treated easily by eating sugar.

Melatonin: Melatonin production appears to be related to the amount of light that enters through the eye. People who work at night and sleep during the day have a reversed cycle of melatonin production. The high melatonin levels occur during the day while they are asleep and the low levels are at night when they are working and light is entering the eye. ■

Common Pathology of the Endocrine System

Disease	Signs and Symptoms	Etiology	Diagnosis and Treatment
Myxedema	Thickening and swelling of the skin, lethargy, weight gain, fatigue, depression, sensitivity to cold.	The condition is caused by a deficiency of thyroid hormone in the adult (hypothyroidism).	Diagnosis it based on medical history, physical examination, and thyroid function tests. It is more common in women than men. Myxedema can be treated with thyroid replacement hormones.
Progeria	Symptoms resemble normal human aging but occur in young children; wrinkled face, baldness, large head.	The condition is caused by a gene mutation resulting in unstable cells that lead to the aging process.	Diagnosis is suspected according to signs and symptoms, such as skin changes, abnormal growth, and loss of hair. A genetic test for mutations can confirm the diagnosis of progeria. No treatment has proven effective.
Cushing syndrome	Excessive deposition of fat in the subscapular area and face; commonly called *moon face.*	Typically caused by overuse of oral corticosteroid medications. In a minority of cases, the cause is a hypersecretion of glucocorticoids from the adrenal cortex that may be the result of a tumor.	Diagnosis includes indications of high blood pressure, loss of muscle mass, glucose intolerance, and weight gain. Treatment is directed at reducing the levels of glucocorticoids with medications.
Type 1 diabetes mellitus	Symptoms include excessive thirst, frequent urination, and extreme hunger. There also may be weight loss, fatigue, blurred vision, sores that heal slowly, erectile dysfunction, and numbness in feet and hands.	Type 1 diabetes is a chronic condition in which the beta cells of the pancreatic islets produce little or no insulin. Also called *insulin-dependent diabetes mellitus* (IDDM) or *juvenile-onset diabetes mellitus.*	Diagnosis relies on various blood tests to evaluate glucose metabolism. Treatment protocol includes monitoring blood sugar levels, taking insulin, exercising regularly, maintaining an optimum weight, and eating a healthy diet. There is no cure.
Type 2 diabetes mellitus	Symptoms include excessive thirst, frequent urination, and extreme hunger accompanied by fatigue, blurred vision, infections that heal slowly, erectile dysfunction, and numbness in the feet and hands.	In this type, the receptors for insulin become resistant so the hormone has a reduced effect. Excess weight and inactivity appear to be contributing factors. Also called non–insulin-dependent diabetes mellitus (NIDDM) or adult-onset diabetes mellitus.	Diagnosis relies on various blood tests to evaluate glucose metabolism. Many individuals are able to manage type 2 diabetes with a healthy diet and regular exercise, whereas others need some form of insulin therapy. There is no cure.

Common Pathology of the Endocrine System—cont'd

Disease	Signs and Symptoms	Etiology	Diagnosis and Treatment
Diabetes insipidus	Patient experiences extreme thirst and produces a large quantity of urine.	Diabetes insipidus occurs when the body is unable to regulate fluids. In the central type, there is damage to the posterior pituitary gland that disrupts the normal production and release of antidiuretic hormone (ADH). In the nephrogenic type, the kidney tubules do not respond to ADH.	Diagnosis is confirmed by a water deprivation test and urinalysis. The central type can be treated with synthetic ADH. The nephrogenic type is managed by a low-salt diet and drinking only sufficient water to avoid dehydration. Complications that may arise from all type are dehydration and electrolyte imbalance.
Hyperthyroidism	Symptoms include sudden weight loss, rapid heartbeat, increased appetite, anxiety, tremor, sweating, frequent bowel movements, and an enlarged thyroid gland.	There are several causes of hyperthyroidism. Most often, the thyroid gland is overproducing thyroid hormone.	Diagnosis is based on a physical examination, blood tests, radioactive iodine uptake test, and thyroid scans. Treatment may involve antithyroid drugs and oral radioactive iodine.
Graves disease	The thyroid significantly enlarges, with increased heartbeat, muscle weakness, disturbed sleep, tremor, weight loss, anxiety, and irritability. It can also cause the eyes to bulge.	Graves disease is caused by a malfunction in the body's disease-fighting immune system that disrupts the normal regulation of the thyroid, resulting in an overproduction of thyroid hormones (hyperthyroidism).	Diagnosis is usually made on the basis of symptoms, although thyroid hormone tests may be useful. The primary treatment goals are to inhibit the overproduction of thyroid hormones and to block the hormonal effects on the body. Protocols include radioactive iodine therapy, antithyroid medications, beta-blockers, and surgery.
Addison disease	The symptoms develop slowly and may include muscle weakness and fatigue, weight loss, decreased appetite, skin darkening, low blood pressure, salt craving, low blood sugar, nausea, joint pain, and depression.	Addison disease results when the adrenal glands produce insufficient amounts of the hormone cortisol (adrenal insufficiency). This may be occur because of damaged cells in the adrenal cortex (primary renal insufficiency) or because of inadequate amounts of adrenocorticotropic hormone (ACTH) from the pituitary gland (secondary renal insufficiency). Cortisol influences the body's ability to convert food fuels into energy, plays a role in the inflammatory response, and helps the body respond to stress. Aldosterone from the adrenal may also be involved.	Diagnosis is based on several tests, including blood levels of sodium, potassium, cortisol, and ACTH. Computed tomography (CT) maybe used to check the size of the adrenal glands. Treatment involves hormone replacement therapy to correct the levels of steroid hormones the body is not producing.

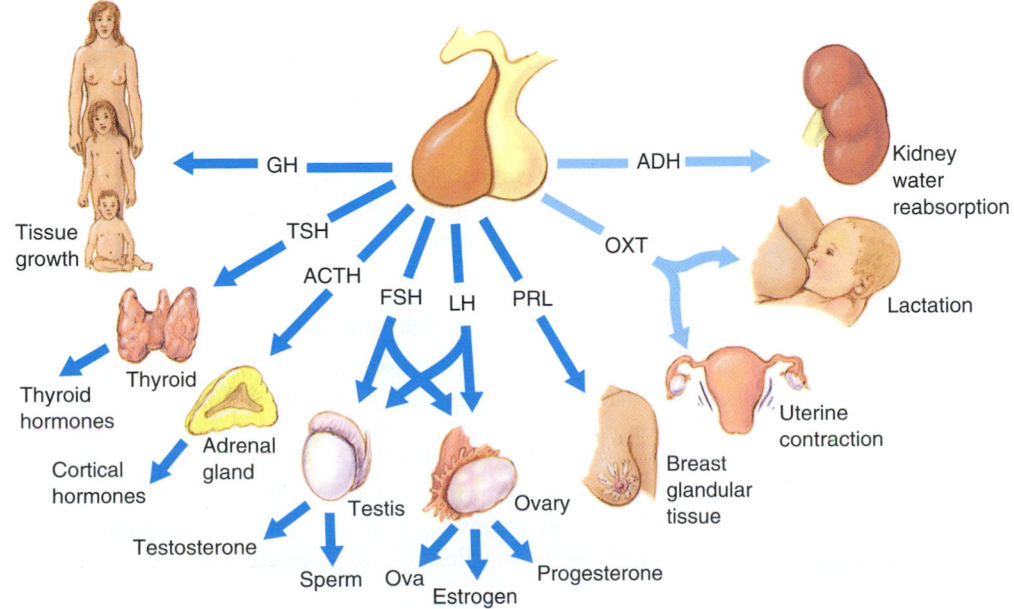

Figure 11-3 Effects of hormones from the pituitary gland. (From Applegate E: *The anatomy and physiology learning system*, ed 4, St Louis, 2011, Saunders.)

pigmentation. Hypersecretion and hyposecretion of ACTH are reflected in the activity of the adrenal cortex.

Gonadotropic Hormones

Gonadotropic hormones react with receptor sites in the gonads—ovaries and testes—to regulate the development, growth, and function of these organs. Follicle-stimulating hormone (FSH) stimulates the development of eggs or ova in the ovaries and of sperm in the testes. In addition, it stimulates estrogen production in the female. Luteinizing hormone (LH) causes ovulation and the production and secretion of progesterone and estrogen. In the male, LH is sometimes called *interstitial cell–stimulating hormone* (ICSH) because it stimulates the interstitial cells of the testes to produce and secrete the male sex hormone testosterone. Without FSH and LH, the ovaries and testes decrease in size, ova and sperm are not produced, and sex hormones are not secreted.

Prolactin

Prolactin (PRL), or lactogenic hormone, promotes the development of glandular tissue in the female breast during pregnancy and stimulates milk production after the birth of the infant. This hormone does not cause the milk to be ejected from the breast. A hormone from the posterior pituitary and other neural influences are responsible for the ejection of the milk.

Hormones of the Posterior Lobe (Neurohypophysis)
Antidiuretic Hormone

Antidiuretic hormone (ADH) promotes the reabsorption of water by the kidney tubules, with the result that less water is lost as urine. This mechanism conserves water for the body. Insufficient amounts of ADH cause excessive water loss in the urine. Large amounts of a dilute urine are produced. This condition is called *diabetes insipidus*. ADH, especially in large amounts, also causes blood vessels to constrict, which increases blood pressure. For this reason, ADH is sometimes called *vasopressin*.

Oxytocin

Oxytocin (OXY) causes contraction of the smooth muscle in the wall of the uterus. It also stimulates the ejection of milk from the lactating breast. A commercial preparation of this hormone, *Pitocin*, is sometimes used to induce labor.

THYROID GLAND

The thyroid gland is a vascular organ that is located in the neck (see Figure 11-2). It consists of two lobes, one on each side of the trachea, just below the larynx or voice box. The two lobes are connected by a narrow band of tissue called the *isthmus*.

Thyroxine and Triiodothyronine

About 95% of the active thyroid hormone is thyroxine, and the remaining 5% is triiodothyronine. Both of these require iodine for their synthesis. The iodine is actively transported into the thyroid gland, and then it is incorporated into the hormone molecules.

If there is an iodine deficiency, the thyroid cannot make sufficient hormone. This stimulates the thyroid gland to increase in size in a vain attempt to produce more hormone. However, it cannot produce more hormone because it does not have the necessary raw materials, namely, iodine. This type of thyroid enlargement is called *simple goiter* or *iodine deficiency goiter*. The use of iodized salt has reduced the incidence of simple goiter.

Thyroxine and triiodothyronine help to regulate the metabolism of carbohydrates, proteins, and lipids in the body. They do not have a single target organ; instead, they affect most of the cells in the body. Thyroid hormones increase the rate at which cells release energy from carbohydrates, enhance protein synthesis, are necessary for normal growth and development, and stimulate the nervous system.

Calcitonin

Calcitonin is secreted by the thyroid gland and reduces the calcium level in the blood. If the blood calcium level becomes too high, calcitonin is secreted until the calcium ion level decreases to normal.

PARATHYROID GLANDS

Four small masses of epithelial tissue are embedded in the connective tissue capsule on the posterior surface of the thyroid glands. These are the parathyroid glands, and they secrete parathyroid hormone (PTH), or parathormone. PTH is the most important regulator of blood calcium levels. The hormone is secreted in response to low blood calcium levels, and its effect is to increase those levels. PTH is antagonistic to calcitonin from the thyroid gland. Calcitonin reduces blood calcium levels, and PTH increases blood calcium. The two hormones work together to maintain calcium homeostasis.

ADRENAL (SUPRARENAL) GLANDS

The adrenal, or suprarenal, glands are paired, with one gland located near the upper portion of each kidney. The glands are embedded in the fat that surrounds the kidneys. Each gland is divided into an outer region called the *adrenal cortex* and an inner region called the *adrenal medulla* (Figure 11-4).

Hormones of the Adrenal Cortex

The adrenal cortex consists of three different regions, with each region producing a different group or type of hormones. Chemically, all the cortical hormones are steroids.

Mineralocorticoids are secreted by the outermost region of the adrenal cortex. As a group, these hormones help regulate blood volume and the concentration of mineral electrolytes in the blood. The principal mineralocorticoid is

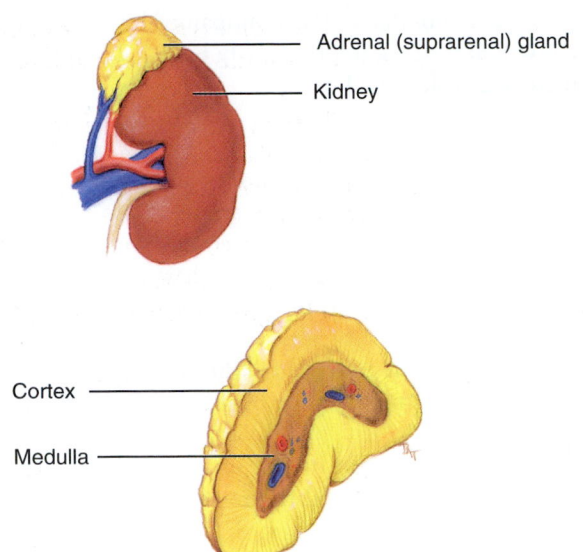

Figure 11-4 Adrenal gland. The cortex produces mineralocorticoids, glucocorticoids, and gonadocorticoids. The medulla produces epinephrine and norepinephrine. (From Applegate E: *The anatomy and physiology learning system*, ed 4, St Louis, 2011, Saunders.)

aldosterone, which primarily affects the kidneys. In general, the primary effect of aldosterone is to conserve sodium ions and water in the body and to eliminate potassium ions. The levels of sodium and potassium ions are important in maintaining blood pressure, nerve impulse conduction, and muscle contraction. **Glucocorticoids** are secreted by the middle region of the adrenal cortex. The principal glucocorticoid is *cortisol*, also called *hydrocortisone*. The overall effect of the glucocorticoids is to increase blood glucose levels. This helps to maintain appropriate blood glucose levels between meals. In times of prolonged stress, cortisol is secreted in greater than normal amounts to help increase glucose levels to provide energy to respond to the stress. Cortisol also helps to counteract the inflammatory response. For this reason it may be used clinically to reduce the inflammation in certain allergic reactions, bursitis and arthritis, infections, and some types of cancer.

Gonadocorticoids, or sex hormones, are the third group of steroids secreted by the adrenal cortex. These are secreted by the innermost region. Male hormones, **androgens**, and female hormones, **estrogens**, are secreted in minimal amounts in both sexes by the adrenal cortex, but their effect is usually masked by the hormones from the testes and ovaries. In females the masculinization effect of androgen secretion may become evident after menopause, when estrogen levels from the ovaries decrease.

Hormones of the Adrenal Medulla

The adrenal medulla secretes two hormones: *epinephrine* (adrenaline) and *norepinephrine* (noradrenaline). About 80% of the medullary secretion is epinephrine. These two hormones are secreted in response to stimulation by sympathetic

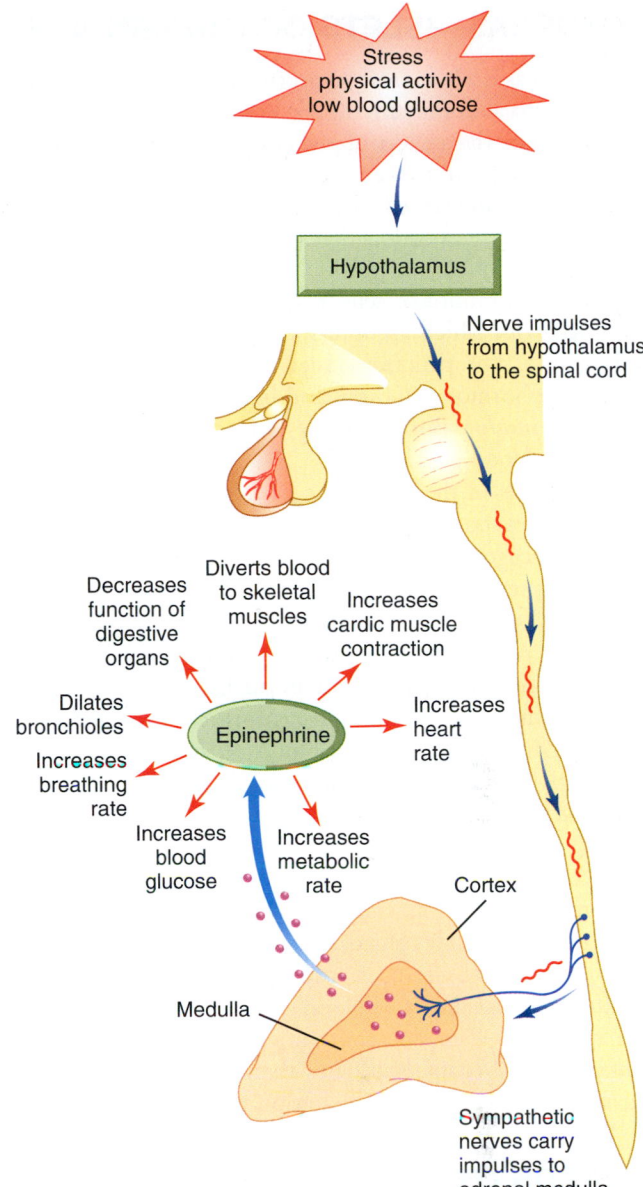

Figure 11-5 Epinephrine—its effects and control of its secretion. (From Applegate E: *The anatomy and physiology learning system*, ed 4, St Louis, 2011, Saunders.)

nerves, particularly during stressful situations. Epinephrine, a cardiac stimulator, and norepinephrine, a vasoconstrictor, together cause increases in heart rate, the force of cardiac muscle contraction, and blood pressure. They divert blood supply to the skeletal muscles and decrease the activity of the digestive tract, dilate the bronchioles and increase the breathing rate, and increase the rate of metabolism to provide energy. They prepare the body for strenuous activity and are sometimes called the *fight-or-flight hormones*. Their effect on the body is similar to effects of the sympathetic nervous system but lasts up to 10 times longer because the hormones are removed from the tissues slowly. The effects of epinephrine are summarized in Figure 11-5.

PANCREAS—ISLETS OF LANGERHANS

The pancreas is a long, soft organ that lies transversely along the posterior abdominal wall, posterior to the stomach, and extends from the region of the duodenum to the spleen. This gland has an exocrine portion that secretes digestive enzymes that are carried through a duct to the duodenum and an endocrine portion that secretes hormones into the blood. The endocrine portion consists of more than 1 million small groups of cells, called *pancreatic islets* or *islets of Langerhans*, which are interspersed throughout the exocrine tissue. The pancreatic islets contain alpha cells that secrete the hormone *glucagon* and beta cells that secrete the hormone *insulin*. Both of these hormones have a role in regulating blood glucose levels.

Alpha cells in the pancreatic islets secrete the hormone glucagon in response to a low concentration of glucose in the blood. Glucagon's principal action is to raise blood glucose levels to prevent hypoglycemia from occurring between meals or when glucose is being used rapidly. Beta cells in the pancreatic islets secrete the hormone insulin in response to a high concentration of glucose in the blood. The action of insulin is the opposite of, or antagonistic to, the action of glucagon. Insulin decreases the blood glucose concentration. Hypoactivity of insulin may be caused by insufficient insulin secretion, insufficient receptor sites on target cell membranes, or defective receptor sites that do not recognize insulin. These dysfunctions lead to diabetes mellitus, which is characterized by abnormally high blood glucose levels.

Maintaining blood glucose levels within a normal range is important because this is the primary source of energy for the nervous system. If blood glucose levels fall too low, the nervous system does not function properly. If blood glucose levels become too high, the kidneys produce large quantities of urine, and dehydration may result.

GONADS (TESTES AND OVARIES)

The gonads, the primary reproductive organs, are the testes in the male and ovaries in the female. These organs are responsible for producing the sperm and ova, but they also secrete hormones and are considered to be endocrine glands. A brief description of their endocrine functions is given here. Information regarding reproductive functions and a more thorough discussion of the hormones appear in Chapter 16.

Testes

Male sex hormones, as a group, are called **androgens**. The principal androgen is *testosterone*, which is secreted by the testes. A small amount is also produced by the adrenal cortex. Production of testosterone begins during fetal development, continues for a short time after birth, nearly ceases during childhood, and then resumes at puberty. This steroid hormone is responsible for the following:

- Growth and development of the male reproductive structures
- Increased skeletal and muscular growth

- Enlargement of the larynx accompanied by voice changes
- Growth and distribution of body hair
- Increased male sexual drive

Ovaries

Two groups of female sex hormones are produced in the ovaries: the **estrogens** and **progesterone**. These steroid hormones contribute to the development and function of the female reproductive organs and sex characteristics. At the onset of puberty, estrogens promote the following:

- Development of the breasts
- Distribution of fat evidenced in the hips, legs, and breasts
- Maturation of reproductive organs, such as the uterus and vagina

Progesterone causes the uterine lining to thicken in preparation for pregnancy. Together, progesterone and estrogens are responsible for the changes that occur in the uterus during the female menstrual cycle.

PINEAL GLAND

The *pineal gland*, also called *pineal body* or *epiphysis cerebri*, is a small cone-shaped structure that extends posteriorly from the third ventricle of the brain. The gland consists of portions of neurons, neuroglial cells, and specialized secretory cells called **pinealocytes**. The pinealocytes synthesize the hormone *melatonin* and secrete it directly into the cerebrospinal fluid, which takes it into the blood. Melatonin secretion is rhythmic in nature, with high levels secreted at night and low levels secreted during the day.

The function of the pineal gland and melatonin in humans has been the subject of controversy and speculation for centuries. Even the ancient Greeks wrote about it. Evidence accumulated during the 1980s indicates that melatonin has a regulatory role in sexual and reproductive development. Melatonin acts on the hypothalamus to inhibit gonadotropin-releasing hormone (GnRH), which then inhibits gonadal development.

Another function of melatonin involves the organization and regulation of **circadian rhythms**, or daily changes in physiologic processes that follow a regular pattern. An example of this is the sleepiness-wakefulness cycle. Increased plasma melatonin levels, which occur at night, are associated with sleepiness. The hormone also seems to play a role in hunger-satiety cycles, mood changes, and jet lag. The high nighttime level of melatonin seems to be a mechanism to "reset" the biologic clock daily.

THYMUS GLAND

The thymus gland is located near the midline, posterior to the sternum and slightly superior to the heart. Through the production of the hormone *thymosin*, the thymus gland assists in the development of certain blood cells that help protect the body against foreign organisms. In this way the thymus gland plays an important role in the body's immune mechanism.

AGING OF THE ENDOCRINE SYSTEM

With age, most endocrine glands show some degree of glandular atrophy, with increased amounts of fibrous tissue and fat deposits. However, the glands remain responsive to stimulation and secrete adequate amounts of hormones. Exceptions to this generalization are the gonads, which are discussed in Chapter 16. There is some evidence of a decline in the rate of hormone secretion, but this may be caused by changes in the target tissues that decrease the cellular need for the hormone. There is also evidence of a reduction in target-tissue receptor sites or in their sensitivity. Whatever the reason for the decline in hormone secretion, it is accompanied by a decreased rate of metabolic destruction so that the blood levels of circulating hormones remain relatively constant throughout senescence. There is no evidence that age-related structural changes in endocrine glands have functional significance or contribute to the overall aging process.

↻ TERMINOLOGY REVIEW

Key Term	Word Parts	Definition
Adenohypophysis	*aden/o:* gland *hypo-:* beneath, below *-physis:* to grow	Anterior portion of the pituitary gland; the gland that grows below the brain.
Androgens	*andr/o:* male, maleness	Steroid hormones that promote male characteristics.
Circadian rhythms		Biologic clock or a person's 24-hour rhythm such as a natural sleep-wake cycle.
Endocrine glands	*endo-:* in, within *-crine:* to secrete	Glands that secrete their products directly into the blood; opposite of exocrine glands.
Endocrinology	*endo-:* in, within *-crine:* to secrete *-ology:* study	Study of the endocrine glands.
Estrogens		Group of hormones that stimulate the development of female secondary sex characteristics.
Exocrine glands	*exo-:* out, away from *-crine:* to secrete	Glands that secret their products to a surface or cavity through ducts; opposite of endocrine glands.
Glucocorticoids	*gluc/o:* sugar *cortic-:* outer region, cortex	Hormones from the adrenal cortex that raise blood sugar levels.
Gonadocorticoids	*gonad/o:* gonad, primary sex organ *cortic-:* outer region, cortex	Sex hormones secreted by the adrenal cortex.
Hormones	*hormon/o:* hormone	Substances secreted by endocrine glands.
Mineralocorticoids	*mineral/o:* pertaining to minerals *cortic-:* outer region, cortex	A group of hormones secreted by the adrenal cortex that regulates electrolyte balance in the body.
Neurohypophysis	*neur/o:* nerve *hypo-:* beneath, below *-physis:* to grow	Posterior portion of pituitary gland; the gland that grows beneath the brain and contains axons of neurons.
Pinealocytes	*-cyte:* cell	Secretory cells of the pineal gland; secrete melatonin
Progesterone	*pro-:* prepares, for, promotes *-gest-:* pregnancy	A hormone secreted by the ovaries that causes the uterine lining to thicken in preparation for pregnancy and then maintains pregnancy.
Target tissue		A tissue (cells) that responds to a particular hormone because it has receptor sites for that hormone.

ON THE WEB

For information on the endocrine system:

Endocrine Diseases: www.mic.ki.se/diseases/C19.html

Endocrine System: www.emc.maricopa.edu/faculty/farabee/BIOBK/BiobookENDOCR.html

Endocrine Web: www.endocrineweb.com

Inner Body: www.innerbody.com

12

Circulatory System

 Check out the Evolve site at http://evolve.elsevier.com/Bonewit/today/ to access additional interactive activities and exercises to help you study and prepare for success.

CHAPTER OUTLINE

INTRODUCTION TO THE CIRCULATORY SYSTEM
HEART
Overview of the Heart
Form, Size, and Location of the Heart
Coverings of the Heart
Structure of the Heart
Layers of the Heart Wall
Chambers of the Heart
Valves of the Heart
Pathway of Blood Through the Heart
Blood Supply to the Myocardium

Physiology of the Heart
Conduction System
Cardiac Cycle
Heart Sounds
BLOOD
Functions and Characteristics of Blood
Composition of Blood
Plasma
Formed Elements
Hemostasis
Vascular Constriction

Platelet Plug Formation
Coagulation
Blood Types
ABO Blood Groups
Rh Blood Groups
BLOOD VESSELS
Classification and Structure of Blood Vessels
Arteries
Capillaries
Veins
Circulatory Pathways
Pulmonary Circuit

Systemic Circuit
LYMPHATIC SYSTEM
Lymph
Lymphatic Vessels
Lymphatic Organs
RESISTANCE TO DISEASE
Nonspecific Defense Mechanisms
Specific Defense Mechanisms
Cell-Mediated Immunity
Antibody-Mediated Immunity
Acquired Immunity
AGING OF THE CIRCULATORY SYSTEM

KEY TERMS

agranulocytes (ay-GRAN-yoo-loh-sytes)
antibodies (AN-tih-bahd-eez)
antibody-mediated immunity (AN-tih-bahd-ee ih-MYOO-nih-tee)
antigens (AN-tih-jenz)
atria (singular atrium) (AY-tree-ah)
atrioventricular valves (ay-tree-oh-ven-TRIK-yoo-lar VALVES)
cardiac cycle (KAR-dee-ak SYE-kul)
cell-mediated immunity (SELL MEE-dee-ate-ed ih-MYOO-nih-tee)
coagulation (koh-ag-yoo-LAY-shun)
conduction myofibers (kon-DUCK-shun my-o-FYE-bers)
diapedesis (dye-ah-peh-DEE-sis)
diastole (dye-AS-toh-lee)
endocardium (end-oh-KAR-dee-um)
epicardium (eh-pih-KAR-dee-um)
erythrocytes (ee-RITH-roh-sytes)

erythropoiesis (ee-rith-roh-POY-ee-sis)
erythropoietin (ee-rith-roh-POY-ee-tin)
granulocytes (GRAN-yoo-loh-sytes)
hematopoiesis (hee-ma-to-poy-EE-sis)
hemocytoblast (hee-moh-SYTE-oh-blast)
hemoglobin (hee-moh-GLOH-bin)
hemostasis (hee-moh-STAY-sis)
immunoglobulins (ih-myoo-noh-GLAHB-yoo-lins)
leukocytes (LOO-koh-sytes)
macrophages (MACK-roh-fayj-es)
megakaryocytes (meg-ah-KAIR-ee-oh-sytes)
myocardium (my-oh-KAR-dee-um)
nonspecific defense mechanisms (non-speh-SIF-ik dee-FENS MECK-ah-nizms)
pericardial cavity (pair-ih-KAR-dee-ull CAV-ih-tee)

pericardium (pair-ih-KAR-dee-um)
pulmonary circulation (PULL-mon-air-ee sir-kyoo-LAY-shun)
renal erythropoietic factor (REE-null ee-rith-roh-POY-eh-tic FACK-tor)
resistance (ree-SIS-tans)
right lymphatic duct (RYTE lim-FAT-ik DUKT)
semilunar valves (seh-mee-LOO-nar VALVES)
specific defense mechanisms (speh-SIF-ik dee-FENS MECK-ah-nizms)
susceptibility (sus-sep-tih-BILL-ih-tee)
systemic circulation (sis-TEM-ik sir-kyoo-LAY-shun)
systole (SIS-toh-lee)
thoracic duct (tho-RAS-ik DUKT)
thrombocytes (THROM-boh-sytes)
ventricles (VEN-trih-kulls)

INTRODUCTION TO THE CIRCULATORY SYSTEM

The circulatory system is made up of the heart, blood, and blood vessels in the cardiovascular component and the lymph, lymphatic vessels, and lymphatic organs in the lymphatic component. In the cardiovascular component, a central pump, the heart, provides the force to move the blood through a system of blood vessels that extend throughout the body. Blood is the primary transport medium that is responsible for meeting the demands of the cells. The lymphatic system may be included with the circulatory system because it has a fluid (lymph) that flows (circulates) through a system of vessels and then drains into venous blood. The lymphatic system also has a major role in the body's defense against disease or immunology. This chapter focuses on the components that make up the circulatory system: heart, blood, blood vessels, lymph, lymphatic vessels, and lymphatic organs. At the end of the chapter, there is a discussion of the body's defense mechanisms and immunity.

HEART

The heart is a muscular pump that provides the force necessary to circulate the blood to all the tissues in the body. Its function is vital because to survive, the tissues need a continuous supply of oxygen and nutrients, and metabolic waste products must be removed. Deprived of these necessities, cells soon undergo irreversible changes that lead to death. Although blood is the transport medium, the heart is the organ that keeps the blood moving through the vessels. The normal adult heart pumps about 5 L of blood every minute throughout life. If it loses its pumping effectiveness for even a few minutes, the individual's life is jeopardized.

OVERVIEW OF THE HEART

Form, Size, and Location of the Heart

Knowledge of the heart's position in the thoracic cavity is important in hearing heart sounds, obtaining electrocardiograms (ECGs), and performing cardiopulmonary resuscitation (CPR). The heart, illustrated in Figure 12-1, is located in the thoracic cavity between the two lungs. It is posterior to the sternum and anterior to the vertebral column, and it rests on the diaphragm. About two thirds of the heart mass is to the left of the body's midline, and one third is to the right. The *apex*, or pointed end of the heart, extends downward to the level of the fifth intercostal space. The opposite end, the *base*, is larger and less pointed than the apex and has several large vessels attached to it. Its most superior portion is at the level of the second rib. The size of the heart varies with the size of the individual. On average, it is about 9 cm wide and 12 cm long, which is about the size of a closed fist.

Coverings of the Heart

The heart is enclosed by a loose-fitting, double-layered sac called the **pericardium** or *pericardial sac.* The outer layer of the pericardium consists of tough, white fibrous connective tissue and is called the *fibrous pericardium.* The fibrous pericardium is lined with a serous membrane called the *parietal pericardium.* Where the pericardium is attached to the vessels at the base of the heart, the parietal pericardium reflects onto the surface of the heart to form the *visceral pericardium.* The small space between the parietal and visceral layers of the pericardium is the **pericardial cavity.** It contains a thin layer of serous fluid that reduces friction

between the membranes as they rub against each other during heart contractions.

STRUCTURE OF THE HEART

Layers of the Heart Wall

The heart wall is formed by three layers of tissue: an outer epicardium, a middle myocardium, and an inner endocardium. The **epicardium** (which is the same as the visceral pericardium) consists of a serous membrane. It is a thin protective layer that is firmly anchored to the underlying muscle. Blood vessels that nourish the heart wall are located in the epicardium.

The thick middle layer is the **myocardium.** It forms the bulk of the heart wall and is composed of cardiac muscle tissue. Refer to Chapter 5 for a review of the different types of muscle tissue. Contraction of the myocardium provides the force that ejects blood from the heart and moves it through the vessels.

The inner lining of the heart wall is the **endocardium.** Its smooth surface permits blood to move easily through the heart. The endocardium also forms the valves of the heart and is continuous with the lining of the blood vessels. Figure 12-2 illustrates the layers of the heart wall.

Chambers of the Heart

The internal cavity of the heart is divided into four chambers (Figure 12-3): right atrium, right ventricle, left atrium, and left ventricle.

The two **atria** are thin-walled chambers that receive blood from the veins. The two **ventricles** are thick-walled chambers that forcefully pump blood out of the heart. Differences in thickness of the heart chamber walls are caused by variations in the amount of myocardium present, which

Figure 12-1 Frontal view of the mediastinum, showing the position of the heart. (From Applegate E: *The anatomy and physiology learning system,* ed 4, St Louis, 2011, Saunders.)

Endocardium

Myocardium

Visceral pericardium
(epicardium)

Parietal pericardium

Fibrous pericardium

Coronary vessels

Pericardial cavity

Figure 12-2 Layers of the heart wall. (From Applegate E: *The anatomy and physiology learning system,* ed 4, St Louis, 2011, Saunders.)

reflects the amount of force each chamber is required to generate.

The *right atrium* receives deoxygenated blood from the superior vena cava and the inferior vena cava. The superior vena cava returns blood to the heart from the head, neck, and upper extremities. The inferior vena cava returns blood to the heart from the thorax, abdomen, pelvis, and lower extremities. The *left atrium* receives oxygenated blood from the lungs through four pulmonary veins, two on the right and two on the left. Because the atria are "receiving" chambers rather than "pumping" chambers, their myocardium is relatively thin. The right and left atria are separated by a partition called the *interatrial septum.* A thin region, the fossa ovalis, is found in the interatrial septum. This represents an opening, the foramen ovale, that is present between the atria in the fetal heart.

The *right ventricle* receives blood from the right atrium and pumps it out to the lungs, where it picks up a new supply of oxygen. The *left ventricle* receives blood from the left atrium and pumps it out to the tissues of the whole body. The ventricles are "pumping" chambers, and this is reflected by a thick myocardium. Because the left ventricle pumps blood to the whole body and the right ventricle sends blood only to the lungs, the left ventricle has to generate a lot more pumping force than the right ventricle. This is reflected in the fact that the left ventricular wall has a thicker myocardium than the right. Both ventricles hold about the same volume of blood. The thick, muscular partition between the right and left ventricles is the *interventricular septum.*

Superior vena cava

Pulmonary artery

Pulmonic valve

Pulmonary veins

Right atrium

Tricuspid (AV) valve

Right ventricle

Inferior vena cava

Trabeculae carneae

Aorta (thoracic)

Aorta (arch)

Pulmonary trunk

Pulmonary artery

Pulmonary veins

Left atrium

Aortic valve

Mitral (AV) valve

Chordae tendineae

Papillary muscle

Left ventricle

Interventricular septum

Figure 12-3 Internal view of the heart showing the chambers and valves. (From Applegate E: *The anatomy and physiology learning system,* ed 4, St Louis, 2011, Saunders.)

Valves of the Heart

Pumps need a set of valves to keep the fluid flowing in one direction, and the heart is no exception. The heart has two types of valves that keep the blood flowing in the correct direction. The valves between the atria and ventricles are called **atrioventricular (AV) valves.** The valves at the base of the large vessels leaving the ventricles are called **semilunar (SL) valves.**

Atrioventricular Valves

The AV valves permit the flow of blood from the atria into the corresponding ventricle. They also prevent the backflow of blood from the ventricles into the atria. Each valve consists of a fibrous connective tissue ring and double folds of endocardium that form the cusps of the valve. The valve cusps are attached to the ventricles by connective tissue strings called *chordae tendineae* (see Figure 12-3). As blood returns to the atria, it pushes the valve cusps open and the blood flows into the ventricles. When the ventricles contract, the force of the blood against the cusps causes them to close and prevents the backward flow of blood into the atria.

The AV valve between the right atrium and right ventricle has three cusps and is called the *tricuspid valve*. The valve between the left atrium and left ventricle has only two cusps and is called the *bicuspid*, or *mitral, valve* (see Figure 12-3).

Semilunar Valves

The SL valves are located at the bases of the large vessels that carry blood from the ventricles (see Figure 12-3). Each valve consists of three cuplike cusps. Contraction of the ventricles increases the pressure of the blood so that it pushes the valves open and the blood leaves the heart. As the ventricles relax and pressure decreases, the blood starts to flow back down the large vessels toward the ventricles. When the blood flows toward the ventricles, it enters the "cups" of the valve cusps. This closes the opening of the valves and prevents the flow of blood back into the ventricles.

The valve at the exit of the right ventricle is in the base of the pulmonary trunk and is called the *pulmonary SL valve*. The valve at the exit of the left ventricle is in the base of the ascending aorta. It is called the *aortic SL valve* (see Figure 12-3).

Pathway of Blood Through the Heart

Although it is convenient to describe the flow of blood through the right side of the heart and then through the left side, it is important to realize that both atria contract at the same time and that both ventricles contract at the same time. The heart functions as two pumps, one on the right and one on the left, that work simultaneously. The "right pump" pumps the blood to the lungs (**pulmonary circulation**) at the same time that the "left pump" pumps blood to the rest of the body (**systemic circulation**). The

Red = oxygenated blood

Blue = deoxygenated blood

1 = capillary beds of lungs
    where gas exchange occurs

2 = capillary beds of body tissues
    where gas exchange occurs

Figure 12-4 Pathway of the blood through the heart: Superior vena cava (SVC) and inferior vena cava (IVC) → Right atrium → Tricuspid valve → Right ventricle → Pulmonary semilunar (SL) valve → Pulmonary trunk → Pulmonary arteries → Capillaries of lungs → Pulmonary veins → Left atrium → Bicuspid valve → Left ventricle → Aortic SL valve → Ascending aorta → Systemic circulation. (From Applegate E: *The anatomy and physiology learning system*, ed 4, St Louis, 2011, Saunders.)

sequence in which the chambers contract is described in more detail with the cardiac cycle.

The arrows in Figure 12-4 depict the direction in which blood flows through the heart. Venous blood from the systemic circulation is relatively low in oxygen and high in carbon dioxide content. This blood enters the *right atrium* through the superior vena cava and inferior vena cava. It then flows through the *tricuspid valve* into the *right ventricle*. From the right ventricle, it passes through the *pulmonary SL valve* into the *pulmonary trunk* and then into the *pulmonary arteries*. The *pulmonary arteries* carry the blood to the *lungs*. In the lungs the blood releases carbon dioxide and picks up a new supply of oxygen. *Pulmonary veins* then carry the blood to the *left atrium*. From the left atrium, the blood flows through the *bicuspid valve* into the *left ventricle*. The blood then flows through the *aortic SL valve* into the *ascending aorta*. Oxygen-rich blood flowing into the aorta is distributed to all parts of the body through the systemic circulation.

Blood Supply to the Myocardium

The myocardium of the heart wall is working muscle that needs a continuous supply of oxygen and nutrients to function with efficiency. Unlike skeletal muscle, cardiac muscle cannot build up an oxygen debt to be repaid at a later time. It needs a continuous oxygen supply or it dies. For this reason, cardiac muscle has an extensive network of blood vessels to bring oxygen to the contracting cells and to remove waste products.

Right and left coronary arteries branch from the ascending aorta just distal to the aortic SL valve. These vessels have numerous branches. Blood flow through the coronary arteries is greatest when the myocardium is relaxed. When the ventricles contract, they compress the arteries, which reduces the flow.

PHYSIOLOGY OF THE HEART

The work of the heart is to pump blood to the lungs through the pulmonary circulation and to the rest of the body through the systemic circulation. This is accomplished by contraction and relaxation of the cardiac muscle in the myocardium.

Conduction System

An effective cycle for productive pumping of blood requires that the heart be synchronized accurately. Both atria need to contract simultaneously, followed by contraction of both ventricles. Contraction of the chambers is coordinated by specialized cardiac muscle cells that make up the conduction system of the heart.

Components of the Conduction System
Sinoatrial Node

The conduction system includes several components (Figure 12-5). The first part of the conduction system is the *sinoatrial (SA) node,* which is located in the right atrium, near the entrance of the superior vena cava. Without any neural stimulation, the SA node rhythmically initiates impulses 70 to 80 times per minute. Because it establishes the basic rhythm of the heartbeat, it is called the pacemaker of the heart. The impulses from the SA node rapidly travel throughout the atrial myocardium and cause the two atria to contract simultaneously. At the same time, the impulses reach the second part of the conduction system.

Atrioventricular Node

The AV node, the second part of the conduction system, is located in the floor of the right atrium, near the interatrial septum. The cells in the AV node conduct impulses more slowly than do other parts of the conduction system, so there is a brief delay as the impulses travel through the node. This allows time for the atria to finish their contraction phase before the ventricles begin contracting.

Atrioventricular Bundle, Bundle Branches, and Conduction Myofibers

From the AV node, the impulses rapidly travel through the *AV bundle* (bundle of His) to the *right* and *left bundle branches.* The bundle branches extend along the right and left sides of the interventricular septum to the apex. These branch profusely to form **conduction myofibers** (Purkinje fibers), which transmit the impulses to the myocardium. The AV bundle, bundle branches, and conduction myofibers rapidly transmit impulses throughout all the ventricular myocardium so that both ventricles contract at the same time. As the ventricles contract, blood is forced out through the SL valves into the pulmonary trunk and the ascending aorta. After the ventricles complete their contraction phase, they relax and the SA node initiates another impulse to start another cardiac cycle.

Cardiac Cycle

The **cardiac cycle** refers to the alternating contraction and relaxation of the heart chambers during one heartbeat (Figure 12-6). The two atria contract at the same time; then they relax while the two ventricles simultaneously contract. The contraction phase of the chambers is called **systole;** the relaxation phase is called **diastole.** When the terms *systole* and *diastole* are used alone, they refer to action of the ventricles.

With a heart rate of 75 beats per minute, one cardiac cycle lasts 0.8 second. The cycle begins with *atrial systole,* when both atria contract (see Figure 12-6). During this time, the AV valves are open, the ventricles are in diastole, and blood is forced into the ventricles. Atrial systole lasts for 0.1 second; then the atria relax for the remainder of the cycle, 0.7 second. This is *atrial diastole.*

When the atria finish their contraction phase, the ventricles begin contracting. *Ventricular systole* lasts for 0.3 second. Pressure in the ventricles increases as they contract. This closes the AV valves and opens the SL valves, and blood is forced into the pulmonary trunk and ascending

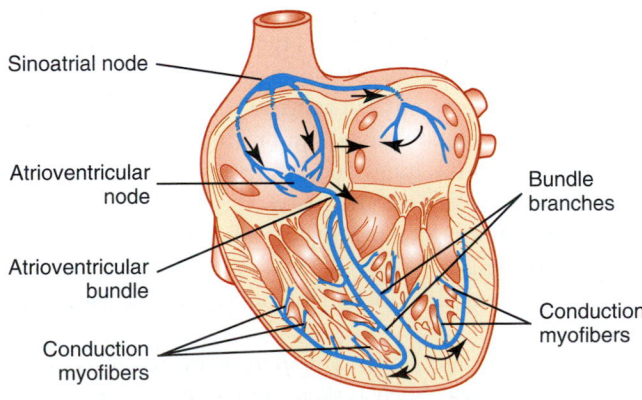

Figure 12-5 Conduction system of the heart. Impulses travel from the sinoatrial (SA) node (pacemaker) → Atrioventricular (AV) node → AV bundle → Right and left bundle branches → Conduction myofibers → Myocardium. (From Applegate E: *The anatomy and physiology learning system,* ed 4, St Louis, 2011, Saunders.)

Sinoatrial node

Atrioventricular node

Atrioventricular bundle

Conduction myofibers

Bundle branches

Conduction myofibers

Atria contract   Ventricles contract   All chambers relaxed

Figure 12-6 Cardiac cycle. Atrial systole is followed by ventricular systole. All chambers are simultaneously in diastole for one half of the cycle. (From Applegate E: *The anatomy and physiology learning system,* ed 4, St Louis, 2011, Saunders.)

aorta, which carry blood away from the heart. During this time the atria are in diastole and are filling with blood that is returned through the venae cavae and pulmonary veins. After ventricular systole, when the ventricles relax, the SL valves close, the AV valves open, and blood flows from the atria into the ventricles. This is *ventricular diastole.* All chambers are in simultaneous diastole for 0.4 second. About 70% of ventricular filling occurs during this period. The remaining blood enters the ventricles during atrial systole.

Heart Sounds

The sounds associated with the heartbeat are caused by the closure of the valves of the heart. A stethoscope is used to listen to these sounds, usually described as *lubb-dupp.* The first heart sound, the *lubb,* is caused by closure of the AV valves. The second heart sound, the *dupp,* is caused by closure of the SL valves. It has a higher pitch than the first heart sound. There is a pause between the *dupp* of the first beat and the *lubb* of the second beat when the entire heart is resting. Therefore the sequence is *lubb-dupp,* pause, *lubb-dupp,* pause, *lubb-dupp,* pause, and so on. Abnormal heart sounds, called *murmurs,* are caused by faulty valves.

BLOOD

The body consists of active cells that need a continuous supply of nutrients and oxygen. Metabolic waste products need to be removed from the cells for maintenance of a stable cellular environment. Blood is the primary transport medium responsible for meeting these cellular demands.

FUNCTIONS AND CHARACTERISTICS OF BLOOD

Blood is one of the connective tissues and is the only liquid tissue in the body. As a connective tissue, it consists of cells and cell fragments *(formed elements)* suspended in an intercellular matrix *(plasma).* The total blood volume in an average adult is 4 to 5 L in women and 5 to 6 L in men. It accounts for approximately 8% of the total body weight. Blood is slightly heavier and four to five times more viscous than water. It is slightly alkaline, with a normal pH range of 7.35 to 7.45.

The activities of the blood may be categorized as *transportation, regulation,* and *protection.* These functional categories overlap and interact as the blood carries out its role in providing suitable conditions for cellular functions. The following activities of blood are transport functions:

- It carries oxygen and nutrients to the cells of the body.
- It transports carbon dioxide and nitrogenous wastes from the tissues to the lungs and kidneys, where these wastes can be removed from the body.
- It carries hormones from the endocrine glands to the target tissues.

The following activities of blood are in the regulation category:

- It helps regulate body temperature by removing heat from active areas, such as skeletal muscles, and transporting it to other regions or to the skin, where it can be dissipated.
- It plays a significant role in fluid and electrolyte balance because the salts and plasma proteins contribute to the osmotic pressure.

HIGHLIGHT on the Circulatory System

Blood doping: Blood doping is a practice reportedly used by some athletes to improve their endurance for aerobic activities such as running, swimming, and cycling. A few weeks before a competition, blood is drawn from the athlete and the red blood cells (RBCs) are separated and frozen. Normal hematopoiesis replaces the lost RBCs and brings the blood cell count back to normal. Then, just before the competition, the frozen RBCs are thawed and injected into the athlete. This creates an artificial polycythemia. The idea is that the additional RBCs are able to deliver more oxygen to the muscles and improve aerobic endurance. Whether this occurs is questionable, and the practice is not without danger. All blood transfusions carry some risk. Furthermore, the additional cells increase the viscosity or thickness of the blood and put a strain on the heart.

Damaged heart valves: Sometimes disease processes damage the heart valves so that they are unable to function properly. Incompetent valves permit a backflow of blood, and the heart has to pump the same blood over and over to get it into the vessels. In valvular stenosis, the valves are stiff and have narrow openings. The heart has to work harder to pump blood out through the small opening. Defective heart valves may result in abnormal heart sounds. For example, if the atrioventricular valves are faulty, a hissing sound may be heard between the first and second heart sounds.

Rising rapidly and dizziness: Sometimes there is a feeling of dizziness when rising rapidly from lying down to a standing position. This is because the body has not had time to respond to the decrease in blood pressure caused by the downward pull of gravity on the blood. The dizziness is a signal that the brain is not receiving enough blood.

Hole in the heart: When the foramen ovale between the two atria fails to close after birth, the result is an interatrial septal defect. Because pressure in the right atrium is lower than in the left, blood flows from the left atrium back into the right atrium without going through the systemic circulation. This defect overloads the pulmonary circulation and puts a strain on the heart as it attempts to pump enough blood to maintain adequate supplies to the body tissues.

Coronary artery blockage: If a branch of a coronary artery becomes blocked, blood supply to that region of the heart is cut off and the muscle cells in that area die because of lack of oxygen. This is a myocardial infarction (MI), also called a *coronary* or a *heart attack*. The extent of the damage and chances of recovery depend on the location of the blockage and the length of time that elapses before medical intervention occurs.

Heart enzymes: When heart muscle is damaged, the dying cells release enzymes into the bloodstream. These enzymes can be measured and are useful in confirming an MI. The enzymes assayed are creatine kinase (CK) and lactate dehydrogenase (LDH).

Dysrhythmias: Variations in normal contraction patterns are called *dysrhythmias* (arrhythmias). One type of dysrhythmia occurs when a conduction myofiber or heart muscle cell independently depolarizes to threshold and triggers a premature heart contraction. The cell responsible for the premature contraction is called an *ectopic focus.* Sometimes ectopic foci form feedback loops within the conduction system, causing myocardial contractions to occur at a rapid rate. If not treated properly, this often leads to ventricular tachycardia, fibrillation, and death.

Smoking: About 20% of a cigarette smoker's hemoglobin is nonfunctional for transporting oxygen because it is bound to carbon monoxide from the cigarette smoke.

Varicose veins: Varicose veins are veins that are twisted and dilated with accumulated blood. These frequently occur in the legs. Conditions that hinder venous return, such as pregnancy, obesity, and standing for long periods of time, allow blood to accumulate in the veins of the extremities. This stretches the veins, so the valve flaps no longer overlap and they permit the backflow of blood. Superficial veins are more susceptible because they receive less support from surrounding tissue.

Sunbathing: When a person remains in the sun for an extended period, the cutaneous blood vessels dilate to bring more blood to the skin's surface, which helps keep the body cool. This action decreases the amount of blood in other parts of the body and may diminish the blood supply to the brain. If one is sunbathing and stands up abruptly, he or she may feel dizzy. This is because the blood momentarily remains in the dilated cutaneous vessels instead of returning to the heart. This causes a decrease in blood pressure. The dizziness is a signal that the brain is not receiving enough oxygen.

Lymphatic system and cancer: The lymphatic system is one route by which cancer cells can spread from a primary tumor site to other areas of the body. As the cells travel with the lymph, they pass through the lymph nodes, where the lymph is filtered. At first, this traps the cancer cells within the lymph node, and the cells are destroyed. Eventually, the number of cancer cells may overwhelm the filtration ability of the lymph nodes and some of the cells pass through the nodes to establish secondary tumors.

Spleen: The spleen is a rather soft and fragile organ, and although it is somewhat protected by the ribs, it is often ruptured in abdominal injuries. Because the spleen is a reservoir for blood, this results in severe internal hemorrhage and shock, which may lead to death if it is not stopped. A splenectomy, surgical removal of the spleen, may be necessary to stop the bleeding. ■

Figure 12-7 Composition of the blood. (From Applegate E: *The anatomy and physiology learning system*, ed 4, St Louis, 2011, Saunders.)

- It functions in pH regulation through the action of buffers in the blood.

Functions of the blood that are in the protection category include the following:

- Its clotting mechanisms prevent fluid loss through hemorrhage when blood vessels are damaged.
- Certain cells in the blood, the phagocytic white blood cells (WBCs), help to protect the body against microorganisms that cause disease by engulfing and destroying the agent.
- Antibodies in the plasma help protect against disease by their reactions with offending agents.

COMPOSITION OF BLOOD

When a sample of blood is spun in a centrifuge, the cells and cell fragments are separated from the liquid part of the blood (Figure 12-7). Because the *formed elements* are heavier than the liquid, they are packed in the bottom of the tube by the centrifugal force. The straw-colored liquid on the top is the *plasma*. Figure 12-7 illustrates that the plasma accounts for about 55% of the blood volume and red blood cells (RBCs) make up the remaining 45% of the volume. The WBCs and platelets form a thin white layer, called the "buffy coat," between the plasma and RBCs.

Plasma

Plasma, the liquid portion of the blood, is about 90% water. The remaining portion consists of more than 100 different organic and inorganic solutes dissolved in the water. Because plasma is a transport medium, its solutes are continuously changing as substances are added or removed by the cells. With a healthy diet, the plasma is normally in a state of dynamic balance that is maintained by various homeostatic mechanisms.

Plasma Proteins

Plasma proteins are the most abundant of the solutes in the plasma. These proteins normally remain in the blood and

interstitial fluid and are not used for energy. The three major classes of plasma proteins are albumins, globulins, and fibrinogen.

Albumins account for about 60% of the plasma proteins. Albumin molecules are produced in the liver and are the smallest of the plasma protein molecules. Because they are so abundant, they contribute to the osmotic pressure of the blood and play an important role in maintaining fluid balance between the blood and interstitial fluid. If the osmotic pressure of the blood decreases, fluid moves from the blood vessels into the interstitial spaces, which results in edema. This also decreases blood volume and in severe cases may reduce blood pressure. When blood osmotic pressure increases, fluid moves from the interstitial spaces into the blood vessels and increases blood volume. This increases blood pressure and decreases the amount of water available to the cells.

Globulins account for about 36% of the plasma proteins. Three types of globulins exist: alpha, beta, and gamma. Alpha and beta globulins are produced in the liver and function in transporting lipids and fat-soluble vitamins in the blood. Gamma globulins are the **antibodies** that function in immunity. These are produced in lymphoid tissue.

The remaining 4% of the plasma proteins consists of *fibrinogen,* which is the largest of the plasma protein molecules. It is produced in the liver and functions in blood clotting. During the clotting process, a series of reactions converts the soluble fibrinogen into insoluble fibrin, which forms the foundation of a blood clot. When blood clots in a test tube, the liquid that remains is called *serum.* It is similar to plasma but has no fibrinogen because the fibrinogen is converted to fibrin.

Other Solutes

Although protein molecules are the most abundant of the solutes in the plasma, there are additional solutes that play a significant role in homeostasis. Urea and uric acid are waste products of protein metabolism and may become toxic if allowed to accumulate. They are transported, as solutes in plasma, to the kidneys for excretion. The simple molecules that are the end products of digestion are transported as solutes in the plasma. Other plasma solutes include the respiratory gases, oxygen and carbon dioxide, and electrolytes that are important in muscle contraction, nerve impulse conduction, and pH of body fluids.

Formed Elements

The formed elements are cells and cell fragments suspended in the plasma. The three classes of formed elements are the **erythrocytes,** or RBCs; the **leukocytes,** or WBCs; and the **thrombocytes,** or platelets.

The production of these formed elements, or blood cells, is called **hematopoiesis** (hemopoiesis). Before birth, hematopoiesis occurs primarily in the liver and spleen. After birth, most production is limited to the red bone marrow in specific regions of the body, but some WBCs are

Erythrocytes
Biconcave disks; no nucleus; 7 to 8 μm in diameter; 4.5 to 6.0 million/mm³
Function to transport oxygen and carbon dioxide

Leukocytes
Nucleated cells; 5000 to 9000/mm³
Function as part of body's defense against disease

Neutrophils
Nucleus with 2 to 5 lobes; indistinct granules in cytoplasm; 12 to 15 μm in diameter 60% to 70% of total WBCs
Function in phagocytosis

Eosinophils
Bilobed nucleus; red-staining granules in cytoplasm; 10 to 12 μm in diameter 2% to 4% of total WBCs
Function to counteract histamine in allergic reactions; destroy parasitic worms

Basophils
U-shaped or bilobed nucleus; granules in cytoplasm stain blue; 10 to 12 μm in diameter
Less than 1% of total WBCs
Function to release histamine and the anticoagulant heparin; called *mast cells*, in the tissues

Lymphocytes
Agranulocyte; small cell with large round nucleus; 6 to 8 μm in diameter
20% to 25% of total WBCs
Function in immunity; produce antibodies

Monocytes
Agranulocyte; large cells with bean-shaped nucleus; may be 20 μm in diameter
3% to 8% of total WBCs
Function in phagocytosis; engulf relatively large particles; called *macrophages* in tissues

Thrombocytes
Cell fragments of megakaryocytes; 2 to 5 μm in diameter
250,000 to 500,000/mm³
Function in hemostasis by forming platelet plug and releasing factors necessary for blood clotting

Figure 12-8 Formed elements in the blood. (From Applegate E: *The anatomy and physiology learning system,* ed 4, St Louis, 2011, Saunders.)

produced in lymphoid tissue. All types of formed elements develop from a single cell type. The precursor cell, or stem cell, is called a **hemocytoblast**. Seven different cell lines develop from the hemocytoblast. Figure 12-8 illustrates the formed elements.

Erythrocytes

Characteristics and Functions

Erythrocytes, or RBCs, are the most numerous of the formed elements. The normal RBC range for a woman is 4 to 5.5 million RBCs per cubic millimeter (mm³) of blood.

The normal RBC range for a man is 4.5 to 6.2 million RBCs/mm³ of blood.

Erythrocytes are tiny biconcave discs about 7.5 micrometers (μm) in diameter. They are thin in the middle and thicker around the periphery. The shape of the RBC provides a combination of flexibility for moving through tiny capillaries along with a maximum surface area for the diffusion of gases. Mature RBCs are anucleate, meaning they do not have a nucleus. During development the nucleus is lost from the cell, presumably to give the cell more room for hemoglobin. Because the mature cells are anucleate, they cannot undergo mitosis, which means that replacement cells have to develop from the stem cells. The primary function of erythrocytes is to transport oxygen and, to a lesser extent, carbon dioxide. This function is directly related to the **hemoglobin** within the RBC.

Production of Erythrocytes

Erythrocyte production, specifically called **erythropoiesis,** is regulated by a negative feedback mechanism that uses the hormone **erythropoietin** to stimulate erythrocyte production (Figure 12-9). The liver produces erythropoietin in an inactive form and secretes it into the blood. The kidneys produce **renal erythropoietic factor** (REF), which activates the erythropoietin. When blood oxygen concentration is low, the kidneys release REF into the blood, which activates the erythropoietin, which then stimulates the red bone marrow to produce RBCs. The additional RBCs combine with oxygen to increase the blood oxygen concentration. As blood oxygen concentration increases, levels of REF and active erythropoietin decrease and RBC production decreases. This is an example of negative feedback.

Iron, vitamin B₁₂, and folic acid are essential to normal RBC production. The iron is necessary for the synthesis of normal hemoglobin. Iron deficiency anemia results when there is a lack of iron in the diet. This results in a reduced amount of hemoglobin, which decreases the blood's

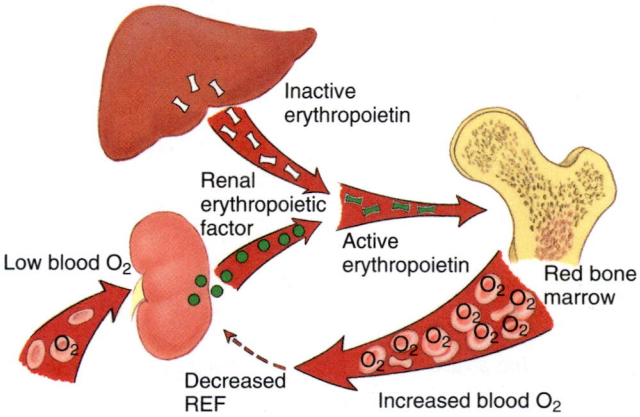

Figure 12-9 Regulation of erythrocyte production. The liver secretes inactive erythropoietin into the blood. In response to low blood O₂, the kidneys release renal erythropoietic factor (REF) into the blood. This activates the erythropoietin, which stimulates the bone marrow to produce red blood cells. (From Applegate E: *The anatomy and physiology learning system,* ed 4, St Louis, 2011, Saunders.)

oxygen-carrying capacity. All cells in the body require vitamins B₁₂ and folic acid for normal formation. This is especially significant in erythrocytes because of the large numbers produced every day. Certain cells in the stomach produce *intrinsic factor,* which is a factor necessary for the absorption of vitamin B₁₂ in the intestines. Without intrinsic factor, vitamin B₁₂ (even though present in the diet) cannot be absorbed. This results in a condition known as *pernicious anemia.*

Destruction of Erythrocytes

Normal erythrocytes live for approximately 120 days. During this time they travel thousands of miles as they circulate throughout the body. Normally the erythrocytes have a flexible cell membrane that allows them to bend and squeeze through the capillaries. As they age, however, their membrane loses its elasticity and becomes fragile. When they are defective or worn out, **macrophages,** which are phagocytic cells in the spleen and liver, remove them from circulation, and they are replaced by an equal number of new cells. Under typical conditions, more than 2 million erythrocytes are destroyed and replaced every second. Bilirubin, a yellow pigment, is a by-product of RBC destruction. It becomes a part of bile and is secreted by the liver.

Leukocytes
Characteristics and Functions

In general, *leukocytes* (WBCs) are larger than erythrocytes, but they are fewer in number. A normal WBC count ranges from 4500 to 11,000/mm³. All leukocytes are derived from hemocytoblast stem cells (see Figure 12-8), but they do not lose their nuclei or accumulate hemoglobin during development. The lack of hemoglobin makes them appear pale in contrast to erythrocytes.

Even though they are considered to be blood cells, leukocytes do most of their work in the tissues. They use the blood as a transport medium. Some are phagocytic, others produce antibodies, some secrete histamine and heparin, and others neutralize histamine. Leukocytes are able to move through the capillary walls into the tissue spaces, a process called **diapedesis.** In the tissue spaces they provide a defense against organisms that cause disease.

Types of Leukocytes

Blood contains two main groups of leukocytes. The cells that develop granules in the cytoplasm are called **granulocytes,** or granular leukocytes, and those that do not have granules are called **agranulocytes,** or nongranular leukocytes. *Neutrophils, eosinophils,* and *basophils* are granular leukocytes. *Monocytes* and *lymphocytes* are nongranular leukocytes. Because WBCs are clear and colorless, they must be stained first with an appropriate dye (usually Wright stain) before they can be identified under the microscope. The nucleus, cytoplasm, and any granules in the cytoplasm take on the characteristic color of their cell type, which aids in proper identification. The five types of WBCs are described here, along with their reactions to Wright stain.

Neutrophils are the most common type of leukocyte and make up 50% to 70% of the total number of WBCs. They are characterized by a purple, multilobed nucleus (usually three to five lobes) and many fine granules in the cytoplasm that stain a violet-pink. Neutrophils are the first leukocytes to respond to tissue damage, by engulfing bacteria by phagocytosis. The number of neutrophils increases during acute infections.

Eosinophils make up 1% to 4% of the WBCs. They are characterized by a segmented nucleus, usually of no more than two lobes. Large granules found in the cytoplasm stain a bright reddish orange. Eosinophils neutralize histamine, and their number increases during allergic reactions. They also destroy parasitic worms.

Basophils are the least numerous of the leukocytes. The normal range for basophils is 0% to 1% of the WBCs. A basophil is about the same size as an eosinophil and has an S-shaped nucleus. The cytoplasm has large, coarse granules that stain a dark bluish-black and almost completely obscure the details of the nucleus. In the tissues, basophils secrete histamine and heparin. Histamine dilates blood vessels to increase blood flow to damaged tissues. It also dilates blood vessels in allergic reactions. Heparin is an anticoagulant that inhibits blood clot formation.

Lymphocytes account for 20% to 35% of the WBCs in the blood. Lymphocytes have a large round or slightly indented nucleus that stains a deep purplish-blue. A small rim of sky-blue cytoplasm around the nucleus contains few or no granules. Lymphocytes are involved with the immune system and the production of antibodies. An increase in lymphocytes usually occurs with certain viral diseases, including infectious mononucleosis, mumps, chickenpox, rubella, and viral hepatitis.

Monocytes are the largest of the WBCs and make up 3% to 8% of the leukocytes in the blood. Monocytes have a U-shaped or kidney-shaped nucleus surrounded by abundant cytoplasm that stains grayish-blue. When monocytes leave the blood and enter the tissues, they are called **macrophages.** In damaged tissues, the macrophages engulf bacteria and cellular debris to finish the cleanup process started by the neutrophils.

Thrombocytes

Thrombocytes, or *platelets,* are not complete cells but small fragments of large cells called **megakaryocytes.** Megakaryocytes develop from hemocytoblasts in the red bone marrow. Platelets are one third to one half the size of an erythrocyte, and an average platelet count ranges from 150,000 to 500,000 platelets/mm³ of blood.

Thrombocytes become sticky and clump together to form platelet plugs that close breaks and tears in blood vessels. They also initiate the formation of blood clots.

HEMOSTASIS

Blood vessels that are torn or cut permit blood to escape into the surrounding tissues or to the outside of the body.

This has damaging effects on the tissues and, in cases of excessive blood loss, may result in death. Whenever blood vessels are injured, several reactions occur that attempt to minimize blood loss and tissue damage. The stoppage of bleeding is called **hemostasis.** It includes three separate but interrelated processes: vascular constriction, platelet plug formation, and coagulation.

Vascular Constriction

The first response to blood vessel injury is contraction of the smooth muscle in the vessel walls. This creates a *vascular constriction* that restricts the flow of blood through the opening in the vessel. The initial constriction lasts for only a few minutes but allows enough time for the other aspects of hemostasis to begin. As platelets accumulate at the site of the injury, they secrete serotonin, a chemical that stimulates smooth muscle contraction and prolongs the vascular constriction.

Platelet Plug Formation

Normally platelets do not stick to one another or to the lining of blood vessel walls. When the lining of the blood vessel breaks, the underlying connective tissue is exposed. The connective tissue attracts platelets and they accumulate in the damaged region, where they adhere to the connective tissue and to one another. This creates a mass of platelets, a *platelet plug,* that obstructs the tear in the vessel. Normal daily activities create numerous tears in minute blood vessels, and these are closed by platelet plugs so that there is no blood loss or damage to surrounding tissues.

Coagulation

The third and most effective mechanism in hemostasis is the formation of a blood clot, or **coagulation.** The blood contains factors called *procoagulants* that promote clotting. It also contains *anticoagulants,* which inhibit clotting. Normally the anticoagulants predominate and override the procoagulants so that the blood remains fluid and does not clot. When vessels are damaged, the procoagulants increase their activity, which results in the formation of a clot.

The formation of a blood clot involves a complex series of chemical reactions and includes numerous clotting factors that are present in the plasma. Even though it is a complex process, it can be summarized in three main steps, as illustrated in Figure 12-10.

1. Platelets and damaged tissues release chemicals that initiate a series of reactions that result in the formation of *prothrombin activator.*
2. In the presence of calcium ions and prothrombin activator, *prothrombin* in the plasma is converted from an inactive form to active *thrombin.*
3. Thrombin, in the presence of calcium ions, acts as an enzyme to convert inactive and soluble *fibrinogen* into active and insoluble *fibrin.* The fibrin threads form a mesh that adheres to the damaged tissue and traps blood cells and platelets to form the clot.

Figure 12-10 Hemostasis. The first response to vessel injury is a vascular spasm. This is followed by platelet plug formation. The third and most effective mechanism of hemostasis is the formation of a blood clot. (From Applegate E: *The anatomy and physiology learning system,* ed 4, St Louis, 2011, Saunders.)

Platelets and all the necessary clotting factors must be available for successful clot formation. The liver produces most of the clotting factors, and many of them require vitamin K for their synthesis. Numerous reactions in the clotting process also require calcium ions. A low platelet count (thrombocytopenia), deficiency of vitamin K or calcium, and liver dysfunction can impair the clotting process.

After a clot has formed, the fibrin strands contract. This process, called *clot retraction,* causes the clot to condense or shrink. Clot retraction pulls the edges of the damaged tissue closer together, reduces the flow of blood to the area, reduces the probability of infection, and enhances healing. Fibroblasts migrate into the clot and form fibrous connective tissue that repairs the damaged area. As healing occurs, the clot is dissolved by a process called *fibrinolysis.*

BLOOD TYPES

ABO Blood Groups

The ABO blood groups are based on the presence or absence of certain antigens called *agglutinogens* on the surface of the

Figure 12-11 Agglutinogens (antigens) and agglutinins (antibodies) involved in the ABO blood groups. (From Applegate E: *The anatomy and physiology learning system,* ed 4, St Louis, 2011, Saunders.)

RBC membrane. These antigens, A and B, are inherited; consequently, blood types are also inherited. Type A blood has type A antigen; type B blood has type B antigen; type AB blood has both type A and type B antigens; and type O blood has neither type A nor type B antigen (Figure 12-11). Certain blood antibodies called *agglutinins* develop in the plasma shortly after birth. Specifically, a person with type A blood develops B antibodies; a person with type B blood develops A antibodies; a person with type AB blood develops neither A nor B antibodies; and a person with type O blood develops both A and B antibodies (see Figure 12-11).

Blood types are important in transfusions. If the blood types are different, the antibodies of the recipient may react with the antigens of the donor and cause hemolysis in the blood. Figure 12-12 illustrates agglutination and hemolysis.

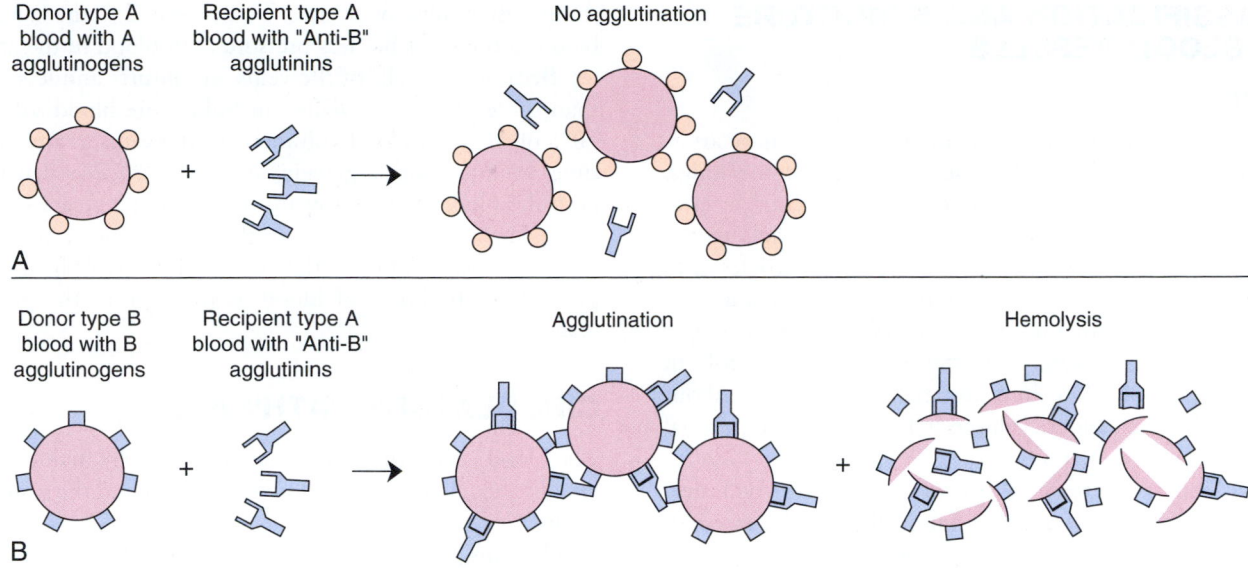

Figure 12-12 Agglutination reactions. **A,** Type A donor and type A recipient results in no agglutination. **B,** Type B donor and type A recipient results in agglutination and hemolysis. (From Applegate E: *The anatomy and physiology learning system,* ed 4, St Louis, 2011, Saunders.)

Rh Blood Groups

Even after the ABO blood groups were well established and accurate blood typing procedures had been developed, there were still unexplained cases of transfusion reactions. This led to more research, which led to the discovery of the *Rh factor,* so named because it was first studied in the rhesus monkey.

People are Rh positive (Rh+) if they have Rh antigens on the surface of their RBCs. About 85% of people are Rh+. The other 15% do not have the Rh antigens and are Rh negative (Rh−). The presence or absence of Rh antigens is an inherited trait. Normally, neither Rh+ nor Rh− individuals have Rh antibodies. If an Rh− person is exposed to Rh+ blood, either through a blood transfusion or by transfer of blood between a mother and fetus, the Rh− individual develops Rh antibodies. If that individual is exposed to Rh+ blood a second time, a transfusion reaction results. When transfusions are given, it is necessary to match both the Rh type and the ABO type.

BLOOD VESSELS

Blood vessels are the channels through which blood is distributed to body tissues. The vessels make up two closed systems of tubes that begin and end at the heart (Figure 12-13). One system, the *pulmonary vessels,* transports blood from the right ventricle to the lungs and back to the left atrium. The other system, the *systemic vessels,* carries blood from the left ventricle to the tissues in all parts of the body and then returns the blood to the right atrium. Based on their structure and function, blood vessels are classified as arteries, capillaries, or veins.

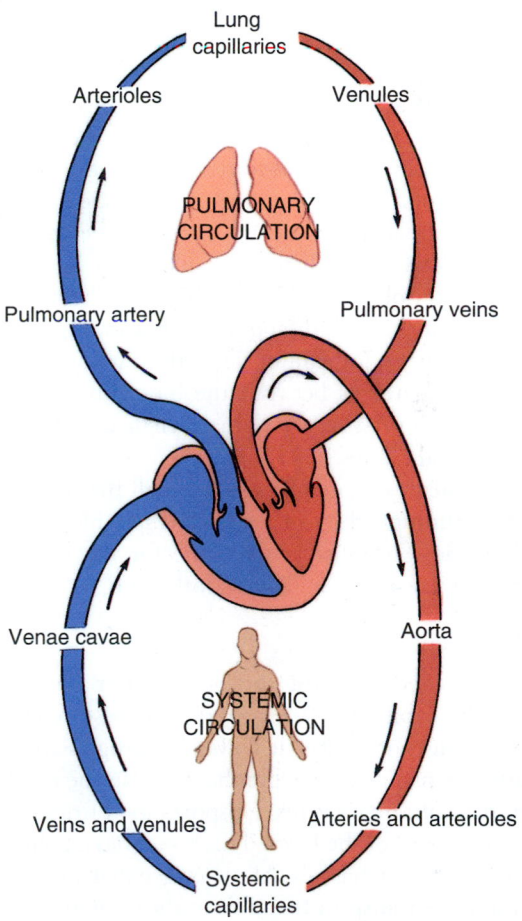

Figure 12-13 Scheme of circulation. In pulmonary circulation, arteries take blood from the right ventricle to the lungs, and veins return the blood to the left atrium. In systemic circulation, arteries take blood from the left ventricle to the body tissues, and veins return the blood to the right atrium. (From Applegate E: *The anatomy and physiology learning system,* ed 4, St Louis, 2011, Saunders.)

CLASSIFICATION AND STRUCTURE OF BLOOD VESSELS

Arteries

Arteries carry blood away from the heart. Pulmonary arteries transport blood from the right ventricle to the lungs. This blood has a low oxygen content. Systemic arteries transport oxygenated blood from the left ventricle to the body tissues. Blood is pumped from the ventricles into large elastic arteries that branch repeatedly into smaller and smaller arteries until the branching results in microscopic arteries called *arterioles*. The arterioles play a key role in regulating blood flow into the tissue capillaries. About 10% of the total blood volume is in the systemic arterial system at any given time.

The wall of an artery consists of three layers. The innermost layer is the *tunica intima* (also called *tunica interna*). The middle layer is the *tunica media,* which consists of smooth muscle and is usually the thickest layer. It not only provides support for the vessel but also changes vessel diameter to regulate blood flow and blood pressure. The outermost layer is the *tunica externa* or *tunica adventitia.*

Capillaries

Capillaries are the smallest and most numerous of the blood vessels. They form the connection between the vessels that carry blood away from the heart (arteries) and the vessels that return blood to the heart (veins). They are the continuation of the smallest arterioles. Arterioles are the smallest vessels that have three distinguishable layers in their wall. When the arterioles branch into capillaries, the middle and outer layers of the wall disappear so that the capillary wall is only a thin endothelium. This thin wall permits the exchange of materials between the blood in the capillary and the adjacent tissue cells. This exchange is the primary function of capillaries.

The diameter of a capillary is so small that erythrocytes must pass through the capillaries in single file. This slows the blood flow to allow ample time for the transport of substances across the capillary endothelium.

Veins

Veins carry blood toward the heart. After blood passes through the capillaries, it enters the smallest veins, called *venules.* From the venules, it flows into progressively larger and larger veins until it reaches the heart. In the pulmonary circuit, the pulmonary veins transport blood from the lungs to the left atrium of the heart. This blood has a high oxygen content because it has just been oxygenated in the lungs. Systemic veins transport blood from the body tissues to the right atrium of the heart. This blood has a reduced oxygen content because the oxygen has been used for metabolic activities in the tissue cells.

The walls of veins have the same three layers as the arteries. Although all the layers are present, there is less smooth muscle and connective tissue. This makes the walls of veins thinner than those of arteries. This is related to the fact that blood in the veins has less pressure than blood in the arteries. Because the walls of the veins are thinner and less rigid than those of arteries, veins can hold more blood. Almost 70% of the total blood volume is in the veins at any given time. Medium and large veins have *venous valves* that help keep the blood flowing toward the heart. These are similar to the SL valves associated with the heart. Venous valves are especially important in the arms and legs, where they prevent the backflow of blood in response to the pull of gravity.

CIRCULATORY PATHWAYS

The blood vessels of the body are functionally divided into two distinct circuits: the pulmonary circuit and the systemic circuit.

The pump for the pulmonary circuit, which circulates blood through the lungs, is the right ventricle. The left ventricle is the pump for the systemic circuit, which provides the blood supply for the tissue cells of the body.

Pulmonary Circuit

The pulmonary circuit takes blood from the right side of the heart to the lungs and then returns it to the left side of the heart (see Figures 12-4 and 12-13). Oxygen-poor blood, which has increased levels of carbon dioxide, is returned to the right atrium from the tissue cells of the body. It passes through the tricuspid valve into the right ventricle. During ventricular systole, the blood is ejected through the pulmonary SL valve into the pulmonary trunk, which divides into the right and left pulmonary arteries. Each pulmonary artery enters a lung and repeatedly divides into smaller and smaller vessels until they become capillaries. The capillaries of the lungs form networks that surround the air sacs, or alveoli, of the lungs. Here CO_2 diffuses from the capillary blood into the alveoli of the lungs, and O_2 diffuses from the alveoli into the blood. The newly oxygenated blood enters pulmonary venules, which form progressively larger veins, until two pulmonary veins emerge from each lung and carry the blood to the left atrium. In the pulmonary circuit, the arteries carry deoxygenated blood away from the heart and the veins carry oxygenated blood to the heart.

Systemic Circuit

The systemic circulation provides the functional blood supply to all body tissues. It carries oxygen and nutrients to the cells and picks up carbon dioxide and waste products. Systemic circulation carries oxygenated blood from the left ventricle, through the arteries, to the capillaries in the tissues of the body. The major systemic arteries are illustrated in Figure 12-14. From the tissue capillaries, the deoxygenated blood returns through a system of veins to the right atrium of the heart. The major systemic veins are illustrated in Figure 12-15.

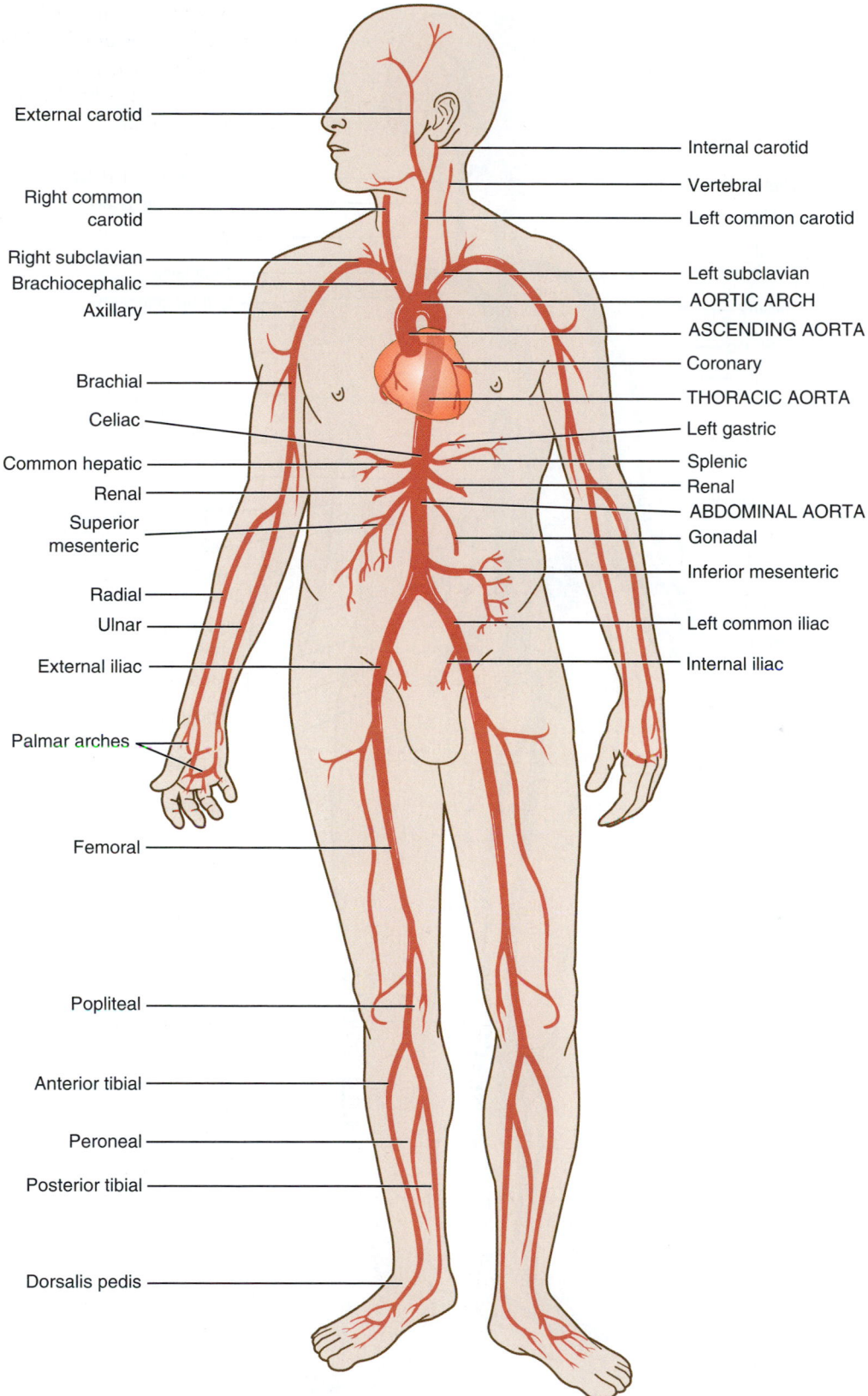

External carotid

Right common
carotid

Right subclavian
Brachiocephalic
Axillary

Brachial

Celiac

Common hepatic
Renal
Superior
mesenteric

Radial
Ulnar

External iliac

Palmar arches

Femoral

Popliteal

Anterior tibial

Peroneal

Posterior tibial

Dorsalis pedis

Internal carotid
Vertebral
Left common carotid

Left subclavian
AORTIC ARCH
ASCENDING AORTA
Coronary
THORACIC AORTA
Left gastric
Splenic
Renal
ABDOMINAL AORTA
Gonadal
Inferior mesenteric

Left common iliac
Internal iliac

Figure 12-14 Major systemic arteries. (From Applegate E: *The anatomy and physiology learning system,*
ed 4, St Louis, 2011, Saunders.)

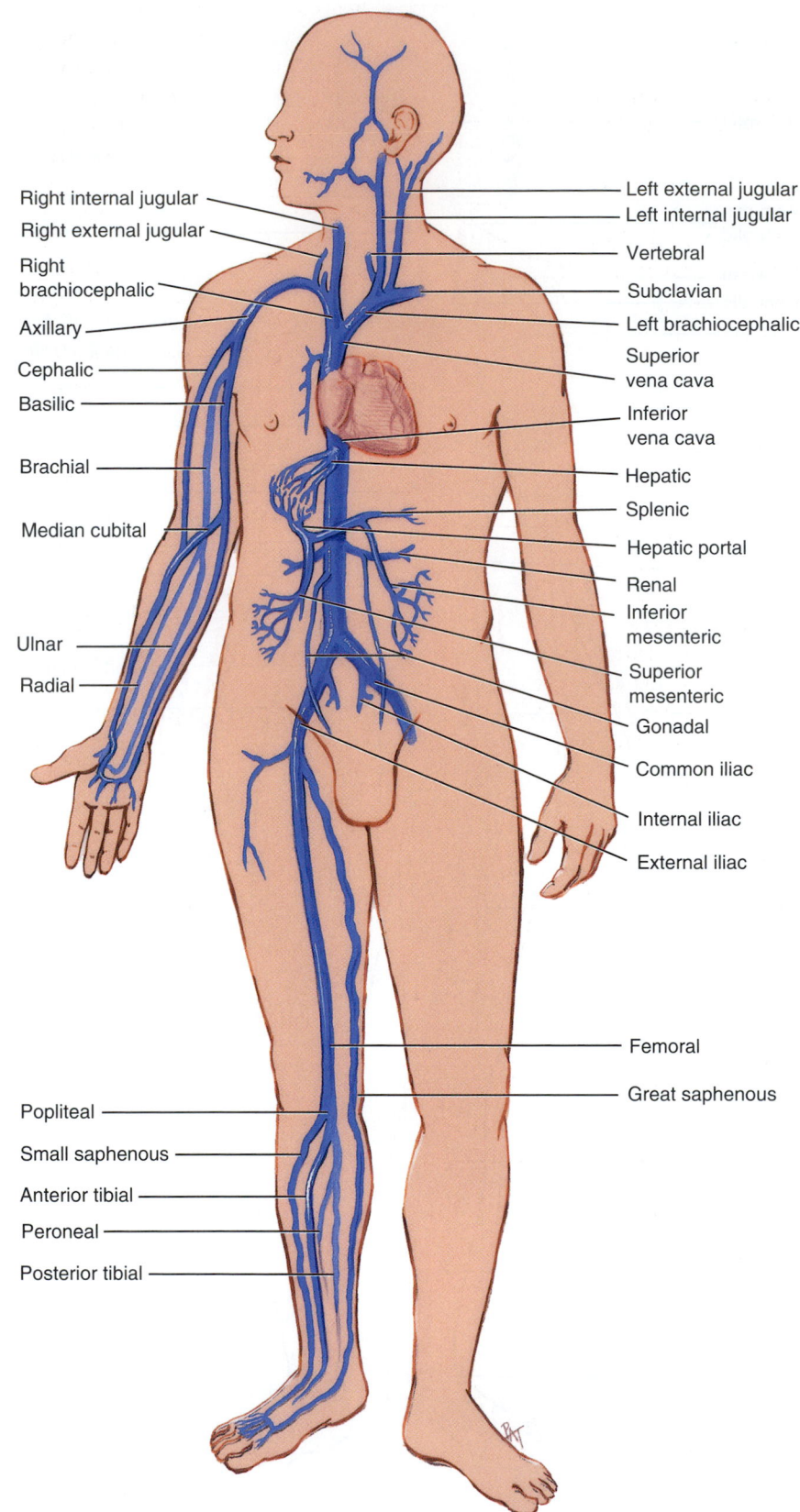

Right internal jugular
Right external jugular
Right brachiocephalic
Axillary
Cephalic
Basilic
Brachial
Median cubital
Ulnar
Radial

Left external jugular
Left internal jugular
Vertebral
Subclavian
Left brachiocephalic
Superior vena cava
Inferior vena cava
Hepatic
Splenic
Hepatic portal
Renal
Inferior mesenteric
Superior mesenteric
Gonadal
Common iliac
Internal iliac
External iliac

Femoral
Great saphenous

Popliteal
Small saphenous
Anterior tibial
Peroneal
Posterior tibial

Figure 12-15 Major systemic veins. (From Applegate E: *The anatomy and physiology learning system,* ed 4, St Louis, 2011, Saunders.)

LYMPHATIC SYSTEM

The lymphatic system has three primary functions. It returns excess interstitial fluid to the blood to maintain homeostasis between the fluid in the blood and the fluid that surrounds tissue cells. The second function deals with the absorption of fats and fat-soluble vitamins. These substances are absorbed from the intestinal tract into specialized lymph capillaries. The third function of the lymphatic system is defense against invading microorganisms and disease.

LYMPH

The fluid in the lymphatic vessels is called *lymph*. It is similar in composition to blood plasma and is derived from it. At the arteriole end of a capillary, some of the plasma escapes from the blood vessel and enters the tissue spaces. About 90% of this fluid reenters the venule end of the capillary. The remaining 10% remains in the tissue spaces as interstitial fluid. As the fluid accumulates, it is picked up by tiny lymph vessels and becomes lymph. This transition of fluid from blood plasma to interstitial fluid to lymph and eventually back to the blood prevents edema and helps maintain blood volume, plasma protein concentration, and blood pressure.

LYMPHATIC VESSELS

Lymphatic vessels carry fluid away from the tissues and return it to the venous system. The smallest lymphatic vessels are the lymph capillaries, which are small blind-ended sacs intertwined with the blood capillaries in the tissue spaces. These tiny lymph capillaries merge to form larger and larger vessels until the lymph enters the two lymphatic ducts. The **right lymphatic duct** receives lymph from the upper right quadrant of the body and empties into the right subclavian vein. The **thoracic duct** drains lymph from the remaining three quadrants of the body and empties into the left subclavian vein. Lymph nodes that filter the lymph are located along the various vessels of the lymphatic system. Like veins, the walls of lymph vessels are thin and have valves. Because there is no pump to provide pressure, the flow of lymph is sporadic and sluggish. The force to create pressure gradients for flow must come from external sources such as skeletal muscle contraction and respiratory movements. Anything that interferes with the flow of lymph, such as an obstruction or surgical ligation, may cause tissue fluid to accumulate, resulting in edema.

LYMPHATIC ORGANS

Lymphatic organs are characterized by clusters of lymphocytes and other cells, such as macrophages, with a meshlike framework of connective tissue fibers. When the body is exposed to foreign substances, the lymphocytes proliferate

then enter the blood and travel to the site of the foreign substance. This is part of the body's immune response that attempts to destroy the invading agent. The lymph nodes, tonsils, spleen, and thymus are lymphatic organs.

Lymph nodes are small bean-shaped structures that are located along the lymphatic vessels. The primary function of lymph nodes is to filter the lymph as it flows through the vessels so that the lymph is cleansed by lymphocytes and macrophages before it enters the blood. Even though lymph nodes are widely distributed in the body, there are three superficial regions where they tend to cluster. These are the *inguinal nodes* in the groin region, the *axillary nodes* in the armpit, and the *cervical nodes* in the neck. These are illustrated in Figure 12-16. There are no lymph nodes in the central nervous system.

Tonsils are clusters of lymphatic tissue just under the mucous membrane of the nose, mouth, and throat. The *pharyngeal tonsils* are near the opening of the nasal cavity in the pharynx. These are sometimes called *adenoids*. The *palatine tonsils* are located near the opening of the oral cavity into the pharynx. These are the ones commonly referred to as "tonsils." The *lingual tonsils* are located near the base of the tongue. Lymphocytes and macrophages in the tonsils help protect against pathogens that may enter the body through the nose and mouth.

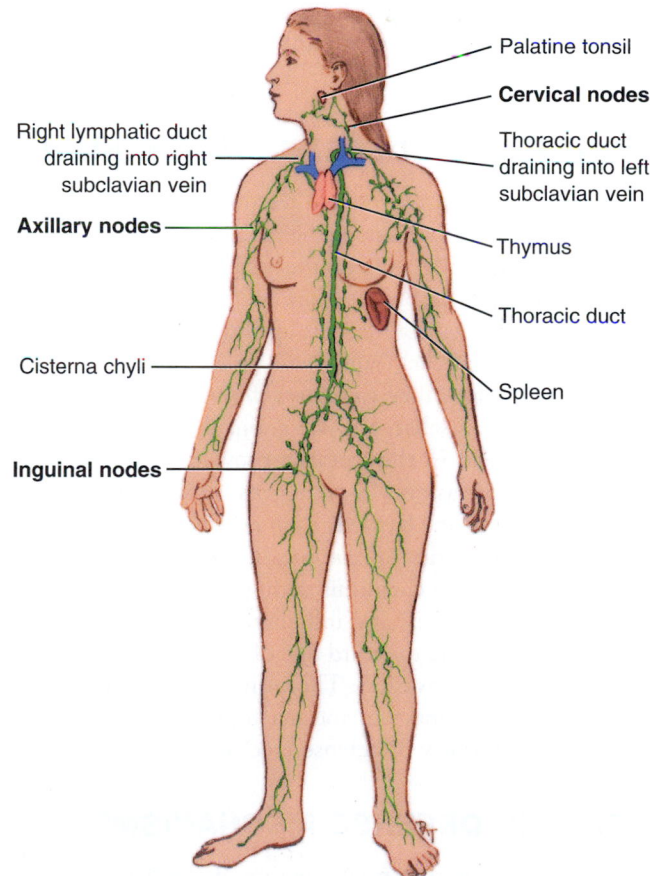

Figure 12-16 Location of the clusters of superficial lymph nodes. (From Applegate E: *The anatomy and physiology learning system,* ed 4, St Louis, 2011, Saunders.)

The *spleen* is located in the upper left quadrant of the abdominal cavity, just under the diaphragm and behind the stomach. It is the largest lymphatic organ. The spleen filters blood in much the same way as a lymph node filters lymph. Lymphocytes and macrophages react with pathogens in the blood and attempt to destroy them. The spleen also acts as a reservoir for blood and destroys old, worn-out erythrocytes.

The *thymus* is a soft, two-lobed organ that is located anterior to the ascending aorta and posterior to the sternum. It is relatively large in infants and children, but after puberty it begins to decrease in size so that in older adults it is quite small. The primary function of the thymus is the maturation of special lymphocytes called *T lymphocytes*. It also produces the hormone *thymosin,* which stimulates the maturation of lymphocytes in other lymphatic organs.

RESISTANCE TO DISEASE

To remain healthy, the body must counteract the effects of pathogens and other harmful substances. This ability is called **resistance,** and the lack of resistance is **susceptibility.** Resistance is dependent on a variety of defense mechanisms. **Nonspecific defense mechanisms** act against all harmful agents; **specific defense mechanisms** are effective against only certain agents. Specific defense mechanisms provide *immunity.* All defense mechanisms act together to maintain a healthy body.

NONSPECIFIC DEFENSE MECHANISMS

Nonspecific mechanisms provide the initial defense against invading agents regardless of their nature. Barriers against entry into the body present the first line of nonspecific defense. Intact or unbroken skin and mucous membranes are effective mechanical barriers against entry. The motion of fluids such as tears, saliva, and urine flushes invading agents away before they can enter the body. Lysozymes in tears and saliva, sebaceous secretions on the skin, and hydrochloric acid in the stomach provide chemical deterrents against invasion. If pathogens succeed in passing through the first-line barriers, then nonspecific second-line barriers attempt to destroy the invading agents. The second-line barriers include chemicals such as interferon and complement, phagocytosis, and inflammation. Specific defense mechanisms provide the third line of defense, or immunity, against microbial invasion. The primary cells involved in immunity are lymphocytes and macrophages. Figure 12-17 provides an overview of defense mechanisms.

SPECIFIC DEFENSE MECHANISMS

In contrast to the nonspecific nature of the first two lines of defense, *specific defense mechanisms* are programmed to be selective and act against specific pathogens. This characteristic is called *specificity.* The second characteristic of

immunity is *memory.* Once the body has been exposed to a particular invading agent, the system "remembers" it and launches a quicker attack when the agent enters the body again.

For the immune system to function properly, lymphocytes must recognize the difference between "self" and "non-self." During development, lymphocytes are programmed to recognize the proteins and other large molecules that belong to the body. Molecules that are not recognized as "self" are interpreted as "non-self," and the immune system attempts to destroy them. These "non-self" molecules are called **antigens** and are usually proteins or large polysaccharide molecules on the surface of the cell membrane. Usually the antigens that cause problems are foreign molecules that originate outside the body, but occasionally the body fails to recognize its own molecules and triggers an immune response against self. This is the basis of autoimmune diseases.

As indicated earlier in this chapter, lymphocytes develop from hemocytoblasts in the bone marrow. During fetal development immature lymphocytes are released into the blood. Some of these immature cells go to the thymus where they acquire the ability to distinguish between self and non-self molecules. These become *T lymphocytes* or *T cells.* Differentiated T cells leave the thymus, enter the blood, and are distributed to lymphoid tissue, especially lymph nodes where they are responsible for **cell-mediated immunity.** About 70% of the circulating lymphocytes are T cells. Developing lymphocytes that differentiate in some place other than the thymus are called *B lymphocytes* or *B cells.* These cells also are distributed to lymphoid tissue and are responsible for **antibody-mediated immunity,** or *humoral immunity.* B cells account for about 30% of circulating lymphocytes.

CELL-MEDIATED IMMUNITY

In **cell-mediated immunity,** T cells directly attack invading antigens. It is most effective against virus-infected cells, cancer cells, foreign tissue cells (transplant rejection), fungi, and protozoan parasites. When a foreign antigen enters the body, it is phagocytized by a macrophage, which presents it to a T cell with receptors for that specific antigen. This activates the T cell and it divides to produce four clones: *killer T cells* that directly destroy the cells with the offending antigen; *helper T cells* that stimulate B cells and promote the immune response; *suppressor T cells* that inhibit B cells and the immune response; and *memory T cells* that promote a faster and more intense response on subsequent exposure to the same antigen. Figure 12-18 illustrates the mechanism of cell-mediated immunity.

ANTIBODY-MEDIATED IMMUNITY

In **antibody-mediated immunity,** B cells are responsible for the production of **antibodies** that inactivate the invading antigens. Because antibodies are found in body fluids, this

Invasion by pathogens

Nonspecific defense   First-line barriers

Skin and mucous membranes   Fluids   Chemicals

Nonspecific defense   Second-line barriers

Chemical action of complement and interferon   Phagocytosis   Inflammation

Specific defense   Lymphocytes and macrophages

Cell-mediated immunity   Antibody-mediated immunity

Figure 12-17 Overview of defense mechanisms. Pathogens that are stopped from entering the body by the first-line barriers of nonspecific defense are represented by green dots. Others get through the first-line barriers but are stopped by nonspecific second-line barriers. These pathogens are represented by blue dots. Those that penetrate nonspecific defense mechanisms are subject to specific defense mechanisms. These pathogens are represented by the red dots. (From Applegate E: *The anatomy and physiology learning system,* ed 4, St Louis, 2011, Saunders.)

type of immunity is sometimes called *humoral immunity.* Antibody-mediated immunity is most effective against bacteria, viruses that are outside body cells, and toxins. It is also involved in allergic reactions. Like T cells, each type of B cell can respond to only one specific type of antigen. There must be a match between the receptor on the B cell and the antigen. When a foreign antigen enters the body, a macrophage engulfs and processes it, then presents it to specific B cells and helper T cells with receptors for that specific antigen. This activates the cells, and the helper T cells further stimulate the B cells to divide and form two clones: *plasma cells* that produce **antibodies,** and *memory B cells* that promote a faster and more intense response on subsequent exposure to the same antigen. Figure 12-19 illustrates the mechanism of antibody-mediated immunity.

All antibodies have a similar structure, but one part of the molecule differs so that each antibody is capable of reacting with only a specific antigen. Antibodies belong to a class of proteins called *globulins,* and because they are involved in immune reactions, they are called **immunoglobulins,** abbreviated Ig. There are five types of immunoglobulins: IgA, IgG, IgM, IgE, and IgD. IgG immunoglobulins

are called *gamma globulins.* Each class of immunoglobulin has a specific role in immunity. These are summarized in Table 12-1.

ACQUIRED IMMUNITY

There are four ways to acquire immunity. The terms *active* and *passive* refer to whose immune system responds to an antigen. Active immunity occurs when an individual's own body responds and produces memory cells. Passive immunity results when the immune agents develop in another person (or animal) and are transferred to an individual who was not previously immune. The terms *natural* and *artificial* refer to how the immunity is obtained. Natural immunity occurs when the immunity is acquired through normal everyday living without any deliberate action. Artificial immunity results when some deliberate action is taken, such as a vaccination. Combining these terms gives four types of acquired immunity: active natural immunity, active artificial immunity, passive natural immunity, and passive artificial immunity. These four types of immunity are summarized in Figure 12-20.

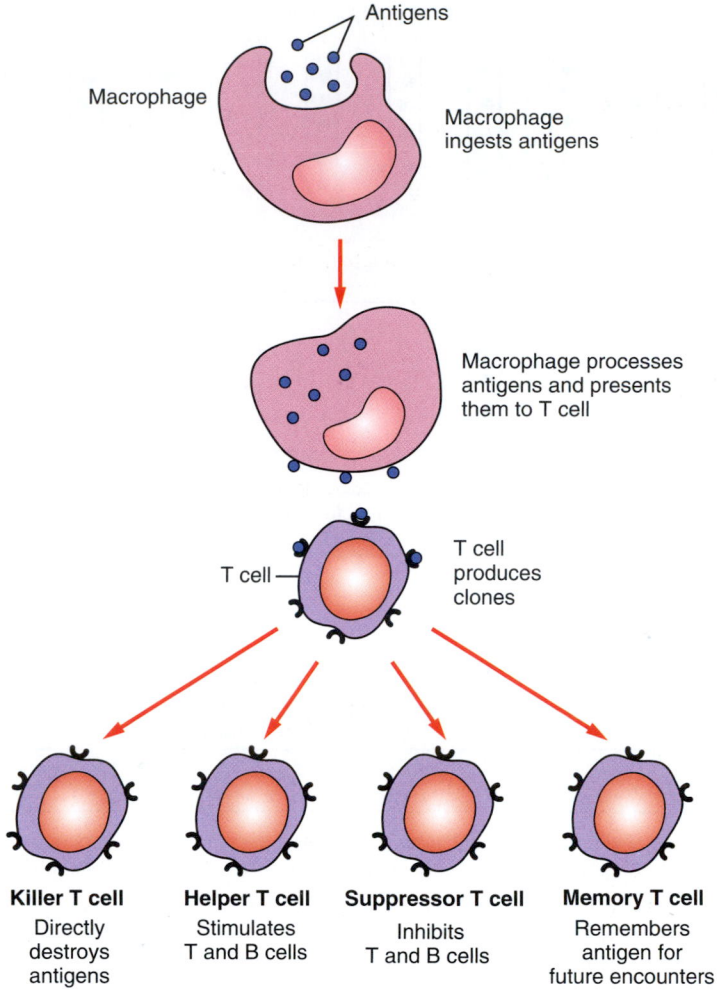

Figure 12-18 Cell-mediated immunity. Macrophage ingests antigens, processes them, and presents them to the T cell. The T cell produces four clones. (From Applegate E: *The anatomy and physiology learning system,* ed 4, St Louis, 2011, Saunders.)

AGING OF THE CIRCULATORY SYSTEM

Numerous "age-related" changes occur in the heart. How many of these are caused by an actual aging process and how many are caused by other factors are questions worth considering. Is it possible to lessen the effects of aging by adjusting lifestyle? Cardiac changes that were once thought to be the result of aging are now believed to be the consequence of a sedentary lifestyle that many consider their "reward" after retirement. Other cardiac changes are caused by a lifetime of habits that, although enjoyable at the time, take their toll later in life. It is difficult to isolate the aging process of the heart because it is so closely related to diet, exercise, and disease processes, but even when these factors are excluded, a clinical pattern of cardiac aging emerges.

In the absence of cardiovascular disease, the heart, particularly the left ventricle, tends to become slightly smaller in elderly people. This results partially from a decrease in the number and size of cardiac muscle cells and partially from the reduced demands placed on it by decreasing physical activity. However, because of cardiovascular disease, the heart is often enlarged.

A general thickening of the endocardium and valves of the heart occurs as part of the aging process. The valves tend to become more rigid and incompetent. Thus heart murmurs are detected more frequently in the elderly. Structural changes also occur throughout the conduction system as conducting myofibers are replaced with fibrous tissue. Usually this does not alter the resting pulse rate, but there is a greater-than-normal increase in heart rate in response to activity. Dysrhythmias are also more frequent.

Numerous disease processes that occur more frequently in the aging individual have an effect on the heart. Most notable of these is arteriosclerosis, or hardening of the arteries. This puts additional stress on the heart and aggravates the normal age-related changes. Although some degree of arteriosclerosis is probably inevitable in the aging process, a significant amount of vascular disease can be prevented by a proper diet, regular walking or other aerobic exercise, and the elimination of cigarette smoking. In other words, lifestyle probably has more effect on the cardiovascular system than aging.

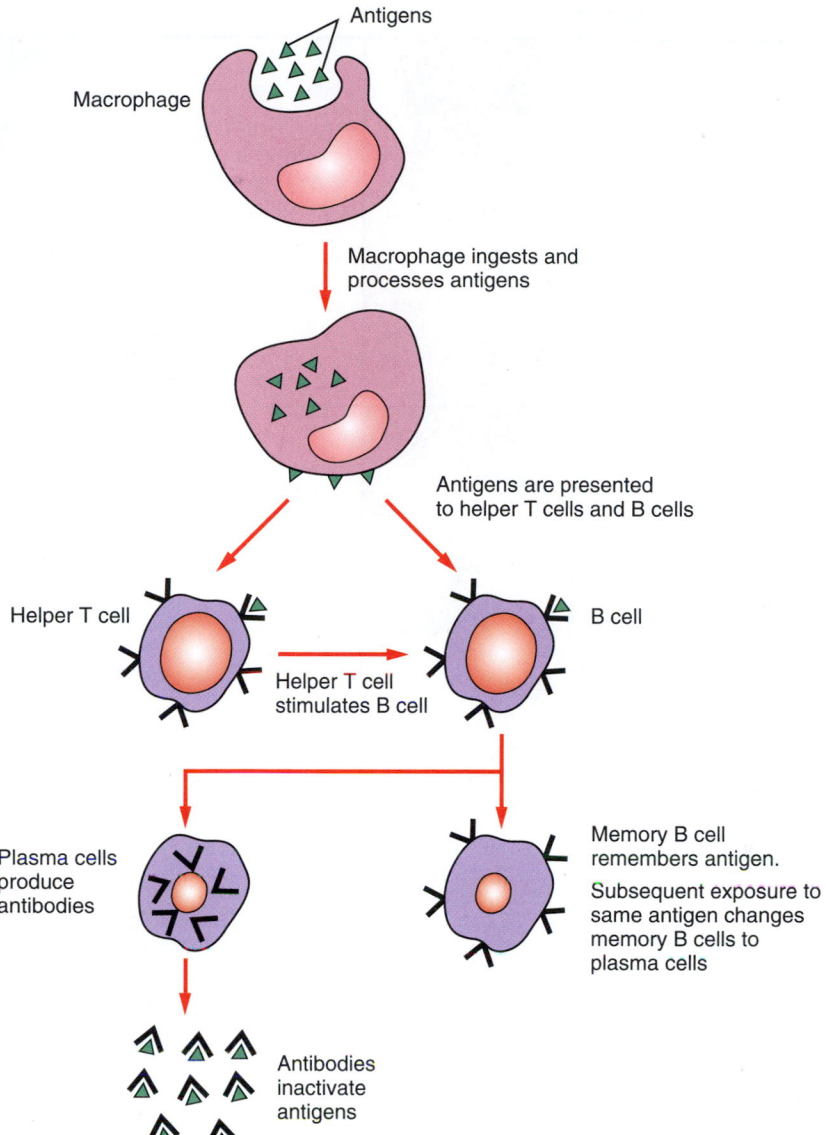

Figure 12-19 Antibody-mediated immunity. Macrophage ingests and processes antigen, then presents it to helper T cells and B cells. Helper T cells stimulate B cells to divide and produce two clones consisting of memory B cells and plasma cells. Plasma cells produce antibodies that inactivate the antigen. (From Applegate E: *The anatomy and physiology learning system,* ed 4, St Louis, 2011, Saunders.)

Table 12-1 Classes of Antibodies

Class	Percentage of Total	Location	Function
IgG	75% to 85%	Blood plasma	Major antibody in primary and secondary immune responses; inactivates antigen; neutralizes toxins; crosses placenta to provide immunity for newborn; responsible for Rh reactions
IgA	5% to 15%	Saliva, mucus, tears, breast milk	Protects mucous membranes for body surfaces; provides immunity for newborn
IgM	5% to 10%	Attached to B cells; released into plasma during immune response	Causes antigen to clump together; responsible for transfusion reactions in ABO blood typing system
IgD	0.2%	Attached to B cells	Receptor sites for antigens on B cells; binding with antigen results in B-cell activation
IgE	0.5%	Produced by plasma cells in mucous membranes and tonsils	Binds to mast cells and basophils, causing release of histamine; responsible for allergic reactions

(From Applegate E: *The anatomy and physiology learning system,* ed 4, St Louis, 2011, Saunders.)

Figure 12-20 Acquired immunity. (From Applegate E: *The anatomy and physiology learning system,* ed 4, St Louis, 2011, Saunders.)

Common Pathology of the Circulatory System

Disease	Signs and Symptoms	Etiology	Diagnosis and Treatment
Acquired immunodeficiency syndrome (AIDS)	Immune system is badly damaged, making an individual vulnerable to infections and opportunistic illnesses. The helper T cell (CD4) number falls below 200 cells/mm^3 in the blood.	Cause is the human immunodeficiency virus (HIV). AIDS is the final stage in the course of the disease.	Diagnosis relies on the HIV enzyme-linked immunosorbent assay (ELISA) and the HIV Western blot test. The helper T cell (CD4) number is below 200 cells/mm^3 in the blood. Early stages of HIV may be treated with antiretroviral therapy (ART). There is no cure. By the time HIV has progressed to AIDS, life expectancy is about 3 years.
Anemia	Fatigue and lethargy, pale skin, dizziness, cold hands and feet, headache, irregular heartbeat.	Most common cause is blood loss; dysfunction in syntheses of hemoglobin; excessive destruction of red blood cells.	Typically diagnosed by a routine blood test, but further testing may be necessary to determine underlying cause. Treatment depends on underlying cause. May need to replace blood cells through transfusion or increase iron or vitamin K in the diet.
Anemia, iron deficiency	Fatigue and lethargy, pale skin, dizziness, cold hands and feet, headache, irregular heartbeat.	Deficiency of iron in the diet, blood loss, ulcers, cancer, prolonged use of aspirin.	Typically diagnosed by a routine blood test, but further testing may be necessary to determine underlying cause. Common treatments are to replace blood cells through transfusion and increase iron in the diet.
Anemia, pernicious	Fatigue and lethargy, pale skin, dizziness, cold hands and feet, headache, irregular heartbeat.	Lack of intrinsic factor from the parietal cells in the stomach interferes with the absorption of vitamin B$_{12}$, which is necessary for production of healthy red blood cells. The most likely cause of the parietal cell dysfunction is an autoimmune response.	Diagnosis is made by use of a combination of medical history, physical examination, and blood tests. Treatment is aimed at restoring vitamin B$_{12}$ levels, usually through pills or injections.

Common Pathology of the Circulatory System—cont'd

Disease	Signs and Symptoms	Etiology	Diagnosis and Treatment
Angina pectoris	Chest pain.	Reduced blood flow to the cardiac muscle.	Some of the tests used to diagnose angina are the electrocardiogram (ECG), stress test, echocardiogram, nuclear stress test, coronary angiography, cardiac magnetic resonance imaging (MRI), and computed tomography (CT). Treatment aims to restore blood flow through rest, angioplasty, stents, or coronary artery bypass grafting (CABG).
Atherosclerosis	In the heart, chest pain; in the brain, transient ischemic attacks (TIAs); in the arms and legs, peripheral artery disease (PAD); in the kidneys, kidney dysfunction.	Specific type of arteriosclerosis (hardening of the arteries) in which fatty deposits narrow the lumen of the vessels. May be caused by high blood pressure, high cholesterol, high triglycerides, smoking, diabetes, infections from other diseases.	Diagnosis is based on physical examination, medical history, blood tests, Doppler ultrasound, ECG, stress test, angiogram, CT, and/or MRI. Treatment options include a healthy diet, exercise regimen, cholesterol medications, beta-blockers, angiotensin-converting-enzyme (ACE) inhibitors, antiplatelet medications (blood thinners), diuretics, and calcium channel blockers. In some patients, angioplasty and stents, endarterectomy, or bypass surgery may be necessary.
Cardiomyopathy	Chest pain, dyspnea, peripheral edema, ECG abnormalities.	Causes include ischemia, drug and alcohol toxicity, certain infections. May be secondary to other conditions such as diabetes mellitus, acromegaly, and muscular dystrophy.	Diagnosis is based on a combination of medical history, blood tests, physical examination, ECG, echocardiogram, cardiac cauterization and biopsy, and cardiac MRI. Treatment depends on the type of cardiomyopathy and condition of the disease but may include one of more of the following: pacemakers, defibrillators, left ventricular assist devices (LVADs), and ablation. Some patients may require a heart transplant.
Congestive heart failure (CHF)	Fatigue, lethargy, peripheral edema, dyspnea.	Heart's pumping ability is impaired; may be caused by coronary artery disease, high blood pressure, cardiomyopathy, valvular disease, or heart defects.	Diagnosis is based on medical history and physical examination; procedures that may aid in diagnosis include ECG, chest x-ray examination, blood tests, and echocardiography. Treatment goal is to have the heart beat more efficiently. Specific treatment depends on underlying cause but may include weight loss, exercise program, and controlling high blood pressure. ACE inhibitors and beta-blockers help heart beat more effectively.
Coronary artery disease (CAD)	Chest pain, dyspnea, arrhythmias, fatigue.	Coronary arteries become narrow or blocked because of the accumulation of fatty deposits in the wall. Risk factors include high blood pressure, high cholesterol, high triglycerides, smoking, diabetes, lack of exercise, and obesity.	Diagnosis is based on physical examination, medical history, blood tests, echocardiography, nuclear imaging, cardiac CT, stress tests, heart cauterization. Treatment options include aspirin, beta-blockers, calcium channel blockers, and angioplasty and stents. Bypass surgery may be necessary in some cases. The best treatment is prevention by maintaining a healthy lifestyle, controlling high blood pressure, cholesterol levels, and diabetes.
Hemophilia	Excessive bleeding and frequent bruising.	The cause is an absence of clotting factors in the blood as a result of a gene defect of the X chromosome.	Diagnosis is based on family history, physical examination, and blood tests. Primary treatment is replacement therapy in which clotting factors are slowly infused into a vein.
Hodgkin lymphoma	Swelling of lymph nodes, fatigue, fever and chills, night sweats, weight loss, dyspnea, loss of appetite, and itching.	Occurs when a B cell develops a mutation in its DNA. Mutation causes a large number of abnormal B cells to accumulate in the lymphatic system, where they crowd out healthy cells.	Diagnostic tools include physical examination, blood tests, imaging tests, lymph node biopsy, and bone marrow testing. Treatment modalities include chemotherapy, radiation therapy, and stem cell transplant.

Continued

Common Pathology of the Circulatory System—cont'd

Disease	Signs and Symptoms	Etiology	Diagnosis and Treatment
Hypertension	Typically is asymptomatic.	No identifiable cause for primary (essential) hypertension; secondary hypertension may be caused by kidney disease, tumors of the adrenal gland, or thyroid dysfunction.	Systolic pressure above 140 mm Hg and diastolic pressure above 90 mm Hg is typically considered hypertension. Treatment may include lifestyle changes to include a healthy diet and exercise. Medications that lower blood pressure include diuretics, beta-blockers, ACE inhibitors, and calcium channel blockers.
Infectious mononucleosis	Fever, sore throat, swollen lymph nodes, fatigue.	Epstein-Barr virus (EBV) spread through saliva.	Diagnosis is primarily from observation of symptoms. Differential tests may be used to distinguish it from cytomegalovirus and *Toxoplasma gondii* infections. The condition is usually self-limiting and little treatment is required. Medications may be used to reduce pain and fever.
Leukemia	Swollen lymph nodes, frequent nosebleeds, bleeding from the gums or rectum, frequent bruising, heavy menstrual bleeding, fever, loss of appetite, fatigue.	Leukemia occurs when the bone marrow starts to produce an abundance of abnormal white blood cells. Cause is unclear. Risk factors include exposure to high levels of radiation and toxic chemicals.	Diagnostic tools include medical history, physical examination, blood tests, bone marrow aspiration and biopsy, lymph node biopsy. The treatment goal is to destroy leukemia cells and allow normal cells to form in the bone marrow. Treatment modalities depend on the type of leukemia but may include chemotherapy, radiation therapy, corticosteroids, and stem cell transplant.
Mitral valve prolapse	Most individuals have no symptoms. When symptoms occur, they may include chest pain, shortness of breath, swelling in the legs and feet, and heart palpitations.	In most patients the cause of mitral valve prolapse is unknown. During ventricular systole a portion of the mitral valve slips backward, allowing some of the blood to flow back into the left atrium instead of exiting the heart through the aorta (mitral regurgitation). Common cause of heart murmurs.	Heart murmurs and abnormal heart sounds heard through a stethoscope may indicate mitral valve prolapse. Diagnosis can be confirmed with echocardiography. Treatment usually is not necessary. Severe cases of mitral regurgitation may benefit from surgery to repair or replace the faulty valve.
Multiple myeloma	No symptoms in the early stages. May progress to include bone pain, weakness and fatigue, weight loss, opportunistic infections, and kidney problems.	The underlying cause is unknown. Plasma cells multiply abnormally within the bone marrow. These release unhealthy levels of immunoglobulin into the blood, which accumulates to cause organ damage, bone lesions, and red blood cell dysfunction, resulting in anemia.	Diagnosis is based on blood and urine tests, imaging tests, and bone marrow biopsy. Treatment modalities may include chemotherapy, radiation therapy, and stem cell transplant.
Myocardial infarction (MI)	Acute chest pain, nausea, vomiting, profuse sweating, heartburn or indigestion.	The typical cause is atherosclerosis in which a coronary artery becomes occluded so that cardiac muscle becomes ischemic and dies.	Diagnosis confirmed by ECG and blood tests to assay for enzymes that are released into the blood by dying heart muscle. The typical treatment protocol is fibrolytic agents, diagnostic angiogram, percutaneous coronary intervention (PCI; also called *stenting*). Some cases may require CABG.
Non-Hodgkin lymphoma	Swollen lymph nodes, weight loss, fever, and night sweats.	Cause is unknown. Occurs when the body produces too many T cell and B cell lymphocytes. Risk factors include medications that suppress the immune system, toxic chemicals, and some viral or bacterial infections.	Diagnosis relies on physical examination, medical history, blood tests, chest x-ray examination, CT and/or positron emission tomography (PET) scan, lymph node and bone marrow biopsies. Treatment depends on the type and stage of the lymphoma, its growth rate, and patient's age and health. Modalities include chemotherapy, radiation therapy, drugs to enhance the immune system, and stem cell transplant.

Common Pathology of the Circulatory System—cont'd

Disease	Signs and Symptoms	Etiology	Diagnosis and Treatment
Peripheral arterial disease (PAD)	Leg pain when walking or climbing stairs; leg numbness; sores on the toes, feet, or legs that do not heal; coldness in lower leg or foot; shiny skin on the legs; change in the color of the legs.	Most frequent cause is atherosclerosis that narrows the blood vessels supplying the legs and reduces blood flow to the legs.	Diagnostic tools include physical examination, ankle-brachial index (ABI) to compare blood pressure in the ankle with blood pressure in the arm, ultrasound, angiography, blood tests. Many patients can be treated with lifestyle changes including diet and exercise. Others may require medications to alleviate pain, prevent blood clots, lower cholesterol, and lower blood pressure. Angioplasty or bypass grafting may be necessary in severe cases.
Polycythemia	Weakness, fatigue, headache, joint pain, dizziness.	In primary polycythemia, a gene mutation results in abnormally high production of red blood cells. In secondary polycythemia, the cause is hypoxia as a result of chronic obstructive pulmonary disease (COPD), chronic heart disease, or renal hypoxia. Temporary polycythemia may occur at high altitudes.	Usually detected by routine blood tests that evaluate hemoglobin, hematocrit, and red blood cell concentration. Other tests may be needed to determine the underlying cause. For primary polycythemia, treatment is phlebotomy and antiplatelet agents. For secondary polycythemia, treatment is directed at the underlying cause.
Rheumatic heart disease (RHD)	Fatigue, lethargy, peripheral edema, dyspnea. Signs and symptoms are caused by heart failure resulting from failure of heart valves to open and close properly.	RHD is caused by faulty mitral and/or aortic valves as a result of endocarditis secondary to rheumatic fever. There may be either stenosis so the valves do not open or regurgitation because the valves do not close.	Diagnosis is based on medical history, chest x-ray examination and/or MRI, echocardiogram, and ECG. Many patients require no treatment. If valve damage is severe, valvuloplasty or valve replacement may be necessary.
Shock	Cool and clammy skin, weak and rapid pulse, nausea, lack of brilliance in eyes, feelings of weakness and confusion.	Trauma, heart failure, bleeding, dehydration, infection, severe allergic reactions. Shock is a life-threatening medical condition as a result of insufficient blood flow through the body.	Diagnosis is based on signs and symptoms. Treatment: call 911 immediately. Administer intravenous fluids to raise blood pressure. Medications such as epinephrine, norepinephrine, and dopamine raise blood pressure. After the patient's condition has been stabilized, treat the underlying cause.
Systemic lupus erythematosus (SLE)	Fever, malaise, joint pain, myalgia, fatigue. There may be skin rash, photosensitivity, mucous membrane ulcers, arthritis, pleuritis or pericarditis, kidney abnormalities, seizures, blood count abnormalities, and antinuclear antibodies in the blood. These are intermittent, and not all are present in any one individual.	SLE is an autoimmune connective tissue disease that can affect any part of the body. There is no single cause. Triggers include heredity, viruses, UV light, and drugs.	Diagnosis depends on physical examination and blood tests. There is no cure. Treatment is directed at relieving symptoms. Some patients may be treated with immunosuppressants.
Thrombophlebitis	Redness, swelling, pain, and warmth in the affected area.	Occurs when a blood clot (thrombus) blocks one or more veins, usually in the leg, with subsequent inflammation of the vessel. May be near the surface or deep within the muscles (deep vein thrombosis [DVT]).	Diagnosis is based on patient history, examination, blood tests, ultrasound, and CT scans. Treatment involves application of heat to the affected area, elevation of the leg, and antiinflammatory drugs. Blood thinning and clot dissolving medications, compression stockings, varicose vein stripping, and insertion of a filter in the inferior vena cava (IVC) to trap emboli before they reach the lungs or heart may be necessary.

TERMINOLOGY REVIEW

Key Term	Word Parts	Definition
Agranulocytes	*a:* without *granul/o:* granules *cyte:* cell	White blood cells that lack granules in the cytoplasm.
Antibodies	*anti:* against	Substances produced by the body that inactivate or destroy other substances that are introduced into the body; immunoglobulins.
Antibody-mediated immunity		Immunity that is the result of B-cell action and the production of antibodies; also called *humoral immunity.*
Antigens		Substances that trigger an immune response when they are introduced into the body.
Atria (singular atrium)		Thin-walled chambers of the heart that receive blood from veins.
Atrioventricular valves	*atri/o:* atrium *ventricul/o:* ventricle	Valves between the atria and the ventricles in the heart.
Cardiac cycle		A complete heartbeat consisting of contraction and relaxation of both atria and both ventricles.
Cell-mediated immunity		Immunity that is the result of T-cell action.
Coagulation	*coagul/o:* clotting *-tion:* process	The process of blood clotting.
Conduction myofibers	*my/o:* muscle	Cardiac muscle cells specialized for conducting action potentials to the myocardium; part of the conduction system of the heart; also called *Purkinje fibers.*
Diapedesis	*dia-:* through	The process by which white blood cells squeeze between the cells in a vessel wall to enter the tissue spaces outside the blood vessel.
Diastole		Relaxation phase of the cardiac cycle; opposite of systole.
Endocardium	*endo:* within *card/i:* heart *-um:* tissue	The thin, smooth inner lining of each chamber of the heart.
Epicardium	*epi:* around, outside *card/i:* heart *-um:* tissue	The outer layer of the heart wall; the visceral pericardium.
Erythrocytes	*erythr/o:* red *-cyte:* cell	Red blood cells.
Erythropoiesis	*erythr/o:* red *-poieses:* formation	The process of red blood cell formation.
Erythropoietin	*erythr/o:* red *-poietin:* substance that forms	A hormone released by the kidneys that stimulates red blood cell production.
Granulocytes	*granul/o:* granules *-cyte:* cell	
Hematopoiesis	*hemat/o:* blood *-poieses:* formation	Blood cell production, which occurs in the red bone marrow; also called *hemopoiesis.*
Hemocytoblast	*hem/o:* blood *-cyt-:* cell *-blast:* to form	A stem cell in the bone marrow from which the blood cells arise.
Hemoglobin	*hem/o:* blood *-globin:* protein	The iron-containing protein in red blood cells that is responsible for the transport of oxygen.
Hemostasis	*hem/o:* blood *-stasis:* control	The control or stoppage of bleeding.
Immunoglobulins	*immun/o:* immunity or protection *globulin:* a class of protein	Substances produced by the body that inactivate or destroy other substances that are introduced into the body; antibodies.
Leukocytes	*leuk/o:* white *-cyt-:* cell	White blood cells.
Macrophages	*macr/o:* large *-phag-:* to eat, devour	Large phagocytic connective tissue cell that functions in immune responses; name given to a monocyte after it leaves the blood and enters the tissues.

TERMINOLOGY REVIEW—cont'd

Key Term	Word Parts	Definition
Megakaryocytes	*mega:* large *kary/o:* nucleus *cyte:* cell	A large cell that contributes to the formation of platelets.
Myocardium	*my/o:* muscle *card/i-:* heart *-um:* tissue	Middle layer of the heart wall; composed of cardiac muscle tissue.
Nonspecific defense mechanisms		Body's ability to counteract all types of harmful agents.
Pericardial cavity	*peri:* around *card/i:* heart	Small space around the heart, between the parietal pericardium and visceral pericardium, that contains a small amount of serous fluid for lubrication.
Pericardium	*per/i:* around *card/i:* heart	Membrane that surrounds the heart; usually refers to the pericardial sac.
Pulmonary circulation	*pulmon-:* lung	The pathway that takes blood from the right side of the heart to the lungs and then returns it to the left side of the heart.
Renal erythropoietic factor	*ren/o:* kidney *erythr/o:* red *poie:* formation of blood cells	A substance produced by the kidneys that activates erythropoietin to stimulate the production of red blood cells.
Resistance		Body's ability to counteract the effects of pathogens and other harmful agents.
Right lymphatic duct		The collecting duct of the lymphatic system that collects lymph from the upper right quadrant of the body.
Semilunar valves		Valves between the ventricles of the heart and the vessels that carry blood away from the ventricles; also pertains to the valves in veins.
Specific defense mechanisms		Activities of the body that counteract only certain types of harmful agents.
Susceptibility		Lack of resistance to disease.
Systemic circulation		Pathways that transport blood from the left side of the heart to all parts of the body and return the blood to the right atrium; excludes pulmonary circulation.
Systole		Contraction phase of the cardiac cycle; opposite of diastole.
Thoracic duct		The primary collecting duct of the lymphatic system that collects lymph from all regions of the body except the upper right quadrant.
Thrombocytes	*thromb/o:* clot *-cyte:* cell	A class of formed elements of the blood; function in blood clotting; also called *platelets.*
Ventricle		Pumping chambers of the heart; right ventricle pumps blood to the lungs and left ventricle pumps blood into systemic circulation.

ON THE WEB

For information on the circulatory system:

America's Blood Centers: www.americasblood.org

Cardio Guide: www.mymedline.com/cardio

The Franklin Institute—Blood: www.fi.edu/learn/heart/blood/blood.html

The Franklin Institute—The Human Heart: www.fi.edu/learn/heart

Heart Point: www.heartpoint.com

Human Blood: anthro.palomar.edu/blood

Inner Body: www.innerbody.com/html/body.html

The Internet Pathology Laboratory for Medical Education—Hematopathology: library.med.utah.edu/WebPath/ORGAN.html *(Click on "Hematopathology")*

from the higher brain centers are ignored and the respiratory center resumes regular breathing.

Involuntary impulses from higher brain centers may stimulate rapid breathing in response to emotions, such as anxiety or excitement. Chronic pain also may result in involuntary stimulation from the higher brain centers. In contrast, sudden pain or sudden cold may cause a gasp or a momentary cessation of breathing.

Temperature

An increase in body temperature caused by a fever or strenuous physical exercise increases the breathing rate. The increased body temperature is associated with increased metabolism, which uses more oxygen and generates more carbon dioxide. When body temperature decreases, metabolic rate diminishes and breathing rate also decreases.

NONRESPIRATORY AIR MOVEMENTS

In addition to normal air movements that occur during breathing and result in pulmonary ventilation, there are a number of modifications called *nonrespiratory air movements.* Some of these are reflexes that clear air passages, others are voluntary, and some express emotions. These nonrespiratory air movements are outlined in Table 13-1.

Table 13-1 Nonrespiratory Air Movements

Movement	Description
Sneezing	Spasmodic contraction of exhalation muscles that forces air through nose and mouth.
Coughing	Long inhalation followed by closure of glottis; then a strong exhalation forces glottis open and sends a blast of air through upper respiratory tract.
Sighing	Long inhalation followed by a shorter but forceful exhalation.
Hiccupping	Spasmodic contraction of diaphragm followed by sudden closure of glottis to produce a sharp sound.
Crying	An inhalation followed by many short exhalations; glottis remains open and vocal cords vibrate; usually accompanied by tears and characteristic facial expressions.
Laughing	Same basic movements as crying but facial expressions differ; may be indistinguishable from crying.
Yawning	A deep inhalation through a widely opened mouth.

From Applegate E: *The anatomy and physiology learning system,* ed 4, St Louis, 2011, Saunders.

AGING OF THE RESPIRATORY SYSTEM

Various harmful substances, including cigarette smoke, air pollution, and pathogens, continually bombard the respiratory system and take their toll. There is no way to avoid all of these irritants except to stop breathing! Some irritants, such as cigarette smoke, can be decreased, but others are inescapable.

Because of the continual contact between the respiratory system and the environment, it is difficult to distinguish between the changes in the tissues of the breathing apparatus, including the lungs, that are the result of aging and those that are the result of disease or other factors outside the body. Modifications in the lining of the respiratory tract probably are caused by environmental rather than solely aging-related factors. Long-term exposure to irritants results in deterioration of the cilia, which hinders their cleansing action and movement of mucus. As a consequence, the occurrence of emphysema and chronic bronchitis increases with age. Diminishing effectiveness of the immune system makes the elderly more susceptible to pneumonia and other microbial diseases. However, excluding external influences, there are changes that take place as a result of "normal" aging.

One of the most common signs of respiratory aging, in general, is when a person is unable to maintain the same level of physical activity that was experienced in younger years. This is a gradual decline and may not be noticeable until phrases such as "I used to be able to…" become part of the conversation. The cardiovascular and muscular systems have an effect on endurance, and the skeletal system has an effect on thoracic volume, but the major change is a decreased ability of the respiratory system to acquire and deliver oxygen to the blood.

The impairment in oxygen delivery is the result of structural changes that take place in the respiratory tissues. One type of change is a loss of elasticity in the tissues of the respiratory system. The cartilage in the walls of the trachea and bronchi undergoes a progressive calcification. Smooth muscle fibers in the bronchioles are replaced by fibrous tissue, so they are less able to stretch and contract. Modifications in lung tissue cause the alveoli to lose some of their elastic recoil. The cumulative effect of these changes is a gradual decrease in respiratory volume and capacity and an increase in the volume of residual air in the lungs. Another change is deterioration of the walls between adjacent alveoli. This increases the size of each individual alveolus but reduces the total surface area of the respiratory membrane for diffusion of gases. A lower percentage of the oxygen in alveolar air is able to diffuse into the lung capillaries. These changes result in a decreased ability to acquire and deliver oxygen to the blood, which reduces the capacity for physical activity.

Common Pathology of the Respiratory System

Disease	Signs and Symptoms	Etiology	Diagnosis and Treatment
Acute respiratory distress syndrome (ARDS)	After an acute lung injury, patient experiences difficulty in breathing, low blood pressure, rapid breathing, and shortness of breath.	ARDS typically occurs in people who are already critically ill or who have had traumatic injuries, such as a pulmonary contusion, aspiration of gastric contents, multiple blood transfusions, or drug overdose. Fluid buildup in the alveoli prevents oxygen from passing into the bloodstream.	An arterial blood gas analysis and chest x-ray examination provide the diagnosis. The overall goal is to maintain acceptable gas exchange. ARDS is typically treated with oxygen therapy, mechanical ventilation, and the administration of antibiotics.
Asthma	Wheezing, shortness of breath, chest tightness, and coughing.	An asthma attack is preceded by airway inflammation, causing the lining of the air passages to swell and the muscles surrounding the airways to tighten. This reduces the amount of air that can pass through the airways. Triggers for the attack are varied and include pollen, pet hair, mold, dust mites, tobacco smoke, air pollution, and many other irritants.	Pulmonary function tests measure how well the lungs are functioning and are used to diagnose and manage asthma. Several types of medications may be prescribed, some inhaled and some taken as pills. All asthma attacks require treatment with a quick-acting inhaler such as albuterol.
Bronchitis	Shortness of breath, often accompanied by fever, chills, fatigue, coughing, and/or the production of mucus (sputum).	Bronchitis may be acute or chronic. Acute bronchitis is usually caused by viruses similar to the cold and flu viruses. Chronic bronchitis is typically the result of smoking. Initially it can be difficult to distinguish the signs and symptoms of bronchitis from those of a common cold.	During a physical examination, a health professional will use a stethoscope to listen closely to lung sounds. A chest x-ray examination and/or pulmonary function tests may be required. Sputum analysis may be needed. Most cases of acute bronchitis resolve without medical treatment. Chronic bronchitis may benefit from pulmonary rehabilitation.
Chronic obstructive pulmonary disease (COPD)	Common signs and symptoms of COPD include chest tightness, a cough that produces mucus, shortness of breath with activity, and wheezing during breathing.	Smoking is the primary cause of COPD. It can also be caused by air pollution and occupational exposures. It is a disease that blocks airflow in and out of the lungs. It usually is a combination of chronic bronchitis and emphysema.	A key factor in diagnosis is the patient history. Pulmonary function tests, along with x-ray examination and computed tomography (CT) scans confirm and evaluate the progression of the disease. Treatment aims to slow the progress and relieve the symptoms. Medications and oxygen therapy may be needed. The most essential step in treatment is to stop smoking.
Croup	Croup is characterized by a barking cough, hoarseness, and strained breathing, which usually worsens at night. It is more common in children.	Croup is caused by a virus and is an infection of the upper airway which obstructs breathing. It is the result of inflammation around the vocal cords, trachea, and bronchial tubes.	Croup is typically diagnosed by observing breathing patterns, listening to chest sounds, and examining the throat. Sometimes x-ray studies or other tests are used to rule out other possible illnesses. Aggressive treatment is rarely needed. If symptoms persist, a type of steroid to reduce inflammation in the airway may be prescribed.
Emphysema	The main symptom of emphysema is shortness of breath, which usually begins gradually but continues to get worse until breathing is difficult even at rest.	The main cause of emphysema is long-term exposure to tobacco smoke. It may also be caused by other airborne irritants. The alveoli at the end of the airways in the lungs are damaged or destroyed and unable to adequately function in oxygen and carbon dioxide exchange.	A variety of tests may be required to diagnose emphysema, including imaging with x-rays and CT scans, blood laboratory analysis, and lung function evaluation. It cannot be cured, but treatments may relieve symptoms and slow the progression of the disease. Depending on the severity, inhaled steroids, bronchodilators, and/or antibiotics may be prescribed. Pulmonary rehabilitation may be required.

Continued

Common Pathology of the Respiratory System—cont'd

Disease	Signs and Symptoms	Etiology	Diagnosis and Treatment
Laryngitis	Laryngitis symptoms may include hoarseness, a weak voice, a tickling sensation with rawness of the throat, and a dry cough.	Laryngitis may be acute or chronic. Causes of acute laryngitis include viral infections and vocal strain from yelling. Chronic laryngitis may be caused by inhaled irritants such as tobacco smoke, acid reflux, chronic sinusitis, or excessive alcohol use.	Diagnosis involves examining the vocal cords with a laryngoscope and may include a biopsy of tissue for examination under a microscope. Sometimes, corticosteroids help reduce vocal cord inflammation.
Lung cancer	Lung cancer typically doesn't produce signs and symptoms in the early stages. Symptoms typically occur only when the disease is advanced, and may include a cough that does not go away, shortness of breath, coughing up blood, chest pain, and wheezing.	Smoking causes the majority of lung cancers. It is believed that smoking causes lung cancer by damaging the DNA in the cells that line the lungs. The mutated abnormal cells proliferate to form malignant tumors.	The diagnosis of lung cancer may require various tests, including x-ray and CT scans, sputum cytology, and tissue biopsy with a bronchoscope. Treatment options typically include one or more of the following; surgery, chemotherapy, radiation therapy, or targeted drug therapy.
Pharyngitis	Pharyngitis is an inflammation of the throat. The throat may be sore, dry, and/or scratchy, accompanied by sneezing, runny nose, cough, headache, fatigue, fever, and chills.	Most cases are caused by an infectious organism, either a virus or a bacterium, acquired from close contact with an infected individual. Like many types of inflammation, pharyngitis can be acute (a condition that is characterized by a rapid onset and typically a relatively short course) or chronic.	Diagnosis is by physical examination of the throat and checking for swollen lymph nodes. The examination may include a throat swab to rule out a streptococcal infection. If the pharyngitis is caused by a bacterial infection, antibiotics may be prescribed. If the cause is a virus, home care can help relieve symptoms.
Pleurisy	Symptoms of pleurisy include chest pain that worsens with breathing, coughing, or sneezing. It may also include shortness of breath and sometimes a cough with fever.	Pleurisy occurs when the pleura around the lung becomes irritated and inflamed. As a result, the two layers of the pleural membrane rub against each other like two pieces of sandpaper, producing pain during breathing.	Diagnosis is by physical examination of the chest with a stethoscope. Various imaging modalities may be used to observe the pleural space. A blood test may identify an infection. The outcome of pleurisy treatment depends on the seriousness of the underlying disease. If the condition that caused pleurisy is diagnosed and treated early, there is likely to be a full recovery.
Pneumoconiosis	Pneumoconiosis, in early stages, may not show any symptoms. When symptoms develop, they include a dry cough, wheezing, and shortness of breath with exercise. As the disease progresses, breathing can become extremely difficult.	Pneumoconiosis is a lung condition that is caused by inhaling particles of mineral dust, usually while working in a high-risk, mineral-related industry. The damaging particles may be asbestos, silica, coal dust, or other agents. At first, the irritating material triggers lung inflammation, causing areas of the lung to be damaged. Over time, these areas can form tough, fibrous tissue that is not effective for oxygen and carbon dioxide exchange.	Diagnosis is based on patient history, physical examination, x-ray films, CT scans, and pulmonary function tests. The outlook for this disease depends on the specific type of pneumoconiosis, the length of exposure to mineral dust, the level of exposure, and whether the patient is a smoker. Medications may be prescribed to make breathing easier.
Pneumonia	Symptoms of pneumonia include fever, cough with fluid, chest pain, shortness of breath, fatigue, muscle aches, headache, nausea, vomiting, and/or diarrhea.	Pneumonia is caused by infections primarily with bacteria or viruses in the air and is classified by the type of infectious agent. Conditions and risk factors that predispose to pneumonia include smoking, immunodeficiency, alcoholism, COPD, chronic kidney disease, and liver disease.	Diagnosis starts with the patient history and physical examination. Chest x-ray films can confirm the presence of pneumonia and determine the extent and location of the infection. Blood tests, pulse oximetry, and a sputum test may be ordered. Oral antibiotics, rest, simple analgesics, and fluids usually suffice for complete resolution. Antibiotics, antiviral medications, and fever reducers may be prescribed.

Common Pathology of the Respiratory System—cont'd

Disease	Signs and Symptoms	Etiology	Diagnosis and Treatment
Pneumothorax	The primary symptoms of a pneumothorax include sudden chest pain and shortness of breath.	A pneumothorax is an abnormal collection of air or gas in the pleural space that separates the lung from the chest wall, often causing the lung to collapse. It can be caused by a puncture trauma to the chest or by rupture of numerous alveoli.	Diagnosis of pneumothorax by physical examination is difficult. A chest x-ray examination or CT scan is usually needed to confirm its presence. The goal in treating a pneumothorax is to relieve the pressure on the lung, allowing it to reexpand, and to prevent recurrences. Often it is self-resolving. A needle may be used to withdraw air from the pleural space. Occasionally surgery is required to close the wound in the chest wall.
Pulmonary edema	The primary symptom of pulmonary edema is difficulty breathing, but signs and symptoms may also include coughing up blood, a feeling of suffocation, and chest pain.	Pulmonary edema is a condition caused by excess fluid in the lungs. This fluid collects in the alveoli of the lungs, making it difficult to breathe. It is often the result of high pressures within the pulmonary circulation caused by congestive heart failure.	Because pulmonary edema requires prompt treatment, initial diagnosis is based on the symptoms, a physical examination, electrocardiogram, and a chest x-ray examination. Providing oxygen therapy is the first step in the treatment of pulmonary edema. Diuretics may be prescribed to reduce the amount of fluid in the lungs, and medications that increase the effectiveness of the heart may reduce the pulmonary hypertension.
Rhinitis	Symptoms of rhinitis include sneezing, coughing, runny nose, watery eyes, and pressure in the ears.	Rhinitis is irritation and inflammation of the mucous membrane inside the nose, accompanied by excessive production of mucus. The most common kind of rhinitis is allergic rhinitis, which is usually triggered by airborne allergens such as pollen and dander. Rhinitis also accompanies viral infections such as cold and flu.	An allergist can diagnose the specific allergens that trigger the illness or determine if symptoms have nonallergic causes. For allergic rhinitis, intranasal corticosteroids and antihistamines can be used to suppress inflammation and control symptoms.
Tuberculosis (TB)	The general symptoms of tuberculosis include fever, chills, night sweats, loss of appetite, weight loss, and fatigue.	Tuberculosis is a potentially serious infectious disease that mainly affects the lungs. The bacteria that cause tuberculosis are spread from one person to another through tiny droplets released into the air via coughs and sneezes.	Diagnosis of active TB is based on chest x-ray films as well as microscopic examination and microbiologic culture of body fluids. Medications are the cornerstone of tuberculosis treatment. But treating TB takes much longer than treating other types of bacterial infections.

⟳ TERMINOLOGY REVIEW

Key Term	Word Parts	Definition
Alveoli	*alveol-:* tiny cavity	Microscopic dilations of terminal bronchioles in the lungs, where diffusion of gases occurs; air sacs in the lungs.
Bronchi	*bronchi-:* bronchi	The airways that are formed when the trachea branches.
Bronchial tree	*bronchi-:* bronchi	The bronchi and all their branches that function as passageways between the trachea and the alveoli.
External respiration		Exchange of gases between the lungs and the blood.
Fauces		Opening from the oral cavity into the oropharynx.
Internal respiration		Exchange of gases between the blood and tissue cells.
Laryngopharynx	*laryng/o-:* larynx	Portion of the pharynx that is behind the larynx and extends from the level of the hyoid bone to the lower margin of the larynx.
Larynx		Passageway for air between the pharynx and trachea; commonly called the *voice box.*
Lower respiratory tract		Portion of the respiratory tract that is inferior to the larynx; includes the trachea, bronchial tree, and lungs.
Nasopharynx	*nas/o:* nose	Portion of the pharynx that is posterior to the nasal cavities; extends from the base of the skull to the uvula.
Oropharynx	*or/o:* mouth	Portion of the pharynx that is posterior to the oral cavity; extends from the uvula to the hyoid bone.
Pharynx	*pharyn/o:* pharynx	Passageway for air and food; extends from the base of the skull to the larynx and esophagus; throat.
Pleura	*pleur/o:* ribs	Serous membrane that lines the ribs (parietal layer) and surrounds the lungs (visceral layer).
Pleural cavity	*pleur/o:* ribs, pleura	The small space between the parietal and visceral layers of the pleura.
Respiration	*respir/o:* breath	Exchange of oxygen and carbon dioxide between the atmosphere and the body cells.
Respiratory membrane		Any surface in the lungs where diffusion occurs; consists of the layers that the gases must pass through to get into or out of the alveoli.
Surfactant		A substance, produced by certain cells in lung tissue, that reduces surface tension between fluid molecules that line the respiratory membrane and helps keep the alveolus from collapsing.
Trachea		Passageway for air that extends inferiorly to the carina where it branches into the bronchi; commonly called the *windpipe.*
Upper respiratory tract		Portion of the respiratory tract that includes the nose, pharynx, and larynx.
Ventilation		Movement of air into and out of the lungs; breathing.

ON THE WEB

For information on the respiratory system:

Chronic Obstructive Pulmonary Disease: www.priory.com/cmol/copd.htm

The Internet Pathology Laboratory for Medical Education—Gastrointestinal Pathology: library.med.utah.edu/WebPath/ORGAN.html *(Click on "Pulmonary Pathology")*

Digestive System

14

Check out the Evolve site at http://evolve.elsevier.com/Bonewit/today/ to access additional interactive activities and exercises to help you study and prepare for success.

LEARNING OBJECTIVES

1. Identify the components of the digestive tract and the accessory organs.
2. List six functions of the digestive system.
3. Describe the general histology of the four layers in the digestive tract wall.
4. Describe the features and function of the oral cavity, teeth, pharynx, and esophagus.
5. List and describe the location of the three salivary glands.
6. Explain the function of saliva.
7. Describe the structure and features of the stomach and its role in digestion.
8. Describe the structure and features of the small intestine and its role in digestion and absorption.
9. Describe the structure, features, and function of the large intestine.
10. Describe the structure and function of the liver, gallbladder, and pancreas.
11. Explain how substances are absorbed into the body through the small intestine.
12. Describe ways in which the aging of an individual affects the digestive system.
13. Identify pathology related to the digestive system.

CHAPTER OUTLINE

INTRODUCTION TO THE DIGESTIVE SYSTEM
FUNCTIONS OF THE DIGESTIVE SYSTEM
GENERAL STRUCTURE OF THE DIGESTIVE TRACT
Mucosa
Submucosa
Muscular Layer
Serosa or Adventitia
COMPONENTS OF THE DIGESTIVE TRACT
Mouth
Lips and Cheeks
Palate
Tongue
Teeth
Salivary Glands
Pharynx
Esophagus
Stomach
Structure
Gastric Secretions
Regulation of Gastric Secretions
Stomach Emptying

Small Intestine
Structure
Secretions of the Small Intestine
Large Intestine
Characteristics
Regions of the Large Intestine
Functions of the Large Intestine
ACCESSORY ORGANS OF DIGESTION
Liver
Structure of the Liver
Blood Supply to the Liver
Functions of the Liver
Bile
Gallbladder
Pancreas
CHEMICAL DIGESTION
Carbohydrate Digestion
Protein Digestion
Lipid Digestion
ABSORPTION
AGING OF THE DIGESTIVE SYSTEM

INTRODUCTION TO THE DIGESTIVE SYSTEM

The digestive system includes the *digestive tract* and its *accessory organs* (Figure 14-1). The function of the digestive system is to process food into molecules that can be absorbed and used by the cells of the body. Food is broken down, bit by bit, until the molecules are small enough to be absorbed and the waste products are eliminated. The digestive tract (also called the *alimentary canal* or *gastrointestinal* [GI] *tract*) consists of a long, continuous tube that extends from the mouth to the anus. It includes the mouth, pharynx, esophagus, stomach, small intestine, and large intestine. The tongue and teeth are accessory structures located in the mouth. The salivary glands, liver, gallbladder, and pancreas are not part of the digestive tract but are major accessory organs that have a role in digestion. These secrete fluids into the digestive tract.

FUNCTIONS OF THE DIGESTIVE SYSTEM

Food undergoes three types of processes in the body:
- Digestion
- Absorption
- Metabolism

Digestion and absorption occur in the digestive tract. After the nutrients have been absorbed, they are available to all cells in the body and are used by the cells in metabolism.

The digestive system prepares nutrients for use by the body's cells through the following six activities:
- Ingestion—The first activity of the digestive system is to take in food. This process is called *ingestion*. Ingestion has to take place before anything else can happen.
- Mechanical digestion—The large pieces of food that are ingested have to be broken into smaller particles that can be acted on by various enzymes. This is called *mechanical digestion*. Mechanical digestion begins in the mouth with chewing, or **mastication**, and continues with churning and mixing actions in the stomach.
- Chemical digestion—The complex molecules of carbohydrates, proteins, and fats are transformed by chemical digestion into smaller molecules that can be absorbed and used by the cells. Chemical digestion uses water to break down the complex molecules. This process is known as **hydrolysis**. Digestive enzymes speed up the hydrolysis process, which is otherwise slow.
- Movements—After ingestion and mastication, the food particles move from the mouth into the pharynx and then into the esophagus. This movement is called **deglutition**, or swallowing. Mixing movements occur in the stomach as a result of smooth muscle contraction. These repetitive contractions mix the food particles with enzymes and other fluids. The movements that propel the food particles through the digestive tract are called **peristalsis**. These are rhythmic waves of contractions that move the food particles through the various regions in which mechanical and chemical digestion takes place.
- Absorption—The simple molecules that are produced from chemical digestion pass through the lining of the small intestine into the blood. This process is called **absorption**.
- Elimination—The food molecules that cannot be digested need to be eliminated from the body. The removal of indigestible wastes through the anus, in the form of feces, is **defecation**.

GENERAL STRUCTURE OF THE DIGESTIVE TRACT

The digestive tract is a long, continuous tube that is about 9 m (30 ft) in length. It opens to the outside at both ends, through the mouth at one end and through the anus at the other. Although there are variations in each region, the basic structure of the wall is the same throughout the entire length of the tube.

The wall of the digestive tract has four layers or tunics (Figure 14-2): mucosa, submucosa, muscular layer (muscularis), and serous layer (serosa).

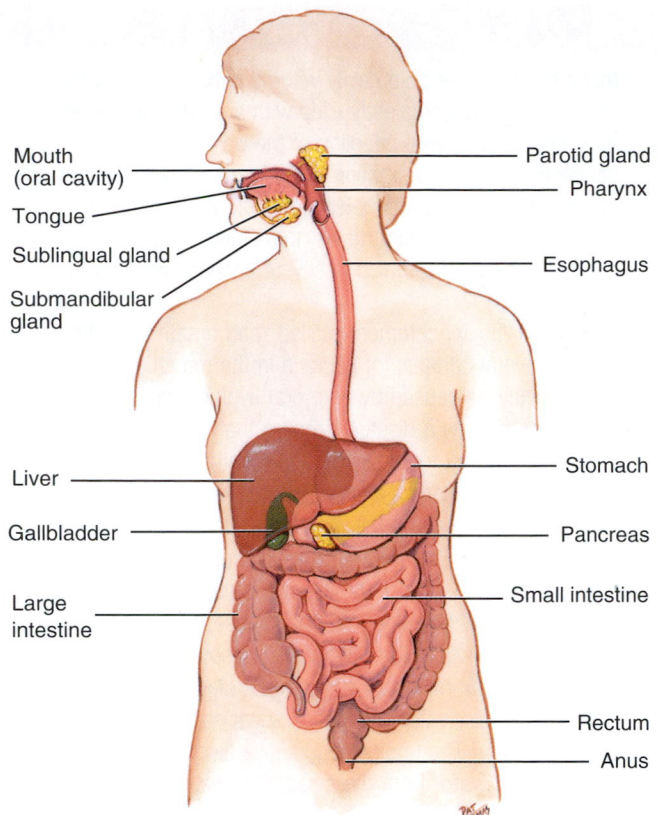

Figure 14-1 Organs of the digestive system. (From Applegate E: *The anatomy and physiology learning system,* ed 4, St Louis, 2011, Saunders.)

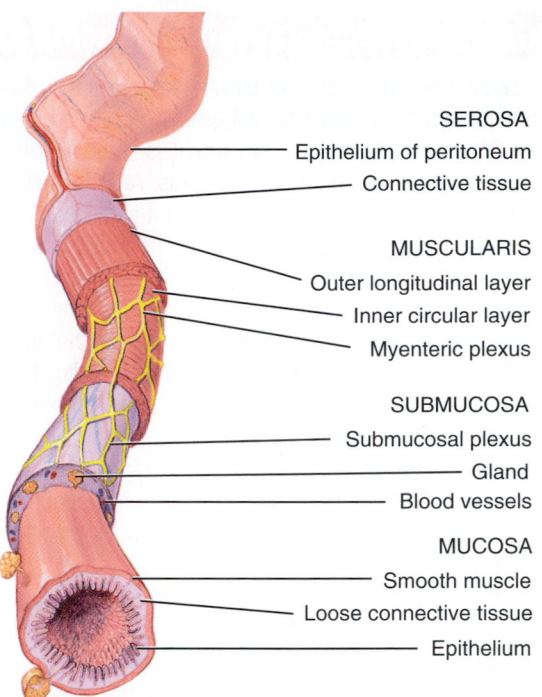

Figure 14-2 Basic histology of the digestive tract. Progressing from the inner to outer, the tissue layers of the digestive tract are the mucosa, submucosa, muscularis, and serosa (adventitia if above the diaphragm). (From Applegate E: *The anatomy and physiology learning system,* ed 4, St Louis, 2011, Saunders.)

MUCOSA

The mucosa, or mucous membrane layer, is the innermost tunic of the wall. It lines the lumen of the digestive tract. The mucosa consists of epithelium, an underlying loose connective tissue layer, and a thin layer of smooth muscle. In certain regions the mucosa develops folds that increase the surface area. Certain cells in the mucosa secrete mucus, digestive enzymes, and hormones. Ducts from other glands pass through the mucosa to the lumen of the digestive tract.

SUBMUCOSA

The submucosa is a thick layer of loose connective tissue that surrounds the mucosa. This layer also contains blood and lymphatic vessels, nerves, and some glands. Abundant blood vessels supply necessary nourishment to the surrounding tissues. Blood and lymph carry away absorbed nutrients that are the end products of digestion. The nerves in the submucosa form a network called the *submucosal plexus* that provides autonomic nerve impulses to the muscle layers of the digestive tract.

MUSCULAR LAYER

The muscular layer (labeled *muscularis* in Figure 14-2) consists of two layers of smooth muscle. The inner circular layer has fibers arranged in a circular manner around the circumference of the tube. When these muscles contract, the diameter of the tube is decreased. In the outer longitudinal layer the fibers run lengthwise along the long axis of the tube. When these fibers contract, their length decreases and the tube shortens. A network of autonomic nerve fibers, called the *myenteric plexus,* exists between the circular and longitudinal muscle layers. The myenteric plexus, along with the submucosal plexus, is important for controlling the movements and secretions of the digestive tract. In general, parasympathetic impulses stimulate movement and secretion in the GI tract, and sympathetic impulses inhibit these activities.

SEROSA OR ADVENTITIA

The fourth and outermost layer in the wall of the digestive tract is called the *adventitia* if it is above the diaphragm and the *serosa* if it is below the diaphragm. The adventitia is composed of connective tissue. The serosa, which is below the diaphragm, has a layer of epithelium covering the connective tissue. It is actually the visceral peritoneum and secretes serous fluid for lubrication. The serous fluid allows the abdominal organs to move smoothly against one another without friction.

HIGHLIGHT on the Digestive System

Cold sores: Cold sores, or fever blisters, are small fluid-filled blisters that itch and are painful, usually appearing around the lips and in the mouth. They are caused by recurring infections with the herpes simplex virus. After the initial infection, the virus remains dormant in a cutaneous nerve until it is activated by stress, fever, or ultraviolet radiation.

Cleft palate: Cleft palate is a condition in which the bones in the hard palate do not fuse completely during prenatal development. This leaves an opening between the nasal and oral cavities. An infant with this problem has difficulty creating enough suction for proper feeding. Cleft palate can usually be corrected surgically.

Tongue-tied: A person with a short lingual frenulum is said to be "tongue-tied." The movement of the tongue is abnormally limited, which causes difficulties in speech. Surgically cutting the frenulum corrects this problem.

Wisdom teeth: The third molars are the last teeth to erupt. These are sometimes called "wisdom teeth" because they usually erupt between the ages of 17 and 25 years, when one is supposed to be wise. These teeth may remain embedded in the jawbone. If this happens, they are said to be impacted. In some cases, wisdom teeth are absent altogether.

Gingivitis: Gingivitis is an inflammation of the gingiva, or gum. The gums become sore and red and may bleed. This condition is reversible if it is not neglected and if corrective action is taken. Periodontal disease results when gingivitis is neglected and bacteria invade the bone around the tooth. This is a major cause of tooth loss in adults.

Cavities: Caries, or dental cavities, are caused by the demineralization of the teeth resulting from the action of bacteria that live in the mouth. The bacteria metabolize sugars in the mouth, producing acids that dissolve the calcium salts of the tooth. If the bacteria reach the pulp cavity, it is necessary to perform a root canal procedure. In this procedure, the pulp cavity with its nerve is destroyed, and the cavity is completely filled with a solid filling material.

Mumps: Mumps is a viral infection of the parotid glands. The infection causes inflammation in the gland, which makes opening the mouth and chewing difficult. If the disease occurs in postadolescent males, the infection may spread to the testes, which in severe cases may result in sterility.

Bad breath: Halitosis, commonly called "bad breath," results from an overabundance of bacteria in the mouth. In some cases it may be caused by poor oral hygiene. In others, it may be caused by a disease process that reduces the secretion of saliva for cleansing the mouth and moving food particles to the pharynx for swallowing. As a result, some food particles remain in the mouth and decompose, which provides a growth medium for the bacteria.

Lactose intolerance: Lactose intolerance is caused by a deficiency of the intestinal enzyme lactase, which acts on lactose, a sugar found in milk. When people with lactose intolerance drink milk, this sugar is not digested properly. Bacterial action on the undigested sugar causes gas and a bloated feeling. The undigested lactose also prevents absorption of water from the small intestine, which leads to diarrhea. The solution to this problem is to avoid milk and milk products.

Appendicitis: Appendicitis is an inflammation that sometimes occurs when infectious material becomes trapped inside the appendix. If the inflamed appendix ruptures and releases the infectious contents into the abdominal cavity, the peritoneum may become involved, resulting in a potentially life-threatening inflammation of the peritoneum, called *peritonitis.* Treatment for appendicitis is usually the surgical removal of the appendix.

Borborygmus: Borborygmus is the rumbling noise caused by the propulsion of gas through the intestines. ∎

COMPONENTS OF THE DIGESTIVE TRACT

MOUTH

The mouth, or *oral cavity,* is the first part of the digestive tract. It is adapted to perform the following: receive food by ingestion, break it into small particles by **mastication,** and mix it with saliva. The lips, cheeks, and palate form the boundaries of the mouth. The oral cavity contains the teeth and tongue and receives the secretions from the salivary glands.

Lips and Cheeks

The lips and cheeks help hold food in the mouth and keep it in place for chewing. They are also used in the formation of words for speech. The lips contain numerous sensory receptors that are useful for judging the temperature and texture of foods. The cheeks form the lateral boundaries of the oral cavity. The main components of the cheeks are the *buccinator muscle* and other muscles of facial expression. On the outside, the muscles are covered by skin and subcutaneous tissue.

Palate

The **palate** is the roof of the oral cavity. It separates the oral cavity from the nasal cavity. The anterior portion, the *hard palate,* is supported by bone. The posterior portion, the *soft palate,* is skeletal muscle and connective tissue. The soft palate ends in a projection called the *uvula.* During swallowing, the soft palate and uvula move upward to direct food away from the nasal cavity and into the oropharynx.

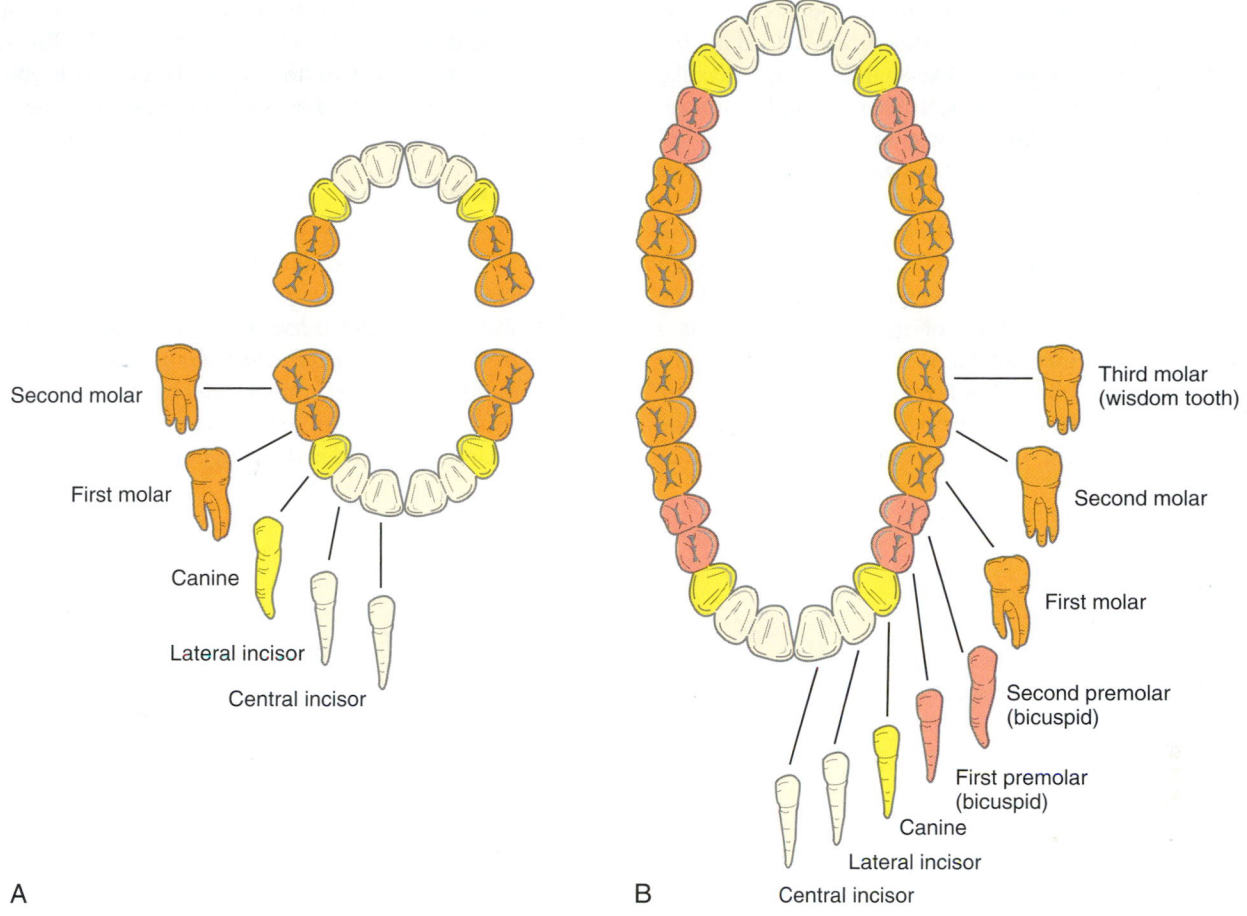

Figure 14-3 Deciduous **(A)** and permanent **(B)** teeth. The deciduous dentition on the left has 20 teeth. The permanent dentition on the right contains 32 teeth. (From Applegate E: *The anatomy and physiology learning system,* ed 4, St Louis, 2011, Saunders.)

Tongue

The largest and most movable organ in the oral cavity is the *tongue.* Most of the tongue consists of skeletal muscle. The major attachment for the tongue is the posterior region, or root, which is anchored to the hyoid bone. The anterior portion is relatively free but is connected to the floor of the mouth, in the midline, by a membranous fold of tissue called the *lingual frenulum.* The dorsal surface of the tongue is covered by tiny projections called *papillae.* The papillae provide friction for manipulating food in the mouth, and they also contain the taste buds (see Chapter 10). The *lingual tonsils* are embedded in the posterior surface of the tongue. The lingual tonsils provide a defense against bacteria that enter the mouth.

The muscles in the tongue allow the tongue to perform the following: manipulate the food in the mouth for mastication, move the food around to mix it with saliva, shape it into a ball-like mass called a *bolus,* and direct it toward the pharynx for swallowing. It is a major sensory organ for taste and is one of the major organs used in speech.

Teeth

Two different sets of teeth develop in the mouth. The first set begins to appear at approximately 6 months of age and continues to develop until about 2½ years of age. This set is known as the *primary* or *deciduous teeth.* The primary teeth contain 10 teeth in each jaw for a total of 20 teeth. Figure 14-3, A illustrates the types of primary teeth. Starting at 6 years of age, the primary teeth begin to fall out and are replaced by the *secondary* or *permanent teeth.* This set contains 16 teeth in each jaw for a total of 32 teeth. These teeth are illustrated in Figure 14-3, B.

Different teeth are shaped to handle food in different ways. The *incisors* are chisel-shaped and have sharp edges for biting food. *Cuspids (canines)* are cone-shaped and have points for grasping and tearing food. *Bicuspids (premolars)* and *molars* have flat surfaces with rounded projections for crushing and grinding. Note the location of each type of tooth in Figure 14-3.

Although the different types of teeth have different shapes, each tooth has three parts: crown, neck, and root.

The *crown* is the visible portion of the tooth, covered by enamel. The *root* is the portion that is embedded in the sockets (alveolar processes) of the mandible and maxilla. The *neck* is a small region in which the crown and root meet and is adjacent to the **gingiva,** or gum.

The central core of a tooth is the *pulp cavity.* It contains the *pulp,* which consists of connective tissue, blood vessels, and nerves. In the root, the pulp cavity is called the *root canal.* Nerves and blood vessels enter the root through an *apical foramen.* The pulp cavity is surrounded by dentin, which forms the bulk of the tooth. Dentin is a living cellular substance similar to bone. In the root, the dentin is surrounded by a thin layer of calcified connective tissue called *cementum,* which attaches the root to the periodontal ligaments. The ligaments have fibers that firmly anchor the root in the alveolar process. Enamel surrounds the dentin in the crown of the tooth. Enamel is the hardest substance in the body. Figure 14-4 shows a longitudinal section of a tooth and illustrates the major features.

Salivary Glands

Three pairs of salivary glands secrete saliva into the oral cavity. The saliva is mixed with food during mastication (Figure 14-5). The *parotid glands* are the largest of the salivary glands. One gland is located on each side of the head just in front of the ear. *Submandibular glands* are located on the floor of the mouth. Small *sublingual glands* are also located in the floor of the mouth, anterior to the submandibular glands, and under the tongue.

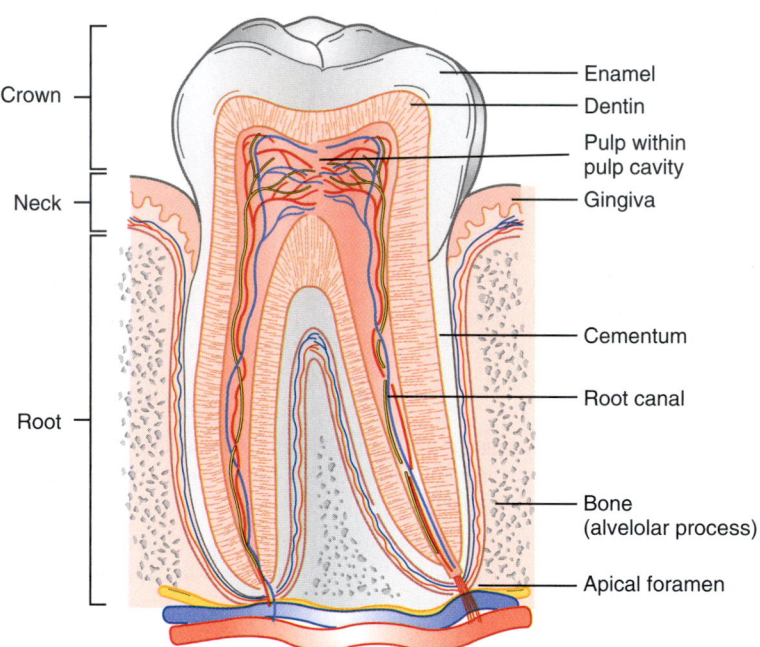

Figure 14-4 Longitudinal section of a tooth. (From Applegate E: *The anatomy and physiology learning system,* ed 4, St Louis, 2011, Saunders.)

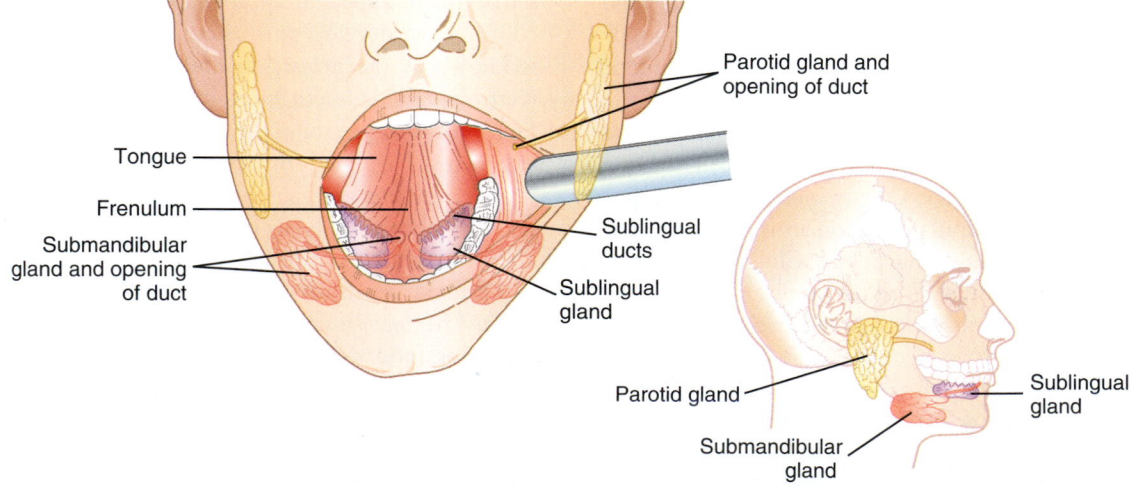

Figure 14-5 Locations of the salivary glands. (From Applegate E: *The anatomy and physiology learning system,* ed 4, St Louis, 2011, Saunders.)

Saliva contains water, mucus, and the enzyme *amylase.* Functions of saliva include the following:

- It has a cleansing action on the teeth.
- It moistens and lubricates food during mastication and swallowing.
- It dissolves certain molecules so that foods can be tasted.
- It begins the chemical digestion of starches.

PHARYNX

The pharynx is a passageway that connects the nasal and oral cavities to the larynx and esophagus (see Figure 13-2). It serves both the respiratory and digestive systems as a channel for air and food. The upper region is the *nasopharynx* and is posterior to the nasal cavity. It contains the pharyngeal tonsils, also known as the adenoids. The nasopharynx functions as a passageway for air but has no function in the digestive system. The middle region posterior to the oral cavity is the *oropharynx.* This is the region food enters when it is swallowed. The opening from the oral cavity into the oropharynx is called the **fauces.** Masses of lymphoid tissue, the palatine tonsils, are near the fauces. The lower region of the pharynx is the *laryngopharynx.* The laryngopharynx opens into both the esophagus and the larynx.

Food is forced into the pharynx by the tongue. When food reaches the opening (fauces), sensory receptors around the fauces respond and initiate an involuntary swallowing reflex. Peristaltic movements propel the food from the pharynx into the esophagus.

ESOPHAGUS

The esophagus is a collapsible muscular tube, about 25 cm (10 inches) long, and it serves as a passageway for food between the pharynx and stomach. It lies behind the trachea and in front of the vertebral column. It passes through an opening in the diaphragm and then empties into the stomach. The mucosa has glands that secrete mucus to keep the lining of the esophagus moist and well lubricated. This eases the passage of food through the esophagus. The **lower esophageal sphincter** (sometimes called the *cardiac sphincter*) controls the movement of food between the esophagus and the stomach.

STOMACH

The stomach receives food from the esophagus and is located in the upper left quadrant of the abdomen. Its capacity varies; in the adult it averages about 1.5 L, although in some individuals it may hold up to 4 L.

Structure

The stomach is divided into the cardiac, fundus, body, and pyloric regions (Figure 14-6). The *cardiac region* is a small region around the opening from the esophagus. The *fundus* is the most superior region. It balloons above the cardiac region to form a temporary storage area. The *body* is the main portion of the stomach. The body of the stomach curves to the right, creating two curvatures. The *lesser curvature* is concave and the *greater curvature* is convex. As the body approaches the exit from the stomach, it narrows into the *pyloric region.* A circular band of smooth muscle forms the **pyloric sphincter,** which acts as a valve between the stomach and small intestine.

The muscular layer in the wall of the stomach provides mixing movements to mix the food with enzymes and other fluids. When the stomach is empty, the mucosa and submucosa exhibit longitudinal folds, called **rugae.** These folds allow the stomach to expand, and as it fills the rugae become less apparent.

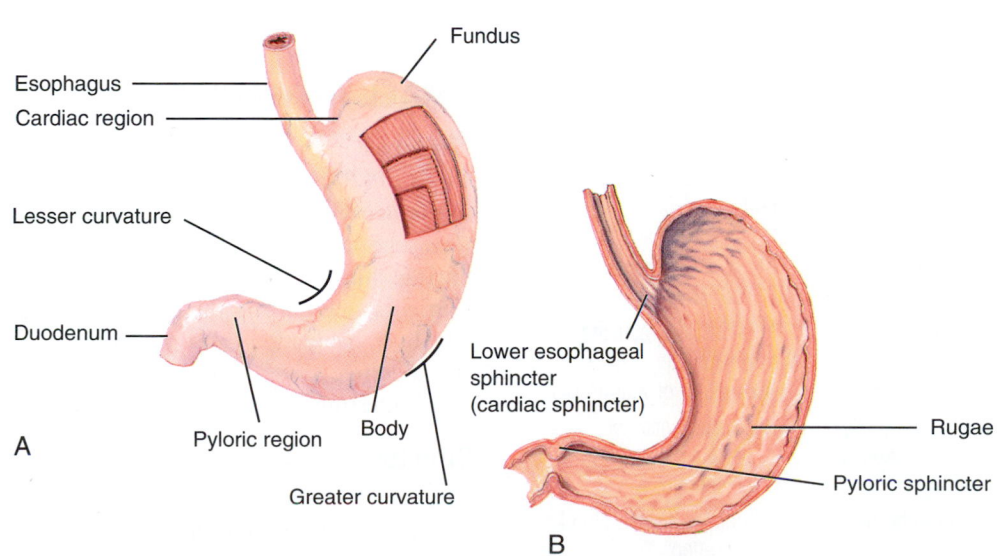

Figure 14-6 Features of the stomach. **A,** External view. **B,** Internal view. Note the rugae. (From Applegate E: *The anatomy and physiology learning system,* ed 4, St Louis, 2011, Saunders.)

Gastric Secretions

The mucosal lining of the stomach contains numerous gastric glands. The gastric glands open to the surface of the mucosa through tiny holes called *gastric pits.* Four different types of cells make up the gastric glands: mucous cells, parietal cells, chief cells, and endocrine cells.

Exocrine gastric glands are composed of mucous cells, parietal cells, and chief cells. The secretions of the exocrine gastric glands make up the **gastric juice.** Approximately 2 to 3 L of gastric juice are produced every day. The products of the endocrine cells are secreted directly into the bloodstream and are not a part of the gastric juice.

Mucous cells produce two types of mucus in the stomach. One type is thick and alkaline and forms a protective coating for the stomach lining. The other type is thin and watery. It mixes with the food and creates a fluid medium for chemical reactions. *Parietal cells* secrete hydrochloric acid and intrinsic factor. The hydrochloric acid kills bacteria and provides an acidic environment for the action of enzymes in the stomach. Intrinsic factor aids in the absorption of vitamin B_{12}. *Chief cells* secrete pepsinogen. Pepsinogen is an inactive form of the enzyme pepsin. Hydrochloric acid converts the inactive pepsinogen into the active enzyme pepsin, which begins the chemical digestion of proteins.

The *endocrine cells* secrete the hormone **gastrin,** which functions in the regulation of gastric activity. Table 14-1 summarizes the various cells and secretions of the gastric glands.

The churning action of the muscles in the stomach wall breaks the food particles of the bolus that was swallowed into smaller sizes and mixes them with the gastric juice. This produces a semifluid mixture called **chyme,** which leaves the stomach through the pyloric sphincter and enters the small intestine.

Regulation of Gastric Secretions

The regulation of gastric secretions is accomplished through neural and hormonal mechanisms. Gastric juice is produced all the time, but the amount varies based on certain factors. Regulation of gastric secretions may be divided into cephalic, gastric, and intestinal phases.

The *cephalic phase* begins when an individual thinks pleasant thoughts about food or sees, smells, or tastes food. This phase anticipates food and prepares the stomach to receive it by increasing the secretion of gastric juice. The *gastric phase* accounts for more than two thirds of the gastric juice secretion. The gastric phase begins when food reaches the stomach. The presence of food in the stomach and the distention of the stomach wall stimulate reflexes that result in gastrin secretion. Gastrin, in turn, stimulates the secretion of gastric juice, which contains hydrochloric acid and pepsinogen. The hydrochloric acid acidifies the stomach contents and activates the pepsinogen into pepsin, which breaks down proteins.

The passage of chyme through the pyloric sphincter into the first part (duodenum) of the small intestine triggers the *intestinal phase* of regulation. Distention and the presence of acid chyme in the duodenum stimulate the secretion of intestinal hormones, which in turn inhibit gastric secretions. These inhibitory responses help prevent excess acid chyme from entering the small intestine. The intestinal phase regulates the entry of chyme into the small intestine.

Stomach Emptying

Peristalsis in the stomach pushes chyme toward the pyloric region. As the chyme accumulates, the pyloric sphincter relaxes and a small amount of chyme is pumped into the small intestine. The rate at which the stomach empties depends on the nature of the contents and the receptivity of the small intestine. The stomach is usually empty within 4 hours after a meal. Liquids tend to pass through the stomach quickly. Solids stay in the stomach until they are well mixed with gastric juice. Carbohydrates move through rather quickly, proteins take a little longer, and fatty foods may stay in the stomach as long as 4 to 6 hours.

SMALL INTESTINE

The small intestine is about 2.5 cm (1 inch) in diameter and 6 m (20 ft) long. It extends from the pyloric sphincter to the **ileocecal valve,** where it empties into the large intestine. The function of the small intestine includes the following: finishing the process of digestion, absorbing the nutrients, and passing the residue on to the large intestine. The liver, gallbladder, and pancreas are accessory organs of the digestive system that are closely associated with the small intestine. These are described later in this chapter.

Structure

The small intestine follows the general structure of the digestive tract in that the wall has four layers: mucosa, submucosa, smooth muscle, and serosa. The mucosa and submucosa have circular folds, called **plicae circulares,** which increase the surface area for absorption (Figure 14-7).

Table 14-1 Secretions of Gastric Glands

Cell Type	Secretion	Function
Mucous cells	Mucus (thick, alkaline)	Protects stomach lining
	Mucus (thin, watery)	Medium for chemical reactions
Parietal cells	Hydrochloric acid	Kills bacteria; activates pepsinogen
	Intrinsic factor	Absorption of vitamin B_{12}
Chief cells	Pepsinogen (active form is pepsin)	Begins digestion of proteins into polypeptides
Endocrine cells	Gastrin (a hormone)	Stimulates gastric gland secretion

From Applegate E: *The anatomy and physiology learning system,* ed 4, St Louis, 2011, Saunders.

Figure 14-7 Wall of the small intestine. (From Applegate E: *The anatomy and physiology learning system,* ed 4, St Louis, 2011, Saunders.)

Finger-like extensions of the mucosa, called *villi,* project from the circular folds, and this further increases the surface area. Each villus surrounds a blood capillary network and a lymph capillary, or *lacteal.* These function in the absorption of nutrients. *Intestinal glands* extend downward between adjacent villi. The surface epithelium on the villi has tiny hairlike cytoplasmic extensions, called *microvilli,* that form a *brush border,* which again increases surface area.

Although the structure is similar throughout, the length of the small intestine is divided into three regions: duodenum, jejunum, and ileum.

The *duodenum* is the first part and is about 25 cm (10 inches) long. It begins at the pyloric sphincter and continues in a C-shaped curve to the jejunum. The duodenum receives the chyme from the stomach and secretions from the liver and pancreas.

The second portion of the small intestine is the *jejunum,* which is about 2.5 m (8 ft) long. This is continuous with the third portion, the *ileum,* which is about 3.5 m (11.5 ft) long. No distinct separation exists between the jejunum and ileum. They are similar in structure and are suspended from the abdominal wall by a fold of peritoneum, called **mesentery.** There is a gradual decrease in the number and length of the villi and an increase in the number of goblet cells in the mucosa from the beginning of the jejunum to the terminal portion of the ileum.

Secretions of the Small Intestine

Intestinal glands secrete large amounts of watery fluid that is neutral or slightly alkaline in pH. It keeps the chyme in a liquid form and provides both an appropriate environment for the many chemical reactions of digestion and a fluid medium for the absorption of nutrients. The fluid is readily reabsorbed by the capillaries in the microvilli.

Mucus is secreted by the wall of the small intestine. The alkaline mucus protects the intestinal wall from the acid chyme and digestive enzymes.

Digestive enzymes are located in the microvilli of the mucosal epithelial cells. These enzymes include the following: *peptidase,* which acts on segments of proteins called *peptides; maltase, sucrase,* and *lactase,* which act on disaccharides (double sugars); and an *intestinal lipase,* which acts on neutral fats. *Enterokinase,* although not actually a digestive enzyme, is produced by the mucosal epithelial cells. This enzyme activates a protein-splitting enzyme from the pancreas.

In addition to mucus and digestive enzymes, intestinal cells secrete at least two hormones—secretin and cholecystokinin. *Secretin* stimulates the pancreas to secrete a fluid that has a high bicarbonate ion concentration. This fluid helps to neutralize chyme so that the intestinal enzymes can function. *Cholecystokinin* stimulates the release of bile from the

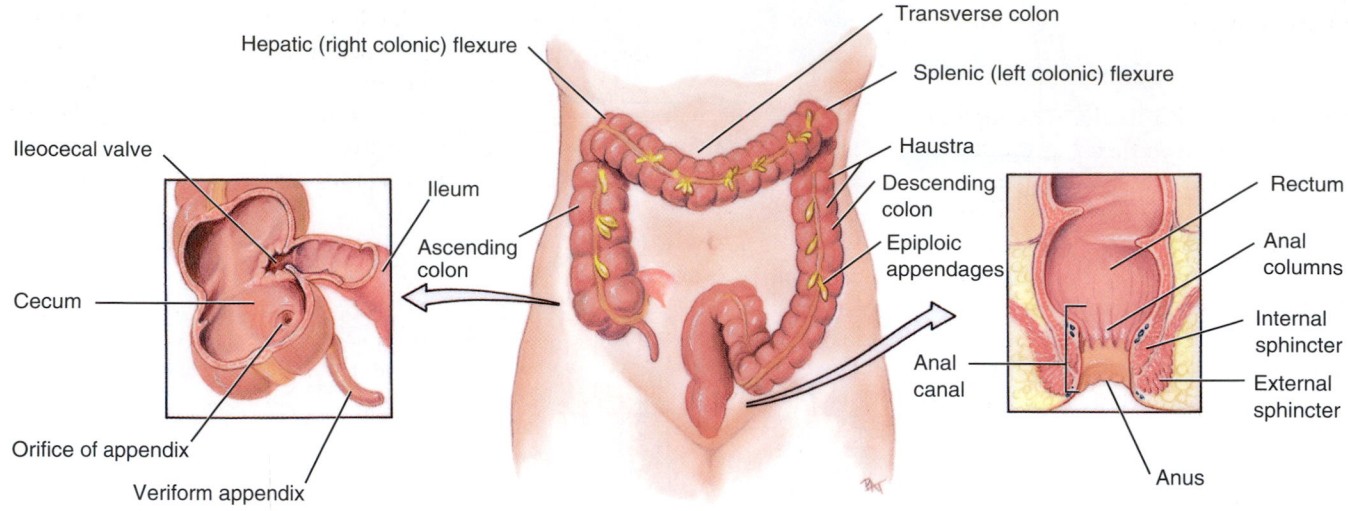

Figure 14-8 Features of the large intestine. (From Applegate E: *The anatomy and physiology learning system,* ed 4, St Louis, 2011, Saunders.)

gallbladder and the secretion of digestive enzymes from the pancreas. It also inhibits gastric motility and secretions.

The most important factor for regulating secretions in the small intestine is the presence of chyme. This is largely a local reflex action in response to chemical and mechanical irritation from the chyme and in response to distention of the intestinal wall. This is a direct reflex action; thus the greater the amount of chyme, the greater the secretion.

LARGE INTESTINE

The *large intestine* is larger in diameter (6.25 cm or 2.5 inches) than the small intestine but is only about 1.5 m (5 ft) long (Figure 14-8). It begins at the ileocecal junction, where the ileum enters the large intestine, and ends at the anus. The ileocecal junction has a circular band of smooth muscle fibers—the ileocecal sphincter—and a valve—the ileocecal valve.

Characteristics

The wall of the large intestine has the same types of tissue that are found in other parts of the digestive tract, but there are some distinguishing characteristics. The mucosa has large numbers of goblet cells but does not have any villi. The longitudinal muscle layer, although present, is incomplete. The longitudinal muscle is limited to three distinct bands, called **teniae coli,** that run the entire length of the colon. Contraction of the teniae coli exerts pressure on the wall and creates a series of pouches, called *haustra,* along the colon. *Epiploic appendages,* pieces of fat-filled connective tissue, are attached to the outer surface of the colon.

Regions of the Large Intestine

The large intestine consists of the cecum, colon, rectum, and anal canal (see Figure 14-8).

Cecum

The cecum is the proximal portion of the large intestine. It is a blind pouch that extends from the ileocecal junction. The vermiform appendix is attached to the cecum. In humans the appendix has no function in digestion but does contain some lymphatic tissue.

Colon

The colon is the longest portion of the large intestine and is divided into ascending, transverse, descending, and sigmoid portions. The *ascending colon* begins at the ileocecal junction and travels upward on the right side, until it reaches the liver. Here it turns to the left, becomes the *transverse colon,* and continues across the abdomen toward the spleen on the left side. Here the colon turns sharply downward and travels along the posterior abdominal wall as the *descending colon.* The descending colon makes an S-shaped curve, called the *sigmoid colon,* and then becomes the rectum. The curve between the ascending and transverse portions is the hepatic flexure. The curve between the transverse and descending portions is the splenic flexure.

Rectum

The rectum continues from the sigmoid colon to the anal canal and has a thick muscular layer.

Anal Canal

The last 2 to 3 cm (1 inch) of the digestive tract make up the anal canal, which opens to the outside at the anus. The mucosa of the anal canal is folded to form longitudinal anal columns. The smooth muscle layer is thick and forms the internal anal sphincter at the superior end of the anal canal. This sphincter is under involuntary control. At the inferior end of the anal canal is the external anal sphincter. This sphincter is composed of skeletal muscle and is under voluntary control.

Functions of the Large Intestine

The large intestine produces no digestive enzymes. Chemical digestion is completed in the small intestine before the chyme reaches the large intestine. There are no villi for the absorption of nutrients. This process is also accomplished in the small intestine. The primary functions of the large intestine are the absorption of fluid and electrolytes and the elimination of waste products.

The chyme that enters the large intestine contains materials that were not digested or absorbed in the small intestine—water, electrolytes, and bacteria. Some of the water and electrolytes are absorbed in the cecum and ascending colon. Although the quantity is relatively small, this absorptive function of the large intestine is important in maintaining fluid balance in the body. The residue that remains from the chyme becomes the feces.

The large intestine has the same types of mixing and peristaltic movements as occur in other parts of the digestive tract, but they are more sluggish and occur less frequently. They are more likely to occur after a meal as a result of reflexes initiated in the small intestine. As the rectum fills with feces, the defecation reflex is triggered and the waste products are eliminated.

The only secretory product in the large intestine is mucus from the numerous goblet cells. The mucus protects the intestinal wall against abrasion and irritation from the chyme. It also helps hold the particles of fecal matter together.

ACCESSORY ORGANS OF DIGESTION

The salivary glands, liver, gallbladder, and pancreas are not part of the digestive tract, but they have a role in digestive activities and are considered accessory organs. Because the salivary glands are so closely associated with the mouth and their primary function is performed in the mouth, they are considered part of the oral cavity. The liver and pancreas have functions in addition to digestion, and the gallbladder is closely related to the liver; thus these three organs are described as separate accessory organs in this section.

LIVER

The liver is a large, reddish-brown organ. It is the largest gland in the body and is located in the right hypochondriac and epigastric regions of the abdomen, just beneath the diaphragm.

Structure of the Liver

The liver is divided into two major lobes and two minor lobes. The *falciform ligament* attaches the liver to the abdominal wall and separates the right lobe from the left lobe. Two additional small lobes are evident on the visceral surface: the caudate lobe and the quadrate lobe (Figure 14-9). The *porta* is also on the visceral surface. The porta is where the hepatic artery and hepatic portal vein enter the liver and where the hepatic ducts exit.

The substance of the liver is divided into functional units called *liver lobules*. A liver lobule consists of *hepatocytes* (liver cells) that radiate outward from the *central vein* like spokes of a wheel. Tiny channels, called *bile canaliculi*, are interwoven with the liver cells and carry the bile that is produced by the hepatocytes toward the periphery of the lobule. Bile canaliculi merge to form larger right and left hepatic ducts. These two ducts combine to form the *common hepatic duct*, which transports bile out of the liver. The plates of hepatocytes are separated from one another by venous channels, called *sinusoids*, which carry blood from the periphery of the lobule toward the central vein. The sinusoids are lined with

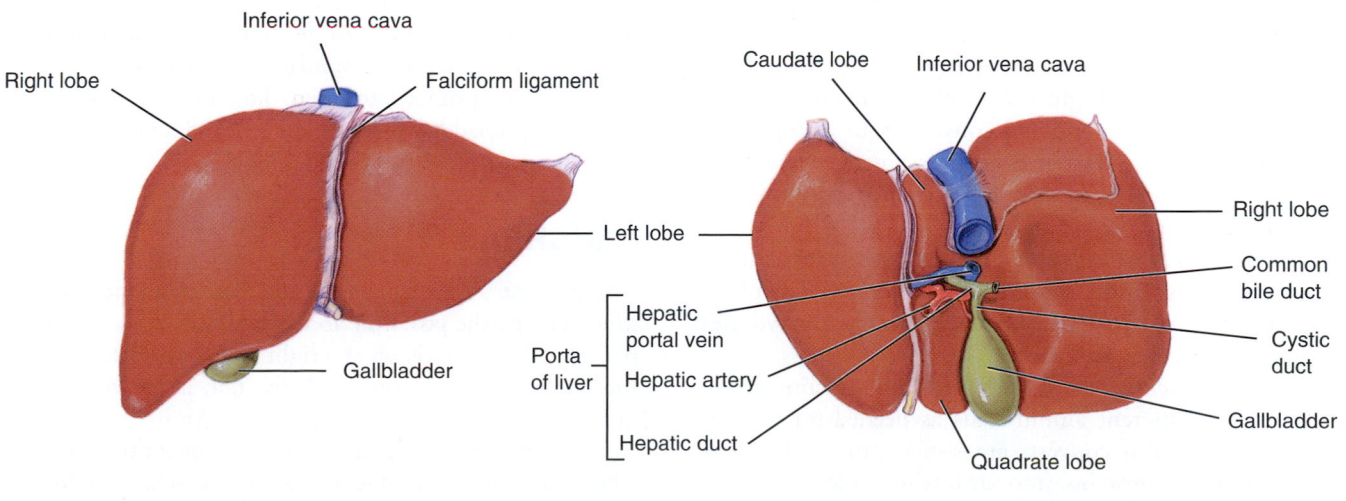

Figure 14-9 Features of the liver. (From Applegate E: *The anatomy and physiology learning system,* ed 4, St Louis, 2011, Saunders.)

special phagocytic cells, called *Kupffer cells,* that remove foreign particles from the blood as it flows through the sinusoids. *Portal triads,* which consist of a branch of the hepatic portal vein, a branch of the hepatic artery, and a branch of a hepatic duct, are located around the periphery of the lobule.

Blood Supply to the Liver

The liver receives blood from two sources. Freshly oxygenated blood is brought to the liver by the *common hepatic artery.* Blood that is rich in nutrients from the digestive tract is carried to the liver by the *hepatic portal vein.* Venous blood from the hepatic portal vein and arterial blood from the hepatic arteries mix together as the blood flows through the sinusoids toward the central vein. The central veins of the liver lobules merge to form larger *hepatic veins* that drain into the inferior vena cava.

Functions of the Liver

The liver has a wide variety of functions, many of which are vital to life. Hepatocytes (liver cells) perform most of the functions attributed to the liver, but the phagocytic Kupffer cells that line the sinusoids are responsible for cleansing the blood. Liver functions include the following:

- *Secretion:* The liver produces and secretes bile.
- *Synthesis of bile salts:* Bile salts are produced in the liver and facilitate fat digestion and the absorption of fats and fat-soluble vitamins.
- *Synthesis of plasma proteins:* The liver synthesizes albumin, fibrinogen, globulins, and clotting factors.
- *Storage:* The liver stores glucose in the form of glycogen and also stores iron and vitamins A, B_{12}, D, E, and K.
- *Detoxification:* The liver alters the chemical composition of toxic compounds to make them less harmful. It also changes the configuration of certain drugs, such as penicillin, and excretes them in the bile to remove them from the body.
- *Excretion:* Hormones, drugs, cholesterol, and bile pigments from the breakdown of hemoglobin are excreted in the bile.
- *Carbohydrate metabolism:* The liver has a major role in maintaining blood glucose levels. It removes excess glucose from the blood and converts it to glycogen for storage; it breaks down glycogen into glucose when more is necessary; and it converts noncarbohydrate molecules into glucose.
- *Lipid metabolism:* The liver functions in the breakdown of fatty acids, in the synthesis of cholesterol and phospholipids, and in the conversion of excess carbohydrates and proteins into fats.
- *Protein metabolism:* The liver converts certain amino acids into different amino acids as needed for protein synthesis. It also converts ammonia, produced in the breakdown of proteins, into urea, which is less toxic and can be excreted in the bile.
- *Filtering:* The phagocytic Kupffer cells that line the sinusoids remove bacteria, damaged red blood cells, and other particles from the blood.

Bile

About 1 L of bile, a yellowish-green fluid, is produced by liver cells each day. Bile is slightly alkaline, with a pH of 7.6 to 8.6, so it helps neutralize the acid chyme. The main components of bile are water, bile salts, bile pigments, and cholesterol. The bile salts are useful secretory products of the liver, but the bile pigments and cholesterol are waste products excreted in the bile and eliminated from the body.

Bile salts function in the digestion of fats. They act as emulsifying agents that break large fat globules into tiny fat droplets. This increases the surface area of the fat and allows for more efficient enzyme action in fat digestion. Bile salts also facilitate the absorption of fat-soluble vitamins and the end products of fat digestion.

Bile pigments are produced in the breakdown of hemoglobin from damaged red blood cells. They are responsible for the color of the urine and feces. The principal bile pigment is *bilirubin.* Cholesterol is a product of lipid metabolism. Bile salts act on cholesterol to make it soluble; then it is excreted in the bile.

GALLBLADDER

The *gallbladder* is a pear-shaped sac that is attached to the liver by the cystic duct (see Figure 14-9). The cystic duct joins the hepatic duct from the liver to form the *common bile duct.* The common bile duct empties into the duodenum. When the gallbladder contracts, bile is ejected from the gallbladder into the cystic duct.

The principal functions of the gallbladder are to store and concentrate bile. Bile is continuously produced by the liver and then travels through the hepatic duct and common bile duct to the duodenum. There is a sphincter (sphincter of Oddi) where the common bile duct enters the duodenum. If the small intestine is empty, the sphincter is closed and the bile backs up through the cystic duct into the gallbladder for concentration and storage until it is needed. When chyme with fatty contents enters the duodenum, the hormone *cholecystokinin* stimulates the gallbladder to contract and the sphincter to open. This permits bile to flow from the gallbladder, through the cystic duct and common bile duct, and then into the duodenum.

PANCREAS

The *pancreas* is an elongated and flattened organ that is located along the posterior abdominal wall. One end of the pancreas, the head, is on the right side within the curve of the duodenum; the other end, the tail, is on the left side next to the spleen.

The pancreas has both endocrine and exocrine functions. The endocrine portion consists of the scattered *islets of Langerhans,* which secrete the hormones insulin and glucagon into the blood. These hormones and their functions are discussed in Chapter 11. The exocrine portion is the major part of the gland. It consists of *pancreatic acinar cells,* which secrete digestive enzymes into tiny ducts interwoven between the cells. These tiny ducts merge to form the main *pancreatic duct,* which extends the full length of the pancreas and empties into the duodenum. The pancreatic duct usually joins the common bile duct to form a single point of entry into the duodenum. Both ducts are controlled by the hepatopancreatic sphincter (sphincter of Oddi).

Pancreatic juice has a high concentration of bicarbonate ions and contains digestive enzymes that act on carbohydrates, proteins, and lipids. *Pancreatic amylase* acts on starch and other complex carbohydrates to break them into simpler sugars called *disaccharides.* Protein-splitting enzymes from the pancreas include *trypsin.* This enzyme breaks the proteins into shorter chains of amino acids, called *peptides.* Like other enzymes that act on proteins, trypsin is secreted in an inactive form, *trypsinogen.* This is activated by enterokinase when it reaches the duodenum. The pancreas also secretes peptidase enzymes that break peptides into amino acids. *Pancreatic lipase* breaks fats into fatty acids and monoglycerides.

Pancreatic secretion of digestive juice is regulated by the nervous system and by hormones. When parasympathetic impulses from the nervous system stimulate secretion of gastric juice, some impulses go to the pancreas and stimulate the secretion of pancreatic juice. When acid chyme enters the duodenum, the intestinal mucosa produces the hormone *secretin,* which travels in the blood to the pancreas. Secretin stimulates the pancreas to produce a fluid that has a high concentration of bicarbonate ions to neutralize the acids in the duodenum. Proteins and fats in the chyme stimulate the intestinal mucosa to secrete the hormone *cholecystokinin,* which also travels in the blood to the pancreas. This hormone stimulates the pancreas to produce a pancreatic juice that is rich in digestive enzymes. These digestive enzymes travel through the pancreatic duct to the duodenum, where they perform their actions.

CHEMICAL DIGESTION

Chemical digestion breaks down large complex molecules into smaller molecules that can be absorbed by the cells of the intestinal mucosa. The reactions in chemical digestion are **hydrolysis** reactions, which use water to split molecules. These reactions proceed at a slow rate. The purpose of the various digestive enzymes is to speed up the hydrolysis reactions of chemical digestion. The enzymes do not alter the reactions; they just make them occur more rapidly. Table 14-2 reviews the hormones and digestive enzymes that are discussed in previous sections of this chapter.

CARBOHYDRATE DIGESTION

Starches and other complex carbohydrates are first broken down into disaccharides, or double sugars, by the action of salivary amylase and pancreatic amylase. The disaccharides *sucrose, maltose,* and *lactose* are the result of this stage of

Table 14-2 Enzymes and Hormones of the Digestive System

Secretion	Source	Action
Enzymes		
Amylase	Salivary glands Pancreas	Digestion of complex carbohydrates into disaccharides
Pepsin	Stomach	Digestion of proteins into polypeptides
Sucrase Maltase Lactase	Small intestine	Digestion of disaccharides into glucose, fructose, and galactose
Peptidase	Small intestine Pancreas	Digestion of peptides into amino acids
Lipase	Small intestine Pancreas	Digestion of fats into monoglycerides and fatty acids
Enterokinase	Small intestine	Activates trypsinogen
Hormones		
Gastrin	Stomach	Stimulates activity of gastric glands
Secretin	Small intestine	Stimulates pancreas to secrete bicarbonate ions to neutralize acid chyme
Cholecystokinin	Small intestine	Stimulates gallbladder to contract and release bile; stimulates pancreas to secrete digestive enzymes

From Applegate E: *The anatomy and physiology learning system,* ed 4, St Louis, 2011, Saunders.

digestion. Sucrase, maltase, and lactase—enzymes from the small intestine—act on the disaccharides to convert them to monosaccharides, or simple sugars, that can be absorbed. The digestion of maltose yields two molecules of glucose; sucrose produces one molecule of glucose and one of fructose; lactose yields one molecule each of glucose and galactose. The end products of complete carbohydrate digestion are the monosaccharides *glucose, fructose,* and *galactose.*

PROTEIN DIGESTION

The first digestive enzyme to act on proteins is pepsin in the stomach. Pepsin is secreted by the gastric glands in an inactive form, pepsinogen, which is activated by hydrochloric acid. When chyme reaches the duodenum, trypsin from the pancreas acts on the proteins. Trypsin is secreted in the inactive form, trypsinogen, which is activated by enterokinase in the small intestine. Pepsin and trypsin break down proteins into shorter chains of amino acids called *peptides.* Peptidase enzymes from the small intestine and pancreas break the peptide bonds to produce *amino acids.* The amino acids are the absorbable end products of protein digestion.

LIPID DIGESTION

The small intestine is the only place in which lipid (fat) digestion occurs because the necessary enzymes are produced by the pancreas and enter the small intestine through the pancreatic duct. Triglycerides are the most abundant dietary fats. Fat molecules tend to attract one another to form large globules, which reduces the surface area for enzyme action. After the fats enter the duodenum, they are emulsified by bile. Emulsification does not break any chemical bonds, but it reduces the attraction between molecules so that they disperse. Pancreatic lipases act on the surfaces of the emulsified fat droplets. Lipase action breaks two fatty acid chains from the triglyceride molecules, yielding *monoglycerides* and *free fatty acids.*

ABSORPTION

Approximately 10 L of food, beverage, and secretions enter the digestive tract every day. Usually less than 1 L enters the large intestine. The other 9 L or more are absorbed in the small intestine. Absorption takes place along the entire length of the small intestine, but most of it occurs in the jejunum. By the time the chyme reaches the distal part of the ileum and large intestine, all that remains are some water, indigestible materials, and bacteria.

AGING OF THE DIGESTIVE SYSTEM

Throughout life the digestive system normally functions day after day with relatively few problems. There may be an occasional episode of GI tract inflammation, called *gastroenteritis,* caused by eating something that "doesn't agree," by irritation from excessively spicy foods, or by eating food that is contaminated by bacteria or toxins. Appendicitis tends to be fairly common in teenagers, but the prevalence decreases with age because the opening into the appendix tends to become smaller and possibly eventually closes. Ulcers and gallbladder problems are associated with middle age, often considered to be the high-stress time of life. Most of the difficulties in the digestive system before old age are caused by external problems rather than by structural changes within the system itself.

Structural changes in the digestive system occur as part of the normal aging process. These changes affect the overall operation of the system and may influence the nutritional state of the aging individual. In the mouth, teeth may become loose as a result of periodontal disease and have to be extracted. Because of dental problems, chewing may be uncomfortable. Salivary glands decrease their production of saliva, which reduces the salivary cleansing action and leads to a dry mouth (xerostomia). Thus food is not adequately moistened for chewing and swallowing. Taste sensations diminish, partially because there is less saliva to dissolve the taste particles and partially because there are fewer taste receptors. Loneliness and the problems in the oral cavity associated with aging may make eating a chore rather than a pleasure.

The mucosa in the stomach and intestines undergoes some atrophy with advancing age. In the stomach this may lead to a deficiency in hydrochloric acid and gastric juice for digestion. Pernicious anemia may develop because there is a lack of intrinsic factor from the gastric mucosa. In the small intestine, mucosal atrophy may lead to fewer enzymes and shorter villi; however, this does not appear to impair digestion and absorption in normal healthy people. The wall of the large intestine becomes thinner and weakens. This makes older people more susceptible to diverticulosis, in which the wall bulges outward to form balloon-like pockets. Constipation is a common complaint in the elderly; statistically, however, there seems to be no basis for it. This is more likely caused by lifestyle and habits rather than by structural changes in the digestive system.

Although structural and functional changes take place in the digestive system as part of the aging process, digestion and absorption are not altered noticeably in healthy older persons. A balanced diet, exercise, and a positive outlook on life will keep the digestive system in good working order for a long time.

Common Pathology of the Digestive System

Disease	Signs and Symptoms	Etiology	Diagnosis and Treatment
Anorexia	Extreme weight loss, thin appearance, abnormal blood count, fatigue, insomnia, dehydration, osteoporosis, and obsession with weight, exercise, and calorie intake.	An eating disorder. Exact cause is unknown. It is probably a combination of biologic, psychological, and environmental factors.	Criteria for diagnosis are refusal to maintain a body weight that is at or above minimum normal, intense fear of gaining weight, denying the seriousness of low body weight, and the absence of menstrual periods for at least 3 consecutive cycles. Treatment involves medical care to restore body weight combined with psychotherapy.

Common Pathology of the Digestive System—cont'd

Disease	Signs and Symptoms	Etiology	Diagnosis and Treatment
Appendicitis	Pain in the lower right abdomen, loss of appetite, nausea and/or vomiting, abdominal swelling, fever.	Occurs when the opening cecum into the appendix becomes blocked. Bacteria inside the appendix multiply rapidly and cause inflammation. A ruptured appendix is a medical emergency because the bacteria can diffuse throughout the abdomen, causing extensive peritonitis.	Diagnosis relies on patient history, blood and urine tests, and imaging techniques. Treatment is surgical removal of the appendix (appendectomy).
Bulimia	Characterized by binge eating and purging. Signs and symptoms include chronic gastric reflux, dehydration, electrolyte imbalance, esophagitis, depression, low self-esteem, obsession with weight and calorie intake.	An eating disorder. Exact cause is unknown, but probably includes environmental factors in the form of social expectations, genetic predisposition, and psychological factors.	Diagnosis relies on physical examination, blood and urine tests, and psychological evaluation. Diagnostic criteria include repeated binging; getting rid of extra calories by vomiting, use of laxatives or diuretics, or excessive exercise; binging and purging at least twice per week for at least 3 months; excessive importance of body weight and shape to feelings of self-esteem. Treatment of choice is cognitive-behavioral therapy to break the binge-purge cycle, solve emotional issues, and change attitudes about weight, diet, and body shape.
Caries	Dental caries (cavities) may present no signs or symptoms in the early stages. As decay continues, there may be sensitivity to heat and cold, and finally a toothache begins.	Caries is the result of poor dental care. Acids from oral bacteria slowly erode the enamel of the teeth until a cavity forms.	Diagnosis is made by a dentist who uses direct observation and dental x-rays. Once a cavity has developed, the dentist may fill it with an amalgam. Prevention is the best treatment. Routine prophylactic dental care and good dental hygiene are the keys to healthy teeth.
Celiac disease	Anemia, diarrhea, gas and bloating, weight loss, fatigue.	Exact cause is unknown, but evidence indicates genetic factors may be involved. Gluten triggers an immune response that damages the small intestine and interferes with the absorption of nutrients.	Physical examination, medical history, blood tests, antibody tests, and endoscopy are used in diagnosis. Treatment is to avoid eating gluten in any form. Nutritional supplements may be necessary.
Cholecystitis	Pain in upper right abdomen, nausea, vomiting, fever, and abdominal bloating.	Inflammation of the gallbladder is most often caused by gallstones that block the cystic duct.	Ultrasound and/or computed tomography (CT) scan are used to confirm diagnosis. Common treatment is surgical removal of the gallbladder (cholecystectomy).
Cholelithiasis	May be asymptomatic for years. When one or more become lodged in a duct, symptoms appear, including sudden and intense pain in upper right abdomen often accompanied by nausea and vomiting.	Cholelithiasis (gallstones) occurs when cholesterol and other substances in the bile precipitate and form crystals in the gallbladder. These may aggregate to form stones.	Diagnosis relies on patient history, abdominal ultrasound, and CT scans. The most reliable treatment, when necessary, is surgery to remove the gallbladder (cholecystectomy).
Cirrhosis	Signs and symptoms are directly related to liver functions and include bruising and bleeding, accumulation of toxins in the blood, jaundice, malnutrition, portal hypertension, splenomegaly, esophageal varices, dilated periumbilical veins, ascites.	The most common causes of cirrhosis are chronic alcohol abuse, hepatitis B, and hepatitis C.	Tests and procedures used to diagnose cirrhosis include liver function tests; imaging procedures such as ultrasound, CT, and magnetic resonance imaging (MRI); and liver biopsy. Treatment protocols are directed at the underlying cause. The goals of treatment are to slow the development of scar tissue and to prevent or alleviate the symptoms.

Continued

Common Pathology of the Digestive System—cont'd

Disease	Signs and Symptoms	Etiology	Diagnosis and Treatment
Cleft palate or lip	Split or opening in the roof of the mouth (palate) or in the upper lip.	Cause is unknown; probably has genetic and environmental factors. Birth defect that occurs early in pregnancy. Smoking and diabetes in the mother appear to increase the risk.	During pregnancy, ultrasound can detect the deformity. After birth the condition is obvious. Treatment is plastic surgery to close the openings.
Cold sores (fever blisters)	Small blisters on the lip, often red, swollen, and sore.	Caused by the herpes simplex virus (HSV), which enters through a break in the skin around the mouth; spread by coming in contact with infected fluid such as saliva.	The occurrence of the blisters is diagnostic. Sores are usually self-resolving within a few days, but skin creams may relieve the discomfort. The virus cannot be "cured"; it remains in the body. Recurrent outbreaks can be minimized by avoiding triggers such as stress.
Colitis	Inflammation of the lining of the colon with abdominal pain, diarrhea, fever, bloating, and blood in feces.	May be caused by bacterial invasion of the lining, loss of blood supply to the colon, or inflammatory bowel disease.	Diagnostic tools include patient history and physical examination, blood tests, urinalysis, and colonoscopy. Treatment is directed at the underlying cause of the inflammation.
Colorectal cancer	May be several years before symptoms develop and then they are nonspecific: fatigue, irregular bowel habits, blood in feces, abdominal pain, cramps, bloating, and weight loss.	Cause is unknown but risk factors include high-fat diet, family history of colorectal cancer, and inflammatory bowel disease.	Diagnosis is by colonoscopy and/or lower gastrointestinal (GI) series (barium enema). Treatment depends on the stage; early stages may be treated by surgery alone, more advanced cancer may require chemotherapy. Early detection through screening is a key factor.
Crohn disease	A type of inflammatory bowel disease; not limited to colon, may affect any part of the digestive tract and may extend into the deeper tissues of the tract. Signs and symptoms are nonspecific: diarrhea, abdominal pain, cramps, ulcers, loss of appetite, weight loss, malnutrition, fever, fatigue, and blood in feces.	Cause is unknown, but heredity and altered immune response seem to be involved. Risk factors include family history and cigarette smoking.	Diagnostic tools include fecal occult blood test, colonoscopy, sigmoidoscopy, and CT and/or MRI scans. There is no cure. Treatment is directed at managing symptoms and may include antiinflammatory medications, immunosuppressants, and antibiotics.
Diverticulosis	Characterized by pouchlike herniations through the muscular wall of the colon; usually asymptomatic unless they become inflamed (diverticulitis), which may cause symptoms of pain in the lower left abdomen, fever and chills, and nausea and vomiting.	Cause is not completely understood. It occurs when high pressure inside the colon pushes against weak areas in the colon wall. Studies have shown links between diverticulosis and obesity, lack of exercise, and smoking.	Diverticulosis is usually discovered during screening such as colonoscopy and needs no treatment. Diverticulitis is usually treated with oral antibiotics.
Dumping syndrome	Abdominal cramps, nausea, diarrhea	Dumping syndrome occurs when stomach contents move into the small intestine too rapidly. Most likely to develop after stomach surgery.	A gastric emptying test measures how quickly food moves into the small intestine. Alterations in diet may be sufficient treatment. For some individuals, medications may slow the passage of food from the stomach. As a last resort, a feeding tube may be necessary.

Common Pathology of the Digestive System—cont'd

Disease	Signs and Symptoms	Etiology	Diagnosis and Treatment
Gastroenteritis	Commonly called *stomach flu,* signs and symptoms include watery diarrhea, abdominal cramps, nausea and vomiting, and fever.	Viruses and/or bacteria are the most common cause of the inflammation in the stomach and small intestine.	Usually is self-limiting, and no tests are needed for diagnosis. Patients should have plenty of fluids to prevent dehydration. In some cases, medications may be necessary to stop the diarrhea and vomiting.
Gastroesophageal reflux disease (GERD)	Heartburn, nausea after eating, difficulty swallowing, regurgitation of stomach contents.	Stomach contents leak back into the esophagus because the lower esophageal sphincter (LES) does not close properly and the stomach acid damages the esophageal lining. Risk factors include obesity, pregnancy, hiatal hernia, use of alcohol, smoking, certain foods and medications.	If symptoms are severe, tests to measure the amount of acid in the esophagus and/or upper endoscopy may be necessary. Treatment involves lifestyle changes, antacids for short-term relief, avoiding foods and medications that trigger reflux. If the condition cannot be controlled, surgery to strengthen the LES may be necessary.
Gingivitis	Inflammation of gum tissue evidenced by red, swollen, tender gums, bleeding during brushing, and bad breath (halitosis).	Plaque is the cause of gingivitis. Plaque creates small pockets of bacteria around the teeth resulting in inflammation of the gums. Risk factors include hormonal changes, illnesses, some medications, diabetes, smoking, human immunodeficiency virus and acquired immunodeficiency syndrome (HIV/AIDS), poor oral hygiene, and a family history of dental disease.	Dentists usually diagnose gingivitis based on symptoms and examination of the oral cavity. Treatment involves removing all traces of plaque and tartar, proper oral hygiene, and regular professional dental checkups and cleaning.
Hemorrhoids	Swollen veins around the anus (external) or in the lower rectum (internal); also called *piles.* Signs and symptoms include itching, discomfort, or pain around the anus; painful bowel movements; blood on tissue after bowel movement.	The cause is increased pressure in the lower rectum. Risk factors include straining during bowel movements, sitting for long periods, chronic diarrhea or constipation, obesity, pregnancy, and a low-fiber diet.	Diagnosis is by visual examination of the area around the anus and a digital rectal examination. Treatments at home are often sufficient, including sitting in a warm water bath, applying creams to relieve itching, and increasing dietary fiber. The doctor may use rubber band ligation or sclerotherapy as a treatment. As a last resort, surgery to remove the hemorrhoids (hemorrhoidectomy) may be advised.
Hepatitis	Swelling and inflammation of the liver; signs and symptoms may be subtle and include fatigue, flulike symptoms, dark urine, pale feces, abdominal pain, loss of appetite, jaundice, and weight loss.	Five types of viral hepatitis, each caused by a different virus. Hepatitis A virus (HAV) is transmitted through contaminated food or water; hepatitis B virus (HBV) through puncture wounds or contact with infectious body fluids; hepatitis C virus (HCV) through direct contact with body fluids, usually through injection drugs or sexual contact. Hepatitis D virus (HDV) occurs in conjunction with hepatitis B and is uncommon in the United States; hepatitis E virus (HEV) is waterborne and occurs in areas of poor sanitation; uncommon in the United States. Nonviral hepatitis may be caused by excessive alcohol consumption, exposure to poisons, overuse of certain medications, and an inappropriate reaction by the immune system.	Diagnosis is by palpation of the liver, liver biopsy, liver function tests, ultrasound, and blood tests. Treatment depends on the type of hepatitis.

Continued

Common Pathology of the Digestive System—cont'd

Disease	Signs and Symptoms	Etiology	Diagnosis and Treatment
Hiatal hernia	By itself, a hiatal hernia causes no symptoms. When symptoms do occur, they are usually due to GERD and include heartburn, chest pain, burping, nausea, vomiting, and large amounts of saliva in the mouth.	A hiatal hernia occurs when a portion of the stomach pushes upward through the diaphragm into the mediastinum. In general, this happens if the diaphragm opening is too large or the surrounding muscle is too weak.	Most cases are discovered during a test or procedure to determine the cause of heartburn; may include barium x-rays, CT scan, and endoscopy. Treatment is aimed at minimizing acid reflux and may include antacids and medications to reduce acid production.
Inflammatory bowel disease (IBD)	A group of inflammatory conditions of the small intestine and colon. Crohn disease and ulcerative colitis are the most common forms. Signs and symptoms are nonspecific: diarrhea, abdominal pain, cramps, ulcers, loss of appetite, weight loss, malnutrition, fever, fatigue, and bloody diarrhea.	Cause is unknown, but heredity and altered immune response seem to be involved.	Diagnostic tools include fecal occult blood test, colonoscopy, sigmoidoscopy, and CT and/or MRI scans. There is no cure. Treatment is directed at managing symptoms and may include antiinflammatory medications, immunosuppressants, and antibiotics.
Irritable bowel syndrome (IBS)	Common disorder of the colon characterized by chronic abdominal pain, bloating, and alterations of bowel habits.	IBS has no known cause; disruptions in the muscle activity and nerve supply of the colon may have a role in the condition. Certain foods, stress, hormone fluctuations, and other illnesses may aggravate the condition.	Diagnosis is based on symptoms and tests to rule out other conditions. Treatment focuses on the relief of symptoms. Dietary adjustments and medications may be advised.
Lactose intolerance	Abdominal pain, gas, bloating, diarrhea, rumbling sounds in the abdomen after eating dairy products.	Occurs when the small intestine does not produce enough lactase enzyme to digest the lactose sugar in milk and dairy products.	Diagnosis is based on symptoms and confirmed by a lactose tolerance test. Treatment involves avoiding the consumption of lactose-containing dairy products or taking lactase supplements.
Leukoplakia	Thick white patches on the tongue and the mucosa of the mouth.	Exact cause is unknown, but evidence suggests the condition results from irritants such as tobacco, whether smoked or chewed, excessive alcohol use, or rough places on the teeth.	A biopsy of the patches confirms the diagnosis. A biopsy may find changes that indicate oral cancer. Treatment is to remove the source of the irritation. Surgical removal may be necessary in some cases.
Malabsorption syndrome	Malabsorption syndrome is an inability of the small intestine to absorb nutrients into the bloodstream. Signs and symptoms vary according to the nutrients not being absorbed, but usually there will be chronic diarrhea, abnormal stools, weight loss, and gas.	Causes include the absence of certain digestive enzymes, lactose intolerance, celiac disease, short bowel syndrome, genetic diseases, and certain medications.	Diagnosis is based on the presence of fat in the feces (steatorrhea). Treatment depends on the cause but may include dietary changes and nutritional supplements.
Mumps	Also called *epidemic parotitis;* most obvious sign is swelling of the parotid glands, which may be accompanied by fever, headache, and muscle aches. Postpubescent males may develop orchitis. In rare cases mumps may lead to hearing loss.	A contagious disease caused by the mumps virus, it was common until mumps vaccination became routine.	Diagnosis is by physical examination and possibly a blood test to detect mumps antibodies. Mumps is usually self-resolving within 2 weeks and no treatment is necessary.

TERMINOLOGY REVIEW

Key Term	Word Parts	Definition
Absorption		The passage of digestive end products from the gastrointestinal tract into the blood or lymph.
Chyme		The semifluid mixture of food and gastric juice that leaves the stomach through the pyloric sphincter.
Defecation		The expulsion of indigestible wastes, or feces, through the anus.
Deglutition		The process of swallowing.
Fauces		Opening from the oral cavity into the oropharynx.
Gastric juice	*gastr/o:* stomach	The secretions of the exocrine gastric glands.
Gastrin	*gastr/o:* stomach	Hormone secreted by the endocrine glands in the stomach.
Gingiva	*gingiv/o:* gums	Soft tissue that covers the alveolar processes of the mandible and maxillae; also called *gums.*
Hydrolysis	*hydr/o:* water *-lysis:* breaking apart	Chemical breakdown of complex molecules by the addition of water.
Ileocecal valve	*ile/o:* ileum *-cec-:* cecum	The valve between the small intestine and large intestine.
Lower esophageal sphincter		Valve between the esophagus and stomach.
Mastication		The process of chewing.
Mesentery		Extensions of peritoneum that are associated with the intestine.
Palate		Roof of the mouth; separates the oral cavity from the nasal cavity.
Peristalsis	*-stalsis:* contraction	Rhythmic contractions of the intestine that move food along the digestive tract.
Plicae circulares		Circular folds in the mucosa and submucosa of the small intestine.
Pyloric sphincter		Valve between the stomach and first part of the small intestine.
Rugae		Longitudinal folds in the mucosa of the stomach.
Teniae coli	*col-:* colon or large intestine	Bands of longitudinal muscle fibers in the large intestine

ON THE WEB

For information on the digestive system:

American Dietetic Association: www.eatright.org

Atlas of Gastrointestinal Endoscopy: www.endoatlas.com

Inner Body: www.innerbody.com/html/body.html

National Institute of Health Digestive Diseases: digestive.niddk.nih.gov

National Institute of Health—Office of Dietary Supplements: dietary-supplements.info.nih.gov

Pathophysiology of the Digestive System: arbl.cvmbs.colostate.edu/hbooks/pathphys/digestion/

The Helicobacter Foundation: www.helico.com

The Internet Pathology Laboratory for Medical Education—Gastrointestinal Pathology: library.med.utah.edu/WebPath/ORGAN.html *(Click on "Gastrointestinal Pathology")*

The Internet Pathology Laboratory for Medical Education—Hepatic Pathology: library.med.utah.edu/WebPath/ORGAN.html *(Click on "Hepatic Pathology")*

15

Urinary System

Check out the Evolve site at http://evolve.elsevier.com/Bonewit/today/ to access additional interactive activities and exercises to help you study and prepare for success.

LEARNING OBJECTIVES

1. State six functions of the urinary system.
2. Describe the location and structural features of the kidneys.
3. Label the parts of a nephron.
4. State the two parts of the juxtaglomerular apparatus.
5. Describe the location, structure, and function of the ureters, urinary bladder, and urethra.
6. List and describe the three steps in urine formation.
7. Identify the hormones that affect kidney function, and explain how they do so.
8. Explain the function of renin.
9. Describe ways in which the aging of an individual affects the urinary system.
10. Identify pathology related to the urinary system.

CHAPTER OUTLINE

INTRODUCTION TO THE URINARY SYSTEM
COMPONENTS OF THE URINARY SYSTEM
Kidneys
Location
Macroscopic Structure
Nephrons
Collecting Ducts
Juxtaglomerular Apparatus
Blood Flow Through the Kidney
Ureters

Urinary Bladder
Urethra
URINE FORMATION
Glomerular Filtration
Tubular Reabsorption
Tubular Secretion
Regulation of Urine Concentration and Volume
Micturition
AGING OF THE URINARY SYSTEM

KEY TERMS

detrusor muscle (dee-TROO-sor MUH-sull)
erythropoietin (ee-rith-roh-poy-EE-tin)
glomerular capsule (gloh-MER-yoo-lar KAP-sool)
glomerular filtration (gloh-MER-yoo-lar fil-TRAY-shun)
glomerulus (gloh-MER-yoo-lus)
juxtaglomerular apparatus (juks-tah-gloh-MER-yoo-lar ap-pah-RAT-us)

micturition (mik-too-RISH-un)
nephrons (NEFF-rahns)
nephron loop (NEFF-rahn LOOP)
renal corpuscle (REE-nal KOAR-pu-sell)
renal cortex (REE-nal KOAR-teks)
renal medulla (REE-nal meh-DOO-lah)
renal pelvis (REE-nal PELL-vis)
renal tubule (REE-nal TOOB-yool)
renin (REE-nin)

trigone (TRYE-goan)
tubular reabsorption (TOOB-yoo-lar ree-ab-SORP-shun)
tubular secretion (TOOB-yoo-lar see-KREE-shun)
ureter (yoo-REE-ter)
urethra (yoo-REE-thrah)
urinary bladder (YOO-rin-air-ee blad-der)

INTRODUCTION TO THE URINARY SYSTEM

The overall function of the urinary system is to maintain the volume and composition of body fluids within normal limits. The urinary system accomplishes this by excreting the waste products that accumulate as a result of cellular metabolism. Because of this, the urinary system is sometimes referred to as the *excretory system.* Although the urinary system has a major role in excretion, other organs contribute to the excretory function. Some waste products, such as carbon dioxide and water, are excreted by the lungs through the respiratory system. The skin excretes wastes through the sweat glands. The liver and intestines excrete bile pigments that result from the destruction of hemoglobin. The major task of excretion, however, still belongs to the urinary system. If the urinary system fails, the other organs cannot take over and compensate adequately. In addition to eliminating waste products, the urinary system maintains an appropriate fluid volume. It does this by regulating the amount of water that is excreted in the urine. Other functions of the urinary system include regulating the concentrations of various electrolytes in the body fluids and maintaining normal pH of the blood.

In addition to maintaining fluid balance in the body, the urinary system controls red blood cell production by secreting the hormone **erythropoietin.** The urinary system also plays a role in maintaining normal blood pressure by secreting the enzyme **renin.**

COMPONENTS OF THE URINARY SYSTEM

The urinary system consists of the kidneys, ureters, urinary bladder, and urethra. The kidneys produce the urine. The ureters transport the urine away from the kidneys to the urinary bladder. The urinary bladder stores the urine until it is excreted from the body. The urethra is a tubular structure that carries the urine from the urinary bladder to the outside of the body. The components of the urinary system are illustrated in Figure 15-1.

KIDNEYS

The *kidneys* are the primary organs of the urinary system. They are the organs that filter the blood, remove the wastes, and excrete the wastes into the urine. They are the organs that perform the functions of the urinary system. The other components of the urinary system are accessory structures to help eliminate the urine from the body.

Location

The kidneys are located between the twelfth thoracic and third lumbar vertebrae, one on each side of the vertebral column. The right kidney is usually slightly lower than the left because the liver displaces it downward. The kidneys are partially protected by the lower ribs and lie in shallow depressions against the posterior abdominal wall behind the peritoneum (retroperitoneal). Each kidney is held in place by connective tissue, called *renal fascia.*

HIGHLIGHT on the Urinary System

Hangover: Alcohol inhibits the secretion of antidiuretic hormone, so when people drink alcohol, they experience diuresis, or excessive urination. Experts believe that the dehydration caused by diuresis contributes to "hangover" symptoms.

Nephrons: The number of nephrons does not increase after birth. Growth of the kidney occurs from enlargement of the individual nephrons. When nephrons are damaged they are not replaced.

Nephroptosis: Nephroptosis, commonly referred to as a *floating kidney,* occurs when the kidney is no longer held in place by the renal fascia and it drops out of its normal position. This may make the kidney more vulnerable to injury if it is no longer protected by the ribs. Another danger is that the ureter may become twisted and block the flow of urine. Nephroptosis occurs more frequently in horseback riders, truck drivers, and people who ride motorcycles.

Uremia: When the kidneys do not function properly and fail to remove the waste products from the blood, uremia may result. Uremia is a condition in which there is a toxic level of urea in the blood.

Urinary incontinence: Urinary incontinence is the inability to control urination and to retain urine in the bladder. Temporary incontinence may result when the muscles around the bladder and urethra become weakened and lose muscle tone. This is sometimes caused by stretching of the muscles during childbirth. Because these muscles help restrict the outlet of the bladder, their weakness contributes to a leakage of urine. A cough or sneeze may increase pressure within the bladder sufficiently to force urine to escape. Permanent incontinence is usually caused by damage to the central nervous system or by extensive damage to the bladder or urethra.

Urinary tract infection (UTI): UTIs occur more frequently in women than in men because of differences in the urethra. In females the urethral opening is in close proximity to the anal opening, which gives intestinal bacteria easier access to the urethra. The female urethra is short, which allows any infection to spread to the urinary bladder. An infection of the urethra is called *urethritis,* and one of the urinary bladders is called *cystitis.* ■

A thick layer of adipose tissue surrounds each kidney. This is called *perirenal fat,* and it helps to protect the kidney. A tough, fibrous connective tissue encases each kidney and is called the *renal capsule.* The renal capsule provides support for the soft tissue that is inside.

Macroscopic Structure

In the adult, each kidney is approximately 3 cm thick, 6 cm wide, and 12 cm long (1.2 × 2.5 × 5 inches). The kidney is bean-shaped with an indentation, called the *hilum.* The hilum leads to a large cavity within the kidney called the *renal sinus.* The *ureter* and *renal vein* leave the kidney at the hilum, and the *renal artery* enters the kidney at the hilum.

The macroscopic internal structure of the kidney is illustrated in Figure 15-2. The outer, reddish region is the **renal cortex.** The renal cortex surrounds a darker reddish-brown region called the **renal medulla.** The renal medulla consists of a series of *renal pyramids.* The renal pyramids appear striated because they contain straight tubular structures and blood vessels. The wide bases of the pyramids are adjacent to the cortex. The pointed ends of the pyramids, called *renal papillae,* are directed toward the center of the kidney. Portions of the renal cortex extend into the spaces between adjacent pyramids to form *renal columns.* The cortex and medulla make up the functional tissue of the kidney.

Figure 15-1 Components of the urinary system. (From Applegate E: *The anatomy and physiology learning system,* ed 4, St Louis, 2011, Saunders.)

Figure 15-2 Coronal (frontal) section through the kidney. (From Applegate E: *The anatomy and physiology learning system,* ed 4, St Louis, 2011, Saunders.)

Common Pathology of the Urinary System

Disease	Signs and Symptoms	Etiology	Diagnosis and Treatment
Acute renal failure	Symptoms of acute renal failure may include decreased urine output, fluid retention, fatigue, drowsiness, shortness of breath, confusion, and nausea.	Acute kidney failure occurs when the kidneys suddenly become unable to filter waste products from the blood, allowing dangerous levels of toxic wastes to accumulate. It may occur when there is direct damage to the kidneys or from other causes.	Diagnosis is based on observation of the urine output, urinalysis, blood tests, and imaging diagnostics. Treatment for acute kidney failure involves identifying the illness or injury that originally damaged the kidneys and correcting it. Often, medications are prescribed to restore normal function. In severe cases, hemodialysis may be required.
Chronic renal failure	Chronic renal failure is initially without specific symptoms. As the disease progresses, blood pressure increases and waste products accumulate in the blood resulting in a general ill feeling and fatigue.	Chronic renal failure is a medical condition in which the kidneys fail to adequately filter waste products from the blood. The three most common causes of chronic renal failure are diabetes mellitus, hypertension, and glomerulonephritis.	It is important to differentiate between acute and chronic renal failure. Sometimes it is necessary to treat for acute failure until it can be determined to be chronic. Controlling blood pressure will slow further kidney damage. Ultimately, frequent hemodialysis is indicated.

Common Pathology of the Urinary System—cont'd

Disease	Signs and Symptoms	Etiology	Diagnosis and Treatment
Bladder cancer	Blood or blood clots in the urine, pain during urination, need for frequent urination, urinary tract infections, pain in the lower back.	It is not always clear what causes bladder cancer. Bladder cancer develops when cells in the bladder begin to grow abnormally. It has been linked to smoking, parasitic infection, radiation, and chemical exposure.	Diagnosis may be based on laboratory and imaging tests, sometimes using a dye to highlight the kidneys, ureters, and bladder. The bladder can be visually examined and tissue removed for biopsy by cystoscopy. There are many treatment options, including radiation therapy, biologic therapy, chemotherapy, and surgery.
Kidney cancer	Blood in the urine, back pain, abdominal swelling, swelling of the veins around a testicle, flank pain, and weight loss.	Kidney cancer starts in the lining of the kidney tubules. It occurs most often in men aged 50 to 70. It is not clear what causes the DNA mutation that results in renal cell carcinoma, but some of the risk factors are dialysis treatments, high blood pressure, polycystic kidney disease, and smoking.	Diagnosis is based on symptoms, imaging scans, blood chemistry, intravenous pyelogram (IVP), and renal arteriography. Surgery to remove all or part of the kidney is recommended. This may include removing the bladder, surrounding tissues, or lymph nodes. A cure is unlikely unless all of the cancer can be removed.
Cystitis	Burning sensation when urinating, persistent urge to urinate, passing small amount of urine, blood in the urine, discomfort in the pelvic area, and fever.	Cystitis is an inflammation of the bladder usually caused by a urinary tract infection (UTI) and involving *Escherichia coli* bacteria. It may also be caused by an infection in a kidney.	Diagnostic tools include urine analysis, cystoscopy, and imaging tests. Antibiotics are the first line of treatment for cystitis caused by bacteria.
Cystocele	Discomfort when coughing, lifting, or straining; repeated bladder infections; a bulge of tissue that protrudes through the vaginal wall or opening; pain or urinary leakage during sexual intercourse.	Cystocele occurs when the supporting tissue between the female bladder and vaginal wall weakens and stretches, allowing the bladder to bulge into the vagina. It can be caused by obesity, heavy lifting, childbirth.	Diagnosis is based on history, pelvic examination, urinalysis, bladder emptying tests. Treatment may include a ring (pessary) inserted into the vagina to support the bladder, and estrogen therapy. In some cases surgery is necessary.
Glomerulonephritis	Foamy, pink or brown urine with red blood cells. High blood pressure, fluid retention, fatigue.	Glomerulonephritis is an inflammation of the glomeruli in the kidneys. Glomeruli remove waste products from the bloodstream and pass them in the urine. Glomerulonephritis may develop after a strep throat infection, or from bacterial, viral, or human immunodeficiency virus (HIV) infections.	Diagnosis is based on urinalysis, blood tests, and imaging examinations. In general, the goal of treatment is to protect the kidneys from further damage. Controlling blood pressure is vital.
Hydronephrosis	Common symptoms include flank pain, abdominal mass, nausea and vomiting, urinary tract infection, fever, painful urination, increased urinary frequency, and increased urinary urgency.	Hydronephrosis describes the situation in which the urine collecting system of the kidney is dilated. This may be a normal variant or it may be the result of an underlying illness or medical condition. It can be caused by an obstruction to the free flow of urine from the kidney, sometimes called a *kidney stone*.	Diagnosis begins with patient history and physical examination. Often, laboratory tests of the urine and blood are required. Treatment of hydronephrosis focuses on the removal of the obstruction and drainage of the urine that has accumulated behind the obstruction.

Continued

Common Pathology of the Urinary System—cont'd

Disease	Signs and Symptoms	Etiology	Diagnosis and Treatment
Interstitial cystitis	Chronic pelvic pain, persistent urge to urinate frequently, pain when bladder is full, pain during sexual intercourse.	Interstitial cystitis is a chronic condition causing frequent painful urination. The exact cause in unknown but may relate to a defect in the protective lining of the bladder.	Diagnosis is based on medical history including a bladder diary, pelvic examination, urinalysis, cystoscopy, and bladder biopsy. Treatment includes physical therapy, nerve stimulation, and oral medications.
Nephroptosis	Asymptomatic in most patients. Some may feel pain when standing that subsides when lying down, along with nausea and chills.	Nephroptosis, also known as *floating kidney,* occurs when a kidney falls from its normal location into the pelvis. It is usually a congenital defect but also can be caused by a hard blow to the abdomen or by lifting a heavy object.	Diagnosis is based on physical examination and imaging studies, including intravenous urography. Usually no treatment is necessary. In some cases, laparoscopic nephropexy surgery is performed.
Nephrotic syndrome	Foamy urine, fluid retention, swelling around the eyes, ankles, and feet. Usually accompanied by high blood pressure.	Nephrotic syndrome is a kidney disorder that causes the kidney to excrete too much protein in the urine. It is usually caused by damage to glomeruli in the kidneys.	Diagnosis includes urinalysis, blood tests, and kidney biopsy. Drugs called *angiotensin-converting enzyme inhibitors* reduce blood pressure and also reduce the amount of protein released in urine.
Neurogenic bladder	Urinary incontinence, small volume during voiding, dribbling, loss of sensation of bladder fullness, urinary tract infections.	Neurogenic bladder is a condition in which a person lacks bladder control because of a brain, spinal cord, or nerve injury.	Urinary incontinence is diagnostic. Because neurogenic bladder involves the nervous system and bladder, a variety of tests are conducted to determine their status. Catheterization is often necessary. Sometimes a stoma is created to bypass the urethra.
Peyronie disease	Penis has a curvature during an erection; a lump of scar tissue may be present under the skin of the penis, and erections are painful.	Peyronie disease normally results from repeated injury to the penis. During healing, a lump of scar tissue forms.	Physical examination is usually sufficient to identify the condition. Interferon, a type of protein that disrupts the production of fibrous tissue and helps break it down, may provide improvement.
Polycystic kidney disease	Blood in urine, high blood pressure, back pain, headaches, abdominal extension, frequent urination, kidney stones, UTIs.	Polycystic kidney disease is an inherited disorder in which clusters of cysts develop within the kidneys. As the cysts accumulate fluid, they can become very large and destroy functioning kidney tissue.	Ultrasound, computed tomography (CT), and magnetic resonance imaging (MRI) examinations detect the size and number of cysts. Medications are prescribed to control blood pressure and pain. Diet and lifestyle changes are often recommended. Dialysis and/or kidney transplant may be necessary as the disease progresses.
Pyelonephritis	Back pain, fever, chills, malaise, nausea, blood in urine, cloudy urine, urination pain, increased urination frequency and urgency.	Pyelonephritis is the result of a urinary tract infection that progresses to involve the upper urinary system. Kidney stones may contribute to the condition.	Diagnosis starts with a physical examination including checking the area over the kidneys for tenderness. Urinalysis and blood tests are required. If kidney stones are suspected, imaging tests are ordered. The condition is treated with antibiotics.
Renal calculi	Severe waves of back and side pain, pain on urination, dark or foul-smelling urine, nausea, frequent urination, fever, chills.	Renal calculi, known as *kidney stones,* are hard crystalline deposits that precipitate from the urine. They occur when the urine contains too much of substances that form crystals. Passing a kidney stone can be very painful.	Diagnosis relies on blood, urine, and imaging tests. Passed stones may be analyzed to determine composition. Drinking large amounts of water can help flush out the system. Pain relievers are often needed. Large stones may be broken up with shock wave lithotripsy.

Common Pathology of the Urinary System—cont'd

Disease	Signs and Symptoms	Etiology	Diagnosis and Treatment
Uremia	Abdominal pain, dry mouth, easy bruising, edema, confusion, excessive thirst, fatigue, skin pallor, low blood pressure, tremors, nausea, weakness, tachycardia.	In uremia, blood urea nitrogen (BUN) is elevated because of the kidney's failure to remove the substances. This may be caused by any condition that damages the kidneys.	Patient history is required to determine if condition is chronic or acute. Diagnosis is based on the blood's basic metabolic panel, showing BUN, creatinine, potassium, phosphate, calcium, and sodium levels. The ultimate treatment for uremia is dialysis.
Urethritis	*For men:* Painful or difficult urination, blood in urine or semen, discharge from penis, frequent urination, swelling of penis, pain with ejaculation. *For women:* Burning pain during urination, abdominal pain, fever, chills, pelvic pain, frequent urination.	Urethritis is inflammation of the urethra. It may be caused by a bacterial or viral infection. It can also be caused by an injury or by sensitivity to chemicals used in spermicides.	*For men:* The medical examination includes the abdomen, bladder area, penis, and scrotum. *For women:* The medical examination includes evaluation of abdominal, pelvic, and urethral tenderness. Urinalysis and blood chemistry tests are performed. The goals of treatment are to eliminate the cause of infection and lessen symptoms.
Urinary incontinence	The primary symptom is the leakage of urine.	Urinary incontinence is the loss of bladder control resulting in the leakage of urine. It may be triggered by coughing, sneezing, or lifting. In some cases the urge to urinate is so sudden that the patient is unable to reach a toilet.	Diagnosis begins with urinalysis, medical history, and physical examination. A postvoid residual measurement may be performed. Kegel exercises to strengthen the muscles that control urination may be suggested as treatment.
Urinary tract infection (UTI)	Persistent urge to urinate, burning sensation during urination, strong-smelling cloudy urine, pelvic or rectal pain.	A UTI is an infection in some part of the urinary system. The most common infecting agent is *E. coli.* Catheterization or the use of spermicides increases the risk of infection.	Diagnostic procedures include urinalysis, laboratory cultures of tract bacteria, intravenous pyelogram, and other imaging modalities. For patients with recurrent infections, a course of antibiotics is effective.
Vesicoureteral reflux	Constipation, high blood pressure, protein in urine, and for children, bedwetting.	Vesicoureteral reflux is the abnormal flow of urine from the bladder back up the ureters. It is often caused by a urinary blockage, typically a UTI that causes swelling in a ureter.	Urinalysis can show the presence of a UTI. Ultrasound studies of the kidney and bladder can detect abnormalities. A voiding cystourethrogram can determine bladder emptying problems. Severe cases may require surgery to repair the valve between the bladder and ureter.

The central region of the kidney contains the **renal pelvis,** a large cavity that collects the urine as it is produced. The periphery of the renal pelvis is interrupted by cuplike projections called *calyces.* A *minor calyx* surrounds the renal papillae of each pyramid and collects urine from that pyramid. Several minor calyces converge to form a *major calyx.* From the major calyces the urine flows into the renal pelvis and from there into the ureter.

Nephrons

Each kidney contains more than 1 million functional units, called **nephrons,** located in the cortex and medulla. The nephron is where the blood is filtered and urine is formed. A nephron consists of a renal corpuscle and a renal tubule (Figure 15-3).

The **renal corpuscle** consists of the **glomerulus** and the **glomerular capsule** (Bowman capsule). The glomerulus is a cluster of capillaries. Blood enters the glomerulus through an *afferent arteriole* and is filtered. The blood then leaves the glomerulus through an *efferent arteriole* (Figure 15-4). As the blood is filtered, the filtrate enters the glomerular capsule, which continues as the renal tubule. Renal corpuscles are located in the cortex of the kidney and give it a granular appearance.

The **renal tubule,** which carries fluid away from the glomerular capsule, consists of a proximal convoluted tubule, a nephron loop (Henle loop), and a distal convoluted tubule.

The first portion of the tubule, located in the cortex, is highly coiled and is known as the *proximal convoluted*

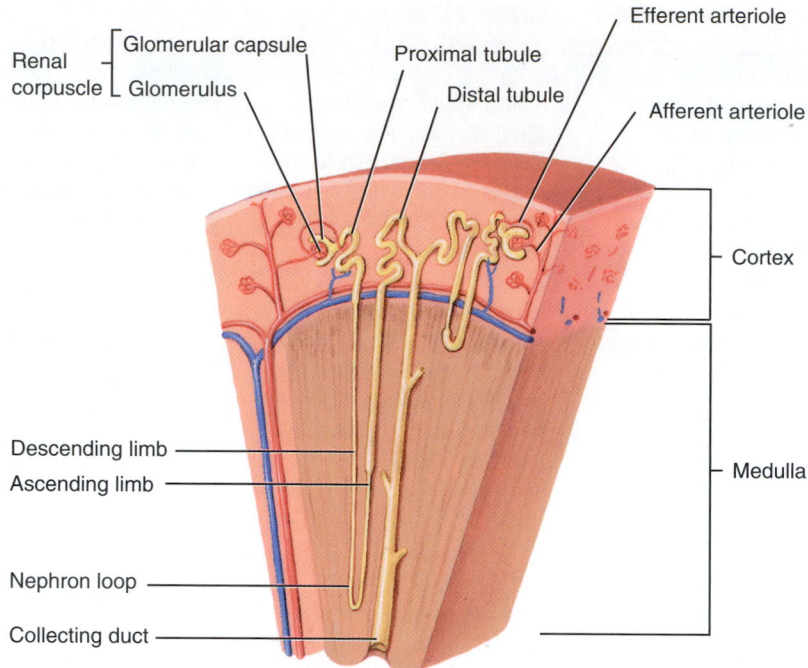

Renal corpuscle — Glomerular capsule / Glomerulus
Proximal tubule
Distal tubule
Efferent arteriole
Afferent arteriole
Cortex
Medulla
Descending limb
Ascending limb
Nephron loop
Collecting duct

Figure 15-3 A section of a kidney showing the structures in the cortex and those in the medulla. The renal pyramids in the medulla contain the nephron loops and collecting ducts. (From Applegate E: *The anatomy and physiology learning system,* ed 4, St Louis, 2011, Saunders.)

tubule. Next the tubule straightens and dips into the medulla, makes a U-turn, and ascends back toward the cortex. This forms the **nephron loop** (Henle loop). The portion of the loop that descends from the proximal convoluted tubule into the medulla is the *descending limb,* and the part that ascends back toward the cortex is the *ascending limb.* The final region of the tubule, which is also coiled and found in the cortex, is known as the *distal convoluted tubule* (see Figure 15-4).

Collecting Ducts

Urine passes from the distal convoluted tubules of the nephrons into *collecting ducts.* These straight tubules, with the nephron loops and blood vessels, give the medulla its striated appearance. Fluid flows from the collecting ducts into the minor calyces that surround the renal papillae.

Juxtaglomerular Apparatus

The ascending limb of the nephron loop, in the region where it continues into the distal convoluted tubule, comes into contact with the glomerular afferent arteriole of the same nephron (see Figure 15-4). In the region of contact, the cells of the ascending limb are modified to form the *macula densa,* and those in the afferent arteriole are modified to form the *juxtaglomerular cells.* The macula densa monitors sodium chloride concentration in the urine and also influences the juxtaglomerular cells. In the afferent arteriole, the juxtaglomerular cells produce the enzyme **renin,** which has a role in the regulation of blood pressure.

Together, the macula densa and juxtaglomerular cells make up the **juxtaglomerular apparatus.**

Blood Flow Through the Kidney

Blood flows through the kidneys at an approximate rate of 1200 mL/min. This is about one fourth of the total cardiac output. Blood is brought to the kidneys by the renal arteries, which are branches from the abdominal aorta. The blood flows through the arteries of the kidney until it enters the afferent arterioles. Each of these tiny vessels continues into a glomerulus, where the blood is filtered. The blood leaves the glomerulus through an efferent arteriole and enters a series of veins. The renal vein exits the kidney and takes blood to the inferior vena cava.

URETERS

Each **ureter** is a small tube, about 25 cm (10 inches) long, that carries urine from the renal pelvis to the urinary bladder. It descends from the renal pelvis and enters the urinary bladder on the posterior inferior surface.

The wall of the ureter consists of three layers (Figure 15-5). The outer layer is a supporting layer of fibrous connective tissue known as the *fibrous coat.* The middle layer is known as the *muscular coat.* It consists of smooth muscle. The main function of this layer is peristalsis to propel the urine through the ureter. The inner layer is the *mucosa.* This layer secretes mucus, which coats and protects the surface of the cells.

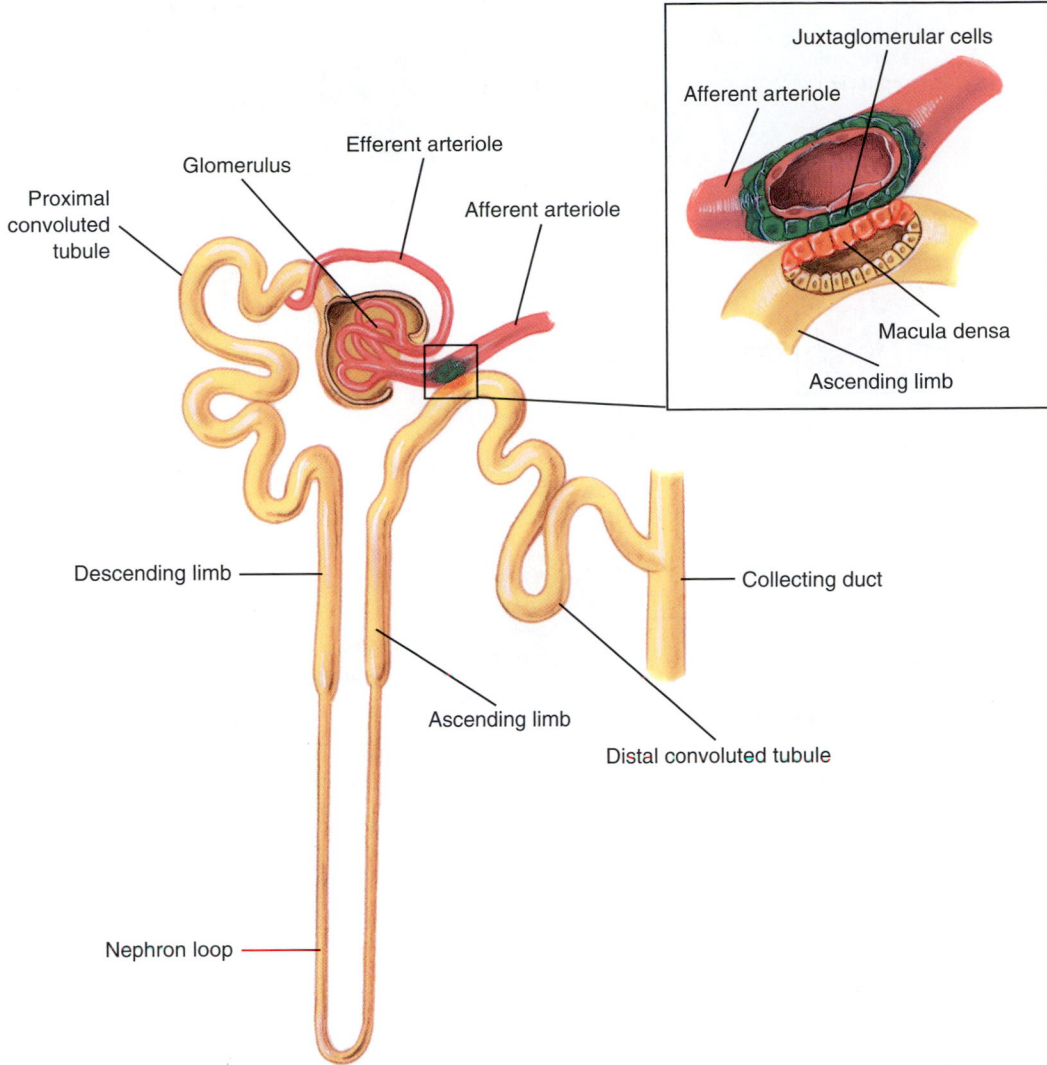

Figure 15-4 Juxtaglomerular apparatus and its relationship to the nephron. The juxtaglomerular apparatus is in the boxes. In the region of contact, the cells of the ascending limb are modified to form the macula densa, and the cells of the afferent arteriole are modified to form the juxtaglomerular cells. Together, these modified regions are the juxtaglomerular apparatus. (From Applegate E: *The anatomy and physiology learning system,* ed 4, St Louis, 2011, Saunders.)

URINARY BLADDER

The **urinary bladder** is located in the pelvic cavity and is a temporary storage reservoir for urine (see Figure 15-5). The size and shape of the urinary bladder vary with the amount of urine it contains and with the pressure from surrounding organs.

The inner lining of the urinary bladder consists of a *mucous membrane.* When the bladder is empty, the mucosa has numerous folds called *rugae.* The rugae allow the bladder to expand as it fills. The next layer is the *muscularis,* which is composed of smooth muscle. The smooth muscle fibers in the muscular layer are interwoven in all directions, and collectively these are called the **detrusor muscle.** Contraction of this muscle expels urine from the bladder.

A triangular area, called the **trigone,** is formed by three openings in the floor of the urinary bladder. Two of the openings are from the ureters and form the base of the trigone. Small flaps of mucosa cover these openings and act as valves that allow urine to enter the bladder but prevent it from backing up from the bladder into the ureters. The third opening, at the apex of the trigone, is the opening into the urethra. A band of the detrusor muscle encircles this opening to form the *internal urethral sphincter.*

URETHRA

The final passageway for the flow of urine is the **urethra.** The urethra consists of a thin-walled tube that conveys urine from the floor of the urinary bladder to outside of the body (see Figure 15-5). The opening to the outside is known as the *external urethral orifice.*

The beginning of the urethra, where it leaves the urinary bladder, is surrounded by the *internal urethral sphincter.*

Figure 15-5 Ureter, urinary bladder, and urethra. **A,** Urinary tract. **B,** Cross section through the ureter. **C,** Cross section of the bladder wall. **D,** Regions of the male urethra. (From Applegate E: *The anatomy and physiology learning system,* ed 4, St Louis, 2011, Saunders.)

This sphincter is smooth (involuntary) muscle. Another sphincter, the *external urethral sphincter,* is skeletal (voluntary) muscle and encircles the urethra where it passes through the pelvic floor. These two sphincters control the flow of urine through the urethra.

In females the urethra is short, only 3 to 4 cm (about 1½ inches) long. The external urethral orifice opens to the outside just anterior to the opening for the vagina.

In males the urethra is much longer, about 20 cm (7 to 8 inches) in length, and transports both urine and semen. The first part of the male urethra passes through the prostate gland and is called the *prostatic urethra.* The second part is a short region that penetrates the pelvic floor and enters the penis. This short region is known as the *membranous urethra.* The third part of the male urethra is the longest region and is called the *spongy urethra.* This portion of the urethra extends the entire length of the penis, and the external urethral orifice opens to the outside at the tip of the penis.

URINE FORMATION

The work of the kidneys, performed by the nephrons, is to maintain the volume and composition of body fluids, regulate the pH of the blood, and remove waste products from the blood. The result of this work is the formation of urine. As urine is excreted to the outside of the body, it carries with it the wastes, excess water, and excess electrolytes. At the same time the kidneys conserve other electrolytes to maintain the appropriate balance. The formation of urine involves glomerular filtration, tubular reabsorption, and tubular secretion, which are illustrated in Figure 15-6.

GLOMERULAR FILTRATION

The first step in the formation of urine is **glomerular filtration.** During this process, blood plasma leaves the glomerulus and enters the glomerular capsule. The force that moves the fluid across the membrane is *filtration pressure,* and the fluid that enters the capsule is the *filtrate.*

Blood flows through the kidneys at an average rate of 1200 mL/min. As the blood passes through the glomeruli, about 19% of the plasma enters the glomerular capsule as filtrate. This is equivalent to forming filtrate at a rate of 125 mL/min, or 180 L (45 gallons) per day. This is the total value for all the nephrons in both kidneys. The filtration membrane acts as a barrier that prevents blood cells and protein molecules from entering the capsule; therefore they are absent from the filtrate.

TUBULAR REABSORPTION

If the volume and composition of the filtrate in the glomerular capsule are compared with the volume and

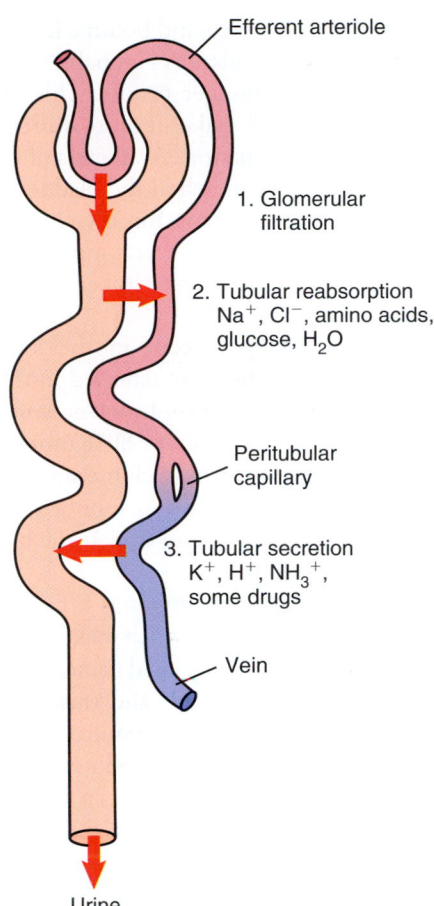

Efferent arteriole

1. Glomerular filtration

2. Tubular reabsorption
   Na^+, Cl^-, amino acids, glucose, H_2O

Peritubular capillary

3. Tubular secretion
   K^+, H^+, NH_3^+, some drugs

Vein

Urine

Figure 15-6 Steps in urine formation. Urine consists of the substances that enter the tubules in glomerular filtration minus substances that are reabsorbed in the tubules plus substances that are secreted into the tubules. (From Applegate E: *The anatomy and physiology learning system,* ed 4, St Louis, 2011, Saunders.)

composition of urine, it is obvious that changes occur after filtration. First of all, about 180 L (45 gallons) of filtrate are formed in a 24-hour period. This volume is reduced to 1 to 2 L of urine. Glucose is present in the filtrate but normally absent in the urine. Urea and uric acid are present in higher concentrations in the urine than in the filtrate.

Tubular reabsorption is the first process that changes the volume and composition of the filtrate. Tubular reabsorption is the movement of substances from the filtrate in the kidney tubules into the blood. Only about 1% of the filtrate remains in the tubules and becomes urine. In general, water and other substances that are useful to the body are reabsorbed. Wastes remain in the filtrate and are excreted in the urine.

TUBULAR SECRETION

The final process in the formation of urine is the transport of molecules and ions into the filtrate. This is called **tubular secretion.** Most of these substances are waste products of cellular metabolism that become toxic if allowed to accumulate in the body. Tubular secretion is the method by which some drugs, such as penicillin, are removed from the body.

The tubular secretion of hydrogen ions plays an important role in regulating the pH of the blood. Other molecules and ions that may enter the filtrate by tubular secretion include potassium ions, creatinine, and histamine.

The final product, urine, produced by the nephrons of the kidney consists of the substances that are filtered, minus the substances that are reabsorbed in the tubules, plus the substances that are added by tubular secretion. If kidney function is impaired by disease or injury, dialysis may be necessary to maintain body fluid composition. Dialysis is a procedure used to separate waste material from the blood and to maintain fluid, electrolyte, and acid-base balance in the body.

REGULATION OF URINE CONCENTRATION AND VOLUME

The concentration and volume of urine depend on conditions in the internal environment of the body. Cells in the hypothalamus are sensitive to changes in the composition of the blood and initiate appropriate responses that affect the kidneys. If the concentration of solutes in the blood increases above normal, the kidneys excrete a small volume of concentrated urine. This conserves water in the body and gets rid of solutes to restore the blood to normal. If the blood solute concentration decreases below normal, the kidneys conserve solutes and get rid of water by producing large quantities of dilute urine. Urine production plays an important role in maintaining homeostasis of blood concentration and volume. By regulating blood volume, the kidneys also play a role in regulating blood pressure because volume is directly related to pressure.

Under average conditions, the kidneys produce about 1500 mL of urine in a 24-hour period, but the volume may vary from 1 to 2 L. The pH may vary from 4.6 to 8, with an average of about 6. This means that urine is usually slightly acidic but may become alkaline under certain conditions such as vegetarian diets.

Three hormones—*aldosterone, antidiuretic hormone (ADH),* and *atrial natriuretic hormone*—influence urine concentration and volume. Aldosterone, secreted by cells of the adrenal cortex, acts on the kidney tubules to increase the reabsorption of sodium. When sodium is reabsorbed, water follows by osmosis. This reduces urine output.

ADH is produced by cells in the hypothalamus and is released from the posterior lobe of the pituitary gland. ADH makes the kidney tubules more permeable to water. When ADH is present, more water is reabsorbed, which reduces the volume of urine and makes it more concentrated. Water is conserved in the body. In the absence of ADH, the tubules are less permeable to water and there is less reabsorption. This results in large quantities of dilute urine, and water is lost from the body.

Special cells in the heart produce a hormone called *atrial natriuretic hormone,* or *atriopeptin,* which is secreted when the atrial cells are stretched. This hormone promotes the excretion of sodium and water by acting directly on the kidney tubules and by inhibiting the secretion of ADH, renin, and aldosterone. The result of atrial natriuretic hormone is a decrease in both blood volume and blood pressure.

Renin is an enzyme that is produced by the juxtaglomerular cells in the kidney in response to low blood pressure or decreased blood sodium concentration. Renin promotes the production of *angiotensin II* in the blood. Angiotensin II is a powerful vasoconstrictor, a substance that increases the blood pressure. Angiotensin II also stimulates the adrenal gland to secrete aldosterone, which acts on the kidney tubules to conserve sodium and water. This increases blood volume and consequently increases blood pressure.

MICTURITION

Micturition, commonly called *urination* or *voiding,* is the act of expelling urine from the bladder. The bladder can hold up to a liter of urine, but normally when it contains 200 to 400 mL, stretch receptors in the bladder wall trigger impulses that initiate the *micturition reflex.* This is an automatic and involuntary response that is coordinated in the spinal cord. Impulses are transmitted along parasympathetic nerves to the detrusor muscle. Even though the micturition reflex is involuntary, it can be inhibited or stimulated by higher brain centers.

It is desirable to completely empty the bladder when urinating. Residual urine is what remains in the bladder if an individual is unable to completely empty the bladder. This may be indicative of a pathologic condition such as a urinary tract infection or, in males, an enlarged prostate.

AGING OF THE URINARY SYSTEM

Some of the more obvious and familiar aging changes occur in the urinary bladder and urethra. Muscles in the walls of these structures tend to weaken and become less elastic with age. As a person ages, the bladder is unable to expand or contract as much as in younger people. This reduces the capacity of the bladder and makes it more difficult to completely empty it during urination. Awareness of the need to urinate, which usually occurs when the bladder is half full in younger people, may be delayed in the elderly until the bladder is nearly full. Thus urgency accompanies awareness. The external urethral sphincter also weakens, which adds to the problems.

Several anatomic changes occur in the kidneys as a person ages, and these changes are reflected in their related functions. There is a general atrophy of nephrons so that by the age of 80, the kidney is about 80% of its young but mature size. Some of the remaining glomeruli are modified, and this, along with the decrease in number, results in a decreased glomerular filtration rate so that the blood is not filtered as quickly as before.

The tubules also undergo changes as a person ages. In general, the tubule walls thicken, which makes them less able to reabsorb water to form concentrated urine. The collecting ducts are less responsive to ADH, and this, along with a diminished thirst mechanism, may result in dehydration. The ability to reabsorb glucose and sodium is also diminished. The tubules become less efficient in the secretion of ions and drugs. They have a diminished ability to compensate for drastic changes in acid-base balance. Drugs that are normally eliminated from the body by tubular secretion may accumulate to toxic levels because they are not cleared from the blood as quickly as they are in younger people.

Amazingly, even with the changes caused by aging, the kidneys of elderly persons are capable of maintaining relatively stable balances in the blood and body fluids under normal conditions. However, their ability to compensate for drastic changes and abnormal conditions is diminished.

TERMINOLOGY REVIEW

Key Term	Word Parts	Definition
Detrusor muscle		The smooth muscle in the wall of the urinary bladder.
Erythropoietin	*erythr/o:* red	A hormone released by the kidneys that stimulates red blood cell production.
Glomerular capsule		Double-layered epithelial cup that surrounds the glomerulus in a nephron; also called *Bowman capsule.*
Glomerular filtration		The movement of blood plasma across the filtration membrane in the renal corpuscle.
Glomerulus		Cluster of capillaries in the nephron through which blood is filtered.
Juxtaglomerular apparatus	*juxta-:* near to	Complex of modified cells in the afferent arteriole and the ascending limb and distal tubule in the kidney; helps regulate blood pressure by secreting renin; consists of the macula densa and juxtaglomerular cells.
Micturition	*mict-:* to pass	Act of expelling urine from the bladder; also called *voiding* or *urination.*
Nephrons	*nephr/o:* kidney	Functional units of the kidney consisting of a renal corpuscle and a renal tubule.
Nephron loop	*nephr/o:* kidney	The hairpin loop of the renal tubule that extends into the renal pyramids.
Renal corpuscle	*ren/o:* kidney	Portion of the nephron where filtration occurs; consists of the glomerulus and glomerular capsule.

TERMINOLOGY REVIEW—cont'd

Key Term	Word Parts	Definition
Renal cortex	*ren/o:* kidney	Outer portion of the kidney that appears granular.
Renal medulla	*ren/o:* kidney	Inner portion of the kidney consisting of renal pyramids.
Renal pelvis	*ren/o:* kidney	Large cavity in the central region of the kidney that collects the urine as it is produced.
Renal tubule	*ren/o:* kidney	Tubular portion of the nephron that carries the filtrate away from the glomerular capsule; site where tubular reabsorption and secretion occur.
Renin	*ren/o:* kidney	An enzyme secreted by the kidneys that functions in blood pressure regulation by stimulating the formation of angiotensin.
Trigone	*tri-:* three	Triangular area in the floor of the urinary bladder formed by the openings for the urethra and the two ureters.
Tubular reabsorption		The movement of filtrate from the renal tubules back into the blood in response to the body's needs during urine formation.
Tubular secretion		The movement of substances from the blood into the renal tubules in response to the body's needs during urine formation.
Ureter	*-ur-:* urine	Tubular structure that carries urine from the renal pelvis to the urinary bladder.
Urethra	*-ur-:* urine	Passageway that conveys urine from the urinary bladder to the exterior.
Urinary bladder	*-ur-:* urine	Storage reservoir for urine: located in the pelvic cavity.

ON THE WEB

For information on the urinary system:

Inner Body: www.innerbody.com/html/body.html

The Internet Pathology Laboratory for Medical Education—Renal Pathology: library.med.utah.edu/WebPath/ORGAN.html *(Click on "Renal Pathology")*

Urinary Incontinence: www.seekwellness.com/incontinence

16 Reproductive System

 Check out the Evolve site at http://evolve.elsevier.com/Bonewit/today/ to access additional interactive activities and exercises to help you study and prepare for success.

CHAPTER OUTLINE

INTRODUCTION TO THE REPRODUCTIVE SYSTEM
MALE REPRODUCTIVE SYSTEM
Testes
Structure
Spermatogenesis
Duct System
Epididymis
Ductus Deferens
Ejaculatory Duct
Urethra
Accessory Glands
Seminal Vesicles
Prostate
Bulbourethral Glands
Seminal Fluid
Penis
Male Sexual Response

Hormonal Control
FEMALE REPRODUCTIVE SYSTEM
Ovaries
Structure
Oogenesis
Ovarian Follicle Development
Ovulation
Genital Tract
Uterine Tubes
Uterus
Vagina
External Genitalia
Female Sexual Response
Hormonal Control
Ovarian Cycle
Uterine (Menstrual) Cycle
Menopause

Mammary Glands
DEVELOPMENT
Prenatal Development

Parturition and Lactation
Postnatal Development
AGING OF THE REPRODUCTIVE SYSTEM

KEY TERMS

clinical age (KLIN-ih-kull AGE)
corpora cavernosa (KOR-por-ah kav-er-NOH-sah)
corpus albicans (KOR-pus AL-bih-kans)
corpus luteum (KOR-pus LOO-tee-um)
corpus spongiosum (KOR-pus spun-jee-OH-sum)
developmental age (dee-VEL-op-men-tul AGE)
ductus deferens (DUCK-tus DEFF-er-enz)
embryonic period (em-bree-ON-ik PEER-ee-ud)
endometrium (end-oh-MEE-tree-um)
epididymis (ep-ih-DID-ih-mis)
fetal period (FEE-tal PEER-ee-ud)
gametes (GAM-eets)

gestation (jes-TAY-shun)
gonads (GO-nads)
interstitial cells (in-ter-STISH-al SELZ)
lactation (lak-TAY-shun)
menarche (meh-NAHR-kee)
myometrium (my-oh-MEE-tree-um)
oogenesis (oh-oh-JEN-eh-sis)
oogonia (oh-oh-GO-nee-ah)
ovarian cycle (oh-VAIR-ee-an SYE-kul)
ovarian follicles (oh-VAIR-ee-an FAHL-ih-kuls)
parturition (par-too-RIH-shun)
perimetrium (pair-ih-MEE-tree-um)
postnatal development (POST-nay-tal dee-VELL-op-ment)
preembryonic period (pree-em-bree-AHN-ik PEER-ee-ud)

prenatal development (PREE-nay-tal dee-VELL-op-ment)
seminiferous tubules (she-mih-NIFF-er-us TOOB-yools)spermatogenesis (spur-mat-oh-JEN-eh-sis)
spermatogonia (spur-mat-oh-GOH-nee-ah)
spermiogenesis (spur-mee-oh-JEN-eh-sis)
stratum basale (STRAY-tum BAY-sah-lee)
stratum functionale (STRAY-tum FUNK-shun-al-ee)
uterine cycle (YOO-ter-in SYE-kul)
uterine tubes (YOO-ter-in TOOBS)
vulva (VUL-vah)
zygote (ZYE-goht)

INTRODUCTION TO THE REPRODUCTIVE SYSTEM

The major function of the reproductive system is to produce offspring. The reproductive system is responsible for the following four functions:

- To produce egg and sperm cells
- To transport and sustain the egg and sperm cells
- To nurture the developing offspring
- To produce hormones

These functions are divided between the primary reproductive organs and the secondary (or accessory) reproductive organs. The primary reproductive organs are called **gonads.** They include the ovaries and testes. These gonads are responsible for producing the egg and sperm cells, known as **gametes.** They are also responsible for producing hormones that function in the maturation of the reproductive system and the development of sexual characteristics. The hormones also play important roles in regulating the normal physiology of the reproductive system. All other organs, ducts, and glands in the reproductive system are considered secondary, or accessory, reproductive organs. These structures transport and sustain the gametes and nurture the developing offspring.

MALE REPRODUCTIVE SYSTEM

The male reproductive system produces, sustains, and transports sperm; introduces the sperm into the female vagina; and produces hormones. Figure 16-1 illustrates the organs of the male reproductive system.

TESTES

The *testes* (or *testicles*) are the male gonads. The testes begin their development high in the abdominal cavity, near the kidneys. During the last 2 months before birth, or shortly after birth, the testes descend into the *scrotum*. The scrotum is a pouch that extends below the abdomen and behind the penis. The location of the testes outside the abdominal cavity may make them vulnerable to injury. However, this location provides a temperature about 3°C below normal body temperature. This lower temperature is necessary for the production of viable sperm. The scrotum consists of skin and subcutaneous tissue. A vertical septum, or partition, of subcutaneous tissue in the center of the scrotum divides it into two parts, each containing one testis. Smooth muscle fibers, called the *dartos muscle,* are located in the subcutaneous tissue. The dartos muscle contracts to give the scrotum its wrinkled appearance. When this muscle is

Figure 16-1 Structures in the male reproductive system. The testes are the primary reproductive organs in the male. The ducts and glands are accessory organs. (From Applegate E: *The anatomy and physiology learning system,* ed 4, St Louis, 2011, Saunders.)

relaxed, the scrotum is smooth. Another muscle known as the *cremaster muscle* is located in the spermatic cord. The cremaster controls the position of the scrotum and testes. When it is cold or a man is sexually aroused, this muscle contracts to pull the testes closer to the body for warmth.

Structure

Each testis is an oval structure about 5 cm long and 3 cm in diameter (Figure 16-2). A tough, white fibrous connective tissue capsule, known as the *tunica albuginea,* surrounds each testis. The tunica albuginea extends inward to form *septa* that partition the testis into *lobules.* Each testis contains about 250 lobules. Each lobule contains one to four highly coiled **seminiferous tubules** that converge into a series of ducts that exit the testes and enter the epididymis. **Interstitial cells** (cells of Leydig) are located between the seminiferous tubules within a lobule. Interstitial cells produce male sex hormones.

Spermatogenesis

Sperm are produced within the seminiferous tubules. The process of sperm formation is **spermatogenesis,** a form of meiosis. The seminiferous tubules are packed with cells in various stages of spermatogenesis (Figure 16-3). Interspersed with these cells are large cells that extend from the periphery of the tubule to the lumen. These large cells are the *supporting cells* (Sertoli cells), which support and nourish the other cells.

Early in embryonic development, *primordial germ cells* enter the testes and differentiate into **spermatogonia.** Spermatogonia are immature cells that remain dormant until puberty. These cells are located around the periphery of the seminiferous tubules. They are diploid cells, meaning that they contain 46 chromosomes (23 pairs). At puberty,

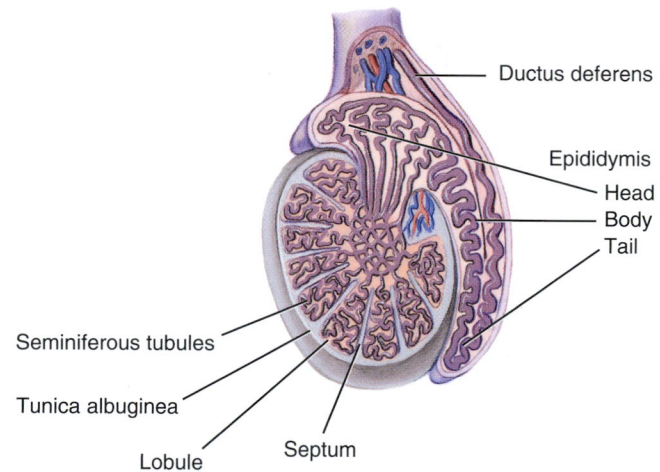

Figure 16-2 Sagittal section of a testis. (From Applegate E: *The anatomy and physiology learning system,* ed 4, St Louis, 2011, Saunders.)

hormones stimulate these cells to begin dividing by mitosis. Some of the daughter cells produced by mitosis remain at the periphery as spermatogonia. Others are pushed toward the lumen and undergo some changes to become *primary spermatocytes.* Because they are produced by mitosis, primary spermatocytes are diploid and have 46 chromosomes.

Each primary spermatocyte goes through the first meiotic division (meiosis I) to produce two *secondary spermatocytes.* In the second meiotic division (meiosis II), each secondary spermatocyte divides to produce two *spermatids.* As a result of the two meiotic divisions, each primary spermatocyte produces four spermatids (Figure 16-4). During spermatogenesis there are two cellular divisions but only one replication of DNA, so each spermatid has 23 chromosomes

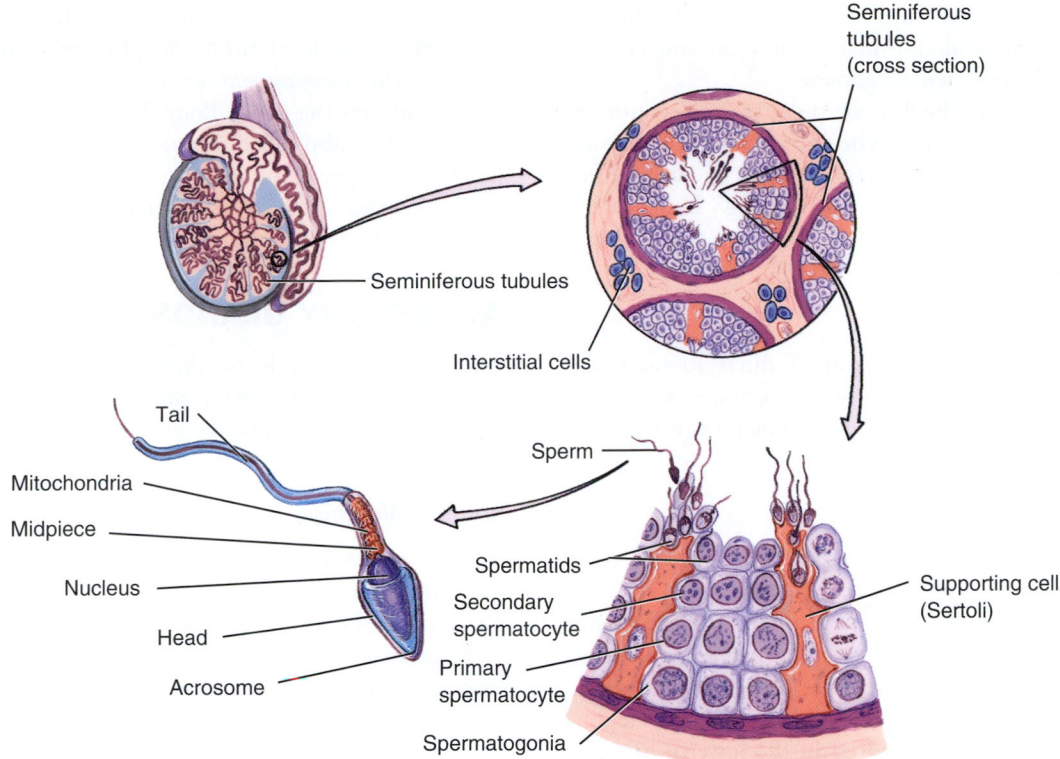

Seminiferous tubules (cross section)

Seminiferous tubules

Interstitial cells

Tail

Mitochondria

Midpiece

Nucleus

Head

Acrosome

Sperm

Spermatids

Secondary spermatocyte

Primary spermatocyte

Spermatogonia

Supporting cell (Sertoli)

Figure 16-3 Cross section of a seminiferous tubule showing the different cell types. Interstitial cells that produce testosterone are between the seminiferous tubules. Spermatids in the lumen become sperm by a process called *spermiogenesis*. (From Applegate E: *The anatomy and physiology learning system,* ed 4, St Louis, 2011, Saunders.)

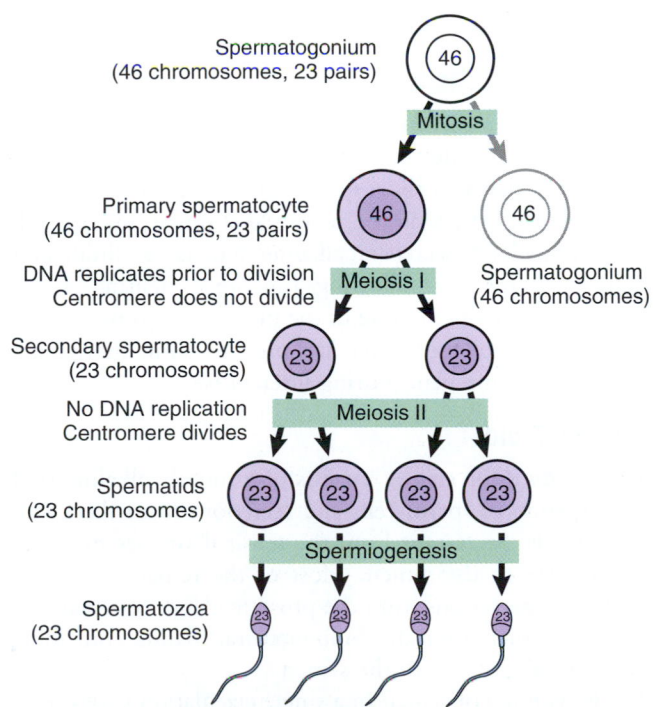

Spermatogonium (46 chromosomes, 23 pairs)

Mitosis

Primary spermatocyte (46 chromosomes, 23 pairs)

DNA replicates prior to division Centromere does not divide

Meiosis I

Spermatogonium (46 chromosomes)

Secondary spermatocyte (23 chromosomes)

No DNA replication Centromere divides

Meiosis II

Spermatids (23 chromosomes)

Spermiogenesis

Spermatozoa (23 chromosomes)

Figure 16-4 Spermatogenesis. Each primary spermatocyte yields four spermatids by meiosis. (From Applegate E: *The anatomy and physiology learning system,* ed 4, St Louis, 2011, Saunders.)

(haploid), one from each pair in the original primary spermatocyte. Each successive stage in spermatogenesis is pushed toward the center of the tubule. This results in the more immature cells being at the periphery, and the more differentiated cells are nearer the center (see Figure 16-3).

Spermatogenesis (and oogenesis in the female) differs from mitosis (review Chapter 5) because the resulting cells have only half the number of chromosomes as the original cell. When the sperm cell nucleus unites with an egg cell nucleus, the full number of chromosomes is restored. If sperm and egg cells were produced by mitosis, then each successive generation would have twice the number of chromosomes as the preceding one.

The final step in the development of sperm is called **spermiogenesis.** In this process, the spermatids formed from spermatogenesis become mature spermatozoa, or sperm. The mature sperm cell has a head, midpiece, and tail (see Figure 16-3). The head contains the 23 chromosomes surrounded by a nuclear membrane. The tip of the head is covered by an *acrosome.* The acrosome contains enzymes that help the sperm penetrate the female gamete. The midpiece contains mitochondria that provide adenosine triphosphate (ATP). The tail, also called the *locomotor region,* is a typical flagellum for locomotion. The sperm are released into the lumen of the seminiferous tubule, where they leave the testes and enter the epididymis. In the epididymis the sperm undergo final maturation and become capable of fertilizing a female gamete.

Sperm production begins at puberty and continues throughout the life of a male. The entire process, beginning with a primary spermatocyte, takes about 74 days. After ejaculation, the sperm can live for about 48 hours in the female reproductive tract.

DUCT SYSTEM

Sperm cells pass through a series of ducts to reach the outside of the body. After they leave the testes, the sperm pass through the epididymis, ductus deferens, ejaculatory duct, and urethra.

Epididymis

Sperm leave the testes through a series of ducts that enter the **epididymis** (see Figure 16-2). The epididymis is a long tube that is tightly coiled to form a comma-shaped organ. When the sperm leave the testes, they are immature and incapable of fertilizing ova. They complete their maturation process and become fertile as they move through the epididymis. Mature sperm are stored in the lower portion of the epididymis.

Ductus Deferens

The **ductus deferens** (also called *vas deferens*) is a tube that is continuous with the epididymis (see Figure 16-2). The ductus deferens enters the abdominopelvic cavity, then descends along the posterior wall of the bladder toward the prostate gland (see Figure 16-1). Sperm are stored in the ductus deferens, near the epididymis, and peristaltic movements propel the sperm through the tube.

The proximal portion of the ductus deferens is a component of the *spermatic cord,* which contains vascular and neural structures that supply the testes. The spermatic cord contains the ductus deferens, testicular artery and veins, lymph vessels, testicular nerve, cremaster muscle (which elevates the testes for warmth and at times of sexual stimulation), and a connective tissue covering.

Ejaculatory Duct

Each ductus deferens joins the duct from the adjacent seminal vesicle to form a short *ejaculatory duct* (see Figure 16-1). Each ejaculatory duct passes through the prostate gland and empties into the urethra.

Urethra

The *urethra* extends from the urinary bladder to the external urethral orifice at the tip of the penis. It is a passageway for sperm and fluids from the reproductive system and for urine from the urinary system. While reproductive fluids are passing through the urethra, sphincters contract tightly to keep urine from entering the urethra.

The male urethra is divided into three regions (see Figure 16-1). The *prostatic urethra* is the portion that passes

through the prostate gland. It receives the ejaculatory duct and numerous ducts from the prostate gland. The next portion, the *membranous urethra,* is a short region that passes through the pelvic floor. The longest portion is the *penile urethra* (also called *spongy urethra*), which extends the length of the penis and opens to the outside at the external urethral orifice. The ducts from the bulbourethral glands open into the penile urethra.

ACCESSORY GLANDS

The accessory glands of the male reproductive system include the seminal vesicles, prostate gland, and bulbourethral glands. These glands secrete fluids that enter the urethra.

Seminal Vesicles

The paired *seminal vesicles* are saclike glands located between the urinary bladder and the rectum (see Figure 16-1). Each gland has a short duct that joins with the ductus deferens to form an ejaculatory duct. The ejaculatory ducts empty into the urethra. The seminal vesicles secrete a fluid that is viscous and contains fructose. The fructose provides an energy source for the spermatozoa.

Prostate

The *prostate gland* is a firm, dense structure that is located just inferior to the urinary bladder (see Figure 16-1). It is about the size of a walnut and encircles the urethra as it leaves the urinary bladder. Numerous short ducts from the prostate gland empty into the prostatic urethra. The secretions of the prostate are thin, milky colored, and alkaline. They enhance the motility of the sperm.

Bulbourethral Glands

The paired *bulbourethral (Cowper) glands* (see Figure 16-1) are small, about the size of a pea, and are located near the base of the penis. A short duct from each gland enters the penile urethra. In response to sexual stimulation, the bulbourethral glands secrete an alkaline, mucus-like fluid. This fluid performs the following functions: neutralizes the acidity of the urine residue in the urethra, helps to neutralize the acidity of the vagina, and provides some lubrication for the tip of the penis during intercourse.

Seminal Fluid

Seminal fluid (or *semen*) consists of a slightly alkaline (pH 7.5) mixture of sperm cells and secretions from the accessory glands. Secretions from the seminal vesicles make up about 60% of the semen. Most of the remaining semen consists of secretions from the prostate gland. Spermatozoa and secretions from the bulbourethral glands contribute only a small volume to the semen.

The volume of semen in a single ejaculation varies from 1.5 to 6 mL. There are usually between 50 and 150 million sperm per milliliter of semen. Sperm counts below 10 to 20 million per milliliter usually cause fertility problems.

Although only one spermatozoon actually penetrates and fertilizes an ovum, it takes several million spermatozoa in an ejaculation to ensure that fertilization will take place.

PENIS

The *penis* is the male copulatory organ located in front of the scrotum. The penis functions in transferring sperm to the vagina. It consists of three columns of erectile tissue that are wrapped in connective tissue and covered with skin (Figure 16-5). There are two dorsal columns known as the **corpora cavernosa.** A single, midline ventral column surrounds the urethra and is called the **corpus spongiosum.**

The penis has a root, body, and glans penis. The root of the penis attaches it to the pubic arch. The body (or shaft) of the penis is the visible, pendant portion. The corpus spongiosum expands at the end of the penis to form the glans penis. The urethra opens through the external urethral orifice at the tip of the glans penis. A loose fold of skin, called the *prepuce,* or foreskin, covers the glans penis.

MALE SEXUAL RESPONSE

In the absence of sexual arousal, the erectile tissue of the penis contains only a small volume of blood, causing the penis to be flaccid. During sexual excitement, arterioles that supply blood to the erectile tissue dilate. As a result, the spaces in the erectile tissue become engorged with blood, causing the penis to enlarge and become rigid. This is called *erection* and is necessary to allow the penis to enter the vagina. The erection reflex may be initiated by stimuli such as anticipation, memory, and visual sensations. It may also be the result of stimulation of touch receptors on the glans penis and skin of the genital area. Emotions and thoughts can inhibit erection.

Continued sexual stimulation causes the reflexes that promote an erection to become more and more intense until a level is reached that prompts a surge of impulses to the genital organs. These impulses stimulate rhythmic contractions of the epididymides, vasa deferentia, and ejaculatory ducts. The impulses also cause contractions of the accessory glands. This results in *emission,* which is the forceful discharge of semen into the urethra. *Ejaculation* immediately follows emission and is the forceful expulsion of semen from the urethra to the exterior. Concurrently with emission and ejaculation, the sphincters of the urinary bladder constrict to prevent semen from entering the bladder and to inhibit the flow of urine from the bladder.

The rhythmic muscle contractions of ejaculation are accompanied by feelings of intense pleasure, increased heart rate, elevated blood pressure, and increased respiration. Together, these physiologic activities are referred to as *climax* or *orgasm.* This is quickly followed by relaxation, and blood leaves the penis so that it becomes flaccid. After orgasm, there is a latent period, lasting from several minutes to several hours, during which another erection is impossible.

HORMONAL CONTROL

The hypothalamus, anterior pituitary, and testes have significant roles in the hormonal control of male reproductive functions. Puberty in males usually begins at ages 10 to 12 and continues until ages 16 to 18. During this period the male reproductive organs become sexually mature. The sequence of events that triggers the onset of puberty is unknown. It begins when certain unknown stimuli cause the hypothalamus to start secreting *gonadotropin-releasing hormone* (GnRH), which enters the blood and goes to the anterior pituitary gland.

In response to GnRH, the anterior pituitary secretes luteinizing hormone (LH) and follicle-stimulating hormone (FSH). *Luteinizing hormone* promotes the growth of the interstitial cells in the testes and stimulates the cells to secrete *testosterone. Follicle-stimulating hormone* acts with testosterone to stimulate spermatogenesis in the seminiferous tubules. Figure 16-6 summarizes the hormonal control of testicular functions.

Male sex hormones are collectively called *androgens.* The most abundant androgen is testosterone. Before birth, testosterone from the adrenal cortex stimulates the development of the male reproductive organs. Between birth and

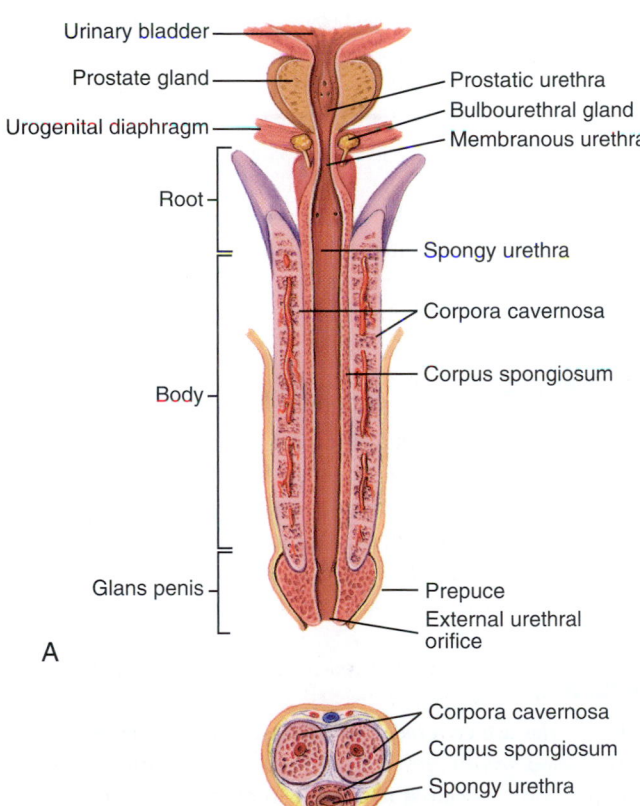

Urinary bladder

Prostate gland

Urogenital diaphragm

Root

Body

Glans penis

Prostatic urethra

Bulbourethral gland

Membranous urethra

Spongy urethra

Corpora cavernosa

Corpus spongiosum

Prepuce

External urethral orifice

A

Corpora cavernosa

Corpus spongiosum

Spongy urethra

Skin

B

Figure 16-5 Structure of the penis. **A,** Longitudinal section. **B,** Cross section. Note that the penis has three regions: root, body, and glans penis. There are two dorsal columns of corpora cavernosum and a ventral column of corpus spongiosum. (From Applegate E: *The anatomy and physiology learning system,* ed 4, St Louis, 2011, Saunders.)

HIGHLIGHT on the Reproductive System

Undescended testicles: The condition in which the testes do not descend into the scrotum is called *cryptorchidism*. *Crypt* means "hidden" and *orchid* refers to the testis, so the term literally means "hidden testis." Cryptorchidism results in sterility if it is not corrected before puberty because the cooler temperature of the scrotum is necessary for sperm production.

Vasectomy: A vasectomy is a surgical procedure, usually accomplished through a tiny incision in the scrotum, that severs the vas deferens. A bilateral vasectomy results in sterility because it interrupts the pathway of the sperm to the outside of the body.

Enlarged prostate gland: Benign prostatic hyperplasia is a common condition in older men. In this condition, the prostate enlarges and compresses the urethra, making urination difficult. This situation results in urine retention in the bladder, which makes the individual more susceptible to urinary tract infections.

Circumcision: Circumcision is the surgical removal of the prepuce of the penis. Sometimes this is done to correct phimosis, a condition in which the prepuce is too tight and obstructs urine flow. In certain cultures, circumcision is performed as a religious rite or an ethnic custom. For others, it is a matter of family preference. The medical benefits of circumcision are a subject of debate in the medical community. Some believe it is practical for hygienic reasons. Evidence indicates that circumcision may reduce the risk of penile cancer.

Ovarian cancer: Carcinomas of the ovary account for more deaths than do cervical and uterine cancers together. Because there are no screening tests and few symptoms in the early stages, ovarian carcinomas are usually in an advanced stage when they are discovered. Surgery, radiation therapy, and chemotherapy are used as therapeutic measures.

Tubal ligation: Tubal ligation is a surgical procedure in which the uterine tubes are burned or severed and tied off. This is a permanent method of birth control because sperm are unable to reach the egg for fertilization. The technique involves making a small incision in the abdomen and inserting a small tube through which the ligation instruments can be introduced.

Mittelschmerz: Mittelschmerz is a term to describe one-sided lower abdominal pain, which may switch sides from one month to another, at or around the time of ovulation. The pain is usually described as sharp or cramping and lasts from 24 to 48 hours. There is no known prevention, and treatment consists of analgesics.

Fibrocystic disease: Fibrocystic disease is a common benign condition of the breast. Small sacs of tissue and fluid develop in the breast tissue and the patient notices lumps in the breast, often associated with premenstrual tenderness. Mammography and surgical biopsy may be indicated to differentiate between fibrocystic disease and carcinoma of the breast. ■

---

puberty, testosterone levels are low. Then at puberty, under the influence of LH, the interstitial cells begin secreting high levels of testosterone. The adrenal cortex continues to secrete small amounts of androgens. The increase in testosterone levels at puberty promotes the maturation of the male reproductive organs, stimulates spermatogenesis, and promotes the development of the male secondary sex characteristics.

After puberty, testosterone production is controlled by a negative feedback mechanism that involves the hypothalamus (see Figure 16-6). High blood testosterone levels inhibit GnRH. This removes the stimulus for LH, which reduces the testosterone level back to normal. Testosterone production continues from puberty throughout the rest of a man's life, although there is some decline in quantity in old age.

FEMALE REPRODUCTIVE SYSTEM

The organs of the female reproductive system perform the following functions: produce and sustain the female sex cells (*egg cells,* or *ova*), transport these cells to a site where they may be fertilized by sperm, provide a favorable environment for the developing offspring, move the offspring to the

outside at the end of the development period, and produce the female sex hormones. The female reproductive system includes the ovaries, uterine tubes, uterus, vagina, accessory glands, and external genital organs (Figure 16-7).

OVARIES

The primary reproductive organs in the female are the paired *ovaries.* Each ovary is a solid, ovoid structure about the size and shape of an almond (approximately 3.5 cm long, 2 cm wide, and 1 cm thick). The ovaries are located in shallow depressions, called *ovarian fossae,* one on each side of the uterus. They are held loosely in place by peritoneal ligaments.

Structure

The ovaries are covered on the outside by a layer of epithelium called *germinal (ovarian) epithelium* (Figure 16-8) and a dense connective tissue capsule known as the *tunica albuginea.* The substance of the ovaries is indistinctly divided into an outer cortex and an inner medulla. The cortex appears more dense and granular because of the presence of numerous **ovarian follicles** in various stages of development. Each of the follicles contains a female germ cell known as an *oocyte.* The medulla consists of loose connective tissue with abundant blood vessels, lymphatic vessels, and nerve fibers.

Oogenesis

Female sex cells (or gametes) develop in the ovaries by a form of meiosis called **oogenesis.** The sequence of events in oogenesis is similar to the sequence in spermatogenesis, but the timing and final result are different (Figure 16-9). Early in fetal development, primitive germ cells in the ovaries differentiate into **oogonia.** The oogonia divide rapidly to form thousands of cells that have a full complement of 46 chromosomes (23 pairs). Oogonia then enter a growth phase, enlarge, and become *primary oocytes.* The primary oocytes (with 46 chromosomes) replicate their DNA and begin the first meiotic division. This process stops in prophase, and the cells remain in this suspended state until puberty. Many of the primary oocytes degenerate before birth. Even with this decline, the two ovaries together contain approximately 700,000 oocytes at birth. This is the lifetime supply, and no more will develop. This is quite different than in the male, in whom spermatogonia and primary spermatocytes continue to be produced throughout the reproductive lifetime. By puberty the number of primary oocytes has further declined to about 400,000.

Beginning at puberty, several primary oocytes start to grow again each month. One of the primary oocytes seems to outgrow the others, and it resumes meiosis I. The other cells degenerate. The large cell undergoes an unequal division so that nearly all the cytoplasm, the organelles, and half the chromosomes go to one cell, which becomes a *secondary oocyte.* The remaining half of the chromosomes go to a smaller cell called the *first polar body.* The secondary oocyte

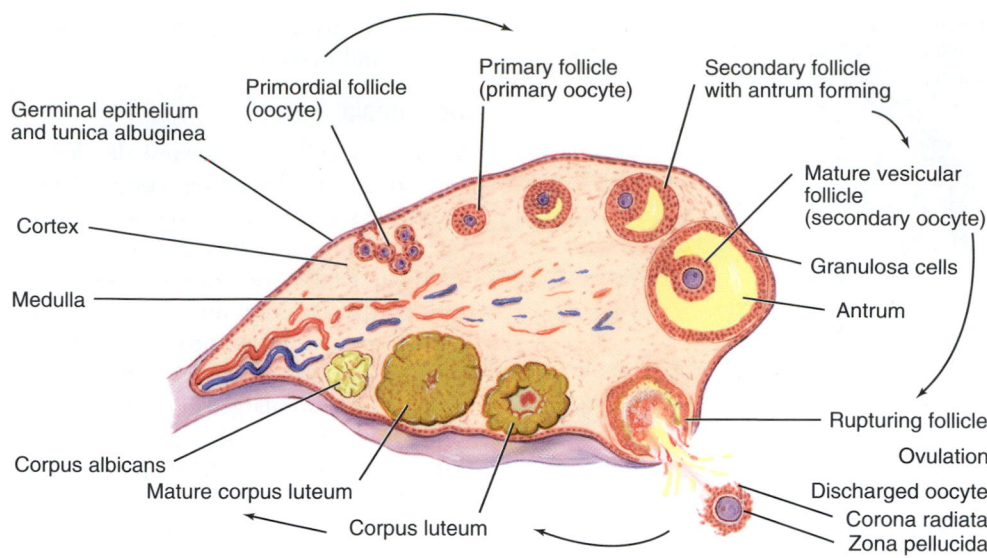

Figure 16-8 Structure of an ovary illustrating the stages in follicle development and corpus luteum formation. (From Applegate E: *The anatomy and physiology learning system,* ed 4, St Louis, 2011, Saunders.)

begins the second meiotic division, but the process stops in metaphase. At this point, ovulation occurs. If fertilization occurs, meiosis II continues. Again, this is an unequal division, with all of the cytoplasm going to the ovum, which has 23 single-stranded chromosomes. The smaller cell from this division is a *second polar body.* The first polar body also usually divides in meiosis II to produce two even smaller polar bodies. If fertilization does not occur, the second meiotic division is never completed and the secondary oocyte degenerates. Here again there are obvious differences between the male and female. In spermatogenesis, four functional spermatozoa develop from each primary spermatocyte. In oogenesis, only one functional fertilizable cell develops from a primary oocyte. The other three cells are polar bodies and they degenerate.

Ovarian Follicle Development

An ovarian follicle consists of a developing oocyte surrounded by one or more layers of cells called *follicular cells.* While the oocyte is progressing through meiosis, corresponding changes are taking place in the follicular cells (see Figure 16-8). *Primordial follicles,* which consist of a primary oocyte surrounded by a single layer of flattened cells, develop in the fetus and are the stage that is present in the ovaries at birth and throughout childhood.

Beginning at puberty FSH stimulates changes in the primordial follicles. The follicular cells become cuboidal, the primary oocyte enlarges, and a *primary follicle* is created. The follicles continue to grow under the influence of FSH, and the follicular cells proliferate to form several layers of *granulosa cells* around the primary oocyte. Most of these primary follicles degenerate along with the primary oocytes within them, but usually one continues to develop each month. The granulosa cells start secreting estrogen. In addition, a cavity known as the *antrum* forms within the follicle. When the antrum starts to develop, the follicle becomes a *secondary follicle.* The granulosa cells also secrete a substance that forms a clear membrane, known as the *zona pellucida,* around the oocyte. After about 10 days of growth the follicle is a mature vesicular (graafian) follicle, which forms a "blister" on the surface of the ovary. It contains a secondary oocyte ready for ovulation.

Ovulation

Ovulation occurs when the mature follicle at the surface of the ovary ruptures and releases the secondary oocyte into the peritoneal cavity. The ovulated secondary oocyte is ready for fertilization. It is still surrounded by the zona pellucida and a few layers of cells called the *corona radiata.* If it is not fertilized, the secondary oocyte degenerates in a couple of days. If a spermatozoon passes through the corona radiata and zona pellucida and enters the cytoplasm of the secondary oocyte, the second meiotic division resumes to form a polar body and a mature ovum.

After ovulation, the portion of the follicle that remains in the ovary enlarges and is transformed into a **corpus luteum** (see Figure 16-8). The corpus luteum is a glandular structure that secretes progesterone and some estrogens. Its fate depends on whether fertilization occurs. If fertilization does not take place, the corpus luteum remains functional for about 10 days and then begins to degenerate into a **corpus albicans.** This structure is primarily scar tissue, and its hormone output ceases. If fertilization occurs, the corpus luteum persists. The corpus luteum continues its hormone functions until the placenta develops sufficiently to secrete the necessary hormones. Again, the corpus luteum ultimately degenerates into a corpus albicans; it just remains functional for a longer period of time.

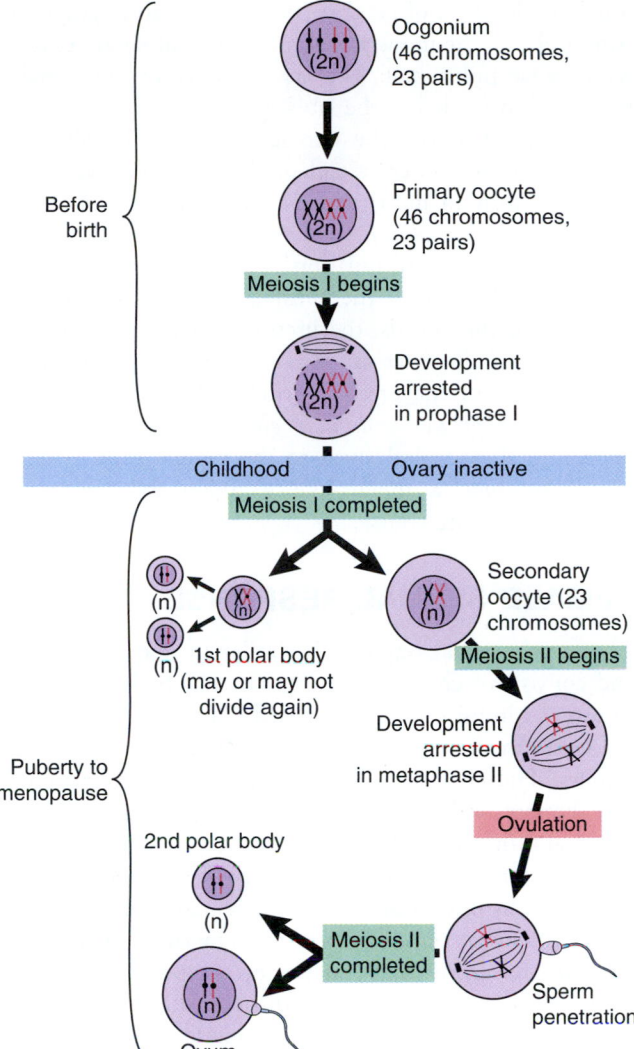

Figure 16-9 Oogenesis. The first meiotic division is interrupted in prophase before birth and does not resume until after puberty. The second meiotic division is interrupted in metaphase and does not resume unless a sperm penetrates the cell. (From Applegate E: *The anatomy and physiology learning system,* ed 4, St Louis, 2011, Saunders.)

GENITAL TRACT

Uterine Tubes

There are two **uterine tubes** (also called *fallopian tubes*). Each tube is about 4 cm long and about 1 cm in diameter and extends laterally from the upper portion of the uterus to the region of the ovary on that side (Figure 16-10). One tube is associated with each ovary. The end of the tube near the ovary expands to form a funnel-shaped *infundibulum,* which is surrounded by finger-like extensions called *fimbriae.* Because there is no direct connection between the infundibulum and the ovary, the oocyte enters the peritoneal cavity before it enters the uterine tube. At the time of ovulation, the fimbriae increase their activity and create currents in the peritoneal fluid that help propel the oocyte into the uterine tube. Once inside the uterine tube, the oocyte is moved along by the rhythmic beating of cilia on the epithelial lining and by the peristaltic action of the smooth muscle in the wall of the tube. The journey through the uterine tube takes about 7 days. Because the oocyte is fertile for only 24 to 48 hours, fertilization usually occurs in the uterine tube.

Uterus

The *uterus* is a muscular organ that receives the fertilized oocyte and provides an appropriate environment for the developing offspring. It is located in the pelvic cavity, between the rectum and urinary bladder (see Figure 16-7). Before the first pregnancy, the uterus is about the size and shape of a pear, with the narrow portion directed inferiorly. After childbirth the uterus is usually larger, and then it regresses after menopause.

The upper, bulging surface of the uterus, above the entrance of the uterine tubes, is known as the *fundus* (see Figure 16-10). The large main portion of the uterus is the *body.* The narrow region of the uterus that is directed into the vagina is the *cervix.* The opening between the body and

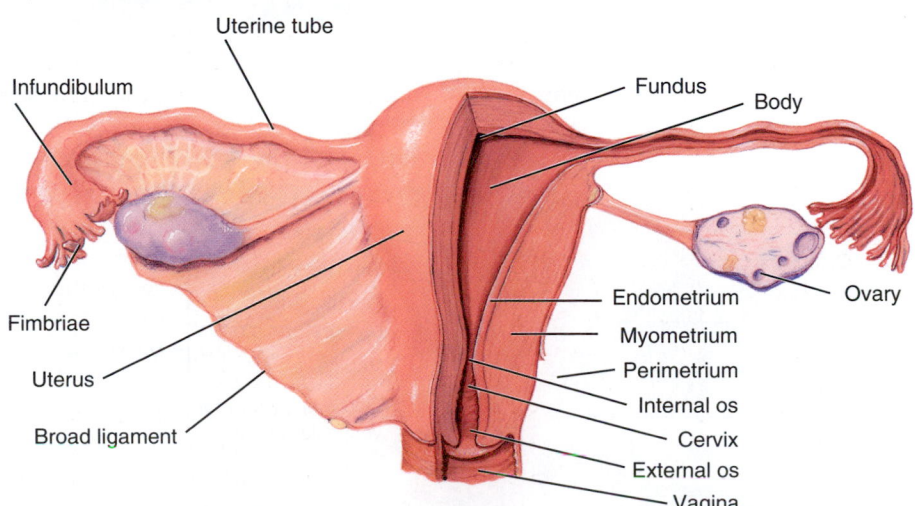

Figure 16-10 Uterus and uterine tubes. (From Applegate E: *The anatomy and physiology learning system,* ed 4, St Louis, 2011, Saunders.)

cervix is known as the *internal os,* and the opening from the cervix into the vagina is the *external os.* Several ligaments hold the uterus in place. The largest of these is the *broad ligament,* which drapes over the uterus like a sheet and extends laterally to the lateral pelvic wall. The broad ligament also encloses the uterine tubes.

The wall of the uterus consists of perimetrium, myometrium, and endometrium. The outer serous layer is known as the **perimetrium.** The thick middle layer is known as the **myometrium.** The myometrium consists of smooth muscle and makes up the bulk of the uterine wall. The inner layer is called the **endometrium.** It is a mucous membrane that is subdivided into two regions. The **stratum functionale** of the endometrium is the portion that is sloughed off during menstruation. The deeper, thinner **stratum basale** is more constant and provides the materials to rebuild the stratum functionale after menstruation.

Vagina

The *vagina* is a fibromuscular tube, about 10 cm long, that extends from the cervix of the uterus to the outside. It is located between the rectum and urinary bladder. The vagina provides a passageway for menstrual flow to reach the outside, receives the penis and semen during sexual intercourse (coitus), and serves as the birth canal during the birth of a baby. The smooth muscle and mucosal lining of the vaginal wall are capable of stretching to accommodate the erect penis and to permit passage of a baby. The opening of the vagina to the outside is known as the *vaginal orifice.* The vaginal orifice may be incompletely covered by a thin fold of mucous membrane called the *hymen.*

EXTERNAL GENITALIA

The external genitalia are accessory structures of the female reproductive system that are outside the vagina. They are also referred to as the **vulva.** The external genitalia include the labia majora, mons pubis, labia minora, clitoris, and glands within the vestibule (Figure 16-11).

The *labia majora* are two large fat-filled folds of skin that enclose the other external genitalia. Anteriorly the labia majora merge to form the *mons pubis.* The mons pubis is a rounded elevation of fat that overlies the pubic symphysis. After puberty the mons pubis and labia majora are covered with coarse pubic hair. The *labia minora* are two smaller folds of skin medial to the labia majora.

The area between the two labia minora is called the *vestibule.* At the anterior end of the vestibule (where the two labia minora meet), there is a small mass of erectile tissue called the *clitoris.* The clitoris becomes erect in response to sexual stimulation. The labia minora merge and form a hood over the clitoris, known as the *prepuce.* Posterior to the clitoris, the urethra and vagina open into the vestibule. *Paraurethral glands* open into the vestibule on each side of the urethral orifice. These glands secrete mucus. The *greater vestibular glands* (Bartholin glands) open into the vestibule next to the vaginal orifice. These glands produce a mucus-like secretion for lubrication during sexual intercourse.

FEMALE SEXUAL RESPONSE

The female sexual response is similar to that of the male and consists of erection and orgasm. The body's responses to sexual stimuli produce increased blood flow to the erectile tissue in the clitoris, the vaginal mucosa, breasts, and nipples. The clitoris and nipples become rigid and erect. The breasts and vaginal mucosa enlarge. Glands in the cervix and the vestibular glands secrete fluids that lubricate the vaginal mucosa and aid the entry of the penis.

With continued stimulation, the female response culminates in orgasm. This is accompanied by rhythmic contractions of the uterus and muscles of the pelvic floor. This helps the movement of sperm through the uterus toward the uterine tubes. The rhythmic muscle contractions are accompanied by feelings of intense pleasure, increased heart rate, elevated blood pressure, and increased respiration rate. This is followed by a general relaxation and feeling of warmth throughout the body.

HORMONAL CONTROL

As in the male, the hypothalamus, anterior pituitary, and gonads secrete hormones that have significant roles in the

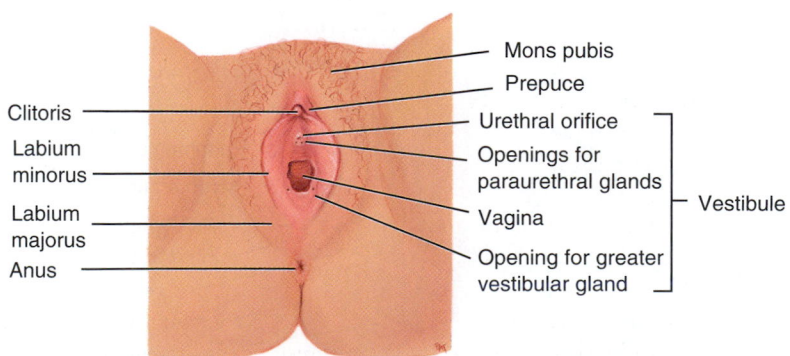

Figure 16-11 Female external genitalia. The area between the two labia minora is the vestibule. (From Applegate E: *The anatomy and physiology learning system,* ed 4, St Louis, 2011, Saunders.)

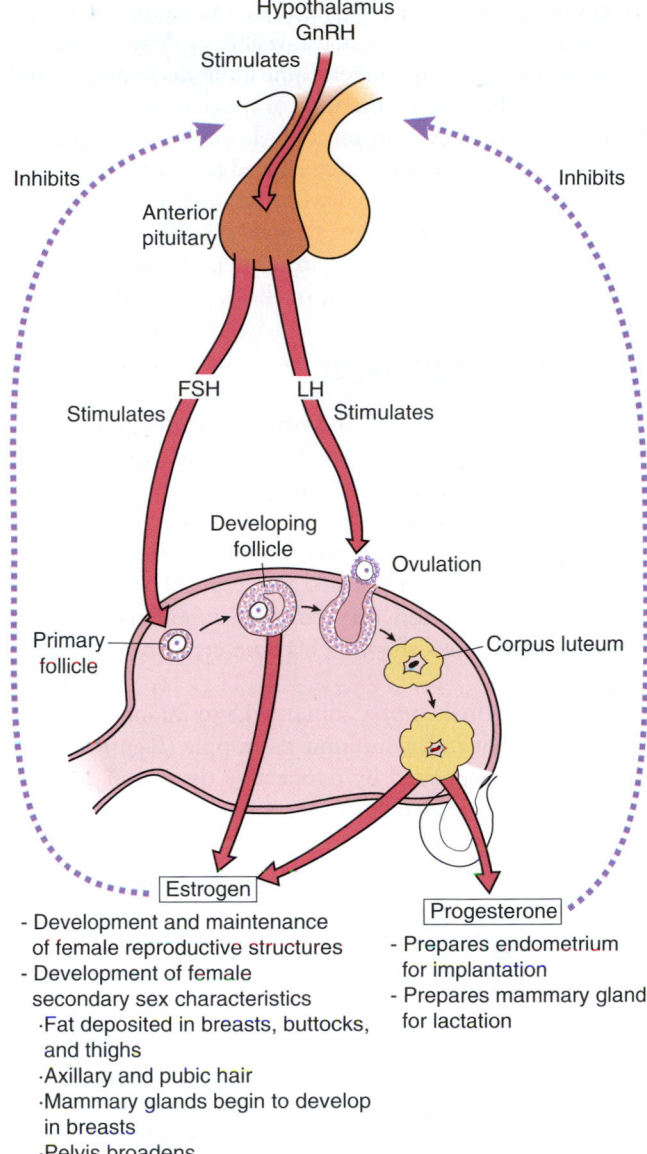

Figure 16-12 Hormonal regulation of ovarian functions. (From Applegate E: *The anatomy and physiology learning system,* ed 4, St Louis, 2011, Saunders.)

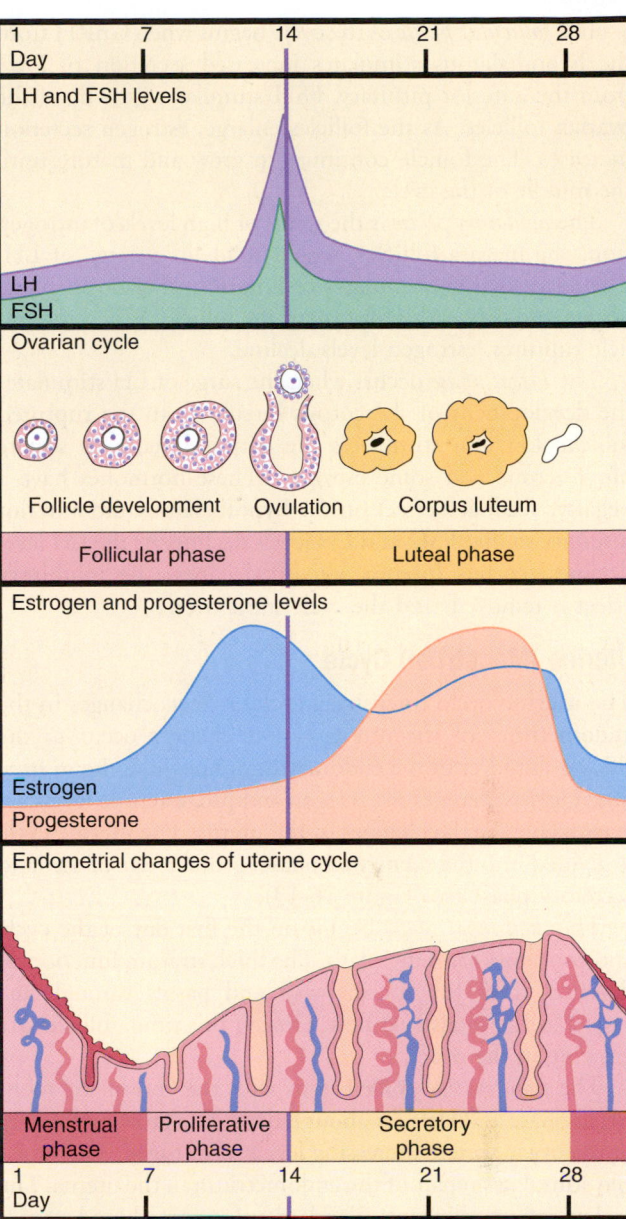

Figure 16-13 Correlation of events in the ovarian and uterine cycles. The menstrual and proliferative phases of the uterine cycle correspond to the follicular phase of the ovarian cycle. The secretory phase of the uterine cycle corresponds to the luteal phase of the ovarian cycle. Note the relative hormone levels in each phase. (From Applegate E: *The anatomy and physiology learning system,* ed 4, St Louis, 2011, Saunders.)

control of reproductive functions (Figure 16-12). The hypothalamus secretes GnRH, the anterior pituitary secretes FSH and LH, and the ovaries secrete the sex hormones *estrogen* and *progesterone*. Unlike in the male, the secretion of these hormones follows monthly cyclic patterns that affect the ovaries and uterus. These cycles, referred to as the **ovarian cycle** and the **uterine cycle** (menstrual cycle), begin at puberty and continue for about 40 years.

At puberty certain stimuli cause the hypothalamus to start secreting GnRH. This hormone enters the blood and goes to the anterior pituitary gland, where it stimulates the secretion of FSH and LH. These hormones, in turn, affect the ovaries and uterus, and the monthly cycles begin. In females the beginning of puberty is marked by the first period of menstrual bleeding, called **menarche.** After this

the cycles continue, more or less regularly, until the late 40s or early 50s. At this time the cycles become increasingly irregular until they finally stop. *Menopause* is the cessation of the reproductive cycles.

Ovarian Cycle

The ovarian cycle includes the changes that occur within the ovaries as the follicles develop (follicular phase), ovulation occurs (ovulatory phase), and the corpus luteum develops (luteal phase) (Figure 16-13).

The *follicular phase* of the cycle begins when GnRH from the hypothalamus stimulates increased secretion of FSH from the anterior pituitary. FSH stimulates growth of the ovarian follicles. As the follicles enlarge, estrogen secretion increases. The follicle continues to grow and mature until the middle of the cycle.

The *ovulatory phase* is the result of high levels of estrogen from the mature follicles, which result in a surge of LH. The surge of LH stimulates resumption of meiosis in the oocyte and causes the rupture of the follicle. When the follicle ruptures, estrogen levels decline.

The *luteal phase* occurs when the surge of LH stimulates the development of the corpus luteum from the ruptured follicle. LH also stimulates the corpus luteum to secrete progesterone and some estrogen. These hormones have a negative feedback effect on the hypothalamus and anterior pituitary so that FSH and LH levels decline. As the LH level declines, corpus luteum activity declines, the inhibitory effect is removed, and the cycle starts over.

Uterine (Menstrual) Cycle

The **uterine cycle** (menstrual cycle) reflects changes in the endometrium of the uterus. These changes occur to the thick outer layer of the endometrium, known as the *stratum functionale.* Changes in estrogen and progesterone levels are responsible for the changes in the uterus. The uterine cycle is divided into the menstrual phase, proliferative phase, and secretory phase (see Figure 16-13).

The *menstrual phase* begins on the first day of the cycle and continues for 3 to 5 days. The thick stratum functionale detaches from the uterine wall and passes through the vagina as the menstrual flow. During this time, follicles are growing in the ovary.

The *proliferative phase* begins with the end of the menstrual phase and lasts for about 8 days. The growing follicles in the ovary secrete increasing levels of estrogen. The estrogen stimulates repair of the endometrium in the uterus. The endometrium thickens, glands develop, and blood vessels grow in the new tissue. Ovulation in the ovary occurs at the end of this uterine phase.

During the *secretory phase,* the corpus luteum secretes progesterone, which stimulates continued growth and thickening of the endometrium. Arteries and glands grow and enlarge. The glands secrete glycogen, which will nourish a developing embryo if fertilization occurs. If fertilization does not occur, the corpus luteum in the ovary begins to degenerate. This leads to menstruation, and the cycle starts over again.

Menopause

Menopause is the cessation of the female reproductive cycles. Even though menopause is marked by the lack of menstrual cycles, the first changes occur in the ovary. By the age of 45 or 50, ovarian follicles cease responding to FSH and LH from the pituitary gland. As a result, the follicle cells do not produce estrogen and there is no ovulation, no corpus luteum, and no progesterone. Without estrogen and progesterone, the cyclic changes in the uterus stop and menstruation ceases. This is the visible evidence of menopause. As estrogen and progesterone levels decline, FSH and LH increase because of the lack of ovarian hormone feedback. These high levels of pituitary hormones with the low levels of ovarian hormones are believed to be responsible for a variety of effects associated with the onset of menopause. Some women experience hot flashes, sweating, depression, headaches, irritability, and insomnia. However, many women experience few, if any, of these.

MAMMARY GLANDS

The mammary glands are the organs of milk production. Mammary glands are located in the breast, overlying the pectoralis major muscles. They are present in both sexes but usually functional only in the female.

Each breast has a raised *nipple,* which is surrounded by a circular pigmented area called the *areola.* The nipples are sensitive to touch, and they contain smooth muscle that contracts and causes them to become erect in response to stimulation.

The adult female breast contains 15 to 20 lobes of glandular tissue that radiate around the nipple (Figure 16-14). The lobes are separated by connective tissue and adipose. The connective tissue helps support the breast. Some bands

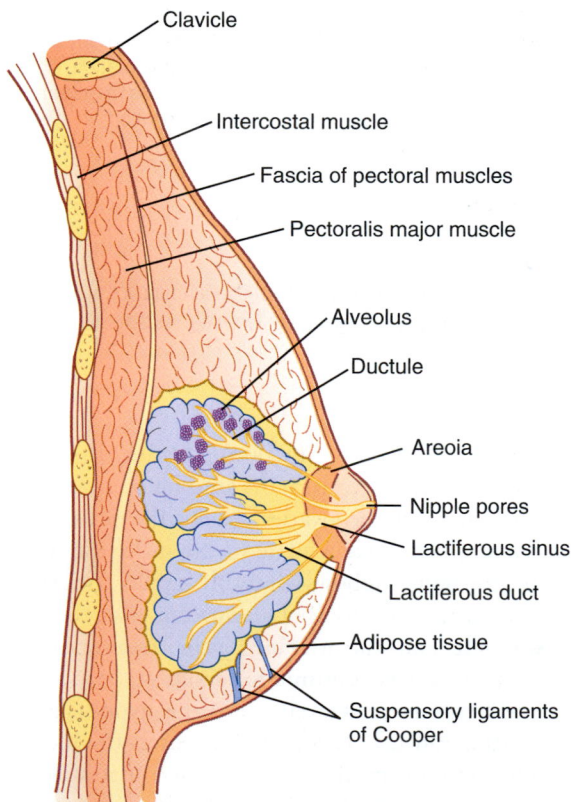

Figure 16-14 Breast and mammary glands. (From Applegate E: *The anatomy and physiology learning system,* ed 4, St Louis, 2011, Saunders.)

of connective tissue, called *suspensory* (Cooper) *ligaments,* extend through the breast from the skin to the underlying muscles. The amount and distribution of the adipose tissue determines the size and shape of the breast. Each lobe consists of *lobules* that contain the glandular units. A *lactiferous duct* collects the milk from the lobules within each lobe and carries it to the nipple. Just before the nipple, the lactiferous duct enlarges to form a *lactiferous sinus (ampulla),* which serves as a reservoir for milk. After the sinus, the duct again narrows and each duct opens independently on the surface of the nipple.

Mammary gland function is regulated by hormones. At puberty, increasing levels of estrogen stimulate the development of glandular tissue in the female breast. Estrogen also causes the breasts to increase in size through the accumulation of adipose tissue. Progesterone stimulates the development of the duct system. During pregnancy these hormones further enhance development of the mammary glands. Prolactin from the anterior pituitary stimulates the production of milk within the glandular tissue, and oxytocin causes the ejection of milk from the glands.

DEVELOPMENT

Development is a continuous process that starts with fertilization (conception) and ends with death. Birth is an awesome event that divides the total span of development into two portions. It is the culmination of 38 weeks of **prenatal development** within the uterus. The period of **postnatal development** begins with birth and lasts until death.

Fertilization, or conception, is the union of the sperm cell nucleus with an egg cell nucleus. The resulting cell is called a **zygote.** Because the egg cells are fertile for only about 24 hours, fertilization usually occurs in the uterine tube near the infundibulum. The zygote is the first cell of the future offspring and has a full complement of 46 chromosomes; 23 from the sperm and 23 from the egg.

PRENATAL DEVELOPMENT

The period of prenatal development, or pregnancy, is referred to as **gestation.** Embryologists describe the timing of events in prenatal development by using the term **developmental age,** which begins at fertilization. The medical community uses **clinical age,** which begins at the date of the last menstrual period (LMP). Developmental age is 2 weeks less than clinical age. In humans, the normal gestation period is 266 days from fertilization (developmental age) or 280 days from the beginning of the LMP (clinical age). Prenatal development is divided into preembryonic, embryonic, and fetal periods.

The **preembryonic period** lasts for about 2 weeks after fertilization. During this time the zygote undergoes numerous cell divisions and moves through the uterine tube into the cavity of the uterus. By the seventh day after fertilization

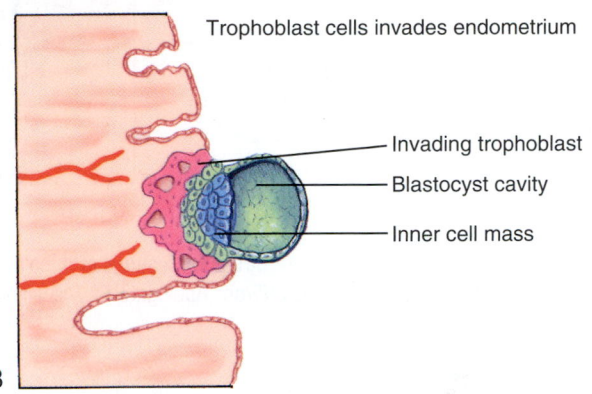

Figure 16-15 Process of implantation. (From Applegate E: *The anatomy and physiology learning system,* ed 4, St Louis, 2011, Saunders.)

(twenty-first day of a menstrual cycle), the zygote has developed into a hollow mass of cells called a *blastocyst.* The cavity is called the *blastocele,* the flattened cells around the cavity make up the *trophoblast,* and the mass of cells on one side is the *inner cell mass.* The blastocyst approaches the endometrium, usually high in the uterus, and attaches to it. This begins the process of *implantation* (Figure 16-15). The trophoblast cells secrete enzymes that erode the endometrium to form a hole, and the blastocyst "burrows" into the thick endometrial tissue. The blastocyst saves itself from being aborted by secreting *human chorionic gonadotropin* (HCG), a hormone that causes the corpus luteum to remain functional and secrete progesterone to maintain the endometrium. Pregnancy tests are based on the presence of HCG in the blood or urine because it is not produced in a woman unless she is pregnant.

The **embryonic period** lasts from the beginning of the third week to the end of the eighth week. The developing offspring is called an embryo during this time. Significant changes during this 6-week period include the formation of the *placenta* and all of the *organ systems.* The placenta is a highly vascular disc that develops from both embryonic and maternal tissue. It is usually formed and fully functioning by the end of the embryonic period. After the infant is born, the placenta is expelled from the uterus as part of the afterbirth. By diffusion of substances across the membranes, the placenta functions as a nutritive, respiratory, and excretory

Figure 16-16 Structural features of the placenta and exchange of nutrients and gases between maternal and fetal blood. (From Applegate E: *The anatomy and physiology learning system,* ed 4, St Louis, 2011, Saunders.)

organ. It also secretes hormones and thus functions as a temporary endocrine gland. The formation of body organs and organ systems is called *organogenesis.* The skin, one of the earliest organs to develop, forms during the third week. By the end of the fourth week, the heart is pumping blood to all parts of the embryo. By the end of the eighth week, all the main internal body organs are established and the embryo has a humanlike appearance, even though it is only about 25 mm (1 inch) long and weighs about 1 gram.

The **fetal period** of development starts at the beginning of the ninth week and lasts until birth. The developing offspring is called a *fetus* during this time. Because all the organ systems are formed during the embryonic period, the fetus is less vulnerable than the embryo to malformations caused by radiation, viruses, and drugs. The fetal period is a time of growth and maturation.

The fetus obtains oxygen and nutrients from maternal circulation and also depends on maternal circulation to remove carbon dioxide and other wastes. This exchange occurs through the placenta, which is attached to the uterine wall of the mother and connected to the umbilicus (navel) of the fetus by the umbilical cord (Figure 16-16). The umbilical cord contains two umbilical arteries and one umbilical vein. Umbilical arteries, branches of the fetal internal iliac arteries, carry blood that is loaded with carbon dioxide and waste products from the fetus to the placenta where they diffuse into the maternal blood. At the same time, oxygen and nutrients diffuse from maternal blood into the umbilical vein, which carries them to fetal circulation. Normally, membranes within the placenta keep the fetal and maternal blood from actually mixing. Because the fetal liver and lungs are immature and nonfunctional, there are special adaptations in fetal circulation that permit most

of the blood to bypass these organs. These adaptations are the *ductus venosus,* which is between the umbilical vein and inferior vena cava and bypasses the immature liver; the *foramen ovale,* which is an opening in the interatrial septum that allows blood to bypass pulmonary circulation; and the *ductus arteriosus,* which is a shunt between the pulmonary trunk and aorta to bypass the lungs. Figure 16-17 illustrates fetal circulation and Table 16-1 provides a summary of the specialized structures. At or shortly after birth, when the lung and liver functions are established, the adaptations in the fetal circulatory pathway are no longer necessary, and changes occur that make the structures nonfunctional. The circulatory pathway becomes like that of an adult.

PARTURITION AND LACTATION

Parturition refers to the birth of an infant, and *labor* is the process by which forceful contractions expel the fetus from the uterus. The onset of *true labor* is characterized by rhythmic contractions, dilation of the cervix, and a discharge of bloody mucus from the cervix and vagina. The onset of labor appears to be the interaction of progesterone, estrogen, oxytocin, and prostaglandins. Labor is divided into three periods: dilation stage, expulsion stage, and placental stage. These are illustrated in Figure 16-18. The *dilation stage* begins with the onset of true labor and lasts until the cervix is fully dilated to a diameter of 10 cm. This is the longest stage and may last 24 hours or longer. The *expulsion stage* lasts from full dilation of the cervix until the delivery of the fetus. This stage usually lasts less than an hour. The final stage is the *placental stage.* Usually within 10 or 15 minutes after the delivery of the fetus, the placenta separates from the uterine wall and forceful contractions expel the

Figure 16-17 Circulation patterns before and after birth. **A,** Fetal circulation. **B,** Circulation after birth. Before birth, the two umbilical arteries transport blood to the placenta and a single umbilical vein returns blood from the placenta to the fetus. The ductus venosus bypasses the nonfunctional fetal liver. The ductus arteriosus and foramen ovale permit blood to bypass the lungs, which are nonfunctional. After birth, the circulatory patterns change to include the liver and lungs. (From Applegate E: *The anatomy and physiology learning system,* ed 4, St Louis, 2011, Saunders.)

Table 16-1 Summary of Special Features in Fetal Circulation

Feature	Location	Before Birth	After Birth
Umbilical arteries (2)	Umbilical cord	Transport blood from fetus to placenta	Degenerate to become lateral umbilical ligaments
Umbilical vein (1)	Umbilical cord	Transports blood from placenta to fetus	Becomes ligamentum teres (round ligament) of liver
Ductus venosus	Between umbilical vein and inferior vena cava	Carries blood directly from umbilical vein to inferior vena cava; bypasses liver	Becomes ligamentum venosum of liver
Foramen ovale	Interatrial septum	Allows blood to go directly from right atrium into left atrium to bypass pulmonary circulation	Closes after birth to become fossa ovalis
Ductus arteriosus	Between pulmonary trunk and aorta	Permits blood in pulmonary trunk to go directly into descending aorta and bypass pulmonary circulation	Becomes a fibrous cord; ligamentum arteriosum

From Applegate E: *The anatomy and physiology learning system,* ed 4, St Louis, 2011, Saunders.

placenta and attached membranes as the afterbirth. The contractions also constrict the torn blood vessels to prevent hemorrhage. Normally less than half a liter of blood is lost during delivery.

Lactation refers to the production of milk by the mammary glands and the ejection of the milk from the breast. Prolactin is the most important hormone that stimulates the production of milk. Prolactin levels increase during pregnancy; however, the hormone's activity is inhibited by the estrogen and progesterone from the placenta. After

parturition, when the placenta is expelled, this inhibition is removed and milk production begins. The infant's suckling stimulates the release of oxytocin from the posterior pituitary gland. Oxytocin causes the ejection of milk from the breast.

POSTNATAL DEVELOPMENT

Development after birth is called **postnatal development** and lasts from parturition until death. It is divided into the during this time. There is an increase in the production of myelin within the nervous system, and this results in improved muscle coordination. The baby learns to sit, crawl, stand, and walk during this period. Teeth begin to erupt, and the baby starts to communicate by smiling, laughing, and making sounds.

Childhood lasts from the end of the first year until puberty. Bone ossification is rapid. Growth is rapid and then slows until puberty, then increases again. Deciduous teeth are shed and replaced by permanent teeth. Language skills develop, motor coordination becomes more refined, and intellect develops.

Adolescence lasts from puberty until adulthood. The individual becomes capable of reproduction during this time. Secondary sex characteristics appear. The adolescent shows increasing levels of motor skills, intellectual ability, and emotional maturity.

Adulthood is the period between adolescence and senescence. The beginning and ending of adulthood are somewhat vague. In general, adulthood is characterized by a maintenance of existing body tissues so that the body remains unchanged anatomically and physiologically for many years.

Senescence is the period of older adulthood that ends in death; the transition from adulthood to senescence is vague. This period is marked by degenerative changes that make the body less capable of coping with the demands placed on it. Changes related to aging and senescence occur in all body systems; however, the rate at which they occur varies from system to system and from individual to individual. Even though there are degenerative changes in all body systems, death usually results from cardiovascular disorders, failure of the immune system, or disease processes that affect vital organs.

AGING OF THE REPRODUCTIVE SYSTEM

Men normally do not experience a sudden decline in reproductive function comparable to menopause in women. Instead, they experience a gradual and subtle decline over many years. After age 50, men have some testicular atrophy, partially caused by a decrease in the size of the seminiferous tubules and partially a result of a reduction in the number of interstitial cells. These changes are accompanied by a decline in sperm and testosterone production. Both the seminal vesicles and the prostate show a decrease in secretory activity, which results in a reduction in the volume of semen. The portion of the prostate gland that surrounds the urethra often enlarges and may constrict the urethra, making urination difficult. The penis may undergo some atrophy and become smaller with age. The blood vessels and erectile tissue in the penis become less elastic, which hinders the ability to attain an erection. Although there is a general decline in the aging male reproductive system, many men are capable of achieving erection and ejaculation into old age.

Figure 16-18 Three stages of labor. **A,** Before labor begins. **B,** Dilation stage begins with onset of true labor and lasts until the cervix is fully dilated. **C,** Expulsion stage is from full cervical dilation until delivery of the fetus. **D,** Placental stage lasts from delivery of the fetus until the placenta and extraembryonic membranes are expelled. (From Applegate E: *The anatomy and physiology learning system,* ed 4, St Louis, 2011, Saunders.)

neonatal period, infancy, childhood, adolescence, adulthood, and senescence.

The *neonatal period* encompasses the first 4 weeks after parturition. During this time the baby is called a *neonate.* This period is critical because the neonate has to make numerous adjustments to life outside the uterus including changes in respiration and in the circulatory pathways. Temperature regulating mechanisms and the immune system are not yet fully developed, so the neonate is vulnerable to environmental temperature changes and infections.

Infancy lasts from the end of the first month until the end of the first year. Many developmental changes occur

After menopause, there is a gradual decline in the female reproductive system. Most of the changes are believed to be caused by the reduction in estrogen. The ovaries undergo progressive atrophy. The uterus becomes smaller, and fibrous connective tissue replaces much of the myometrium. The vagina becomes narrower and shorter, and its walls become thin and less elastic. Glands that lubricate the vagina reduce their secretory activity, and the vagina becomes dry. The vaginal secretions that remain are less acidic, which makes older women more susceptible to vaginal infections. The external genitalia and mammary glands undergo atrophic changes. The lack of estrogen also affects nonreproductive organs. This is particularly true in the case of bone metabolism, which is indicated by the increased prevalence of osteoporosis in postmenopausal women. There is also increased cardiovascular disease.

Estrogen replacement therapy is prescribed for many women to combat osteoporosis and other effects of menopause. However, there is controversy about the risks involved with this treatment, particularly the risks of uterine and breast cancer. Consideration should be given to the risks and benefits before beginning estrogen replacement therapy. Current practice often involves prescription of progesterone in conjunction with estrogen, which seems to reduce some of the risks.

There is a growing awareness that elderly people have sexual needs and enjoy sexual relations. Although age-related physical and hormonal changes that take place in the reproductive system may alter these needs and sexual functioning, studies demonstrate that sexuality remains important to many older people.

Common Pathology of the Reproductive System

Disease	Signs and Symptoms	Etiology	Diagnosis and Treatment
Abruptio placentae	Also called *placental abruption;* premature separation of placenta from the uterine wall. Signs and symptoms include bleeding, uterine contractions, and fetal distress.	Exact cause is unknown. Risk factors include maternal hypertension, maternal trauma, cigarette smoking, cocaine use, alcohol consumption, and blood clotting disorders.	Diagnosis is based on symptoms combined with ultrasound, fetal monitoring, and blood tests. Treatment includes intravenous (IV) fluids and blood transfusion if bleeding has been severe. An emergency Cesarean section may be needed. If the baby is very premature and there is little separation, mother may be kept on bed rest for several days.
Benign prostatic hypertrophy (BPH)	Also called *benign prostatic hyperplasia;* especially common; estimated that 90% of men over age of 70 have some degree of BPH. Symptoms include difficulty in urinating, dribbling at the end of urination, and being unable to completely empty the bladder.	Symptoms occur when the prostate enlarges and compresses the urethra enough to interfere with urine flow. The reason for the hypertrophy is unknown.	Diagnosis is based on medical history, physical examination, digital rectal examination (DRE), and urinalysis. Other tests may be required to rule out other conditions such as prostate cancer and infections. Medications may be sufficient for mild to moderate symptoms. The standard surgical procedure is transurethral resection of the prostate (TURP).
Cancer, breast	Lump or mass in the breast tissue, tenderness in the breast, skin changes in the breast, and changes in the nipple.	Cause is unknown. Occurs when some cells in the breast begin growing abnormally to accumulate and form a mass. Cells may spread to nearby lymph nodes and to other parts of the body. A family history of breast cancer increases the risk.	Diagnosis is based on a breast examination, mammogram, breast ultrasound, and biopsy of the tumor. Treatment involves surgical removal of either the tumor and a small amount of breast tissue (lumpectomy) or the entire breast (mastectomy). Depending on the type of breast cancer and the stage, further treatment by radiation therapy, chemotherapy, or hormone therapy may be necessary.
Cancer, cervical	Early cervical cancer usually produces no signs or symptoms; later stages may cause abnormal vaginal bleeding or other vaginal discharge and pelvic pain.	Occurs when healthy cells undergo a genetic mutation that turns them into abnormal cells that grow and multiply out of control. The accumulating cells form a tumor that can spread to nearby tissues, or pieces can break off and spread to other parts of the body. The cause of the mutation is unknown, but various strains of human papillomavirus (HPV) appear to have a role in many cases.	Diagnosis is accomplished by visual examination of the cervix (colposcopy) and by a cytologic examination of a tissue sample for abnormal cells. Imaging modalities are used to determine the stage of the cancer. Treatment depends on the stage and personal preference. Treatment options include surgery, radiation, and chemotherapy. Early detection through a Papanicolaou (Pap) smear and/or HPV DNA test is key to successful treatment.

Continued

Common Pathology of the Reproductive System—cont'd

Disease	Signs and Symptoms	Etiology	Diagnosis and Treatment
Cancer, ovarian	Early ovarian cancer is usually asymptomatic. Advanced cancer symptoms are nonspecific. They include abdominal bloating or swelling, weight loss, discomfort in the pelvic area, changes in bowel habits, and a frequent need to urinate.	As with most other cancers, there is no specific known cause. A genetic mutation turns normal healthy cells into rapidly growing cancer cells of the ovary. The accumulating cancer cells form a tumor that may spread to surrounding tissue and to other parts of the body.	Diagnosis is based on a pelvic examination, imaging tests, blood tests, and a biopsy. Treatment is a combination of surgery and chemotherapy.
Cancer, uterine	Vaginal bleeding after menopause, an abnormal discharge from the vagina, pelvic pain, and pain during intercourse.	As with most other cancers, there is no specific known cause. A genetic mutation turns normal healthy uterine cells into rapidly growing cancer cells. The accumulating cancer cells form a tumor that may spread to surrounding tissue and to other parts of the body.	There are no screening methods for uterine cancer. Diagnosis is by pelvic examination, transvaginal ultrasound, hysteroscopy, and tissue biopsy. Treatment depends on characteristics of the cancer and the stage. The recommended treatment is surgery to remove the uterus (hysterectomy). Usually the uterine tubes and ovaries are also removed (salpingo-oophorectomy). Additional treatments are radiation therapy, chemotherapy, and hormone therapy.
Cancer, prostate	Prostate cancer may cause no symptoms and go undetected in the early stages. As it progresses, it produces a lump on the surface of the gland. There may be difficulty in urinating, some discomfort in the pelvic region, blood in the urine and/or semen, and erectile dysfunction.	The initial cause is unknown. A mutation in a few cells, usually in one of the secretory glands of the prostate, causes them to become abnormal. These cells grow rapidly and also destroy normal cells. The accumulating abnormal cells form a tumor that may invade surrounding tissue.	Diagnosis is based on DRE, prostate-specific antigen (PSA) test, and tissue biopsy of the prostate. Imaging techniques are useful to determine the stage of the cancer and how far it has spread, then treatment protocols may be established. Options include surgery to remove the prostate (prostatectomy), radiation therapy, chemotherapy, and hormone therapy.
Cancer, testicular	Lump in either testicle, feeling of heaviness in scrotum, sudden collection of fluid in scrotum, pain or discomfort in scrotum. Signs and symptoms usually affect only one side.	As with most other cancers, there is no specific known cause. A genetic mutation turns normal healthy cells into rapidly growing cancer cells. The accumulating cancer cells form a tumor that may spread to surrounding tissue and to other parts of the body. Nearly all testicular cancers begin in the germ cells.	Most men discover the lump in the testicle themselves. Ultrasound and blood tests help determine if the lump is cancer. Typically the testicle is surgically removed (orchiectomy) and cells examined to confirm diagnosis. Computed tomography (CT) and blood tests determine the type and stage. Surgical removal is usually sufficient for early stage cancer. More advanced stages may require radiation therapy and chemotherapy.
Candidiasis	Vaginal itching, burning sensation when urinating, white vaginal discharge.	Caused by an overgrowth of the fungal microorganism *Candida albicans*.	Testing a sample of the vaginal discharge confirms diagnosis. Over- the-counter and prescription medications are usually sufficient treatment.
Cryptorchidism	Absence of one or both testicles in the scrotum.	Cause is unknown. The testicles develop in the abdominal cavity, then shortly before birth they descend into the scrotum. For some reason, one (or both) may not descend all the way. The condition will cause sterility if not corrected.	Not finding a testicle in the scrotum is sufficient for diagnosis. A minor surgical procedure will correct the problem.

Common Pathology of the Reproductive System—cont'd

Disease	Signs and Symptoms	Etiology	Diagnosis and Treatment
Ectopic pregnancy	Often the first indication is abdominal or pelvic pain and light vaginal bleeding. Severe pain and bleeding indicate a crisis.	The zygote implants somewhere other than the uterine wall, often in the uterine tubes. Risk factors include a history of pelvic inflammatory disease (PID), sexually transmitted disease (STD), a previous ectopic pregnancy, or scarring from previous pelvic surgery.	Diagnosis is based on physical examination and ultrasound. The embryo or fetus cannot develop outside the uterus so an ectopic pregnancy must be terminated. The early stages of pregnancy can be terminated using medications. A ruptured uterine tube is a medical crisis and requires emergency surgery.
Endometriosis	Pelvic pain associated with menstruation (dysmenorrhea), pain with intercourse, pain with bowel movements and urination, infertility.	Endometriosis occurs when pieces of endometrial tissue grow in places other than the lining of the uterus; usually on the ovaries, intestines, or pelvic wall. The cause is unknown, but it is most likely the result of retrograde menstruation when pieces of endometrium pass through the uterine tubes into the pelvic cavity instead of passing out of the uterus with the menstrual flow.	A pelvic examination, ultrasound, and laparoscopy may be used in diagnosis. Treatment consists of pain medications and possibly hormone therapy or laparoscopic surgery.
Erectile dysfunction, impotence	Inability to develop or maintain an erection of the penis during sexual activity.	Male sexual arousal is a complex interaction of many factors; consequently dysfunction has numerous causes. Most causes are physical secondary to other health conditions—for example, heart disease, atherosclerosis, diabetes, and treatment for prostate cancer; other causes may be psychological, such as depression, anxiety, and stress.	The condition is not difficult to diagnose, but it may be difficult to determine the underlying cause. A variety of medications are available to promote an erection. If these are insufficient, penis pumps and penile implants are available; and if the difficulty is of a psychological nature, then counseling may be recommended.
Fibrocystic disease	Lumps in the breast, aches in the breast, tenderness of breast tissue, thickened areas of breast tissue, cysts.	Exact cause is unknown.	Tests are used to differentiate between fibrocystic disease and breast cancer. These include a clinical breast examination, mammography, ultrasound, fine needle aspiration of fluid in cysts, and breast biopsy. Mild symptoms usually require no treatment. If the cysts are large and painful, fine needle aspiration to remove the fluid will reduce the size. Rarely is surgery necessary.
Genital herpes	Pain, itching, and sores in the genital area. The initial infection may produce flulike symptoms.	Caused by the herpes simplex virus. It is a common sexually transmitted disease spread by sexual contact.	The physician can usually diagnose by looking at the sores but may test a sample from the sores for confirmation. There is no cure. Once the virus is present in the body, it remains there, but it may remain dormant until a recurrent outbreak. Medications can prevent or shorten outbreaks.
Genital warts	Small flesh-colored or pink growth in the genital area, itching and discomfort in the genital area, and bleeding during intercourse.	Genital warts are caused by HPV, which is easily transmitted by sexual contact.	Diagnosis is by visual examination. A mild acetic acid solution may be used to whiten the warts to make them more visible. Usually no treatment is needed. If the warts are causing discomfort, there are medications to relieve an outbreak. There is no cure. Once the virus is present in the body, it remains there.

Continued

Common Pathology of the Reproductive System—cont'd

Disease	Signs and Symptoms	Etiology	Diagnosis and Treatment
Gonorrhea	Many patients have no symptoms. For men, symptoms may include painful urination, puslike discharge from the tip of the penis, and pain or swelling in the testicles. For women, there may be painful urination, vaginal discharge, abdominal or pelvic pain, and vaginal bleeding. The disease can also affect the rectum, eyes, throat, and joints.	Gonorrhea is a sexually transmitted disease caused by the bacterium *Neisseria gonorrhoeae*. Babies can be infected during childbirth.	Diagnostic tools include a urine test to detect bacteria in the urethra and a swab of the affected area to detect the bacteria. This is a bacterial disease, so antibiotics are an effective treatment.
Gynecomastia	Enlarged breast gland tissue, breast tenderness, feelings of embarrassment.	Gynecomastia is enlarged breast tissue in boys or men, caused by an imbalance of the hormones estrogen and testosterone. It also occurs in Klinefelter syndrome.	Diagnosis is by physical examination with careful evaluation of breast tissue, assisted by blood tests, imaging scans, biopsies, and mammograms. If the condition is very bothersome, surgery may be required to remove the breast tissue.
Hypospadias	Hooded appearance of the penis with a downward curve, abnormal spraying during urination.	Hypospadias is a condition in which the opening of the urethra is on the underside of the penis instead of at the tip. It is a congenital defect that may be inherited.	Hypospadias may be diagnosed by physical appearance. In some cases, treatment involves surgery to reposition the urethral opening and to straighten the shaft of the penis if necessary.
Inguinal hernia	A bulge in the pubic bone area with an aching sensation; pain when lifting, coughing, or bending over; and weakness or pressure in the groin.	In an inguinal hernia, a portion of the intestines protrudes through a weak point of the abdominal wall. If the intestine becomes trapped in the abdominal wall, its blood supply may be cut off. This is called a *strangulated hernia*.	An inguinal hernia can usually be diagnosed with only a physical examination. An enlarged or painful hernia will usually require surgery to relieve discomfort and prevent serious complications.
Mastitis	Breast tenderness and swelling, pain while breast feeding, skin redness, fever, malaise.	Mastitis is a breast tissue infection. It may be caused by a blocked milk duct or by bacteria entering the breast.	Mastitis diagnosis is based on patient history and physical examination, looking for a tender wedge-shaped area on the breast that points toward the nipple. Treatment is with antibiotics and pain relievers.
Ovarian cysts	Menstrual irregularities, pelvic pain at the start and end of the period, pain during bowel movements, nausea, breast tenderness.	Most ovarian cysts develop from the follicles that develop each month. For some unknown reason some of the follicles may continue to grow and form fluid-filled cysts on the surface of the ovary instead of degenerating with the monthly cycle. Typically, ovarian cysts cause little or no discomfort and are harmless. Cysts that have ruptured can lead to severe pain and internal bleeding.	An ovarian cyst diagnosis may be achieved with pelvic ultrasound or laparoscopy. The physician may suggest removal of a large cyst if it is growing or persists through two or three menstrual cycles. Cysts that cause pain or other symptoms may also be removed.

Common Pathology of the Reproductive System—cont'd

Disease	Signs and Symptoms	Etiology	Diagnosis and Treatment
Placenta previa	Vaginal bleeding without pain during the second half of pregnancy is the main sign of placenta previa.	Placenta previa is an obstetric complication in which the placenta is inserted partially or wholly over the cervix. The exact cause is unknown. It has been suggested that it may be the result of irregularities in the vascularization of the endometrium.	Placenta previa can be diagnosed with ultrasound. If the patient has little or no bleeding, bed rest at home may be recommended. If the bleeding is heavy, a cesarean delivery is scheduled for as soon as the baby can be delivered safely.
Polycystic ovary syndrome (PCOS)	Infertility, infrequent or prolonged menstrual periods, facial hair, cysts of the ovaries, obesity, pelvic pain, depression, sleep apnea.	PCOS is a varied disorder of uncertain cause. There is strong evidence that it is a genetic disease. The condition name comes from the appearance of the ovaries, which contain numerous small cysts.	There is no single test for diagnosing PCOS. Medical history, physical examination, pelvic examination, blood tests, and vaginal ultrasound are typical procedures. There is no cure for PCOS. Management includes lifestyle modifications, use of birth control pills, and fertility medications.
Preeclampsia and eclampsia	Increase in blood pressure, signs of kidney problems, severe headaches, blurred vision, abdominal pain, nausea, decreased urine output, edema, shortness of breath.	Preeclampsia is a disorder in pregnancy in which the patient has high blood pressure and proteinuria. The exact cause of preeclampsia is unknown. During pregnancy, new blood vessels develop to provide blood to the placenta. In women with preeclampsia, these blood vessels do not seem to develop properly, limiting the blood flow.	Preeclampsia is diagnosed when a pregnant woman's blood pressure abruptly increases. The only known definitive treatment for preeclampsia is delivery of the fetus and placenta. Women with severe hypertension during pregnancy should receive treatment with antihypertensive agents. Eclampsia is the development of convulsions in a patient with preeclampsia.
Syphilis	The first sign of syphilis is a small sore, called a *chancre,* that appears at the spot where the bacteria entered the body. A few weeks later a rash appears. If untreated the disease enters a latent stage.	Syphilis is an STD that can have very serious complications when left untreated. It is caused by the spirochete *Treponema pallidum.*	A blood test can be used to test for syphilis. Syphilis can be cured with the proper antibiotics, but it is important to receive treatment at the first sign of the chancre.
Trichomoniasis	Most infected people do not have symptoms. When symptoms appear, they can range from mild irritation to severe inflammation and include a foul-smelling vaginal discharge in women; a discharge from the urethra in men; redness, burning, and itching in the genital area; and painful urination or intercourse. Pregnant women with trichomoniasis are more likely to have their babies prematurely.	Trichomoniasis is a common STD caused by a protozoan parasite, *Trichomonas vaginalis.* Although symptoms of the disease vary, most women and men who have the parasite are not aware that they are infected. The parasite is passed from an infected person to an uninfected person during sex.	Trichomoniasis is diagnosed by collecting a specimen and visually observing the trichomonads via a microscope. It can be cured with a single dose of antibiotic medication.

⟲ TERMINOLOGY REVIEW

Key Term	Word Parts	Definition
Clinical age		Method of timing in development that begins with the last menstrual period; 2 weeks more than developmental age.
Corpora cavernosa	*corpor/o-:* body *cav/o-:* hollow, cavity	Two dorsal columns of erectile tissue found in the penis.
Corpus albicans	*corp/o-:* body *alb/o-:* white	Scar tissue in the ovary that forms when the corpus luteum degenerates.
Corpus luteum	*corp/o-:* body *lute/o-:* yellow	The yellow structure that develops from the mature follicle after ovulation.
Corpus spongiosum	*corp/o-:* body	Ventral column of erectile tissue found in the penis.
Developmental age		Method of timing in development that begins with fertilization; 2 weeks less than clinical age.
Ductus deferens	*duct/o-:* to lead or carry	Tubular structure that is continuous with the epididymis; it ascends through the inguinal canal and transports sperm to the ejaculatory duct.
Embryonic period	*embry/o-:* embryo	Stage of development that lasts from the beginning of the third week until the end of the eighth week after fertilization; period during which the organ systems develop in the body.
Endometrium	*endo-:* in; within *metri/o-:* uterus	Innermost mucous membrane layer of the uterine wall.
Epididymis		Tightly coiled tubule along the posterior margin of each testicle; functions in the maturation and storage of sperm.
Fetal period		Stage of development that starts at the beginning of the ninth week after fertilization and lasts until birth.
Gametes		Sex cells: sperm and ova.
Gestation	*gest/o-:* pregnancy	Time of prenatal development; pregnancy.
Gonads		Primary reproductive organs; organs that produce the gametes: testes in the male and ovaries in the female.
Interstitial cells	*inter-:* between	Cells between the seminiferous tubules in the testes; produce testosterone; also called *cells of Leydig.*
Lactation	*lact/o-:* milk	Milk production and ejection from the mammary glands.
Menarche	*men/o-:* menses; menstruation *-arche:* beginning	First period of menstrual bleeding at puberty.
Myometrium	*my/o-:* muscle *-metri-:* uterus	Thick middle layer of the uterus; it is composed of smooth muscle.
Oogenesis	*oo-:* egg, ovum *-genesis:* producing, forming	Process of meiosis in the female in which one ovum and three polar bodies are produced from one primary oocyte.
Oogonia	*oo-:* egg, ovum *-gon-:* seed	Stem cells that give rise to ova or egg cells.
Ovarian cycle	*ovary/o:* ovary	Monthly cycle of events that occur in the ovary from puberty to menopause; occurs concurrently with the uterine cycle.
Ovarian follicles	*ovary/o:* ovary	Oocytes surrounded by one or more layers of cells within the ovaries.
Parturition	*partum:* birth; labor	Act of giving birth to an infant.
Perimetrium	*metri-:* uterus	Outermost layer of the uterus.
Postnatal development	*-nat/i-:* birth	Development that begins with birth and lasts until death.
Preembryonic period	*pre-:* before; in front of *embry/o:* embryo	First 2 weeks after fertilization; period of cleavage, implantation, and formation of primary germ layers.
Prenatal development	*pre-:* before; in front of *nat/i-:* birth	Development within the uterus.
Seminiferous tubules	*semin/i:* semen; seed *tub/o-:* tube	Tightly coiled structures within which sperm are produced in the testes.
Spermatogenesis	*spermat/o:* spermatozoa, sperm cells	Process of meiosis in the male in which four spermatids are produced from one primary spermatocyte.

⟲ TERMINOLOGY REVIEW—cont'd

Key Term	Word Parts	Definition
Spermatogonia	*spermat/o:* spermatozoa, sperm cells *-gon-:* seed	Stem cells that give rise to sperm cells.
Spermiogenesis	*spermi/o:* spermatozoa, sperm cells *-genesis:* producing, forming	Morphologic changes that transform a spermatid into a mature sperm.
Stratum basale	*strat-:* layer	Bottom layer of the endometrium that is responsible for rebuilding the stratum functionale after menstruation.
Stratum functionale	*strat-:* layer	Portion of the endometrium that is sloughed off during menstruation.
Uterine cycle	*uter/o:* uterus, womb	Monthly cycle of events that occur in the uterus from puberty to menopause; also called the *menstrual cycle;* occurs concurrently with the ovarian cycle.
Uterine tubes	*uter/o:* uterus	The tubes that extend laterally from the upper portion of the uterus to the region of the ovaries; also called *fallopian tubes* or *oviducts.*
Vulva	*vulv/o-:* vulva	Collective term for the external accessory structures of the female reproductive system; also called the *pudendum.*
Zygote	*zyg/o-:* union; pair; tied together	The single diploid cell that is a fertilized ovum.

ON THE WEB

For information on the reproductive system:

Department of Health and Human Services, Office of Women's Health: www.4women.gov/COE

Gene School: library.thinkquest.org/28599/index.htm

Inner Body: www.innerbody.com/html/body.html

The Internet Pathology Laboratory for Medical Education—Female Reproductive Pathology: library.med.utah.edu/WebPath/ORGAN.html *(Click on "Female Genital Tract Pathology")*

The Internet Pathology Laboratory for Medical Education—Male Reproductive Pathology: library.med.utah.edu/WebPath/ORGAN.html *(Click on "Male Reproductive Pathology")*

The Visible Embryo: visembryo.com

17

Medical Asepsis and the OSHA Standard

ℯ Check out the Evolve site at http://evolve.elsevier.com/Bonewit/today/ to access additional interactive activities and exercises to help you study and prepare for success.

LEARNING OBJECTIVES	PROCEDURES
Microorganisms and Medical Asepsis	
1. Define microorganism and give examples of types of microorganisms.	Handwashing.
2. Explain the difference between a nonpathogen and a pathogen.	
3. Define medical asepsis.	
4. List the six basic requirements for growth and multiplication of microorganisms.	
5. Outline the infection process cycle, including the following:	
• Give examples of the means of entry of microorganisms into the body.	
• Give examples of the means of transmission of microorganisms from one person to another.	
• Give examples of the means of exit of microorganisms from the body.	
• List and explain the protective mechanisms the body uses to prevent the entrance of microorganisms.	
6. Explain the difference between resident flora and transient flora.	
7. State when each of the following is performed: handwashing, antiseptic handwashing, and use of an alcohol-based hand rub.	Applying an alcohol-based hand rub.
8. Identify medical aseptic practices that should be followed in the medical office.	
9. Explain how proper handwashing helps prevent the transmission of microorganisms.	
10. List examples of when to wear clean disposable gloves.	Application and removal of clean disposable gloves.
OSHA Bloodborne Pathogens Standard	
11. Explain the purpose of the Occupational Safety and Health Administration (OSHA).	Adhere to the OSHA Bloodborne Pathogens Standard.
12. Describe the purpose of the Needlestick Safety and Prevention Act.	
13. List and describe the elements that must be included in the OSHA exposure control plan.	
14. Explain the purpose of each of the following OSHA requirements: labeling requirements and sharps injury log.	
15. Define and give examples of each of the following: engineering controls, work practice controls, personal protective equipment, and housekeeping procedures.	
16. Identify the guidelines for use of personal protective equipment.	
Regulated Medical Waste	
17. List examples of medical waste and explain how to discard each type of waste.	Prepare regulated waste for pickup by an infectious waste service.
18. Explain how to handle and dispose of regulated medical waste.	
Bloodborne Diseases	
19. Explain how hepatitis B and C are transmitted in the health care setting.	
20. Describe postexposure prophylaxis for hepatitis B.	
21. Explain what occurs when the human immunodeficiency virus (HIV) gains entrance into the body.	

CHAPTER OUTLINE

INTRODUCTION TO MEDICAL ASEPSIS AND THE OSHA STANDARD
MICROORGANISMS AND MEDICAL ASEPSIS
Growth Requirements for Microorganisms
Infection Process Cycle
Protective Mechanisms of the Body
Medical Asepsis in the Medical Office
Hand Hygiene
Infection Control
Gloves
OSHA BLOODBORNE PATHOGENS STANDARD
Purpose of the Standard
Needlestick Safety and Prevention Act
OSHA Terminology
Components of the OSHA Standard
Exposure Control Plan
Labeling Requirements
Communicating Hazards to Employees

Record Keeping
Control Measures
Engineering Controls
Work Practice Controls
Personal Protective Equipment
Housekeeping
Hepatitis B Vaccination
Universal Precautions
REGULATED MEDICAL WASTE
Handling Regulated Medical Waste
Disposal of Regulated Medical Waste
BLOODBORNE DISEASES
Hepatitis B
Postexposure Prophylaxis
Hepatitis C
Acquired Immunodeficiency Syndrome
Transmission of AIDS

KEY TERMS

aerobe (AIR-obe)
anaerobe (AN-er-obe)
antiseptic
cilia (SIL-ee-ah)
hand hygiene
infection
medical asepsis
microorganism
  (MYE-kroe-OR-gan-iz-um)

nonintact (NON-in-takt) skin
nonpathogen (non-PATH-oh-jen)
opportunistic (OP-pore-tune-IS-tik)
  infection
optimum (OP-tuh-mum) growth
  temperature
parenteral (pare-EN-ter-al)
pathogen (PATH-oh-jen)

postexposure prophylaxis
  (proe-fil-ACKS-is)
regulated medical waste
resident flora (FLOE-ruh)
transient (TRAN-zee-ent) flora

INTRODUCTION TO MEDICAL ASEPSIS AND THE OSHA STANDARD

Medical asepsis and infection control are crucial in preventing the spread of disease. The medical assistant should always practice good medical aseptic techniques to provide a safe and healthy environment in the medical office. The Occupational Safety and Health Administration (OSHA) Bloodborne Pathogens Standard is important for infection control. This standard is required by the federal government to reduce the exposure of health care employees to infectious diseases. This chapter presents a thorough discussion of medical asepsis, infection control, and the OSHA Bloodborne Pathogens Standard.

MICROORGANISMS AND MEDICAL ASEPSIS

Microorganisms are tiny living plants or animals that cannot be seen with the naked eye, but instead must be viewed with the aid of a microscope. Common types of microorganisms include bacteria, viruses, protozoa, fungi, and animal parasites. Most microorganisms are harmless and do not cause disease. They are termed **nonpathogens.** Other microorganisms, known as **pathogens,** are harmful to the body and can cause disease.

In the medical office, practices must be employed to inhibit the growth and hinder the transmission of pathogenic microorganisms to prevent the spread of infection.

These practices are known as *medical asepsis*. **Medical asepsis** means that an object or area is clean and free from disease-producing microorganisms. Nonpathogens would still be present on a clean or medically aseptic object or surface, but all the pathogens would have been eliminated.

GROWTH REQUIREMENTS FOR MICROORGANISMS

For microorganisms to survive, certain growth requirements must be present in the environment, as follows:

1. *Proper nutrition.* Microorganisms that use inorganic or nonliving substances as sources of food are known as *autotrophs.* Microorganisms that use organic or living substances for food are known as *heterotrophs.*
2. *Oxygen.* Most microorganisms need oxygen to grow and multiply and are termed **aerobes.** Other microorganisms, known as **anaerobes,** grow best in the absence of oxygen.
3. *Temperature.* Each microorganism has a temperature at which it grows best, known as the **optimum growth temperature.** Most microorganisms grow best at 98.6° F (37° C), the human body temperature.
4. *Darkness.* Microorganisms grow best in darkness.

5. *Moisture.* Microorganisms need moisture for cell metabolism and to carry away wastes.
6. *pH.* The pH is the degree to which a solution is acidic or basic. Most microorganisms prefer a neutral pH. If the environment of the microorganisms becomes too acidic or too basic, they die.

If growth requirements are taken away from the environment of microorganisms, they are unable to survive. Eliminating these conditions is one way to reduce the growth and transmission of pathogens in the medical office.

INFECTION PROCESS CYCLE

Infection is the condition in which the body, or part of it, is invaded by a pathogen. For a pathogen to survive and produce disease, a continuous cycle must be followed; this is known as the *infection process cycle* (Figure 17-1). If the cycle is broken at any point, the pathogen dies. The medical assistant has a responsibility to help break this cycle in the medical office by practicing good techniques of medical asepsis. These techniques are discussed in the next section.

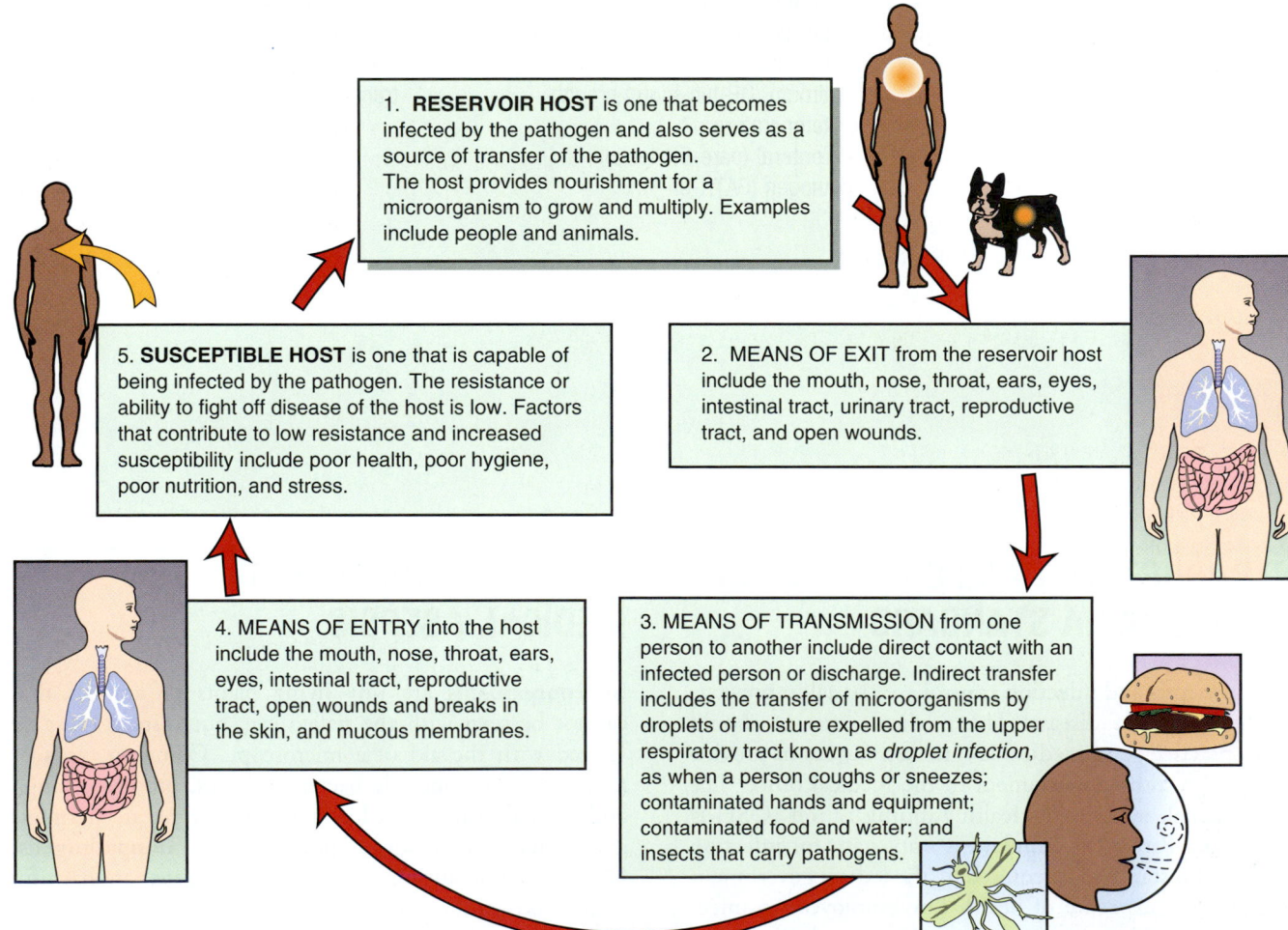

1. **RESERVOIR HOST** is one that becomes infected by the pathogen and also serves as a source of transfer of the pathogen. The host provides nourishment for a microorganism to grow and multiply. Examples include people and animals.

5. **SUSCEPTIBLE HOST** is one that is capable of being infected by the pathogen. The resistance or ability to fight off disease of the host is low. Factors that contribute to low resistance and increased susceptibility include poor health, poor hygiene, poor nutrition, and stress.

2. MEANS OF EXIT from the reservoir host include the mouth, nose, throat, ears, eyes, intestinal tract, urinary tract, reproductive tract, and open wounds.

4. MEANS OF ENTRY into the host include the mouth, nose, throat, ears, eyes, intestinal tract, reproductive tract, open wounds and breaks in the skin, and mucous membranes.

3. MEANS OF TRANSMISSION from one person to another include direct contact with an infected person or discharge. Indirect transfer includes the transfer of microorganisms by droplets of moisture expelled from the upper respiratory tract known as *droplet infection*, as when a person coughs or sneezes; contaminated hands and equipment; contaminated food and water; and insects that carry pathogens.

Figure 17-1 The infection process cycle.

PROTECTIVE MECHANISMS OF THE BODY

The body has protective mechanisms to help prevent the entrance of pathogens, and these help break the infection process cycle. Protective mechanisms of the body are as follows:

1. The skin is the body's most important defense mechanism; it serves as a protective barrier against the entrance of microorganisms.
2. The mucous membranes of the body, which line the nose and throat and respiratory, gastrointestinal, and genital tracts, help protect the body from invasion by microorganisms.
3. Mucus and cilia in the nose and respiratory tract fight off pathogens. Mucus traps the smaller microorganisms that enter the body, and the hairlike **cilia** constantly beat toward the outside to remove them from the body.
4. Coughing and sneezing help force pathogens from the body.
5. Tears and sweat are secretions that aid in the removal of pathogens from the body.
6. Urine and vaginal secretions are acidic. Pathogens cannot grow in an acidic environment.
7. The stomach secretes hydrochloric acid, which helps in the process of digestion. This acidic environment discourages the growth of pathogens that enter the stomach.

MEDICAL ASEPSIS IN THE MEDICAL OFFICE

Hand Hygiene

Hand hygiene refers to the process of cleansing or sanitizing the hands. Hand hygiene is considered the most important medical aseptic practice in the medical office for preventing the spread of infection. Specific techniques for sanitizing the hands in the medical office include the following:

- Handwashing with plain (nonmicrobial) soap and water
- Handwashing with an antimicrobial soap and water
- Applying an alcohol-based hand rub

The Centers for Disease Control and Prevention (CDC) has established recommendations for hand hygiene in health care settings. The purpose of these guidelines is to promote improved hand hygiene practices and to reduce transmission of pathogenic microorganisms to patients and employees in health care settings. The CDC guidelines for hand hygiene as they apply to the medical office are outlined in Box 17-1. They are also discussed further in this section.

Resident and Transient Flora

Microorganisms on the hands are classified into the following categories: resident flora and transient flora. **Resident flora** (also known as *normal flora*) normally resides and grows in the epidermis and deeper layers of the skin known as the *dermis*. Resident flora is usually harmless and nonpathogenic. Because resident flora is attached to the deeper skin layers, it is difficult to remove from the skin.

Transient flora lives and grows on the superficial skin layers, or epidermis. It is picked up on the hands during the course of daily activities. In the medical office, this may include contact with an infected patient, contaminated equipment, or contaminated surfaces. Transient flora is often pathogenic, but because it is attached loosely to the skin, it can be removed easily with proper handwashing or by applying an alcohol-based hand rub.

BOX 17-1   CDC Guidelines for Hand Hygiene in Health Care Settings

Wash Hands with Plain Soap or an Antimicrobial Soap

- When the hands are visibly soiled with dirt or body fluids (e.g., blood, feces, urine, respiratory secretions)
- Before eating
- After using the restroom

Apply an Alcohol-Based Hand Rub (or Wash Hands)

- Before having direct patient contact
- After contact with a patient's intact skin (e.g., measuring pulse or blood pressure)
- Before applying and after removing gloves
- After contact with body fluids or excretions, mucous membranes, nonintact skin, and wound dressings as long as the hands are not visibly soiled
- When moving from a contaminated body site to a clean body site during patient care
- After contact with inanimate objects (e.g., medical equipment) when providing health care to a patient

General Recommendations

- Keep natural nail tips less than $\frac{1}{4}$ inch long. Avoid wearing artificial nails.
- Do not add soap to a partially empty liquid soap dispenser. The practice of "topping off" dispensers can lead to bacterial contamination of the soap. The correct procedure is either to dispose of an empty dispenser or to rinse an empty dispenser thoroughly and then refill it.
- Use hand lotions or creams to minimize the occurrence of dermatitis associated with frequent handwashing.
- Wear gloves if contact with blood or other potentially infectious materials, mucous membranes, and nonintact skin could occur.
- Change gloves during patient care if moving from a contaminated body site to a clean body site.
- Remove gloves after caring for a patient. Do not wear the same pair of gloves for the care of more than one patient.

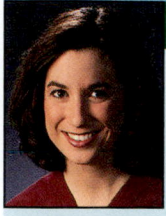

Putting It All Into Practice

My name is Jennifer Hawk, and I work for a large group of physicians in a multispecialty clinic. I work in both the front and back areas of the office. I really enjoy experiencing all of these areas of the office, and I definitely never get bored.

The most interesting experience I have had as a practicing medical assistant is seeing the impact that I make in patients' lives. They rely on you and look to you first for help in their health care situation. You are most often the first person they come into contact with in the office, and they look to you for understanding and empathy. Especially patients who come to your office on a regular basis see you as a kind of family member. They appreciate a familiar face and a smile. Most often, you are the individual giving patients instructions concerning testing they will be having done or medication they will be taking. Patients truly do count on your knowledge and assistance throughout their course of care. I was genuinely surprised at what an impact I could have on others. ∎

Figure 17-2 A, Antimicrobial soap. **B,** Alcohol-based hand rubs.

Handwashing

Handwashing refers to washing the hands with plain (nonmicrobial) soap and water. Plain soap contains agents that help break down and emulsify dirt and oil present on the skin. Soap is used to sanitize the hands through the physical removal of dirt and transient flora. It is important to use adequate friction during handwashing to ensure the removal of all transient flora. The CDC recommends that the hands be rubbed together vigorously for at least 15 seconds, making sure to cover all surfaces and to focus on the fingertips and fingernails. Procedure 17-1 outlines the handwashing procedure.

The CDC hand hygiene guidelines recommend that handwashing be performed when the hands are visibly soiled with dirt or body fluids, before eating, and after using the restroom (see Box 17-1). If the hands are not visibly soiled, the CDC recommends that an alcohol-based hand rub, rather than handwashing, be used to sanitize the hands. This is because repeated handwashing tends to dry out the hands, leading to irritation, chapping, and dermatitis.

Antiseptic Handwashing

Washing the hands with an antimicrobial soap is termed *antiseptic handwashing.* Antimicrobial soaps contain an **antiseptic,** which is an agent that functions to kill or inhibit the growth of microorganisms (Figure 17-2, *A*). Antiseptic handwashing sanitizes the hands through the mechanical scrubbing action and through the action of the antiseptic. Proper handwashing with an antimicrobial soap removes all soil and transient flora from the hands. Most antimicrobial soaps also deposit an antibacterial film on the skin that discourages bacterial growth. Antiseptic handwashing should be performed by the medical assistant before assisting with

minor office surgery. Examples of antiseptics contained in antimicrobial soaps include triclosan, chlorhexidine, hexachlorophene, iodine, and chloroxylenol.

Alcohol-Based Hand Rubs

CDC guidelines recommend the use of an alcohol-based hand rub for sanitizing the hands when they are not visibly soiled (see Box 17-1). Alcohol-based hand rubs, also known as alcohol-based *hand sanitizers,* consist of 60% to 90% alcohol (ethanol or isopropanol) and come in the forms of gels, lotions, and foams (Figure 17-2, *B*). Studies have shown that hand rubs are more effective than traditional soap and water handwashing in removing transient flora and reducing bacterial counts on the hands. The advantages that alcohol-based hand rubs offer over traditional handwashing are as follows:

- Alcohol-based hand rubs are usually more accessible than sinks.
- They do not require rinsing; water or hand drying with a towel is not needed.
- Less time is required to perform hand hygiene. It takes approximately 30 seconds to sanitize the hands with an alcohol-based hand rub compared with 1 to 2 minutes to perform proper handwashing.
- They are less damaging to the skin, resulting in less dryness and irritation. Most alcohol-based hand rubs contain emollients, which help prevent the skin of the hands from overdrying. As the alcohol dries, protective fats and oils remain on the hands.

Alcohol-based hand rubs have disadvantages. They are more expensive than plain soap. They also cause a brief stinging sensation if they are applied to broken skin, such as a cut or abrasion on the hand. Procedure 17-2 describes the proper steps for performing an alcohol-based hand rub.

Infection Control

In addition to hand hygiene, other good aseptic practices in the medical office include the following:

1. Follow the OSHA Bloodborne Pathogens Standard (presented in this chapter).

2. Keep the medical office free from dirt and dust, which can collect and carry microorganisms.
3. Ensure that the reception area and examining rooms are well ventilated. Stuffy rooms encourage microorganisms to settle on objects.
4. Keep the reception area and examining rooms bright and airy. Light discourages the growth of microorganisms.
5. Eliminate insects by the use of insecticides or window screens. Insects are a means of transmission of microorganisms.
6. Carefully dispose of wastes, such as urine, feces, and respiratory secretions; all wastes should be handled as though they contain pathogens.
7. Do not let soiled items touch clothing.
8. Avoid coughs and sneezes of patients. Moisture droplets expelled from the lungs with coughing and sneezing may contain pathogens.
9. Use discretion in the amount of jewelry worn; wear minimal jewelry or no jewelry at all. Microorganisms can become lodged in the grooves and crevices of jewelry and serve as a means of transmission of pathogens.
10. Teach patients aseptic practices to control the spread of infection at home.

Gloves

Gloves reduce hand contamination by 70% to 80%, reduce cross-contamination between patients, and protect patients and health care workers from infection. The CDC recommends that clean disposable gloves be worn when the medical assistant is likely to come in contact with any body substance, such as blood, urine, feces, mucous membranes, and nonintact skin. Clean disposable gloves should be worn when administering an injection, performing a venipuncture, or performing a urinalysis. Clean disposable gloves come in the following sizes: small, medium, large, and extra large, and sometimes extra small. Procedure 17-3 presents the proper method for applying and removing clean disposable gloves.

Sterile gloves are used to perform sterile procedures, such as a dressing change, or to assist the physician during minor office surgery, which is described in greater detail in Chapter 25.

Types of Gloves

There are two general types of gloves: latex and nonlatex. Latex gloves are made from natural rubber latex (NRL), which is a milky liquid that is extracted from rubber trees. Nonlatex gloves are made from synthetic rubber. Examples of nonlatex gloves include nitrile, vinyl, and polychloroprene (neoprene) gloves.

NRL gloves have a number of advantages over non-latex gloves. Latex gloves are soft and elastic and therefore stretch to fit more comfortably, whereas some nonlatex gloves (e.g., vinyl gloves) are stiffer and are not as comfortable to wear. Latex gloves are thin, which allows the health care worker better feel, dexterity, and grip, and they are lower in cost than most nonlatex gloves. In addition, latex has been in use for more than 100 years and has proven barrier protective capability, whereas the barrier effectiveness of nonlatex gloves is not as well established at this time. The primary disadvantage of latex gloves is that they can cause an allergic reaction in individuals with a hypersensitivity to latex.

Latex Glove Allergy

The primary substance causing a latex glove allergy is a protein present within the latex that enters the body through direct contact or through inhalation. When latex gloves are donned by an allergic individual, the protein comes in direct contact with the skin. The protein is absorbed into the skin, which then triggers an allergic reaction known as a *latex hypersensitivity reaction*. The allergic reaction may range from mild to severe. A mild allergic reaction causes the following symptoms: redness of the skin, urticaria (hives), and itching (Figure 17-3). A more severe allergic reaction causes sneezing, itchy red eyes, runny nose, and asthma symptoms (shortness of breath, coughing, and wheezing). Symptoms typically begin within minutes after contact with the latex.

The National Institute for Occupational Safety and Health (NIOSH) has issued the following recommendations to help prevent the development of latex allergies in the workplace:

1. Use nonlatex gloves for tasks that are not likely to involve contact with infectious materials (e.g., use nonlatex gloves to perform an ear irrigation for the removal of cerumen). Because of their proven barrier protective capability, latex gloves are recommended for tasks that are likely to involve contact with infectious materials.
2. Appropriate barrier protection is necessary when handling infectious materials. If you choose latex gloves, use powder-free gloves with a reduced protein content.
3. Use appropriate work practices to reduce the chance of a reaction to latex:
   - After removing latex gloves, wash hands with a mild soap and dry thoroughly.
4. Use good housekeeping practices to remove latex-containing dust from the workplace:

Figure 17-3 Latex glove allergy. (From Goodman CC: Pathology: implications for the physical therapist, ed 3, St Louis, 2010, Saunders.)

PROCEDURE 17-1

- Frequently clean areas contaminated with latex dust (e.g., upholstery, carpets, and ventilation ducts).
- Frequently change ventilation filters and vacuum bags used in latex-contaminated areas.
5. Take advantage of any latex allergy education and training provided by your employer:
  - Become familiar with procedures for preventing latex allergy.
  - Learn to recognize the symptoms of latex allergy.

Glove Guidelines

The medical assistant should adhere to the following glove guidelines:

1. Keep fingernails trimmed short (less than $\frac{1}{4}$ inch long) to reduce the risk of tearing the gloves during application and use.
2. Wear the correct size glove. Gloves that are too small may rip as they are applied or may become uncomfortable to wear. Gloves that are too large may make it difficult to perform tasks.
3. Do not use oil-based hand lotions or creams because they can damage and deteriorate NRL gloves.
4. Do not store gloves in areas where there are extremes in temperatures (e.g., near a heater or air conditioner). These conditions can cause deterioration of the gloves.

PROCEDURE 17-1   Handwashing

Outcome Perform handwashing

Equipment/Supplies

- Liquid soap
- Paper towels
- Waste container

1. **Procedural Step.** Remove your watch or push it up on the forearm so that the wrist is clear. Avoid wearing rings. If you wear rings, remove all except a plain wedding band and put them in a safe place.
   Principle. Microorganisms can lodge in the crevices and grooves of rings.
2. **Procedural Step.** Stand at the sink, making sure clothing does not touch the sink.
   Principle. The sink is considered contaminated, and if the uniform touches the sink, it may pick up microorganisms and transfer them.
3. **Procedural Step.** Turn on the faucets, using a paper towel.
   Principle. The faucets are considered contaminated because they harbor microorganisms.

Turn on the faucet using a paper towel.

4. **Procedural Step.** Adjust the water temperature. The water should be warm to make the best suds.
   Principle. Water that is too hot or too cold tends to dry the skin, causing chapping and cracking and making it easy for pathogens to enter the body or be transferred to patients.
5. **Procedural Step.** Discard the paper towel in the waste container.
   Principle. The paper towel is considered contaminated after touching the faucets.
6. **Procedural Step.** Wet the hands and forearms thoroughly with water. The hands should be held lower than the elbows at all times. Do not touch the inside of the sink because it is also contaminated.
   Principle. When you hold the hands lower than the elbows, bacteria and debris are carried away from the arms and body and into the sink.
7. **Procedural Step.** Apply soap to the hands. Apply 1 teaspoon of liquid soap (approximately the size of a nickel) to the palm of one hand.

Apply soap to the hands.

8. Procedural Step. Wash the palms and backs of the hands with 10 circular motions. Use friction along with the circular motions to wash the palm and back of each hand.
Principle. Friction helps to dislodge and remove microorganisms from the hands.

Wash the palms and backs of the hands.

9. Procedural Step. Wash the fingers with 10 circular motions while focusing on the fingertips and fingernails. Interlace the fingers and thumbs, and use friction and circular motions while rubbing the fingers back and forth.

Principle. This kind of movement helps remove microorganisms and debris that have accumulated between the fingers.

Interlace the fingers and thumbs, and use friction.

10. Procedural Step. Rinse well, making sure to hold the hands lower than the elbows.
Principle. Running water helps to rinse away dirt and microorganisms.

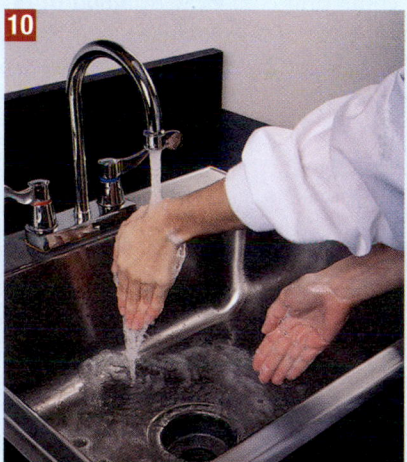

Rinse well, holding the hands lower than the elbows.

11. Procedural Step. Wash the wrists and forearms, using friction along with circular motions.
(*Note:* The hands are washed first because they are the most contaminated; microorganisms and dirt are washed away and do not spread to the wrists and forearms.)

Continued

PROCEDURE 17-1

PROCEDURE 17-2

PROCEDURE 17-1   Handwashing—cont'd

Wash wrists and forearms using friction.

12. **Procedural Step.** Clean the fingernails with a manicure stick. The fingernails should be cleaned at least once daily, preferably during initial handwashing (i.e., handwashing performed just after arriving at the medical office to begin your day). *Principle.* Dirt and microorganisms collect underneath the fingernails.

13. **Procedural Step.** Rinse the arms and hands. *Principle.* The running water rinses away the dirt and microorganisms.

14. **Procedural Step.** Repeat the handwashing procedure. For initial handwashing or when the hands come into contact with blood or other potentially infectious materials, the handwashing procedure should be repeated to ensure removal of all pathogens.

15. **Procedural Step.** Dry the hands gently and thoroughly, and discard the paper towel. *Principle.* Gently drying the hands prevents them from becoming chapped. Microorganisms can lodge in the crevices of chapped hands. Ensure that the hands are dried completely, because wet skin also may cause chapping.

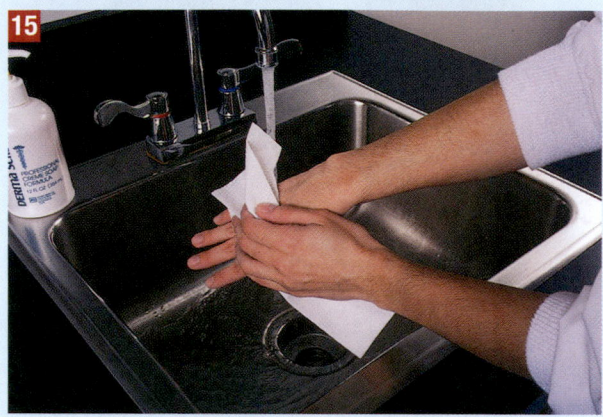

Dry the hands gently and thoroughly.

16. **Procedural Step.** Turn off the water, using a paper towel, and discard the paper towel in a waste container. *Principle.* The faucet is considered contaminated, whereas the hands are medically aseptic or clean.

17. **Procedural Step.** Do not touch the sink with the bare hands. *Principle.* The hands are now medically aseptic, and the sink is considered contaminated.

PROCEDURE 17-2   Applying an Alcohol-Based Hand Rub

Outcome   Apply an alcohol-based hand rub

Equipment/Supplies

• Alcohol-based hand rub

1. **Procedural Step.** Inspect the hands to ensure that they are not visibly soiled. Hands that are visibly soiled must be washed with soap and water. *Principle.* Alcohol-based hand rubs are not intended for the removal of visible soil.

2. **Procedural Step.** Remove your watch or push it up on the forearm. Avoid wearing rings. If you wear rings, remove all except a plain wedding band and put them in a safe place.

Principle. Microorganisms can lodge in the crevices and grooves of rings.

3. **Procedural Step.** Apply the alcohol-based hand rub to the palm of one hand as follows: *Gel or lotion.* Apply approximately 1 mL of the gel or lotion to the palm of one hand; this amount is approximately equal to the size of a dime.

PROCEDURE 17-2   **Applying an Alcohol-Based Hand Rub—cont'd**

Apply lotion or gel equal to the size of a dime.

Foam. Apply 3 grams of foam to the palm of one hand; this amount is approximately equal to the size of a walnut.

Principle. The proper amount of hand rub must be applied to ensure coverage of all surfaces of both hands. Using more than the recommended amount results in a prolonged (and unnecessary) period of time for your hands to dry.

Apply foam equal to the size of a walnut.

4. Procedural Step. Thoroughly spread the hand rub over all surfaces of both hands (and fingers) up to ½ inch above the wrist. Spread the hand rub around the fingertips and around and under your fingernails.

Principle. Failure to cover all surfaces can leave areas of the hands contaminated. Microorganisms tend to collect around and underneath the fingernails.

5. Procedural Step. Rub the hands together until they are dry; this usually takes up to 30 seconds. Allow your hands to dry completely before touching anything. The hands are now medically aseptic. *Note:* After cleaning your hands 5 to 10 times with a hand rub, a buildup of emollients may occur on your hands. The emollients can be easily removed by washing your hands with soap and water.

Principle. If you have applied a sufficient amount of hand rub, it should take up to to 30 seconds for your hands to feel dry. Your hands will still feel a little wet at first. Let them dry completely before touching anything.

PROCEDURE 17-2

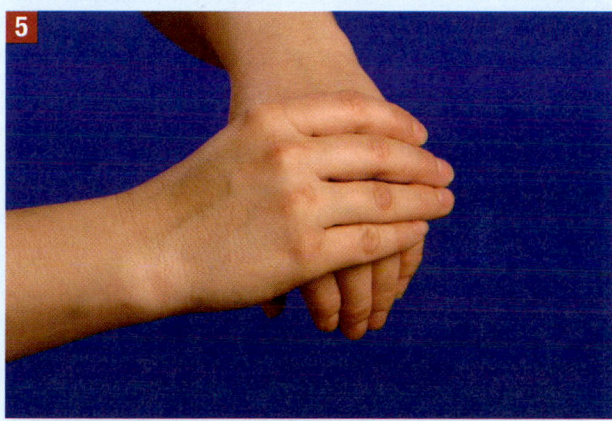

Rub the hands together until they are dry.

PROCEDURE 17-3   Application and Removal of Clean Disposable Gloves

Outcome Apply and remove clean disposable gloves

Equipment/Supplies

- Clean disposable gloves

Applying Clean Disposable Gloves

No special technique is required when clean disposable gloves are applied. This is because the hands are clean and the gloves are clean; the medical assistant can touch any part of the gloves during application without contaminating them.

1. **Procedural Step.** Remove all rings, and sanitize your hands. Handwashing should be performed if the hands are visibly soiled. If this is not the case, use an alcohol-based hand rub to sanitize the hands. Ensure that your hands are completely dry.
   Principle. Rings may cause the gloves to tear. The warm, moist environment inside gloves provides ideal growing conditions for the multiplication of transient microorganisms present on the hands. Sanitizing the hands removes these microorganisms and prevents the transmission of pathogens. Moisture encourages the growth of microorganisms.
2. **Procedural Step.** Choose the appropriate size of gloves; they should not be too small or too large. The gloves should fit snugly but not be too tight. Apply the gloves, and adjust them so they fit comfortably.
   Principle. If your gloves are too small, they may rip as you are applying them or may become uncomfortable to wear. If they are too large, you may find it difficult to perform your tasks.

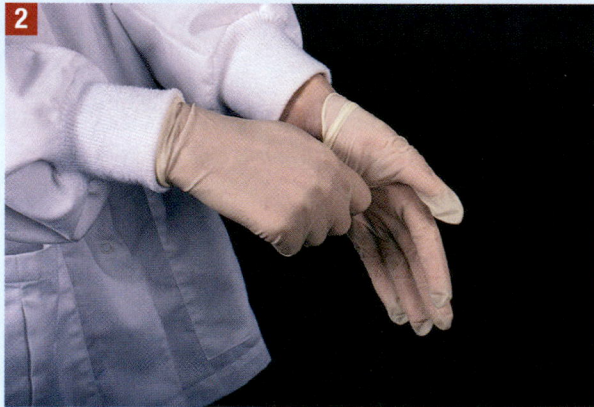

Apply the gloves.

3. **Procedural Step.** Inspect the gloves for tears. If a tear is present, remove the torn glove and apply a new one.

Removing Clean Disposable Gloves

Gloves must be removed in a manner that protects the medical assistant from contaminating his or her clean hands with pathogens that may be present on the outsides of the gloves. This is accomplished by not allowing the bare hands to come in contact with the outsides of the gloves.

1. **Procedural Step.** Grasp the outside of the left glove 1 to 2 inches from the top with your gloved right hand. (*Note:* It does not matter which glove is removed first. You may start with the right glove if you prefer.)

Grasp the glove 1 to 2 inches from the top of the glove.

2. **Procedural Step.** Slowly pull the left glove off the hand. It will turn inside out as it is removed from your hand.
3. **Procedural Step.** Pull the left glove free, and scrunch it into a ball with your gloved right hand.

Scrunch the glove into a ball.

PROCEDURE 17-3   Application and Removal of Clean Disposable Gloves—cont'd

4. Procedural Step. Place the index and middle fingers of the left hand on the inside of the right glove. Do not allow your clean hand to touch the outside of the glove.

Place the index and middle fingers inside the glove.

5. Procedural Step. Pull the glove off the right hand. It will turn inside out as it is removed from your hand, enclosing the balled-up left glove. Discard both gloves in an appropriate container. If your gloves are visibly contaminated with blood or other potentially infectious materials, discard them in a biohazard waste container. Otherwise, they can be discarded in a regular waste container.

Discard both gloves in an appropriate container.

6. Procedural Step. Sanitize your hands to remove any microorganisms or other contaminants that may have come in contact with your hands during glove removal.

OSHA BLOODBORNE PATHOGENS STANDARD

PURPOSE OF THE STANDARD

The federal government established OSHA (Occupational Safety and Health Administration) to assist employers in providing a safe and healthy working environment for their employees. To provide a safe working environment for health care workers, OSHA developed a comprehensive set of regulations known as the *OSHA Occupational Exposure to Bloodborne Pathogens Standard.*

These regulations went into effect in 1992 and are designed to reduce the risk to employees of exposure to infectious diseases.

The OSHA Bloodborne Pathogens Standard must be followed by any employee with occupational exposure to pathogens, regardless of the place of employment. In addition to medical assistants, employees with occupational exposure include physicians, nurses, dentists, dental hygienists, medical laboratory personnel, and emergency medical technicians. Employees who may have less obvious occupational exposure are correctional and law enforcement officers, firefighters, hospital laundry workers, morticians, and custodians.

Failure by employers to comply with the OSHA standard could result in a citation carrying a maximum penalty of $7000 for each violation and a maximum penalty of $70,000 for repeat violations.

NEEDLESTICK SAFETY AND PREVENTION ACT

Since the adoption of the OSHA Bloodborne Pathogens Standard, needlestick injuries among health care workers have continued to be a problem because of their high frequency of occurrence and the severity of the health effects associated with exposure to bloodborne pathogens. To address this problem, Congress passed the Needlestick Safety and Prevention Act (NSPA). The NSPA directed OSHA to revise the Bloodborne Pathogens Standard to incorporate stronger measures to reduce needlesticks and

What Would You Do? What Would You *Not* Do?

Case Study 1

Petra Meyer has come in for her annual gynecologic examination. Because Petra has been feeling tired and run-down, the physician orders blood to be drawn for a complete blood count (CBC) and a comprehensive blood chemistry profile. Petra indicates that she wears rubber latex gloves when house-cleaning to protect her hands from the chemicals in her cleaning solution. Petra says that the last two times she cleaned her house, she experienced redness and itching of her hands along with a runny nose and red itchy eyes. She wants to know if this might be caused by breathing in the cleaning solution or getting some of it on her hands after taking off her gloves. Petra says she also experienced redness and itching of her feet the last time she wore her rubber flip flops. ■

other sharps injuries among health care workers. In response to this mandate, the primary measure instituted by OSHA was to establish detailed requirements that employers identify and make use of safer medical devices. This revised OSHA Bloodborne Pathogens Standard went into effect in 2001 and is described in detail in this chapter.

OSHA TERMINOLOGY

The following definitions help clarify terms related to the OSHA Bloodborne Pathogens Standard.

Occupational exposure: Occupational exposure is reasonably anticipated skin, eye, mucous membrane, or parenteral contact with blood or other potentially infectious materials (OPIM) that may result from the performance of an employee's duties.

Sharps: Sharps are objects that can penetrate the skin, including (but not limited to) needles, lancets, scalpels, broken glass, and glass capillary tubes.

Parenteral: Parenteral refers to the piercing of the skin barrier or mucous membranes, such as through needlesticks, human bites, cuts, and abrasions.

Blood: Blood means human blood, human blood components, and products made from blood. Blood components include plasma, serum, platelets, and serosanguineous fluid (e.g., exudates from wounds). An example of a blood product is a medication derived from blood, such as immune globulins.

Bloodborne pathogens: Bloodborne pathogens are pathogenic microorganisms in human blood that can cause disease in humans. Bloodborne pathogens include, but are not limited to, hepatitis B virus (HBV), hepatitis C virus (HCV), and human immunodeficiency virus (HIV).

Other potentially infectious materials: OPIM include the following:
- Semen and vaginal secretions
- Cerebrospinal, synovial, pleural, pericardial, peritoneal, and amniotic fluids
- Any body fluid that is visibly contaminated with blood
- Any body fluid that has not been identified
- Saliva in dental procedures
- Any unfixed human tissue
- Any tissue culture, cells, or fluid known to be HIV infected

Contaminated: Contaminated is defined as the presence or reasonably anticipated presence of blood or OPIM on an item or surface.

Decontamination: Decontamination is the use of physical or chemical means to remove, inactivate, or destroy pathogens on a surface or item to the point where they are no longer capable of transmitting infectious particles, and the surface or item is rendered safe for handling, use, or disposal.

Nonintact skin: Nonintact skin is skin that has a break in the surface. It includes, but is not limited to, skin with dermatitis, abrasions, cuts, burns, hangnails, chapping, and acne.

Exposure incident: An *exposure incident* is defined as a specific eye, nose, mouth, or other mucous membrane, nonintact skin, or parenteral contact with blood or OPIM that results from an employee's duties.

COMPONENTS OF THE OSHA STANDARD

The OSHA Bloodborne Pathogens Standard is presented on the following pages as it pertains to the medical office and includes the following categories:
- Exposure control plan
- Safer medical devices
- Labeling requirements
- Communication of hazards to employees
- Record keeping

Exposure Control Plan

The OSHA standard requires that the medical office develop an exposure control plan (ECP) (Figure 17-4). The ECP is a written document stipulating the protective measures that must be followed in that medical office to eliminate or minimize employee exposure to bloodborne pathogens and OPIM. The ECP must be made available for review by all medical office staff. The ECP must include the following elements:

1. *An exposure determination.* The purpose of this section of the ECP is to identify employees who must receive training, protective equipment, hepatitis vaccination, and other protections required by the OSHA Bloodborne Pathogens Standard. The exposure determination must include (1) a list of all job classifications in which *all* employees are likely to have occupational exposure, such as physicians, medical assistants, and laboratory technicians, and (2) a list of job classifications in which only *some* employees have occupational exposure, such as custodians. For the second classification of jobs, the

determination must include a list of tasks in which occupational exposure may occur, such as emptying the trash.

2. *The method of compliance.* The method of compliance section of the ECP must document the specific health and safety control measures that are taken in the medical office to eliminate or minimize the risk of occupational

Figure 17-4 Example of an exposure control plan.

exposure. These measures are extremely important in reducing the risk of infectious disease for the medical assistant and are discussed in greater detail later in this section (see Control Measures).

3. *Postexposure evaluation and follow-up procedures.* Postexposure evaluation and follow-up must specify the procedures to follow in the event of an exposure incident in the medical office, including the method of documenting and investigating an exposure incident and the postexposure evaluation, medical treatment, and follow-up that would be made available to the employee. (Refer to the OSHA Postexposure Evaluation and Follow-up Procedures box.)

OSHA requires employers to review and update their ECP at least annually to ensure that the plan remains current with the latest information on eliminating or reducing exposure to bloodborne pathogens. The ECP also must be updated whenever necessary to reflect new or modified tasks and procedures that affect occupational exposure.

Labeling Requirements

The OSHA Bloodborne Pathogens Standard requires that containers and appliances containing biohazardous materials be labeled with a *biohazard warning label*. The biohazard warning label must be fluorescent orange or orange-red and must contain the biohazard symbol and the word *BIOHAZARD* in a contrasting color (Figure 17-5, *A*).

A warning label must be attached to the following: (1) containers of regulated waste; (2) refrigerators and freezers

OSHA Postexposure Evaluation and Follow-up Procedures

An exposure incident is a specific eye, nose, mouth, or other mucous membrane, nonintact skin, or parenteral contact with blood or other potentially infectious materials that results from an employee's duties. In the event of an exposure incident involving bloodborne pathogens or other potentially infectious materials (OPIM), OSHA requires the following steps to be performed:

1. Perform initial first aid measures immediately (e.g., wash a needlestick injury thoroughly with soap and water).
2. Document the route of exposure and the conditions and circumstances of the exposure incident. This includes such information as the engineering controls, the work practice controls, and personal protective equipment being used at the time of the incident.
3. Identify and document the source individual (unless the employer can establish that identification is not feasible or is prohibited by state or local law). A source individual is any person, living or dead, whose blood or OPIM may be a source of occupational exposure to the health care worker.
4. Obtain consent to test the source individual's blood. Test it as soon as possible to determine hepatitis B virus (HBV), hepatitis C virus (HCV), and human immunodeficiency virus (HIV) infectivity. The following guidelines apply to this requirement:

- If consent is not obtained, the employer must document that legally required consent cannot be obtained.
- If the source individual's consent is not required by law, the source individual's blood (if available) must be tested and the results documented.
- If the source individual is already known to be infected with HBV, HCV, or HIV, testing does not need to be repeated.

5. Provide the exposed employee with the source individual's test results. Inform the employee of applicable laws and regulations concerning disclosure of the identity and infectious status of the source individual.
6. Obtain consent to test the employee's blood. Collect and test the blood of the employee as soon as possible for HBV, HCV, and HIV serologic status. If the employee does not give consent for HIV serologic testing, the baseline blood sample must be preserved for at least 90 days. If the employee elects to have the baseline sample tested during the 90-day waiting period, such testing must be done as soon as feasible.
7. When medically indicated, provide the employee with appropriate postexposure prophylaxis, as recommended by the U.S. Public Health Service.

Figure 17-5 A, Biohazard warning label. **B,** Biohazard bag used to hold and transport blood or other potentially infectious materials.

used to store blood and OPIM; and (3) containers and bags used to store, transport, or ship blood or OPIM (Figure 17-5, *B*). Red bags or red containers may be substituted for biohazard warning labels. The labeling requirement is designed to alert employees to possible exposure, particularly in situations in which the nature of the material or contents is not readily identifiable as blood or OPIM.

Communicating Hazards to Employees

According to the OSHA standard, employers must ensure that all medical office employees with risk of occupational exposure participate in a training program. This program must present the ECP for the medical office while focusing on the measures that employees are to take for their safety. Training must be provided at the time an employee is

initially assigned to tasks in which occupational exposure may occur and at least annually thereafter.

The employer must maintain records of the training sessions, which must include presentation dates, content of the sessions, names and qualifications of the trainers, and names and job titles of employees who attended. These records must be maintained for 3 years from the date of the training session.

Record Keeping

The OSHA Bloodborne Pathogens Standard requires that the following records be maintained:

1. *OSHA medical record.* The OSHA standard requires that the employer maintain an accurate OSHA record of every medical office employee at risk for occupational exposure. These records must be kept confidential except for review by OSHA officials and as required by law. The record must include the following: employee's name; social security number; hepatitis B vaccination status, including dates of vaccination; results of any postexposure examinations, medical testing, and follow-up procedures; and a written evaluation of any exposure incident along with a copy of the exposure incident report. The employer is required to maintain records for the duration of employment plus 30 years.

2. *Sharps injury log.* Employers with more than 10 employees at risk for occupational exposure are required to maintain a log of injuries from contaminated sharps. The log must be maintained in a way that protects the confidentiality of injured employees (e.g., removal of personal identification). The purpose of the log is to help employers and employees keep track of all needlestick injuries. This tracking helps in identifying problem areas that need attention and ineffective devices that need to be replaced. The sharps injury log must contain the following information:
   - Type and brand of device involved in the injury
   - Location of the incident (i.e., work area)
   - Explanation of how the incident occurred

CONTROL MEASURES

Specific health and safety control measures are required by OSHA to eliminate or minimize the risk of occupational exposure in the medical office. These measures are divided into six categories: engineering controls, work practice controls, personal protective equipment, housekeeping, hepatitis B vaccination, and universal precautions.

Engineering Controls

The medical office must use engineering controls to eliminate or minimize the risk of occupational exposure. *Engineering controls* include all measures and devices that isolate or remove the bloodborne pathogens hazard from the workplace. Engineering controls must be examined and maintained or replaced as required to ensure their effectiveness. Examples of engineering controls include the following:

Figure 17-6 **A** and **B,** Safety-engineered syringes. **C,** Safety-engineered phlebotomy device.

- Readily accessible handwashing facilities
- Safer medical devices
- Biohazard sharps containers and biohazard bags
- Autoclaves

Safer Medical Devices

Safer medical devices are one example of an engineering control. A *safer medical device* is a device that, based on reasonable judgment, would make an exposure incident involving a contaminated sharp less likely. *Reasonable judgment* refers to the judgment of the health care worker who would be using the device.

Safer medical devices include sharps with engineered sharps injury protection and needleless systems. A *sharp with engineered sharps injury protection (SESIP)* is a non-needle sharp or a needle device with a built-in safety feature used for procedures that involve the risk of sharps injury. Examples of SESIPs include safety-engineered syringes and phlebotomy devices (Figure 17-6).

A *needleless system* is a device that does not use a needle for (1) the administration of medication or other fluids, (2) the collection or withdrawal of body fluids after initial access to a vein or artery has been established, or (3) any other procedure involving the potential for occupational exposure to bloodborne pathogens as a result of percutaneous injuries from contaminated sharps. An example of a needleless system is a jet injection syringe, which uses compressed air rather than a needle to administer an injection.

Employers are required to evaluate and implement commercially available safer medical devices and other engineering controls that eliminate occupational exposure to the lowest extent feasible. Input from employees involved in direct patient care must be taken into consideration in making this determination. This helps to ensure that the individuals who are using the devices have the opportunity

for input. As part of the annual review of the ECP, the following information must be documented: (1) safer medical devices that reflect changes in technology are being evaluated and implemented in the workplace, and (2) input was obtained from employees in selecting safer medical devices.

Work Practice Controls

Work practice controls reduce the likelihood of exposure by altering the manner in which the technique is performed. It is important that the medical assistant consistently adhere to these safety rules, which include the following:

1. Perform all procedures involving blood or OPIM in a manner that minimizes splashing, spraying, spattering, and generation of droplets of these substances.
2. Observe warning labels on biohazard containers and appliances. Bags or containers that bear a biohazard warning label or are color-coded red indicate that they hold blood or OPIM. Refrigerators, freezers, and other appliances that contain hazardous materials also must bear a biohazard warning label.
3. Bandage cuts and other lesions on the hands before gloving.
4. Sanitize the hands after removing gloves, regardless of whether or not the gloves are visibly contaminated.
5. If your hands or other skin surfaces come in contact with blood or OPIM, thoroughly wash the area as soon as possible with soap and water.
6. If your mucous membranes (e.g., eyes, mouth, nose) come in contact with blood or OPIM, flush them with water as soon as possible.
7. Do not break or shear contaminated needles.
8. Do not remove, recap, or bend a contaminated needle except in unusual circumstances when no other alternative is possible, or when this is required by a specific medical procedure. Such actions must be performed by

a method other than the traditional two-handed procedure. Needle removal can be accomplished with a one-handed technique using a sharps container with a well-designed unwinder. Recapping must be performed through the use of a one-handed technique; using a two-handed technique is strictly prohibited. The one-handed recapping technique involves holding the syringe in the dominant hand and picking up the needle with the cap, using a scooping motion. The cap is secured onto the needle by pushing it against a hard surface. (*Note:* Sterile needles may be recapped, such as after the withdrawal of medication from a vial or ampule.)

9. Immediately after use, place contaminated sharps in a puncture-resistant, leakproof container that is appropriately labeled or color-coded. *Contaminated sharps* are contaminated objects that can penetrate the skin, including (but not limited to) needles, lancets, scalpels, broken glass, and capillary tubes.

10. Do not eat, drink, smoke, apply cosmetics or lip balm, or handle contact lenses in areas where you may be exposed to blood or OPIM.

11. Do not store food or drinks in refrigerators, freezers, or cabinets or on shelves or countertops where blood or OPIM are present.

12. Place blood specimens or OPIM in containers that prevent leakage during collection, handling, processing, storage, transport, or shipping. Ensure that the containers are closed before they are stored, transported, or shipped, and are labeled or color-coded for easy identification.

13. Before any equipment that might be contaminated is serviced or shipped for repair or cleaning, such as a centrifuge, it must be inspected for blood or OPIM. If such material is present, the equipment must be decontaminated. If it cannot be decontaminated, it must be appropriately labeled to indicate clearly the contamination site, to enable those coming into contact with the equipment to take appropriate precautions.

14. If you are exposed to blood or OPIM, perform first aid measures immediately (e.g., wash a needlestick injury thoroughly with soap and water). After taking these measures, report the incident to your physician-employer as soon as possible so that postexposure procedures can be instituted. (See the box entitled OSHA Postexposure Evaluation and Follow-up Procedures.) The most obvious exposure incident is a needlestick, but any eye, mouth, or other mucous membrane, nonintact skin, or parenteral contact with blood or OPIM constitutes an exposure incident and should be reported.

Personal Protective Equipment

The OSHA standard specifies that personal protective equipment must be used in the medical office whenever occupational exposure remains after engineering and work practice controls have been instituted. *Personal protective equipment* is clothing or equipment that protects an individual from

Figure 17-7 Jennifer wears a combination mask and eye-protection device and a laboratory coat to protect against splashes, spray, spatter, and droplets of blood.

contact with blood or OPIM; examples include gloves, chin-length face shields, masks, protective eyewear, laboratory coats, and gowns. The type of protective equipment appropriate for a given task depends on the degree of exposure that is anticipated, as outlined here:

1. Wear gloves when it is reasonably anticipated that your hands will have contact with blood and OPIM, mucous membranes, or nonintact skin; when performing vascular access procedures; and when handling or touching contaminated surfaces or items. Gloves cannot prevent a needlestick or other sharps injury, but they can prevent a pathogen from entering the body through a break in the skin, such as a cut, abrasion, burn, or rash.

2. Wear chin-length face shields or masks in combination with eye-protection devices whenever splashes, spray, spatter, or droplets of blood or OPIM may be generated, posing a hazard through contact with the eyes, nose, or mouth (e.g., removing a stopper from a tube of blood, transferring serum from whole blood) (Figure 17-7).

3. Wear appropriate protective clothing, such as gowns, aprons, and laboratory coats, when gross contamination can reasonably be anticipated during performance of a task or procedure (e.g., laboratory testing procedure). The type of protective clothing needed depends on the task and degree of exposure anticipated.

Personal Protective Equipment Guidelines

Certain guidelines must be followed when using protective equipment:

1. Protective equipment must not allow blood or OPIM to pass through or reach the skin, underlying garments (e.g., scrubs, street clothes, undergarments), eyes, mouth, or other mucous membranes under normal conditions of use and for the duration of time the protective equipment is used.

2. The employer must provide appropriate personal protective equipment at no cost to you. The employer is

Figure 17-8 Examples of eye-protection devices. *Left,* Face shield; *center,* goggles; *right,* glasses with solid side shields.

Figure 17-9 Clean and decontaminate work surfaces with an appropriate disinfectant after completing procedures involving blood and other potentially infectious materials.

responsible for ensuring that the equipment is available in appropriate sizes, is readily accessible, and is used correctly. In addition, the employer must ensure that the equipment is cleaned, laundered, repaired, replaced, or disposed of as necessary to ensure its effectiveness.

3. Alternatives must be provided for employees who are allergic to latex gloves. Examples of alternatives include nonlatex gloves and powderless gloves.
4. If gloves become contaminated, torn, or punctured, replace them as soon as practical.
5. All eye-protection devices must have solid side shields; chin-length face shields, goggles, and glasses with solid side shields are acceptable (Figure 17-8); standard prescription eyeglasses are unacceptable as eye protection.
6. If a garment is penetrated by blood or OPIM, it must be removed as soon as possible and placed in an appropriately designated container for washing.
7. All personal protective equipment must be removed before you leave the medical office.
8. When protective equipment is removed, it must be placed in an appropriately designated area or container for storage, washing, decontamination, or disposal.
9. Utility gloves may be decontaminated and reused unless they are cracked, peeling, torn, or punctured or no longer provide barrier protection.
10. If you believe that using protective equipment would prevent proper delivery of health care or would pose an increased hazard to your safety or that of a coworker, in extenuating circumstances you may temporarily and briefly decline its use. After such an incident, the circumstances must be investigated to determine whether the situation could be prevented in the future.

Housekeeping

The OSHA standard requires that specific housekeeping procedures be followed to ensure that the work site is maintained in a clean and sanitary condition. The medical office must develop and implement a written schedule for cleaning and decontaminating each area where exposure occurs. The cleaning and decontamination method must be specified for each task and should be based on the type of surface to be cleaned, the type of soil present, and the tasks or procedures being performed in that area. Housekeeping procedures include the following:

1. Clean and decontaminate equipment and work surfaces after completing procedures that involve blood or OPIM. Cleaning is accomplished using plain soap, and decontamination is performed using an appropriate disinfectant (Figure 17-9).
2. Clean and decontaminate all equipment and work surfaces as soon as possible after exposure to blood or OPIM. For decontamination of blood spills, OSHA recommends the use of a 10% solution of sodium hypochlorite (household bleach) in water (1 part bleach to 9 parts water).
3. Inspect and decontaminate all reusable receptacles, such as bins, pails, and cans, on a regular basis. If contamination is visible, the item must be cleaned and decontaminated as soon as possible.
4. Do not pick up broken, contaminated glassware with the hands, even if gloves are worn. Use mechanical means, such as a brush and dustpan, tongs, and forceps (Figure 17-10).
5. Protective coverings, such as plastic wrap and aluminum foil, may be used to cover work surfaces or equipment, but they must be removed or replaced if contamination occurs.
6. Handle contaminated laundry as little as possible and with appropriate personal protective equipment. Place all contaminated laundry in leakproof bags that are properly labeled or color-coded. Contaminated laundry must not be sorted or rinsed at the medical office.
7. If the outside of a biohazard container becomes contaminated, it must be placed in a second suitable container.
8. Biohazard sharps containers (Figure 17-11) must be closable, puncture resistant, and leakproof. They must bear

What Would You Do? What Would You *Not* Do?

Case Study 2

Tracy Smith is pregnant and is at the medical office to have her blood drawn for a prenatal profile. Tracy says she has been reading information about the hepatitis B vaccine because she knows her baby will be given this vaccine soon after birth. She wants to know why it is recommended that an infant be immunized for hepatitis B. Tracy says that infants are not at risk for contracting hepatitis B because the way it is transmitted is mostly through sexual contact and illegal drug use. ∎

HIGHLIGHT on OSHA Bloodborne Pathogens Standard

General Information

The exposure control plan must be made available to OSHA on request.

OSHA inspectors are responsible for determining whether the medical office meets the Bloodborne Pathogens Standard. This is accomplished through careful review of the exposure control plan, interviews with the medical office employer and employees, and observation of work activities.

Feces, nasal secretions, saliva, sputum, sweat, tears, urine, and vomitus are not considered by OSHA to be potentially infectious materials unless they contain blood.

Control Measures

Employees must be trained in proper use of the following: engineering controls (including safer medical devices), work practice controls, and personal protective equipment.

General work clothes, such as scrubs, uniforms, pants, shirts, and blouses, are not intended to function as protection against a hazard and are not considered personal protective equipment.

Employees are not permitted to launder contaminated clothing at home; it is the employer's responsibility to have contaminated clothing laundered.

If an employee is allergic to standard latex gloves, the employer must provide a suitable nonlatex alternative.

Needlestick Injuries

The CDC estimates that every year, 600,000 to 800,000 health care workers in the United States experience needlestick and other sharps injuries, and 1000 of these individuals contract serious infections as a result of these injuries. The CDC estimates that 62% to 88% of sharps injuries can be prevented by the use of safer medical devices.

A wide variety of commercially available safer medical devices has been developed to reduce the risk of needlestick and other sharps injuries.

Safer medical devices that eliminate exposure to the lowest extent feasible must be evaluated and implemented in the health care setting. Lack of injuries on the sharps injury log does *not* exempt the employer from this provision. ∎

---

a biohazard warning label and must be color-coded red to ensure identification of the contents as hazardous. To ensure effectiveness, the following guidelines must be observed:

- Locate the sharps container as close as possible to the area of use to avoid the hazard of transporting a contaminated needle through the workplace.
- Maintain sharps containers in an upright position to keep liquid and sharps inside.
- Do not reach into the sharps container with your hand.
- Replace sharps containers on a regular basis, and do not allow them to overfill. (It is recommended that sharps containers be replaced when they are three-quarters full.)

Hepatitis B Vaccination

The OSHA standard requires employers to offer the hepatitis B vaccination series free of charge to all medical office personnel who have occupational exposure. The vaccination must be offered within 10 working days of initial assignment to a position with occupational exposure, unless the following factors exist: (1) the individual has previously received the hepatitis B vaccination series, (2) antibody testing has revealed that the individual is immune to

Figure 17-10 Use mechanical means to pick up broken contaminated glass.

hepatitis B, or (3) the vaccine is contraindicated for medical reasons.

Medical office personnel who decline vaccination must sign a hepatitis B waiver form documenting refusal. This form must be filed in the employee's OSHA record

(Figure 17-12). Employees who decline vaccination may request the vaccination later; the employer must then provide it, according to the aforementioned criteria.

Universal Precautions

Before the release of the OSHA standard, the CDC issued recommendations for health care workers known as the *Universal Precautions.* According to the concept of Universal Precautions, all human blood and certain human body fluids are treated as though they are known to be infectious for HIV, HBV, HCV, and other bloodborne pathogens. The OSHA standard states that the Universal Precautions must be observed; these precautions form the heart of the OSHA standard itself.

REGULATED MEDICAL WASTE

Medical waste is generated in the medical office through the diagnosis, treatment, and immunization of patients. Some of this waste poses a threat to health and safety and is known as **regulated medical waste** (RMW). The OSHA Bloodborne Pathogens Standard defines RMW as follows:

- Any liquid or semiliquid blood or OPIM
- Items contaminated with blood or OPIM that would release these substances in a liquid or semiliquid state if compressed
- Items that are caked with dried blood or OPIM and are capable of releasing these materials during handling
- Contaminated sharps
- Pathologic and microbiologic wastes that contain blood or OPIM

RMW must be discarded properly so as not to become a source of transfer of disease. According to the OSHA definition, a dressing saturated with blood is considered RMW and must be discarded in a biohazard bag. A bandage with a spot of blood on it is not considered RMW and can be discarded in a regular waste container. Box 17-2 gives the guidelines for discarding medical waste in the medical office.

Figure 17-11 Biohazard sharps container.

HEPATITIS B VACCINE REFUSAL

I understand that due to my occupational exposure to blood or other potentially infectious materials, I may be at risk of acquiring hepatitis B virus (HBV) infection. I have been given the opportunity to be vaccinated with hepatitis B vaccine at no charge to myself. However, I decline hepatitis B vaccination at this time. I understand that by declining this vaccine I continue to be at risk of acquiring hepatitis B, a serious disease. If in the future I continue to have occupational exposure to blood or to other potentially infectious materials and I want to be vaccinated with hepatitis B vaccine, I can receive the vaccination series at no charge to me.

_____
Employee Name (printed)

_____   _____
Employee Signature   Date

_____   _____
Witness Signature   Date

Figure 17-12 Hepatitis B declination form. This form must be signed by an employee with occupational exposure who declines hepatitis B vaccination.

HIGHLIGHT on Hepatitis B Vaccine

The hepatitis B vaccine became available in 1982 and is 95% effective in providing immunity. The hepatitis B vaccine is administered intramuscularly in a series of three doses. The hepatitis B vaccine is well tolerated by most patients. The most common side effect is soreness at the injection site, including induration, erythema, and swelling. Occasionally, a low-grade fever, headache, and dizziness occur.

Approximately 5% of the population does not form antibodies to the hepatitis B vaccine. Because of this, the CDC recommends that an antibody titer test be performed on all health care workers between 1 and 2 months after the last dose of the hepatitis B vaccine. The titer test is performed to determine if the health care worker has developed protective antibodies to hepatitis B and has immunity to hepatitis B virus (HBV) infection. Health care workers who do not respond to the primary vaccination series, as indicated by a negative titer test, must be revaccinated with a second three-dose vaccination series and then undergo a repeat titer test. If the titer test is still negative, this means that the health care worker probably lacks immunity to HBV infection.

Current data show that vaccine-induced antibodies may decline over time, but the immune system memory that programs the body to produce these antibodies remains intact indefinitely. Because of this, an individual with declining antibodies is still protected against hepatitis B. At present, the CDC does not recommend a booster dose once an individual has received the initial (three-dose) vaccine series.

The hepatitis B vaccine is recommended for all infants and children, and for adolescents who are 18 years old or younger. It also is recommended for adults older than 18 years who are at increased risk for developing hepatitis B. This population includes employees with occupational exposure (e.g., health care workers), hemodialysis patients, hemophiliacs, individuals with multiple sex partners, homosexually active men, injection drug users, individuals with HIV infection, household and sexual contacts of individuals infected with HBV, individuals with chronic liver or kidney disease, residents and staff in institutions for the developmentally disabled, and people who travel to countries where hepatitis B is common.

The number of individuals contracting hepatitis B has decreased sharply since the development of the hepatitis B vaccine. As more people become immune to hepatitis B through the immunization of infants, the goal of eliminating hepatitis B in the United States may be realized. ■

BOX 17-2 Guidelines for Discarding Medical Waste in the Medical Office

Regular Waste Container

The following items that have been used for health care *are not* considered regulated medical waste and can be discarded in a covered waste container lined with a regular trash bag.

- Disposable drapes
- Disposable patient gowns
- Examining table paper
- Disposable clean or sterile gloves
- Gauze tinged with blood or other body fluids
- Disposable probe covers for thermometers
- Tongue depressors
- Tissues with respiratory secretions
- Disposable ear speculums
- Empty urine containers
- Urine testing strips
- Disposable diapers
- Feminine hygiene products

Biohazard Sharps Container

The following items are sharps. They *are* considered regulated medical waste and must be discarded in a biohazard sharps container.

- Hypodermic syringes and needles
- Venipuncture needles
- Lancets
- Razor blades
- Scalpel blades
- Suture needles
- Blood tubes
- Capillary pipets
- Microscope slides and coverslips
- Broken glassware

Biohazard Bag Waste Container

The following items *are* considered regulated medical waste. They are not sharps and can be discarded in a covered waste container lined with a biohazard bag.

- Any item saturated or dripping with blood or other potentially infectious materials (OPIM) (e.g., dressings, gauze, cotton balls, paper towels, tissues that are saturated or dripping with blood)
- Any item caked with dried blood or OPIM, such as dressings and sutures
- Disposable clean or sterile gloves contaminated with blood or OPIM
- Disposable vaginal speculums and collection devices (e.g., swabs, spatulas, brushes)
- Tissue or fluid removed during minor office surgery
- Microbiologic waste, such as specimen cultures and collection devices
- Discarded live and attenuated vaccines

Sanitary Sewer

Disposal of small quantities of blood and other body fluids to the sanitary sewer is considered a safe method of disposing of these waste materials. The following fluids can be carefully poured down a utility sink, drain, or toilet. (*Note:* State regulations may dictate the maximum volume allowable for discharge of blood or body fluids into the sanitary sewer.)

- Blood
- Body excretions such as urine
- Body secretions such as sputum

HANDLING REGULATED MEDICAL WASTE

RMW must be handled carefully to prevent an exposure incident. The OSHA Bloodborne Pathogens Standard outlines specific actions to take when handling RMW, as follows:

1. Separate regulated waste from the general refuse at its point of origin. Disposable items containing RMW should be placed directly into biohazard containers and should not be mixed with the regular trash.
2. Ensure that biohazard containers are closable, leakproof, and suitably constructed to contain the contents during handling, storage, and transport. These containers include biohazard bags and sharps containers.
3. To prevent spillage or protrusion of the contents, close the lid of a sharps container before removing it from an examining room. Never open, empty, or clean a contaminated sharps container. If there is a chance of leakage from the sharps container, the medical assistant should place it in a second container that is closable, leakproof, and appropriately labeled or color-coded.
4. Securely close biohazard bags before removing them from an examining room. To provide additional protection, some medical offices double-bag by placing the primary bag inside a second biohazard bag.
5. Transport full biohazard containers to a secured area away from the general public, using personal protective equipment (e.g., gloves).

DISPOSAL OF REGULATED MEDICAL WASTE

Each state is responsible for developing policies for disposal of RMW. To avoid noncompliance, it is important for the medical assistant to know and understand the specific regulated waste policies and guidelines set forth in his or her state. Regulated waste policies and guidelines for each state can be found at the following website: www.envcap.org/statetools/rmw/rmwlocator.html.

Most medical offices use a commercial medical waste service to dispose of RMW. This service is responsible for picking up and transporting the medical waste to a treatment facility for incineration to destroy pathogens and render them harmless. The waste can then be safely disposed of in a sanitary landfill. Regulated waste treatment facilities must be licensed and hold permits issued by the Environmental Protection Agency (EPA), allowing them to dispose of RMW.

A series of steps must be followed for preparing and storing RMW for pickup by the service. Although these steps may vary slightly from state to state, general measures required by most states include the following:

1. Place biohazard bags and sharps containers into a receptacle provided by the medical waste service. The receptacle is usually a cardboard box (Figure 17-13). The box should be securely sealed with packing tape, and a biohazard warning label must appear on two opposite sides of the box.

Figure 17-13 Jennifer places a biohazard bag inside a cardboard box in preparation for pickup by the medical waste service.

2. Store the biohazard boxes in a locked room inside the facility or in a locked collection container outside for pickup by the medical waste service. This step is aimed at preventing unauthorized access to items such as needles and syringes. The regulated waste storage area should be labeled with one of the following:
   • "Authorized Personnel Only" sign
   • International biohazard symbol
3. Many states require that a tracking record be completed when the waste is picked up by the medical waste service. This form includes such information as the type and quantity of waste (weighed in pounds) and where it is being sent. The form must be signed by a representative of the medical waste service and the medical office. After the waste has been destroyed at the regulated waste treatment facility, a record documenting its disposal is mailed to the medical office.

What Would You Do? What Would You *Not* Do?

Case Study 3

Giles Lee is 55 years old and is at the medical office. Thirty years ago, he was in a serious car accident and had to have a blood transfusion. He says that he donated blood for the first time 2 months ago. Last week he received a letter saying that his blood tested positive for hepatitis C and that he should see his physician. Giles says that he must have gotten hepatitis C from the blood transfusion he received when he was 25. He does not understand how that could have happened because the blood supply is tested for these types of diseases. Giles wants to know why he has not had any symptoms. He also wants to know if he can give hepatitis C to his wife. ■

BLOODBORNE DISEASES

The biggest threats to health care workers from occupational exposure are HBV, HCV, and HIV. Hepatitis is much easier to transmit than HIV. After a needlestick exposure to blood infected with HBV, health care workers who are not immune to hepatitis B have a 6% to 30% chance of developing the disease. The risk of infection after a needlestick exposure to blood infected with HCV is approximately 2%. After a needlestick exposure to HIV-infected blood, a health care worker has a 0.3% chance of developing HIV; he or she has a 0.1% chance of developing HIV after a mucous membrane exposure of the eyes, nose, or mouth.

HEPATITIS B

Hepatitis B is an infection of the liver caused by HBV. The most common means of transmitting hepatitis B in the health care setting are blood and blood components, such as serum and plasma.

Health care workers are most likely to contract hepatitis B through needlesticks and cuts with contaminated sharps. The virus also is spread in the health care setting, but less effectively, through blood splashes to the eyes, mouth, and nonintact skin and through body fluids such as semen and vaginal secretions.

The number of health care workers who contract hepatitis B in the workplace has declined dramatically since the development of the OSHA standard and the hepatitis B vaccine. Statistics show that in 1983 there were more than 10,000 health care workers who contracted hepatitis B in the workplace, but by 2001, that number had decreased to fewer than 400 health care workers. Preventive treatment is available for individuals exposed to hepatitis B who have not been vaccinated.

Postexposure Prophylaxis

Postexposure prophylaxis (PEP) refers to treatment administered to an individual after exposure to an infectious disease, to prevent the disease. PEP for unvaccinated individuals exposed to hepatitis B involves the administration of a passive and an active immunizing agent. It is important to administer both of these agents as soon as possible after an exposure incident—preferably within 24 hours, but no later than 7 days.

The passive immunizing agent provides temporary immunity to hepatitis B, giving the active agent a chance to take effect. The passive agent is hepatitis B immune globulin (HBIG), which contains antibodies that provide immunity to hepatitis B for 1 to 3 months.

The active immunizing agent in the hepatitis B vaccine (Figure 17-14) is produced from genetically altered yeast cells; brand names are Recombivax HB and Engerix-B. The hepatitis B vaccine is administered intramuscularly in a series of three doses. The second dose is given 1 month after the first dose, and the third dose is administered 6 months

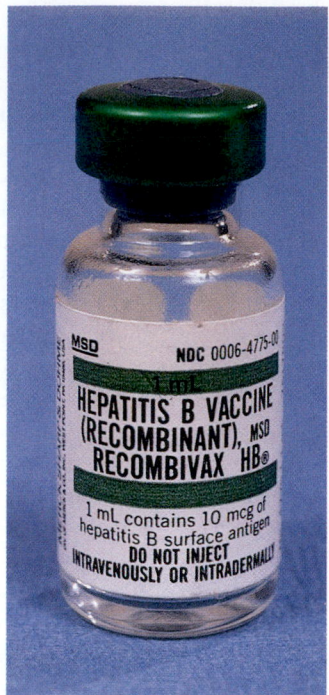

Figure 17-14 Hepatitis B vaccine.

after the first dose (i.e., 0, 1 month, and 6 months). Mild side effects, such as soreness at the injection site, may occur, but serious reactions to the vaccine are extremely rare.

As previously discussed, the OSHA standard recommends that all health care workers receive the hepatitis B vaccine (an active immunizing agent) as a preventive measure against hepatitis B. After an exposure incident, a medical assistant who has previously been vaccinated probably would not require further treatment.

HEPATITIS C

Hepatitis C is an infection of the liver caused by HCV. Currently, no vaccine is available for the prevention of hepatitis C. In the medical office the most likely means of contracting hepatitis C is through parenteral exposure to contaminated blood such as through needlesticks and other sharps injuries. The chance of contracting hepatitis C in the health care setting is much lower than that of contracting hepatitis B.

Most individuals with acute hepatitis C have no symptoms; if symptoms do occur, they are mild and flulike. Approximately 70% to 85% of individuals with acute hepatitis C develop chronic hepatitis C. After 10 to 30 years, about 20% of these individuals develop serious liver disease, including cirrhosis of the liver and cancer of the liver. Ultimately, 1% to 5% of individuals with chronic hepatitis C die from liver failure (see the Highlight on Viral Hepatitis box). Antiviral drugs have been developed to treat chronic hepatitis C and are effective in 40% of cases.

Memories *from* Practicum

Jennifer Hawk: As a student, I was extremely nervous to go out on practicum. I was so scared to think that I was actually going to be in a medical office setting and would have to put everything I had learned into practice. Would I remember everything? Would I do something wrong and hurt the patient? It was such an overwhelming feeling! But to my relief, I had a very good experience. The office staff was so friendly and helpful to me, and I surprised myself at how easily everything I had learned stayed with me. It was so exciting to see that I was actually functioning as a team member in the health care field. I could not have had better training. ■

HIGHLIGHT on Viral Hepatitis

In 2010 there were an estimated 72,000 new cases of viral hepatitis in the United States. Approximately 52% of these infections were caused by the hepatitis B virus, 24% were caused by the hepatitis A virus, and 24% were caused by the hepatitis C virus.

Symptoms common to all types of hepatitis include fatigue, nausea, loss of appetite, abdominal pain, and jaundice.

Hepatitis A, B, and C are designated by the CDC as nationally notifiable diseases. When the physician diagnoses a case of hepatitis A, B, or C, a reportable disease form must be completed and filed with the local public health department.

In recent years, antiviral drugs have been developed to treat chronic forms of hepatitis B and C; however, not all infected individuals are candidates for treatment. These drugs, which must be taken for a prolonged time, are effective in removing the virus from approximately 40% of chronically infected patients.

Hepatitis B

The virus that causes hepatitis B is found in the blood and in certain body fluids (e.g., semen, vaginal secretions) of HBV-infected individuals. The most common means of transmission of hepatitis B is through sexual contact with an infected individual, by sharing needles for injection drug use with an infected individual, and perinatally from an infected mother to her infant during birth. Other modes of transmission include contact with blood or open sores of an infected individual and sharing of items such as razors or toothbrushes with an infected individual. Hepatitis B is not spread by sneezing, coughing, hugging, kissing, casual contact, breast-feeding, food, water, or sharing eating utensils or drinking glasses.

The highest rate of new hepatitis B infection occurs in adults, particularly among males 20 to 49 years of age. The greatest decline has occurred among children and adolescents as a result of routine hepatitis B immunization.

It is estimated that 800,00 to 1.4 million people in the United States are infected with chronic hepatitis B; this means that these individuals are carriers of hepatitis B and are capable of transmitting the disease to others. Many of these individuals do not know that they are carriers.

Every year, approximately 3000 Americans die as a result of the long-term consequences of chronic hepatitis B, such as cirrhosis and liver cancer.

Whether or not an HBV-infected individual goes on to develop chronic hepatitis B depends primarily on age. After infection with acute viral hepatitis B occurs, chronic infection develops in 90% of infants infected by their mothers at birth, 30% of children infected from age 1 to 5 years, and 6% of individuals infected after age 5 years.

Hepatitis B can survive outside the body in a dried state for at least 1 week and still can be capable of causing infection. Examples of surfaces that could harbor dried blood or body fluids infected with HBV include contaminated worktables, equipment, and instruments.

Hepatitis C

Chronic hepatitis C is the most common chronic viral infection in the United States. Approximately 4 million Americans have been diagnosed with chronic hepatitis C, and each year it causes an estimated 12,000 deaths resulting from cirrhosis and liver cancer.

The most common means of transmission of hepatitis C is by sharing needles for injection drug use with an infected individual. Hepatitis C is not spread by casual contact, such as sneezing, coughing, hugging, sharing food or water, or sharing eating utensils or drinking glasses. It is rarely transmitted through sexual contact.

Individuals infected with hepatitis C should not share with other members of the household personal items that may have blood on them (e.g., toothbrushes, nail-grooming equipment, razors).

Chronic hepatitis C is known as "an epidemic that occurred in the past." Numerous individuals became infected with hepatitis C more than 30 years ago and are now being diagnosed with it. This is because the symptoms of chronic hepatitis C often do not appear until 10 to 30 years after infection, and many times the first symptoms come only with advanced liver disease. Chronic hepatitis C surpasses alcoholism as the leading cause of liver cirrhosis and liver transplantation in the United States.

Before 1992, a blood test to determine the presence of hepatitis C did not exist. Because of this, a significant number of people contracted hepatitis C from HCV-infected blood transfusions. The CDC encourages people who received blood transfusions before July 1992 to ask their physicians if they should be tested for hepatitis C.

Postexposure prophylaxis with immune globulin is not effective in preventing hepatitis C, and no vaccine exists yet to prevent hepatitis C. Vaccines for hepatitis C are difficult to develop because the virus mutates so frequently. The only way to control the disease is by preventing exposure to the hepatitis C virus. ■

ACQUIRED IMMUNODEFICIENCY SYNDROME

Acquired immunodeficiency syndrome (AIDS) is a chronic disorder of the immune system that eventually destroys the body's ability to fight off infection. AIDS is caused by a retrovirus known as *human immunodeficiency virus (HIV)*. The following description helps to clarify the difference between these two terms. The virus and the infection itself are known as *HIV,* whereas the term *AIDS* is used to refer to the last stage of HIV infection. Simply put, the terms *HIV infection* and *AIDS* refer to different stages of the same disease.

When HIV gains entrance into the body, it begins to attack and destroy certain white blood cells known as *CD4+ T cells,* which are involved in protecting the body against viral, fungal, and protozoal infections. As more and more CD4+ T cells are destroyed, the immune system is gradually weakened. After a period of time, which may last 10 years or longer, the body's immune system becomes so ravaged by the attack that it succumbs to the diseases associated with AIDS.

AIDS is characterized by the presence of severe and life-threatening opportunistic infections and unusual cancers that rarely affect individuals with healthy immune systems. An **opportunistic infection** is an infection that results from a defective immune system that cannot defend itself from pathogens normally found in the environment. Opportunistic infections are extremely difficult to treat because the infection tends to recur quickly after a course of therapy is completed.

Transmission of AIDS

Research has shown that HIV is not transmitted through casual contact or even extensive contact, such as occurs among family members of AIDS patients. In the general population, HIV is spread primarily through sexual contact with an infected person and by sharing drug injection needles with someone who is infected. Untreated HIV-infected women also can transmit the virus to their infants during pregnancy and birth and through their breast milk.

Because HIV is not easily transmitted, the risk to health care workers is low. Since reporting began in 1985, the CDC has received reports of 57 documented cases and 138 possible cases of HIV infection from occupational exposure to health care workers. Despite the low risk of infection, however, the serious nature of HIV infection warrants the use of the OSHA Bloodborne Pathogens Standard by all health care workers. Because most HIV carriers are asymptomatic and may be unaware of their infection, precautions minimizing the risk of exposure to blood and body fluids should be taken with all patients at all times. These precautions also are recommended as a means of protection against other bloodborne pathogens, such as hepatitis B, hepatitis C, and syphilis.

HIGHLIGHT on AIDS

Prevalence

AIDS was first reported in the United States in 1981, but most likely it existed here and in other parts of the world for many years before that. Since 1981, more than 1.7 million cases of AIDS have been reported in the United States, and every year approximately 50,000 people in the United States are newly infected with HIV. Since 1981, there have been an estimated 600,000 deaths from AIDS in the United States.

Currently, almost 75% of those individuals newly diagnosed with HIV are adolescent and adult males, and the largest proportions of these are men who have sex with men, followed by individuals infected through high-risk heterosexual contact.

Transmission

HIV is spread primarily through sexual contact with an infected individual and by sharing drug injection needles with infected individuals. Scientific evidence shows that HIV is not spread through casual, everyday contact. There is no evidence that HIV is spread by sharing facilities or equipment, such as telephones, computers, food utensils, bedding, doorknobs, and bathrooms. Because HIV is not passed through the air, it is not spread through coughing and sneezing. HIV also is not spread through tears or sweat, or by shaking hands, hugging, or donating blood.

Most individuals infected with HIV show no symptoms and may not develop full-blown AIDS for 10 years or longer. After infection with HIV, the individual is infected for life.

Women can transmit HIV to their fetuses during pregnancy or birth. Approximately one quarter to one third of pregnant women infected with HIV who are not being treated with antiretroviral drugs pass the infection to their infants. HIV also can be spread to infants through the breast milk of mothers infected with the virus. Because of this, the CDC recommends that testing for HIV be included in the routine panel of prenatal screening tests for all pregnant women, and that separate written consent not be required. The CDC further recommends that the patient should be notified that HIV testing will be performed unless the patient declines the test (known as *opt-out screening*). The CDC recommends that repeat HIV screening be performed in the third trimester in areas that have elevated rates of HIV infection among pregnant women.

Worldwide, more than 400,000 infants are infected with HIV each year. If antiretroviral drugs are taken during pregnancy and the infant is delivered by cesarean section, the chance of transmitting HIV to the infant is reduced significantly. In developing countries, such as sub-Saharan Africa, women seldom know their HIV status, and treatment is often unavailable.

HIV Testing

The CDC recommends HIV screening for patients in all health care settings after the patient is notified that the testing will be performed, and separate written consent is not required. HIV screening should be performed unless the patient declines (known as *opt-out screening*). The CDC further recommends that individuals at high risk for HIV infection undergo HIV screening at least annually.

The enzyme immunoassay (EIA) test and the enzyme-linked immunosorbent assay (ELISA) test are used as screening tests for

HIGHLIGHT on AIDS—cont'd

the presence of HIV. Newer rapid HIV testing kits are also commercially available; brand names include Uni-Gold Recombigen HIV (Trinity Biotech, County Wicklow, Ireland), Clearview HIV (Inverness Medical, Princeton, New Jersey), and OraQuick Rapid HIV test (OraSure Technologies, Bethlehem, Pennsylvania). Because of the possibility of a false-positive result, a second screening test is always performed if a blood specimen tests positive. If the second test result also is positive, a more specific test, such as the Western blot test, is performed to confirm the test results. An individual who tests positive for HIV is seropositive.

A negative HIV test is not conclusive for the absence of HIV infection. If an individual has recently been infected with HIV, the antibodies may not have had time to develop. In general, it takes 2 to 12 weeks (but possibly as long as 6 months) for the HIV antibodies to appear in the blood.

CDC Definition of AIDS

As scientists have learned more about the disease, the CDC's definition of AIDS has changed several times since the beginning of the AIDS epidemic. The current AIDS definition includes the presence of one or both of the following conditions:

1. HIV-positive status and a CD4+ T-cell count below 200 cells/μL (normal CD4+ T-cell count for a healthy individual ranges from 500 to 1500 cells/μL)
2. Presence of one or more AIDS-defining conditions

Kaposi sarcoma is an example of an AIDS-defining condition. (From Forbes CD: *Color atlas and text of clinical medicine,* ed 3, St Louis, 2003, Mosby.)

Treatment

There is no known cure for AIDS; there is no vaccine to prevent it. Powerful antiviral drugs have been developed that slow the reproduction of the virus and reduce the viral load in the body. In many patients these drugs have dramatically delayed HIV from progressing to full-blown AIDS, thereby allowing the patients to live longer. These drugs can have serious side effects, and they do not prevent the spread of the disease to someone else. Numerous drugs also are available to treat the opportunistic infections and cancers that occur with AIDS. ∎

What Would You Do? | What Would You *Not* Do? | RESPONSES

Case Study 1
Page 302

What Did Jennifer Do?
❑ Told Petra that the physician would need to determine what is causing her symptoms.
❑ Documented Petra's symptoms in her medical record. Made sure to document that Petra's symptoms occur after she has contact with rubber latex gloves and rubber flip flops.
❑ As a precaution, made sure to use nonlatex gloves and a nonlatex tourniquet when drawing Petra's blood.
❑ If instructed to do so by the physician, provided Petra with latex allergy education and training.

What Did Jennifer Not *Do?*
❑ Did not tell Petra that she has a latex allergy, because only the physician is qualified to make a diagnosis.

Case Study 2
Page 308

What Did Jennifer Do?
❑ Told Tracy that having her infant immunized for hepatitis B is an investment in her child's future. Explained that her child could come into contact with the virus anytime in his or her life. Stressed that if a young child becomes infected with hepatitis B, the child has a higher risk of developing chronic hepatitis, which can cause serious liver problems later in life.
❑ Gave Tracy a brochure on hepatitis B to take home.

What Did Jennifer Not *Do?*
❑ Did not discourage Tracy from having her baby immunized for hepatitis B.

Case Study 3
Page 311

What Did Jennifer Do?
❑ Explained to Giles that the blood supply was not tested for hepatitis C until 1992 because a test to detect the presence of hepatitis C was not developed until then.
❑ Told Giles that it is possible for someone to have hepatitis C and not exhibit any symptoms.
❑ Told Giles that he should ask the physician his question about giving hepatitis C to others.

What Did Jennifer Not *Do?*
❑ Did not automatically assume that Giles had hepatitis C, because he had not yet been seen by the physician. It would be up to the physician to make a diagnosis of hepatitis C.
❑ Did not tell Giles about the serious complications of hepatitis C. If Giles is diagnosed with hepatitis C, it would be the physician's responsibility to relay this information.

↻ TERMINOLOGY REVIEW

Key Term	Word Parts	Definition
Aerobe	*aer/o:* air	A microorganism that needs oxygen to live and grow.
Anaerobe	*an-:* without *aer/o:* air	A microorganism that grows best in the absence of oxygen.
Antiseptic	*anti-:* against *-septic:* infection	An agent that inhibits the growth of or kills microorganisms.
Cilia		Slender, hairlike projections that constantly beat toward the outside to remove microorganisms from the body.
Hand hygiene		The process of cleansing or sanitizing the hands.
Infection		The condition in which the body, or part of it, is invaded by a pathogen.
Medical asepsis	*a-:* without *sepsis:* infection	Practices that are employed to inhibit the growth and hinder the transmission of pathogenic microorganisms to prevent the spread of infection.
Microorganism	*micro-:* small *organism:* organism	A microscopic plant or animal.
Nonintact skin	*non-:* not	Skin that has a break in the surface. It includes, but is not limited to, abrasions, cuts, hangnails, paper cuts, and burns.
Nonpathogen	*non-:* not *path/o:* disease *-gen:* producing	A microorganism that does not normally produce disease.
Opportunistic infection		An infection that results from a defective immune system that cannot defend the body from pathogens normally found in the environment.
Optimum growth temperature		The temperature at which an organism grows best.
Parenteral	*para-:* apart from *enter/o:* intestine *-al:* pertaining to	Taken into the body through piercing of the skin barrier or mucous membranes, such as through needlesticks, human bites, cuts, and abrasions.
Pathogen	*path/o:* disease *-gen:* producing	A disease-producing microorganism.
Postexposure prophylaxis	*post-:* after *pro-:* before *phylaxis:* prevention of disease	Treatment administered to an individual after exposure to an infectious disease to prevent the disease.
Regulated medical waste		Medical waste that poses a threat to health and safety.
Resident flora		Harmless, nonpathogenic microorganisms that normally reside on the skin and usually do not cause disease. Also known as *normal flora.*
Transient flora		Microorganisms that reside on the superficial skin layers and are picked up in the course of daily activities. They are often pathogenic but can be removed easily from the skin by sanitizing the hands.

ON THE WEB

For information on federal regulations and recommendations for infection control:

Occupational Safety and Health Administration (OSHA): www.osha.gov

Centers for Disease Control and Prevention (CDC): www.cdc.gov

CDC National Institute for Occupational Safety and Health (NIOSH): www.cdc.gov/niosh

CDC Recommendations for Hand Hygiene in the Healthcare Setting: www.cdc.gov/handhygiene

Food and Drug Administration (FDA): www.fda.gov

Environmental Protection Agency: www.epa.gov

Association for the Advancement of Medical Instrumentation (AAMI): www.aami.org

CDC Healthcare-Associated Infections: www.cdc.gov/hai

CDC Epidemiology Program Office: www.cdc.gov/epo

CDC *Morbidity and Mortality Weekly Report:* www.cdc.gov/mmwr

For information on hepatitis:

CDC Viral Hepatitis: www.cdc.gov/hepatitis

Hepatitis Foundation International: www.hepfi.org

Hepatitis B Foundation: www.hepb.org

National Institute of Allergy and Infectious Diseases: www.niaid.nih.gov

About Hepatitis: hepatitis.about.com

For information on AIDS:

AIDS.gov: www.aids.gov

CDC HIV/AIDS: www.cdc.gov/hiv

AIDS.org: www.aids.org

AIDS Education Global Information System: www.aegis.com

AIDS Information: www.aidsinfo.nih.gov

The Body—AIDS and HIV Information Resource: www.thebody.com

About AIDS: aids.about.com

18 Sterilization and Disinfection

 Check out the Evolve site at http://evolve.elsevier.com/Bonewit/today/ to access additional interactive activities and exercises to help you study and prepare for success.

<table>
<tr><td>

LEARNING OBJECTIVES

</td><td>

PROCEDURES

</td></tr>
<tr><td>

Hazard Communication Standard
1. Explain the purpose of the Hazard Communication Standard.
2. List and describe the information that must be included on the label of a hazardous chemical.
3. List and describe the information that must be included in a safety data sheet (SDS).

</td><td>

Read and interpret an SDS.

</td></tr>
<tr><td>

Sanitization
4. State the purpose of sanitization.
5. State the advantages of using an ultrasonic cleaner to clean instruments.
6. List and describe the guidelines that should be followed when sanitizing instruments.

</td><td>

Sanitize instruments.

</td></tr>
<tr><td>

Disinfection
7. State the uses of the three levels of disinfection: high, intermediate, and low.
8. Explain the differences among the following: critical item, semicritical item, and noncritical item.
9. List and describe the primary use of disinfectants in the medical office.

</td><td></td></tr>
<tr><td>

Sterilization
10. Explain how the autoclave functions to sterilize articles.
11. List the components of a sterilization monitoring program.
12. List and describe types of sterilization indicators.
13. Identify the advantages and disadvantages of each of the following types of wraps: sterilization paper, sterilization pouches, and muslin.
14. List the guidelines that should be followed when the autoclave is loaded.
15. Identify the sterilization times for each of the following categories: unwrapped articles, wrapped articles, liquids, and large wrapped packs.
16. Describe the method for storing wrapped articles.
17. Describe the daily, weekly, and monthly maintenance of the autoclave.

</td><td>

Wrap articles to be autoclaved.
Sterilize articles in the autoclave.

Maintain the autoclave.

</td></tr>
<tr><td>

Other Sterilization Methods
18. State the primary use of each of the following types of sterilization methods: dry heat, ethylene oxide gas, chemicals, and radiation.

</td><td></td></tr>
</table>

CHAPTER OUTLINE

INTRODUCTION TO STERILIZATION AND DISINFECTION
DEFINITIONS OF TERMS
HAZARD COMMUNICATION STANDARD
Hazard Communication Program
Inventory of Hazardous Chemicals
Labeling of Hazardous Chemicals
Container Label Requirements
Safety Data Sheets
Safety Data Sheet Requirements
Employee Information and Training

SANITIZATION
Sanitizing Instruments
Cleaning Instruments
Guidelines for Sanitizing Instruments
DISINFECTION
Levels of Disinfection
High-Level Disinfection
Intermediate-Level Disinfection
Low-Level Disinfection
STERILIZATION

Sterilization Methods
Autoclave
Monitoring Program
Wrapping Articles
Operating the Autoclave
Handling and Storing Packs

Maintaining the Autoclave
Other Sterilization Methods
Dry Heat Oven
Ethylene Oxide Gas Sterilization
Cold Sterilization
Radiation

KEY TERMS

autoclave (AU-toh-klave)
critical item
detergent
disinfectant (dis-in-FEK-tant)
hazardous chemical

incubate (IN-kyoo-bate)
load
noncritical item
safety data sheet
sanitization (san-ih-tih-ZAY-shun)

semicritical item
spore
sterilization (stare-ill-ih-ZAY-shun)
thermolabile (ther-moh-LAH-bul)

INTRODUCTION TO STERILIZATION AND DISINFECTION

The air and all objects around us contain microorganisms. The medical assistant is responsible for helping to reduce and eliminate microorganisms to prevent the spread of disease. This can be accomplished by practicing good techniques of medical and surgical asepsis (see Chapters 17 and 25).

Physical and chemical agents are used to destroy microorganisms in the medical office. The agent selected depends on the intended use of the article. Articles that penetrate sterile tissue or the vascular system, such as surgical instruments, must be sterilized. Articles that come in contact with the skin, such as stethoscopes, blood pressure cuffs, and percussion hammers, should be disinfected.

Sanitization, disinfection, and sterilization involve hazardous chemicals. It is essential for the medical assistant to know the precautions that are required when working with hazardous chemicals.

DEFINITIONS OF TERMS

Terms that aid in understanding this chapter are listed and defined here.

Sanitization *Sanitization* is a process that removes organic material and reduces the number of microorganisms to a safe level as determined by public health requirements. Sanitization removes all organic material, such as blood, body fluids, and tissue, from an article. For articles that are used in examinations, treatments, and office surgery to be properly sterilized or disinfected, they must first be sanitized.

Decontamination *Decontamination* refers to the use of physical or chemical means to remove or destroy pathogens on an item so that it is no longer capable of transmitting disease; this makes the item safe to handle.

Detergent A *detergent* is an agent that cleanses by emulsifying dirt and oil.

Disinfectant A *disinfectant* is an agent used to destroy pathogenic microorganisms; however, it does not kill the resistant bacterial spores. Disinfectants are usually applied to inanimate objects.

Spore A *spore* is a hard, thick-walled capsule that some bacteria form by losing moisture and condensing their contents to contain only the essential parts of the protoplasm of the cell. Spores represent a resting and protective stage of the bacterial cell and are more resistant to drying, sunlight, heat, and disinfectants than is the vegetative form of the bacterium. Favorable conditions cause the spore to germinate into a vegetative bacterium again that is capable of reproducing. Two examples of species of bacteria that form spores are *Clostridium botulinum,* which causes botulism, and *Clostridium tetani,* which causes tetanus.

Sterilization *Sterilization* is the process of destroying all forms of microbial life, including bacterial spores. An object that is *sterile* is free of all living microorganisms and spores. There can be no relative degrees of sterility—an object is either sterile or not sterile. The device most commonly used to sterilize articles in the medical office is the autoclave.

HAZARD COMMUNICATION STANDARD

The Hazard Communication Standard (HCS), first established in 1983, is a requirement of the Occupational Safety and Health Administration (OSHA). The purpose of the

HCS is to ensure that employees are informed of the hazards associated with chemicals in their workplace and the precautions to take to protect themselves when working with hazardous chemicals. A **hazardous chemical** is any chemical that is classified as a health or physical hazard, a simple asphyxiant, a combustible dust, a pyrophoric gas, or a hazard not otherwise classified. *Health hazards* include the potential of the chemical to cause acute toxicity, skin corrosion or irritation, serious eye damage or irritation, respiratory or skin sensitization, germ cell mutagenicity, cancer, or reproductive toxicity, or is an aspiration hazard. *Physical hazards* include the potential of the chemical to catch fire, explode, or react with other chemicals or materials.

In 2012 the HCS was revised to incorporate the Globally Harmonized System of Classification and Labeling of Chemicals (GHS) set forth by the United Nations. The GHS is an international standard that provides consistency in the classification and labeling of chemicals through the use of pictograms, signal words, and hazard warnings. The GHS classifies chemicals according to their health and physical hazards. The GHS also requires the use of a standardized format for labeling containers and the development of safety data sheets (SDSs).

The GHS revisions to the HCS enable employees to quickly obtain and more easily understand information regarding the safe handling and use of hazardous chemicals. This, in turn, assists in preventing injury and illness associated with exposure to hazardous chemicals.

In the medical office, sanitization, disinfection, and sterilization procedures involve the use of hazardous chemicals; the medical assistant must have a thorough knowledge of the HCS. The HCS consists of the following components:

- Development of a hazard communication program
- Inventory of hazardous chemicals
- Labeling requirements
- SDS requirements
- Employee information and training

HAZARD COMMUNICATION PROGRAM

As part of the HCS, employers are required to develop a hazard communication program. The hazard communication program consists of a written plan that describes what the facility is doing to meet the requirements of the HCS. The information in the plan must be made available and communicated to all employees who work with hazardous chemicals.

INVENTORY OF HAZARDOUS CHEMICALS

The employer must develop and maintain a list of hazardous chemicals that are used and stored in the workplace. The list must be updated as new chemicals are introduced into the workplace. In the medical office, hazardous chemicals often include the following:

Figure 18-1 Hazardous chemical used as a disinfectant in the medical office.

- Products used for sanitization, disinfection, and sterilization (e.g., chemical disinfectants, autoclave cleaners) (Figure 18-1)
- Chemicals used for laboratory testing (e.g., laboratory testing reagents, developing solutions, controls)
- Pharmaceutical products such as local anesthetics (e.g., lidocaine [Xylocaine])
- Front office products (e.g., toner for copying machine and laser printer)
- Cleaning products (e.g., drain cleaner)

LABELING OF HAZARDOUS CHEMICALS

The HCS requires that each container of a hazardous chemical be labeled by the manufacturer with a warning to alert the user that the chemical is dangerous. This label must include the possible hazards of the chemical and the steps that can be taken to protect against those risks. The label on a hazardous chemical must not be removed or defaced. If a label falls off a product or is damaged or obscured, a replacement label must be applied. If a chemical is transferred to a new container, a label with all the required information must be attached to the new container.

Container Label Requirements

The HCS requires that manufacturers label the containers of hazardous chemicals they produce according to GHS guidelines The information on the container label allows the user of the chemical to tell at a glance the hazards of using the chemical and how to prevent or lessen exposure

PRODUCT IDENTIFIER
Code: 7489
Product Name: Glutaraldehyde Solution

SUPPLIER IDENTIFICATION
Poston Corporation
2010 East Main Street
Camden, New Jersey 08106

PRECAUTIONARY STATEMENTS
Do not breathe dust/fumes/gas/mist/
vapors/spray
Avoid release to the environment
Wear protective gloves/ eye protection/
face protection
IF ON SKIN: Wash with plenty of soap
and water
IF ON EYES: Rinse cautiously with water
for several minutes. Remove contact lenses,
if present and easy to do. Continue rinsing
IF SWALLOWED: Immediately call a POISON
CENTER or doctor/physician

HAZARD PICTOGRAMS

SIGNAL WORD
DANGER

HAZARD STATEMENTS
Toxic if swallowed
May be harmful in contact with skin
Causes skin irritation
Causes serious eye damage
May cause allergy or asthma
symptoms or breathing difficulties
May cause respiratory irritation
Very toxic to aquatic life

SUPPLEMENTAL INFORMATION
Storage: Store at room temperature
Disposal: Discard residual solution
in drain. Flush thoroughly with water

Expiration Date: 10/15/xx

Figure 18-2 Hazardous chemical container label following the GHS system.

to the chemical (Figure 18-2). Information required by the GHS includes the following:

- *Product identifier:* The product identifier specifies how the hazardous chemical is identified. This can be (but is not limited to) the chemical name and the code number or batch number.
- *Supplier identification:* Supplier information includes the name, address, and telephone number of the chemical manufacturer.
- *GHS signal word:* A signal word is a word used to indicate the relative degree of severity of the hazardous chemical and to alert the user to a potential hazard on the label. There are two possible signal words under GHS:
  Danger: Denotes a more severe hazard possible
  Warning: Denotes a less serious hazard possible but potentially harmful
- *GHS hazard statement(s):* A hazard statement is a phrase that describes the types of hazards associated with a hazardous chemical, including, when appropriate, the degree of the hazard (e.g., Causes damage to kidneys through prolonged or repeated exposure when absorbed through the skin).
- *GHS hazard pictograms:* Pictograms consist of standardized graphic symbols that allow employees to quickly identify the types of hazards associated with a hazardous chemical. There are eight different pictograms representing the health and physical hazards covered in the GHS (Figure 18-3).
- *GHS precautionary statement(s):* A precautionary statement is a phrase that describes recommended measures to be taken to minimize or prevent adverse effects resulting from exposure to the hazardous chemical or from improper

storage or handling (e.g., Wear protective gloves/ protective clothing/eye protection/face protection).

- *Supplementary information:* The manufacturer may provide additional information that it deems helpful, such as directions for use and the expiration date of the chemical.

SAFETY DATA SHEETS

A **safety data sheet** (SDS), previously known as a *material safety data sheet* (MSDS), provides more detailed information than the container label regarding the chemical, its hazards, and measures to take to prevent injury and illness when handling the chemical (Figure 18-4). The HCS requires that a current SDS be kept on file for each hazardous chemical used or stored in the workplace. SDSs must be readily accessible to employees and provided to them on request. It is important that the medical assistant review the SDS before working with a hazardous chemical.

Companies that manufacture and distribute hazardous chemicals must provide an SDS with every product. A hazardous chemical should never be used unless an SDS is available. In the event of an accidental exposure, information on the SDS must be readily available as a reference for emergency treatment. If an SDS is missing, it must be replaced. This can be accomplished by contacting the supplier or the manufacturer of that chemical for a replacement or by going to the manufacturer's website; most manufacturers post their SDSs on their websites for easy access.

An SDS does not have to be kept on file for a hazardous chemical that is used in the workplace in the same way that a household consumer would use it. For example,

PICTOGRAM	MEANING OF PICTOGRAM	TYPE OF HAZARD(S) (Associated with this pictogram)
Health Hazard	The chemical is a risk to health if used improperly	• Carcinogen • Mutagenicity • Reproductive Toxicity • Respiratory Sensitizer • Target Organ Toxicity • Aspiration Toxicity
Severe Toxic	The chemical is a serious health or physical hazard or poison. It will produce adverse effects following a single dose. This pictogram is usually used in combination with the Health Hazard Pictogram.	• Acute Toxicity (fatal or toxic) if inhaled or swallowed, or if it comes in contact with the skin.
Acute Toxic	The chemical may cause immediate, serious health effects but it is less severe than the Severe Toxic pictogram (skull and crossbones). This pictogram is usually used in combination with the Health Hazard Pictogram.	• Irritant (skin and eye) • Skin Sensitizer • Acute Toxicity • Narcotic Effects • Respiratory Tract Irritant
Flammable	The chemical may burst into flame. Be careful to keep away from ignition sources and combustible materials.	• Flammables • Pyrophorics • Self-Heating • Emits Flammable Gas • Self-Reactive • Organic Peroxides
Corrosive	The chemical is a physical or health hazard that can easily damage skin or eyes. Be aware of PPE and storage requirements.	• Skin Corrosion/Burns • Eye Damage • Corrosive to Metals
Oxidizer	The chemical may cause other materials to ignite or burn faster. It can create an increased fire risk in work or storage environment.	• Oxidizers
Gas Under Pressure	This chemical consist of pressurized gas that would explode, rocket, or damage health if heated, ruptured or leaking.	• Gases Under Pressure
Explosive	This material can blow up or otherwise create an uncontrolled reaction. Should be treated with extreme caution.	• Explosives • Self-Reactives • Organic Peroxides

Figure 18-3 GHS Hazard Pictograms. (Pictograms from U.S. Department of Labor, Occupational Safety and Health Administration.)

SAFETY DATA SHEET
(SDS)

SECTION 1: IDENTIFICATION

Product name:	Glutaraldehyde Solution	**Telephone:** 1 (800) 331-0766	
Brand:	Aldecyde	**Emergency phone number:** 1 (800) 773-8690	
Manufacturer:	Poston Corporation 2010 East Main Street Camden, New Jersey 08106	**Recommended Use:** High Level Disinfectant	
		Restrictions on Use: Not recommended for drug, food, or household use.	

SECTION 2: HAZARDS IDENTIFICATION

Hazard Classification

Acute toxicity, oral:	GHS Category 3	Respiratory sensitization:	GHS Category 1
Skin irritation:	GHS Category 2	Skin sensitization:	GHS Category 1
Serious eye damage:	GHS Category 1	Acute aquatic toxicity:	GHS Category 1

Signal Word

Danger

Hazard Statements

H301	Toxic if swallowed
H313	May be harmful in contact with skin
H315	Causes skin irritation
H318	Causes serious eye damage
H334	May cause allergy or asthma symptoms or breathing difficulties if inhaled
H335	May cause respiratory irritation
H400	Very toxic to aquatic life

Hazard Pictograms

Precautionary Statements

P260	Do not breathe dust/fumes/gas/mist/vapors/spray
P273	Avoid release to the environment
P280	Wear protective gloves/eye protection/face protection
P302 + P352	IF ON SKIN: Wash with plenty of soap and water
P305 + P351 + P338	IF ON EYES: Rinse cautiously with water for several minutes. Remove contact lenses, if present and easy to do. Continue rinsing.
P310	IF SWALLOWED: Immediately call a POISON CENTER or doctor/physician

SECTION 3: COMPOSITION/INFORMATION ON INGREDIENTS

CAS NUMBER	CHEMICAL NAME OF INGREDIENTS	PERCENT
111-30-8	Glutaraldehyde	2.5
7732-18-5	Water	97.4
7632-00-0	Sodium Nitrite	<1

SECTION 4: FIRST AID MEASURES

Skin Contact: Rinse with water. Remove contaminated clothing and wash before reuse. Consult a physician if skin redness or irritation persist.

Eye Contact: Immediately flush with water for 15 minutes. Seek medical attention.

Inhalation: Remove to fresh air immediately. If experiencing difficulty breathing, seek medical attention.

Ingestion: Call a physician or Poison Control Center immediately. Do not ingest emetic.

SECTION 5: FIRE FIGHTING MEASURES

Suitable Extinguishing Media: Use extinguishing agent which is suitable for the surrounding fire.

Hazardous Combustion Products: Carbon monoxide and carbon dioxide.

Special Protective Equipment for Firefighters: Wear self-contained breathing apparatus for fire fighting if necessary.

Figure 18-4 Safety data sheet (SDS).

Continued

SAFETY DATA SHEET
(SDS)

SECTION 6: ACCIDENTAL RELEASE MEASURES

Personal Precautions: Ventilate area. Avoid breathing vapors or mist. Wear eye and skin protection while handling material for clean-up.

Cleanup Procedures: Contain spill by placing suitable absorbent material around the edges of the spill and work inward. Carefully scoop up into waste container for disposal. Dispose of in accordance with applicable Federal, State and Local regulations.

SECTION 7: HANDLING AND STORAGE

Precautions for Safe Handling: Use in a well-ventilated area. Avoid breathing vapors or mist. Avoid contact with skin, eyes and clothing. Remove contaminated clothing and launder before use.

Conditions for Safe Storage: Store in a cool, dry area (59-86º F) away from direct sunlight or sources of intense heat. Keep container tightly closed when not in use.

SECTION 8: EXPOSURE CONTROLS/PERSONAL PROTECTION

Exposure Control Limits:

PEL: 0.2 ppm
TLV: 0.2 ppm

Engineering Controls and Personal Protective Equipment:

Ventilation: Ensure adequate ventilation.

Respiratory Protection: None normally required for routine use.

Skin Protection: Wear protective chemical resistant gloves. Wear suitable protective clothing.
Eye Protection: Eye protection required.

SECTION 9: PHYSICAL AND CHEMICAL PROPERTIES

APPEARANCE: Bluish-green liquid	BOILING POINT: 212º F
PHYSICAL STATE: Liquid	EVAPORATION RATE: 0.98
ODOR: Sharp odor	VAPOR PRESSURE (mm Hg): 0.20 at 20º C
ODOR THRESHOLD: 0.04 ppm	VAPOR DENSITY (AIR = 1): 1.1
pH: 7.5-8.5	SPECIFIC GRAVITY: 1.004
FREEZING POINT: 32º F	SOLUBILITY IN WATER: Complete (100%)

SECTION 10: STABILITY AND REACTIVITY

STABILITY: Stable under recommended storage conditions.

CONDITIONS TO AVOID: Avoid temperatures above 200º F

INCOMPATIBILITY (MATERIAL TO AVOID): Strong acids, bases and oxidizing agents.

HAZARDOUS DECOMPOSITION BY PRODUCTS: None

HAZARDOUS POLYMERIZATION: Will not occur

SECTION 11: TOXICOLOGICAL INFORMATION

Acute Health Hazards:

Inhalation: Inhalation of mist or vapors may be severely irritating to the nose, throat and lungs.

Skin Contact: May cause skin irritation. May aggravate pre-existing dermatitis.

Eye Contact: Severe irritant and corrosive to the eyes.

Ingestion: Ingestion of this material may cause oral thrush, nausea, vomiting, epigastric distress, diarrhea, headache, fatigue, dizziness, insomnia, mental confusion, and impairment.

Chronic Health Hazards:

No adverse effects expected based on the available data.

Medical Conditions Aggravated By Exposure:

Inhalation of vapor may cause asthma-like symptoms (chest discomfort and tightness, difficulty with breathing) as well as aggravate pre-existing asthma and inflammatory or fibrotic pulmonary disease.

Carcinogen:

None of the components is listed as a carcinogen or potential carcinogen by NTP, IARC, or OSHA.

SECTION 12: ECOLOGICAL INFORMATION

This product is classified as toxic to the aquatic environment.

Figure 18-4, cont'd

SAFETY DATA SHEET (SDS)

SECTION 13: DISPOSAL CONSIDERATIONS

Container must be triple rinsed and disposed of in accordance with Federal, State, and/or Local regulations. Used solution should be flushed thoroughly with water into sewage disposal in accordance with Federal, State, and/or Local regulations.

SECTION 14: TRANSPORT INFORMATION

Restrictions:	None. Not regulated.
UN Number:	None
UN Proper Shipping Name:	N/A
Transport Hazard Class:	N/A
Packing Group Number:	N/A

SECTION 15: REGULATORY INFORMATION

EPA SARA 311/312 Hazard Classification: Acute Health, Chronic Health

SECTION 16: OTHER INFORMATION

Issue Date:	4/28/02
Revision Date:	10/10/2014

Figure 18-4, cont'd

correction fluids, such as Wite-Out and Liquid Paper, contain a hazardous chemical. However, if the medical assistant uses these products in the same way that a household consumer would use them (i.e., to correct errors on a document), an SDS does not need to be kept on file. If household bleach (sodium hypochlorite) is used to decontaminate blood spills in the medical office, an SDS would need to be kept on file because the bleach is not being used in the same way that a household consumer would use it.

What Would You Do? What Would You *Not* Do?

Case Study 1

Elba Cordera has brought her daughter Maria in for a well-baby visit. Maria is 9 months old and is just starting to crawl. Mrs. Cordera is taking precautions to baby-proof her house to protect Maria from accidents. Mrs. Cordera wants to know how to tell whether a cleaning product is poisonous. She also wants to know what she should do if Maria gets into a cleaning product and spills it on herself or swallows it. ■

Safety Data Sheet Requirements

The Hazard Communication Standard requires that manufacturers of hazardous chemicals follow GHS guidelines in preparing an SDS. GHS guidelines require that the information on the SDS be presented using a standardized 16-section format that follows a specified sequence. The information on the SDS must be presented using the following 16 headings in the order outlined below (Figure 18-4 is an example of an SDS that follows the GHS system):

1. *Identification:* This section provides information used to identify the hazardous chemical and must include the product name and brand name and the name, address, phone number, and emergency phone number of the manufacturer. This section must also include the recommended use of the chemical and any restrictions on use.

2. *Hazards Identification:* This section includes the hazards of the chemical and the appropriate warning information associated with those hazards and includes the following:
   - GHS hazard classification of the chemical
   - GHS signal word
   - GHS hazard statement(s)
   - GHS hazard pictograms
   - GHS precautionary statement(s)

3. *Composition/Information on Ingredients:* This section provides a list of the ingredients in the hazardous chemical.

4. *First-Aid Measures:* This section describes the initial care that should be given by an untrained responder to an individual who has been exposed to the hazardous chemical. It is subdivided according to the different routes of exposure (e.g., skin contact, inhalation).

5. *Fire-Fighting Measures:* Some hazardous chemicals may cause a fire if used improperly. This section provides recommendations for fighting a fire caused by the chemical, including suitable extinguishing agents.

6. *Accidental Release Measures:* This section provides recommendations on the appropriate response to spills, leaks, or releases including containment and cleanup practices to prevent or minimize exposure to people, properties, or the environment. It also identifies the personal precautions that should be taken during the cleanup such as wearing skin and eye protection.

7. *Handling and Storage:* This section identifies precautions that should be taken for safe handling of the

chemical and conditions for safe storage of the chemical.

8. *Exposure Controls/Personal Protection:* This section indicates the exposure control limits, engineering controls, and personal protective measures that should be used to protect oneself from the hazardous chemical. The exposure control limits include OSHA's Permissible Exposure Limit (PEL) and the Threshold Limit Value (TLV).

9. *Physical and Chemical Properties:* This section lists the physical and chemical properties associated with the hazardous chemical such as appearance, physical state, odor, pH, and boiling point.

10. *Stability and Reactivity:* Some chemicals react when combined with other chemicals or materials. This section lists the substances and conditions that the hazardous chemical should be kept away from to prevent a dangerous reaction.

11. *Toxicological Information:* This section identifies the toxicological effects that can result from overexposure to the chemical and includes the following:
    - Route of entry, which indicates how the hazardous chemical can enter the body, including inhalation, skin contact, eye contact, and ingestion
    - Signs and symptoms of overexposure (e.g., skin irritation, eye damage, lung damage) categorized according to acute and chronic health hazards
    - Medical conditions that are aggravated by exposure to the hazardous chemical (e.g., asthma, dermatitis)
    - Indication of whether the hazardous chemical has been identified as a potential carcinogen by the National Toxicology Program (NTP), the International Agency for Research on Cancer (IARC), and OSHA.

12. *Ecological Information:* This section provides information to help determine the environmental impact of the hazardous chemical if it were released into the environment.

13. *Disposal Considerations:* This section provides guidance on proper disposal of the hazardous chemical.

14. *Transport Information:* This section provides guidance to suppliers for shipping and transporting the hazardous chemical.

15. *Regulatory Information:* This section identifies the safety, health, and environmental regulations specific for the hazardous chemical that is not indicated anywhere else on the SDS.

16. *Other Information:* This section includes other important information related to the hazardous chemical such as when the SDS was prepared or when the last known revision was made.

EMPLOYEE INFORMATION AND TRAINING

The HCS requires that employees be provided with information and training regarding hazardous chemicals in the

Putting It All Into Practice

My name is Kara VanDyke, and I work for two physicians in a family practice medical office. As a medical assistant, one of the situations you deal with on an almost-daily basis is drug representatives who come to the office to promote their products. Their job is anything but easy. The waiting and the frequent rejections would make most people think twice before applying for the job.

One winter day, I am sure I made one drug representative really think twice about his career choice. As the representative stopped at our office, he, being a polite young man, let a patient enter the building first with wet, snow-covered feet. Trying to make a good impression with a new suit and dress shoes, he soon found himself doing a "Spanish fandango" while trying to maintain his balance and eventually crashed to the floor.

I thought I would help by mopping up the snow-tracked floor. What I did not know was the mop had wax on it. Needless to say, when he returned with the requested drug samples, we were not able to keep him from falling a second time! ∎

workplace. The training session must be offered at the time of an employee's initial assignment to a work area where hazardous chemicals are present, and whenever a new chemical hazard is introduced into the work area. The training program must be an ongoing activity, and each training session must be documented. The HCS requires that the following information be relayed to employees who work with hazardous chemicals:

1. Requirements making up the HCS
2. Physical and health hazards associated with exposure to chemicals in the workplace
3. Measures employees can take to protect themselves from hazardous chemicals in the workplace
4. Emergency procedures to carry out in the event of exposure to a hazardous chemical or a chemical spill
5. The meaning of the information on container labels, including signal words, hazard statements, and precautionary statements, and how to use that information
6. The meaning of the information on the SDS and how to use that information
7. The location of the following: hazard communication program plan, list of hazardous chemicals in the workplace, and SDS for each chemical in the workplace

SANITIZATION

Sanitization involves a series of steps designed to remove organic material from an article and to reduce to a safe level the number of microorganisms on the article (Procedure 18-1). Organic material on an article may result in incomplete sterilization or disinfection. This is because the organic material acts as a physical barrier preventing the physical or chemical agent from reaching the surface of the article to kill microorganisms.

SANITIZING INSTRUMENTS

Items most frequently sanitized in the medical office are medical and surgical instruments. This section focuses on the theory and procedure for sanitizing instruments. The general steps in the sanitization procedure of instruments are as follows:

1. *Rinse* the instruments to prevent organic material from drying on the instruments.
2. *Decontaminate* the instruments with a chemical disinfectant to remove pathogenic microorganisms, making the instrument safe to handle.
3. *Clean* the instruments to remove all organic matter.
4. *Thoroughly rinse* the instruments to remove all detergent residue.
5. *Dry* the instruments to prevent stains on the instruments.
6. *Check the instruments* for defects and working condition.
7. *Lubricate* hinged instruments to make the instruments function well and last longer.

Cleaning Instruments

Two methods can be used to perform the cleaning step (step 3 in the preceding list) of the sanitization procedure: the manual method and the ultrasound method.

Manual Method

The manual method is used most often in the medical office. It involves the manual cleaning of instruments with a cleaning solution and a brush. Manual cleaning is recommended for delicate instruments because vibrations that occur with the ultrasound method may damage these instruments.

Ultrasound Method

The ultrasound method uses a machine known as an *ultrasonic cleaner* (Figure 18-5). The ultrasound method offers a safety advantage in that instruments do not have to be handled during the cleaning process. This decreases the incidence of an accidental puncture or cut from a sharp instrument. An ultrasonic cleaner works by converting sound waves into mechanical energy, which creates small bubbles all over the instruments. When the bubbles burst, vibrations occur that loosen and remove debris from the instruments. Ultrasonic cleaners are especially good at removing debris from hard-to-reach areas, such as box locks of hemostats and screw locks of scissors.

Before the instruments are placed in the ultrasonic cleaner, they should be separated according to the type of metal (e.g., stainless steel, aluminum, brass). Instruments made of dissimilar metals should not be cleaned together in the ultrasonic cleaner. When different metals are in close contact, the ions from one metal can flow to another. This

Figure 18-5 Ultrasonic cleaner.

may result in a permanent blue-black stain on an instrument, which can be removed only by having the instrument refinished.

GUIDELINES FOR SANITIZING INSTRUMENTS

The following guidelines should be followed when sanitizing surgical instruments:

1. *Wear gloves during the sanitization process.* While following the OSHA Bloodborne Pathogens Standard, the medical assistant should wear disposable gloves during the entire sanitization procedure. This protects the medical assistant from bloodborne pathogens and other potentially infectious materials. The medical assistant should be especially careful when working with hazardous chemicals and when handling sharp instruments. Heavy-duty utility gloves should be worn over the disposable gloves to provide protection from the irritating effects of chemical agents and accidental punctures or cuts from sharp instruments.

2. *Handle instruments carefully.* Instruments are expensive and delicate, yet durable. They can last for many years if handled and maintained properly. Dropping an instrument on the floor or throwing an instrument into a basin may damage it. Instruments should never be piled in a heap because they become entangled and may be damaged when separated. Keep sharp instruments separate from other instruments to prevent damaging or dulling the cutting edge. Also, keep delicate instruments separate to protect them from damage.

3. *Follow instructions on labels of chemical agents.* Before using a chemical agent such as a chemical disinfectant, an instrument cleaner, or an autoclave cleaner, review the product's SDS, and carefully read the label on the container. Check the label to determine the use, mixing, and storage of the chemical agent. Read and observe precautions listed on the label regarding personal safety, such as the use of gloves and eye protection (Figure 18-6).

PROCEDURE 18-1 **Sanitization of Instruments—cont'd**

Principle. Decontaminating the instruments removes pathogenic microorganisms from them, making them safe to handle. A disinfectant past its expiration date loses its potency and should not be used. An EPA-approved disinfectant has been determined by the U.S. Environmental Protection Agency to be effective when used as directed, without causing an unreasonable risk to the public or the environment. The container must be kept covered to prevent the escape of toxic fumes and to prevent evaporation of the disinfectant, which could change its potency.

7. Procedural Step. Clean the instruments. The instruments can be cleaned using the manual method or the ultrasound method as follows.

Manual Method for Cleaning Instruments

a. Obtain the instrument cleaning solution; check its expiration date.

b. Observe all personal safety precautions listed on the label of the cleaning agent.

c. Follow the directions on the manufacturer's label for proper mixing and use of the cleaning agent. The detergent may need to be diluted with water.

d. Remove the articles from the chemical disinfectant and place them in the basin containing the cleaning solution.

e. Use a stiff nylon brush to clean the surface of each instrument. Scrub all parts of the instrument thoroughly. Brush delicate instruments carefully to prevent damaging them.

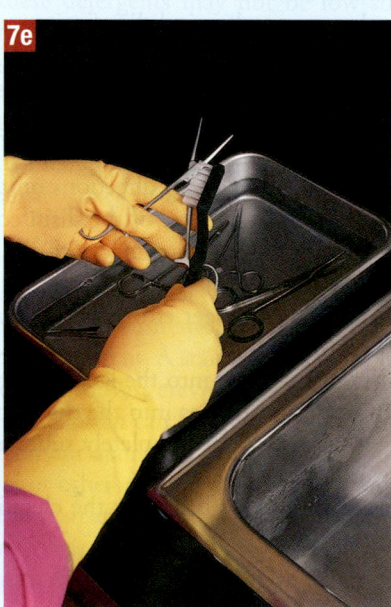

Clean the surface of the instrument with a stiff nylon brush.

f. Use a stainless-steel wire brush to clean grooves, crevices, or serrations where contaminants such as blood and tissue may collect.

Clean gloves, crevices, or serrations with a wire brush.

g. If there is a stain on the instrument, attempt to remove it with a damp cloth or sponge to which a commercial stain remover has been applied.

h. Scrub each instrument until it is visibly clean and free from organic material and stains.

Principle. A cleaning agent past its expiration date loses its potency and should not be used. Taking appropriate precautions with cleaning agents prevents harm to the medical assistant from hazardous chemicals. All organic material must be removed from the instruments to ensure complete sterilization in the autoclave.

Ultrasound Method for Cleaning Instruments

a. Using a cleaning agent recommended by the manufacturer, prepare the cleaning solution in the ultrasonic cleaner. Observe all personal safety precautions listed on the label.

b. Remove the articles from the chemical disinfectant and separate instruments made of dissimilar metals, such as stainless steel, aluminum, and bronze.

c. Place the instruments in the ultrasonic cleaner with hinged instruments in an open position.

d. Ensure that sharp instruments do not touch other instruments.

e. Ensure that all instruments are fully submerged in the cleaning solution.

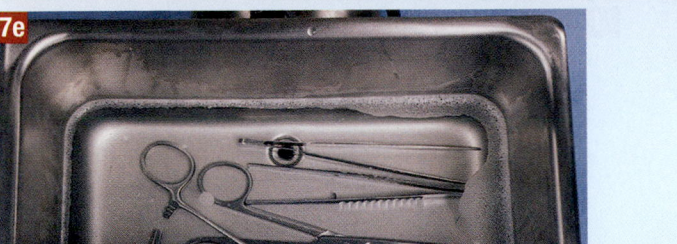

Completely submerge instruments in the cleaning solution.

f. Place the lid on the ultrasonic cleaner.

Place the lid on the ultrasonic cleaner.

g. Turn on the ultrasonic cleaner, and clean the instruments for the length of time recommended by the manufacturer.
h. After completion of the cleaning cycle, remove the instruments from the machine.
Principle. Taking appropriate precautions with chemical agents prevents harm to the medical assistant from hazardous chemicals. Mixing dissimilar metals together could result in permanent stains on the instruments. Instruments must be completely submerged with hinged instruments in an open position so the solution can reach all parts of the instrument.

8. Procedural Step. Rinse each instrument thoroughly with warm, not hot, water (110°F [44°C]) for at least 20 to 30 seconds to remove all traces of the detergent. Open and close hinged instruments while rinsing to ensure the solution is completely rinsed out of every part of the instrument.

Principle. Detergent residue left on the instrument could cause stains, which could build up and interfere with proper functioning of the instrument. Using warm water helps to remove the cleaning solution and facilitates the drying process.

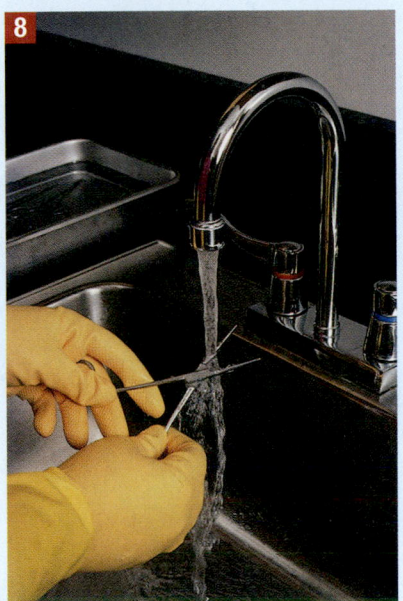

Rinse thoroughly with warm water.

9. Procedural Step. Dry each instrument with a paper towel, and place the instrument on a cloth towel for additional air drying.
Principle. If the instrument is not completely dry, stains may occur on the instrument.

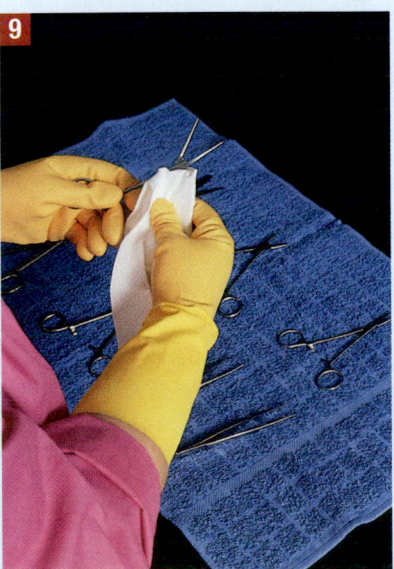

Dry the instrument with a paper towel.

Continued

PROCEDURE 18-1

10. Procedural Step. Check each instrument for defects and proper working condition. Scissors should cut all the way to the end of a thin piece of gauze without catching. If defects are noted or the instrument is not working properly, it must be discarded or sent to the manufacturer for repair. *Principle.* Instruments that have defects or are not in proper working condition are unsafe to use on a patient during a medical or surgical procedure.

10 (1)

Check the instrument for defects and proper working order.

10 (2)

Scissors should cut through gauze without catching.

11. Procedural Step. Lubricate hinged instruments using a steam-penetrable lubricant as follows:
a. Apply the lubricant to a hinged instrument in its open position.
b. Open and close the instrument after applying the lubricant so it reaches all parts of the hinged area.
c. Place the instrument back on the towel and allow it to drain. Rinsing or wiping is unnecessary.
Principle. Lubricating an instrument makes it function better and last longer.

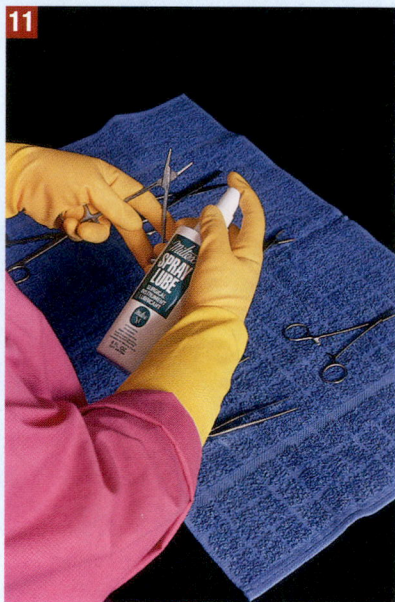

11

Lubricate hinged instruments.

12. Procedural Step. Dispose of the cleaning solution according to the manufacturer's instructions. Remove both sets of gloves, and sanitize your hands.

13. Procedural Step. Wrap the instruments and sterilize them in the autoclave according to the medical office policy.

DISINFECTION

Disinfection is the process of destroying pathogenic microorganisms, but it does not kill bacterial spores. Disinfection is accomplished in the medical office through the use of liquid chemical agents that are applied to inanimate objects. Chemical disinfection has been discussed with respect to its role in the sanitization process to decontaminate surgical instruments and make them safe to handle. This section discusses the use of chemical disinfection to disinfect semicritical and noncritical items so they can be used for patient care.

Table 18-1 lists disinfectants most frequently used in the medical office, along with common names and uses for each.

LEVELS OF DISINFECTION

Based on killing action, disinfection can be classified according to three levels.

High-Level Disinfection

High-level disinfection is a process that destroys all microorganisms with the exception of bacterial spores. High-level disinfection is used to disinfect semicritical items. A semicritical item is an item that comes in contact with nonintact skin or intact mucous membranes, such as a flexible fiberoptic sigmoidoscope. A frequently used high-level disinfectant is 2% glutaraldehyde (e.g., Cidex, MetriCide). A high-level disinfectant that is growing in popularity is Cidex OPA (*ortho*-phthalaldehyde). Cidex OPA does not contain glutaraldehyde, which means it is less toxic and is safer to handle.

Intermediate-Level Disinfection

Intermediate-level disinfection is a process that inactivates tubercle bacilli (the causative agents of tuberculosis), all vegetative bacteria, most viruses, and most fungi, but it does not kill bacterial spores. Intermediate-level disinfection is used to disinfect noncritical items. **Noncritical items** are items that come in contact with intact skin but not with mucous membranes, including stethoscopes, blood pressure cuffs, tuning forks, percussion hammers, and crutches. A common intermediate-level disinfectant is isopropyl alcohol, which is frequently used in the form of alcohol wipes.

Low-Level Disinfection

Low-level disinfection is a process that kills most bacteria, some viruses, and some fungi, but it cannot be relied on to

Table 18-1	Disinfectants Used in the Medical Office	
Disinfectant	**Common Names**	**Use in the Medical Office**
Glutaraldehyde	Cidex MetriCide ProCide Omnicide Wavicide	Disinfection of flexible fiberoptic sigmoidoscopes.
Alcohol	Isopropyl alcohol	Disinfection of stethoscopes, blood pressure cuffs, tuning forks, and percussion hammers; isopropyl alcohol wipes are used to disinfect rubber stoppers of multiple-dose medication vials.
Chlorine and chlorine compounds	Sodium hypochlorite (household bleach)	Recommended by OSHA for decontamination of blood spills.
Phenolics	Carbolic acid Hydroxybenzene Phenic acid Phenyl hydroxide Phenylic acid	Disinfection of walls, furniture, floors, and laboratory work surfaces.
Quaternary ammonium compounds	Benzalkonium chloride	Disinfection of walls, furniture, floors, and laboratory work surfaces.

OSHA, Occupational Safety and Health Administration.

What Would You Do? | What Would You *Not* Do?

Case Study 2

Alecia Scout brings in her 2-year-old son, Benjamin, for a preschool physical examination. Benjamin is very unhappy and is crying loudly. Mrs. Scout says that Benjamin is upset because she wouldn't let him play with the toys in the waiting room. She is afraid that he will catch a disease from a sick child who has played with the toys. Mrs. Scout is visibly annoyed and says that medical offices should not keep toys in the waiting room because they might spread disease and cause problems for parents who do not want their children to play with the toys. ■

Memories *from* Practicum

Kara VanDyke: During my practicum experience, I was placed in a pediatrician's office. I wanted to go to a pediatric site because I love being around children. One day I was in the examining room with my patient, a 4-year-old boy who was there with his mother. It was standard procedure at this office to take every patient's temperature. I started getting out our electronic thermometer to take his temperature when I noticed he looked a little frightened. He was looking at the thermometer funny, and he said, "Can you do it in my ear?" I said I was sorry but we didn't have that kind of thermometer. I told him I could do it under his arm or under his tongue. His mom looked at him, and he said, "But I want it in my ear." He finally agreed to let me do it under his arm. When I was finished taking his temperature, he smiled and said, "You are so nice!" ■

kill resistant microorganisms, such as tubercle bacilli, and it cannot kill bacterial spores. Low-level disinfectants typically are used to disinfect surfaces such as examining tables, laboratory countertops, and walls. Low-level disinfectants used in the medical office include sodium hypochlorite (household bleach) and phenolics.

Items Sterilized in the Autoclave	
Surgical instruments	Brushes
Medical instruments	Dressings
Minor office surgery trays	Glassware
Liquids	Reusable syringes

STERILIZATION

Sterilization is the process of destroying all forms of microbial life, including bacterial spores. An item that is sterile is free of all living microorganisms and spores. Sterilization must be used to process all critical items. A **critical item** is an item that comes in contact with sterile tissue or the vascular system.

As previously described, a semicritical item (one that comes in contact with nonintact skin or with intact mucous membranes) can be chemically disinfected with a high-level disinfectant. Most offices prefer instead to sterilize semicritical items (e.g., vaginal specula, nasal specula) in the autoclave. The autoclave provides a convenient, efficient, safe, and inexpensive method for destroying microorganisms. Chemical disinfectants not only are more expensive to use, but also are more hazardous and create problems regarding their proper disposal. The exception is any semicritical item that is heat sensitive. Flexible fiberoptic sigmoidoscopes would be damaged by the heat of an autoclave and must be chemically disinfected.

STERILIZATION METHODS

Sterilization involves the use of physical or chemical methods. Each method of sterilization has advantages and disadvantages. The method used to achieve sterility depends primarily on the nature of the item to be sterilized. The most common physical and chemical sterilization methods include the following:

Physical Methods	Chemical Methods
Steam under pressure (autoclave)	Ethylene oxide gas
Hot air (dry heat oven)	Cold sterilization (chemical agents)
Radiation	

The most common method for sterilizing articles in the medical office is steam under pressure using an autoclave. The autoclave is discussed in detail in this chapter; the other methods of sterilization are briefly described.

AUTOCLAVE

The autoclave is dependable, efficient, and economical and can be used to sterilize items that are not harmed by moisture or high temperature. Refer to the box *Items Sterilized in the Autoclave* for a list of heat-resistant items that can be sterilized in the autoclave.

An **autoclave** consists of an outer jacket surrounding an inner sterilizing chamber. Under pressure, distilled water is converted to steam, which fills the inner sterilizing chamber. The pressure plays no direct part in killing microorganisms; rather, it functions to attain a higher temperature than could be reached by the steam from boiling water (212°F [100°C]). The cooler, drier air already in the chamber is forced out through the air exhaust valve.

It is important that all the air in the chamber be replaced by steam. When air is present, the temperature in the autoclave is reduced, and a temperature that is adequate for sterilization is not reached. When all the air has been removed, the air exhaust valve seals off the inner chamber, and the temperature in the autoclave begins to increase.

During the sterilization process, the steam penetrates the materials in the sterilizing chamber. The materials are cooler, so the steam condenses into moisture on them, giving up its heat. This heat serves to kill all microorganisms and their spores.

The autoclave is usually operated at approximately 15 pounds of pressure per square inch (psi) at a temperature of 250°F (121°C). Vegetative forms of most microorganisms are killed in a few minutes at temperatures ranging from 130°F to 150°F (54°C to 65°C), but certain bacterial spores can withstand a temperature of 240°F (115°C) for longer than 3 hours. No organism, however, can survive direct exposure to saturated steam at 250°F (121°C) for 15 minutes or longer.

The sterilization process using the autoclave is discussed in this section (with the exception of sanitization, which was already presented). The sterilization process consists of the following components:
- Monitoring program
- Sanitizing articles
- Wrapping articles
- Operating the autoclave (autoclave cycle)
- Handling and storing packs
- Maintaining the autoclave

Monitoring Program

To ensure that instruments and supplies are sterile when used, the Centers for Disease Control and Prevention (CDC) recommends that the medical office establish and maintain a monitoring program of the sterilization process. The monitoring program should consist of the following:
1. Written policies and procedures for each step of the sterilization process

AUTOCLAVE LOG						
Date/Time	Description of the Load	Cycle Time (min)	Temperature (°F)	Indicator* (+/−)	Initials	Comments
7/25/XX 4:00 PM	Surgical instruments	20	250	−	KV	
7/26/XX 3:00 PM	MOS tray setups	30	250	−	KV	

*Indicator Interpretation:
Positive (+): Spores not killed, indicating sterilization conditions have not been met.
Negative (−): Spores killed, indicating sterilization conditions have been met.

MAINTENANCE: (Indicate date, vendor name, service, etc.)

Figure 18-8 Example of an autoclave log.

2. Sterilization indicators to ensure that minimum sterilizing conditions have been achieved
3. Records for each cycle, maintained in an autoclave log (see Figure 18-8)

The information that should be recorded for each autoclave cycle includes the following:
- Date and time of the cycle
- Description of the load
- Exposure time
- Exposure temperature
- Results of the sterilization indicator
- Initials of the operator

Some autoclaves have recorders that automatically print out a portion of this information at the end of the cycle (Figure 18-9).

Sterilization Indicators

Materials that are being sterilized must be exposed to steam at a sufficient temperature and for a proper length of time. Sterilization indicators are available to determine the effectiveness of the procedure and to check against improper wrapping of articles, improper loading of the autoclave, and faulty operation of the autoclave.

An article is not considered sterile unless the steam has penetrated to its center; most sterilization indicators are placed in the center of the pack. The medical assistant should carefully read the instructions that come with the sterilization indicators. The most reliable indicators check for the attainment of the proper temperature and indicate the duration of the temperature.

If an indicator does not change properly, a problem may be present in the sterilization technique or in the working condition of the autoclave. The manufacturer's guidelines for proper sterilization techniques should be reviewed, and the articles should be resterilized, following these guidelines. If the indicator still does not change properly, the autoclave is in need of repair and should not be used until it has been serviced.

READY			
BEGIN			
SET TEMP:	270 F		Temperature
SET TIME:	015	←	Time
RUN #	011	←	Cycle number
DATE	7/25/XX		

HEAT UP			
DEG	PSI	MIN	
066	00.0	000	
066	00.0	002	
074	00.0	004	Heat-up phase
164	00.0	006	
219	04.1	008	
234	09.4	010	
261	22.6	012	

STERILIZE			
DEG	PSI	MIN	
272	30.2	000	
272	30.7	001	
273	31.3	002	
274	31.0	003	
273	30.7	004	
273	30.4	005	
273	30.1	006	
272	30.0	007	Sterilization phase
272	30.1	008	
272	30.4	009	
272	30.4	010	
272	30.7	011	
273	31.0	012	
273	30.8	013	
274	31.0	014	
273	30.7	015	

VENT			
COMPLETE			

Figure 18-9 Example of a printout of an autoclave cycle.

Sterilization indicators should be stored in a cool, dry area. Excessive heat or moisture can damage the indicator. The most common sterilization indicators are chemical indicators and biologic indicators, which are described next.

Figure 18-10 Autoclave tape. *Top*, Autoclave tape as it appears before the sterilization process. *Bottom*, Diagonal lines appear on the tape during autoclaving and indicate that the wrapped article has been autoclaved.

Chemical Indicators

Chemical indicators are impregnated with a **thermolabile** dye that changes color when exposed to the sterilization process. If the chemical reaction of the indicator does not show the expected results, the item may not be sterile and must be resterilized. Chemical indicators include autoclave tape and sterilization strips.

Autoclave Tape

Autoclave tape contains a chemical that changes color if it has been exposed to steam. The tape is available in a variety of colors, can be written on, and is useful for closing and identifying the wrapped article (Figure 18-10). Autoclave tape has some limitations as an indicator. Because it is placed on the outside of the pack, it cannot ensure that steam has penetrated to the center of the pack. It also does not ensure that the item has been sterilized; it merely indicates that an article has been in the autoclave and that a high temperature has been attained.

Sterilization Strips

Sterilization strips are commercially prepared paper or plastic strips that contain a thermolabile dye and that change color when exposed to steam under pressure for a certain length of time (Figure 18-11). Most sterilization strips are designed to change color after being exposed to a temperature of 250° F (121° C) for 15 minutes. The indicator strip should be placed in the center of the wrapped pack, with the end containing the dye placed in an area of the pack considered to be the hardest for steam to penetrate.

Biologic Indicators

Biologic indicators are the best means available for determining the effectiveness of the sterilization procedure. The CDC recommends that medical office personnel use a biologic indicator to monitor all autoclaves at least once a week.

A biologic indicator is a preparation of living bacterial spores. Biologic indicators are commercially available in the form of dry spore strips in small glassine envelopes. Biologic monitoring of an autoclave requires the use of a preparation

Figure 18-11 Sterilization strips. Sterilization strips contain a thermolabile dye and change color when exposed to steam under pressure for a certain length of time.

Figure 18-12 Biologic indicator. A biologic indicator includes two spore tests that are sterilized *(top right)* and one spore control that is not sterilized *(bottom right)*.

of spores of *Geobacillus stearothermophilus,* which is a microorganism whose spores are particularly resistant to moist heat and are not harmful to humans.

Each biologic testing unit includes two spore tests that are sterilized and one spore control that is not sterilized (Figure 18-12). The biologic indicator is placed in the center of two wrapped articles. The articles are placed in areas of the autoclave that are the least accessible to steam penetration, such as on the bottom tray of the autoclave, near the front of the autoclave, and in the back of the autoclave.

After the indicators have been exposed to sterilization conditions, they must be processed before the results can be obtained. The two methods for processing results are the in-house method and the mail-in method.

In-House Method

The in-house method involves processing and interpreting the results at the medical office. After sterilization, the processed spores are incubated for 24 to 48 hours. If sterilization conditions have been met, the color or condition of

Figure 18-13 Sterilization paper wraps. Sterilization paper consists of square sheets of paper that are available in different sizes.

the processed spores is different from those of the control, and the spore test result is interpreted as negative. If sterilization conditions have not been met, the processed spores and the unprocessed control display the same color or condition, and the spore test result is interpreted as positive.

Mail-in Method

With this method, the processed bacterial spores and the (unprocessed) control are mailed to a processing laboratory. The test is performed by the laboratory, and the results are returned to the medical office.

If spores are not killed in routine spore tests, the autoclave should be checked immediately for proper use and function, and the spore test should be repeated. If the spore test result remains positive, the autoclave should not be used until it is serviced.

Wrapping Articles

Articles to be sterilized in the autoclave first must be thoroughly sanitized (see Procedure 18-1). Next, the articles are prepared for autoclaving by wrapping them. The purpose of wrapping articles is to protect them from recontamination during handling and storage. Articles that are wrapped and handled correctly remain sterile after autoclaving until the package seal is broken.

The wrapping material should be made of a substance that is not affected by the sterilization process and should allow steam to penetrate while preventing contaminants, such as dust, insects, and microorganisms, from entering during handling and storage. It should not tear or puncture easily and should allow the sterilized package to be opened without contamination of the contents. A wrapper should not be used if it is torn or has a hole. Examples of wrapping materials used for autoclaving are sterilization paper, sterilization pouches, and muslin.

Sterilization Paper

Sterilization paper is a disposable and inexpensive wrapping material. It consists of square sheets of paper of different sizes (Figure 18-13). The most common sizes (in inches) are 12 × 12, 15 × 15, 18 × 18, 24 × 24, 30 × 30, and 36 × 36.

Articles must be wrapped in such a way that they do not become contaminated when the pack is opened. The proper method for wrapping instruments using sterilization paper is outlined in Procedure 18-2. This method of wrapping can be used for all types of instruments and supplies.

The disadvantage of sterilization paper is that it is difficult to spread open for removal of the contents. It has a "memory" and tends to flip back easily, so it may not open flat to provide a sterile field. (*Memory* is the ability of a material to retain a specific shape or configuration.) Because sterilization paper is opaque, it is impossible to view the contents of a pack before opening it.

Sterilization Pouches

Sterilization pouches typically consist of a combination of paper and plastic; paper makes up one side of the pouch, and a plastic film makes up the other side (Figure 18-14). Sterilization pouches are available in different sizes; the most common sizes (in inches) are 3×9, 5×10, and 7×12.

Most pouches have a peel-apart seal on one end that is used later to open the pouch for removal of the sterile item. The other end of the pouch is open and is used to insert the item into the pouch. When the article has been inserted, this end is sealed with heat or adhesive tape. The proper

---

PROCEDURE 18-2   Wrapping Instruments Using Paper or Muslin

Outcome Wrap an instrument for autoclaving.

Equipment/Supplies

- Sanitized instrument
- Appropriate-sized wrapping material (sterilization paper or muslin)

- Sterilization indicator strip
- Autoclave tape
- Permanent marker

1. **Procedural Step.** Sanitize your hands.
2. **Procedural Step.** Assemble the equipment. Select the appropriate-sized wrapping material for the instrument being wrapped. Check the expiration date on the sterilization indicator box. If the sterilization strips are outdated, do not use them.
   Principle. Instruments are wrapped so they are protected from recontamination after they have been sterilized. Outdated strip indicators may not provide accurate test results.
3. **Procedural Step.** Place the wrapping material on a clean, flat surface. Turn the wrap in a diagonal position to your body so that it resembles a diamond shape.

4. **Procedural Step.** Place the instrument in the center of the wrapping material with the longest part of the instrument pointing toward the two side corners. If the instrument has a movable joint, place it on the wrap in a slightly open position. If necessary, a gauze square can be used to hold the instrument in an open position.
   Principle. Instruments with movable joints must be in an open position to allow steam to reach all parts of the instrument. If the instrument is in a closed position, heat exposure could cause the instrument to crack at its weakest part, such as the lock area.
5. **Procedural Step.** Place a sterilization indicator in the center of the pack next to the instrument.
   Principle. Sterilization indicators assess the effectiveness of the sterilization process.

Turn the wrap in a diagonal position.

Place a sterilization indicator in the center of the pack next to the instrument.

PROCEDURE 18-2 Wrapping Instruments Using Paper or Muslin—cont'd

6. Procedural Step. Fold the wrapping material up from the bottom, and double-back a small corner, creating a flap. This flap will later be used to open the sterile pack without contaminating the instrument.

Fold the wrapping material up from the bottom, and double-back a small corner.

7. Procedural Step. Fold over one edge of the wrapping material, and double-back the corner.

8. Procedural Step. Fold over the other edge of the wrapping material, and double-back the corner.

Fold over the other edge of the wrapping material, and double-back the corner.

9. Procedural Step. Fold the pack up from the bottom, pull the top flap down, and secure it with autoclave tape. Ensure that the pack is firm enough for handling but loose enough to permit proper circulation of steam.

Principle. Instruments must be wrapped properly to permit full penetration of steam and to prevent contaminating them when the wrap is opened. Using autoclave tape indicates that the pack has been through the autoclave cycle and prevents mix-ups with packs that have not been processed.

Fold the pack up from the bottom.

10. Procedural Step. Label the pack according to its contents. Mark the pack with the date of sterilization and your initials.

Principle. Dating the pack helps in ensuring that the most recently sterilized packs are stored behind previously sterilized packs.

Label and date the pack. Include your initials.

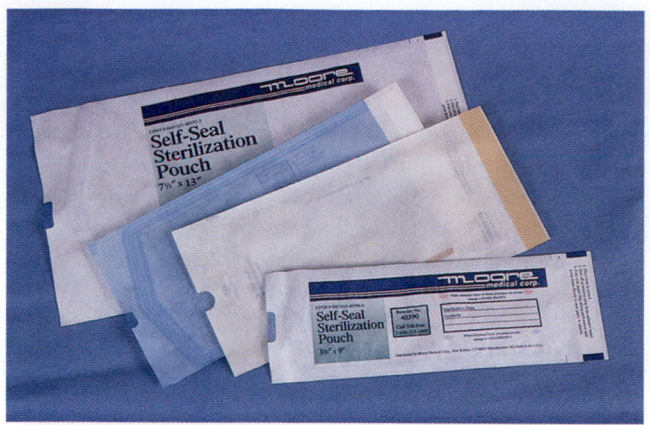

Figure 18-14 Sterilization pouches. Sterilization pouches consist of a combination of paper and plastic and are available in different sizes.

method for wrapping an instrument by using a pouch is outlined in Procedure 18-3.

Sterilization pouches provide good visibility of the contents on the plastic side. Most manufacturers include a sterilization indicator on the outside of the pouch. After removing a pouch from the autoclave, the medical assistant should check the indicator for the proper color change. If the indicator does not change to the appropriate color (as specified by the manufacturer), the contents of the pouch must be resterilized.

Muslin

Muslin is a reusable woven fabric that is available in different sizes. Muslin is flexible and easy to handle and is considered the most economical sterilization wrap because it can be reused. Because of its durability, muslin is frequently used to wrap large packs, such as tray setups for minor office surgery. Muslin is "memory free," so it lies flat when opened. A pack wrapped in muslin may be opened on a table so that the wrapper becomes a sterile field. The procedure for wrapping an article with muslin is the same as that for sterilization paper (see Procedure 18-2).

Operating the Autoclave

The autoclave must be operated according to the manufacturer's instructions. The medical assistant should read the operating manual carefully before running the autoclave for the first time. Thereafter, the manual should be kept in an accessible location so that it is available if needed as a reference. Procedure 18-4 outlines a general procedure for sterilizing articles in the autoclave.

The steps involved in achieving sterilization using an autoclave are known as the *autoclave cycle*. Accomplishment of each step varies based on whether the autoclave is operated manually or automatically. Figure 18-15 illustrates the autoclave cycle for manual and automatic autoclave operation.

PROCEDURE 18-3　Wrapping Instruments Using a Pouch　

Outcome Wrap an instrument for autoclaving.

Equipment/Supplies

- Sanitized instrument
- Appropriate-sized sterilization pouch
- Permanent marker

1. **Procedural Step.** Sanitize your hands.
2. **Procedural Step.** Assemble the equipment. Select the appropriate-sized sterilization pouch for the instrument being wrapped. For hinged instruments, use a bag wide enough so the instrument can be placed in a slightly open position inside the bag.
   Principle. Instruments are wrapped so they are protected from recontamination after they have been sterilized.
3. **Procedural Step.** Place the sterilization pouch on a clean, flat surface.
4. **Procedural Step.** Label the pack according to its contents. Mark the pack with the date of sterilization and your initials.
   Principle. Dating the pack helps in ensuring that the most recently sterilized packs are stored behind previously sterilized packs.

Label and date the pack. Include your initials.

PROCEDURE 18-3   Wrapping Instruments Using a Pouch—cont'd

5. Procedural Step. Insert the instrument to be sterilized into the unsealed, open end of the pouch. If the instrument has a movable joint, place it in the pouch in a slightly open position.

Insert the instrument into the pouch.

6. Procedural Step. Seal the open end of the pouch as follows:

Adhesive Closure. Peel off the paper strip located above the perforation to expose the adhesive. Fold along the perforation and press firmly to seal the paper to the plastic. Ensure that the seal is secure by running your fingers back and forth on both sides of the pouch over the entire sealing area.

Heat Closure. Seal the pouch using a heat-sealing device.

Peel off the paper strip.

Press firmly to seal the pack.

7. Procedural Step. Sterilize the pack in the autoclave.

Guidelines for Autoclave Operation
Location of the Autoclave

The autoclave must be placed on a level surface to ensure that the chamber fills correctly. The front of the autoclave should be near the front of the support surface so that water can be easily drained from the drain tube into a container when the autoclave is being flushed.

Filling the Water Reservoir

Distilled water is used to fill the water reservoir of the autoclave. Normal tap water contains minerals, such as chlorine, which have corrosive effects on the stainless-steel chamber of the autoclave. In addition, using tap water may cause a mineral buildup that can block the air exhaust valve. This causes air pockets, which prevent the temperature from increasing in the autoclave. The water reservoir is filled to the proper level as indicated in the operating manual. An autoclave malfunction may occur if the reservoir is overfilled or if there is not enough water in the reservoir.

Loading the Autoclave

For an item to attain sterility, steam must penetrate every fiber and reach every surface of the item at a required temperature and for a specified time. To accomplish this, all packs must be positioned in the chamber to allow free circulation and penetration of steam. The following guidelines should be followed when loading the autoclave:

1. Small packs are best because steam penetrates them more easily; it takes longer for steam to reach the center of a large pack to ensure sterilization. A pack should be no larger than $12 \times 12 \times 20$ inches.
2. To allow for proper steam penetration, the packs should be packed as loosely as possible inside the autoclave, with approximately 1 to 3 inches between small packs and 2 to 4 inches between large packs. Packs should not be allowed to touch surrounding walls, and at least 1 inch should separate the autoclave trays. Placing the articles too close together retards the flow of steam (Figure 18-16).

AUTOMATIC OPERATION

MANUAL OPERATION

The autoclave is turned on

Set the sterilization program

Press start button

Chamber automatically fills with water

The chamber is filled with water

Fill manually using control

The automatic timer begins a timing countdown

Temperature reaches desired temperature and pressure (usually 250° F, 15 lb pressure)

Set timer using control

Packs are subjected to steam at a specified temperature and duration of time

Autoclave automatically vents

Steam is vented from the chamber

Manually vent steam using control

Door automatically opens slightly, and audible beep sounds when completed

The load is dried

Crack the door

Set timer for appropriate drying time

Figure 18-15 The autoclave cycle for manual and automatic operation.

Wrong method   Right method

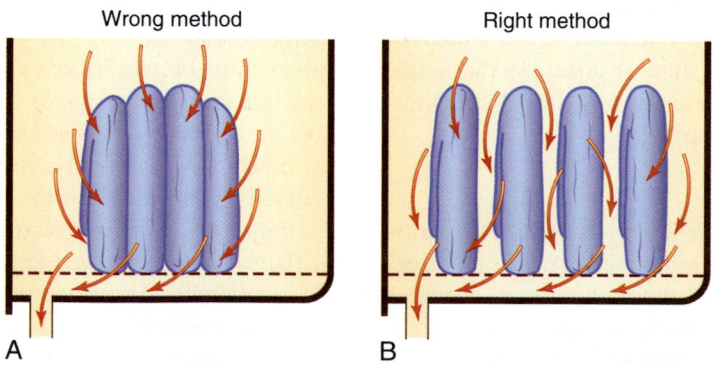

A   B

Figure 18-16 Arrangement of packs in the autoclave. **A,** Improper arrangement of packs in the autoclave. This arrangement prevents adequate penetration of steam, resulting in failure to sterilize the portions in the center of the mass. **B,** Proper arrangement of packs in the autoclave. The packs are separated from each other, and steam can now permeate each pack quickly and in the much shorter period of exposure needed. (Courtesy of and modified from AMSCO/American Sterilizer Company, Erie, Pa.)

Figure 18-17 Jars and glassware should be placed on their sides in the autoclave with their lids removed. (Courtesy AMSCO/American Sterilizer Company, Erie, Pa.)

Table 18-2 Minimum Sterilizing Times

Items (Manual Operation)*	Program (Automatic Operation)†	Time (Min at 250° F [121° C])
Unwrapped nonsurgical instruments	Unwrapped	15
Open glass or metal canisters		
Nonsurgical rubber tubing		
Wrapped instruments	Wrapped	20
Fabric or muslin		
Wrapped trays of loose instruments		
Rubber tubing		
Minor office surgery tray setup (wrapped)	Packs	30
Liquids or gels	Liquids	30

*Manual operation: The sterilizing time is selected on the basis of the items being sterilized, as indicated in this column. The sterilizing time is set by using the manual timing control when the autoclave has reached a temperature of 250° F (121° C).

†Automatic operation: The sterilization program selected from this column is based on the item being autoclaved. This program is selected by pressing the appropriate program button on the front of the autoclave (i.e., unwrapped, wrapped, packs, liquids). The autoclave automatically begins the proper timing countdown when it reaches 250° F (121° C).

3. Jars and glassware should be placed on their sides in the autoclave with their lids removed. If they are placed upright, air may be trapped in them, and they would not be sterilized. Trapped air must flow out and be replaced by steam during the sterilization process (Figure 18-17).
4. Packs that contain layers of fabric, such as dressings, should be placed in a vertical position. Because steam flows from top to bottom, this method allows the steam to penetrate the layers of fabric.
5. Sterilization pouches should be positioned on their sides to maximize steam circulation and to facilitate the drying process. Pouches can also be placed on the autoclave tray with the paper side up and the plastic side down.

Timing the Load

The autoclave is operated at approximately 15 psi with a temperature of 250° F (121° C). The length of time required for sterilization varies according to the item that is being sterilized (Table 18-2). Steam can easily reach the surfaces of hard, nonporous items such as unwrapped instruments (e.g., vaginal specula) to kill microorganisms; these items require approximately 15 minutes of sterilization time. A large minor office surgery pack requires a longer sterilization time, about 30 minutes, because more time is needed for steam to penetrate to the center of the pack. Rubber goods may be damaged, however, by exposure to excessive heat. To prevent this, the medical assistant should sterilize rubber items for only the prescribed length of time.

The sterilizing time should not begin until the desired temperature in the autoclave has been reached. Timing the load is accomplished automatically or manually. Autoclaves with automatic operation begin timing the load automatically when the desired temperature has been reached. With the manual method of operation, the medical assistant must set the timer by hand using a timing control on the front of the autoclave. The medical assistant should not set the timer until the temperature gauge has reached the desired temperature. The articles in the load are not considered sterile unless they have been subjected to steam for the proper length of time at the proper temperature.

Drying the Load

The sterilized articles are moist and must be allowed to dry before they are removed from the autoclave. Microorganisms can move quickly through the moisture on a wet wrap and onto the sterile article inside, resulting in contamination.

When the load has been subjected to steam for the proper length of time and temperature, the chamber must be vented of steam. Venting the chamber permits the pressure in the autoclave to decrease to zero and the chamber to cool, making it safe for the door to be opened. Most autoclaves are designed to vent automatically, which eliminates having to vent them manually.

The door of the autoclave should be opened approximately ½ inch but no more than 1 inch. Opening the door more than 1 inch causes cold air from the outside to rush into the autoclave, resulting in condensation of water on the packs. Cracking the door allows the moisture on the articles to change from a liquid to a vapor and to escape through the crack. The residual heat in the inner chamber also helps to dry the articles. The load should be allowed to dry for 15 to 60 minutes, depending on the type of autoclave and the load. Loads that contain large packs require a longer drying time than loads with smaller packs. The medical assistant should follow the manufacturer's recommendations for proper drying times of various loads.

Handling and Storing Packs

Sterilized wrapped articles should be handled carefully and as little as possible. If a wrapped article is crushed, compressed, or dropped, the sterility of the contents cannot be assumed, and the pack must be resterilized. This is known as *event-related sterility*, meaning that a sterile pack is considered sterile indefinitely unless an event occurs that interferes with the sterility of the article.

Sterilized packs should be stored in clean, dry areas that are free from dust, insects, and other sources of contamination. Wrapped articles should be stored with the most recently sterilized articles placed in the back. The medical assistant should thoroughly check each sterilized pack at least twice: before storing it and before using it. If the pack is torn or opened or if it is wet, it is no longer sterile and must be rewrapped and resterilized.

Maintaining the Autoclave

For the autoclave to work efficiently, it must be maintained properly. The operating manual that accompanies the autoclave provides specific information for the care and maintenance of that type of autoclave.

Safety precautions should be followed when performing maintenance procedures. Before proceeding with preventive maintenance, the autoclave must be cool, the pressure gauge at zero, and the power cord disconnected from the wall socket. Autoclave maintenance is performed on a daily, weekly, and monthly basis as follows.

Daily Maintenance

1. Wipe the outside of the autoclave with a damp cloth and a mild detergent.
2. Wipe the interior of the autoclave and the trays with a damp cloth.
3. Clean the rubber gasket on the door of the autoclave with a damp cloth.
4. Inspect the rubber door gasket for damage that could prevent a good seal.

Weekly Maintenance

1. Wash the inside of the chamber and the trays with a commercial autoclave cleaner according to the manufacturer's instructions, while observing all personal safety precautions. This usually involves the following steps: The water reservoir must be drained first. A soft cloth or a soft brush should be used to clean the chamber. Do not use steel wool, a steel brush, or other abrasive agents because they can damage the chamber. When the chamber is clean, it should be rinsed thoroughly with distilled water. The chamber must be dried thoroughly and the door left open overnight.
2. Wash the metal shelves with an autoclave cleaner, and rinse them thoroughly with distilled water.

Monthly Maintenance

1. Flush the system to remove any buildup of residue, which could cause corrosion of the chamber lines. Carefully follow the manufacturer's directions in the instruction manual to perform this procedure.
2. Check the air trap jet to ensure it is functioning properly. The air trap jet prevents air pockets from occurring in the chamber, to ensure adequate sterilization.
3. Check the safety valve to ensure it is functioning properly. The safety valve releases pressure in the chamber if it gets too high.

OTHER STERILIZATION METHODS

In addition to the autoclave, other methods can be used to sterilize articles. These methods are not usually used in the medical office and are discussed only briefly in this chapter.

Dry Heat Oven

Dry heat ovens are used to sterilize articles that cannot be penetrated by steam or may be damaged by it. Dry heat is less corrosive than moist heat for instruments with sharp edges; it does not dull their sharp edges. Oil, petroleum jelly, and powder cannot be penetrated by steam and must be sterilized in a dry heat oven. Moist heat sterilization tends to erode the ground-glass surfaces of reusable syringes, whereas dry heat does not.

Dry heat ovens operate similarly to ordinary cooking ovens. A longer exposure period is needed with dry heat because microorganisms and spores are more resistant to dry heat than to moist heat and because dry heat penetrates more slowly and unevenly than moist heat. The most commonly used temperature for dry heat sterilization is 320° F (160° C) for 1 to 2 hours, depending on the article being sterilized. The recommended wrapping material for dry heat sterilization is aluminum foil because it is a good conductor of heat, and it protects against recontamination during handling and storage. Dry heat sterilization indicators are available to determine the effectiveness of the sterilization process.

Ethylene Oxide Gas Sterilization

Ethylene oxide is a colorless gas that is toxic and flammable. It is used to sterilize heat-sensitive items that cannot be sterilized in an autoclave. After items are sterilized with this gas, they must be aerated to remove the toxic residue of the ethylene oxide.

Ethylene oxide sterilization is a more complex and expensive process than steam sterilization. It frequently is used in the medical manufacturing industry for producing prepackaged, presterilized disposable items, such as syringes, sutures, catheters, and surgical packs.

Cold Sterilization

Cold sterilization involves the use of a chemical agent for an extended length of time. Only chemicals that are designated *sterilants* by the U.S. Environmental Protection

Agency (EPA) can be used for sterilizing articles. If a chemical agent holds this status, the word *sterilant* is printed on the front of the container.

The item to be sterilized must be completely submerged in the chemical for a long time (6 to 24 hours depending on the manufacturer's instructions). Prolonged immersion of instruments can damage them. In addition, each time an instrument is added to the instrument container, the clock must be restarted for the entire amount of time. For these reasons, and because this method involves the use of a hazardous chemical, cold sterilization should be used only when an autoclave, gas, or a dry heat oven is not indicated or is unavailable.

Radiation

Radiation uses high-energy ionizing radiation to sterilize articles. Medical manufacturers use radiation to sterilize prepackaged surgical equipment and instruments that cannot be sterilized by heat or chemicals.

PROCEDURE 18-4   Sterilizing Articles in the Autoclave

Outcome Sterilize a load of contaminated articles in the autoclave.

Equipment/Supplies

- Autoclave and instruction manual
- Distilled water
- Wrapped articles
- Heat-resistant gloves

---

1. **Procedural Step.** Assemble the equipment.
2. **Procedural Step.** Check the level of water in the autoclave and add distilled water, if needed.
   Principle. Water contained in the water reservoir of the autoclave is converted to steam during the sterilization process. Distilled water is used to prevent corrosion of the stainless-steel chamber of the autoclave.

If needed, add distilled water to the autoclave.

3. **Procedural Step.** Properly load the autoclave while following these guidelines:
   a. Do not overload the chamber. Small packs should be placed 1 to 3 inches apart, and large packs should be placed 2 to 4 inches apart. The packs should not touch the chamber walls.
   b. Ensure that at least 1 inch separates the autoclave trays.
   c. Place jars and glassware on their sides.

   d. Place dressings in a vertical position.
   e. When sterilizing dressings and hard goods together, place dressings on the top shelf and hard goods on the lower shelf.
   f. When using sterilization pouches, set the pouches on their sides to maximize steam circulation and to facilitate drying.
   Principle. The autoclave must be loaded properly to ensure adequate steam penetration of all articles.

Properly load the autoclave.

4. **Procedural Step.** Operate the autoclave according to the procedure described in the instruction manual. A general procedure for the manual and the automatic methods of operation follows.

Manually Operated Autoclave

   a. Determine the sterilizing time for the types of articles being autoclaved (see Table 18-2).
   b. Turn on the autoclave.

Continued

PROCEDURE 18-4   Sterilizing Articles in the Autoclave—cont'd

c. Fill the chamber with water using the appropriate control.

d. Securely close and latch the door of the autoclave.

e. Set the timing control when the temperature gauge reaches the desired temperature (usually 250°F [121°C]). At the end of the steam exposure time, an indicator light usually comes on or a beeper sounds.

Set the timing control.

f. If the autoclave does not vent automatically, use the appropriate control to release steam from the chamber.

g. Dry the load by cracking open the door approximately ½ inch but no more than 1 inch. Set the drying time using the timing control. The drying time varies between 15 and 60 minutes, depending on the autoclave and the type of load.

Principle. To ensure sterilization, the load should not be timed until the proper temperature has been reached. The sterility of wrapped packs cannot be ensured unless the wrapped articles are allowed to dry fully. Microorganisms can move through the moisture on a wet wrap and contaminate the sterile article inside.

Crack the door to dry the load.

Automatically Operated Autoclave

a. Securely close and latch the door of the autoclave.

b. Turn on the autoclave.

c. Determine the sterilization program according to what is being autoclaved (see Table 18-2). Press the appropriate program button on the front of the autoclave to select the program. Press the start button.

d. Indicators on the front of the autoclave tell you what is happening (automatically) in the autoclave:

Filling Indicator. Lights up when the chamber is filling with water

Sterilizing Indicator. Lights up during the heat-up and sterilization phases of the cycle

Temperature Display. Digital display of the temperature in the autoclave

Time Display. Digital countdown of the time remaining in the sterilization program

Drying Indicator. Lights up during the drying phase of the cycle

Complete or Ready Indicator. Illuminates when the autoclave has completed the cycle and sterilized articles can be removed from the autoclave

Automatic autoclave buttons and indicators.

5. Procedural Step. Turn off the autoclave. Wearing heat-resistant gloves, remove the load. Do not touch the inner chamber of the autoclave with your bare hands.

Principle. Heat-resistant gloves protect the medical assistant's hands when the warm packs from the chamber of the autoclave are being removed. The inner chamber of the autoclave is hot and could burn bare skin.

PROCEDURE 18-4   Sterilizing Articles in the Autoclave—cont'd

PROCEDURE 18-4

Remove the load with heat-resistant gloves.

6. Procedural Step. Inspect the packs as you take them out of the autoclave. If the packs show any damage, such as holes or tears, the articles should be rewrapped and resterilized.

7. Procedural Step. Check the sterilization indicators located on the outside of the pack to ensure the proper response has occurred.
Principle. Autoclave tape indicates only that the article has been through the autoclave cycle; it does not ensure that sterilization has taken place. Sterilization is confirmed when the pack is opened for use and the sterilization strip indicator in the center of the pack is checked for its proper response.

Check the sterilization indicator on the outside of the pack.

8. Procedural Step. Record monitoring information in the autoclave log. Include the date and time of the cycle, a description of the load, and the exposure time and temperature. If a biologic indicator has been included in the load, process it according to the medical office policy, and record results on the autoclave log.

9. Procedural Step. Store the packs in a clean, dustproof area with the most recently sterilized packs placed behind previously sterilized packs.

10. Procedural Step. Maintain appropriate daily care of the autoclave, following the manufacturer's recommendations. Daily care of the autoclave includes the following:
a. Wipe the outside of the autoclave with a damp cloth and a mild detergent.
b. Wipe the interior of the autoclave and the trays with a damp cloth.
c. Clean the rubber gasket located on the door of the autoclave with a damp cloth.
d. Inspect the rubber door gasket for damage that could prevent a good seal.
Principle. For the autoclave to work efficiently, it must be properly maintained.

Clean the rubber gasket with a damp cloth.

What Would You Do? What Would You *Not* Do? RESPONSES

Case Study 1
Page 325

What Did Kara Do?
❑ Complimented Mrs. Cordera for her concern and efforts to baby-proof her home.
❑ Gave Mrs. Cordera a patient information brochure on baby-proofing the home.
❑ Told Mrs. Cordera that she should assume that all cleaning products are poisonous. Got out a disinfectant container to show Mrs. Cordera the information on the label that tells what to do in case of an accidental poisoning.
❑ Gave the Poison Help Line number (1-800-222-1222) to Mrs. Cordera and told her that was the fastest way to obtain information on what to do in case of an accidental poisoning. Told her to keep this number by her phone.

What Did Kara Not Do?
❑ Did not take Mrs. Cordera's question lightly.

Case Study 2
Page 333

What Did Kara Do?
❑ Explained to Mrs. Scout that toys are in the waiting room for children to play with to make their visit more comfortable and less stressful.
❑ Reassured Mrs. Scout that the medical office personnel do everything they can to prevent the spread of germs in the office and that the toys are sanitized every day.
❑ Relayed to Mrs. Scout that only toys that can be sanitized are kept in the medical office.

❑ Told Mrs. Scout that her concern would be brought up at the weekly office meeting.

What Did Kara Not Do?
❑ Did not get defensive because Mrs Scout was just being concerned about her child's health.

Case Study 3
Page 336

What Did Kara Do?
❑ Told Cassie through verbal and nonverbal behavior that her concern was valid.
❑ Told Cassie that hepatitis C can be transmitted through dirty instruments.
❑ Reassured Cassie that all instruments are sterilized in the autoclave, which has special indicators to ensure all germs have been killed.
❑ Gave Cassie a patient information brochure on hepatitis C. Told her that individuals with chronic hepatitis C can develop liver cancer and that the best way to avoid hepatitis C is through measures and behaviors recommended for prevention.
❑ Told Cassie that a vaccine is available to prevent hepatitis B, but not hepatitis C.

What Did Kara Not Do?
❑ Did not dismiss Cassie's concern about dirty instruments as unimportant.
❑ Did not overly alarm Cassie about the consequences of chronic hepatitis C.

TERMINOLOGY REVIEW

Autoclave	An apparatus for the sterilization of materials, using steam under pressure.
Critical item	An item that comes in contact with sterile tissue or the vascular system.
Detergent	An agent that cleanses by emulsifying dirt and oil.
Disinfectant	An agent used to destroy pathogenic microorganisms but not their spores. Disinfectants are usually applied to inanimate objects.
Hazardous chemical	Any chemical that is classified as a health or physical hazard, a simple asphyxiant, a combustible dust, a pyrophoric gas, or a hazard not otherwise classified.
Incubate	To provide proper conditions for growth and development.
Load	The articles that are being sterilized.
Noncritical item	An item that comes into contact with intact skin but not with mucous membranes.
Safety data sheet	A sheet that provides information regarding a chemical, its hazards, and measures to take to prevent injury and illness when handling the chemical.
Sanitization	A process to remove organic matter from an article and to reduce the number of microorganisms to a safe level as determined by public health requirements.
Semicritical item	An item that comes into contact with nonintact skin or intact mucous membranes.
Spore	A hard, thick-walled capsule formed by some bacteria that contains only the essential parts of the protoplasm of the bacterial cell.
Sterilization	The process of destroying all forms of microbial life, including bacterial spores.
Thermolabile	Easily affected or changed by heat.

ON THE WEB

For information on infection control in the health care setting:

Centers for Disease Control and Prevention: www.cdc.gov

Environmental Protection Agency: www.epa.gov

National Institute of Environmental Health Sciences: www.niehs.nih.gov

National Institute for Occupational Safety and Health: www.cdc.gov/niosh

Infection Control Today: www.infectioncontroltoday.com

Association for Professionals in Infection Control and Epidemiology: www.apic.org

To locate a safety data sheet:

MSDS-Search: www.msdssearch.com

HazCom: www.hazard.com/msds

19 Vital Signs

LEARNING OBJECTIVES	PROCEDURES

Temperature

1. Define a *vital sign*.
2. Explain the reasons for taking vital signs.
3. Explain how body temperature is maintained.
4. List examples of how heat is produced in the body.
5. List examples of how heat is lost from the body.
6. State the normal body temperature range and the average body temperature.
7. List and explain factors that can cause variation in the body temperature.
8. List and describe the three stages of a fever.
9. List the sites for taking body temperature, and explain why these sites are used.

Measure oral body temperature.
Measure axillary body temperature.
Measure rectal body temperature.
Measure aural body temperature.
Measure temporal artery body temperature.

Pulse

10. Explain the mechanism of pulse.
11. List and explain the factors that affect the pulse rate.
12. Identify a specific use for each of the eight pulse sites.
13. State the normal range of pulse rate for each age group.
14. Explain the difference between pulse rhythm and pulse volume.

Measure radial pulse.
Measure apical pulse.

Respiration

15. Explain the purpose of respiration.
16. State what occurs during inhalation and exhalation.
17. State the normal respiratory rate for each age group.
18. List and explain the factors that affect the respiratory rate.
19. Explain the difference between rhythm and depth of respiration.
20. Describe the character of each of the following abnormal breath sounds: crackles, rhonchi, wheezes, and pleural friction rub.

Measure respiration.

Pulse Oximetry

21. Explain the purpose of pulse oximetry.
22. State the normal oxygen saturation level of a healthy individual.
23. List and describe the functions of the controls, indicators, and displays on a pulse oximeter.
24. Describe the difference between a reusable and a disposable oximeter probe.
25. List and describe factors that may interfere with an accurate pulse oximetry reading.

Perform pulse oximetry.

Blood Pressure

26. Define blood pressure.
27. State the normal range of blood pressure for an adult.
28. List and describe factors that affect the blood pressure.
29. Identify the different parts of a stethoscope and a sphygmomanometer.
30. Identify the Korotkoff sounds.
31. State the advantages and disadvantages of an automatic blood pressure monitor.
32. Explain how to prevent errors in blood pressure measurement.

Measure blood pressure.
Determine systolic pressure by palpation.

CHAPTER OUTLINE

INTRODUCTION TO VITAL SIGNS
TEMPERATURE
Regulation of Body Temperature
Heat Production
Heat Loss
Body Temperature Range
Alterations in Body Temperature
Variations in Body Temperature
Fever
Assessment of Body Temperature
Assessment Sites
Types of Thermometers
PULSE
Mechanism of the Pulse
Factors Affecting Pulse Rate
Pulse Sites
Assessment of Pulse
Pulse Rate
Pulse Rhythm and Volume
RESPIRATION
Mechanism of Respiration
Control of Respiration
Assessment of Respiration

Respiratory Rate
Rhythm and Depth of Respiration
Color of the Patient
Respiratory Abnormalities
Breath Sounds
PULSE OXIMETRY
Assessment of Oxygen Saturation
Mechanism of Action
Interpretation of Results
Purpose of Pulse Oximetry
Components of the Pulse Oximeter
Factors Affecting Pulse Oximetry
Pulse Oximeter Care and Maintenance
BLOOD PRESSURE
Mechanism of Blood Pressure
Interpretation of Blood Pressure
Factors Affecting Blood Pressure
Assessment of Blood Pressure: Manual Method
Stethoscope
Manual Sphygmomanometer
Korotkoff Sounds
Assessment of Blood Pressure: Automatic Method

KEY TERMS

adventitious (ad-ven-TISH-us) sounds
afebrile (uh-FEB-ril)
alveolus (al-VEE-oh-lus)
antecubital (AN-tih-CYOO-bi-tul) space
antipyretic (AN-tih-pye-REH-tik)
aorta (ay-OR-tuh)
apical-radial pulse
apnea (AP-nee-uh)
axilla (aks-ILL-uh)
bounding pulse
bradycardia (BRAY-dee-CAR-dee-uh)
bradypnea (BRAY-dip-NEE-uh)
Celsius (SELL-see-us) scale
conduction (kon-DUK-shun)
convection (kon-VEK-shun)
crisis
cyanosis (sye-an-OH-sus)
diastole (dye-AS-toh-lee)
diastolic (DYE-uh-STOL-ik) pressure
dyspnea (DISP-nee-uh)
dysrhythmia (dis-RITH-mee-uh)

eupnea (YOOP-nee-uh)
exhalation (EKS-hal-AY-shun)
Fahrenheit (FAIR-en-hite) scale
febrile (FEH-bril)
fever
frenulum linguae (FREN-yoo-lum
   LIN-gway)
hyperpnea (HYE-perp-NEE-uh)
hyperpyrexia (HYE-per-pye-REK-see-uh)
hypertension (HYE-per-TEN-shun)
hyperventilation
   (HYE-per-ven-til-AY-shun)
hypopnea (hye-POP-nee-uh)
hypotension (HYE-poe-TEN-shun)
hypothermia (HYE-poe-THER-mee-uh)
hypoxemia (hye-pok-SEE-mee-uh)
hypoxia (hye-POKS-ee-uh)
inhalation (IN-hal-AY-shun)
intercostal (IN-ter-KOS-tul)
Korotkoff (kuh-ROT-kof) sounds
malaise (mal-AYZE)

manometer (man-OM-uh-ter)
meniscus (men-IS-kus)
orthopnea (orth-OP-nee-uh)
pulse deficit
pulse oximeter
pulse oximetry
pulse pressure
pulse rhythm
pulse volume
radiation (RAY-dee-AY-shun)
Sao_2
sphygmomanometer
   (SFIG-moe-man-OM-uh-ter)
SpO_2
stethoscope (STETH-uh-skope)
systole (SIS-toh-lee)
systolic (sis-TOL-ik) pressure
tachycardia (TAK-ih-KAR-dee-uh)
tachypnea (TAK-ip-NEE-uh)
thready pulse

INTRODUCTION TO VITAL SIGNS

Vital signs are objective guideposts that provide data to determine a person's state of health. Vital signs include temperature, pulse, and respiration (collectively called *TPR*) and blood pressure. Another indicator of a patient's health status is pulse oximetry. Although some physicians order this measurement routinely for all patients as part of the patient workup, most physicians order measurement of this vital sign only when the patient complains of respiratory problems (e.g., shortness of breath).

The normal ranges of the vital signs are finely adjusted, and any deviation from normal may indicate disease. During the course of an illness, variations in the vital signs may occur. The medical assistant should be alert to any significant changes and report them to the physician because they indicate a change in the patient's condition. When patients visit the medical office, vital signs are routinely checked to establish each patient's usual state of health and to establish baseline measurements against which future measurements can be compared. The medical assistant should have a thorough knowledge of the vital signs and should attain proficiency in taking them to ensure accurate findings.

General guidelines that the medical assistant should follow when measuring the vital signs are as follows:

1. Be familiar with the normal ranges for all vital signs. Keep in mind that normal ranges vary based on the different age groups (infant, child, adult, elder).
2. Make sure that all equipment for measuring vital signs is in proper working condition to ensure accurate findings.
3. Eliminate or minimize factors that affect the vital signs, such as exercise, food and beverage consumption, smoking, and emotional state.
4. Use an organized approach when measuring the vital signs. If all of the vital signs are ordered, they are usually measured starting with temperature, followed by pulse, respiration, blood pressure, and pulse oximetry.

TEMPERATURE

REGULATION OF BODY TEMPERATURE

Body temperature is maintained within a fairly constant range by the hypothalamus, which is located in the brain. The hypothalamus functions as the body's thermostat. It normally allows the body temperature to vary by only about 1° to 2° Fahrenheit (F) throughout the day.

Body temperature is maintained through a balance of the heat produced in the body and the heat lost from the body (Figure 19-1). A constant temperature range must be maintained for the body to function properly. When minor changes in the temperature of the body occur, the hypothalamus senses this and makes adjustments as necessary to ensure that the body temperature stays within a normal and safe range. If an individual is playing tennis on a hot day,

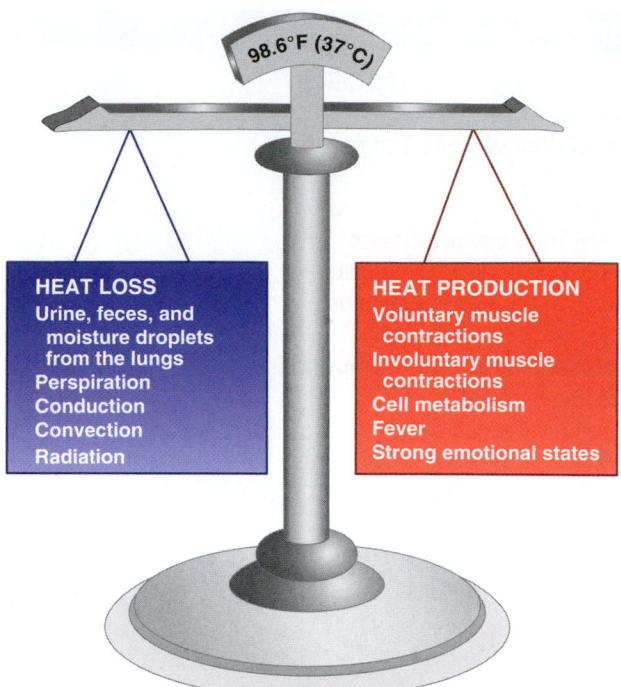

Figure 19-1 Body temperature represents a balance between the heat produced in the body and the heat lost from the body.

the body's heat-cooling mechanism is activated to remove excess heat from the body through perspiration.

Heat Production

Most of the heat produced in the body is through voluntary and involuntary muscle contractions. Voluntary muscle contractions involve the muscles over which a person has control, for example, the moving of legs or arms. Involuntary muscle contractions involve the muscles over which a person has no control; examples are physiologic processes such as digestion, the beating of the heart, and shivering.

Body heat also is produced by cell metabolism. Heat is produced when nutrients are broken down in the cells. Fever and strong emotional states also can increase heat production in the body.

Heat Loss

Heat is lost from the body through the urine, feces, and in water vapor during exhalation. Perspiration also contributes to heat loss. Perspiration is the excretion of moisture through the pores of the skin. When the moisture evaporates, heat is released and the body is cooled.

Radiation, conduction, and convection all cause loss of heat from the body. **Radiation** is the transfer of heat in the form of waves; body heat is continually radiating into cooler surroundings. **Conduction** is the transfer of heat from one object to another by direct contact; heat can be transferred by conduction from the body to a cooler object it touches. **Convection** is the transfer of heat through air currents; cool air currents can cause the body to lose heat. These processes are illustrated in Figure 19-2.

Radiation

Conduction

Convection

Figure 19-2 Heat loss from the body. With **radiation,** the body gives off heat in the form of waves to the cooler outside air. With **conduction,** the chair becomes warm as heat is transferred from the individual to the chair. With **convection,** air currents move heat away from the body.

BODY TEMPERATURE RANGE

The purposes of measuring body temperature are to establish the patient's baseline temperature and to monitor an abnormally high or low body temperature. The normal body temperature range is 97°F to 99°F (36.1°C to 37.2°C), the average temperature being 98.6°F (37°C). Body temperature is usually recorded using the Fahrenheit system of measurement. Table 19-1 lists comparable **Fahrenheit** and **Celsius** temperatures and explains how to convert temperatures from one scale to the other.

Alterations in Body Temperature

A body temperature greater than 100.4°F (38°C) indicates a **fever,** or *pyrexia.* If the body temperature falls between 99°F (37.2°C) and 100.4°F (38°C), this is called a *low-grade fever.* When an individual has a fever, the heat the body is producing is greater than the heat the body is losing. A temperature reading greater than 105.8°F (41°C) is known as **hyperpyrexia.** Hyperpyrexia is a serious condition, and a temperature greater than 109.4°F (43°C) is generally fatal.

A body temperature less than 97°F (36.1°C) is classified as subnormal, or **hypothermia.** This means that the heat the body is losing is greater than the heat it is producing. A person usually cannot survive with a temperature below 93.2°F (34°C). Terms used to describe alterations in body temperature are illustrated in Figure 19-3.

Variations in Body Temperature

During the day-to-day activities of an individual, normal body temperature may fluctuate. The body temperature rarely stays the same throughout the course of a day. The medical assistant should take the following points into consideration when evaluating a patient's temperature.

Table 19-1 Equivalent Fahrenheit and Celsius Temperatures	
Fahrenheit	**Celsius**
93.2	34
95	35
96.8	36
97.7	36.5
98.6	37
99.5	37.5
100.4	38
101.3	38.5
102.2	39
104	40
105.8	41
107.6	42
109.4	43
111.2	44

Temperature Conversion

1. *Celsius to Fahrenheit:* To convert Celsius to Fahrenheit, multiply by $\frac{9}{5}$ and add 32:

$$°F = (°C \times \tfrac{9}{5}) + 32$$

2. *Fahrenheit to Celsius:* To convert Fahrenheit to Celsius, subtract 32 and multiply by $\frac{5}{9}$:

$$°C = (°F - 32) \times \tfrac{5}{9}$$

1. *Age.* Infants and young children normally have a higher body temperature than adults because their thermoregulatory system is not yet fully established. Elderly individuals usually have a lower body temperature owing to factors such as loss of subcutaneous fat, lack of exercise, and loss of thermoregulatory control. Table 19-2

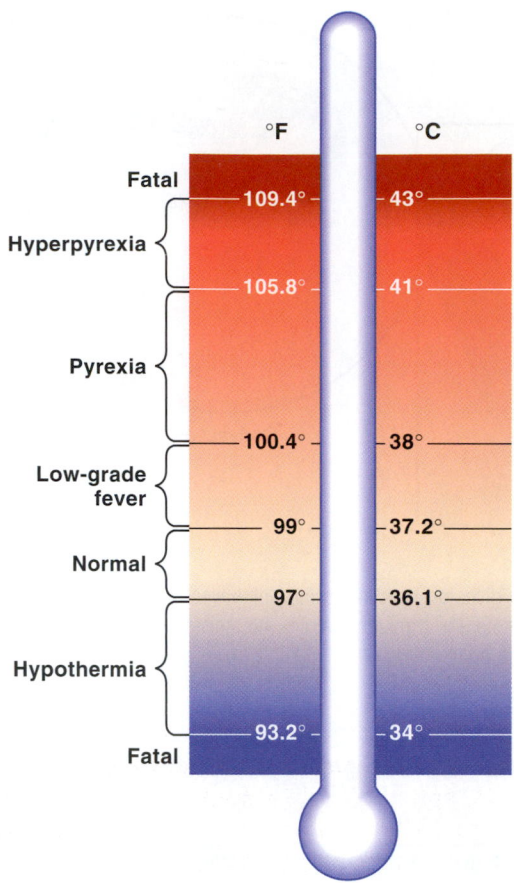

Figure 19-3 Terms that describe alterations in body temperature (adult oral temperature).

Table 19-2 Variations in Body Temperature by Age			
Age	**Site**	**Average Temperature**	
Newborn	Axillary	97° F-100° F	36.1° C-37.8° C
1 yr	Oral	99.7° F	37.6° C
5 yr	Oral	98.6° F	37° C
Adult	Oral	98.6° F	37° C
	Rectal	99.6° F	37.5° C
	Axillary	97.6° F	36.4° C
	Aural	98.6° F	37° C
Elderly (over 70 yr)	Oral	96.8° F	36° C

shows the normal ranges of body temperature according to age group.

2. *Diurnal variations.* During sleep, body metabolism slows down, as do muscle contractions. The body's temperature is lowest in the morning before metabolism and muscle contractions begin increasing.

3. *Emotional states.* Strong emotions such as extreme anger and crying can increase the body temperature. This is important to consider when working with young children, who frequently cry during examination procedures or when they are ill.

4. *Environment.* Cold weather tends to decrease the body temperature, whereas hot weather increases it.

5. *Exercise.* Vigorous physical exercise causes an increase in voluntary muscle contractions, which elevates the body temperature.

6. *Patient's normal body temperature.* Some patients normally run a low or high temperature. The medical assistant should review the patient's past vital sign recordings.

7. *Pregnancy.* Cell metabolism increases during pregnancy, and this elevates body temperature.

Fever

Fever, or pyrexia, denotes that a patient's temperature has increased to higher than 100.4° F (38° C). An individual who has a fever is said to be **febrile;** one who does not have a fever is **afebrile.**

Fever is a common symptom of illness, particularly inflammation and infection. When there is an infection in the body, the invading pathogen functions as a *pyrogen,* which is any substance that produces fever. Pyrogens reset the hypothalamus, causing the body temperature to increase to above normal. Fever is not an illness itself, but rather a sign that the body may have an infection. Most fevers are self-limited, that is, the body temperature returns to normal after the disease process is complete.

Stages of a Fever

A fever can be divided into the following three stages:

1. The *onset* is when the temperature first begins to increase. This increase may be slow or sudden, the patient often experiences coldness and chills, and the pulse and respiratory rate increase.

2. During the *course of a fever,* the temperature rises and falls in one of the following three fever patterns: continuous, intermittent, or remittent. Fever patterns are described and illustrated in Table 19-3. During this stage the patient has an increased pulse and respiratory rate and feels warm to the touch. The patient also may experience one or more of the following: flushed appearance, increased thirst, loss of appetite, headache, and malaise. **Malaise** refers to a vague sense of body discomfort, weakness, and fatigue.

3. During the *subsiding stage,* the temperature returns to normal. It can return to normal gradually or suddenly (known as a **crisis**). As the body temperature is returning to normal, the patient usually perspires and may become dehydrated.

ASSESSMENT OF BODY TEMPERATURE

Assessment Sites

There are five sites for measuring body temperature: mouth, **axilla,** rectum, ear, and forehead. The locations in which temperatures are taken should have an abundant blood supply so that the temperature of the entire body is obtained, not the temperature of only a part of the body. In addition,

Table 19-3 Fever Patterns

Pattern	Description	Illustration
Continuous fever	Body temperature fluctuates minimally but always remains elevated. *Occurs with:* Scarlet fever Pneumococcal pneumonia	
Intermittent fever	Body temperature alternately rises and falls and at times returns to normal or becomes subnormal. *Occurs with:* Bacterial infections Viral infections	
Remittent fever	Wide range of temperature fluctuations occur, all of which are above normal. *Occurs with:* Influenza Pneumonia Endocarditis	

the site must be as closed as possible to prevent air currents from interfering with the temperature reading. The site chosen for measuring a patient's temperature depends on the patient's age, condition, and state of consciousness; the type of thermometer available; and the medical office policy.

HIGHLIGHT on Fever

Although most fevers indicate an infection, not all do. Noninfectious causes of fever include heatstroke, drug hypersensitivity, neoplasms, and central nervous system damage.

A fever usually is not harmful if the temperature remains below 102° F (38.9° C). Research suggests that fever may serve as a defense mechanism to destroy pathogens that are unable to survive above the normal body temperature range.

The level of the fever is not related to the seriousness of the infection. A patient with a temperature of 104° F (40° C) may not be any sicker than a patient with a temperature of 102° F (38.9° C).

In children, fever often is one of the first signs of illness and has a tendency to become highly elevated. In contrast, in elderly patients, fever may be elevated to only 1° F to 2° F above normal, even with a severe infection.

During a fever, the body's basal metabolism increases by 7% for each degree of temperature elevation. Heart and respiratory rates also increase to meet this metabolic demand.

Chills during a fever result when the hypothalamus has been reset at a higher temperature. In an attempt to reach this temperature, involuntary muscle contractions (chills) occur, which produce heat, causing the temperature of the body to increase. After the higher temperature has been reached, the chills subside, and the individual then feels warm.

Increased perspiration during a fever occurs when the hypothalamus has been reset at a lower temperature, for example, after an individual takes an **antipyretic** or after the cause of the fever has been removed. To cool the body and reach this lower temperature, the body perspires, often profusely; profuse perspiration is known as *diaphoresis.* ∎

Putting It All Into Practice

My name is Sergio Martinez, and I am a Registered Medical Assistant. I work in a large clinic that is associated with a medical school. At present, I work in the family medicine department, but I also have worked in dermatology and internal medicine. Family medicine is the area I enjoy most because of the wide variety of tasks that are performed. There is rarely a dull moment.

I focus primarily on clinical medical assisting. Taking vital signs is a big part of my job responsibilities. It is routine at my clinic to take height, weight, TPR, and blood pressure on every patient seen at the clinic, no matter what the reason for his or her visit. I assist the physician with various procedures, examinations, and minor office surgery, and I administer injections, run electrocardiograms, and perform various laboratory tests.

Taking vital signs and length and weight on small children can be very challenging at times. Some children start to cry as soon as they are put on the scale. Taking a temperature on an uncooperative toddler can be very difficult. I try to calm the child as much as possible, and for good behavior, I give a lot of praise. Stickers also are a great reward for cooperative behavior. Usually when small children learn that they can trust you, they are not as frightened by the experience. It is rewarding when a child learns not to be afraid of being evaluated for routine vital signs. ∎

Oral Temperature

The oral method is a convenient and one of the most common means for measuring body temperature. When the medical assistant records a temperature, the physician assumes it has been taken through the oral route unless otherwise noted. There is a rich blood supply under the tongue in the area on either side of the **frenulum linguae.** The thermometer should be placed in this area to obtain the most accurate reading. The patient must keep the mouth closed during the procedure to provide a closed space for the thermometer.

Axillary Temperature

Axillary temperature is recommended as a site for measuring temperature in toddlers and preschoolers. The axillary site also should be used for mouth-breathing patients and for patients with oral inflammation or who have had oral surgery.

The temperature obtained through the axillary method measures approximately 1°F lower than the same person's temperature taken through the oral route (see Table 19-2). The medical assistant should make a notation to tell the physician that the temperature was taken through the axillary route.

Rectal Temperature

The rectal temperature provides an extremely accurate measurement of body temperature because few factors can alter the results. The rectum is highly vascular and, of the five sites, provides the most closed cavity. The temperature obtained by the rectal route measures approximately 1°F higher than the same person's temperature taken by the oral route (see Table 19-2). The medical assistant should make a notation on the patient's chart if the temperature has been taken rectally.

In general, the rectal method is used for infants and young children, unconscious patients, and mouth-breathing patients and when greater accuracy in body temperature is desired. The rectal site should not be used with newborns because of the danger of rectal trauma.

Aural Temperature

The aural (ear) site is used with the tympanic membrane thermometer. The ear provides a closed cavity that is easily accessible. Tympanic membrane thermometers provide instantaneous results, are easy to use, and are comfortable for the patient. They make it easier to measure the temperature of children younger than 6 years, uncooperative patients, and patients who are unable to have their temperatures taken orally.

Forehead Temperature

The temporal artery is a major artery of the head that runs laterally across the forehead and down the side of the neck. In the area of the forehead, it is located approximately 2 mm below the surface of the skin. Because the temporal artery is located so close to the skin surface and is easily accessible, the forehead provides an ideal site for obtaining a body temperature measurement. In addition, the temporal artery has a constant steady flow of blood, which assists in providing an accurate measurement of the patient's body temperature.

The forehead site can be used to measure body temperature using a temporal artery thermometer in individuals of all ages (newborns, infants, children, adults, elderly). The results compare in accuracy with other methods used to measure body temperature. The temperature obtained from the forehead site is about the same as a rectal temperature measurement. The temporal artery reading measures approximately 1° higher than oral body temperature and 2° higher than axillary temperature on the Fahrenheit scale.

Types of Thermometers

The four types of thermometers available for measuring body temperature are electronic thermometers, tympanic membrane thermometers, temporal artery thermometers, and chemical thermometers. Mercury glass thermometers are no longer used in the medical office because they break easily and release mercury. Mercury is a chemical that is dangerous to the human body because it can cause damage to the nervous system. If mercury is released into the environment, it can be harmful to wildlife. Many cities have banned the sale or use of mercury because of its potential hazards.

Electronic Thermometer

An electronic thermometer is often used in the medical office to measure body temperature. Electronic thermometers are portable and measure oral, axillary, and rectal temperatures ranging from 84°F to 108°F (28.9°C to 42.2°C).

An electronic thermometer measures body temperature in a brief time—between 4 and 20 seconds depending on the brand of thermometer used. The temperature results are digitally displayed on a liquid crystal diode (LCD) screen. An electronic thermometer consists of interchangeable oral and rectal probes attached to a battery-operated portable unit (Figure 19-4). The probes are color-coded for ease in identifying them. The oral probe is color-coded with blue on its collar and is used to take oral and axillary temperatures; the rectal probe is color-coded with red on its collar and is used to take rectal temperatures only.

A disposable plastic cover is placed over the probe to prevent the transmission of microorganisms among patients. Depending on the method of taking the temperature, the probe may be inserted into the mouth, axilla, or rectum and is left in place until an audible tone is emitted from the thermometer. When the tone sounds, the patient's temperature in degrees Fahrenheit is displayed on the screen. The medical assistant ejects the plastic probe cover into a regular waste container.

The casing, probes, and attached cords of the electronic thermometer should be periodically cleaned with a soft cloth slightly dampened with a solution of warm water and a disinfectant cleaner.

Procedures 19-1, 19-2, and 19-3 outline the methods for measuring oral, axillary, and rectal temperatures using an electronic thermometer.

Tympanic Membrane Thermometer

The tympanic membrane thermometer is used at the aural site. The tympanic membrane thermometer functions by detecting thermal energy that is naturally radiated from the body. As with the rest of the body, the tympanic membrane

Figure 19-4 Electronic thermometer.

gives off heat waves known as *infrared waves*. The tympanic thermometer functions like a camera by taking a "picture" of these infrared waves, which are considered a documented indicator of body temperature (Figure 19-5). The thermometer calculates the body temperature from the energy generated by the waves and converts it to an oral or rectal equivalent.

The tympanic membrane thermometer is battery operated and consists of a small handheld device with a sensor probe (Figure 19-6). To operate the thermometer, the probe is covered with a disposable soft plastic cover and is placed in the outer third of the external ear canal. An activation button is depressed momentarily, and the results are displayed in 1 to 2 seconds on a digital screen. The probe cover is ejected into a regular waste container. The procedure for taking aural body temperature using a tympanic membrane thermometer is presented in Procedure 19-4.

Temporal Artery Thermometer

Use of a temporal artery thermometer is the newest method for assessing body temperature. A temporal artery thermometer is an electronic device consisting of a probe attached to a portable unit (Figure 19-7).

To perform the procedure, a scan button is continually depressed while the probe is gently and slowly moved across the patient's forehead. During this process the probe sensor scans the forehead for the infrared heat given off by the temporal artery. The probe sensor captures the highest temperature or *peak temperature* in the area being scanned. The peak temperature represents the temperature given off by the temporal artery, or body temperature.

Along with measuring the peak temperature, the probe sensor automatically measures the *ambient temperature*, which is the surrounding air temperature. This is done because there is a small heat loss from the forehead that occurs as a result of cooling by ambient temperature. The thermometer's computer determines and automatically corrects for any effect from ambient temperature. An accurate

Figure 19-5 The tympanic membrane thermometer functions by detecting thermal energy that is naturally radiated from the tympanic membrane.

Figure 19-6 Tympanic membrane thermometer.

Figure 19-7 Temporal artery thermometer.

body temperature reading is digitally displayed on the screen on the thermometer. The procedure for measuring temperature with a temporal artery thermometer is presented in Procedure 19-5.

Earlobe Temperature Measurement

Sweating of the forehead can cause an inaccurate temporal artery temperature reading. This is because perspiration causes the skin of the forehead to cool, resulting in a falsely low temperature reading. Sweating of the forehead occurs when a patient's fever breaks. It also occurs when a patient's skin is clammy; in this instance, forehead sweating may be present but not readily visible. To avoid this problem, the temperature of the neck area located just behind the earlobe also must be measured.

The area behind the earlobe is less affected by sweating than the forehead. During sweating, the blood vessels behind the earlobe dilate, resulting in a constant, steady flow of blood, which provides an accurate measurement of body temperature. After scanning the forehead, the medical assistant must place the probe of the thermometer in the soft depression of the neck just below the mastoid process of the ear. If the patient's forehead has cooled from sweating, the earlobe temperature automatically registers as the peak temperature, thereby overriding the forehead temperature.

The area behind the earlobe does not normally provide an accurate body temperature measurement and supersedes the forehead measurement only when the patient is in a diaphoretic state. Additional guidelines for temporal artery temperature measurement are presented in Box 19-1.

Care and Maintenance

The temporal artery thermometer should be stored in a clean, dry area. The thermometer must be protected from extremes in temperature, direct sunlight, and dust. The casing of the thermometer should be cleaned periodically with a soft cloth moistened with a solution of warm water and a disinfectant cleaner; never splash water on or immerse the unit in water because this could damage the internal components of the thermometer.

To obtain an accurate measurement, the probe lens must be clean and shiny. Dust and other minute particles of environmental debris can build up on the probe lens during normal use, preventing the probe sensor from getting an accurate "view" of the heat emitted by the temporal artery and resulting in a falsely low reading. The lens should be cleaned if it becomes dirty and as a part of routine maintenance. The lens is cleaned by gently wiping its surface with an antiseptic wipe and immediately wiping it dry with a cotton-tipped applicator stick.

Chemical Thermometers

Chemical thermometers contain chemicals that are heat sensitive and include disposable chemical single-use thermometers and temperature-sensitive strips. They are used most often by patients at home to measure body temperature. Although chemical thermometers are less accurate than other types of thermometers, they assist in providing a general assessment of body temperature. Because of their chemical makeup, they should be stored in a cool area, preferably colder than 86° F (30° C), and should not be exposed to direct sunlight because heat may cause the thermometer to register a higher temperature. Each type of chemical thermometer is described here.

Disposable Chemical Single-Use Thermometers

The disposable chemical single-use thermometer has small chemical dots at one end that respond to body heat by changing color (Figure 19-8, *A* and *B*). Each thermometer comes in its own wrapper. The protective wrapper must be peeled back to expose the handle of the thermometer. The thermometer is removed from the wrapper by pulling on the handle, taking care not to touch the dotted area. The thermometer is inserted under the tongue and is left in place for the duration of time recommended by the manufacturer (usually 60 seconds). After removal of the thermometer, the dots are observed for a change in color. The thermometer is read by noting the highest reading among the dots that have changed color (Figure 19-8, *C*). The thermometer is discarded after use.

Temperature-Sensitive Strips

A temperature-sensitive strip consists of a reusable plastic strip that contains heat-sensitive liquid crystals designed to measure body temperature. The plastic strip is pressed onto the forehead and is held in place until the colors stop changing, usually for 15 seconds. The results are read by observing the color change and noting the corresponding temperature indicated on the strip (Figure 19-9).

Text continued on p. 370

PROCEDURE 19-1   Measuring Oral Body Temperature—Electronic Thermometer

Outcome Measure oral body temperature

Equipment/Supplies

- Electronic thermometer
- Oral probe (blue collar)
- Plastic probe cover
- Waste container

1. **Procedural Step.** Sanitize your hands, and assemble the equipment.

2. **Procedural Step.** Remove the thermometer unit from its storage base, and attach the oral (blue collar) probe to it. This is accomplished by inserting the latching plug (at the end of the coiled cord of the oral probe) to the plug receptacle on the thermometer unit until it clicks into place. Insert the probe into the face of the thermometer.
Principle. The oral probe is color-coded with a blue collar for ease in identifying it.

3. **Procedural Step.** Greet the patient and introduce yourself. Identify the patient and explain the procedure. If the patient has recently ingested hot or cold food or beverages or has been smoking, you must wait 15 to 30 minutes before taking the temperature.
Principle. Ingestion of hot or cold food or beverages and smoking change the temperature of the mouth, which could result in an inaccurate reading.

4. **Procedural Step.** Grasp the probe by the collar, and remove it from the face of the thermometer. Slide the probe into a disposable plastic probe cover until it locks into place.
Principle. Removing the probe from the thermometer automatically turns on the thermometer. The probe cover prevents the transfer of microorganisms from one patient to another.

Attach the oral probe to the thermometer.

Continued

PROCEDURE **19-1**   **Measuring Oral Body Temperature—
Electronic Thermometer—cont'd**

Slide the probe into a probe cover.

5. **Procedural Step.** Take the patient's temperature by inserting the probe under the patient's tongue in the pocket located on either side of the frenulum linguae. Instruct the patient to keep the mouth closed.
Principle. There is a good blood supply in the tissue under the tongue. The mouth must be kept closed to prevent cooler air from entering and affecting the temperature reading.

Insert the probe under the patient's tongue.

6. **Procedural Step.** Hold the probe in place until you hear the tone. At that time, the patient's temperature appears as a digital display on the screen. Make a mental note of the temperature reading. (The temperature indicated on this thermometer is 98.2° F [36.8° C].)

The patient's temperature appears as a digital display on the screen.

7. **Procedural Step.** Remove the probe from the patient's mouth. Discard the probe cover by firmly pressing the ejection button while holding the probe over a regular waste container. Do not allow your fingers to come in contact with the probe cover.
Principle. The probe cover should not be touched, to prevent the transfer of microorganisms from the patient to the medical assistant. Saliva is not considered regulated medical waste; the probe can be discarded in a regular waste container.

PROCEDURE 19-1   **Measuring Oral Body Temperature—Electronic Thermometer—cont'd**

7

Discard the probe cover by pressing the ejection button.

8. **Procedural Step.** Return the probe to its stored position in the thermometer unit. Return the thermometer unit to its storage base.
   Principle. Returning the probe to the unit automatically turns off and resets the thermometer.
9. **Procedural Step.** Sanitize your hands.
10. **Procedural Step.** Chart the results in the patient's medical record.
    a. *Paper-based patient record:* Record the date, the time, and the temperature reading (refer to the PPR charting example).
    b. *Electronic medical record:* In SimChart® for the Medical Office, record the temperature reading and site. The temperature can be recorded in either Fahrenheit or Celsius, and the software will convert the temperature so that both are displayed (refer to the SimChart® for the Medical Office example).
    Principle. Patient data must be recorded properly to aid the physician in the diagnosis and to provide future reference.

PPR CHARTING EXAMPLE

Date	
10/15/XX	2:15 p.m. T: 98.2° F.——— S. Martinez, RMA

EMR CHARTING EXAMPLE

Add Vital Signs   ✕

Temperature

Fahrenheit: [98.2]   Site: [Oral ▼]
                                     -Select-
                                     Forehead
Celsius: [36.8]   Oral
                                     Rectal
Pulse   Tympanic

Pulse: [   ]   Site: [-Select- ▼]

Respiration

Respiration: [   ]

Blood Pressure

Systolic: [   ]   Site: [-Select- ▼]

Diastolic: [   ]   Mode: [-Select- ▼]

Position: [-Select- ▼]

Oxygenation

Saturation %: [   ] Site: [-Select- ▼]

Oxygen Delivery: ○ Room Air

                  ○ Oxygen in Use (Amount in L/min)

Charting a temperature reading in SimChart® for the Medical Office.

PROCEDURE 19-2   Measuring Axillary Body Temperature—Electronic Thermometer

Outcome Measure axillary body temperature. *Note:* Many of the principles for taking a temperature already have been stated and are not included in this procedure.

Equipment/Supplies

- Electronic thermometer
- Oral probe (blue collar)
- Plastic probe cover
- Waste container

1. **Procedural Step.** Sanitize your hands, and assemble the equipment.
2. **Procedural Step.** Remove the thermometer unit from its storage base, and attach the oral (blue collar) probe to it. This is accomplished by inserting the latching plug (on the end of the coiled cord of the oral probe) to the plug receptacle on the thermometer unit until it locks into place. Insert the probe into the face of the thermometer.
3. **Procedural Step.** Greet the patient and introduce yourself. Identify the patient and explain the procedure.
4. **Procedural Step.** Remove clothing from the patient's shoulder and arm. Ensure that the axilla is dry. If it is wet, pat it dry with a paper towel or a gauze pad.
   Principle. Clothing removal provides optimal exposure of the axilla for proper placement of the thermometer. Rubbing the axilla causes an increase in the temperature in that area owing to friction, resulting in an inaccurate temperature reading.
5. **Procedural Step.** Grasp the probe by the collar, and remove it from the face of the thermometer. Slide the probe into a disposable probe cover until it locks into place.
6. **Procedural Step.** Take the patient's temperature by placing the probe in the center of the patient's axilla. Instruct the patient to hold the arm close to the body. Hold the arm in place for small children and other patients who cannot maintain the position themselves.
   Principle. Interference from outside air currents is reduced when the arm is held in the proper position.

Place the probe in the center of the patient's axilla.

7. **Procedural Step.** Hold the probe in place until you hear the tone. At that time, the patient's temperature appears as a digital display on the screen. Make a mental note of the temperature reading.
8. **Procedural Step.** Remove the probe from the patient's axilla. Discard the probe cover by firmly pressing the ejection button while holding the probe over a regular waste container. Do not allow your fingers to come in contact with the probe cover.

PROCEDURE 19-2   Measuring Axillary Body Temperature— Electronic Thermometer—cont'd

9. Procedural Step. Return the probe to its stored position in the thermometer unit. Return the thermometer unit to its storage base.

Return the thermometer to its base.

10. Procedural Step. Sanitize your hands.

11. Procedural Step. Chart the results in the patient's medical record.

   a. *Paper-based patient record:* Record the date, the time, and the axillary temperature reading. The symbol Ⓐ must be charted next to the temperature reading to tell the physician that an axillary reading was taken (refer to the PPR charting example).

   b. *Electronic medical record:* In SimChart® for the Medical Office, record the temperature reading and site. The temperature can be recorded in either Fahrenheit or Celsius and the software will convert the temperature so that both are displayed.

PPR CHARTING EXAMPLE

Date	
10/15/XX	9:30 a.m. T: 97.4° F Ⓐ —S. Martinez, RMA

PROCEDURE 19-3 (side tab)

PROCEDURE 19-3   Measuring Rectal Body Temperature— Electronic Thermometer

Outcome Measure rectal body temperature

Equipment/Supplies

- Electronic thermometer
- Rectal probe (red collar)
- Plastic probe cover
- Lubricant
- Disposable gloves
- Tissues
- Waste container

1. Procedural Step. Sanitize your hands, and assemble the equipment.

2. Procedural Step. Remove the thermometer unit from its storage base. Attach the rectal (red collar) probe to it. This is accomplished by inserting the latching plug (on the end of the coiled cord of the rectal probe) to the plug receptacle on the thermometer unit. Insert the probe into the face of the thermometer.

   Principle. The rectal probe is color-coded with a red collar for ease in identifying it.

3. Procedural Step. Greet the patient and introduce yourself. Identify the patient and explain the procedure. If the patient is a child or an adult, provide him or her with a patient gown. Instruct the patient to remove enough clothing to provide access to the anal area and to put on the gown with the opening in the back. If the patient is

an infant, ask the parent to remove the infant's diaper.

   Principle. It is important to explain what you will be doing, because body temperature may be higher in a fearful or apprehensive patient. The patient gown provides the patient with modesty and comfort.

4. Procedural Step. Apply gloves. Position the patient. *Adults and children:* Position the patient in the Sims position, and drape the patient to expose only the anal area. *Infants:* Position the infant on his or her abdomen.

   Principle. Gloves protect the medical assistant from microorganisms in the anal area and feces. Correct positioning allows clear viewing of the anal opening and provides for proper insertion of the thermometer. Draping reduces patient embarrassment and provides warmth.

Continued

PROCEDURE 19-3   Measuring Rectal Body Temperature—Electronic Thermometer—cont'd

PROCEDURE 19-3

5. Procedural Step. Grasp the probe by the collar, and remove it from the face of the thermometer. Slide the probe into a disposable plastic probe cover until it locks into place. Apply a lubricant to the tip of the probe cover up to a level of 1 inch.
Principle. A lubricated thermometer can be inserted more easily and does not irritate the delicate rectal mucosa.

Apply a lubricant to the tip of the probe cover.

6. Procedural Step. Instruct the patient to lie still. Separate the buttocks to expose the anal opening, and gently insert the thermometer probe approximately 1 inch into the rectum of an adult, ⅝ inch in children, and ½ inch in infants. Do not force insertion of the probe. Hold the probe in place until the temperature registers.
Principle. The probe must be inserted correctly to prevent injury to the tissue of the anal opening. The probe should be held in place to prevent damage to the rectal mucosa.

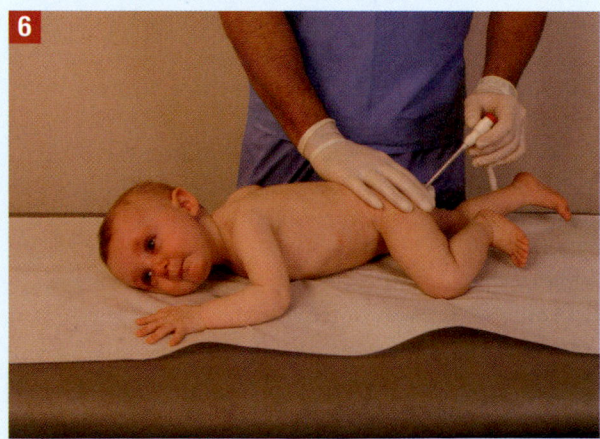

Gently insert the probe ½ inch into the rectum.

7. Procedural Step. Hold the probe in place until you hear the tone. At that time, the patient's temperature appears as a digital display on the screen. Make a mental note of the temperature reading.

8. Procedural Step. Gently remove the probe from the rectum in the same direction as it was inserted. Avoid touching the probe cover. Discard the probe cover by firmly pressing the ejection button while holding the probe over a regular waste container. Return the probe to its stored position in the thermometer unit. Return the thermometer unit to its storage base.
Principle. Fecal material is not considered regulated medical waste; the probe can be discarded in a regular waste container.

9. Procedural Step. Wipe the patient's anal area with tissues to remove excess lubricant. Dispose of the tissues in a regular waste container.
Principle. Wiping the anal area makes the patient more comfortable.

10. Procedural Step. Remove gloves, and sanitize your hands.

11. Procedural Step. Chart the results in the patient's medical record.

a. *Paper-based patient record:* Record the date, the time, and the rectal temperature reading. The symbol Ⓡ must be charted next to the temperature reading to tell the physician that a rectal reading was taken (refer to the PPR charting example).

b. *Electronic medical record:* In SimChart® for the Medical Office, record the temperature reading and site. The temperature can be recorded in either Fahrenheit or Celsius and the software will convert the temperature so that both are displayed.

PPR CHARTING EXAMPLE

Date	
10/15/XX	11:15 a.m. T: 99.8° F Ⓡ — S. Martinez, RMA

PROCEDURE 19-4 Measuring Aural Body Temperature— Tympanic Membrane Thermometer

Outcome Measure aural body temperature

Equipment/Supplies

- Tympanic membrane thermometer
- Probe cover
- Waste container

1. **Procedural Step.** Sanitize your hands, and assemble the equipment.
   Principle. Your hands should be clean and free from contamination.

2. **Procedural Step.** Greet the patient and introduce yourself. Identify the patient and explain the procedure.
   Principle. It is important to explain what you will be doing, because body temperature may be higher in a fearful or apprehensive patient.

3. **Procedural Step.** Remove the thermometer from its storage base. Ensure that the probe lens is clean and intact. To clean the lens, gently wipe its surface with an antiseptic wipe and immediately wipe it dry with a cotton swab. After cleaning, allow at least 5 minutes before taking a temperature.
   Principle. A dirty or damaged probe lens could result in a falsely low temperature reading.

4. **Procedural Step.** Attach a cover on the probe by pressing the probe tip straight down into the cover box. You will be able to see and feel the cover snap securely into place on the probe. This procedure automatically turns on the thermometer.
   Principle. The probe cover protects the lens and provides infection control. The cover must be seated securely on the probe to activate the thermometer.

Place a cover on the probe.

5. **Procedural Step.** Pull the probe straight up from the cover box. Look at the digital display to see if the thermometer is ready to use.

When the thermometer is ready, it displays the word *READY*.

6. **Procedural Step.** Hold the thermometer in your dominant hand. If you are right-handed, you should take the temperature in the patient's right ear. If you are left-handed, take the temperature in the patient's left ear.
   Principle. Taking the temperature with the dominant hand assists in the proper placement of the probe in the patient's ear.

7. **Procedural Step.** Straighten the patient's external ear canal with your nondominant hand, as follows:
   Adults and children older than 3 years: Gently pull the ear auricle upward and backward.
   Children younger than 3 years: Gently pull the ear pinna downward and backward.
   Principle. Straightening the ear canal allows the probe sensor to obtain a clear picture of the tympanic membrane, resulting in an accurate temperature measurement.

Continued

PROCEDURE **19-4** Measuring Aural Body Temperature—
Tympanic Membrane Thermometer—cont'd

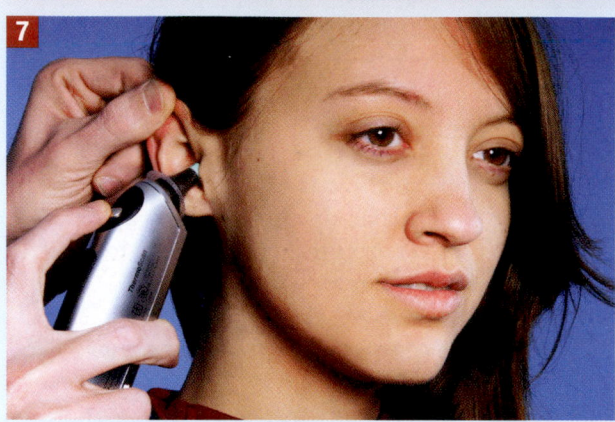

Straighten the canal of adults and children older than 3 years by pulling the ear auricle upward and backward.

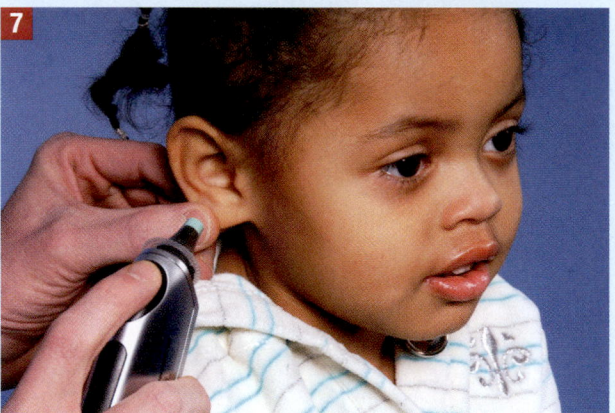

Straighten the canal of children younger than 3 years by pulling the ear auricle downward and backward.

8. **Procedural Step.** Insert the probe into the patient's ear canal tightly enough to seal the opening, but without causing patient discomfort. Point the tip of the probe toward the opposite temple (approximately midway between the opposite ear and eyebrow).
   Principle. Sealing the ear canal prevents cooler external air from entering the ear, which could result in a falsely low reading. Correct positioning of the probe optimizes the sensor's view of the tympanic membrane, leading to an accurate temperature reading.

9. **Procedural Step.** Ask the patient to remain still. Hold the thermometer steady, and depress the activation button. Depending on the brand of the thermometer, perform one of the following:
   a. Hold the button down for 1 full second and then release it, or
   b. Hold down the button down until an audible tone is heard.

Principle. The thermometer cannot take a temperature unless the activation button is depressed for 1 full second. When the button is depressed, the infrared sensor in the probe scans the thermal energy radiated by the tympanic membrane.

10. **Procedural Step.** Remove the thermometer from the ear canal. Turn the digital display of the thermometer toward you, and read the temperature. Make a mental note of the temperature reading. If the temperature seems to be too low, repeat the procedure to ensure that you have used the proper technique. The temperature indicated on this thermometer is 99.8° F (37.7° C). The temperature remains on the display screen for 30 to 60 seconds or until another cover is inserted on the probe (whichever occurs first).
    Principle. The temperature remains on the display screen until another cover is inserted on the probe. Improper technique can result in a falsely low temperature reading.

Read the temperature on the digital display.

11. Procedural Step. Dispose of the probe cover by ejecting it into a regular waste container.

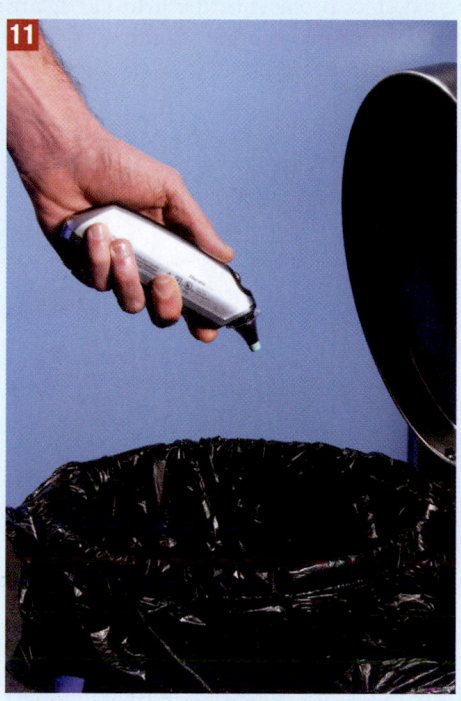

Dispose of the probe cover.

12. Procedural Step. Replace the thermometer in its storage base.
Principle. The thermometer should be stored in its base to protect the probe lens from damage and dirt.

13. Procedural Step. Sanitize your hands.

14. Procedural Step. Chart the results in the patient's medical record.

   a. *Paper-based patient record:* Record the date, the time, the aural temperature reading, and which ear was used to take the temperature. Indicating which ear was used alerts the physician that the temperature was taken through the aural route (refer to the PPR charting example).

   b. *Electronic medical record:* In SimChart® for the Medical Office, record the temperature reading and site. The temperature can be recorded in either Fahrenheit or Celsius and the software will convert the temperature so that both are displayed.

PPR CHARTING EXAMPLE

Date	
10/15/XX	3:00 p.m. T: 99.8° F, Ⓡ ear—S. Martinez, RMA

PROCEDURE 19-5   Measuring Temporal Artery Body Temperature

Outcome   Measure temporal artery body temperature

Equipment/Supplies

- Temporal artery thermometer
- Probe cover
- Antiseptic wipe
- Waste container

1. Procedural Step. Sanitize your hands, and assemble the equipment.

2. Procedural Step. Greet the patient and introduce yourself. Identify the patient and explain the procedure.

3. Procedural Step. Examine the probe lens of the temporal artery thermometer to ensure that the lens is clean and intact.
Principle. A dirty or damaged probe lens could result in a falsely low temperature reading.

4. Procedural Step. Place a disposable cover over the probe. If the thermometer does not use disposable covers, clean the probe with an antiseptic wipe, and allow it to dry.
Principle. Applying a probe cover or cleaning the probe with an antiseptic wipe provides infection control.

Place a disposable probe cover on the thermometer.

Continued

PROCEDURE 19-5   Measuring Temporal Artery Body Temperature—cont'd

5. Procedural Step. Select an appropriate site; the right or left side of the forehead can be used. The site selected should be fully exposed to the environment.
Principle. The temporal artery is located in the center of each side of the forehead, approximately 2 mm below the surface of the skin.

6. Procedural Step. Prepare the patient by brushing away any hair that is covering the side of the forehead to be scanned and the area behind the earlobe on the same side.
Principle. Hair covering the area to be measured traps body heat, resulting in a falsely high temperature reading.

7. Procedural Step. Hold the thermometer in your dominant hand with your thumb on the scan button.

8. Procedural Step. Gently position the probe of the thermometer on the center of the patient's forehead, midway between the eyebrow and the hairline.

Position the probe on the center of the patient's forehead.

9. Procedural Step. Depress the scan button, and keep it depressed for the entire measurement.
Principle. Not keeping the scan button depressed can result in a falsely low temperature reading.

10. Procedural Step. Slowly and gently slide the probe straight across the forehead, midway between the eyebrow and the upper hairline. Continue until the hairline is reached. Keep the scan button depressed and the probe flush (flat) against the forehead. During this time, a beeping sound occurs and a red light blinks to indicate that a measurement is taking place. Rapid beeping and blinking indicate a rise to a higher temperature. Slow beeping indicates that the thermometer is still scanning but is not finding a higher temperature.

Principle. The thermometer continually scans for the peak temperature as long as the scan button is depressed. The probe must be held flat against the forehead to ensure accurate scanning of the temporal artery.

Slowly slide the probe straight across the patient's forehead.

11. Procedural Step. Keeping the button depressed, lift the probe from the forehead, and gently place the probe behind the earlobe in the soft depression of the neck just below the mastoid process. Hold the probe in place for 1 to 2 seconds.
Principle. Taking the patient's temperature behind the earlobe prevents an error in temperature measurement in the event that the patient is sweating.

Place the probe behind the earlobe.

PROCEDURE 19-5   Measuring Temporal Artery Body Temperature—cont'd

12. Procedural Step. Release the scan button on the digital display, and read the temperature. Make a mental note of the temperature reading. (The temperature indicated on this thermometer is 99.1° F [37.3° C].) The reading remains on the display for approximately 15 to 30 seconds after the button is released. The thermometer shuts off automatically after 30 seconds. To turn the thermometer off immediately, press and release the scan button quickly. If the patient's temperature needs to be taken again, wait 60 seconds or use the opposite side of the forehead.
Principle. Taking a measurement cools the skin, and taking another measurement too soon may result in an inaccurate reading.

13. Procedural Step. Dispose of the probe cover by pushing it off the probe with your thumb and ejecting it into a regular waste container. Wipe the probe with an antiseptic wipe, and allow it to dry.

Wipe the probe with an antiseptic wipe.

14. Procedural Step. Sanitize your hands.
15. Procedural Step. Chart the results in the patient's medical record.
  a. *Paper-based patient record:* Record the date, the time, and the temperature reading. The symbol (TA) must be charted next to the temperature reading to tell the physician that a temporal artery reading was taken (refer to the PPR charting example).
  b. *Electronic medical record:* In SimChart® for the Medical Office, record the temperature reading and site. The temperature can be recorded in either Fahrenheit or Celsius and the software will convert the temperature so that both are displayed.
16. Procedural Step. Store the thermometer in a clean, dry area.

Read the temperature.

PPR CHARTING EXAMPLE	
Date	
10/15/XX	9:15 a.m. T: 99.1° F (TA)— S. Martinez, RMA

PROCEDURE 19-5

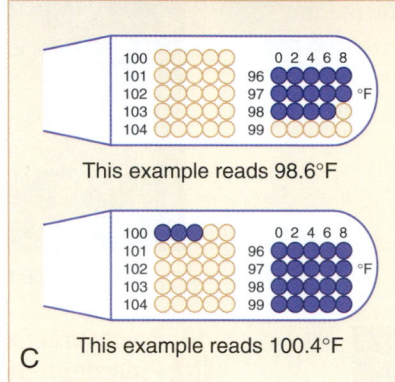

Figure 19-8 Disposable chemical single-use thermometers. **A,** The thermometer is removed from the wrapper by pulling on the handle. **B,** The thermometer is inserted under the tongue and is left in place for 60 seconds. **C,** The thermometer is read by noting the highest reading among the dots that have changed color.

Figure 19-9 Temperature-sensitive strip. The plastic strip is pressed onto the forehead and is held in place until the color stops changing (in general for 15 seconds). The results are read by observing the color and noting the corresponding temperature indicated on the strip.

PULSE

MECHANISM OF THE PULSE

When the left ventricle of the heart contracts, blood is forced from the heart into the **aorta,** which is the major trunk of the arterial system of the body. The aorta is already filled with blood and must expand to accept the blood being pushed out of the left ventricle. This creates a pulsating wave that travels from the aorta through the walls of the arterial system. This wave, known as the *pulse,* can be felt as a light tap by an examiner. The pulse rate is measured by counting the number of taps, or beats, per minute. The heart rate can be determined by taking the pulse rate.

Factors Affecting Pulse Rate

Pulse rate can vary depending on many factors. The medical assistant should take each of the following into consideration when measuring pulse:

1. *Age.* The pulse varies inversely with age. As age increases, the pulse rate gradually decreases. Table 19-4 lists the pulse rates of various age groups.
2. *Gender.* Women tend to have a slightly faster pulse rate than men.
3. *Physical activity.* Physical activity, such as jogging and swimming, increases the pulse rate temporarily.

Table 19-4 Pulse Rates of Various Age Groups

Age Group	Pulse Range (beats/min)	Average Pulse (beats/min)
Infant (birth to 1 yr)	120-160	140
Toddler (1-3 yr)	90-140	115
Preschool child (3-6 yr)	80-110	95
School-age child (6-12 yr)	75-105	90
Adolescent (12-18 yr)	60-100	80
Adult (after 18th yr)	60-100	80
Adult (after 60th yr)	67-80	74
Well-trained athletes	40-60	50

4. *Emotional states.* Strong emotional states, such as anxiety, fear, excitement, and anger, temporarily increase the pulse rate.
5. *Metabolism.* Increased body metabolism, such as occurs during pregnancy, increases the pulse rate.
6. *Fever.* Fever increases the pulse rate.
7. *Medications.* Medications may alter the pulse rate. For example, digitalis decreases the pulse rate, and epinephrine increases it.

What Would You Do? What Would You *Not* Do?

Case Study 1

Marcela Mason comes in with Olivia, her 5-year-old daughter. Olivia has had a fever and sore throat for the past 2 days. Olivia's aural temperature is taken in her left ear, and it measures 103.3° F. Mrs. Mason says that she has an ear thermometer at home, but when she took Olivia's temperature with it, the readings were always below 97° F. She knew that could not be right because Olivia felt so warm. Mrs. Mason would like to be able to use her ear thermometer, but she thinks that it might be broken because of the low readings. Mrs. Mason says that she is thinking of switching back to a mercury glass thermometer, but she has heard that it isn't a good idea to use this type of thermometer anymore and wants to know why. ∎

Pulse Sites

The pulse is felt most strongly when a superficial artery is held against a firm tissue, such as bone. The locations of sites used for measuring the pulse are shown in Figure 19-10 and are described next.

Radial

The most common site for measuring the pulse is the radial artery, which is located in a groove on the inner aspect of the wrist just below the thumb. The radial pulse is easily accessible and can be measured with no discomfort to the patient. This site is also used by individuals at home monitoring their own heart rates, such as athletes, patients

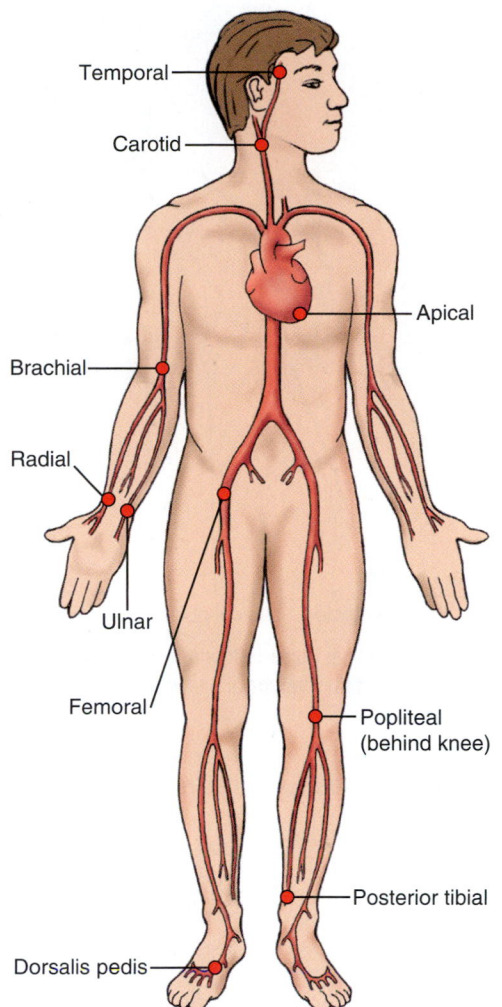

Figure 19-10 Pulse sites.

taking heart medication, and individuals starting an exercise program. The procedure for measuring radial pulse is outlined in Procedure 19-6.

Apical

The apical pulse has a stronger beat and is easier to measure than the other pulse sites. If the medical assistant is having difficulty feeling the radial pulse, or if the radial pulse is irregular or abnormally slow or rapid, the apical pulse should be taken (Procedure 19-7). This pulse site is often used to measure pulse in infants and in children up to 3 years old because the other sites are difficult to palpate accurately in these age groups. The apical pulse is measured using a stethoscope. The chest piece of the stethoscope is placed lightly over the apex of the heart, which is located in the fifth **intercostal** (between the ribs) space at the junction of the left midclavicular line (Figure 19-11).

Brachial

The brachial pulse is in the **antecubital space,** which is the space located at the front of the elbow. This site is used to take blood pressure, to measure pulse in infants during

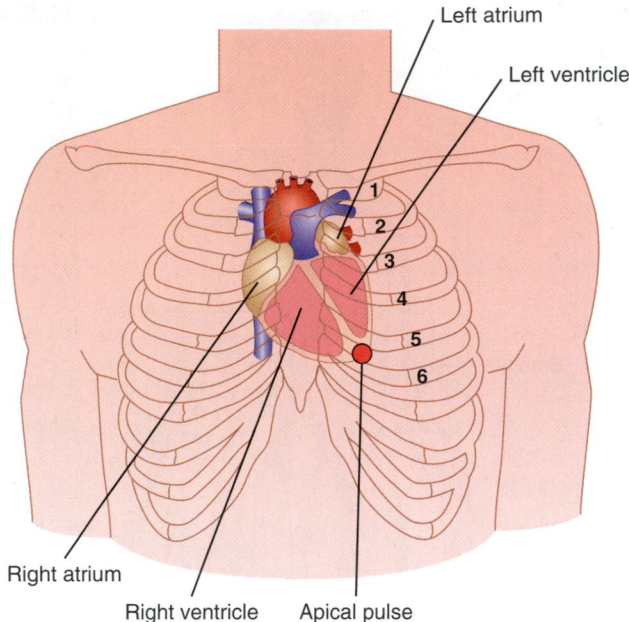

Figure 19-11 The apical pulse is found over the apex of the heart, which is located in the fifth intercostal space at the junction of the left midclavicular line.

cardiac arrest, and to assess the status of the circulation to the lower arm.

Ulnar

The ulnar pulse is located on the ulnar (little finger) side of the wrist. It is used to assess the status of circulation to the hand.

Temporal

The temporal pulse is located in front of the ear and just above eye level. This site is used to measure pulse when the radial pulse is inaccessible. It is also an easy access site to assess pulse in children.

Carotid

The carotid pulse is located on the anterior side of the neck, slightly to one side of the midline, and is the best site to find a pulse quickly. This site is used to measure pulse in children and adults during cardiac arrest. The carotid site also is commonly used by individuals to monitor pulse during exercise.

Femoral

The femoral pulse is in the middle of the groin. This site is used to measure pulse in infants and children and in adults during cardiac arrest and to assess the status of circulation to the lower leg.

Popliteal

The popliteal pulse is at the back of the knee and is detected most easily when the knee is slightly flexed. This site is used to measure blood pressure when the brachial pulse is inaccessible and to assess the status of circulation to the lower leg.

Posterior Tibial

The posterior tibial pulse is located on the inner aspect of the ankle just posterior to the ankle bone. This site is used to assess the status of circulation to the foot.

Dorsalis Pedis

The dorsalis pedis pulse is located on the upper surface of the foot, between the first and second metatarsal bones. This site is used to assess the status of circulation to the foot.

Memories *from* **Practicum**

Sergio Martinez: One experience that really stands out in my memory occurred during my practicum at a family practice medical office. I needed to take the blood pressure of a small 6-year-old boy. After I put the cuff on his arm, his eyes started filling up with tears. I stopped, removed the cuff, and asked him if something was wrong. He said he was afraid that when I started squeezing that thing around his arm, his hand would fall off. I sat down next to him, spent some time talking with him, and reassured him that his hand would be perfectly fine and would not fall off. I put the cuff on my arm and pumped it up to show him that he would be safe. He then agreed to let me take his blood pressure. After I took his blood pressure, he wiggled his hand, gave me a big smile, and said that it didn't hurt at all. That situation made me realize that children may have a lot of fears about what might happen to them at the medical office. Since that experience, I always take the time to explain procedures to children before I perform them. ∎

ASSESSMENT OF PULSE

The purpose of measuring pulse is to establish the patient's baseline pulse rate and to assess the pulse rate after special procedures, medications, or disease processes that affect heart functioning. Pulse is measured using palpation at all of the pulse sites except the apical site.

Pulse is palpated by applying moderate pressure with the sensitive pads located on the tips of the three middle fingers. The pulse should not be taken with the thumb because the thumb has a pulse of its own. This could result in measurement of the medical assistant's pulse rather than the patient's pulse. Excessive pressure should not be applied when measuring pulse because this could obliterate, or close off, the pulse. It may not be possible to detect the pulse if too little pressure is applied, however. An accurate assessment of pulse includes determinations of the pulse rate, the pulse rhythm, and the pulse volume.

Pulse Rate

The pulse rate is the number of heart pulsations or heartbeats that occur in 1 minute; therefore pulse rate is measured in beats per minute. Normal pulse rates vary widely in the various age groups, as shown in Table 19-4. For a healthy adult, the normal resting pulse rate ranges from 60 to 100 beats per minute, with the average falling between 70 and 80 beats per minute.

An abnormally fast heart rate of more than 100 beats per minute is known as **tachycardia.** Tachycardia may indicate disease states such as hemorrhaging or heart disease. Tachycardia usually occurs when an individual is involved in vigorous physical exercise or is experiencing strong emotional states.

Bradycardia is an abnormally slow heart rate—less than 60 beats per minute. A pulse rate of less than 60 beats per minute may occur normally during sleep. Trained athletes often have low pulse rates. If a patient exhibits tachycardia or bradycardia during radial pulse measurement, the apical pulse should also be measured.

Pulse Rhythm and Volume

In addition to measuring the pulse rate, the medical assistant should determine the rhythm and volume of the pulse. The **pulse rhythm** denotes the time interval between heartbeats; a normal rhythm has the same time interval between beats. Any irregularity in the heart's rhythm is known as a **dysrhythmia** (also termed *arrhythmia*) and is characterized by unequal or irregular intervals between the heartbeats. If a dysrhythmia is present, the physician may order one or more of the following:

an apical-radial pulse, an electrocardiogram, or Holter monitoring.

An **apical-radial pulse** is measured to determine whether a pulse deficit is present. Taking an apical-radial pulse involves measuring the apical pulse at the same time as the radial pulse for a duration of 1 full minute. A **pulse deficit** exists when the radial pulse rate is less than the apical pulse rate. If one medical assistant measures an apical pulse rate of 88 beats per minute while another medical assistant simultaneously measures a radial pulse rate of 76 beats per minute, this results in a pulse deficit of 12 beats. A pulse deficit means that not all of the heartbeats are reaching the peripheral arteries. A pulse deficit is caused by an inefficient contraction of the heart that is not strong enough to transmit a pulse wave to the peripheral pulse site. A pulse deficit frequently occurs with atrial fibrillation, which is a type of dysrhythmia.

The **pulse volume** refers to the strength of the heartbeat. The amount of blood pumped into the aorta by each contraction of the left ventricle should remain constant, making the pulse feel strong and full. If the blood volume decreases, the pulse feels weak and may be difficult to detect. This type of pulse is usually accompanied by a fast heart rate and is described as a **thready pulse.** An increase in the blood volume results in a pulse that feels extremely strong and full, known as a **bounding pulse.**

PATIENT TEACHING | **Aerobic Exercise**

Answer questions patients have about aerobic exercise.

What is aerobic exercise?
Aerobic exercise increases, sustains, and decreases your pulse over time. Aerobic exercise is accomplished through steady, nonstop activity, such as walking, jogging, cycling, or swimming. Each workout should include warm-up and cool-down periods of at least 5 minutes each. This is needed to prevent muscle or joint injuries.

What are the benefits of an aerobic exercise program?
The benefits of an aerobic exercise program include strengthening of the heart, a slower resting pulse rate, reduction of stress, increased energy, lowering of body fat, decreased "bad" (low-density lipoprotein) cholesterol, and increased "good" (high-density lipoprotein) cholesterol. The key to a safe and effective aerobic exercise program is the target heart rate (THR).

What is target heart rate?
Your THR is a safe and effective exercise pulse range that indicates that you are exercising at the right level for your age and for what you are trying to accomplish with exercise. Exercising at a level below your THR does little to promote fitness; exercising at a level above your THR may not be safe.

How do I determine my target heart rate?
The following formula is used to determine your THR:
1. Subtract your age from 220 to determine your maximum heart rate (MHR), which is the fastest your heart can beat

safely for your age. The MHR of a 40-year-old person is calculated as follows:
220 − 40 years old = 180 (MHR)
2. Determine the lower end of your THR range by multiplying your MHR by 0.6. For our example:
180 × 0.60 = 108 (low end of THR)
3. Determine the upper end of your THR range by multiplying your MHR by 0.8. For our example:
180 × 0.80 = 144 (upper end of THR)

Always exercise within your THR range. The 40-year-old person in our example should exercise with a THR between 108 and 144.

How often should aerobic exercise be performed?
To promote and maintain health, the American Heart Association (AHA) recommends that healthy adults aged 18 to 65 spend at least 30 minutes a day, 5 days a week, in moderately intense aerobic exercise (e.g., brisk walking), or 20 minutes, 3 days each week, in vigorous-intensity exercise (e.g., jogging), or a combination of moderate and vigorous exercise. These moderate- and vigorous-intensity recommendations should be added to the light-intensity activities of daily living such as washing dishes and taking out the trash. In addition, the AHA recommends that adults perform activities that maintain or increase muscular strength and endurance a minimum of 2 days each week. The AHA further recommends that children and adolescents engage in at least 60 minutes of moderate to vigorous physical activity per day. ■

RESPIRATION

MECHANISM OF RESPIRATION

The purpose of respiration is to provide for the exchange of oxygen and carbon dioxide between the atmosphere and the blood. Oxygen is taken into the body to be used for vital body processes, and carbon dioxide is given off as a waste product.

Each respiration is divided into two phases: **inhalation** and **exhalation** (Figure 19-12). During inhalation, or inspiration, the diaphragm descends and the lungs expand, causing air containing oxygen to move from the atmosphere into the lungs. Exhalation, or expiration, involves the removal of carbon dioxide from the body. The diaphragm ascends, and the lungs return to their original state so that air containing carbon dioxide is expelled. One complete respiration is composed of one inhalation and one exhalation.

Respiration can be classified as *external* or *internal.* External respiration involves the exchange of oxygen and carbon dioxide between the **alveolus** (thin-walled sacs) of the lungs and the blood (Figure 19-13). The blood, located in small capillaries, comes in contact with the alveoli, picks up oxygen, and carries it to the cells of the body. At this point, the oxygen is given off to the cells, and carbon dioxide is picked up by the blood to be transported as a waste product to the lungs. The exchange of oxygen and carbon dioxide between the body cells and the blood is known as *internal respiration.*

Control of Respiration

The medulla oblongata, located in the brain, is the control center for involuntary respiration. A buildup of carbon dioxide in the blood sends a message to the medulla, which triggers respiration to occur automatically.

To a certain extent, respiration is also under voluntary control. An individual can control respiration during activities such as singing, laughing, talking, eating, and crying. Voluntary respiration is ultimately under the control of the medulla oblongata. The breath can be held for only a certain length of time, after which carbon dioxide begins to build up in the body, resulting in a stimulus to the medulla that causes respiration to occur involuntarily. Small children may voluntarily hold their breath during a temper tantrum. A parent who does not understand the principles of

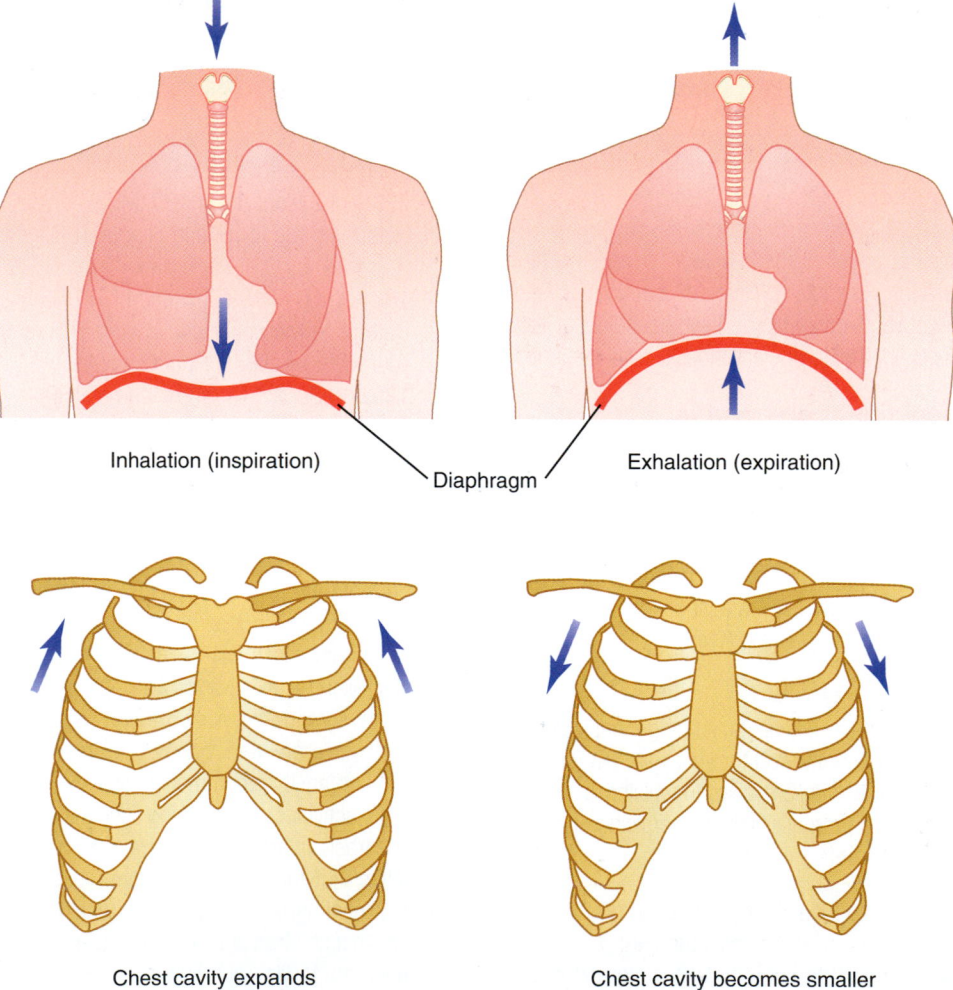

Inhalation (inspiration)   Diaphragm   Exhalation (expiration)

Chest cavity expands   Chest cavity becomes smaller

Figure 19-12 Inhalation and exhalation.

External Respiration

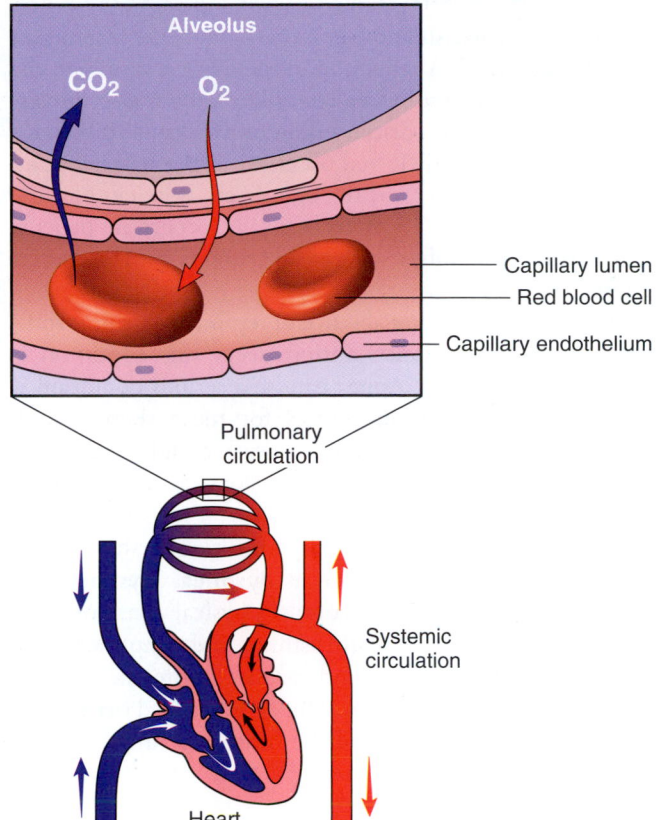

Figure 19-13 Exchange of oxygen and carbon dioxide between the alveoli of the lungs and the blood.

respiration may be concerned that the child would cease to breathe. The medical assistant should be able to explain that involuntary respiration would eventually occur and the child would resume breathing.

| What Would You Do? | What Would You *Not* Do? |

Case Study 2

Alex Jacoby is 18 years old and a senior in high school. He comes to the office complaining of severe pain in his left shoulder. Alex is an outstanding competitive swimmer and is currently ranked first in the state in the 100-yard butterfly. Alex has a big meet coming up and must do well because he has a chance of getting an athletic scholarship to the University of Florida. He says he thinks he can take 2 seconds off his best time at this meet and he doesn't want anything to interfere with that. Alex wants the physician to do whatever he can to make his shoulder better and thinks that a steroid injection and OxyContin might be the answer. His vital signs are as follows: temperature 98.5° F, pulse 48 beats per minute, respirations 12 breaths per minute, and blood pressure 108/68 mm Hg. Alex asks why his pulse is so slow and wants to know if there is any medication that he can take to make it faster. ■

ASSESSMENT OF RESPIRATION

Because an individual can control his or her respiration, the medical assistant should measure respirations without the patient's knowledge. Patients may change their respiratory rate unintentionally if they are aware that they are being measured. An ideal time to measure respiration is after the pulse is taken. Procedure 19-6 outlines the procedures for taking pulse and respiration in one continuous procedure.

Respiratory Rate

The respiratory rate of a normal healthy adult ranges from 12 to 20 respirations per minute. With most adults, there is a ratio of one respiration for every four pulse beats. If the respiratory rate is 18, the pulse rate would be approximately 72 beats per minute. An abnormal increase in the respiratory rate of more than 20 respirations per minute is referred to as **tachypnea.** An abnormal decrease in the respiratory rate of less than 12 respirations per minute is known as **bradypnea.** When measuring the respiratory rate, the medical assistant should take into consideration the following factors:

1. *Age.* As age increases, the respiratory rate decreases. The respiratory rate of a child would be expected to be faster than that of an adult. Table 19-5 provides a chart of the respiratory rates for various age groups.
2. *Physical activity.* Physical activity increases the respiratory rate temporarily.
3. *Emotional states.* Strong emotional states temporarily increase the respiratory rate.
4. *Fever.* A patient with a fever has an increased respiratory rate. One way that heat is lost from the body is through the lungs; a fever causes an increased respiratory rate as the body tries to rid itself of excess heat.
5. *Medications.* Certain medications increase the respiratory rate, and others decrease it. If the medical assistant is unsure of what effect a particular drug may have on the respiratory rate, he or she should consult a drug reference, such as the *Physician's Desk Reference* (PDR).

Table 19-5 Respiratory Rates of Various Age Groups		
	Average Respiratory Range, Breaths per Minute	Respiratory Average, Breaths per Minute
Infant (birth to 1 yr)	30-40	35
Toddler (1-3 yr)	23-35	30
Preschool child (3-6 yr)	20-30	25
School-age child (6-12 yr)	18-26	22
Adolescent (12-18 yr)	12-20	16
Adult (after 18th yr)	12-20	16

Rhythm and Depth of Respiration

The *rhythm* and *depth* should be noted when measuring respiration. Normally the rhythm should be even and regular, and the pauses between inhalation and exhalation should be equal. The depth of respiration indicates the amount of air that is inhaled or exhaled during the process of breathing. Respiratory depth is typically described as normal, deep, or shallow and is determined by observing the amount of movement of the chest. For normal respirations, the depth of each respiration in a resting state is approximately the same. Deep respirations are those in which a large volume of air is inhaled and exhaled, whereas shallow respirations involve the exchange of a small volume of air. Normal respiration is referred to as **eupnea.** The rate is approximately 12 to 20 breaths per minute, the rhythm is even and regular, and the depth is normal.

Hyperpnea is an abnormal increase in the rate and depth of respirations. A patient with hyperpnea exhibits a very deep, rapid, and labored respiration. Hyperpnea occurs normally with exercise and abnormally with pain and fever. It also can occur with any condition in which the supply of oxygen is inadequate, such as heart disease and lung disease.

Hyperventilation is an abnormally fast and deep type of breathing that is usually associated with acute anxiety conditions, such as panic attacks. An individual who is hyperventilating is "overbreathing," which usually causes dizziness and weakness.

Hypopnea is a condition in which a patient's respiration exhibits an abnormal decrease in rate and depth. The depth is approximately half that of normal respiration. Hypopnea often occurs in individuals with sleep disorders.

Color of the Patient

The patient's color should be observed while the respiration is being measured. A reduction in the oxygen supply to the tissues (**hypoxia**) results in a condition known as **cyanosis,** which causes a bluish discoloration of the skin and mucous membranes. Cyanosis is first observed in the nail beds and lips because in these areas the blood vessels lie close to the surface of the skin. Cyanosis typically occurs in patients with advanced emphysema and in patients during cardiac arrest.

Apnea is a temporary absence of respirations. Some individuals experience apnea during sleep; this condition is known as *sleep apnea.* Apnea can be a serious condition if the individual's breathing ceases for more than 4 to 6 minutes because brain damage or death could occur.

Respiratory Abnormalities

A patient who is having difficulty breathing or shortness of breath has a condition known as **dyspnea.** Dyspnea may occur normally during vigorous physical exertion and abnormally in patients with asthma and emphysema. A patient with dyspnea may find it easier to breathe while in a sitting or standing position. This state is called **orthopnea** and occurs with disorders of the heart and lungs, such as asthma, emphysema, pneumonia, and congestive heart failure.

Breath Sounds

Breath sounds are caused by air moving through the respiratory tract. Normal breath sounds are quiet and barely audible. Abnormal breath sounds are referred to as **adventitious sounds** and typically signify the presence of a

---

PATIENT TEACHING | **Chronic Obstructive Pulmonary Disease**

Answer questions that patients have about chronic obstructive pulmonary disease (COPD).

What is COPD?
COPD is a chronic airway obstruction that results from emphysema or chronic bronchitis or a combination of these conditions. COPD is a chronic, debilitating, irreversible, and sometimes fatal disease.

How many people have COPD?
More than 12 million Americans have been diagnosed with COPD; however, it is estimated that an additional 12 million Americans have the disease but remain undiagnosed. COPD is the fourth leading cause of death in the United States behind heart disease, cancer, and stroke. Although COPD is much more common in men than in women, the greatest increase in death rates is occurring in women.

What causes COPD?
Cigarette smoking over a period of many years is the leading cause of COPD. Other causes include air pollution and occupational exposure to irritating inhalants, such as noxious dusts, fumes, and vapors.

What types of tests might the physician order?
Respiratory tests to diagnose COPD include various types of pulmonary function tests. Examples of pulmonary function tests are spirometry, lung volumes, diffusion capacity, arterial blood gas studies, pulse oximetry, and cardiopulmonary exercise tests.

What treatment might the physician prescribe?
Treatment is focused on improving breathing difficulties and may include bronchodilator drug therapy, breathing exercises, and oxygen therapy.
1. Encourage patients with COPD to comply with the therapy prescribed by the physician.
2. Provide the patient with information about smoking, emphysema, and chronic bronchitis. Educational materials are available from the American Lung Association, the American Heart Association, and the American Cancer Society. ■

Table 19-6 Abnormal Breath Sounds

Type	Cause	Character
Crackles* (rales)	Air moving through airways that contain fluid	Dry or wet intermittent sounds that vary in pitch (this sound can be duplicated by rubbing hair together next to ear)
Rhonchi*	Thick secretions, tumors, or spasms that partially obstruct air flow through large upper airways	Deep, low-pitched, rumbling sound more audible during expiration
Wheezes	Severely narrowed airways caused by partial obstruction in smaller bronchi and bronchioles; common symptom of asthma	Continuous, high-pitched, whistling musical sounds heard during inspiration and expiration
Pleural friction rub*	Inflamed pleurae rubbing together	High, grating sound similar to rubbing leather pieces together, heard on inspiration and expiration

*Audible only through a stethoscope.

respiratory disorder. The causes and characters of abnormal breath sounds are presented in Table 19-6.

PULSE OXIMETRY

Pulse oximetry is a painless and noninvasive procedure used to measure the oxygen saturation of hemoglobin in arterial blood. Hemoglobin is a complex compound found in red blood cells that functions in transporting oxygen in the body. Pulse oximetry provides the physician with information on a patient's cardiorespiratory status—in particular, the amount of oxygen being delivered to the tissues of the body. The procedure for performing pulse oximetry is presented in Procedure 19-8.

A **pulse oximeter** is the device used to measure and display the oxygen saturation of the blood. It is a computerized device that consists of a two-sided, cliplike probe connected by a cable to a monitor (Figure 19-14). A pulse oximeter also measures the patient's pulse rate in beats per minute. A constant-pitched audible beep is emitted with each pulse beat.

ASSESSMENT OF OXYGEN SATURATION

Mechanism of Action

The probe of the pulse oximeter must be attached to a peripheral pulsating capillary bed, such as the tip of a finger. One side of the probe contains a **light-emitting diode (LED)** that transmits infrared light and red light through the patient's tissues to a light detector located on the other side of the probe, known as the *photodetector* (Figure 19-15).

Hemoglobin that is bright red in color has a high oxygen content (*oxygen rich*) and absorbs more of the infrared light emitted by the LED. Hemoglobin that is dark red in color is low in oxygen (*oxygen poor*) and absorbs more of the red light. The computer of the oximeter compares and calculates the light transmitted from the oxygen-rich hemoglobin and the oxygen-poor hemoglobin and from this ratio is able to determine the oxygen saturation of the patient's

Figure 19-14 Pulse oximeter.

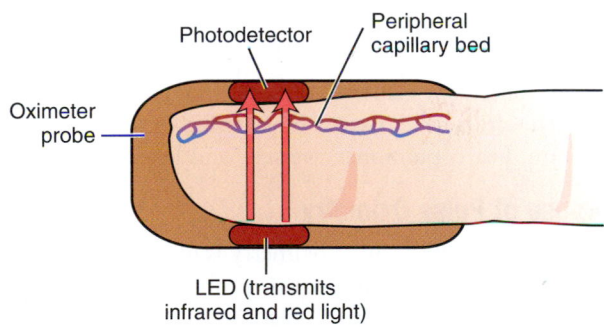

Figure 19-15 The probe of the pulse oximeter is attached to a peripheral capillary bed in the fingertip. The LED transmits light through the capillary bed to a light detector (photodetector) located on the other side of the probe to measure the oxygen saturation of hemoglobin.

hemoglobin. This measurement is converted to a percentage and is displayed as a digital readout on the screen of the monitor. Because the pulse oximeter measures the oxygen saturation of peripheral capillaries, the abbreviation **SpO₂** (*saturation of peripheral oxygen*) is used to record the reading.

A more complete but invasive measurement of oxygen saturation is arterial blood gas analysis, which requires drawing a blood specimen from an artery. The abbreviation for this type of arterial oxygen saturation measurement is **SaO₂** (*saturation of arterial oxygen*).

Interpretation of Results

The pulse oximetry reading represents the percentage of hemoglobin that is saturated (filled) with oxygen. Each molecule of hemoglobin can carry four oxygen molecules. If 100 molecules of hemoglobin were fully saturated with oxygen, they would be carrying 400 molecules of oxygen, and the oxygen saturation reading would be 100%. If these same 100 molecules of hemoglobin were carrying only 360 molecules of oxygen, however, the oxygen saturation reading would be 90%. The more hemoglobin that is saturated with oxygen, the higher the oxygen saturation of the blood.

The oxygen saturation level of most healthy individuals is 95% to 99%. Because the air we breathe is only 21% saturated with oxygen, it is unusual for an individual's hemoglobin to be fully or 100% saturated with oxygen. Patients on supplemental oxygen sometimes have a reading of 100%, however.

An oxygen saturation level of less than 95% typically results in an inadequate amount of oxygen reaching the tissues of the body, although patients with chronic pulmonary disease are sometimes able to tolerate lower saturation levels. Respiratory failure, resulting in tissue damage, usually occurs when the oxygen saturation decreases to a level between 85% and 90%. Cyanosis typically appears when an individual's oxygen saturation reaches a level of 75%, and an oxygen saturation of less than 70% is life-threatening.

A decrease in the oxygen saturation of the blood (less than 95%) is known as **hypoxemia.** Hypoxemia can lead to a more serious condition known as hypoxia. **Hypoxia** is defined as a reduction in the oxygen supply to the tissues of the body, and if not treated it can lead to tissue damage and death. The first symptoms of hypoxia include headache, mental confusion, nausea, dizziness, shortness of breath, and tachycardia. The tissues most sensitive to hypoxia are the brain, heart, pulmonary vessels, and liver.

Purpose of Pulse Oximetry

In the medical office, pulse oximetry is often performed on patients complaining of respiratory problems (e.g., dyspnea). A decreased pulse oximetry reading (along with further testing and the patient's clinical signs and symptoms) assists the physician in proper diagnosis and treatment, which may include drug therapy and oxygen therapy.

Conditions that can cause a decreased SpO_2 value (hypoxemia) include the following:
- Acute pulmonary disease (e.g., pneumonia)
- Chronic pulmonary disease (e.g., emphysema, asthma, bronchitis)
- Cardiac problems (e.g., congestive heart failure, coronary artery disease)

In addition to assisting the physician in diagnosing a patient's condition, pulse oximetry is used to assess the following:
- Effectiveness of oxygen therapy
- Patient's tolerance to activity

- Effectiveness of treatment (e.g., bronchodilators)
- Patient's tolerance to analgesia and sedation

In the medical office, pulse oximetry is most often used as a "spot-check" measurement—in other words, as a single measurement of oxygen saturation. Occasionally, pulse oximetry may be used in the medical office for the short-term *continuous monitoring* of a patient experiencing an asthmatic attack or to monitor a sedated patient during minor office surgery.

Components of the Pulse Oximeter

Most medical offices use a handheld pulse oximeter (see Figure 19-14), which is portable, lightweight, and battery operated. This is in contrast to a stand-alone oximeter, which is more apt to be used in a hospital setting for the continuous bedside monitoring of a patient's oxygen saturation level. A pulse oximeter not only measures oxygen saturation, it also measures the pulse rate in beats per minute. The two main parts of the pulse oximeter—the monitor and the probe—are described in detail next.

Monitor

The monitor contains controls, indicators, and displays (Figure 19-16). These may vary slightly depending on the brand of oximeter. Those that are found on most handheld pulse oximeters include the following:
1. *On/off control.* Turns the oximeter on and off.
2. *SpO_2% display.* A digital display of the patient's oxygen saturation expressed as a percent. This number is updated with each pulse beat.
3. *Pulse rate display.* This display indicates the patient's pulse rate in beats per minute. This number is updated with each pulse beat. Most oximeters emit a constant-pitched audible beep with each pulse beat.
4. *Pulse strength bar-graph indicator.* This indicator provides a visual display of the patient's pulse strength at the probe placement site. The pulse strength indicator consists of a segmented display of bars. The pulse strength indicator "sweeps" with each pulse beat, and the stronger the pulse, the more segments that light up on the bar graph.
5. *Pulse search indicator.* This indicator lights up when the oximeter is searching for the patient's pulse.

Figure 19-16 Pulse oximeter monitor: controls, indicators, and displays.

6. *Adjustable volume control.* This control is used to adjust the beep that sounds with each pulse beat. In most oximeters, the settings are high, low, and off.
7. *Low battery indicator.* This indicator is used to warn that the battery is getting low. The indicator lights up and the monitor sounds an alarm when approximately 30 minutes of battery use remain.
8. *Alarm messages.* Alarm messages indicate a problem or condition that may affect the reading. Alarm messages must not be ignored and must be corrected before continuing.

When the pulse oximeter is turned on, it automatically performs a power-on self-test (POST), which takes approximately 3 to 5 seconds. During the POST, the oximeter checks its internal systems to ensure they are functioning properly. If the oximeter detects a problem, an alarm sounds and the monitor displays an error code. If this occurs, the medical assistant should refer to the troubleshooting section of the user's manual for interpretation of the error code and the necessary action that should be taken.

When the POST is completed, the oximeter begins searching for a pulse. During this time, the pulse search indicator lights up. It takes several seconds for the oximeter to locate a pulse and to calculate and display the SpO_2 reading. If the oximeter is unable to detect a pulse, or if the pulse is too weak to provide the data needed to calculate oxygen saturation, the oximeter is unable to make a measurement. In this case, an alarm sounds and the oximeter may automatically shut off. If this occurs, the medical assistant should reposition the probe or move the probe to another finger and perform the procedure again.

Probe

The probe of the pulse oximeter may be reusable or disposable (Figure 19-17). Most offices use reusable clip-on probes. Reusable probes are convenient to use and easy to apply, but they are more susceptible to inaccurate readings owing to patient movement. Reusable probes must be cleaned and disinfected after each use. Disposable probes are expensive to use and are usually employed for the long-term monitoring of a patient's oxygen saturation level in a hospital setting. Disposable probes are made of an adhesive bandage–like material and are discarded after use.

It is important to handle reusable probes carefully. Hitting a probe against a hard object or dropping it may damage it. It is important to use the probe designed for the pulse oximeter that is being used. Mixing probes from different manufacturers can result in an inaccurate reading.

The probe must be attached to the patient at a peripheral site that is highly vascular and where the skin is thin. The most common site to apply a probe is the tip of a finger (Figure 19-18); other acceptable sites include the toe and earlobe. A specially designed probe is available for application to the earlobe; it is smaller than a finger probe and has a curved ear attachment to hold it in place.

A cable connects the probe to the monitor. The probe may be permanently attached to the cable, or it may be a

Figure 19-17 Disposable *(top)* and reusable *(bottom)* probes for the pulse oximeter.

Figure 19-18 Applying a probe to the tip of a finger.

separate device that requires connection to the cable. The pulse oximeter monitor should never be lifted or carried by the cable because this could damage the cable connections or could cause the cable to disconnect from the monitor and possibly drop on the floor or fall on the patient.

Factors Affecting Pulse Oximetry

Although pulse oximetry is an easy procedure to perform, the medical assistant must be aware of certain factors that may interfere with an accurate reading. These factors are listed, along with guidelines for correcting or preventing them.

1. *Incorrect positioning of the probe.* As previously discussed, the oximeter probe consists of two parts: an LED and a photodetector. Because light is transmitted from the LED through the tissues to the photodetector, it is important that these two components be aligned directly opposite each other during the measurement. In most cases, this automatically occurs when the clip-on probe is applied. Proper alignment of the probe may be impossible, however, with patients who have very small fingers (e.g., a thin individual, a child) or with patients who have very large fingers (e.g., an obese individual). To obtain an accurate reading, another site must be used, such as the earlobe. In addition, pediatric probes are available for use with thin patients or children.

2. *Fingernail polish or artificial nails.* A dark, opaque coating on the fingernail may result in a falsely low reading. This is because the coating interferes with proper light transmission through the finger. The darker the coating, the more likely that the SpO_2 reading will be affected. Blue, black, and green fingernail polishes tend to cause the most problems. If the patient is wearing fingernail polish, it should be removed with acetone or fingernail polish remover. If the patient has artificial fingernails, another site should be used to take the measurement, such as the earlobe or the toe. Oil, dirt, and grime on the fingertip can also interfere with proper light transmission. If the patient's fingertip is dirty, cleanse the site with soap and water and allow it to dry. Areas with bruises, burns, stains, or tattoos should be avoided as a probe placement site. Darkly pigmented skin and jaundice do not usually affect the ability of the oximeter to obtain an accurate reading.

3. *Poor peripheral blood flow.* A pulse oximeter works best when there is a strong pulse in the finger to which the probe is applied. Poor peripheral blood flow may cause the pulse to be so weak that the oximeter cannot obtain a reading. Conditions resulting in poor blood flow include peripheral vascular disease, vasoconstrictor medications, severe hypotension, and hypothermia. In these situations, the medical assistant should try using the earlobe because it is less affected by decreased blood flow. Sometimes patients with cold fingers (but who are not hypothermic) may have enough constriction of the peripheral capillaries that it interferes with obtaining a reading. To solve this problem, the medical assistant should ask the patient to warm his or her fingers by rubbing the hands together. The probe should never be attached to the finger of an arm to which an automatic blood pressure cuff is applied because blood flow to the finger will be cut off when the cuff inflates, resulting in loss of the pulse signal.

4. *Ambient (surrounding) light.* Ambient light shining directly on the probe, such as bright fluorescent light, direct sunlight, or an overhead examination light, may result in an inaccurate reading. This is because some of the ambient light may be picked up by the probe's photodetector and alter the reading. This problem can be corrected by one of the following: turning off the light, moving the patient's hand away from the light source, or covering the probe with an opaque material such as a washcloth.

5. *Patient movement.* Patient movement is a common cause of an inaccurate reading. Motion affects the ability of the light to travel from the LED to the photodetector and prevents the probe from picking up the pulse signal. To avoid this problem, it is important that the medical assistant instruct the patient to remain still during the procedure. Occasionally, patient movement cannot be eliminated, such as when the patient has tremors of the hands. In these instances, the oxygen saturation level should be measured at a site that is less affected by motion, such as the toe or the earlobe.

Pulse Oximeter Care and Maintenance

The pulse oximeter monitor and cable should be cleaned periodically using a cloth slightly dampened with a solution of warm water and a disinfectant cleaner. The medical assistant should make sure that the cloth is not too wet to prevent the solution from running into the monitor, which could damage the internal components. The probe should be cleaned periodically with a soft cloth moistened with warm water and a disinfectant cleaner. Cleaning the probe removes dirt and grime that could interfere with proper light transmission, leading to an inaccurate reading. The probe also should be disinfected after each use by wiping it thoroughly with an antiseptic wipe and allowing it to dry. The probe should never be soaked or immersed in a liquid solution because this would damage it. The probe is heat sensitive and cannot be autoclaved. The pulse oximeter should be stored at room temperature in a dry environment.

PROCEDURE 19-6   Measuring Pulse and Respiration

Outcome Measure pulse and respiration

Equipment/Supplies

• Watch with a second hand

1. **Procedural Step.** Sanitize your hands. Greet the patient and introduce yourself. Identify the patient and explain the procedure. Observe the patient for any signs that might affect the pulse or respiratory rate.
   Principle. Pulse rate can vary according to the factors listed on pages 370-371.

2. **Procedural Step.** Have the patient sit down. Position the patient's arm in a comfortable position. The forearm should be slightly flexed to relax the muscles and tendons over the pulse site.
   Principle. Relaxed muscles and tendons over the pulse site make it easier to palpate the pulse.

3. **Procedural Step.** Place your three middle fingertips over the radial pulse site. Never use your thumb to take a pulse. The radial pulse is located in a groove on the inner aspect of the wrist just below the thumb.
   Principle. The thumb has a pulse of its own; using the thumb results in measurement of the medical assistant's pulse and not the patient's pulse.

4. **Procedural Step.** Apply moderate, gentle pressure directly over the site until you feel the pulse. If you cannot feel the pulse, this may be caused by:
   a. Incorrect location of the radial pulse: Move your fingers to a slightly different location in the groove of the wrist until you feel the pulse.
   b. Applying too much pressure or not enough pressure: Vary the depth of your hold until you can feel the pulse.
   Principle. A normal pulse can be felt with moderate pressure. The pulse cannot be felt if not enough pressure is applied, whereas too much pressure applied to the radial artery closes it off, and no pulse is felt.

5. **Procedural Step.** Count the pulse for 30 seconds and make a mental note of this number. Note the rhythm and volume of the pulse. If abnormalities are present in the rhythm or volume, count the pulse for 1 full minute.
   Principle. A longer time ensures an accurate assessment of abnormalities.

Place the three middle fingers over the radial pulse site.

Count the pulse for 30 seconds.

PROCEDURE 19-6

PROCEDURE 19-6   Measuring Pulse and Respiration—cont'd

6. Procedural Step. After taking the pulse, continue to hold three fingers on the patient's wrist with the same amount of pressure, and measure the respirations. This helps to ensure that the patient is unaware that respirations are being monitored.
Principle. If the patient is aware that respiration is being measured, the breathing may change.

Count the number of respirations for 30 seconds.

7. Procedural Step. Observe the rise and fall of the patient's chest as the patient inhales and exhales.
Principle. One complete respiration includes one inhalation and one exhalation.

8. Procedural Step. Count the number of respirations for 30 seconds and make a mental note of this number; note the rhythm and depth of the respirations. Also observe the patient's color. If abnormalities are present in rhythm or depth, count the respiratory rate for 1 full minute.

9. Procedural Step. Sanitize your hands.

10. Procedural Step. Chart the results in the patient's medical record. If you counted the pulse and respirations for 30 seconds, multiply each of the numbers counted by 2. This will give you the pulse rate and respiratory rate for 1 full minute.

  a. *Paper-based patient record:* Record the date; the time; the pulse rate, rhythm, and volume; and the respiratory rate, rhythm, and depth (refer to the PPR charting example).

  b. *Electronic medical record:* In SimChart® for the Medical Office, record the pulse rate, rhythm, and volume; and the respiratory rate, rhythm, and depth using textboxes, dropdown menus, and/or radio buttons.

PPR CHARTING EXAMPLE	
Date	
10/15/XX	2:30 p.m. P: 74. Reg and strong. R: 18. Even and reg. ——————— S. Martinez, RMA

PROCEDURE 19-7   Measuring Apical Pulse

Outcome Measure apical pulse

Equipment/Supplies

- Watch with a second hand
- Stethoscope
- Antiseptic wipe

1. Procedural Step. Sanitize your hands. Greet the patient and introduce yourself. Identify the patient and explain the procedure. Observe the patient for any signs that might increase or decrease the pulse rate.

2. Procedural Step. Assemble the equipment. If the stethoscope's chest piece consists of a diaphragm and a bell, rotate the chest piece to the bell position. Clean the earpieces and chest piece of the stethoscope with an antiseptic wipe.

Principle. The bell position allows better auscultation of heart sounds. Cleaning the earpieces helps prevent the transmission of microorganisms.

3. Procedural Step. Ask the patient to unbutton or remove his or her shirt. Have the patient sit or lie down (supine).

Principle. A sitting or supine position allows access to the apex of the heart.

PROCEDURE 19-7 Measuring Apical Pulse—cont'd

4. Procedural Step. Warm the chest piece of the stethoscope with your hands. Insert the earpieces of the stethoscope into your ears, with the earpieces directed slightly forward, and place the chest piece over the apex of the patient's heart. The apex of the heart is located in the fifth intercostal space at the junction of the left midclavicular line. *Principle.* Warming the chest piece reduces the discomfort of having a cold object placed on the chest. In addition, a cold chest piece could startle the patient, resulting in an increase in pulse rate. The earpieces should be directed forward to follow the direction of the ear canal, which facilitates hearing.

Insert the earpieces into your ears with the earpieces directed slightly forward.

5. Procedural Step. Listen for the heartbeat, and count the number of beats for 30 seconds (and multiply by 2) if the rhythm and volume are normal or if the apical pulse of an infant or child is being taken. If abnormalities are present in the rhythm or volume, count the pulse for 1 full minute. You will hear a *lubb-dupp* sound through the stethoscope. This sound is the closing of the heart's valves. Each *lubb-dupp* is counted as one beat.

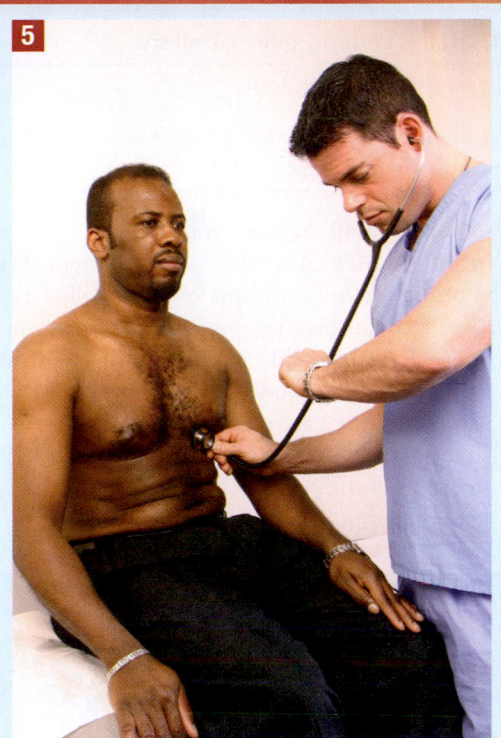

Count the number of beats for 30 seconds, and multiply by 2.

6. Procedural Step. Sanitize your hands.
7. Procedural Step. Chart the results in the patient's medical record.
  a. *Paper-based patient record:* Record the date, the time, and the apical pulse rate, rhythm, and volume (refer to the PPR charting example).
  b. *Electronic medical record:* In SimChart® for the Medical Office, record the rate, rhythm, and volume and the site for taking this pulse using textboxes, drop-down menus, and/or radio buttons.
8. Procedural Step. Clean the earpieces and the chest piece of the stethoscope with an antiseptic wipe.

PPR CHARTING EXAMPLE	
Date	
10/15/XX	10:15 a.m. AP: 68. Reg and strong.————
	———————— S. Martinez, CMA (AAMA)

PROCEDURE 19-7

PROCEDURE 19-8   Performing Pulse Oximetry

Outcome Perform pulse oximetry

Equipment/Supplies

- Handheld pulse oximeter
- Reusable finger probe
- Antiseptic wipe

1. **Procedural Step.** Sanitize your hands.
2. **Procedural Step.** Assemble the equipment. Handle the probe carefully, and perform the following:
   a. Carefully inspect the probe to ensure it opens and closes smoothly. Inspect the probe windows (light-emitting diode [LED] and photodetector) to ensure they are clean and free of lint.
   b. Disinfect the probe windows and surrounding platforms with an antiseptic wipe, and allow them to dry.

Disinfect the probe with an antiseptic wipe.

   c. If necessary, connect the probe to the cable.
   d. Connect the cable to the monitor by plugging it into the port on the monitor. Do not lift or carry the monitor by the cable.

Connect the cable to the monitor by plugging it into the port on the monitor.

Principle. Misuse or improper handling of the probe could damage it. Dirt or lint on the probe windows could interfere with proper light transmission, leading to an inaccurate reading. Cross-contamination between patients is prevented by disinfecting the probe. Lifting the monitor by the cable could damage the cable connections.

3. **Procedural Step.** Greet the patient and introduce yourself. Identify the patient and explain the procedure. Explain to the patient that the clip-on probe does not hurt and feels similar to a clothespin attached to the finger. If the patient seems fearful, place the probe on your own finger first to reassure the patient that it is not painful.

4. **Procedural Step.** Seat the patient comfortably in a chair with the lower arm firmly supported and the palm facing down.
Principle. Supporting the lower arm helps prevent patient movement during the procedure.

5. **Procedural Step.** Select an appropriate finger to apply the probe. Use the tip of the patient's index, middle, or ring finger. If the patient's fingers are very small or very large and the probe cannot seem to be aligned properly, use the earlobe to take the measurement. If the patient exhibits tremors of the hands, use the earlobe to obtain the reading.
Principle. The probe must be applied to a peripheral site with thin skin that is highly vascular. Very small or very large fingers may not allow for proper positioning of the probe on the finger.

6. **Procedural Step.** Observe the patient's fingernail. If the patient is wearing dark fingernail polish, ask him or her to remove it with acetone or nail polish remover. If the patient is wearing artificial nails, choose another probe site, such as the toe or earlobe.
Principle. An opaque coating on the fingernail may interfere with proper light transmission through the finger, leading to an inaccurate reading.

7. **Procedural Step.** Check to ensure that the patient's fingertip is clean. If it is dirty, cleanse the site with soap and water, and allow it to dry. Ensure that the patient's finger is not cold. If it is cold, ask the patient to rub his or her hands together.
Principle. Oils, dirt, or grime on the finger can interfere with proper light transmission through the finger, leading to an inaccurate reading. Sometimes

PROCEDURE 19-8   Performing Pulse Oximetry—cont'd

patients with cold fingers may have enough constriction of the capillaries that it interferes with obtaining a reading.

8. Procedural Step. Ensure that ambient light does not interfere with the measurement. Position the probe securely on the fingertip as follows:

a. Ensure that the probe window is fully covered by placing the finger over the LED window, with the fleshy tip of the finger covering the window. The tip of the finger should touch the end of the probe stop.

Position the probe securely on the fingertip.

b. Ensure that the LED and the photodetector are aligned opposite to each other.

c. Allow the cable to lay across the back of the hand and parallel to the arm of the patient.

Principle. Ambient light can be picked up by the probe and alter the reading. Proper alignment of the LED and photodetector is necessary for an accurate reading.

9. Procedural Step. Instruct the patient to remain still and to breathe normally. Turn on the oximeter by pressing the on/off control. Wait while the oximeter goes through its power-on self-test (POST). If the monitor fails the POST, refer to the troubleshooting section of the user manual for interpretation of the error code and the necessary action that should be taken.

Principle. Patient movement may lead to an inaccurate reading. The monitor automatically conducts a POST to ensure that it is functioning properly.

10. Procedural Step. Allow several seconds for the pulse oximeter to detect the pulse and calculate the oxygen saturation of the blood. Ensure that the pulse strength indicator fluctuates with each

pulsation and that the pulse signal is strong. If the oximeter sounds an alarm indicating that it was unable to locate a pulse, reposition the probe on the patient's finger or move the probe to another finger, and perform the procedure again.

Principle. The reading takes several seconds to display. The pulse strength indicator provides a quick assessment of pulse quality. If the oximeter is unable to locate a pulse, it will be unable to obtain a reading.

Allow several seconds for the pulse oximeter to detect the pulse.

11. Procedural Step. Leave the probe in place until the oximeter displays a reading. Read the oxygen saturation value and pulse rate, and make a mental note of these readings. On this pulse oximeter, the oxygen saturation reading is 100% and the pulse rate is 75. If the SpO_2 reading is less than 95%, reposition the probe on the finger, and perform the procedure again.

Principle. A low SpO_2 reading may be caused by improper positioning of the probe on the finger.

Read the oxygen saturation value and pulse rate.

Continued

PROCEDURE 19-8   Performing Pulse Oximetry—cont'd

12. **Procedural Step.** Remove the probe from the patient's finger, and turn off the oximeter.
13. **Procedural Step.** Sanitize your hands.
14. **Procedural Step.** Chart the results in the patient's medical record.
    a. *Paper-based patient record:* Record the date, the time, the SpO₂ reading, and the pulse rate (refer to the PPR charting example).
    b. *Electronic medical record:* In SimChart® for the Medical Office, enter the SpO₂ reading and the pulse rate using textboxes, drop-down menus, and/or radio buttons.

15. **Procedural Step.** Disconnect the cable from the monitor. Disinfect the probe with an antiseptic wipe. Properly store the monitor in a clean, dry area.

PPR CHARTING EXAMPLE

Date	
10/15/XX	2:30 p.m. SpO₂: 100%. P: 75.
	S. Martinez, RMA

BLOOD PRESSURE

MECHANISM OF BLOOD PRESSURE

Blood pressure is a measurement of the pressure or force exerted by the blood on the walls of the arteries in which it is contained. Each time the ventricles contract, blood is pushed out of the heart and into the aorta and pulmonary trunk, exerting pressure on the walls of the arteries. This phase in the cardiac cycle is known as **systole,** and it represents the highest point of blood pressure in the body, or the **systolic pressure.** The phase of the cardiac cycle in which the heart relaxes between contractions is referred to as **diastole.** The **diastolic pressure** (recorded during diastole) is lower because the heart is relaxed. Contraction and relaxation of the heart result in two different pressures—systolic and diastolic.

Interpretation of Blood Pressure

Blood pressure measurement is expressed as a fraction. The numerator is the systolic pressure, and the denominator is the diastolic pressure. The standard unit for measuring blood pressure is millimeters of mercury (mm Hg). A blood pressure reading of 110/70 mm Hg means that there was enough force to raise a column of mercury 110 mm during systole and 70 mm during diastole.

Based on guidelines from the National Heart, Lung, and Blood Institute (NHLBI), a blood pressure reading of less than 120/80 mm Hg is classified as normal, whereas a blood pressure reading of 120/80 is classified as *prehypertension.* These guidelines were issued as a result of scientific studies showing that the risk of heart disease begins at a blood pressure reading lower than previously thought. The NHLBI guidelines are outlined in Table 19-7.

Blood pressure should be taken during every office visit to allow the physician to compare the patient's readings over time. This is a good preventive measure in guarding against serious illness. A single blood pressure reading taken on one occasion does not characterize an individual's blood pressure accurately. Several readings, taken on different occasions, provide a good index of an individual's baseline blood pressure.

Blood pressure readings always should be interpreted using a patient's baseline blood pressure. An increase or decrease of 20 to 30 mm Hg in a patient's baseline blood pressure is significant, even if it is still within the normal accepted blood pressure range.

The most common condition that causes an abnormal blood pressure reading is **hypertension.** Hypertension, or high blood pressure, results from excessive pressure on the walls of the arteries. Hypertension is determined by a sustained systolic blood pressure reading of 140 mm Hg or greater, or a sustained diastolic reading of 90 mm Hg or greater. See Table 19-7 for the NHLBI classifications for hypertension. **Hypotension,** or low blood pressure, results from reduced pressure on the arterial walls. Hypotension is determined by a blood pressure reading of less than 95/60 mm Hg.

Table 19-7   Classification of Blood Pressure for Adults Age 18 and Older

Blood Pressure Classifications	Systolic Blood Pressure, mm Hg		Diastolic Blood Pressure, mm Hg
Normal	Less than 120	*and*	Less than 80
Prehypertension*	120-139	*or*	80-89
Hypertension*			
Stage 1	140-159	*or*	90-99
Stage 2	160 or higher	*or*	100 or higher

*Based on the average of two or more properly measured, seated blood pressure readings taken at each of two or more visits.
From National Heart, Lung, and Blood Institute: Seventh report of the Joint National Committee on Detection, Evaluation, and Treatment of High Blood Pressure. Bethesda, Md: NIH Publication No. 03-5231, May, 2003, U.S. Department of Health and Human Services.

Pulse Pressure

The difference between systolic and diastolic pressures is the **pulse pressure.** It is determined by subtracting the smaller number from the larger. If the blood pressure is 110/70 mm Hg, the pulse pressure would be 40 mm Hg. A pulse pressure between 30 and 50 mm Hg is considered to be within normal range.

Factors Affecting Blood Pressure

Blood pressure does not remain at a constant value. Numerous factors may affect it throughout the course of the day. An understanding of these factors helps to ensure an accurate interpretation of blood pressure readings.

1. *Age.* Age is an important consideration when determining whether a patient's blood pressure is normal. As age increases, the blood pressure gradually increases. A 6-year-old child may have a normal reading of 90/60 mm Hg, whereas a young, healthy adult may have a blood pressure reading of 116/76 mm Hg, and it would not be unusual for a 60-year-old man to have a reading of 130/90 mm Hg. As an individual gets older, there is a loss of elasticity in the walls of the blood vessels, causing this increase in pressure to occur. Table 19-8 is a chart of the average optimal blood pressure readings for various age groups.
2. *Gender.* After puberty, women usually have a lower blood pressure than men of the same age. After menopause, women usually have a higher blood pressure than men of the same age.
3. *Diurnal variations.* Fluctuations in an individual's blood pressure are normal during the course of a day. When one awakens, the blood pressure is lower as a result of decreased metabolism and physical activity during sleep. As metabolism and activity increase during the day, the blood pressure rises.
4. *Emotional states.* Strong emotional states, such as anger, fear, and excitement, increase the blood pressure. If the

medical assistant observes such a reaction, an attempt should be made to calm the patient before taking his or her blood pressure.
5. *Exercise.* Physical activity temporarily increases the blood pressure. To ensure an accurate reading, a patient who has been involved in physical activity should be given an opportunity to rest for 20 to 30 minutes before blood pressure is measured.
6. *Body position.* The blood pressure of a patient who is in a lying or standing position is usually different from that measured when the patient is sitting. For example, the diastolic pressure of an individual in a sitting position is higher than his or her diastolic pressure in a lying position. A notation should be made on the patient's chart if the reading was obtained in any position other than sitting, by using the following abbreviations: *L* (lying) and *St* (standing).
7. *Medications.* Many medications may increase or decrease the blood pressure. Because of this factor, it is important to record in the patient chart all prescription and over-the-counter medications that the patient is taking.
8. *Other factors.* Other factors that may increase the blood pressure include pain, a recent meal, caffeine, smoking, and bladder distention.

What Would You Do? What Would You *Not* Do?

Case Study 3

Tyrone Jackson, 45 years old, is at the medical office to have his blood pressure checked. Three months ago, Tyrone started taking a diuretic and an antihypertensive prescribed by the physician to reduce his blood pressure. The last recording in his chart indicates that Tyrone's blood pressure decreased from 168/112 mm Hg to 118/78 mm Hg; however, his blood pressure at this visit is 138/98 mm Hg. Tyrone says that he has not been very good at taking his medication lately. He says it is really hard to remember to take all those pills every day. He also says that he felt just fine before being put on blood pressure pills, but when he started taking them, he felt awful. He had to urinate more often; when he got up fast, he felt dizzy; and he had some problems with headaches. Tyrone says that he decided to cut back on his pills to see if these problems got better, and sure enough, they went away altogether. Tyrone wants to know if there's anything he can do to lower his blood pressure other than taking pills. ∎

ASSESSMENT OF BLOOD PRESSURE: MANUAL METHOD

The equipment needed to measure blood pressure using the manual method includes a stethoscope and a sphygmomanometer. This method requires the medical assistant to perform the steps in the procedure manually, or by hand; this includes inflation and deflation of the cuff and determining the blood pressure measurement by listening to the sounds produced by the brachial artery (Korotkoff sounds).

Table 19-8 Average Optimal Blood Pressure for Age	
Age	**Blood Pressure, mm Hg**
Newborn (6.6 lb)	40 (mean)
1 mo	85/54
1 yr	95/65
6 yr*	105/65
10-13 yr*	110/65
14-17 yr*	120/75
Adult	Less than 120/80

*In children and adolescents, hypertension is defined as blood pressure that is, on repeated measurement, at the 95th percentile or greater adjusted for age, height, and gender (NHBPEP, 1997).
From National High Blood Pressure Education Program (NHBPEP); National Heart, Lung, and Blood Institute; National Institutes of Health: The seventh report of the Joint National Committees on Detection, Evaluation, and Treatment of High Blood Pressure, *JAMA* 239:2560, 2003.

Figure 19-20 The parts of an aneroid sphygmomanometer.

Figure 19-19 A, The parts of a stethoscope. **B,** Types of chest pieces.

Figure 19-21 The scale of the gauge of an aneroid sphygmomanometer.

The equipment required for the manual measurement of blood pressure is described in more detail in the following sections.

Stethoscope

A **stethoscope** amplifies sounds produced by the body and allows the medical assistant to hear them. The most common type of stethoscope used in the medical office is the acoustic stethoscope. It consists of four parts: earpieces, sidepieces known as *binaurals,* plastic or rubber tubing, and a chest piece (Figure 19-19, *A*).

Stethoscope Chest Piece

There are two types of chest pieces: a *diaphragm,* which is a large, flat disc, and a bell, which has a bowl-shaped appearance (Figure 19-19, *B*). The chest piece of a stethoscope consists of a diaphragm and a bell, or just a diaphragm. If a chest piece consists of a diaphragm and a bell, the medical assistant must ensure that the desired piece is rotated into position before use. Failure to do so would not allow the medical assistant to hear sound through the earpieces.

The diaphragm chest piece is more useful for hearing high-pitched sounds, such as lung and bowel sounds, whereas the bell chest piece is more useful for hearing low-pitched sounds, such as those produced by the heart and vascular system. Before using a stethoscope, the medical assistant should ensure that it is in proper working condition.

Manual Sphygmomanometer

The **sphygmomanometer** is an instrument that measures the pressure of blood within an artery. A manual sphygmomanometer consists of a **manometer,** an inner inflatable bladder surrounded by a covering known as the *cuff,* and a pressure bulb with a control valve to inflate and deflate the inner bladder. The manometer contains a scale for registering the pressure of the air in the bladder.

Two types of sphygmomanometers are used to manually measure blood pressure—aneroid and mercury. They are described in more detail in the following paragraphs.

Aneroid Sphygmomanometer

The aneroid sphygmomanometer (Figure 19-20) has a manometer gauge with a round scale. The scale is calibrated in millimeters, with a needle that points to the calibrations (Figure 19-21). To ensure an accurate reading, the needle

Answer questions patients have about hypertension.

What is high blood pressure?

Blood pressure is the force of blood against the walls of the arteries. High blood pressure, also called *hypertension,* means the pressure in the arteries is consistently above normal (140/90 mm Hg), resulting in excessive pressure on the walls of the arteries. Hypertension is the most common life-threatening disease among Americans. It is estimated that 68 million adult Americans age 18 and older (one in three adults) have high blood pressure. Another 70 million Americans have blood pressure in the prehypertension range. Prehypertension is a reading higher than 120/80 but below 140/90. Without lifestyle modifications, individuals with prehypertension have an increased risk of developing hypertension. The incidence of hypertension in the United States has increased dramatically as a result of an aging population and an increased incidence of obesity.

What are the symptoms of high blood pressure?

Approximately 20% to 30% of individuals who have high blood pressure are unaware of it because there are few or no symptoms, and as a result an individual with hypertension may go undiagnosed for many years. If symptoms do occur, they may include one or more of the following: headaches, dizziness, flushed face, fatigue, epistaxis (nosebleed), excessive perspiration, heart palpitations, frequent urination, and leg claudication (cramping in the legs with walking). The only way to know for sure whether you have high blood pressure is to have it checked regularly.

What causes high blood pressure?

In 90% to 95% of cases, the precise cause of high blood pressure is unknown. This type of hypertension is known as *essential* or *primary hypertension.* Certain factors seem to increase the risk of developing essential hypertension, however; these include the following.

Uncontrollable Risk Factors

- *Heredity.* A family history of high blood pressure increases an individual's risk of developing high blood pressure.
- *Ethnicity.* Research has shown that more black than white Americans develop high blood pressure.
- *Age.* Blood pressure normally increases as one grows older. High blood pressure occurs most often in individuals over the age of 35. Men tend to develop high blood pressure most often between the ages of 35 and 55, whereas women are more likely to develop it after menopause.

Controllable Risk Factors

- *Obesity.* Individuals with a BMI (body mass index) of 30 or higher are more likely to develop high blood pressure.
- *Sodium intake.* Sodium, found in salt and processed, canned, and most snack foods, does not cause high blood pressure; however, it can aggravate high blood pressure. Most Americans consume more sodium than they need. The current recommendation is to consume less than 2.4 g (2400 mg) of sodium per day. This is equivalent to 6 g (about 1 teaspoon) of salt.

- *Lack of physical exercise.* A sedentary lifestyle makes it easier to gain weight and increases the chance of developing high blood pressure.
- *Chronic stress.* Research indicates that people who are under continuous stress tend to develop more heart and circulatory problems than people who are not under stress.
- *Smoking.* Smoking tobacco constricts blood vessels, causing an increase in blood pressure.
- *Alcohol consumption.* Heavy and regular alcohol consumption can increase blood pressure.

The remaining 5% to 10% of individuals with hypertension have *secondary hypertension.* This means that high blood pressure can be linked to a known cause, such as chronic kidney disease, adrenal and thyroid diseases, narrowing of the aorta, steroid therapy, oral contraceptives, or preeclampsia associated with pregnancy.

What can happen if high blood pressure is not treated?

If high blood pressure is not brought under control, it can cause severe damage to vital organs, such as the heart, brain, kidneys, and eyes. This damage can result in a heart attack or heart failure, stroke, kidney damage, or damaged vision. Early detection and treatment of high blood pressure can prevent these complications. High blood pressure is often discovered during a routine medical examination or (less commonly) when an individual experiences one of the complications of hypertension caused by damage to a vital organ.

Can high blood pressure be cured?

Essential hypertension cannot be cured, but many treatments are used to bring it under control. These include lifestyle modifications, such as weight reduction; a healthy diet rich in fruits and vegetables and low in saturated fat, *trans* fat, and cholesterol, limitation of salt intake; regular aerobic exercise; cessation of smoking; limitation or elimination of alcohol consumption; and stress management. If lifestyle modifications alone are not enough, medications are available for reducing blood pressure, allowing the patient to lead a normal, healthy, active life.

How long will I undergo treatment?

Treatment for essential hypertension is usually lifelong. Even if you feel fine, you'll probably have to continue treatment for the rest of your life to maintain your blood pressure within a healthy range. If you discontinue your diet and lifestyle changes or stop taking your medication, your blood pressure will increase again.

- Encourage patients with hypertension to adhere to the treatment prescribed by the physician. Help patients remember to take their medication by telling them to associate their medication schedule with a daily routine, such as brushing their teeth or with meals.
- Provide the patient with educational materials about high blood pressure, available from sources such as the American Heart Association. ■

Figure 19-22 **A,** Wall-mounted aneroid sphygmomanometer. **B,** Mobile floor-stand aneroid sphygmomanometer. (**A,** Courtesy Holzer Health Systems, Athens, Ohio.)

must be positioned initially at zero. At least once a year an aneroid sphygmomanometer should be recalibrated to ensure its accuracy.

Aneroid sphygmomanometers are available in three different designs:

- Portable aneroid sphygmomanometer (see Figure 19-20)
- Wall-mounted aneroid sphygmomanometer (Figure 19-22, *A*)
- Mobile floor-stand aneroid sphygmomanometer (Figure 19-22, *B*)

Mercury Sphygmomanometer

The mercury sphygmomanometer (Figure 19-23) has a vertical tube calibrated in millimeters that is filled with mercury. Although more accurate than the aneroid sphygmomanometer, use of the mercury sphygmomanometer is being discouraged because mercury is a hazardous chemical that can be dangerous to humans and the environment.

If a mercury manometer is used to measure blood pressure, it must be placed in the correct position for proper viewing. The medical assistant should be no farther than 3 feet from the scale of the manometer. A portable mercury manometer should be placed on a flat surface so the mercury column is in a vertical position. The wall model mercury manometer is mounted securely on a wall, placing the mercury column in a vertical position.

The following guidelines must be followed when measuring blood pressure with a mercury sphygmomanometer. Before the blood pressure reading is obtained, the mercury must be even with the zero level at the base of the calibrated tube. Pressure created by inflation of the inner bladder causes the mercury to rise in the tube. The top portion of the mercury column, the **meniscus,** curves slightly upward. The blood pressure should be read at the top of the meniscus, with the eye at the same level as the meniscus of the mercury column.

Figure 19-23 The parts of a mercury sphygmomanometer.

Figure 19-24 Blood pressure cuffs: child, adult, and thigh.

Table 19-9 Types of Blood Pressure Cuffs

Cuff	Bladder Length, cm	Bladder Width, cm	Acceptable Circumference, cm
Child arm	21	8	16-21
Small adult arm	24	10	22-26
Adult arm	30	13	27-34
Large adult arm	38	16	35-44
Adult thigh	42	20	45-52

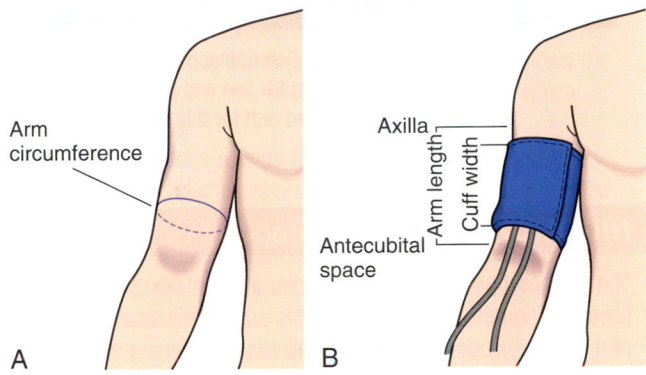

Figure 19-25 Determination of proper cuff size. **A,** The bladder of the cuff should be long enough to encircle 80% of the arm. **B,** The cuff should be wide enough to cover two thirds of the distance from the axilla to the antecubital space.

Cuff Sizes

Blood pressure cuffs come in a variety of sizes and are measured in centimeters (cm) (Figure 19-24). The size of a cuff refers to its inner inflatable bladder, rather than its cloth cover. Table 19-9 lists the types of cuffs available and the size of the inner bladder of each cuff.

For accurate blood pressure measurement, the inner bladder of the cuff should encircle at least 80% (but not more than 100%) of the arm circumference and should be wide enough to cover two thirds of the distance from the axilla to the antecubital space (Figure 19-25). Many blood pressure cuffs are marked with a *range line,* which permits determination of the proper cuff size (Figure 19-26, *A*). When the proper-sized cuff is applied to the patient's arm, an *index line* located at the end of the cuff falls within this range line (Figure 19-26, *B*). If the index line does not fall within the range line, the cuff is not a proper fit for that patient and either a larger or a smaller cuff must be used.

The adult cuff is typically used for the average-sized adult arm while a child cuff often must be used for adults with thin arms. The thigh cuff is used for taking blood pressure from the thigh or for adults with large arms. If the cuff is too small, the reading may be falsely high, as it would be, for example, when an adult cuff is used on a patient with a large arm. If the cuff is too large, the reading may be falsely low, as it would be when an adult cuff is used on a patient with a thin arm. The cuff should fit snugly and should be applied so that the center of the inflatable bag is directly over the brachial artery to allow for complete compression of the artery. The cuff has an interlocking, self-sticking substance (Velcro) that facilitates closing and fastening the cuff in place temporarily.

In obese patients with an arm circumference greater than 50 cm (20 inches), it may not be possible to fit even an adult thigh cuff around the patient's arm. In this situation the American Heart Association (AHA) states that the patient's blood pressure can be measured using the forearm and radial artery; however, the AHA further states that this method may result in a falsely high systolic reading. When this method is used, an appropriate-sized cuff should be positioned midway between the elbow and the wrist, with

Table 19-10 Korotkoff Sounds

Phase	Description	Illustration
	Inflation of cuff compresses and closes off brachial artery so that no blood flows through the artery.	Cuff pressure inflated above systolic pressure (no pulse sounds heard) Brachial artery occluded by cuff, no blood flow No sound
Phase I	First faint but clear tapping sound is heard, and it gradually increases in intensity. First tapping sound is the systolic pressure.	SYSTOLIC PRESSURE Pressure in cuff is released to below systolic but higher than diastolic Blood spurts into constricted artery Sounds first heard 120 mm Hg Korotkoff sounds
Phase II	As cuff continues to deflate, sounds have murmuring or swishing quality.	DIASTOLIC PRESSURE Pressure in cuff below diastolic Blood flows freely 80 mm Hg Sounds disappear
Phase III	With further deflation, sounds become crisper and increase in intensity.	
Phase IV	Sounds become muffled and have soft, blowing quality.	
Phase V	Sounds disappear. This is recorded as the diastolic pressure.	

ASSESSMENT OF BLOOD PRESSURE: AUTOMATIC METHOD

Automatic blood pressure monitors (also known as *digital* or *electronic blood pressure monitors*) are increasingly being used in medical offices to measure blood pressure. They are becoming especially popular for use in home monitoring of blood pressure by patients with high blood pressure. It is important to use an automatic monitor that has undergone a formal clinical validation process to assess its accuracy. A current list of clinically validated automatic blood pressure monitors can be found on the following websites: British Hypertension Society (www.bhsoc.org) and the Association for the Advancement of Medical Instrumentation (www.aami.org).

Automatic monitors are battery operated and do not require the use of a stethoscope to measure blood pressure. The monitor uses an electronic sensor to measure oscillations from the wall of the brachial artery as the cuff gradually deflates. An oscillation is a back-and-forth movement that occurs in the brachial artery as the pulse wave travels through it. The point of maximum oscillation corresponds to the mean arterial pressure, which is an overall index of an individual's blood pressure. A computer in the monitor then uses this information to calculate the systolic blood pressure and the diastolic blood pressure. Results are then displayed digitally on an LED screen. The automatic blood pressure procedure takes approximately 30 seconds to complete from start to finish.

Automatic blood pressure monitors are available in the following designs:
- Portable automatic monitor (Figure 19-27, *A*)
- Mobile floor-stand automatic monitor (Figure 19-27, *B*)

The medical assistant must make sure to follow the manufacturer's instructions for the particular brand and model of automatic monitor used; these instructions are outlined in the user manual that accompanies the monitor. Many of the principles for the accurate measurement of blood pressure using an automatic device are the same as those for manual measurement of blood pressure (refer to the box *Prevention of Errors in Blood Pressure Measurement*). The automatic monitor should be calibrated periodically according to the manufacturer's recommendations. Automatic monitors offer certain advantages and disadvantages, described as follows.

Advantages

1. The automatic monitor can automatically determine how much the cuff should be inflated to reach a pressure that is approximately 30 mm Hg above the systolic pressure.
2. The cuff does not have to be manually inflated and deflated because this function is performed automatically by the device.
3. A stethoscope and user listening skills are not required to obtain the reading because the electronic sensor in the automatic device measures oscillations from the wall of the brachial artery to obtain the reading.

Figure 19-27 Automatic blood pressure monitors. **A,** Portable automatic monitor. **B,** Mobile floor-stand automatic monitor (also includes an electronic thermometer and pulse oximeter). (**B,** Courtesy Holzer Health Systems, Athens, Ohio.)

4. Automatic monitors are less susceptible to external environmental noise than are manual monitors.
5. The blood pressure measurement is easy to read because the systolic and diastolic readings are shown on a digital display screen.

6. Most automatic monitors allow multiple measurements to be taken. The monitor then averages these values and displays them on the screen.
7. Most automatic monitors measure the pulse rate, which is then displayed on the screen along with the blood pressure measurement.
8. Most automatic monitors come equipped with an internal memory for storing multiple blood pressure measurements.

Disadvantages

1. There are certain factors that can cause an automatic monitor to fail to obtain a reading. These include patient movement, muscle tremors, preeclampsia, dysrhythmias (such as atrial fibrillation), and a very weak pulse. If any of these conditions are present, an alternative method of blood pressure measurement should be used.
2. Because the device relies on brachial artery oscillations to obtain a reading, stiff arteries (especially in older patients) can interfere with obtaining an accurate reading.
3. Automatic monitors designed for use in a medical office setting are more expensive than manual monitors.

PROCEDURE 19-9   Measuring Blood Pressure

Outcome   Measure blood pressure

Equipment/Supplies

- Stethoscope
- Portable aneroid sphygmomanometer
- Antiseptic wipe

1. Procedural Step. Sanitize your hands, and assemble the equipment. If the chest piece consists of a diaphragm and a bell, rotate it to the diaphragm position. Clean the earpieces and chest piece of the stethoscope with the antiseptic wipe.
Principle. The chest piece must be rotated to the proper position for sound to be heard through the earpieces.

Rotate the chest piece to the diaphragm position.

2. Procedural Step. Greet the patient and introduce yourself. Identify the patient and explain the procedure. Explain to the patient that measuring blood pressure may normally cause a little numbing and tingling in the arm when the cuff is inflated. While explaining the procedure, observe the patient for signs that might influence the reading, such as anger, fear, pain, and recent physical activity. If it is not possible to reduce or eliminate these influences, list them in the patient's chart. Determine how high to pump the cuff by checking the patient's chart for previously measured systolic readings, or determine the patient's systolic pressure by palpation (see Procedure 19-10).

3. Procedural Step. Have the patient sit quietly in a comfortable position in a chair with the legs uncrossed at the knees and the back supported. The patient should relax in a sitting position for at least 5 minutes before measurement of his or her blood pressure. Roll up the patient's sleeve approximately 5 inches above the elbow so that the cuff can be applied to bare skin. If the sleeve does not roll up or is too tight after being rolled up, remove the arm from the sleeve. The arm should be positioned at heart level and well supported, with the palm facing up.

PROCEDURE **19-9**   Measuring Blood Pressure—cont'd

Principle. Patient anxiety can cause a significant increase in blood pressure. Clothing interferes with the ability to hear Korotkoff sounds, which could result in an inaccurate blood pressure reading. A tight sleeve causes partial compression of the brachial artery, resulting in an inaccurate reading. The position of the arm allows easy access to the brachial artery. Placing the arm above heart level may cause the reading to be falsely low. Not supporting the arm or placing it below heart level and crossing the legs at the knees may cause the reading to be falsely high.

4. **Procedural Step.** Select the proper cuff size. The inner inflatable bladder of the cuff should be long enough to encircle at least 80% (but no more than 100%) of the patient's arm and wide enough to cover two thirds of the distance from the axilla to the antecubital space.

Principle. The appropriate-sized cuff must be used to ensure an accurate measurement. If the cuff is too small, it may come loose as the cuff is inflated, or the reading may be falsely high. If the cuff is too large, the reading may be falsely low.

5. **Procedural Step.** Make sure the cuff is completely deflated and that there is no residual air in the bladder of the cuff. Locate the brachial pulse with the fingertips. The brachial pulse is located near the center of the antecubital space but slightly toward the little finger–side of the arm. Center the inner bladder over the brachial pulse site. (*Note:* Place the cuff on the patient's arm so that the lower edge of the cuff is approximately 1 to 2 inches above the bend in the elbow. Most cuffs are labeled with right and left arrows indicating the center of the bladder. The right arrow should be placed over the brachial pulse site when you are using the right arm, and the left arrow should be placed over the brachial pulse site when you are using the left arm.)

Principle. The cuff should be placed high enough to prevent the stethoscope from touching it; otherwise, extraneous sounds, which could interfere with an accurate measurement, may be picked up. Centering the inner bladder over the pulse site allows complete compression of the brachial artery.

The inner bladder should encircle at least 80% of the patient's arm.

Center the inner bladder over the brachial pulse site.

Continued

PROCEDURE 19-9

ON THE WEB

For information on hypertension:

American Heart Association: www.heart.org

National Heart, Lung, and Blood Institute: www.nhlbi.nih.gov

Health Communities: www.healthcommunities.com

Hypertension Education Foundation: www.hypertensionfoundation.org

American Society of Hypertension: www.ash-us.org

WebMD on Hypertension: www.webmd.com/hypertension-high-blood-pressure/default.htm

MedicineNet Hypertension: www.medicinenet.com/high_blood_pressure/article.htm

Mayo Clinic Hypertension: www.mayoclinic.com/health/high-blood-pressure/ds00100

For information on lung disease:

American Lung Association: www.lung.org

Lung Disease and Respiratory Health: www.webmd.com/lung/lung-diseases-overview

Lung Cancer Online: www.lungcanceronline.org

Medline Plus Lung Diseases: www.nlm.nih.gov/medlineplus/lungdiseases.html

CDC Chronic Obstructive Pulmonary Disease: www.cdc.gov/copd

The Physical Examination

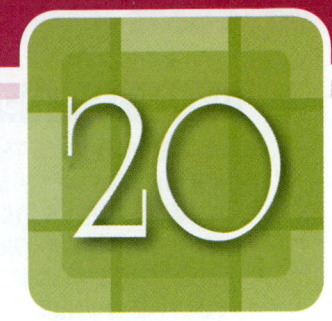

(e) Check out the Evolve site at http://evolve.elsevier.com/Bonewit/today/ to access additional interactive activities and exercises to help you study and prepare for success.

LEARNING OBJECTIVES	PROCEDURES

Preparation for the Physical Examination

1. Identify the three components of a complete patient examination.
2. List the guidelines that should be followed in preparing the examining room.
3. Identify equipment and instruments used during the physical examination.

Prepare the examining room.
Operate and care for equipment and instruments used during the physical examination, according to the manufacturers' instructions.
Prepare a patient for a physical examination.

Measuring Weight and Height

4. Explain the purpose of measuring weight and height.
5. List the guidelines that should be followed when measuring weight and height.

Measure weight and height.

Body Mechanics

6. Explain the importance of using proper body mechanics.
7. State the basic principles related to proper body mechanics that should be followed.

Demonstrate proper body mechanics when standing, sitting, and lifting an object.

Positioning and Draping

8. Explain the purposes of positioning and draping.
9. List one use of each patient position.

Position and drape a patient in each of the following positions:
- Sitting
- Supine
- Prone
- Dorsal recumbent
- Lithotomy
- Sims
- Knee-chest
- Fowler

Wheelchair Transfer

10. Explain the purpose of a wheelchair.
11. Describe the purpose of a transfer belt.

Transfer a patient from a wheelchair to the examining table and back again.

Assessment of the Patient

12. List and define the four techniques of examining the patient.
13. State an example of the use of each examination technique during the physical examination of a patient.

Assisting the Physician

14. Describe the responsibilities of the medical assistant during the physical examination.

Assist the physician during the physical examination of a patient.

CHAPTER OUTLINE

INTRODUCTION TO THE PHYSICAL EXAMINATION
DEFINITIONS OF TERMS
PREPARATION OF THE EXAMINING ROOM
PREPARATION OF THE PATIENT
MEASURING WEIGHT AND HEIGHT
BODY MECHANICS
Principles
Application of Body Mechanics
Standing
Sitting
Lifting

POSITIONING AND DRAPING
WHEELCHAIR TRANSFER
ASSESSMENT OF THE PATIENT
Inspection
Palpation
Percussion
Auscultation
ASSISTING THE PHYSICIAN

KEY TERMS

audiometer (aw-dee-OM-eh-ter)
auscultation (os-kul-TAY-shun)
bariatrics (BAR-ee-AT-riks)
body mechanics
clinical diagnosis
diagnosis

differential (diff-er-EN-shul) diagnosis
inspection
mensuration (men-soo-RAY-shun)
ophthalmoscope (off-THAL-meh-skope)
otoscope (AH-toh-skope)
palpation (pal-PAY-shun)

percussion (per-KUSH-un)
percussion hammer
prognosis
speculum (SPEK-yoo-lum)
symptom

INTRODUCTION TO THE PHYSICAL EXAMINATION

A complete patient examination consists of three parts: the *health history,* the *physical examination* of each body system, and *laboratory and diagnostic tests.* The physician uses the results to determine the patient's general state of health, to arrive at a diagnosis and prescribe treatment, and to observe any change in a patient's illness after treatment has been instituted.

An important and frequent responsibility of the medical assistant is to assist with a physical examination. Because health-promotion and disease-prevention activities have become an important focus of health care, individuals are becoming more aware of the need for a yearly physical examination to detect early signs of illness and to prevent serious health problems. Also, a physical examination may be a prerequisite for employment, participation in sports, attendance at summer camp, and admission to school. The physical examination is explained in detail in this chapter. Taking the health history, collecting specimens, and performing laboratory and diagnostic tests are discussed in other chapters.

DEFINITIONS OF TERMS

The medical assistant should know and understand the following terms related to the patient examination.

Final diagnosis. Often simply called the *diagnosis,* this term refers to the scientific method of determining and identifying a patient's condition through evaluation of the health history, the physical examination, laboratory tests, and diagnostic procedures. A final diagnosis is crucial because it provides a logical basis for treatment and prognosis.

Clinical diagnosis. The clinical diagnosis is an intermediate step in the determination of a final diagnosis. The clinical diagnosis of a patient's condition is obtained through evaluation of the health history and the physical examination without the benefit of laboratory or diagnostic tests. Laboratory and diagnostic imaging facilities provide a space to specify the clinical diagnosis on their request forms; this information assists the facility in correlating data from their test results with the physician's needs. When the physician has analyzed the test results, a final diagnosis can often be established.

Differential diagnosis. Two or more diseases may have similar symptoms. The differential diagnosis involves determining which of these diseases is producing the patient's symptoms so that a final diagnosis can be established. For example, streptococcal sore throat and pharyngitis have similar symptoms. A differential diagnosis is made by obtaining a throat specimen and performing a strep test.

Prognosis. The prognosis consists of the probable course and outcome of a patient's condition and the patient's prospects for recovery.

Risk factor. A risk factor is a physical or behavioral condition that increases the probability that an individual will develop a particular condition; examples are genetic factors, habits, environmental conditions, and physiologic conditions. The presence of a risk factor for a

HIGHLIGHT on Health Screening

The chance of developing certain diseases is greater at different ages. Periodic health screening is recommended for the detection and early treatment of disease.

Test or Procedure	Gender	Recommended Frequency (for Individuals of Average Risk)
Beginning at Age 20 Years		
Blood pressure	M and F	Every year.
Cholesterol levels	M and F	Every 5 years.
Blood glucose level	M and F	Every 3-5 years.
Breast self-examination	F	Every month.
Beginning at the Age Specified		
Clinical breast examination (by a physician)	F	Every 3 years between the ages of 20 and 39 and then every year beginning at age 40.
Cervical cancer screening	F	Every 3 years with a Pap test beginning at age 21 until age 29. Beginning at age 30, preferred screening includes a Pap test and an HPV test every 5 years until age 65.
Testicular self-examination	M	Every month beginning at age 15.
Fecal occult blood test	M and F	Every year starting at age 50.
Colonoscopy	M and F	Every 10 years beginning at age 50.
Prostate cancer screening	M	Should be offered by a health provider every year beginning at age 50 to men with a life expectancy of at least 10 years.
Mammography	F	Every year beginning at age 40.
Electrocardiogram	M and F	One baseline recording starting at age 40. ■

certain disease does not mean that the disease will develop; it means only that a person's chances of developing that disease are greater than those of a person without the risk factor. For example, cigarette smoking is a risk factor for developing lung cancer and heart disease. A person who smokes has a higher risk of developing lung cancer than a person who does not smoke or who has stopped smoking.

Acute illness. An acute illness is characterized by symptoms that have a rapid onset, are usually severe and intense, and subside after a relatively short time. In some cases, the acute episode progresses into a chronic illness. Examples of acute illness include colds, influenza, strep throat, and pneumonia.

Chronic illness. A chronic illness is characterized by symptoms that persist for longer than 3 months and show little change over a long time. Examples of chronic illness include diabetes mellitus, hypertension, and emphysema.

Therapeutic procedure. A therapeutic procedure is performed to treat a patient's condition with the goal of eliminating it or promoting as much recovery as possible. Examples of therapeutic procedures include administration of medication, ear and eye irrigations, and application of heat and cold.

Laboratory testing. Laboratory testing involves the analysis and study of specimens obtained from patients to assist in diagnosing and treating disease. Examples of laboratory testing include the hemoglobin test, glucose test, urinalysis, and strep testing.

Diagnostic procedure. A diagnostic procedure is a procedure performed to assist in the diagnosis of a patient's condition; examples include electrocardiography, colonoscopy, and mammography.

PREPARATION OF THE EXAMINING ROOM

Proper preparation of the examining room provides a comfortable and healthy environment for the patient and facilitates the physical examination. The following guidelines should be followed in preparing the examining room:

1. Ensure that the examining room is free of clutter and well lit.
2. Check the examining rooms daily to ensure there are ample supplies. Restock supplies that are getting low.
3. Empty waste receptacles frequently.
4. Replace biohazard containers as necessary. When removing biohazard containers from the examining room (see Chapter 17), follow the OSHA Bloodborne Pathogens Standard.
5. Make sure the room is well ventilated, and install an air freshener to eliminate odors.
6. Maintain room temperatures that are comfortable not only for a fully clothed individual, but also for an individual who has disrobed.
7. Clean and disinfect examining tables, countertops, and faucets daily.

HIGHLIGHT on Patient Teaching

The purpose of patient teaching is to help the patient develop habits, attitudes, and skills that enable the individual to maintain and improve his or her own health.

Fact: Patients who are active, informed participants in their health care are more apt to follow the physician's instructions than patients who are passive recipients of medical services.

Action: Provide patients with information on health care. Every patient interaction is an opportunity for teaching.

Fact: Adult learners are goal oriented and performance centered. They need and want information that would assist them in managing and improving their health.

Action: Review the information that you provide to patients, and determine whether it is nice to know or necessary to know. Select subject matter that is practical and useful and relates directly to the patient's needs.

Fact: The more information that is presented, the more the patient is likely to forget. Approximately one half of information presented to the patient is forgotten in the first 5 minutes after the patient receives it.

Action: When teaching, use the following pointers to help patients learn and retain information:

- Keep it short and be specific.
- Speak in terms the patient can understand.
- Focus on "how" rather than "why."
- Repeat and reinforce important information.
- Give practical examples, and provide ample time for patient practice.

- Ask for feedback from the patient to determine whether he or she understands the information.
- Provide the patient with written information.

Fact: Each individual has a distinct style of learning and learns best when using his or her preferred learning style. The three main learning styles are reading, listening, and doing. People often use more than one style for learning.

Action: Use a variety of teaching strategies to engage the various learning styles of patients. Examples of teaching strategies include explanations, printed handouts, audiovisual aids, demonstrations, and discussions.

Fact: Only two thirds of patients comply with health care instructions prescribed by the physician. Factors that influence compliance include the patient's adaptation to illness, motivation to change, physical capability, and *support systems.*

Action: The following help increase patient compliance with prescribed treatment:

- Address the patient by his or her name of choice. (Keep in mind that many patients object to being called by their first name by strangers.)
- Encourage the patient to take an active role in personal health care.
- Help the patient set goals and objectives for change.
- Encourage care and support from family members.
- Make the patient aware of outside resources.
- Give positive reinforcement when the patient makes healthy changes. ■

Putting It All Into Practice

My Name is Hope Fauber, and I am a certified medical assistant. I work in a medical clinic with a family medicine department of 10 physicians and 10 residents and interns. My duties cover a broad spectrum, from pediatrics to geriatrics, and include prenatal care, allergy injections, minor office surgery, electrocardiograms, colposcopies, immunizations, and wound care.

At our clinic, many of the patients are elderly. I occasionally come across geriatric patients who are not very cooperative and are "set in their ways." One 90-year-old woman, in particular, had a reputation in the office for being cantankerous and difficult to work with. One day when the physician ordered laboratory work on her, I prepared to draw blood from her tiny, frail body, praying that everything would go smoothly. As I helped her up after a successful "stick," she, of all people, reached to give me a hug and said to me, "I like you. That didn't even hurt!" She continued to hold my hand and talk to me as I walked her out of the office. This turned out to be the last time I would see her because she moved out of town, but not out of my heart, leaving a lasting impression on my life. ■

What Would You Do? | What Would You *Not* Do?

Case Study 1

Abbey Auden, 35 years old, is at the medical office. Her husband got a backyard trampoline for their two school-aged children, and she decided to try it out. Abbey landed wrong on the trampoline and hurt her back and neck. For the past 5 days, she has been having headaches and back pain. Abbey refuses to have her weight taken because she has gained weight over the past several years and does not want to know how much she's gained. She does not understand why weight has to be taken at an office visit in the first place. Abbey says that many times when she should go to the doctor, she doesn't, just to avoid being weighed. She says she would not even be here now except that her husband insisted that she come. ■

BMI	19	20	21	22	23	24	25	26	27	28	29	30	31	32	33	34	35
Height (inches)	Body Weight (pounds)																
58	91	96	100	105	110	115	119	124	129	134	138	143	148	153	158	162	167
59	94	99	104	109	114	119	124	128	133	138	146	147	153	158	163	168	173
60	97	102	107	112	118	123	128	133	138	143	148	153	158	163	168	174	179
61	100	106	111	116	122	127	132	137	143	148	153	158	164	169	174	180	185
62	104	109	115	120	126	131	136	142	147	153	158	164	169	175	180	186	191
63	107	113	118	124	130	135	141	146	152	158	163	169	175	180	186	191	197
64	110	116	122	128	134	140	154	151	157	163	169	174	180	186	192	197	204
65	114	120	126	132	138	144	150	156	162	168	174	180	186	192	198	204	210
66	118	124	130	136	142	148	155	161	167	173	179	186	192	198	204	210	216
67	121	127	134	140	146	153	159	166	172	178	185	191	198	204	211	217	223
68	125	131	138	144	151	158	164	171	177	184	190	197	203	210	216	223	230
69	128	135	142	149	155	162	169	176	182	189	196	203	209	216	223	230	236
70	132	139	143	153	160	167	174	181	188	195	202	209	216	222	229	236	243
71	136	143	150	157	165	172	179	186	193	200	208	215	222	229	236	243	250
72	140	147	154	162	169	177	184	191	199	206	213	221	228	235	242	250	258
73	144	151	159	166	174	182	189	197	204	212	219	227	235	242	250	257	265
74	148	155	163	171	179	186	194	202	210	218	225	233	241	249	256	264	272
75	152	160	168	176	184	192	200	208	216	224	232	240	248	256	264	272	279
76	156	164	172	170	189	197	205	213	221	230	238	246	254	263	271	279	287

Figure 20-2 Body mass index (BMI) table. To use the table, find the appropriate height in the left-hand column labeled Height. Move across to a given weight (in pounds). The number at the top of the column is the BMI at that height and weight. Pounds have been rounded off. (From National Heart, Lung, and Blood Institute, U.S. Department of Health and Human Services.)

Table 20-2 Interpretation of Body Mass Index (BMI)

BMI	Weight Status Category
Less than 15	Very severely underweight
15 to 15.9	Severely underweight
16 to 18.49	Underweight
18.5-24.9	Healthy weight
25-29.9	Overweight
30-34.9	Obese Class I (Moderately obese)
35.0-39.9	Obese Class II (Severely obese)
40 or more	Obese Class III (Very severely obese)

or at the following website: www.nhlbi.nih.gov/health/educational/lose_wt/BMI/bmicalc.htm For adults 20 years and older, BMI is then interpreted using weight status categories. Adult patients with a BMI between 18.5 and 24.9 are considered to be within normal weight. Table 20-2 outlines each of the BMI ranges and the corresponding weight status categories.

Text continued on p. 418

What Would You Do? What Would You *Not* Do?

Case Study 2

Karen Steiner drops her 17-year-old daughter, Mikayla, off at the medical office for her sports physical examination. Mikayla is captain of the varsity cheerleading squad and is getting ready to start her senior year in high school. Mikayla's vital signs are normal, and she measures 5 feet, 6 inches tall and weighs 105 pounds. With some reluctance, Mikayla admits that she's been having problems with heartburn, and she's pretty sure she knows what's causing it. She says that she has to keep her weight down for cheerleading, and after eating dinner with her family, she makes herself vomit to get rid of the food in her stomach. Mikayla is not too concerned about doing this because a lot of the popular girls at school are doing the same thing. She says it's the easy way to stay slim, and she would like to lose another 10 pounds before football season starts. Mikayla wants some prescription drug samples to help with the heartburn because the over-the-counter pills that she's been taking are not working anymore. She does not want her parents to know about any of this because she's afraid that they would not understand and might make her drop out of cheerleading. ∎

mother's health. Procedure 20-1 describes how to measure height and weight using an upright balance scale.

An adult's weight usually is measured during each office visit; an adult's height is typically measured only during the first visit or when a complete physical examination of the patient is requested. Children are weighed and their height (or length) is measured during each office visit to observe their pattern of growth and to calculate medication dosage.

The patient's weight and height are used to determine body mass index (BMI). The BMI strongly correlates with total body fat and therefore is used as a screening tool to identify patients who may be at risk for diseases that occur with overweight and obesity (see the box *Highlight on Body Mass Index*). The BMI can be determined by comparing a patient's weight and height against a BMI table (Figure 20-2). The BMI can also be determined through the use of a BMI calculator available as part of an EMR program

HIGHLIGHT on Cultural Diversity

Culture consists of the values, beliefs, and practices of a particular group of people. Culture is deeply rooted and is passed on from one generation to the next through communication. It includes areas such as religion, dietary practices, family lines of authority, family life patterns, beliefs, and health practices.

As the demographics of the United States continue to change, the medical assistant is faced with the challenge of providing care to an increasing number of cultural groups. It is important for the medical assistant to learn as much as possible about the cultural values of patients coming to the medical office. This is known as *cultural awareness* and can be accomplished by carefully observing and listening to patients to acquire knowledge of their cultural values.

Cultural sensitivity is respect and appreciation for cultural diversity, whereas *cultural competence* is understanding and using the cultural background of a patient to assist with the resolution of a problem. Because health practices are part of a patient's culture, changing them may have a negative impact on the patient. Whenever possible, the medical assistant should incorporate factors from a patient's cultural background into his or her health care.

Guidelines for Achieving Cultural Competence

The following guidelines help the medical assistant in developing cultural awareness and sensitivity and in achieving cultural competence:

1. *Respect the patient's values, beliefs, and practices.* Even if you do not agree with them, it is important to respect the patient's right to hold these values and to not dismiss them as strange or odd. Cultural values play an important role in a patient's lifestyle. Patients from some cultures believe that losing blood depletes the body's strength and provides a route for the soul to leave the body. If a blood specimen is needed, these patients may become highly distressed or refuse to have their blood drawn. Members of some cultural groups believe that illness results when the body's natural balance or harmony is disturbed. To restore the balance, alternative forms of medicine, such as herbal remedies and aromatherapy, are used.

2. *Refrain from cultural stereotypes.* Not all people of a cultural group have the same beliefs, practices, and values. Assuming that all members of a cultural group are alike is known as *stereotyping* and should be avoided. Just as one would never assume that all people in the United States like hamburgers and baseball, every individual must be approached according to his or her specific beliefs and practices.

3. *Always address patients by their last names (and Mr., Mrs., Miss, Ms.) unless they give you permission to use other names.* In many cultures, using a first name to address anyone other than family or friends is considered disrespectful. Most older people in the United States dislike being called by their first name and feel it shows a lack of respect.

4. *Speak slowly and clearly.* Communicating with a patient may be difficult if the patient has a limited knowledge of English. With these patients, you should speak slowly and clearly in a normal tone and volume of voice. Speaking loudly does not help the patient understand any better and may be offensive to the patient.

5. *Show respect for cultural lines of authority.* In many cultures, respect is given based on age and gender. In certain cultures, elders are considered the holders of the culture's wisdom and are highly respected. In other cultures, youth is valued over age. In certain cultures men dominate, and women have very little status. Because of this, a female patient from this type of culture may not be permitted to give her own health history or to answer questions. In addition, a male patient from this culture may not accept instructions from a female medical assistant.

6. *Use appropriate eye contact.* In most cultures, direct eye contact is important and in general shows that the other is attentive and listening. It conveys self-confidence, openness, interest, and honesty, whereas the lack of eye contact may be interpreted as secretiveness, shyness, guilt, or lack of interest. Other cultures consider eye contact impolite or an invasion of privacy; these patients show respect by avoiding direct eye contact.

7. *Be aware of cultural responses to illness.* The conditions under which an individual assumes the role of a (sick) patient and the way he or she performs in that role vary with culture. Individuals of some cultures resist the sick role and blame sickness on external forces as a means of punishment. These individuals may deny their illness and fail to provide much information when the medical assistant takes their symptoms. In other cultures, individuals take an optimistic view of the outcome of health care and because of this are more likely to offer information and to follow the physician's instructions.

8. *Learn to appreciate the richness of diversity as an asset, rather than a hindrance, to communication and effective interaction with patients.* ■

Teach patients the essentials of health promotion and disease prevention. Help patients become aware of the following patterns of behavior that promote and support health:

- Keeping up to date with immunizations
- Eating nutritiously from the food pyramid
- Exercising regularly
- Maintaining normal weight
- Managing stress
- Maintaining high self-esteem
- Avoiding tobacco and drugs
- Using alcohol wisely

- Understanding how the environment affects health and taking appropriate action to improve it
- Knowing the facts about cardiovascular disease, cancer, infections, sexually transmitted diseases, and accidents, and using this knowledge to protect against them
- Understanding the changes that occur through the natural processes of aging
- Developing a sense of responsibility for health by taking an active role in establishing and maintaining a healthy lifestyle ■

Guidelines for Measuring Weight and Height

When using an upright balance scale to measure weight and height, use the following guidelines.

Weight

1. *Locate the scale to provide privacy for the patient.* Place the scale on a hard, level surface in a private location. Many patients are self-conscious about having their weight measured and prefer that it be done in privacy. Do not make weight-sensitive comments during the procedure. This is especially important for patients with weight-control problems such as obesity and eating disorders.
2. *Balance the scale before measuring weight.* If the scale is not balanced, the weight measurement will be inaccurate. The scale is balanced when the upper and lower weights are on zero and the indicator point comes to a rest at the center of the balance area.
3. *Assist the patient.* Assist the patient onto and off of the scale platform. The scale platform moves slightly and may cause the patient to become unsteady.
4. *Obtain an accurate weight.* Always ask the patient to remove his or her shoes. Measure weight with the patient in normal clothing. Ask the patient to remove heavy outer clothing, such as a sweater or a jacket.
5. *Interpret the calibration markings accurately.* The lower calibration bar is divided into 50-lb increments (Figure 20-3, *A*). The upper calibration bar is divided into pounds and quarter pounds. The longer calibration lines indicate pound increments, and the shorter calibration lines indicate quarter-pound and half-pound increments (Figure 20-3, *B*).
6. *Determine the patient's weight correctly.* Add the measurement on the lower scale to the measurement on the upper scale. The result should be rounded to the nearest quarter pound. Occasionally the patient's weight may need to be converted to kilograms, which is the metric unit of measurement for weight. This may be required when determining medication dosage. The following formulas are used to convert weight and height measurements from one system to another.

Upper weight — Upper calibration bar — Lower weight — Lower calibration bar

14 lbs — 1/4 lb — 1/2 lb — 3/4 lb — 15 lbs

Figure 20-3 Calibration markings for measuring weight on an upright balance scale. **A,** The upper calibration bar is divided into pounds and quarter pounds. **B,** The longer calibration lines indicate pound increments, and the shorter calibration lines indicate quarter-pound and half-pound increments.

Weight Conversion

Pounds to kilograms: Divide the number of pounds by 2.2:
    136 lb ÷ 2.2 = 61.8 kg
Kilograms to pounds: Multiply the number of kilograms by 2.2:
    75 kg × 2.2 = 165 lb

Continued

BODY MECHANICS

Daily activities in a medical office sometimes carry the risk of acute or chronic musculoskeletal injury. Because of this, the medical assistant should have a thorough knowledge of the principles of proper body mechanics and know when to use them. **Body mechanics** is the use of the correct muscles to maintain proper balance, posture, and body alignment to accomplish a task safely and efficiently without undue strain on muscles or joints. Proper body mechanics should be used when the medical assistant performs the following: standing, walking, sitting, lifting, positioning a patient on the examining table, and transferring a patient. The medical assistant should also use proper body mechanics at home in his or her activities of daily living. Using proper body mechanics prevents musculoskeletal strains to the back and other body structures such as the knees, neck, shoulders, and wrists.

The primary benefits of proper body mechanics include the following:
1. Allows an individual to conserve energy, which makes it easier to perform a task
2. Protects the body from injury by reducing stress and strain on muscles, nerves, joints, tendons, ligaments, and soft tissues
3. Helps to maintain proper body control and balance
4. Promotes effective, efficient, and safe movement

Studies show that health care workers sustain a significantly higher incidence of back injuries compared with workers in other professions. To help prevent an injury to the back, a primary focus of proper body mechanics is to keep the natural curves of the spine or vertebral column in proper alignment. The vertebral column has four curvatures. These curvatures increase the strength and resilience of the vertebral column and include the cervical curvature, thoracic curvature, lumbar curvature, and sacral curvature (Figure 20-6). The vertebral column extends from the skull to the pelvis and consists of a series of bones known as *vertebrae.* The vertebrae are separated by shock-absorbing *intervertebral discs* (see Figure 20-6). These discs allow an individual to bend and twist. Over time, with improper and repeated bending and twisting (especially while carrying an object), the discs can deteriorate, which causes them to narrow, to harden, and even to crack and tear. This condition is known as *degenerative disc disease.* With degenerative disc disease, the discs lose their shock-absorbing ability and cause the patient to experience localized pain and stiffness in the area of disc deterioration. In addition, once a disc is weakened, it can bulge out or rupture; this is known as a *herniated disc.*

PRINCIPLES

There are some basic principles related to proper body mechanics that should be followed:
1. Movements should be smooth and coordinated rather than jerky.

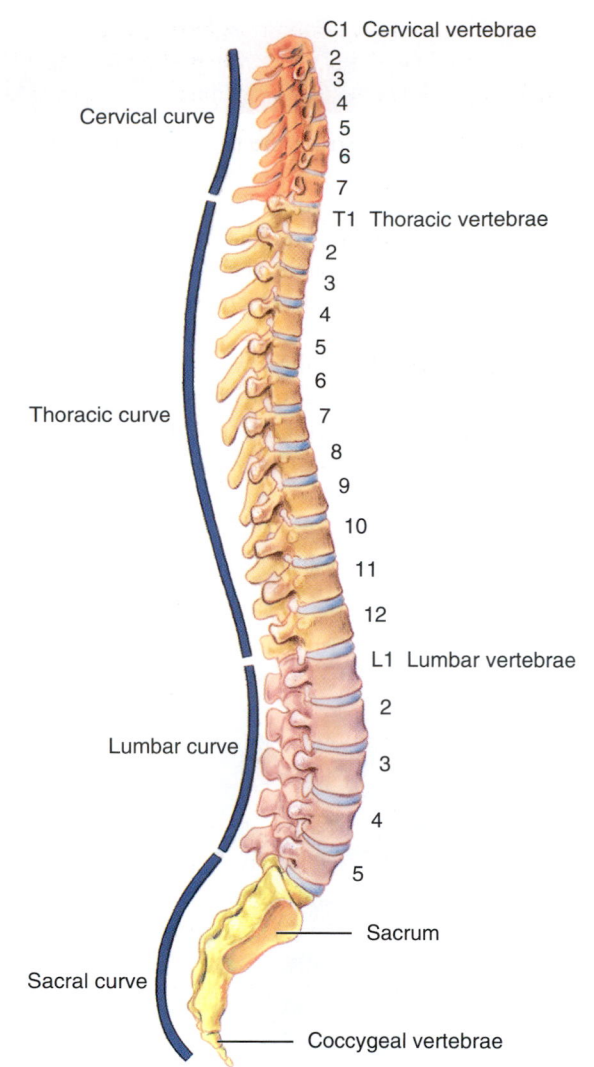

Figure 20-6 Vertebral column. (From Applegate E: *The anatomy and physiology learning system,* ed 4, St Louis, 2011, Saunders.)

2. Keeping the body in good physical condition through exercising, stretching, and weight training helps to prevent musculoskeletal injury.
3. To avoid straining the back, do not reach for something that is farther than 14 to 18 inches away.
4. Work at a comfortable height that avoids having to bend the neck or back forward to perform the task. People are usually most comfortable working at a height that falls between the waist and elbow levels.
5. If possible, push, pull, or slide an object rather than lifting it. This conserves energy and places less strain on the back.
6. Lighter items should be stored on higher shelves or cabinets, and heavier items should be stored at or below waist level.
7. When an object from an overhead shelf or cabinet needs to be retrieved, use a step stool or chair to come up to the level of the object. Reaching for a stored overhead item can produce strain on the back.

8. When lifting an object or transferring a patient, the large muscles of the arms and legs should be used as much as possible and the back muscles as little as possible. The more muscle groups that are used, the more evenly the weight is distributed over the medical assistant's body, which puts less strain on the back.

9. When transferring a patient, encourage the patient to assist as much as possible.

10. If a patient becomes dizzy or faint or starts to fall, do not try to hold the patient in an upright position. Instead, balance yourself with your legs apart to form a wide base of support, and gently and gradually lower the patient to a chair or to the floor.

11. Always ask for assistance if you don't think you can lift a heavy object or transfer a patient.

APPLICATION OF BODY MECHANICS

The medical assistant should practice proper body mechanics when standing, sitting, lifting an object, positioning a patient on the examining table, and transferring a patient from a wheelchair to an examining table and back again, as outlined on the following pages.

Standing

It is important to maintain good posture by positioning the body in the correct standing position as outlined here. This provides the medical assistant with good balance and stability and reduces strain on the back by keeping the vertebral column at its natural alignment.

1. Wear comfortable low-heeled shoes that provide good support.
2. Hold the head erect at the midline of the body, the back as straight as possible with the pelvis tucked inward, the chest forward with the shoulders back, and the abdomen drawn in and kept flat. This helps to maintain appropriate alignment of the vertebral column (Figure 20-7).
3. The knees should be slightly flexed with the feet pointing forward and parallel to each other about 3 inches apart. This provides a broad base of support and improves balance.
4. The arms should be positioned comfortably at the side, and the weight of the body should be evenly distributed over both feet.

Sitting

The medical assistant should use proper body mechanics when in a sitting position (Figure 20-8), as follows:
1. Sit in a chair with a firm back.
2. Sit firmly with the back and buttocks supported against the back of the chair; avoid slumping. The body weight should be evenly distributed over the buttocks and thighs.
3. Use a small pillow or a rolled towel to support the lower back.
4. The feet should be flat on the floor, and the knees should be level with the hips.

Figure 20-7 Proper standing position.

Figure 20-8 Proper sitting position.

5. If you need to sit for a prolonged period of time, use a footstool to raise one knee to reduce strain on the back.
6. Take frequent stretch breaks.

Lifting

The following steps outline the procedure for lifting an object while using proper body mechanics:
1. First determine the weight of the object to determine if you can safely lift it. Pushing the object with one foot can

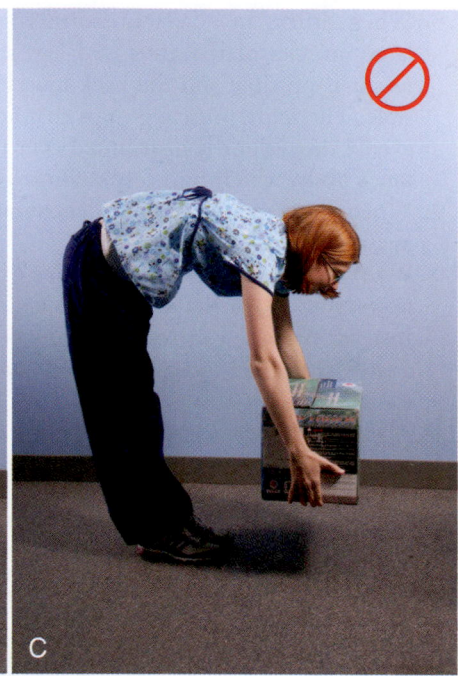

Figure 20-9 **A,** To lift the object, always bend the body at the knees and hips. **B,** Lift with the leg muscles, while keeping the back straight. **C,** Never bend from the waist.

help you determine if you can lift it without assistance. Never lift anything heavier than you can easily manage.

2. Stand in front of the object and balance yourself with the feet about 6 to 8 inches apart, toes pointed outward, and one foot slightly forward to provide a wide base of support. Tighten the stomach and gluteal muscles in preparation for lifting the object.

3. To lift the object, always bend the body at the knees and hips (Figure 20-9, *A*). This helps to maintain your center of gravity and allows the strong muscles of the legs to do the lifting. Never bend from the waist (Figure 20-9, *C*).

4. Grasp the object firmly with both hands.

5. Keeping the back straight, lift the object smoothly with the leg muscles, not the back muscles (Figure 20-9, *B*). The muscles of the back are not as strong and are more easily injured than the leg muscles.

6. Hold the object as close to the body as possible and at waist level. This allows the weight of the object to be lifted by the arm and leg muscles rather than the back muscles. To prevent strain on the back, never lift anything higher than the level of the chest.

7. If you need to turn after lifting the object, don't twist. Turn by pivoting your whole body. Twisting the spine can cause a serious back injury.

8. If you need to carry the object to another location, make sure the area of transport is dry and free of clutter.

9. Lower the object slowly, making sure to bend from the knees to allow the leg muscles to do the work.

POSITIONING AND DRAPING

Correct positioning of the patient facilitates the examination by permitting better access to the part being examined or treated. The basic positions used in the medical office are sitting, supine, prone, dorsal recumbent, lithotomy, Sims, knee-chest, and Fowler.

The position used depends on the type of examination or procedure to be performed. More than one position may be used to examine the same body part during the physical examination. The sitting and supine positions are both used to examine the chest. It is important to know the correct position for each examination or treatment. When positioning a patient, the medical assistant should explain the position to the patient and assist the patient in attaining it. The medical assistant should make sure to use proper body mechanics when positioning a patient to avoid musculoskeletal injuries.

It is important to take the patient's endurance and degree of wellness into consideration when positioning him or her. Patients who are weak or ill may be unable to assume a position or may require special assistance in attaining it. Some positions, such as the lithotomy and knee-chest positions, are embarrassing and uncomfortable. A patient should not be kept in these positions any longer than necessary. Some patients (especially the elderly) become dizzy after a time in certain positions, such as the knee-chest position. These patients should be allowed to rest before they get off the examining table. The medical assistant also should assist patients off the examining table to prevent falls.

The patient is draped during positioning to provide for modesty, comfort, and warmth. Only the part to be examined should be exposed. Patient gowns and drapes used in the medical office are usually made of paper but also may be made of cloth. Procedures 20-2 through 20-9 present proper positioning and draping of the patient.

Text continued on p. 429

PROCEDURE 20-2 Sitting Position

Outcome Position and drape a patient in the sitting position. The sitting position is used to examine the head, neck, chest, and upper extremities and to measure vital signs.

Equipment/Supplies

- Examining table
- Disposable patient gown
- Disposable patient drape

1. **Procedural Step.** Sanitize your hands. Greet the patient and introduce yourself.

2. **Procedural Step.** Identify the patient and explain the type of examination or procedure that will be performed.

3. **Procedural Step.** Provide the patient with a patient gown. Instruct the patient to remove clothing as appropriate for the type of examination being performed and to put on the patient gown with the opening in front. The disrobing facility should provide privacy, a place to sit, and a place to hang clothing.

4. **Procedural Step.** Pull out the footrest of the examining table, and assist the patient into a sitting position. The patient's buttocks and thighs should be firmly supported on the edge of the table.

Sitting position.

5. **Procedural Step.** Place a drape over the patient's thighs and legs to provide warmth and modesty.

Place the drape over the patient's thighs and legs.

6. **Procedural Step.** After completion of the examination, assist the patient down from the table. Return the footrest to its normal position. Instruct the patient to get dressed. Discard the gown and drape in a waste container.

PROCEDURE 20-2

PROCEDURE 20-3 Supine Position

Outcome Position and drape a patient in the supine position. The supine position is used to examine the head, chest, abdomen, and extremities.

Equipment/Supplies

- Examining table
- Disposable patient gown
- Disposable patient drape

1. **Procedural Step.** Sanitize your hands. Greet the patient and introduce yourself.
2. **Procedural Step.** Identify the patient and explain the type of examination or procedure that will be performed.
3. **Procedural Step.** Provide the patient with a patient gown. Instruct the patient to remove clothing as appropriate for the type of examination being performed and to put on the patient gown with the opening in front. The disrobing facility should provide privacy, a place to sit, and a place to hang clothing.
4. **Procedural Step.** Pull out the footrest of the examining table, and assist the patient into a sitting position. Place a drape over the patient's thighs and legs.
5. **Procedural Step.** Ask the patient to move back on the table. As the patient is doing this, pull out the table extension while supporting the patient's lower legs.

Position the patient on the back with the legs together.

7. **Procedural Step.** Position the drape lengthwise over the patient to provide warmth and modesty. As the physician examines the patient, move the drape according to the body parts being examined.

Pull out the table extension while supporting the patient's legs.

6. **Procedural Step.** Ask the patient to lie on his or her back with the legs together. Provide assistance if needed. The patient's arms may be placed above the head or alongside the body.

Place a drape lengthwise over the patient.

8. **Procedural Step.** After completion of the examination, assist the patient into a sitting position. Slide the table extension back into place while supporting the patient's lower legs.
9. **Procedural Step.** Assist the patient down from the table. Instruct the patient to get dressed. Return the footrest to its normal position. Discard the gown and drape in a waste container.

PROCEDURE 20-4   Prone Position

Outcome Position and drape a patient in the prone position. The prone position is used to examine the back and to assess extension of the hip joint.

Equipment/Supplies

- Examining table
- Disposable patient gown
- Disposable patient drape

1. **Procedural Step.** Sanitize your hands. Greet the patient and introduce yourself.

2. **Procedural Step.** Identify the patient and explain the type of examination or procedure that will be performed.

3. **Procedural Step.** Provide the patient with a patient gown. Instruct the patient to remove clothing as appropriate for the type of examination being performed and to put on the patient gown with the opening in back. The disrobing facility should provide privacy, a place to sit, and a place to hang clothing.

4. **Procedural Step.** Pull out the footrest of the examining table, and assist the patient into a sitting position. Place a drape over the patient's thighs and legs.

5. **Procedural Step.** Ask the patient to move back on the table. As the patient is doing this, pull out the table extension while supporting the patient's lower legs.

6. **Procedural Step.** Ask the patient to lie on his or her back. Provide assistance if needed. Position the drape lengthwise over the patient.

7. **Procedural Step.** Ask the patient to turn onto his or her stomach by rolling toward you. Provide assistance for this step by helping him or her turn and adjusting the drape to provide modesty.
   Principle. This step prevents the patient from accidentally rolling off the table.

8. **Procedural Step.** Position the patient with the legs together and the head turned to one side. The arms can be placed above the head or alongside the body.

Position the patient's legs together with the head turned to one side.

9. **Procedural Step.** Adjust the drape as needed so that it is positioned lengthwise over the patient to provide warmth and modesty. As the physician examines the patient, move the drape according to the body parts being examined.

Place a drape lengthwise over the patient.

10. **Procedural Step.** After completion of the examination, ask the patient to turn back over by rolling toward you. Assist the patient into a supine position and then into a sitting position. Slide the table extension back into place while supporting the patient's lower legs.

11. **Procedural Step.** Assist the patient down from the table. Return the footrest to its normal position. Instruct the patient to get dressed. Discard the gown and drape in a waste container.

PROCEDURE 20-4

PROCEDURE 20-6   Lithotomy Position—cont'd

Position the drape diagonally.

12. Procedural Step. After completion of the examination, pull out the footrest and table extension. Ask the patient to slide the buttocks back from the end of the table. Lift the patient's legs out of the stirrups at the same time, and place them on

the table extension (supine position). Remove the stirrup covers and discard them in a waste container. Return the stirrups to their normal position. Assist the patient into a sitting position. Slide the table extension back into place while supporting the patient's lower legs.

Principle. Lifting both the patient's legs out of the stirrups at the same time avoids strain on the back and abdominal muscles.

13. Procedural Step. Assist the patient down from the table. Return the footrest to its normal position. Instruct the patient to get dressed. Discard the gown and drape in a waste container.

PROCEDURE 20-7   Sims Position

Outcome Position and drape a patient in the Sims position. The Sims position, also known as the *left lateral position,* is used to examine the vagina and rectum, to measure rectal temperature, to perform a flexible sigmoidoscopy, and to administer an enema.

Equipment/Supplies

- Examining table
- Disposable patient gown

- Disposable patient drape

1. Procedural Step. Sanitize your hands. Greet the patient and introduce yourself.
2. Procedural Step. Identify the patient and explain the type of examination or procedure that will be performed.
3. Procedural Step. Provide the patient with a patient gown. Instruct the patient to remove clothing from the waist down and to put on the patient gown with the opening in back. The disrobing facility should provide privacy, a place to sit, and a place to hang clothing.
4. Procedural Step. Pull out the footrest of the examining table, and assist the patient into a sitting position. Place a drape over the patient's thighs and legs.

5. Procedural Step. Ask the patient to move back on the table. As the patient is doing this, pull out the table extension while supporting the patient's lower legs.
6. Procedural Step. Ask the patient to lie on his or her back. Provide assistance if needed.
7. Procedural Step. Position the drape lengthwise over the patient to provide warmth and modesty.
8. Procedural Step. Ask the patient to turn onto the left side. Provide assistance during this step to prevent the patient from accidentally rolling off the table and to adjust the drape to provide modesty. The patient's left arm should be positioned behind the body and the right arm forward with the elbow

PROCEDURE 20-7   Sims Position—cont'd

bent. Assist the patient in flexing the legs. The right leg is flexed sharply, and the left leg is flexed slightly.

The right leg is flexed sharply, and the left leg is flexed slightly.

9. **Procedural Step.** Adjust the drape as needed. When the physician is ready to examine the patient, a small portion of the drape is folded back to expose the anal area.

Adjust the drape as needed.

10. **Procedural Step.** After completion of the examination, assist the patient into a supine position and into a sitting position. Slide the table extension back into place while supporting the patient's lower legs.
11. **Procedural Step.** Assist the patient down from the table. Return the footrest to its normal position. Instruct the patient to get dressed. Discard the gown and drape in a waste container.

PROCEDURE 20-8   Knee-Chest Position

Outcome Position and drape a patient in the knee-chest position. The knee-chest position is used to examine the rectum and to perform a proctoscopic examination because it provides maximal exposure to the rectal area. This is a difficult position to maintain; the patient should not be put into this position until just before the examination.

Equipment/Supplies

- Examining table
- Disposable patient gown
- Disposable patient drape
- Pillow

1. **Procedural Step.** Sanitize your hands. Greet the patient and introduce yourself.
2. **Procedural Step.** Identify the patient and explain the type of examination or procedure that will be performed.
3. **Procedural Step.** Provide the patient with a patient gown. Instruct the patient to remove clothing from the waist down and to put on the gown with the opening in back. The disrobing facility should provide privacy, a place to sit, and a place to hang clothing.
4. **Procedural Step.** Pull out the footrest of the examining table, and assist the patient into a sitting position. Place a drape over the patient's thighs and legs.

Continued

PROCEDURE 20-8   Knee-Chest Position—cont'd

5. Procedural Step. Ask the patient to move back on the table. As the patient is doing this, pull out the table extension while supporting the patient's lower legs.

6. Procedural Step. Assist the patient into the supine position and then into the prone position, making sure to have the patient roll toward you. Position the drape diagonally over the patient to provide warmth and modesty.

7. Procedural Step. Ask the patient to bend the arms at the elbows and rest them alongside the head. Ask the patient to elevate the buttocks while keeping the back straight. The patient's head should be turned to one side, and the weight of the body should be supported by the chest. A pillow under the chest can give additional support and aid in relaxation. The knees and lower legs are separated approximately 12 inches.

The buttocks are elevated, and the head is turned to one side.

8. Procedural Step. Adjust the drape diagonally as needed with one corner over the patient's back and the opposite corner over the buttocks and falling between the patient's legs. When the physician is ready to examine the patient, a small portion of the drape is folded back to expose the anal area.

Position the drape diagonally.

9. Procedural Step. After completion of the examination, assist the patient into a prone position and then into a supine position. Allow the patient to rest in the supine position before he or she sits up. *Principle.* Patients (especially elderly ones) frequently become dizzy after being in the knee-chest position and should be allowed to rest before they sit up.

10. Procedural Step. Assist the patient into a sitting position. Slide the table extension back into place while supporting the patient's lower legs.

11. Procedural Step. Assist the patient down from the table. Return the footrest to its normal position. Instruct the patient to get dressed. Discard the gown and drape in a waste container.

PROCEDURE 20-9   Fowler Position

Outcome Position and drape a patient in the Fowler position. The Fowler position is used to examine the upper body of patients with cardiovascular and respiratory problems, such as congestive heart failure, emphysema, and asthma. These patients find it easier to breathe in this position than in a sitting or supine position. This position also is used to draw blood from patients who are likely to faint.

Equipment/Supplies

- Examining table
- Disposable patient gown
- Disposable patient drape

1. Procedural Step. Sanitize your hands. Greet the patient and introduce yourself.

2. Procedural Step. Identify the patient and explain the type of examination or procedure that will be performed.

3. Procedural Step. Provide the patient with a patient gown. Instruct the patient to remove clothing as appropriate for the type of examination being performed and to put on the patient gown with the opening in front. The disrobing facility should

PROCEDURE 20-9 Fowler Position—cont'd

provide privacy, a place to sit, and a place to hang clothing.

4. **Procedural Step.** Position the head of the table as follows:
   a. For the semi-Fowler position, the table should be positioned at a 45-degree angle.
   b. For the full Fowler position, the table should be positioned at a 90-degree angle.

5. **Procedural Step.** Pull out the footrest of the examining table, and assist the patient into a sitting position. Place a drape over the patient's thighs and legs.

6. **Procedural Step.** Pull out the table extension while supporting the patient's lower legs. Ask the patient to lean back against the table head. Provide assistance during this step.

Ask the patient to lean back against the table head.

7. **Procedural Step.** Position the drape lengthwise over the patient to provide warmth and modesty. As the physician examines the patient, move the drape according to the body parts being examined.

Position the table at a 45-degree angle for the semi-Fowler position.

8. **Procedural Step.** After completion of the examination, assist the patient into a sitting position. Slide the table extension back into place while supporting the patient's lower legs.

9. **Procedural Step.** Assist the patient down from the table. Instruct the patient to get dressed. Return the head of the table and the footrest to their normal positions. Discard the gown and drape in a waste container.

WHEELCHAIR TRANSFER

A wheelchair is a chair mounted on wheels designed to make mobility easier for individuals who cannot walk or who are having difficulty walking because of illness or disability. Although some patients who come to the medical office in a wheelchair are able to transfer themselves from a wheelchair to an examining table, others may need assistance. The medical assistant plays an important role in the safe and efficient transfer of a patient from a wheelchair to an examining table and back again.

The Occupational Safety and Health Administration (OSHA) recommends that assistive devices be used whenever possible to transfer patients. A transfer belt (also known as a *gait belt*) is a safety device that is approximately $1\frac{1}{2}$ to 2 inches wide and 48 or 60 inches long and is made of a durable fiber such as canvas, nylon, or leather (Figure 20-10). It can be used to assist in the safe transfer of a

Figure 20-10 Transfer belts. **A,** Transfer belt that is 48 inches in length. **B,** Transfer belt that is 60 inches in length.

patient from a wheelchair to an examining table and back again. The transfer belt is wrapped around the patient's waist over his or her clothing and is securely fastened. The belt provides the medical assistant with a secure grip for holding onto the patient and controlling the patient's movement. This makes the transfer more comfortable for the patient because the medical assistant will not have to grasp the patient around the rib cage or under the axillae to make the transfer. Using a transfer belt also reduces the chance of the medical assistant hurting his or her musculoskeletal system while transferring a patient. Procedure 20-10 outlines the procedure for transferring a patient from a wheelchair to an examining table and back again using a transfer belt.

It is important for the medical assistant to realize that it may not always be possible to transfer a patient from a wheelchair to the examining table, even with the use of a transfer belt. Before transferring a patient, the medical assistant should carefully assess his or her ability to make the transfer. There are certain factors that may place undue strain on the medical assistant's musculoskeletal system. These factors include patients who are overweight or patients who have conditions that limit their mobility (e.g., leg paralysis), making it impossible for the patient to assist with the transfer. If factors exist that might cause strain to the medical assistant's musculoskeletal system, the medical assistant should ask for assistance or notify the physician that it is not possible to transfer the patient to the examining table.

PROCEDURE 20-10 Wheelchair Transfer

Outcome Transfer a patient from a wheelchair to the examining table and from an examining table to a wheelchair.

Equipment/Supplies

- Examining table
- Transfer belt

Transferring the Patient to the Examining Table

1. **Procedural Step.** Sanitize your hands.
2. **Procedural Step.** Greet the patient and introduce yourself. Identify the patient and explain the procedure.
3. **Procedural Step.** Evaluate the patient to determine his or her mental and physical capabilities to perform the transfer. Determine how heavy the patient is and if he or she is able to assist in the transfer. Assess whether or not you are able to perform the transfer safely. Do not perform the transfer if you think you may incur a musculoskeletal injury.
4. **Procedural Step.** Wrap the transfer belt snugly around the patient's waist over the patient's clothing with the buckle in front. Securely fasten the belt by threading it through the teeth of the buckle. Put the belt through the other two openings to lock it. The belt should be snug with just enough space between the belt and the patient's clothing to allow your fingers to be inserted comfortably between the belt and the patient's waist. *Principle.* Placing the transfer belt over the patient's clothing prevents abrasions to the patient's skin. The belt must be snug to prevent it from sliding upward on the patient's body.

5. **Procedural Step.** With the patient's stronger side next to the examining table, position the wheelchair at a 45-degree angle to the end of the examining table.

Position the wheelchair at a 45-degree angle.

6. **Procedural Step.** If the examining table is height adjustable, lower it to the same height as the wheelchair or slightly lower. If it is not height adjustable, pull out the footrest of the examining table.
7. **Procedural Step.** Lock the brakes of the wheelchair and fold back the wheelchair footrests.

PROCEDURE **20-10**   Wheelchair Transfer—cont'd

Principle. The wheels must be locked to prevent the chair from moving during the transfer. The wheelchair footrests must be out of the way to provide an unobstructed path for making the transfer.

Lock the brakes.

8. Procedural Step. Inform the patient of what he or she will be required to do during the transfer. During the transfer, clearly state in a step-by-step manner what the patient should do. Encourage the patient to help as much as possible during the transfer by using the muscles of his or her arms and legs.

9. Procedural Step. Make sure the patient's feet are positioned flat on the floor.
Principle. Making sure the patient's feet are flat on the floor provides the patient with balance and stability when he or she stands.

10. Procedural Step. Stand in front of the patient with the feet apart about 6 to 8 inches, the toes pointed outward, one foot slightly forward, and the knees bent.
Principle. This position conserves energy and provides a wide base of support for the transfer.

11. Procedural Step. Ask the patient to place his or her hands on the armrests of the wheelchair and to lean forward.

12. Procedural Step. Grasp the transfer belt on either side of the patient's waist using an underhand grasp.
Principle. The transfer belt provides a secure handle for holding onto the patient and controlling the patient's movement.

Grasp the transfer belt on either side of the patient's waist.

13. Procedural Step. Tighten your abdominal gluteal muscles in preparation for the transfer. Ask the patient to push off the armrests and into a standing position on the count of 3. At the same time, straighten your knees and assist the patient to a standing position by pulling upward on the transfer belt, making sure to keep your back straight.
Principle. The patient pushing upward with his or her arm and leg muscles provides an additional lifting force and reduces the chance of straining your back muscles. Lifting the patient using your knees and the transfer belt allows the strong muscles of the legs and arms to do the lifting, rather than the back muscles.

Continued

PROCEDURE 20-10   Wheelchair Transfer—cont'd

Assist the patient to a standing position.

14. Procedural Step. Pivot the patient toward the examining table. Position the patient's buttocks and backs of the knees toward the examining table. Instruct the patient to step onto the footrest (backward) one foot at a time.
Principle. Pivoting prevents twisting of the spine, which can result in a serious back injury.

Position the patient toward the table.

15. Procedural Step. Gradually lower the patient into a sitting position on the examining table. Make sure the patient's buttocks and thighs are firmly supported on the table. Remove the transfer belt.

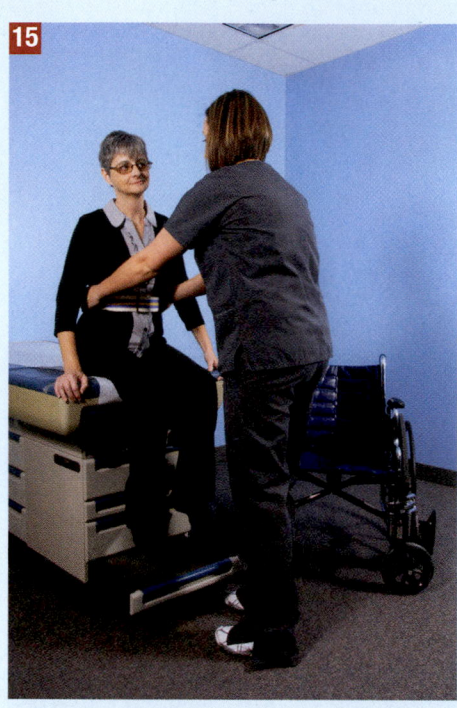

Gradually lower the patient onto the table.

16. Procedural Step. Unlock the wheelchair and move it out of the way of the examining table. Push in the footrest of the examining table.
17. Procedural Step. Stay with the patient to prevent falls.

Transferring the Patient to the Wheelchair

1. Procedural Step. Wrap the transfer belt snugly around the patient's waist and securely fasten it.
2. Procedural Step. Position the wheelchair at a 45-degree angle to the end of the examining table.
3. Procedural Step. If the examining table is height adjustable, lower it to the same height as the wheelchair or slightly lower. If it is not height adjustable, pull out the footrest of the examining table.
4. Procedural Step. Lock the wheelchair into place and fold back the footrests.
5. Procedural Step. Inform the patient of what he or she will be required to do during the transfer.

PROCEDURE 20-10   Wheelchair Transfer—cont'd

6. **Procedural Step.** Stand in front of the patient with the feet apart about 6 to 8 inches, the toes pointed outward, one foot slightly forward, and the knees bent.

7. **Procedural Step.** Ask the patient to place his or her arms on your shoulders. To prevent a neck injury, do not allow the patient to place his or her arms around your neck.

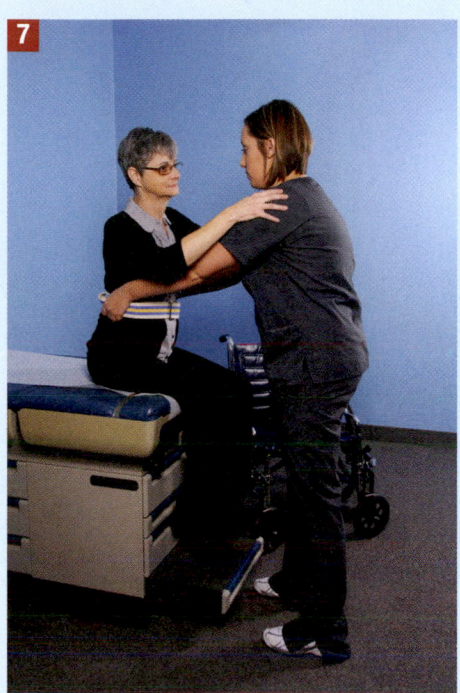

Ask the patient to put his or her arms on your shoulders.

8. **Procedural Step.** Grasp the transfer belt on either side of the patient's waist using an underhand grasp.

9. **Procedural Step.** Ask the patient to push to a standing position using his or her thigh and leg muscles on the count of 3. At the same time, straighten your knees and assist the patient to a standing position by pulling upward on the transfer belt.

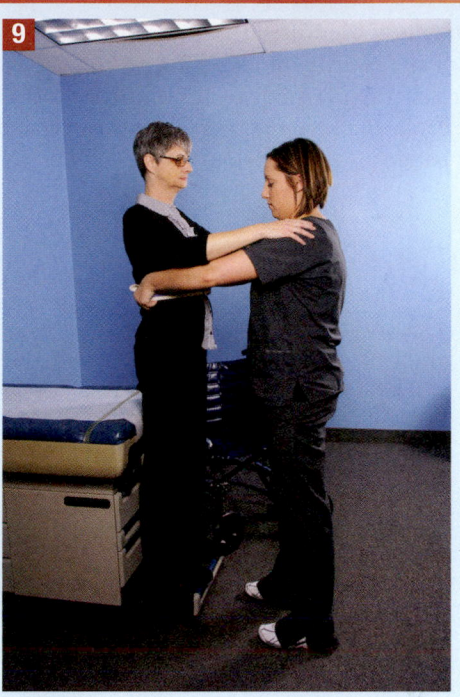

Assist the patient to a standing position.

10. **Procedural Step.** Instruct the patient to step down from the footrest, one foot at a time.

Instruct the patient to step down from the footrest.

11. **Procedural Step.** Pivot the patient toward the wheelchair. Position the backs of the patient's legs against the seat of the wheelchair.

Continued

PROCEDURE 20-10   Wheelchair Transfer—cont'd

12. Procedural Step. Bend at your knees and gradually lower the patient into a sitting position in the wheelchair with the patient's buttocks at the back of the chair. Remove the transfer belt and make sure the patient is comfortable.

13. Procedural Step. Reposition the wheelchair footrests and place the patient's feet in the footrests. Unlock the wheelchair.

14. Procedural Step. Push in the footrest of the examining table.

Gradually lower the patient into the wheelchair.

ASSESSMENT OF THE PATIENT

The extent of patient assessment during the physical examination depends on the purpose of the examination and the patient's condition. A complete physical examination involves a thorough assessment of all body systems. The physician uses an organized and systematic approach in performing a physical examination, starting with the patient's head and proceeding toward the feet. Using this type of approach facilitates the examination process and requires the fewest position changes by the patient.

With a paper-based patient record, the physician notes the results of the physical examination in the patient's medical record, typically on a preprinted form. With an EMR, the physician uses free-text entry, drop-down lists, and checkboxes to record findings on the screen of a computer monitor. The EMR program uses this information to generate the physical examination report. This means that by the end of the examination, the physical examination report is complete, and the physician does not need to dictate his or her findings at a later time. This alleviates the need for transcribing the physician's dictation into a written report.

Patients who exhibit symptoms of illness usually require only select portions of the physical examination. A patient who comes to the medical office with symptoms of bronchitis usually does not require a complete physical examination; rather, the physician examines the body system that is most likely to be associated with the symptoms. Four assessment techniques are used to obtain information during the physical examination: inspection, palpation, percussion, and auscultation.

Memories *from* **Practicum**

Hope Fauber: During my practicum at a student health center at a 4-year college, I was responsible for working up patients for gynecologic examinations. The two-piece drapes had the top opening in the front and the bottom opening in the back. After explaining this to an Asian student who spoke very little English, I noticed that she had the openings opposite of what I had explained. I explained again, with words and gestures, that she needed to reverse the openings. To my surprise, she stood up, turned around in a circle, and sat down! ∎

INSPECTION

Inspection involves observation of the patient for any signs of disease, and of the four assessment techniques, it is the one most frequently used. Good lighting, either natural or artificial, is important for effective observation. The patient's color, speech, deformities, skin condition (e.g., rashes, scars, warts), body contour and symmetry, orientation to the surroundings, body movements, and anxiety level are assessed through inspection. The medical assistant should develop a high level of detailed observational skills to assist the physician in assessing physical characteristics.

PALPATION

Palpation is the examination of the body using the sense of touch (Figure 20-11). The physician uses palpation to determine the placement and size of organs; the presence of lumps; and the existence of pain, swelling, or tenderness. Examining the breasts and taking the pulse are performed by palpation. Palpation often helps verify data obtained by inspection. The patient's verbal and facial expressions also are observed during palpation to assist in the detection of abnormalities.

The two types of palpation—light and deep—are categorized by the amount of pressure applied. *Light palpation* of structures is performed to determine areas of tenderness. The fingertips are placed on the part to be examined and are gently depressed approximately ½ inch. *Deep palpation* is used to examine the condition of organs such as those in the abdomen. Two hands are used for deep palpation. One hand is used to support the body from below, and the other hand is used to press over the area to be palpated. Deep palpation is used by the physician to perform a bimanual pelvic examination.

PERCUSSION

Percussion involves tapping the patient with the fingers and listening to the sounds produced to determine the size, density, and locations of organs. This technique is often used to examine the lungs and abdomen.

The fingertips are used to produce a sound vibration similar to that of tapping a drumstick on a drum. The nondominant hand is placed directly on the area to be assessed, with the fingers slightly separated. The dominant hand is used to strike the joint of the middle finger placed on the patient to produce the sound vibration (Figure 20-12). Structures that are dense, such as the liver, spleen, and heart, produce a dull sound. Empty or air-filled

Figure 20-11 Palpation is examination of the body using the sense of touch.

Figure 20-12 Percussion involves tapping the patient with the fingers. **A,** The nondominant hand is placed directly on the area to be assessed, with the fingers slightly separated. **B,** The fingers of the dominant hand are used to strike the joint of the middle finger to produce a sound vibration.

structures, such as the lungs, produce a hollow sound. Any condition that changes the density of an organ or tissue, such as fluid in the lungs, would change the quality of the sound.

AUSCULTATION

Auscultation is an examination technique that involves listening with a stethoscope to the sounds produced within the body. This technique is used to listen to the heart and lungs or to measure blood pressure. Environmental noise interferes with effective auscultation of body sounds and should be minimized. The diaphragm of the stethoscope chest piece is used to assess high-pitched sounds, such as lung and bowel sounds; the bell of the stethoscope chest piece is used to assess low-pitched sounds, such as those produced by the heart and vascular system. The chest piece

should be cleaned with an antiseptic wipe and warmed with the hands before being placed on the patient.

ASSISTING THE PHYSICIAN

During the patient assessment, the medical assistant should assist the physician as required. This includes helping the patient change positions for the physician's examination of different parts of the body, handing the physician instruments and supplies, and reassuring the patient to reduce apprehension. When the examination is completed, the medical assistant should assist the patient off the examining table and provide additional information if needed, such as scheduling a return visit or patient education to promote wellness. Procedure 20-11 describes the procedure for assisting with the physical examination.

What Would You Do? What Would You *Not* Do?

Case Study 3

Ben-Yi Sun has brought his father, Chang-Yi Sun, to the medical office. Chang-Yi Sun is 76 years old and lives with Ben-Yi and his family. Because there is a large Asian population in the community, the medical office personnel have learned two things about the Asian culture: (1) They are brought up to respect elders, and elders are always considered first, and (2) Asians have a great respect

for harmony. If they do not understand something, they may not admit it to avoid disrupting harmony. Ben-Yi Sun speaks very good English, but his father understands only a few words of English. Chang-Yi Sun has been diagnosed with hypertension, and he needs education about going on a low-sodium diet. He also needs instructions on taking his blood pressure at home and recording the results. ■

PROCEDURE 20-11   Assisting with the Physical Examination

Outcome Prepare the patient and assist with a physical examination.

Equipment/Supplies

- Examining table

- Equipment for the type of examination to be performed

1. **Procedural Step.** Prepare the examining room. Ensure that the room is clean, free of clutter, and well lit and that the room temperature is comfortable for the patient.
2. **Procedural Step.** Sanitize your hands.
3. **Procedural Step.** Assemble the equipment according to the type of examination to be performed and the physician's preference. Arrange the instruments and supplies in a neat and orderly manner on a table or tray. Do not allow one item to be placed on top of another.

Assemble the equipment.

PROCEDURE 20-11   Assisting with the Physical Examination—cont'd

4. Procedural Step. Obtain the patient's medical record. (If an EMR is being used, pull up the record for the appropriate patient, based on his or her name.) Go to the waiting room and ask the patient to come back to the examining room.

5. Procedural Step. Escort the patient to the examining room.

6. Procedural Step. Ask the patient to be seated. Greet the patient and introduce yourself using a calm and friendly manner. Identify the patient by his or her full name and date of birth.

Principle. Identifying the patient correctly avoids mistaking one patient for another. Using a calm and friendly manner helps to put the patient at ease.

Greet and identify the patient by name and date of birth.

7. Procedural Step. Seat yourself so that you face the patient at a distance of 3 to 4 feet.

8. Procedural Step. Obtain essential information from the patient on allergies, current medications, and symptoms and document this information in the patient's medical record (Refer to Chapter 38: Procedure 38-3). If your office uses an EMR, document essential patient information by entering the appropriate data into the computer.

9. Procedural Step. Measure the patient's vital signs, and chart the results.

10. Procedural Step. Measure the weight and height of the patient, and chart the results. If required by the medical office policy, determine the patient's BMI and record this number following the weight and height measurements. (*Note:* The EMR automatically calculates and documents the patient's BMI from the weight and height measurements that are entered into the computer.)

11. Procedural Step. Instruct and prepare the patient for the examination as follows:

a. Ask the patient whether he or she needs to empty the bladder before the examination. If a urine specimen is needed, the patient will be required to void into a urine container.

b. Provide the patient with a patient gown. Instruct the patient to remove all clothing and to put on the patient gown. Offer assistance if you sense the patient may have trouble undressing.

c. Tell the patient to have a seat on the examining table after putting on the patient gown. Inform the patient that the physician will be with him or her soon, and leave the room to provide the patient with privacy.

Principle. An empty bladder makes the examination easier and is more comfortable for the patient.

Instruct and prepare the patient for the examination.

12. Procedural Step. Make the medical record available to the physician. The medical office has a designated location where the record is placed, such as on a small shelf mounted on the wall next to the outside of the examining room door or in a chart holder on the outside of the examining room door. Position the medical record so that patient-identifiable information is not visible. If your office uses an EMR, you do not need to perform this step. With an EMR, the physician accesses the patient's record on the computer.

13. Procedural Step. Check to make sure that the patient is ready to be seen by the physician. Before entering a patient's room, knock lightly on the door to let the patient know that you are getting ready to enter the room. If a patient is ready to be seen, inform the physician. This may be done using a

Continued

PROCEDURE 20-11

PROCEDURE 20-11   Assisting with the Physical Examination—cont'd

color-coded flagging system mounted on the wall next to the examining room.
Principle. HIPAA requires protection of a patient's health information.

14. Procedural Step. Assist the physician with examination of the body systems as follows:

a. Ensure that the patient is positioned correctly in a sitting position on the examining table. This allows the physician to examine the patient's head, eyes, ears, nose, mouth and pharynx, neck, chest, lungs, and heart.

b. Hand the physician the ophthalmoscope, otoscope, and tongue depressor.

c. Dim the light when the physician is ready to use the ophthalmoscope. The dim light helps dilate the patient's pupils, providing the physician better visualization of the interior of the eye.

d. After use, the tongue depressor should be transferred by holding it at the center to prevent contact with the patient's secretions, which may contain pathogens. Dispose of the tongue depressor in a regular waste container.

Transfer the tongue depressor by holding it at the center.

e. Offer reassurance to the patient to reduce apprehension.

15. Procedural Step. Position the patient as required for examination of the remaining body systems. Place and drape the patient in the proper position for examination of a particular part of the body using proper body mechanics.

16. Procedural Step. Assist and instruct the patient as follows:

a. Allow the patient to rest in a sitting position on the examining table before he or she gets off of it. Some patients become dizzy after being positioned on the examining table.

b. Assist the patient off the examining table to prevent falls.

c. Instruct the patient to get dressed. Provide assistance if needed.

d. Provide the patient with any necessary instructions, such as patient education and scheduling a return visit. Give instructions involving medical care in terms the patient can understand; do not use medical terms.

e. Sanitize the hands, and chart in his or her medical record any instructions given to the patient.

f. Escort the patient to the reception area.

17. Procedural Step. Clean the examining room in preparation for the next patient as follows:

a. Discard the paper on the examining table. Then, apply gloves and clean and disinfect the table. Unroll a fresh length of paper on the table.

b. Discard all disposable supplies into an appropriate waste container.

c. Ensure that there are ample numbers of clean gowns and drapes and other supplies.

d. Remove reusable equipment to a work area for sanitization, sterilization, or disinfection as required by the medical office policy.

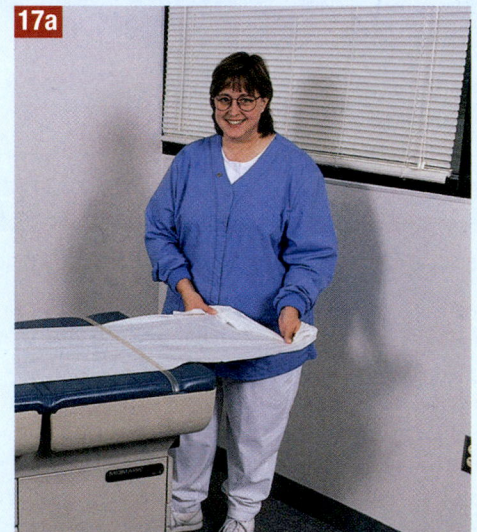

Unroll a fresh length of paper.

PPR CHARTING EXAMPLE	
Date	
11/20/XX	11:30 a.m. CC. Shortness of breath x 2 days.
	T: 98.8° F TA, P: 78 reg and strong, R: 20 even
	and reg, BP: 110/68, Wt: 126, Ht: 5' 6", BM1: 20
	————————— H. Fauber, CMA (AAMA)

What Would You Do? What Would You *Not* Do? RESPONSES

Case Study 1
Page 410

What Did Hope Do?
- ❏ Empathized with Abbey and told her that a lot of patients feel just like she does about having their weight taken. Explained that the information in her medical record is strictly confidential.
- ❏ Told Abbey that weight is important so that the physician can properly diagnose and treat her condition, and that medication dosage is often based on a person's weight.
- ❏ Told Abbey that she could stand on the scale backward while her weight is being measured so that she would not see the reading on the scale.
- ❏ Returned the weights to zero before Abbey got off the scale.
- ❏ Recorded Abbey's weight in her chart without telling her the results.
- ❏ Encouraged Abbey to see the physician when she needs to so that she stays as healthy as possible.

What Did Hope Not *Do*?
- ❏ Did not make any comments about Abbey's body or weight after weighing her.
- ❏ Did not criticize Abbey for letting her weight stand in the way of coming in when she needed health care.

Case Study 2
Page 411

What Did Hope Do?
- ❏ Listened carefully to Mikayla and showed concern verbally and nonverbally.

- ❏ Carefully charted the information relayed by Mikayla so that the physician would be aware of all aspects of Mikayla's problem.
- ❏ Told Mikayla that she needs to talk to the physician about wanting some medicine for heartburn.
- ❏ Encouraged Mikayla to talk to her parents about what's been going on with her.

What Did Hope Not *Do*?
- ❏ Did not agree with Mikayla that she needs to lose more weight.
- ❏ Did not make comments about Mikayla being too thin.

Case Study 3
Page 436

What Did Hope Do?
- ❏ Greeted Chang-Yi first before greeting his son.
- ❏ Spoke clearly and slowly to Ben-Yi in a normal tone of voice.
- ❏ Gave them a brochure on low-sodium diets and go over the foods that are low in sodium.
- ❏ Asked Chang-Yi (via Ben-Yi's translating) to indicate the foods he likes that he thinks would be low in sodium. Determined whether these foods are low in sodium.
- ❏ Showed Ben-Yi how to take his father's blood pressureHad Ben-Yi practice taking his father's blood pressure.
- ❏ Made sure that Chang-Yi and Ben-Yi understood all of the information before they left the office.

What Did Hope Not *Do*?
- ❏ Be careful not to ignore Chang-Yi.

TERMINOLOGY REVIEW

Key Term	Word Parts	Definition
Audiometer	*audi/o:* hearing *-meter:* instrument used to measure	An instrument used to measure hearing.
Auscultation		The process of listening to the sounds produced within the body to detect signs of disease.
Bariatrics	*bar/o:* weight *-iatrics:* a branch of medicine	The branch of medicine that deals with the treatment and control of obesity and diseases associated with obesity.
Body mechanics		Use of the correct muscles to maintain proper balance, posture, and body alignment to accomplish a task safely and efficiently without undue strain on any muscle or joint.
Clinical diagnosis		A tentative diagnosis of a patient's condition obtained through evaluation of the health history and the physical examination, without the benefit of laboratory or diagnostic tests.
Diagnosis	*dia-:* through, complete *-gnosis:* knowledge	The scientific method of determining and identifying a patient's condition.
Differential diagnosis		A determination of which of two or more diseases with similar symptoms is producing a patient's symptoms.

Continued

TERMINOLOGY REVIEW—cont'd

Key Term	Word Parts	Definition
Inspection		The process of observing a patient to detect signs of disease.
Mensuration		The process of measuring a patient.
Ophthalmoscope	*ophthalm/o:* eye *-scope:* to view, to examine	An instrument for examining the interior of the eye.
Otoscope	*ot/o:* ear *-scope:* to view, to examine	An instrument for examining the external ear canal and tympanic membrane.
Palpation		The process of feeling with the hands to detect signs of disease.
Percussion		The process of tapping the body to detect signs of disease.
Percussion hammer		An instrument with a rubber head, used for testing reflexes.
Prognosis	*pro-:* before *-gnosis:* knowledge	The probable course and outcome of a patient's condition and the patient's prospects for recovery.
Speculum		An instrument for opening a body orifice or cavity for viewing.
Symptom		Any change in the body or its functioning that indicates a disease might be present.

ON THE WEB

For information on nutrition:

Academy of Nutrition and Dietetics: www.eatright.org

Ask the Dietitian: www.dietitian.com

For information on weight control and fitness:

American Obesity Association: www.obesity.org

Obesity Action Coalition: www.obesityaction.org

Weight Watchers: www.weightwatchers.com

E-Diets: www.ediets.com

Calorie Control Council: www.caloriecontrol.org

Prevent Obesity: www.preventobesity.net

For information on accessing health information:

InteliHealth: www.intelihealth.com

Mayo Clinic: www.mayoclinic.com

U.S. Department of Health and Human Services: www.hhs.gov

American Academy of Family Physicians: Family Doctor: www.familydoctor.org

Healthfinder: www.health.gov

WebMD: www.webmd.com

Medline Plus: www.nlm.nih.gov/medlineplus

For information on cultural diversity:

National Geographic Society: www.nationalgeographic.com

U.S. Department of the Interior: Workforce Diversity: www.doi.gov/diversity/workforce

Generations United: www.gu.org

Eye and Ear Assessment and Procedures

Check out the Evolve site at http://evolve.elsevier.com/Bonewit/today/ to access additional interactive activities and exercises to help you study and prepare for success.

LEARNING OBJECTIVES

The Eye
1. Define visual acuity.
2. State the cause and visual difficulty of each of the following:
   - Myopia
   - Hyperopia
   - Astigmatism
   - Presbyopia
3. Explain the differences among an ophthalmologist, an optometrist, and an optician.
4. Explain the significance of the top and bottom numbers next to each line of letters on the Snellen eye chart.
5. Explain the difference between congenital and acquired color vision defects.
6. List the reasons to perform an eye irrigation and an eye instillation.

The Ear
7. Identify conditions that may cause conductive and sensorineural hearing loss.
8. List and describe the ways in which hearing acuity can be tested.
9. List the reasons to perform an ear irrigation and an ear instillation.

PROCEDURES

Assess distance visual acuity.
Assess near visual acuity.
Assess color vision.
Perform an eye irrigation.
Perform an eye instillation.

Perform an ear irrigation.
Perform an ear instillation.

CHAPTER OUTLINE

INTRODUCTION TO THE EYE
VISUAL ACUITY
Assessment of Distance Visual Acuity
Conducting a Snellen Test
Assessing Distance Visual Acuity in Preschool Children
Assessment of Near Visual Acuity
ASSESSMENT OF COLOR VISION
Ishihara Test
EYE IRRIGATION
EYE INSTILLATION

INTRODUCTION TO THE EAR
ASSESSMENT OF HEARING ACUITY
Types of Hearing Loss
Hearing Acuity Tests
Gross Screening Test
Tuning Fork Tests
Audiometry
Tympanometry
EAR IRRIGATION
EAR INSTILLATION

KEY TERMS

astigmatism (uh-STIG-muh-tizm)
audiometer (aw-dee-OM-eh-ter)
canthus (KAN-thus)
cerumen
hyperopia (HYE-per-OH-pee-uh)

impacted
instillation (IN-still-AY-shun)
irrigation (EAR-ih-GAY-shun)
myopia (mye-OH-pee-uh)
otoscope (AH-toh-skope)

presbyopia (PRESS-bee-OH-pee-uh)
refraction (ree-FRAK-shun)
tympanic membrane (tim-PAN-ik MEM-brane)

441

INTRODUCTION TO THE EYE

The medical assistant is responsible for performing a variety of assessments and procedures that involve the eye. An understanding of the structure and function of the eye is essential to mastering skills in these areas. Refer to Chapter 10 to review the structure and function of the eye.

A visual acuity test is usually part of the routine physical examination. This test is a screening test to detect deficiencies in vision.

The medical assistant may also be responsible for assessing color vision with the use of specially prepared colored plates. As a result of this testing, color blindness can be detected. Color blindness is an inability to distinguish certain colors; the most common problem is with the colors red and green. Color blindness is particularly significant if the patient is involved in an activity that relies on the ability to distinguish colors, such as electronics or interior decorating.

The medical assistant is responsible for performing or teaching the patient to perform eye irrigations and instillations. **Irrigation** is washing a body canal with a flowing solution. **Instillation** is dropping a liquid into a body cavity. Eye irrigations and instillations should be performed using the important principles of medical asepsis outlined in Chapter 17.

VISUAL ACUITY

Visual acuity refers to acuteness or sharpness of vision. A person with normal visual acuity can see clearly and is able to distinguish fine details close up and at some distance.

Errors of refraction are the most common causes of defects in visual acuity (Figure 21-1). **Refraction** refers to the ability of the eye to bend the parallel light rays coming into it so that they can be focused on the retina. An *error of refraction* means that the light rays are not being refracted or bent properly and are not adequately focused on the retina. A defect in the shape of the eyeball can cause a refractive error. Errors of refraction can be improved with corrective lenses.

A person who is nearsighted has a condition termed **myopia.** The eyeball is too long from front to back, causing the light rays to be brought to a focus in front of the retina. A myopic person has difficulty seeing objects at a distance and may squint and have headaches as a result of eyestrain. Corrective lenses (e.g., eyeglasses, contact lenses) or laser eye surgery can correct this condition, which then allows the light rays to come to a focus on the retina.

A person who is farsighted has a condition known as **hyperopia.** The eyeball is too short from front to back, resulting in a different type of refractive error, in which the light rays are brought to a focus behind the retina. The individual has difficulty viewing objects at a reading or working distance. An individual with hyperopia may

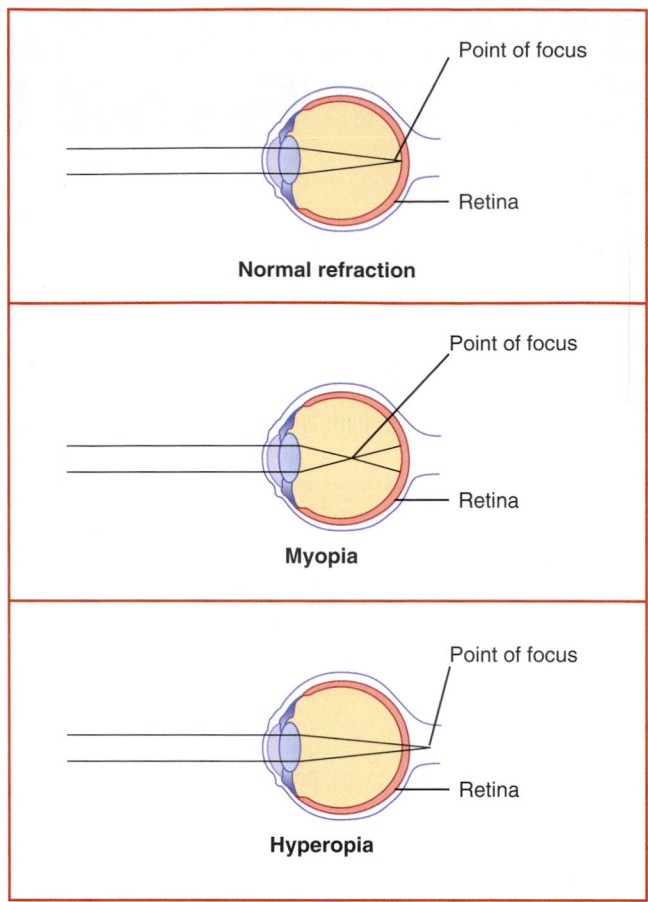

Errors of Refraction

Figure 21-1 Diagram of normal refraction compared with myopia (nearsightedness) and hyperopia (farsightedness), which are errors of refraction that cause visual defects.

experience blurring, headaches, and eyestrain while performing up-close tasks. Corrective lenses can correct this condition by causing the light rays to come to a focus on the retina.

Astigmatism is a refractive error that causes distorted and blurred vision for both near and far objects. A normal cornea has a round or spherical shape and is smooth. With astigmatism, the cornea is curved into an oval shape. This causes the light rays to focus on two different points on the retina, instead of just one, resulting in distorted and blurred vision. Astigmatism often occurs in combination with myopia or hyperopia and can be corrected with corrective lenses.

In most people, a decrease in the elasticity of the lens of the eye begins to occur after age 40 years. This condition, **presbyopia,** results in a decreased ability to focus clearly on close objects.

If a defect in visual acuity is detected, the patient is referred to an eye specialist for further evaluation. Several types of specialists are involved in the care of the eyes. An *ophthalmologist* is a physician who specializes in diagnosing and treating diseases and disorders of the eye. An ophthalmologist is qualified to prescribe ophthalmic and systemic medications and to perform eye surgery. An *optometrist* is a licensed primary health care provider who has expertise in measuring visual acuity and prescribing corrective lenses for the treatment of refractive errors. An optometrist also is qualified to diagnose and treat disorders and diseases of the eye and to prescribe ophthalmic medications. An optometrist is not a physician and is not permitted to prescribe systemic medications or to perform eye surgery. An *optician* is a professional who interprets and fills prescriptions for eyeglasses and contact lenses.

ASSESSMENT OF DISTANCE VISUAL ACUITY

Myopia can be diagnosed (in combination with other tests) by a distance visual acuity (DVA) test. In the medical office, the Snellen eye chart is most often used. Two types of charts are commonly used. One type is used for school-age children and adults and consists of a chart of letters in decreasing sizes (Figure 21-2). The other type is used for preschool children, non–English-speaking people, and nonreaders; it is composed of the capital letter *E* in decreasing sizes and arranged in different directions (Figure 21-3). Visual acuity charts with pictures of familiar objects also are available for use with preschool children. Testing with these charts tends to be less accurate than with the Snellen charts. Some children are unable to identify the objects because of lack of recognition, not because of a defect in visual acuity. It is suggested that the Snellen Big E chart be used with preschool children.

Conducting a Snellen Test

The visual acuity test should be performed in a well-lit room that is free of distractions. The test is usually performed at a distance of 20 feet; this can be conveniently marked off in the medical office with paint or a piece of tape so that it does not have to be remeasured every time the test is performed.

Two numbers, separated by a line, appear at the side of each row of letters on the chart. The number above the line represents the distance (in feet) at which the test is conducted. It is usually 20 feet because most eye tests are conducted at this distance. The number below the line represents the distance from which a person with normal visual acuity can read the row of letters. The line marked 20/20 indicates normal distance visual acuity , or 20/20 vision. This means a person can read what he or she is supposed to read at a distance of 20 feet.

A visual acuity reading of 20/30 means this is the smallest line that the individual can read at a distance of 20 feet. People with normal acuity would be able to read this line at a distance of 30 feet.

A visual acuity reading of 20/15 means this is the smallest line that the individual can read at a distance of 20 feet. It indicates above-average acuity for distance vision.

Figure 21-2 Snellen eye chart consisting of letters in decreasing sizes; this chart is used to measure distance visual acuity.

People with normal acuity would be able to read this line at 15 feet.

The acuity of each eye should be measured separately, traditionally beginning with the right eye. Most physicians prefer that the patient wear his or her contact lenses or glasses, except reading glasses, during the test; the medical assistant should record in the patient's chart that corrective lenses were worn by the patient during the test. An eye occluder should be held over the eye not being tested. The patient's hand should not be used to cover the eye because this may encourage peeking through the fingers,

Figure 21-3 Snellen Big E eye chart consisting of the capital letter *E* in decreasing sizes and arranged in different directions; this chart is used to measure distance visual acuity.

especially in the case of children. The patient should be instructed to leave open the eye not being tested because closing it causes squinting of the eye that is being tested. The procedure for measuring distance visual acuity is outlined in Procedure 21-1.

Assessing Distance Visual Acuity in Preschool Children

With minor variations, Procedure 21-1 can be used to test distance visual acuity in preschool children. The Snellen Big E chart is used for this purpose.

A child needs a complete and thorough explanation of what is expected of him or her before beginning the test.

Tell the child you will be playing a pointing game. Do not force the child to play the game because the results then tend to be inaccurate. Draw the capital letter *E* on an index card, and teach the child to point in the direction of the open part of the *E* by turning the card in different directions (up, down, to the right, and to the left). Using such phrases as "fingers" or "the legs of the table" to describe the open part of the *E* helps the child understand what is expected (Figure 21-4). Allow the child to practice the pointing game with the index card until you are sure this level of skill has been mastered. Be sure to praise the child when the correct response is given.

The child might need help holding the eye occluder in place. The aid of another person such as the parent would then be required.

ASSESSMENT OF NEAR VISUAL ACUITY

Near visual acuity (NVA) testing assesses the patient's ability to read close objects (i.e., at a reading or working distance); the test results are used to detect hyperopia and presbyopia.

The test is conducted with a card similar to the Snellen eye chart; however, the size of the type ranges from the size of newspaper headlines down to considerably smaller print such as would be found in a telephone directory (Figure 21-5). The test card is available in a variety of forms, such as printed paragraphs, printed words, and pictures.

The test should be performed in a well-lit room free of distractions. It is conducted with the patient holding the test card at a distance between 14 and 16 inches. If the patient wears reading glasses, they should be worn during the test. The acuity should be measured in each eye separately, traditionally beginning with the right eye. An eye occluder should be held over the eye not being tested. The patient should be instructed to keep the covered eye open because closing it may cause squinting of the eye that is being tested. The patient is asked to read or identify orally each line or paragraph of type. During the test, the patient should be observed for unusual symptoms, such as squinting, tilting the head, or watering of the eyes, which may indicate that the patient is having difficulty reading the card. The patient continues until reaching the smallest type that can be read.

The results are recorded as the smallest type that the patient could comfortably read with each eye at the distance at which the card was held (i.e., 14 to 16 inches). The recording is based on the type of test card used to conduct the test. One type of card uses a recording method similar to that used with the Snellen eye test. For this type of near visual acuity card, the results would be recorded as 14/14 for a patient with normal near visual acuity . This means the patient read what was supposed to be read at a distance of 14 inches. Also included in the recording should be the date and time, corrective lenses worn, and any unusual symptoms exhibited by the patient.

Figure 21-4 A, Cammie teaches a preschool child to point in the direction of the open part of the capital letter *E.* **B,** Cammie performs the Snellen Big E visual acuity test.

No. 1.
.37M

In the second century of the Christian era, the empire of Rome comprehended the fairest part of the earth, and the most civilized portion of mankind. The frontiers of that extensive monarchy were guarded by ancient renown and disciplined valor. The gentle but powerful influence of laws and manners had gradually cemented the union of the provinces. Their peaceful inhabitants enjoyed and abused the advantages of wealth.

No. 2.
.50M

fourscore years, the public administration was conducted by the virtue and abilities of Nerva, Trajan, Hadrian, and the two Antonines. It is the design of this, and of the two succeeding chapters, to describe the prosperous condition of their empire; and afterwards, from the death of Marcus Antoninus, to deduce the most important circumstances of its decline and fall; a revolution which will ever be remembered, and is still felt by

No. 3.
.62M

the nations of the earth. The principal conquests of the Romans were achieved under the republic; and the emperors, for the most part, were satisfied with preserving those dominions which had been acquired by the policy of the senate, the active emulations of the consuls, and the martial enthusiasm of the people. The seven first centuries were filled with a rapid succession of triumphs; but it was

No. 4.
.75M

reserved for Augustus to relinquish the ambitious design of subduing the whole earth, and to introduce a spirit of moderation into the public councils. Inclined to peace by his temper and situation, it was very easy for him to discover that Rome, in her present exalted situation, had much less to hope than to fear from the chance of arms; and that, in the prosecution of

No. 5.
1.00M

the undertaking became every day more difficult, the event more doubtful, and the possession more precarious, and less beneficial. The experience of Augustus added weight to these salutary reflections, and effectually convinced him that, by the prudent vigor of

No. 6.
1.25M

his counsels, it would be easy to secure every concession which the safety or the dignity of Rome might require from the most formidable barbarians. Instead of exposing his person or his legions to the arrows of the Parthinians, he obtained, by an honor-

No. 7.
1.50M

able treaty, the restitution of the standards and prisoners which had been taken in the defeat of Crassus. His generals, in the early part of his reign, attempted the reduction of Ethiopia and Arabia Felix. They marched near a thou-

No. 8.
1.75M

sand miles to the south of the tropic; but the heat of the climate soon repelled the invaders, and protected the unwarlike natives of those sequestered regions

No. 9.
2.00M

The northern countries of Europe scarcely deserved the expense and labor of conquest. The forests and morasses of Germany were

No. 10.
2.25M

filled with a hardy race of barbarians who despised life when it was separated from freedom; and though, on the first

No. 11.
2.50M

attack, they seemed to yield to the weight of the Roman power, they soon, by a signal

Figure 21-5 Example of a near visual acuity card.

ASSESSMENT OF COLOR VISION

Defects in color vision may be classified as congenital or acquired. *Congenital defects* are more common and refer to a color vision deficiency that is inherited and is present at birth. Congenital color vision deficiencies most often affect males. *Acquired defects* refer to a color vision deficiency that is acquired after birth, resulting from such factors as an eye or brain injury, disease, and certain drugs. Color vision tests, such as the Ishihara test (Figure 21-6), detect congenital color vision disturbances and are commonly performed in the medical office. A basic screening for color vision can be performed by asking the patient to identify the red and green lines on the Snellen eye chart.

What Would You Do? What Would You *Not* Do?

Case Study 1

Nicole Neason brings her daughter, Haley, to the office for a camp physical. Haley has just completed the fourth grade and is going to summer camp for 2 weeks with Tess, her best friend. Tess wears glasses and Haley thinks they are really cool. She often asks to try on Tess's glasses and wishes she could wear glasses just like her best friend. When Haley is measured for visual acuity, she misses a few letters on the 20/70 line, the 20/50 line, the 20/40 line, and the 20/20 line. She is unable to read any of the letters on the 20/15 line. After the examination, Haley wants to know if she's missed enough letters to be able to get glasses. ■

ISHIHARA TEST

The Ishihara test for color blindness is a convenient and accurate method to detect total congenital color blindness and red-green color blindness by assessing an individual's ability to perceive primary colors and shades of color. The Ishihara book contains a series of polychromatic plates of primary colored dots arranged to form a numeral against a background of similar dots of contrasting colors (see Figure 21-6). Patients with normal color vision are able to read the appropriate numeral; however, patients with color vision defects read the dots either as not forming a number at all or as forming a number different from the one identified by the individual with normal color vision. The first plate in the Ishihara book is designed to be read correctly by all individuals (with normal vision and exhibiting color vision deficiencies) and should be used to explain the procedure to the patient.

The book includes plates with winding colored lines for patients who are unable to identify the numbers by name, such as preschool children and non–English-speaking people. The patient should be asked to trace the line formed by the colored dots using a cotton swab or the eraser end of a pencil. The patient's finger should not be used to do the tracing because over time soiled fingers can degrade the polychromatic plates.

Figure 21-6 Ishihara color plates. Polychromatic plates. In the upper figure, a person with normal color vision reads 74, but a person with red-green color blindness reads 21. In the lower figure, a red-blind person (protanope) reads 2, but a green-blind person (deuteranope) reads 4. A normal-vision person reads 42. Reproduced plates are not good for testing for color deficiency. (From Isihara J: *Tests for color blindness,* Tokyo, 1920, Kanehara.)

The Ishihara test should be conducted in a quiet room illuminated by natural daylight. If this is not feasible, a room lit with electric light may be used; however, the light should be adjusted to resemble the effect of natural daylight as much as possible. Using light other than just described, such as bright sunlight, may change the appearance of shades of color on the plates, leading to inaccurate test results.

The medical assistant is responsible for performing the color vision test and for recording results in the patient's chart. The physician assesses the results to determine whether the patient has a deficiency in color vision.

The Ishihara test consists of 14 color plates. Plates 1 through 11 are used to conduct the basic test, and plates 12, 13, and 14 are used to further assess patients who exhibit a red-green color deficiency. It is unnecessary to include these plates (12, 13, and 14) in the test of patients who exhibit normal color vision. In interpreting the results, if 10 or more plates are read correctly, the patient's color vision is considered normal. If 7 or fewer of the 11 Ishihara plates are read correctly, the patient is identified as having a color vision deficiency. It would be unusual for the medical assistant to obtain results in which the patient has read eight or nine plates correctly. The test is structured so that a patient with a color vision defect typically does not read eight or nine plates correctly and the rest incorrectly.

If a defect in color vision is detected, the patient is referred for additional assessment of color vision to an ophthalmologist or optometrist, who would use more precise color vision tests. The procedure for assessing color vision using the Ishihara color plates is outlined in Procedure 21-2.

PROCEDURE 21-1

Putting it all into Practice

My name is Cammie Lindner, and I work for an ear, nose, and throat (ENT) surgeon. There are administrative responsibilities in my job; however, the focus is on the clinical aspects, including vital signs measurements, allergy testing, immuno-therapy, and assisting with minor office surgeries, such as excision of skin lesions and tympanostomy tube insertions. Over past years in an ENT practice, there have been many challenging and rewarding situations. A recent incident was one that certainly falls into the rewards category.

A young girl came into the office from the emergency department for repair of a facial laceration. It had been quite a day for her, so it was understandable that she was a bit nervous and upset.

As the suturing was being performed, she grasped her mother's hand as I tried to discuss interests and school with her. She did fine and was very relieved when the last suture was done.

On her return visit for suture removal, her mother could not accompany her. As I was showing her to the examination room, she quietly asked if I would be in the room. I said, "If you would like, I certainly will." She anxiously nodded yes. As the sutures were removed, she squeezed my hand tighter and tighter. After all of them were out, she first checked her appearance in the mirror, then turned before going out the door and gave me a big hug and a "thank you." Days like this one are truly great rewards and make you feel you really can make a difference in someone's care. ■

PROCEDURE 21-1   Assessing Distance Visual Acuity—Snellen Chart

Outcome Assess distance visual acuity

Equipment/Supplies

- Snellen eye chart
- Eye occluder
- Antiseptic wipe

1. **Procedural Step.** Sanitize your hands.
2. **Procedural Step.** Assemble the equipment. Perform the test in a well-lit room that is free of distractions. Wipe the eye occluder with an antiseptic wipe, and allow it to dry completely.
   Principle. The eye occluder should be disinfected before use.
3. **Procedural Step.** Greet the patient and introduce yourself. Identify the patient and explain the procedure. Tell the patient that he or she will be asked to read several lines of letters. The patient should not have an opportunity to study or memorize the letters before beginning the test.
4. **Procedural Step.** Determine whether the patient wears contact lenses or glasses (other than reading glasses). If the patient wears such aids, he or she should be told to keep them on during the test.
5. **Procedural Step.** Ask the patient to stand on the marked line located 20 feet from the chart.
6. **Procedural Step.** Position the center of the Snellen chart at the patient's eye level. Stand next to the chart during the test to indicate to the patient the line to be identified.
   Principle. Ensure that the chart is at the patient's eye level rather than at your eye level, to provide the most accurate results.
7. **Procedural Step.** Test the acuity of each eye separately. Measure the visual acuity of the right eye first.

Principle. The medical assistant should establish a pattern of beginning with the same eye (traditionally the right eye) every time the test is performed. This helps to reduce errors during the recording of results.

8. **Procedural Step.** Ask the patient to cover the left eye with the eye occluder. If the patient wears eyeglasses, tell him or her to place the occluder in front of the glasses gently to prevent the glasses from being moved out of their normal position. Instruct the patient to keep the left eye open. During the test, the medical assistant should check to make sure the patient is keeping the left eye open.
   Principle. Eyeglasses moved out of normal position may lead to inaccurate test results. Keeping the left eye open prevents squinting of the right eye, which temporarily improves vision, leading to inaccurate test results.
9. **Procedural Step.** Instruct the patient not to squint during the test because squinting temporarily improves vision. Ask the patient to identify orally one line at a time on the Snellen chart, starting with the 20/70 line (or a line that is several lines above the 20/20 line).
   Principle. It is best to start at a line above the 20/20 line to give the patient a chance to gain confidence and to become familiar with the test procedure.

Continued

PROCEDURE 21-1   Assessing Distance Visual Acuity—Snellen Chart—cont'd

Ask the patient to identify one line at a time.

Ask the patient to cover the right eye and to keep the left eye open.

10. **Procedural Step.** If the patient is able to read the 20/70 line, proceed down the chart until reaching the smallest line of letters the patient can read. If the patient is unable to read the 20/70 line, proceed up the chart until the smallest line of letters the patient can read is reached.
11. **Procedural Step.** While the patient is reading the letters, observe him or her for unusual symptoms, such as squinting, tilting of the head, or watering of the eyes.
    Principle. These symptoms may indicate that the patient is having difficulty identifying the letters.
12. **Procedural Step.** On a small piece of paper, jot down the numbers that are displayed next to the smallest line of letters that the patient is able to read. If one or two letters are missed, record the visual acuity with a minus sign next to the bottom number, along with the number of letters missed. If more than two letters are missed, the previous line is recorded.
13. **Procedural Step.** Ask the patient to cover the right eye with the eye occluder and to keep the right eye open. Measure the visual acuity in the left eye as described in steps 9 through 12. During the test, check to make sure the patient is keeping the right eye open.
    Principle. Keeping the right eye open prevents squinting of the left eye.

14. **Procedural Step.** Chart the procedure in the patient's medical record.
    a. *Paper-based patient record:* Record the date and time, the name of the test (Snellen test), the visual acuity results, and any unusual symptoms the patient exhibited during the test (refer to the PPR charting example). Also chart whether the patient was wearing corrective lenses during the test. Use the following abbreviations: $\overline{sc}$ for "without correction" or $\overline{cc}$ for "with correction."
    b. *Electronic medical record:* In SimChart® for the Medical Office, document the visual acuity results and any unusual symptoms the patient exhibited during the test using the correct radio buttons, drop-down menus, and free text fields. It should also be documented if the patient was wearing corrective lenses during the test and what type of corrective lenses were used (glasses or contact lenses).
15. **Procedural Step.** Disinfect the eye occluder with an antiseptic wipe, and sanitize your hands.

PPR CHARTING EXAMPLE

Date	
11/5/XX	3:30 p.m. Snellen test, s̄c: Ⓡ eye: 20/20-1. Ⓛ eye: 20/25. Exhibited squinting, Ⓡ eye.
	——————— C. Lindner, CMA (AAMA)

PROCEDURE 21-2 Assessing Color Vision—Ishihara Test

Outcome Assess color vision

Equipment/Supplies

- Ishihara book
- Cotton swab

1. **Procedural Step.** Sanitize your hands. Assemble the equipment.

2. **Procedural Step.** Conduct the test in a quiet room illuminated by natural daylight.
   Principle. Using unnatural light may change the appearance of the shades of color on the plates, leading to inaccurate test results.

3. **Procedural Step.** Greet the patient and introduce yourself. Identify the patient and explain the procedure. Using the first (practice) plate as an example, instruct the patient to orally identify numbers formed by colored dots. Tell the patient that 3 seconds will be given to identify each plate.
   Principle. The first plate is designed to be read correctly by all individuals and is used to explain the procedure to the patient.

4. **Procedural Step.** Hold the first color plate 30 inches (75 cm) from the patient, at a right angle to the patient's line of vision. The patient should keep both eyes open during the test.

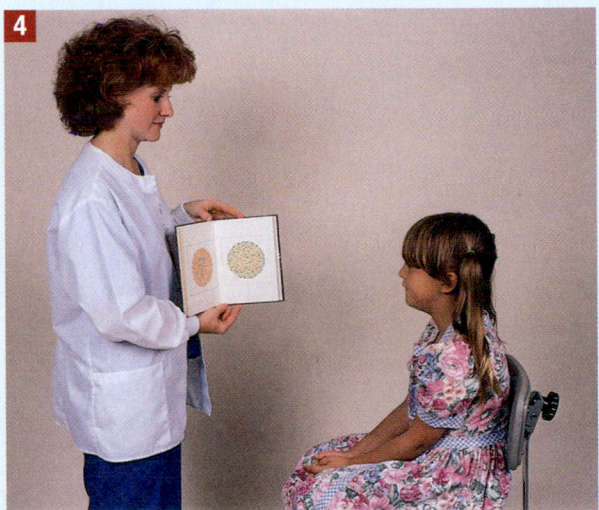

Hold the color plate 30 inches from the patient.

5. **Procedural Step.** Ask the patient to identify the number on the plate. If the plate consists of a traceable winding colored line, ask the patient to trace the line using a cotton swab or the eraser end of a pencil. The patient's finger should not be used to make the tracing.
   Principle. The patient's finger should not be used to trace the line because soiled fingers can degrade the plate over time.

6. **Procedural Step.** Record results after each plate. Continue until the patient has viewed all the plates.

   a. *Paper-based patient record:* To record color vision results, use the plate identification number and the number given by the patient. If the patient is unable to identify a number, the mark X should be recorded to indicate that the patient could not read the plate. Examples:

   Plate 5: 21. This means the patient read the number 21 on plate 5 (instead of 74).

   Plate 6: X. This means the patient could not identify a number on plate 6.

   Plate 11: Traceable. This means that the patient correctly traced a winding line on plate 11.

   As you can see from the results of this patient's color vision test, the patient correctly identified all 11 plates, which indicates normal color vision. Because the patient has normal color vision, the medical assistant did not need to include plates 12, 13, and 14 in the color vision test.

   b. *Electronic medical record:* In SimChart® for the Medical Office, document the color vision results using the correct radio buttons, drop-down menus, and free text fields to indicate the plate identification number and the number given by the patient or to indicate that the patient is unable to identify a number.

Continued

PROCEDURE 21-2

PROCEDURE **21-2**   Assessing Color Vision—Ishihara Test—cont'd

Principle. Reading 10 or more plates correctly indicates normal color vision. If 7 or fewer plates are read correctly, the patient is identified as having a color vision deficiency.

7. Procedural Step. Complete the charting entry.

a. *Paper-based patient record:* Record the date and time, the name of the test (Ishihara test), and any unusual symptoms the patient exhibited during the test, such as squinting or rubbing the eyes.

b. *Electronic medical record:* In SimChart® for the Medical Office, document any unusual symptoms the patient exhibited during the test, such as squinting or rubbing the eyes.

8. Procedural Step. Return the Ishihara book to its proper place. The book of color plates must be stored in a closed position to protect it from light.

Principle. Exposing the plates to excessive and unnecessary light results in fading of the color.

PPR CHARTING EXAMPLE

Plate No.	Normal Person	Results
1	12	12
2	8	8
3	5	5
4	29	29
5	74	21
6	7	X
7	45	45
8	2	2
9	X	X
10	16	16
11	Traceable	Traceable
11/6/XX	10:00 a.m.	
	C. Lindner, CMA (AAMA)	

EYE IRRIGATION

An eye irrigation involves washing the eye with a flowing solution. Eye irrigations are performed for the following purposes: to cleanse the eye by washing away foreign particles, ocular discharges, or harmful chemicals; to relieve inflammation through the application of heat; and to apply an antiseptic solution. Procedure 21-3 shows how to perform an eye irrigation.

EYE INSTILLATION

An eye instillation involves the dropping of a liquid into the lower conjunctival sac of the eye. Eye instillations are performed to treat eye infections (with medication), to soothe an irritated eye, to dilate the pupil, and to anesthetize the eye during an eye examination or treatment. Medication to be instilled in the eye may come in the form of a liquid, as ophthalmic drops, or as an ophthalmic ointment. Eye drops are usually dispensed in a flexible plastic container with an attached dropper. Eye ointment is dispensed in a small metal tube with a small tip for applying the medication. Procedure 21-4 shows how to perform an eye instillation.

Text continued on p. 455

What Would You Do? What Would You *Not* Do?

Case Study 2

Peter Mitchell comes in with his 5-year-old son, Clive. Clive is diagnosed with conjunctivitis (pinkeye), and the physician prescribes Polytrim ophthalmic suspension. Mr. Mitchell says that Clive does not cooperate very well when having drops put in his eyes and asks for any ideas that might make it less of an ordeal. Mr. Mitchell has 7-year-old twin girls at home and wants to know what can be done so they don't get pinkeye. He asks if it would be all right to instill the drops in the twins' eyes as a preventive measure. ■

PATIENT TEACHING | Conjunctivitis

Answer questions that patients have about conjunctivitis.

What is conjunctivitis?

Conjunctivitis, often referred to as *pink eye,* is an inflammation of the conjunctiva (see illustration). The conjunctiva is a thin transparent membrane that covers the white of the eye. Conjunctivitis occurs when the conjunctiva becomes infected with a bacterium or virus. Other causes of conjunctivitis include allergies, prolonged wearing of contact lenses, and irritation from wind, dust, and smoke. Conjunctivitis is almost always harmless and clears up by itself within 2 weeks. If it is caused by a bacterium, the physician may prescribe antibiotic eye drops or ointment.

What are the symptoms of conjunctivitis?

Most types of conjunctivitis are relatively painless. The eye is red or pink because of irritation, and there is a feeling of sandiness or grittiness in the eye. A discharge is usually present, which dries at night when the eyes are closed. This may cause the eyelids to be stuck together in the morning. Other symptoms include tearing, itching, and sensitivity to light.

Is conjunctivitis contagious?

Conjunctivitis caused by a virus or bacterium is highly contagious. It can be spread easily from one eye to another and throughout a family or classroom in a matter of days.

How can we avoid spreading conjunctivitis?

The following measures help prevent the spread of conjunctivitis:
- Avoid touching or rubbing the infected eye, which can spread the infection to the other eye or to other people.
- Sanitize your hands frequently with soap, particularly after touching the eyes or face.
- Do not share washcloths, towels, or pillows with anyone.
- Do not wear contact lenses or eye makeup until the conjunctivitis is completely gone.
- Discard eye makeup that was used while you were infected to prevent reinfection.
- Encourage the patient to practice techniques that prevent the spread of conjunctivitis.
- If the physician has prescribed eye medication, teach the patient (or parent) the proper procedure for performing an eye instillation.
- Give the patient educational materials on conjunctivitis. ∎

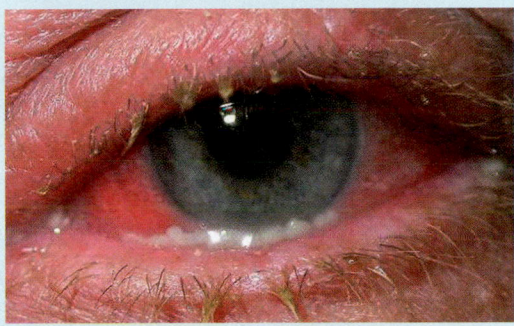

Bacterial conjunctivitis.

PROCEDURE 21-3 Performing an Eye Irrigation

Outcome Perform an eye irrigation

Equipment/Supplies

- Disposable gloves (nonpowdered)
- Irrigating solution
- Solution basin
- Bath thermometer
- Disposable rubber bulb syringe
- Basin
- Moisture-resistant towel
- Gauze pads

---

1. **Procedural Step.** Sanitize your hands.
2. **Procedural Step.** Assemble the equipment. If both eyes are to be irrigated, two sets of equipment must be used to prevent cross-infection from one eye to the other. Normal saline is usually used to irrigate the eye. Perform the following:

   a. Carefully check the label of the irrigating solution three times to make sure you have the correct solution. The first time is after you remove the solution container from the shelf. Compare the label of the solution container with the physician's instructions.

   b. Check the expiration date of the solution.

   c. Warm the irrigating solution to body temperature (98.6° F [37° C]) by placing the solution container in a basin of warm water. Use a bath thermometer to make sure the temperature of the water used to warm the solution does not exceed body temperature.

Continued

PROCEDURE 21-3   Performing an Eye Irrigation—cont'd

d. Check the solution label a second time before pouring the solution.

e. Pour the solution as follows:

f. Palm the label of the container and remove the cap. Place the cap on a flat surface with the open end up. Pour the solution into the basin and replace the cap without contaminating it. Cover the basin to keep the solution warm.

g. Check the solution label a third time before returning the container to its storage area.

Principle. The solution label should be carefully checked three times to prevent an error. Outdated solutions may produce undesirable effects and should be discarded. If the solution is too cold or too warm, it will be uncomfortable for the patient. Palming the label prevents solution from dripping on the label and obscuring it or loosening the label. Placing the cap open end up prevents contamination.

3. **Procedural Step.** Greet the patient and introduce yourself. Identify the patient and explain the procedure and the irrigation. If the patient wears glasses or contact lenses, ask him or her to remove them.

4. **Procedural Step.** Position the patient. The patient may be placed in a sitting or lying position. Place a moisture-resistant towel on the patient's shoulder to protect the patient's clothing. Position a basin tightly against the patient's cheek under the affected eye to catch the irrigating solution, and ask the patient to hold it in place. Ask the patient to tilt the head in the direction of the affected eye.

Principle. The patient is positioned so that the solution flows away from the unaffected eye to prevent cross-infection.

5. **Procedural Step.** Apply nonpowdered gloves. Cleanse the eyelids from inner to outer **canthus** with a moistened gauze pad to remove any discharge or debris on the lids. The inner canthus is the inner junction of the eyelids next to the nose. The outer canthus is the junction of the eyelids farthest from the nose. Normal saline or the solution ordered for the irrigation may be used. Discard the gauze pad after each wipe.

Principle. Nonpowdered gloves avoid irritation of the patient's eye with powder that may have gotten on the outside of the glove. The eyelids should be clean to prevent foreign particles from entering the eye during the irrigation. Cleansing from inner to outer canthus prevents cross-infection.

Cleanse the eyelids from inner to outer canthus.

6. **Procedural Step.** Fill the irrigating syringe with the solution by squeezing the bulb and slowly releasing it until the desired amount of solution enters the bulb. Instruct the patient to keep both eyes open and to find a focal point in the room and focus on it.

Principle. Looking at a focal point helps the patient keep the irrigated eye open during the procedure.

7. **Procedural Step.** Separate the eyelids with the index finger and thumb to expose the lower conjunctiva and to hold the upper eyelid open.

Principle. The medical assistant must hold the eye open during the procedure because the patient has a tendency to close it.

PROCEDURE 21-3 Performing an Eye Irrigation—cont'd

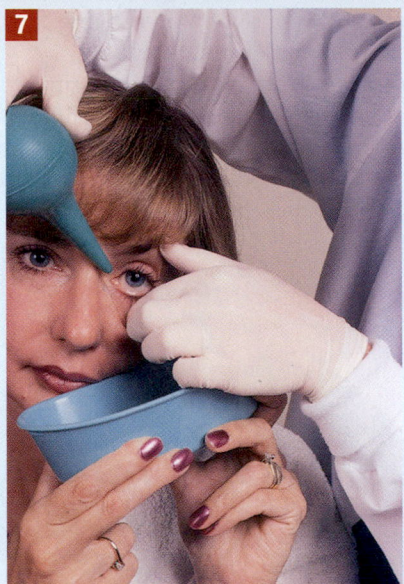

Separate the eyelids, and hold the tip of the syringe 1 inch above the eye.

8. Procedural Step. Hold the tip of the syringe approximately 1 inch above the eye. Gently release the solution onto the eye at the inner canthus. This allows the solution to flow over the eye at a moderate rate from the inner to the outer canthus. Direct the solution to the lower conjunctiva. To prevent injury, do not allow the tip of the syringe to touch the eye.
Principle. The solution flows away from the unaffected eye to prevent cross-infection. The cornea is sensitive and can be harmed easily. The irrigating solution must be directed to the lower conjunctiva to prevent injury to the cornea.

9. Procedural Step. Refill the syringe, and continue irrigating until the desired results have been obtained or all the solution is used, depending on the purpose of the irrigation.
10. Procedural Step. Dry the eyelids from inner to outer canthus with a gauze pad.
11. Procedural Step. Remove the gloves, and sanitize your hands.
12. Procedural Step. Chart the procedure in the patient's medical record.
   a. *Paper-based patient record:* Record the following: the date and time; which eye was irrigated; the type, strength, and amount of solution used; and any significant observations and patient reactions (refer to the PPR charting example).

PPR CHARTING EXAMPLE

Date	
11/5/XX	10:30 a.m. Irrigated (L) eye c̄ sterile saline at 98.6° F. No complaints of discomfort. ———————— C. Lindner, CMA (AAMA)

   b. *Electronic medical record:* In SimChart® for the Medical Office, document, using the correct radio buttons, drop-down menus, and free text fields, which eye was irrigated; the type, strength, and amount of solution used; and any significant observations and patient reactions.
13. Procedural Step. Remove reusable equipment to a work area for sanitization, sterilization, or disinfection as required by the medical office policy.

PROCEDURE 21-4 Performing an Eye Instillation

Outcome Perform an eye instillation

Equipment/Supplies

- Disposable gloves (nonpowdered)
- Ophthalmic drops or ophthalmic ointment as ordered by the physician
- Tissues
- Gauze pads

1. Procedural Step. Sanitize your hands.
2. Procedural Step. Assemble the equipment, and perform the following:
   a. Check the drug label three times to make sure you have the correct medication. The first time should be when you remove the medication from the shelf. The medication label must bear the word *ophthalmic.*
   b. Check the medication label a second time against the physician's instructions. Also check the dose ordered by the physician.

Continued

PROCEDURE 21-4

c. Check the expiration date.

d. Check the medication label a third time before the cap is removed to instill the medication (as indicated in Procedural Step 5).

Principle. The drug label should be carefully checked three times to prevent a medication error. Medication not bearing the word *ophthalmic* must never be placed in the eye because it could injure the eye. An outdated medication may produce undesirable effects and should be discarded.

3. Procedural Step. Greet the patient and introduce yourself. Identify the patient and explain the procedure and the purpose of the instillation. If the patient wears glasses or contact lenses, ask him or her to remove them.

4. Procedural Step. Help the patient into a sitting or supine position.

5. Procedural Step. Apply nonpowdered gloves. Prepare the medication.

Eye drops: If the medication requires mixing, shake the container well. Check the medication label for the third time, and remove the cap from the container.

Eye ointment: Check the medication label for the third time, and remove the cap from the tip of the tube.

Principle. Nonpowdered gloves avoid irritation of the patient's eyes with powder that may have gotten on the outside of the gloves.

6. Procedural Step. Ask the patient to look up at the ceiling, and expose the lower conjunctival sac by using the fingers of the nondominant hand placed over a tissue. The fingers should be placed on the patient's cheekbone just below the eye, and the skin of the cheek should be drawn gently downward.

Principle. Looking up helps keep the patient from blinking when the drops are instilled.

7. Procedural Step. Insert the medication.

Eye drops: Invert the container and hold the tip of the dropper approximately ½ inch above the eye sac. Do not allow the dropper to touch the eye or any other surface. Gently squeeze the container and place the correct number of eye drops in the center of the lower conjunctival sac. Never place the drops directly on the eyeball. Replace the cap on the container.

Eye ointment: Gently squeeze the tube and place a thin ribbon of ointment along the length of the lower conjunctival sac from inner to outer canthus. Be careful not to touch the tip of the ointment tube to the eye or any other surface.

Discontinue the ribbon by twisting the tube. Replace the cap on the tube.

Principle. Touching the dropper or tip of the tube to the eye (or other surfaces) could injure the eye and contaminate the medication. Placing the medication in the conjunctival sac, rather than directly on the eyeball, is more comfortable for the patient.

Ask the patient to look up, and insert the medication.

8. Procedural Step. Ask the patient to close his or her eyes gently and move the eyeballs. Instruct the patient not to shut the eyes tight or to blink and to keep the eyes closed for 1 to 2 minutes. Tell the patient that the instillation may blur the vision temporarily.

Principle. Moving the eyeballs helps distribute the medication over the entire eye. Keeping the eyes closed allows the medication to be absorbed. If the eyes are shut tightly or if the patient blinks, the drops or ointment may be pushed out of the eye.

9. Procedural Step. Dry the eyelid from inner to outer canthus with a gauze pad to remove excess medication.

10. Procedural Step. Remove the gloves, and sanitize your hands.

PROCEDURE 21-4   Performing an Eye Instillation—cont'd

11. Procedural Step. Chart the procedure in the patient's medical record.

a. *Paper-based patient record:* The medication dosage for eye drops is recorded in the number of drops instilled. The recording should include the date and time, the name and strength of the medication, the number of drops or amount of ointment, which eye received the instillation, your observations, and the patient's reaction (refer to the PPR charting example).

b. *Electronic medical record:* In SimChart® for the Medical Office, document, using the correct radio buttons, drop-down menus, and free text fields, the name and strength of the medication, the number of drops or amount of ointment, which eye received the instillation, your observations, and the patient's reaction.

12. Procedural Step. Return the medication to its proper storage area.

PPR CHARTING EXAMPLE

Date	
11/5/XX	2:30 p.m. Atropine sulfate, 1%, 2 drops in each eye.
	Pt states a temporary blurring of vision. ——
	——————————— C. Lindner, CMA (AAMA)

INTRODUCTION TO THE EAR

The medical assistant is responsible for performing a variety of procedures that involve the ear. An understanding of the structure and function of the ear is essential to mastering skills in these areas. Refer to Chapter 10 to review the structure and function of the ear.

Hearing tests also may be part of the routine physical examination. During contact with the patient, the medical assistant should be alert to signs that indicate the patient might be having difficulty hearing what is being said. A whispered voice next to the patient's ear can be a screening test for hearing acuity. The use of tuning forks or an audiometer provides a more accurate determination of hearing acuity. An **audiometer** is an instrument that emits sound waves at various frequencies. The patient is instructed to indicate when a sound at a given frequency can be heard.

The medical assistant is responsible for performing or teaching the patient to perform ear irrigations and instillations. Ear irrigations and instillations should be performed using the important principles of medical asepsis outlined in Chapter 17.

ASSESSMENT OF HEARING ACUITY

The assessment of hearing acuity is an integral part of a complete physical examination. It is possible for an individual to have hearing loss and not be aware of it. Early detection and treatment of hearing problems help prevent permanent hearing loss.

An individual with normal hearing should be able to hear the frequencies of normal speech, which range from 300 to 4000 Hz (hertz, or cycles per second) at a normal sound intensity. Patients who exhibit hearing loss are referred to an otolaryngologist or an audiologist for further evaluation.

What Would You Do? What Would You *Not* Do?

Case Study 3

Willow Basil brings in her 6-year-old daughter, Jade. For the past 3 days, Jade has been running a fever and has had persistent pain and hearing loss in her left ear. Mrs. Basil practices alternative medicine and uses prescription medications as little as possible. She says that she has been trying herbal therapy and aromatherapy to make Jade better, but it does not seem to be helping. Jade is diagnosed with acute otitis media, and the physician prescribes amoxicillin for 10 days. Mrs. Basil wants to know if she has to give Jade the amoxicillin for the entire 10 days. She asks if she can stop using it when Jade starts feeling better. Mrs. Basil also wants to know if the ear infection will cause a permanent problem with Jade's hearing. ■

TYPES OF HEARING LOSS

There are three types of hearing loss: conductive, sensorineural, and mixed. *Conductive hearing loss* results when there is a physical interference with the normal conduction of sound waves through the external and middle ear. Because of the interference, the amount of sound reaching the inner ear is less than normal, resulting in hearing impairment. Conductive loss in the external ear may be caused by an obstruction in the external ear canal, such as swelling from external otitis (swimmer's ear), foreign bodies, benign growths such as polyps, and impacted cerumen. **Cerumen** is a yellowish waxy substance secreted by the glands in the ear canal. **Impacted** cerumen refers to cerumen that is wedged firmly together in the ear canal so as to be immovable. Conductive loss in the middle ear may be caused by serous otitis media (fluid in the middle ear) or acute otitis media (infection in the middle ear), a perforated **tympanic membrane** (eardrum), or otosclerosis. The cause of conductive hearing loss often can be detected by examining the external ear canal with an otoscope. Hearing is frequently restored by removing the obstruction (e.g., impacted cerumen) or treating the disorder (e.g., serous otitis media).

Sensorineural hearing loss results from damage to the inner ear or auditory nerve. With this type of hearing loss, sound is conducted normally through the outer and middle ear structures, but because of a problem with the perception of sound waves, a hearing deficit occurs. Specific causes of sensorineural loss include hereditary factors, degenerative changes from the normal aging process known as *presbycusis,* intense noise exposure over time, tumors, ototoxicity caused by certain medications, and infectious diseases, such as measles, mumps, and meningitis. The most common cause of sensorineural hearing loss in an adult is presbycusis. As an individual ages, nerves and sensory receptor cells in the inner ear deteriorate, leading to a gradual loss of hearing. *Mixed hearing loss* is a combination of conductive and sensorineural loss.

HEARING ACUITY TESTS

Numerous tests can be used to assess hearing acuity. Tests range from the simple gross screening test to qualitative tests using a tuning fork to highly specific quantitative tests using an audiometer. It is important to test only one ear at a time because a hearing deficit can exist in one ear only. The ear not being tested should be blocked by an earplug or masked. *Masking* involves the presentation of sound (usually noise) to the ear not being tested so that the patient's response is based only on hearing in the ear being tested.

Gross Screening Test

The gross hearing test is a simple and quick screening test used to identify a large hearing impairment. The physician performs the screening test during the physical examination. Hearing is assessed by asking the patient to repeat a simple word or series of numbers whispered from a distance of 1 to 2 feet from the ear. When a hearing loss is discovered, a tuning fork or audiometer is used for a more precise assessment of hearing.

Tuning Fork Tests

Tuning fork tests provide a general assessment of hearing acuity and may be part of the physical examination. A tuning

Normal Hearing
The patient hears the sound equally in both ears or in the center of the head.

Conductive Hearing Loss
The patient hears the sound better in the problem ear.

Sensorineural Hearing Loss
The patient does not hear the sound as well in the problem ear.

Figure 21-7 Weber test.

fork with a frequency of 512 Hz or 1024 Hz is usually used because these frequencies fall within the range of normal speech. The Weber and Rinne tests are the tuning fork tests most commonly performed by the physician; they are used to identify conductive and sensorineural hearing loss.

The *Weber test* is a useful assessment of hearing loss when one ear hears better than the other. The tuning fork is set in vibration, and the base of the fork is placed on the center of the patient's head. The patient is asked to indicate where the sound is heard best. A patient with normal hearing would hear the sound equally in both ears or in the center of the head. Figure 21-7 illustrates the Weber test and describes the interpretation of results.

The *Rinne test* compares the duration of sound perception by air conduction with that of bone conduction. The tuning fork is set in vibration, and the base of the fork is placed against the bone of the mastoid process. The patient is instructed to indicate when the sound is no longer heard. The prongs of the fork (still vibrating) are placed in the air about 1 inch from the opening of the patient's ear canal, and the patient indicates when the sound is no longer heard. An individual with normal hearing is able to hear the sound at least twice as long through air conduction as through bone conduction. Figure 21-8 illustrates the Rinne test and describes the interpretation of results.

Audiometry

Audiometry is the measurement of hearing acuity using a special instrument called an **audiometer.** An audiometer quantitatively measures hearing for the various frequencies of sound waves. Audiometry is a more specific hearing acuity test because it provides information on how extensive a hearing loss is and which frequencies are involved. It is important that the test be conducted in a quiet room because outside noise may affect the results, especially in the lower frequencies. The patient wears headphones placed snugly over the ears (Figure 21-9). The audiometer delivers a single frequency at a time at specific intensities, starting with low-frequency tones of 250 to 500 Hz and going to very high frequencies of 6000 to 8000 Hz. The patient is asked to signal when he or she hears a sound so

Bone conduction

Normal Hearing
The patient hears the sound at least twice as long through air conduction as through bone conduction.

Conductive Hearing Loss
The patient hears the sound longer by bone conduction than by air conduction.

Sensorineural Hearing Loss
The sound is reduced. The patient will also hear the sound longer through air conduction than through bone conduction but not twice as long.

Air conduction

Figure 21-8 Rinne test.

Memories *from* Practicum

Cammie Lindner: There is one characteristic that is shared by all patients. I first noticed this during my practicum, and it does not seem to matter what type of practice it is. Patients like to feel special and to be treated that way. They like consistency in their physician and in the office staff, and seeing familiar faces. This is especially hard during practicum. The time spent is too short to truly get to know the patients, but it is a great learning experience.

It is important to observe the staff and patient communication and interaction skills. By doing this, you can decide which ones you admire and those that you do not wish to copy. The following are just a few of the guidelines that have helped me: (1) Call patients by name, and be sure that they know your name. (2) Follow through with what you have told patients you will do, and keep them updated if circumstances change. (3) Smile, and do not let one patient's negative attitude interfere with your care of others. (4) Take time to listen.

When you do begin your career, it does not take long to get into a routine and to start knowing your patients. When patients see a familiar face, they are more willing to share information that can contribute to improved communication and good health care. ■

that the patient's hearing threshold for each frequency can be determined. The hearing acuity in each ear is assessed separately, and the results are plotted on a graph known as an *audiogram.* The medical assistant may be responsible for performing audiometry in the medical office. Before operating an audiometer, however, the medical assistant must receive extensive on-site training from an audiologist to ensure that proper technique is used to conduct the test.

Tympanometry

Tympanometry is not a hearing test, but it does help determine the cause of hearing loss, so it is presented in this section. The tympanometer consists of an earpiece attached to an electronic device (Figure 21-10). The earpiece is placed snugly in the patient's ear, and low-frequency sound waves are directed against the eardrum while pressure is applied in the ear canal. With a normal ear, the eardrum exhibits mobility in response to the pressure, as indicated

Figure 21-9 **A,** Audiometer. **B,** The patient signals when he hears a sound. (Courtesy GSI [Grayson-Stadler], Milford, NH.)

Figure 21-10 **A,** Tympanometer. **B,** The earpiece is placed snugly in the patient's ear. (Courtesy GSI [Grayson-Stadler], Milford, NH.)

on a graphic readout known as a *tympanogram.* If there is fluid in the middle ear, the eardrum does not move but remains stiff, as indicated on the tympanogram. Tympanometry is useful in diagnosing serous otitis media (fluid in the middle ear), which is a common cause of temporary hearing loss in children.

EAR IRRIGATION

Ear irrigation is the washing of the external auditory canal with a flowing solution. Ear irrigations are performed for the following purposes: to cleanse the external auditory canal to remove cerumen, discharge, or a foreign body; to relieve inflammation by applying an antiseptic solution; and to apply heat to the ear. Before irrigating, impacted cerumen must be softened by instilling warm mineral oil or hydrogen peroxide for 10 to 15 minutes. An ear irrigation should not be performed if the tympanic membrane is perforated because this could result in severe irritation or infection of the middle ear.

Ear irrigations are most commonly performed in the medical office using either an ear irrigating syringe or an Elephant Ear Wash System. Procedure 21-5 shows how to perform an ear irrigation using both of these methods..

EAR INSTILLATION

An ear instillation involves dropping a liquid into the external auditory canal. Ear instillations are performed to soften impacted cerumen, to combat infection with the use of antibiotic ear drops, and to relieve pain. The ear drops are usually dispensed in a flexible plastic container with an attached dropper. Procedure 21-6 shows how to perform an ear instillation.

PATIENT TEACHING | Acute Otitis Media

Answer questions that patients have about otitis media.

What is a middle ear infection?

An infection of the middle ear is medically referred to as *acute otitis media*. It is an inflammation of the middle ear caused by an infection and can occur in one or both ears. It is common in young children 3 months to 3 years old, but is unusual in adults. A middle ear infection is not serious if treated promptly and effectively. If not treated, however, middle ear infections can lead to serious complications, such as acute mastoiditis, meningitis, and permanent hearing loss.

What causes a middle ear infection?

A middle ear infection is often the result of an upper respiratory infection or allergy that causes the eustachian tube to swell and become blocked. The blockage causes fluid to build up in the middle ear. This fluid is an ideal place for bacteria to grow. If this occurs, the result is acute otitis media.

What are the symptoms of a middle ear infection?

The most common symptoms are intense pain, fever, and temporary hearing loss. Other symptoms may include dizziness, nausea and vomiting, and (if the eardrum ruptures) drainage from the ear.

How does the physician know whether a middle ear infection is present?

The physician examines the ears with an otoscope. If a middle ear infection is present, the eardrum is red and swollen (see illustration) as a result of irritation from the infection, and pus and mucus can be seen behind the eardrum.

Chronic otitis media. (From Damjanov I, Linder J: *Pathology: a color atlas,* St Louis, 1999, Mosby.)

How is the infection treated?

A middle ear infection is usually treated with an oral antibiotic for 10 to 14 days. It is important to take all of the antibiotic prescribed; otherwise, the ear infection may recur. The physician also may recommend a decongestant to help open the blocked eustachian tube. After the acute infection is over, fluid may remain trapped in the middle ear. This condition is known as *serous otitis media* (see illustration) and, if not treated, may last for days, weeks, months, or even a year. Although fluid in the middle ear is painless, it may result in a feeling of fullness or pressure in the ears and temporary hearing loss.

Serous otitis media. (From Swartz MH: *Textbook of physical diagnosis,* ed 5, Philadelphia, 2006, Saunders.)

Why are middle ear infections so common in children?

In children, the eustachian tube is positioned horizontally and is shorter and narrower than in adults. When a child has an upper respiratory infection, bacteria can travel easily to the middle ear. In addition, swelling from the respiratory infection can block this narrow tube, which causes fluid to build up in the middle ear.

- Encourage the patient to complete the entire prescribed course of antibiotics.
- If the physician has prescribed ear drops, teach the patient (or parent) the proper procedure for performing an ear instillation.
- Encourage early treatment of upper respiratory infections.
- Give the patient educational materials on otitis media. ■

PROCEDURE 21-5   Performing an Ear Irrigation

Outcome Perform an ear irrigation

Equipment/Supplies

- Disposable gloves
- Irrigating solution
- Solution basin
- Bath thermometer
- Ear irrigating syringe or Elephant Ear Wash System

- Ear basin
- Moisture-resistant towel
- Gauze pads
- Ear wick

1. Procedural Step. Sanitize your hands.

2. Procedural Step. Assemble the equipment. If both ears are to be irrigated, two sets of equipment must be used to prevent cross-infection from one ear to the other.

Ear irrigation syringe setup.

Elephant Ear Wash System setup.

3. Procedural Step: Prepare the irrigating solution:

a. Carefully check the label of the irrigating solution three times to make sure you have the correct solution. The first time is after you remove the solution container from the shelf. Compare the label of the solution container with the physician's instructions.

b. Check the expiration date of the solution.

c. Warm the irrigating solution to body temperature (98.6° F [37° C]) by placing the solution container in a basin of warm water. Use a bath thermometer to make sure the temperature of the water used to warm the solution does not exceed body temperature.

d. Check the solution label a second time before pouring the solution.

e. Pour the solution as follows:
Palm the label of the container and remove the cap. Place the cap on a flat surface with the open end up.
Ear irrigating syringe: Pour the solution into the basin and replace the cap without contaminating it. Cover the basin to keep the solution warm.
Elephant Ear Wash System: Remove the top of the spray bottle and pour the solution into the bottle. Replace the top of the spray bottle.

f. Check the solution label a third time before returning the container to its storage area.

Principle. The solution label should be carefully checked three times to prevent an error. An outdated solution may produce undesirable effects. If the solution is too cold or too warm, it might stimulate the inner ear and the patient may become dizzy. Palming the label prevents the solution from dripping on the label and obscuring it or loosening the label. Placing the cap open end up prevents contamination.

PROCEDURE 21-5 Performing an Ear Irrigation—cont'd

4. Procedural Step. Greet the patient and introduce yourself. Identify the patient and explain the procedure. Explain the purpose of performing the irrigation—for example, to remove cerumen. Tell the patient the procedure is not painful; however, he or she may feel a minimal amount of discomfort and occasional dizziness, fullness, and warmth as the ear solution comes in contact with the tympanic membrane.

5. Procedural Step. Position the patient in a sitting position. Place a moisture-resistant towel on the patient's shoulder under the ear to be irrigated to protect clothing and to prevent water from running down the neck. Position a basin tightly against the patient's neck under the affected ear to catch the irrigating solution, and ask the patient to hold it in place. Ask the patient to tilt the head in the direction of the affected ear.

Principle. The patient is positioned so that gravity aids the flow of the solution out of the ear and into the basin.

6. Procedural Step. Apply gloves. Cleanse the outer ear with a moistened gauze pad to remove any discharge or debris present. Normal saline or the solution ordered for the irrigation may be used.

Principle. The outer ear should be clean to prevent foreign particles from entering the ear canal during the irrigation.

7. Procedural Step. Prepare the irrigating device.

a. *Ear irrigating syringe:* Fill the syringe with the irrigating solution (approximately 50 mL). Expel air from the syringe.

Principle. Air forced into the ear is uncomfortable for the patient.

b. *Elephant Ear Wash System:* Twist a disposable tip onto the nozzle of the tubing, making sure to screw it firmly into place.

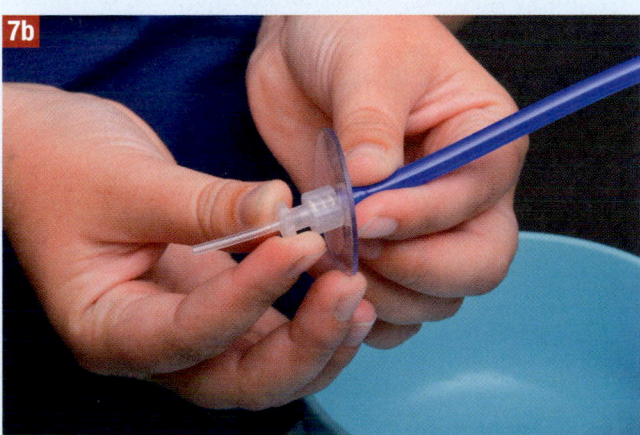

Twist a disposable tip onto the nozzle.

8. Procedural Step. Straighten the external ear canal. The canal is straightened by gently pulling the ear upward and backward for adults and children older than 3 years and downward and backward for children 3 years old or younger.

Principle. Straightening the canal permits the irrigating solution to reach all areas of the canal.

9. Procedural Step. Insert the tip of the irrigating device into the ear, but not too deeply.

(*Note:* With regard to the ear irrigating syringe, make sure that the tip of the ear irrigating syringe does not obstruct the canal opening so that the solution can flow freely out of the canal. Obstruction of the canal causes pressure to build up in the canal, resulting in patient discomfort and possible injury to the tympanic membrane).

Principle. Inserting the tip of the syringe too deeply causes discomfort for the patient and possible injury to the tympanic membrane.

10. Procedural Step. Perform the irrigation.

a. *Ear irrigating syringe:* Inject the irrigating solution toward the roof of the ear canal by slowly depressing the plunger of the irrigating syringe.

Inject the irrigating solution toward the roof of the ear canal.

b. *Elephant Ear Wash System:* Spray the irrigating solution toward the roof of the ear canal by depressing the trigger handle of the ear wash system. Make sure to keep the tubing fairly straight to prevent bending of the tubing. This ensures a good flow of solution into the ear.

Principle. The tip of the irrigating device should be directed at the roof of the canal to prevent injury to the tympanic membrane and to aid in the removal of foreign particles by allowing the solution to flow

Continued

PROCEDURE 21-5 Performing an Ear Irrigation—cont'd

down the length of the canal and out the bottom. In addition, severe patient discomfort and dizziness may occur if the solution is injected directly onto the tympanic membrane.

Spray the irrigating solution toward the roof of the ear canal.

11. Procedural Step. Continue irrigating until the desired results have been obtained or all the solution is used, depending on the purpose of the irrigation. Observe the returning solution to note the material present (e.g., cerumen, discharge, a foreign object) and the amount (small, moderate, or large).

12. Procedural Step. Dry the outside of the ear with a gauze pad. Have the patient lie on the affected side on the treatment table. Tell the patient that the ear will feel sensitive for a short time. Place a cotton wick loosely in the ear canal for 15 minutes if instructed to do so by the physician.

Principle. Any solution remaining in the ear canal should be allowed to drain out. A cotton wick makes the patient's ear feel less sensitive after the irrigation.

13. Procedural Step. Remove the gloves, and sanitize your hands.

14. Procedural Step. Chart the procedure in the patient's medical record.

   a. *Paper-based patient record:* Record the following: the date and time; which ear was irrigated; the type, strength, and amount of solution used; the amount and type of material returned in the irrigating solution; any significant observations; and patient reactions (refer to the PPR charting example).

PPR CHARTING EXAMPLE	
Date	
11/15/XX	2:15 p.m. Irrigated Ⓡ ear c̄ saline, 200 mL at 98.6° F. Mod amt of cerumen present in returned solution. Cotton wick placed in ear canal × 15 min. No complaints of discomfort. ————————— C. Lindner, CMA (AAMA)

   b. *Electronic medical record:* In SimChart® for the Medical Office, document, using the correct radio buttons, drop-down menus, and free text fields, which ear was irrigated; the type, strength, and amount of solution used; the amount and type of material returned in the irrigation solution; any significant observations, and patient reactions.

15. Procedural Step. Remove equipment to a work area for sanitization, sterilization, disinfection, or disposal as required by the medical office policy.

PROCEDURE 21-6 Performing an Ear Instillation

Outcome Perform an ear instillation

Equipment/Supplies

- Disposable gloves
- Otic drops
- Gauze pad

1. **Procedural Step.** Sanitize your hands.
2. **Procedural Step.** Assemble the equipment, and perform the following:
   a. Check the drug label three times to make sure you have the correct medication. The first time should be when you remove the medication from the shelf. The medication label must bear the word *otic*.
   b. Check the medication label a second time against the physician's instructions. Also check the dose ordered by the physician.
   c. Check the expiration date.
   d. Check the medication label a third time before the cap is removed to instill the medication (as indicated in Procedural Step 6).
   Principle. The drug label should be carefully checked three times to prevent a medication error. Medication not bearing the word *otic* must never be placed in the ear because it could injure the ear. An outdated medication may produce undesirable effects and should be discarded.
3. **Procedural Step.** Greet the patient and introduce yourself. Identify the patient and explain the procedure and the purpose of the instillation.
4. **Procedural Step.** Position the patient in a sitting position.
5. **Procedural Step.** Warm the drops to body temperature by holding the medication container in the palms of your hands for a few minutes. Do not warm the drops by placing them in hot water.
   Principle. If the drops are too cold or too warm, they might stimulate the inner ear, causing the patient to become dizzy.
6. **Procedural Step.** Apply gloves. If the medication requires mixing, shake the container well. Check the medication label for the third time, and remove the cap from the container.
7. **Procedural Step.** Ask the patient to tilt his or her head in the direction of the unaffected ear. Straighten the external auditory canal. The canal is straightened by pulling the ear upward and backward for adults and children older than 3 years and downward and backward for children 3 years old and younger. Gravity aids in the flow of medication into the ear canal.

Principle. Straightening the canal permits the medication to reach all areas of the canal.

8. **Procedural Step.** Invert the container and place the tip of the dropper at the opening of the ear canal. Be careful not to touch the tip of the dropper to the ear. Gently squeeze the container and instill the correct number of drops along the side of the canal. Replace the cap on the container.

Instill the medication along the side of the ear canal.

9. **Procedural Step.** Instruct the patient to lie on the unaffected side for 2 to 3 minutes.
   Principle. Lying on the unaffected side prevents the medication from running out and allows complete distribution of the medication.
10. **Procedural Step.** Place a moistened cotton wick loosely in the ear canal for 15 minutes if instructed to do so by the physician.
    Principle. The cotton wick prevents the medication from running out when the patient is upright.

Continued

PROCEDURE 21-6   Performing an Ear Instillation—cont'd

Moistening the wick prevents the medication from being absorbed by the cotton.

11. **Procedural Step.** Remove the gloves, and sanitize your hands.

12. **Procedural Step.** Chart the procedure in the patient's medical record.

   a. *Paper-based patient record:* Record the date and time, the name and strength of the medication, the number of drops, which ear received the instillation, any significant observations, and the patient's reaction (refer to the PPR charting example).

   b. *Electronic medical record:* In SimChart® for the Medical Office, document, using the correct radio buttons, drop-down menus, and free text fields, the strengths of the medication, the number of drops, which ear received the instillation, and any significant observations, as well as the patient's reaction.

13. **Procedural Step.** Return the medication to its storage area.

PPR CHARTING EXAMPLE

Date	
11/20/XX	9:30 a.m. Auralgan, 2 drops, ℞ ear. No discharge present. Pt states a relief of pain.
	——————— C. Lindner, CMA (AAMA)

HIGHLIGHT on Hearing Impairment

The number of individuals with a hearing impairment has gradually increased over the past 20 years. Factors that contribute to this increase include an aging population and a noisier environment.

It is estimated that approximately 28 million people in the United States have a hearing loss severe enough to interfere with their daily activities, and another 2 million individuals are profoundly deaf.

Precise screening of preschool children for hearing loss is difficult. This is because tuning fork tests and audiometry require the ability to signal in response to sound, and children up to age 4 or 5 years have trouble mastering this skill.

Most state, county, and local school systems require hearing screening as a prerequisite for entrance to school and again at periodic intervals, usually during the first, third, fifth, and seventh grades.

Risk factors for hearing impairment in children include family history of deafness, premature birth, low birth weight, measles, mumps, high fevers, meningitis, recurrent or chronic ear infections, and the maternal rubella infection during pregnancy.

Signs of hearing impairment in children are poor attentiveness, delayed speech development, and persistent problems with articulation. Signs of hearing impairment in adults include frequent requests for words or statements to be repeated, leaning toward the speaker, turning the head, cupping the ears, and speaking in a loud or unvaried tone of voice.

The most common cause of conductive hearing loss in children is fluid in the middle ear, which prevents the tympanic membrane from vibrating freely. In adults, the most common cause of conductive loss is otosclerosis, a condition in which the stapes becomes fixed because of calcium deposits and less able to pass on vibrations when sound enters the ear.

The loudness of sound is measured in units called *decibels* (dB). Sounds of less than 75 dB, even after long exposure, are unlikely to cause hearing loss. Normal conversation is approximately 60 dB, and a whisper in a quiet library is 30 to 40 dB.

Permanent sensorineural hearing loss can result when the ear is repeatedly bombarded with loud sounds over time. Standards set by the Occupational Safety and Health Administration (OSHA) indicate that continued exposure to noise louder than 85 dB eventually harms an individual's hearing by damaging the tiny hair cells in the organ of Corti. The organ of Corti is a structure in the cochlea (inner ear) that converts sound waves into nerve impulses for transmission to the brain. This type of sensorineural hearing loss is known as *noise-induced hearing loss.* It is most often seen in individuals who frequently listen to loud music, fire guns without wearing ear protection, or are exposed to loud noise as part of their jobs. The following are examples of common noises and the decibel level of each:

Noise	Decibels
Normal breathing	10
Humming of a refrigerator	40
Television	70
Vacuum cleaner	60 to 85
Motorcycle	95 to 100
Personal stereo system with earphones (on high)	115
Rock concert	120
Chain saw	120
Auto stereo on high	125
Jet taking off	140
Firecracker	150
Firearms	140 to 170

Many hearing impairments can be helped with the use of a hearing aid. Individuals who benefit most from a hearing aid have mild to moderate conductive hearing loss. Individuals with sensorineural or mixed hearing loss have more trouble finding a suitable hearing aid and often get less satisfactory results. ■

What Would You Do? What Would You *Not* Do? RESPONSES

Case Study 1
Page 446

What Did Cammie Do?
❑ Talked with Haley (on her level) about why someone needs to wear glasses.
❑ Retested Haley with the Snellen chart to see if she missed the same letters.
❑ Tested Haley with the Big E chart to give the physician an additional measurement to make an interpretation of Haley's visual acuity.

What Did Cammie Not Do?
❑ Did not tell Haley that she needs glasses.
❑ Did not scold Haley for trying to miss letters on the test.

Case Study 2
Page 450

What Did Cammie Do?
❑ Gave Mr. Mitchell some suggestions on how to put drops in Clive's eyes so it is less scary. One idea is to have Clive lie down flat and close his eyes. Place the drops in the inner corner of his eye next to the bridge of his nose, letting them make a little lake there. When Clive relaxes and opens his eye, the drops will gently flow into his eye.
❑ Talked with Clive (on his level) about why he needs eye drops.
❑ Told Mr. Mitchell that the eye drops were prescribed for Clive, and they should be used only for Clive. Told him that if the twins developed conjunctivitis, he should call the office.
❑ Gave Mr. Mitchell suggestions for preventing the twins from getting conjunctivitis (not touching the infected eye, frequent handwashing, not sharing toys or towels).

What Did Cammie Not Do?
❑ Did not tell Mr. Mitchell to hold Clive down or force drops in his eyes.
❑ Did not tell Mr. Mitchell that he should know better than to think about giving the twins a medication not prescribed for them.

Case Study 3
Page 455

What Did Cammie Do?
❑ Explained to Mrs. Basil that Jade may begin to feel better after several days of antibiotics, but not all of the germs causing her ear infection will have been killed by then. If she does not give Jade the full course of antibiotics, the infection could come back.
❑ Documented all the medications that Mrs. Basil has administered to Jade.
❑ Gave Mrs. Basil a patient information brochure on acute otitis media.
❑ Told Mrs. Basil that she needs to talk to the physician about her concern regarding hearing loss because the physician is most qualified to answer that question.
❑ Encouraged Mrs. Basil to bring Jade in sooner when she develops fever and ear pain.

What Did Cammie Not Do?
❑ Did not criticize Mrs. Basil for waiting so long to bring Jade in.
❑ Did not offer a personal opinion about alternative medicine.

TERMINOLOGY REVIEW

Key Term	Word Parts	Definition
Astigmatism	*a-:* without *stigma/a:* point *-ism:* state of	A refractive error that causes distorted and blurred vision for both near and far objects due to a cornea that is oval shaped.
Audiometer	*audi/o:* hearing *-meter:* instrument used to measure	An instrument used to measure hearing acuity quantitatively for the various frequencies of sound waves.
Canthus		The junction of the eyelids at either corner of the eye.
Cerumen		A yellowish waxy substance secreted by glands in the ear canal which functions to lubricate and protect the ear canal. Earwax.
Hyperopia	*hyper-:* above, excessive *-opia:* vision	Farsightedness.
Impacted		Wedged firmly together so as to be immovable.
Instillation		The dropping of a liquid into a body cavity.
Irrigation		The washing of a body canal with a flowing solution.
Myopia	*-opia:* vision	Nearsightedness.
Otoscope	*ot/o:* ear *-scope:* to view	An instrument used to examine the external ear canal and tympanic membrane.
Presbyopia	*-opia:* vision	A decrease in the elasticity of the lens that occurs with aging, resulting in a decreased ability to focus on close objects.
Refraction		The deflection or bending of light rays by a lens.
Tympanic membrane	*tympan/o:* eardrum *-ic:* pertaining to	A thin, semitransparent membrane between the external ear canal and the middle ear that receives and transmits sound waves. Also known as the *eardrum*.

ON THE WEB

For information on the eye:

American Optometric Association: www.aoa.org

American Academy of Ophthalmology: www.aao.org

National Eye Institute: www.nei.nih.gov

All About Vision: www.allaboutvision.com

Sight and Hearing Association: www.sightandhearing.org

American Academy of Optometry: www.aaopt.org

American Association for Pediatric Ophthalmology and Strabismus: www.aapos.org

About Cataract Surgery: www.aboutcataractsurgery.com

The Eyes Have It: www.kellogg.umich.edu/theeyeshaveit/index.html

Eye Care America: www.eyecareamerica.org

For information on the ear:

American Academy of Audiology: www.audiology.org

National Institute on Deafness and Other Communication Disorders: www.nidcd.nih.gov

Healthy Hearing: www.healthyhearing.com

Hear It: www.hear-it.org

Center for Hearing and Communication: www.chchearing.org

Better Hearing Institute: www.betterhearing.org

Physical Agents to Promote Tissue Healing

22

 Check out the Evolve site at http://evolve.elsevier.com/Bonewit/today/ to access additional interactive activities and exercises to help you study and prepare for success.

LEARNING OBJECTIVES

Local Application of Heat and Cold
1. State examples of moist and dry applications of heat and cold.
2. State the factors to consider when applying heat and cold.
3. List the effects of local application of heat, and state reasons for applying heat.
4. List the effects of local application of cold, and state reasons for applying cold.

Ambulatory Aids
5. List factors that are taken into consideration when ambulatory aids are prescribed.
6. Explain the difference between an axillary crutch and a forearm crutch.
7. State conditions that may result when axillary crutches are not fitted properly.
8. List the guidelines that should be followed by the patient to ensure safe use of crutches.
9. State the use of each of the following crutch gaits: four-point gait, two-point gait, three-point gait, swing-to gait, and swing-through gait.
10. List and describe the three types of canes.
11. Identify the patient conditions that warrant the use of a cane or walker.

PROCEDURES

Apply each of the following heat treatments:
- Heating pad
- Hot soak
- Hot compress
- Chemical hot pack

Apply each of the following cold treatments:
- Ice bag
- Cold compress
- Chemical cold pack

Measure a patient for axillary crutches.
Instruct a patient in the proper use of crutches.
Instruct a patient in the proper procedure for each of the following crutch gaits:
- Four-point
- Two-point
- Three-point
- Swing-to
- Swing-through

Instruct a patient in the use of a cane.
Instruct a patient in the proper use of a walker.

CHAPTER OUTLINE

INTRODUCTION TO TISSUE HEALING
LOCAL APPLICATION OF HEAT AND COLD
Factors Affecting the Application of Heat and Cold
Heat
Local Effects of Heat
Purpose of Applying Heat
Types of Heat Applications
Cold
Local Effects of Cold

Purpose of Applying Cold
Types of Cold Applications
AMBULATORY AIDS
Crutches
Axillary Crutch Measurement
Crutch Guidelines
Crutch Gaits
Canes
Walkers

KEY TERMS

ambulation (AM-byoo-LAY-shun)
ambulatory
compress (KOM-press)
edema (uh-DEE-muh)

erythema (err-uh-THEE-muh)
exudate (EKS-oo-date)
soak
sprain

strain
suppuration (SUP-er-AY-shun)

INTRODUCTION TO TISSUE HEALING

Physical agents are often employed in the medical office to promote tissue healing for individuals who experience a disability as a result of injury, disease, or loss of a body part. Physical agents are used therapeutically to improve circulation, provide support, and promote the return of motion so that the individual can perform the activities of daily living. Physical agents frequently used in the medical office include heat and cold applied locally and ambulatory aids, such as crutches, canes, and walkers.

LOCAL APPLICATION OF HEAT AND COLD

The application of heat and cold is used therapeutically to treat conditions such as infection and trauma. The medical assistant may be responsible for applying various forms of heat and cold at the medical office or for instructing patients in the proper procedure for applying heat or cold at home. The medical assistant should have a basic understanding of the physiologic effects of heat and cold on the body and of possible adverse reactions if they are not administered correctly.

Heat and cold can be applied in moist or dry forms. Common applications of dry and moist heat and cold are as follows:

1. *Dry heat:* heating pad, chemical hot pack
2. *Moist heat:* hot soak, hot compress
3. *Dry cold:* ice bag, chemical cold pack
4. *Moist cold:* cold compress

Heat and cold are applied for short periods (typically 15 to 30 minutes) to produce the desired therapeutic results. The application may be repeated at time intervals specified by the physician. Prolonged application of heat or cold is not recommended because it can result in adverse secondary effects. The type of heat or cold application used for a particular condition depends on the purpose of the application, the location and condition of the affected area, and the age and general health of the patient. The physician instructs the medical assistant to apply a heat or cold treatment based on these factors.

Heat and cold receptors in the skin readily adapt to changes in temperature, eventually resulting in diminished heat or cold sensations. The temperature actually remains the same and is providing the intended therapeutic effects. The patient, not perceiving the same degree of temperature, may want to increase the intensity of the application, however, without realizing the inherent dangers. Excessive heat or cold could result in tissue damage. A common example of this situation is a patient who turns up the setting of a heating pad from medium to high when the heating pad no longer feels warm. The medical assistant should fully explain to the patient the

necessity of maintaining a safe temperature range during the application.

Putting It All Into Practice

My name is Marlyne Cooper, and I am a Certified Medical Assistant. I work in a community health center. My primary responsibilities are to take patients back to the examination rooms and to prepare them for procedures and treatments. I take the patient's chief complaint and the health history. I greet each patient in a kind and calm way. This helps put the patient at ease before the physician goes into the examining room.

I once worked in a private office with a small waiting room and a narrow hall. One of my regular patients was a healthy 20-year-old man who was confined to a wheelchair by a spinal injury from an automobile accident. He had great difficulty maneuvering his motorized chair in tight spaces, and he felt embarrassed and conspicuous sitting in the middle of the waiting room. I began bringing him through the larger back door into the physician's office, directly into an examination room. Talking about things we had in common, such as interests in sports and movies, made him feel more at ease. By making the situation as easy as possible for him, I was able to help him keep his dignity while not drawing attention to his special needs. ■

FACTORS AFFECTING THE APPLICATION OF HEAT AND COLD

Before applying heat or cold, certain factors must be taken into consideration to prevent unfavorable reactions, such as tissue necrosis. The temperature may need to be adjusted based on the following conditions:

1. *The age of the patient.* Young children and elderly patients tend to be more sensitive to the application of heat or cold.
2. *Location of the application.* Certain areas of the body are more sensitive to the application of heat or cold, especially thin areas of the skin and areas that are usually covered by clothing, such as the chest, back, and abdomen. The skin on the hands and face is not as sensitive and is better able to tolerate temperature change. Broken skin, such as is found with an open wound, is more sensitive to heat and cold and is more prone to tissue damage.
3. *Impaired circulation.* Patients with impaired circulation tend to be more sensitive to heat and cold. This impairment may be at the site of the application or may be a systemic problem involving the entire body that is a result of certain conditions, such as peripheral vascular disease, diabetes mellitus, or congestive heart failure.
4. *Impaired sensation.* Patients with impaired sensation, such as diabetic patients, must be watched carefully

because tissue damage may occur from the application of heat or cold without the patient's awareness.

5. *Individual tolerance to change in temperature.* Some individuals cannot tolerate temperature change as easily as others.

The medical assistant should observe the area to which the heat or cold has been applied before, during, and after treatment for signs indicating that a modification of temperature is needed. Prolonged erythema or paleness, pain, swelling, and blisters should be reported to the physician. The medical assistant also should ask the patient whether the application feels comfortable or is too hot or too cold.

HEAT

Local Effects of Heat

The application of moderate heat to a localized area of the body for a short time (approximately 15 to 30 minutes) produces *dilation,* or an increase in diameter, of the blood vessels in the area as the body tries to rid itself of excess heat (Figure 22-1). This results in an increased blood supply to the area, and tissue metabolism increases. Nutrients and oxygen are provided to the cells at a faster rate, and wastes and toxins are carried away faster. The skin in the area

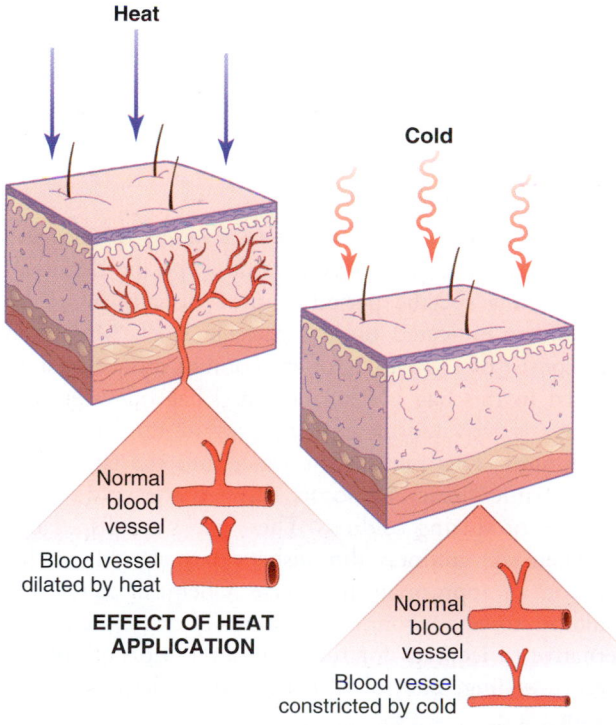

EFFECT OF HEAT APPLICATION

Heat

Cold

Normal blood vessel

Blood vessel dilated by heat

Normal blood vessel

Blood vessel constricted by cold

EFFECT OF COLD APPLICATION

Figure 22-1 Effects of the local application of heat and cold. (From Wood LA, Rambo BJ: *Nursing skills for allied health services,* vol 2, Philadelphia, 1980, Saunders.)

becomes warm and exhibits erythema. **Erythema** is reddening of the skin caused by dilation of superficial blood vessels in the skin.

These physiologic effects of moderate heat applied to a localized area promote healing. Prolonged application of heat (longer than 1 hour) produces secondary effects, however, that reverse this healing process. Blood vessels constrict, and blood supply to the area decreases. The medical assistant must be careful to apply heat for the length of time specified by the physician.

Purpose of Applying Heat

Heat functions in relieving pain, congestion, muscle spasms, and inflammation. Conditions for which the local application of heat is often prescribed are low back pain, arthritis, menstrual cramping, and localized abscesses.

Heat promotes muscle relaxation and is often used for the relief of pain caused by excessive contraction of muscle fibers. **Edema,** or swelling, in the tissues can be reduced through the application of heat because the increased blood supply functions to increase the absorption of fluid from the tissues through the lymphatic system.

Heat, usually in the form of a hot **compress,** can be used to soften exudates. An **exudate** is a discharge produced by the body's tissues. Exudates may sometimes form a hard crust over an area and require removal. Heat also increases **suppuration,** or the process of pus formation, to help in the relief of inflammation by breaking down infected tissues. Heat is not recommended, however, for the initial treatment of acute inflammation or trauma.

Types of Heat Applications

The most common types of heat applications are described next, along with the conditions they are often used to treat.

Heating Pad

The electric heating pad consists of a network of wires that function to convert electric energy into heat to provide a constant and even heat application. The wires must not be bent or crushed. This could damage the pad, resulting in overheating of parts of the pad and leading to burns or fire. Pins must not be inserted into the pad as a means of securing it; if a pin comes in contact with a wire, an electric shock could result. To prevent electric hazards, heating pads should not be used over areas that contain moisture, such as wet dressings. Heating pads are often used to relieve pain and muscle spasms.

Hot Soak

A **soak** is the direct immersion of a body part in water or a medicated solution. A soak can be applied to an extremity or a part of the torso. Hot soaks are often prepared using a ratio (e.g., two parts water to one part medication), and are used to cleanse open wounds, increase suppuration, increase the blood supply to an area to hasten the healing process, and apply a medicated solution to an area.

Hot Compress

A hot compress is a soft, moist, absorbent cloth, such as a washcloth, that is immersed in a warm solution and applied to a body part. Hot compresses are used to increase suppuration, to improve circulation to a body part to aid in healing, to promote drainage from infection, and to soften exudates. Applying a hot compress to an open wound requires the use of sterile technique.

Chemical Hot Pack

Chemical hot packs are available in a variety of sizes and shapes. When activated, they provide a specific degree of heat for a specific period of time (usually 30 to 60 minutes), as indicated on the package label. A chemical hot pack consists of a vinyl bag containing calcium chloride crystals and a smaller bag (encased in the vinyl bag) containing water. Pressure is applied with the hands to break the inner bag. The water in the inner bag combines with the calcium chloride crystals to produce heat. After using the pack, it should be discarded in an appropriate receptacle. Chemical hot packs should be stored at room temperature and are used as an alternative to a heating pad to relieve pain and muscle spasms.

Procedures 22-1, 22-2, 22-3, and 22-6 (see later) present the proper application of heat with a heating pad, a hot soak, a hot compress, and a chemical hot pack.

| What Would You Do? | What Would You *Not* Do? |

Case Study 1

Aaron Collins is at the office. Aaron recently helped a friend move, and the next day he developed intense pain in his lower back. To alleviate the pain, he slept on a heating pad, but when he woke up, his back was red and blistered. Aaron says he turned the setting on the heating pad to high because his back was hurting so much and he thought that it would help his back feel better sooner. Aaron wants to know the best way to apply heat using a heating pad. He also wants to know what he can do to prevent low back pain in the future. ■

COLD

Local Effects of Cold

The application of moderate cold to a localized area produces *constriction,* or a decrease in diameter, of blood vessels in the area as the body attempts to prevent heat loss (see Figure 22-1). This constriction leads to decreased blood supply to the area. Tissue metabolism decreases, less oxygen is used, and fewer wastes accumulate. The skin becomes cool and pale. Prolonged application of cold (longer than 1 hour) has a reverse secondary effect. Blood vessels dilate, and tissue metabolism is increased. To prevent secondary effects, the medical assistant must apply cold for the recommended length of time only.

Purpose of Applying Cold

The application of moderate cold for a short time is used to prevent edema. Cold may be applied immediately after an individual has sustained direct trauma, such as a bruise, minor burn, **sprain, strain,** joint injury, or fracture. The cold limits the accumulation of fluid in the body tissues by constricting blood vessels and reducing the leakage of fluid into the tissues. Through constriction of peripheral blood vessels, cold can be used to control bleeding. Cold temporarily relieves pain through its anesthetic, or numbing, effect, which reduces stimulation of the pain receptors. Cold also slows the movement of blood and tissue fluids in the affected area, resulting in less pressure against pain receptors and therefore less pain. In the early stages of an infection, the local application of cold inhibits the activity of microorganisms. In this way, suppuration is decreased and inflammation is reduced. Cold applications should always be placed in a protective covering because applying cold directly to the skin could result in a skin burn.

Types of Cold Applications

Ice Bag

An ice bag consists of a waterproof bag with a screw-on cap. Before use, it must be filled with small pieces of ice and placed in a protective covering. Ice bags are used to prevent swelling, control bleeding, and relieve pain and inflammation.

Cold Compress

A cold compress is a soft, moist, absorbent cloth, such as a washcloth, that is immersed in a cold solution and applied to a body part. Cold compresses are used to relieve pain and inflammation and to treat conditions such as headache, injury to the eye, and pain after tooth extraction.

Chemical Cold Pack

Chemical cold packs are available in a variety of sizes and shapes. When activated, they provide a specific degree of coldness for a specific period of time (usually 30 to 60 minutes), as indicated on the package label. Most cold packs consist of a vinyl bag of ammonium nitrate crystals. Enclosed in this bag is a smaller vinyl bag of water. The cold pack is activated by applying pressure until the inner bag ruptures. This releases the water into the larger bag, and a chemical reaction occurs between the crystals and the water, producing coldness. These packs are disposable, and when the coldness diminishes, they should be discarded in an appropriate receptacle. Chemical cold packs should be stored at room temperature. They are used as an alternative to ice bags for the local application of cold to prevent swelling, control bleeding, and relieve pain and inflammation.

Procedures 22-4, 22-5, and 22-6 present proper application of cold with an ice bag, a cold compress, and a chemical cold pack.

Text continued on p. 477

PROCEDURE 22-1   Applying a Heating Pad

Outcome Apply a heating pad

Equipment/Supplies

- Heating pad with a protective covering

1. **Procedural Step.** Sanitize your hands.
2. **Procedural Step.** Assemble the equipment.
3. **Procedural Step.** Greet the patient and introduce yourself. Identify the patient and explain the procedure. Explain the purpose of the application (e.g., to relieve pain).
4. **Procedural Step.** Place the heating pad in the protective covering.
   Principle. The protective covering provides more comfort for the patient and absorbs perspiration.

Place the heating pad in a protective covering.

5. **Procedural Step.** Connect the plug to an electric outlet. Set the selector switch at the proper setting, as designated by the physician (usually low or medium).
6. **Procedural Step.** Place the heating pad on the patient's affected body area. Ask the patient how the temperature feels. The heating pad should feel warm but not uncomfortable.
7. **Procedural Step.** Instruct the patient not to lie on the pad or turn the control higher to prevent burns.
   Principle. Lying on the pad causes heat to accumulate and burn the patient. The patient's heat receptors eventually become adjusted to the temperature change, resulting in a decreased heat sensation, and the patient may be tempted to increase the temperature. Turning the control higher results in excessive heat on the patient's skin, which could burn the patient.

8. **Procedural Step.** Check the patient periodically for signs of an increase or decrease in redness or swelling, and ask the patient whether the site is painful. Administer the treatment for the proper length of time as designated by the physician.
9. **Procedural Step.** Sanitize your hands.
10. **Procedural Step.** Chart the procedure in the patient's medical record.
    a. *Paper-based patient record:* Record the date and time, method of heat application (heating pad), temperature setting of the pad, location and duration of the application, appearance of the application site, and the patient's reaction. Also, chart any instructions provided to the patient on applying a heating pad at home (refer to the PPR charting example).
    b. *Electronic Medical Record (EMR):* Using an EMR such as SimChart for the Medical Office, use the

PPR CHARTING EXAMPLE

Date	
12/10/XX	10:15 a.m. Heating pad on medium setting applied to lower back x 20 min. Area appears pink following application. Pt states a relief of pain and better mobility. Provided instructions on the application of a heating pad at home. _____ M. Cooper, CMA (AAMA)

correct radio buttons, drop-down menus, and free text fields to document the method of heat application, the location and duration of the application, the appearance of the application site, and the patient's reaction. Also, document any instructions provided to the patient on applying a heating pad at home.
11. **Procedural Step.** Properly care for equipment, and return it to its storage location. Also, if the protective covering is disposable, throw it away; if it is reusable, either wash it in the washing machine or sanitize it before reusing it.

Outcome Apply a hot soak

Equipment/Supplies

- Soaking solution ordered by the physician
- Bath thermometer
- Basin
- Bath towels

1. **Procedural Step.** Sanitize your hands.
2. **Procedural Step.** Assemble the equipment. Check the label on the solution container to make sure you have the correct solution as ordered by the physician. Place the solution containers in a basin of warm water. Warm the soaking solution to a temperature between 105°F and 110°F (41°C and 44°C).
3. **Procedural Step.** Greet the patient and introduce yourself. Identify the patient and explain the procedure. Explain the purpose of the application (e.g., to apply a medicated solution).
4. **Procedural Step.** Fill the basin one third to two thirds full with the warmed soaking solution.
5. **Procedural Step.** Check the temperature of the solution with a bath thermometer. The temperature for an adult should be 105°F to 110°F (41°C to 44°C).
6. **Procedural Step.** Assist the patient into a comfortable position to avoid fatigue and muscle strain. Pad the side of the basin with a towel for the patient's comfort.
7. **Procedural Step.** Slowly and gradually immerse the patient's affected body part in the solution. Ask the patient how the temperature feels.
   Principle. The affected body part should gradually become accustomed to the change in temperature.
8. **Procedural Step.** Test the temperature of the solution frequently. To keep the solution at a constant temperature, remove cooler fluid every 5 minutes and replace it with hot solution. Pour the hot solution in near the edge of the basin by placing your hand between the patient and the solution. Stir the solution as you pour.
   Principle. The solution should be added away from the patient's body part to prevent splashing hot fluid on the patient. Stirring in the solution helps distribute the heat and keep the temperature constant.

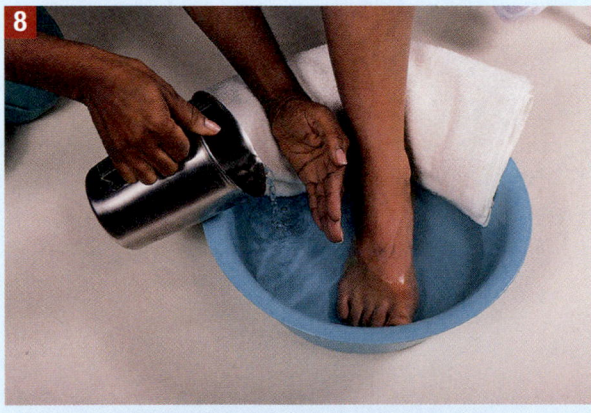

Replace cooler solution with hot solution.

9. **Procedural Step.** Check the patient's skin periodically for signs of an increase or decrease in redness or swelling, and ask the patient whether the site is painful. Apply the hot soak for the proper length of time as designated by the physician (usually 15 to 20 minutes).
10. **Procedural Step.** Dry the affected part completely and gently.
11. **Procedural Step.** Sanitize your hands.
12. **Procedural Step.** Chart the procedure in the patient's medical record.
    a. *Paper-based patient record:* Record the date and time, method of heat application (hot soak), name and strength of the solution, temperature of the soak, location and duration of the application, appearance of the application site, and the patient's reaction (refer to the PPR charting example).

PPR CHARTING EXAMPLE	
Date	
12/12/XX	1:15 p.m. Normal saline hot soak at 105° F applied to ⓇR ankle x 20 min. Area appears pink following application. Pt states less stiffness in ankle. — M. Cooper, CMA (AAMA)

   b. *Electronic medical record (EMR):* Using an EMR such as SimChart for the Medical Office, use the correct radio buttons, drop-down menus, and free text fields to document the method of heat application, name and strength of the solution, temperature of the soak, location and duration of the application, appearance of the application site, and the patient's reaction.
13. **Procedural Step.** Properly care for equipment, and return it to its storage location.

PROCEDURE 22-3   Applying a Hot Compress

Outcome Apply a hot compress

Equipment/Supplies

- Solution ordered by the physician
- Bath thermometer
- Basin
- Washcloths
- Waterproof covering
- Towel

1. **Procedural Step.** Sanitize your hands.
2. **Procedural Step.** Assemble the equipment. Check the label on the solution container to make sure you have the correct solution as ordered by the physician. Place the solution containers in a basin of warm water. Warm the soaking solution to a temperature between 105°F and 110°F (41°C and 44°C).
3. **Procedural Step.** Greet the patient and introduce yourself. Identify the patient and explain the procedure. Explain the purpose of the application (e.g., to soften an exudate).
4. **Procedural Step.** Fill the basin half full with warmed solution. Check the temperature of the solution with the bath thermometer. The temperature for an adult should be 105°F to 110°F (41°C to 44°C).
5. **Procedural Step.** Completely immerse the compress in the solution. Wring the compress to remove excess moisture. The compress should be wet but not dripping. Apply it lightly at first to the affected site to allow the patient to become used to the heat gradually. You may want to cover the compress with a waterproof cover to help hold in the heat. Ask the patient how the temperature feels. The compress should be as hot as the patient can comfortably tolerate.
   Principle. The waterproof cover prevents cool air currents from coming into contact with the compress and reduces the number of times the compress needs to be changed.

Wring out the compress.

Apply the compress to the affected site.

6. **Procedural Step.** Place additional compresses in the solution so that they are ready for use.
7. **Procedural Step.** Repeat the application of the compress every 2 to 3 minutes for the duration of time specified by the physician (usually 15 to 20 minutes). Check the patient's skin periodically for signs of an increase or decrease in redness or swelling, and ask the patient whether the site is painful.
8. **Procedural Step.** Check the temperature of the solution periodically. Remove cooler fluid and replace it with hot solution if needed. Administer the treatment for the proper length of time as designated by the physician.
9. **Procedural Step.** Dry the affected part thoroughly and gently.
10. **Procedural Step.** Sanitize your hands.
11. **Procedural Step.** Chart the procedure in the patient's medical record.
    a. *Paper-based patient record:* Record the date and time, method of heat application (hot compress), name and strength of the solution, temperature of the solution, location and duration of the application, appearance of the application site, and the patient's reaction (refer to the PPR charting example).

PPR CHARTING EXAMPLE

Date	
12/20/XX	10:30 a.m. Normal saline hot compress at 110° F applied to ℞ forearm x 20 min. No complaints of discomfort. ———————————————— M. Cooper, CMA (AAMA)

Continued

PROCEDURE **22-3**   Applying a Hot Compress—cont'd

b. *Electronic medical record (EMR):* Using an EMR such as SimChart for the Medical Office, use the correct radio buttons, drop-down menus, and free text fields to document the method of heat application, name and strength of the solution, temperature of the solution, location and duration of the application, appearance of the application site, and the patient's reaction.

12. **Procedural Step.** Properly care for equipment, and return it to its storage location.

PROCEDURE **22-4**   Applying an Ice Bag

Outcome   Apply an ice bag

Equipment/Supplies

- Ice bag with a protective covering
- Small pieces of ice (ice chips or crushed ice)

1. **Procedural Step.** Sanitize your hands.
2. **Procedural Step.** Assemble the equipment.
3. **Procedural Step.** Greet the patient and introduce yourself. Identify the patient and explain the procedure. Explain the purpose of applying the ice bag (e.g., to prevent swelling).
4. **Procedural Step.** Check the ice bag for leakage.
   Principle. A leaking bag would get the patient wet and cause chilling.
5. **Procedural Step.** Fill the bag one half to two thirds full with small pieces of ice.
   Principle. Small pieces of ice work better than large pieces because they reduce the air spaces in the bag, resulting in better conduction of cold. In addition, small pieces of ice allow the bag to mold better to the body area.
6. **Procedural Step.** Expel air from the bag by squeezing the empty top half of the bag together and screwing on the stopper.
   Principle. Air is a poor conductor of cold and makes it difficult to mold the ice bag to the body area.

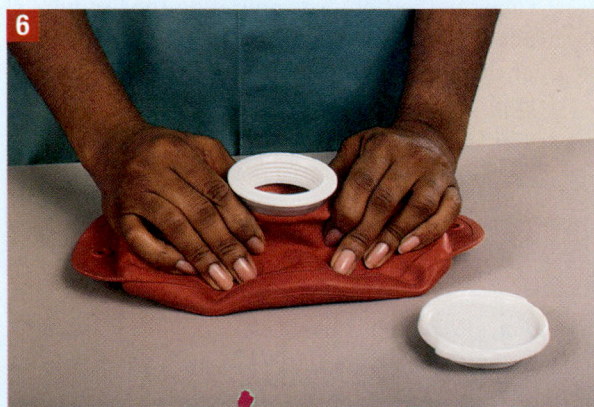
Expel air from the bag.

7. **Procedural Step.** Place the bag in the protective covering.
   Principle. The protective covering provides for patient comfort and absorbs the moisture that condenses on the outside of the bag.
8. **Procedural Step.** Place the bag on the patient's affected body area. Ask the patient how the temperature feels. The application of ice is usually uncomfortable, but most patients tolerate it when they know how much benefit may be derived from it.
   Principle. Individuals vary in their ability to tolerate cold.
9. **Procedural Step.** Check the patient's skin periodically for signs of an increase or decrease in redness or swelling, and ask the patient whether the site is painful. If extreme paleness and numbness or a mottled blue appearance occur at the application site, remove the bag and notify the physician.
10. **Procedural Step.** Refill the bag with ice as necessary, and change the protective covering if needed. Administer the treatment for the proper length of time, as designated by the physician (usually until the area feels numb, approximately 15 to 30 minutes).
11. **Procedural Step.** Sanitize your hands.
12. **Procedural Step.** Chart the procedure in the patient's medical record.
   a. *Paper-based patient record:* Record the date and time, method of cold application (ice bag), location and duration of the application, appearance of the application site, and the patient's reaction. Also, chart any instructions provided to the patient on applying an ice bag at home (refer to the PPR charting example).

PROCEDURE 22-4   Applying an Ice Bag—cont'd

PPR CHARTING EXAMPLE

Date	
12/22/XX	11:30 a.m. Ice bag applied to ⓡ knee x 20 min. Pt complained of slight discomfort during the application. Area appears less swollen following application. Provided instructions on the application of an ice bag at home. ———— M. Cooper, CMA (AAMA)

b. *Electronic medical record (EMR):* Using an EMR such as SimChart for the Medical Office, use the correct radio buttons, drop-down menus, and free text fields to document the method of cold application, location and duration of the

application, appearance of the application site, and the patient's reaction. Also, document any instructions provided to the patient on applying an ice bag at home.

13. Procedural Step. Properly care for the ice bag. Dispose of or launder the protective covering as required. Cleanse the ice bag with a warm detergent solution, rinse thoroughly, and dry by hanging the bag upside down with the top removed. Store the bag by screwing on the stopper, leaving air inside to prevent the sides from sticking together.

PROCEDURE 22-5

PROCEDURE 22-5   Applying a Cold Compress

Outcome Apply a cold compress

Equipment/Supplies

- Ice cubes
- Basin
- Washcloths
- Towel
- Ice bag

1. Procedural Step. Sanitize your hands.
2. Procedural Step. Assemble the equipment. Check the label on the solution container to make sure you have the correct solution as ordered by the physician.
3. Procedural Step. Greet the patient and introduce yourself. Identify the patient and explain the procedure. Explain the purpose of the application (e.g., to treat an eye injury).
4. Procedural Step. Place large ice cubes in the basin. Add the solution until the basin is half full. *Principle.* Using larger pieces of ice prevents them from sticking to the compress and slows the rate at which they melt in the solution.

Place large ice cubes in the basin.

Continued

PROCEDURE 22-5   Applying a Cold Compress—cont'd

5. Procedural Step. Completely immerse the compress in the solution. Wring the compress to rid it of excess moisture. The compress should be wet but not dripping. Apply it lightly at first to the affected site to allow the patient to become used to the cold gradually. The compress can be covered with an ice bag to help keep it cold and to reduce the number of times it needs to be changed. Ask the patient how the temperature feels.

6. Procedural Step. Place additional compresses in the solution to be ready for use.

7. Procedural Step. Repeat the application of the compress every 2 to 3 minutes for the duration of time specified by the physician (usually 15 to 20 minutes). Check the patient's skin periodically for signs of an increase or decrease in redness or swelling, and ask the patient whether the site is painful.

8. Procedural Step. Add ice if needed to keep the solution cold. Administer the treatment for the proper length of time designated by the physician.

9. Procedural Step. Thoroughly dry the affected part.

10. Procedural Step. Sanitize your hands.

11. Procedural Step. Chart the procedure in the patient's medical record.

a. *Paper-based patient record:* Record the date and time, method of cold application (cold compress), location and duration of the application, appearance of the application site, and patient's reaction (refer to the PPR charting example).

PPR CHARTING EXAMPLE

Date	
12/27/XX	9:15 a.m. Normal saline cold compress applied to bridge of nose x 15 min. Nose appears less swollen following application. Tolerated application well.————————————————— M. Cooper, CMA (AAMA)

b. *Electronic medical record (EMR):* Using an EMR such as SimChart for the Medical Office, use the correct radio buttons, drop-down menus, and free text fields to document the method of cold application, location and duration of the application, appearance of the application site, and patient's reaction.

12. Procedural Step. Properly care for equipment, and return it to its storage location.

PROCEDURE 22-6   Applying a Chemical Pack

Outcome Apply a chemical cold pack and a chemical hot pack
The procedure for applying a chemical cold or hot pack is as follows:

1. Procedural Step. Shake the crystals to the bottom of the bag.

2. Procedural Step. Squeeze the bag firmly with your hands to break the inner water bag.

3. Procedural Step. Shake the bag vigorously to mix the contents.

4. Procedural Step. Cover the bag with a protective covering.

5. Procedural Step. Apply the bag to the affected area. Check the patient's skin periodically.

6. Procedural Step. Administer the treatment for the proper length of time.

7. Procedural Step. Discard the bag in an appropriate receptacle.

8. Procedural Step. Sanitize your hands.

9. Procedural Step. Chart the procedure in the patient's medical record.

a. *Paper-based patient record:* Record the date and time, method of application (chemical cold or hot pack), location and duration of the application, appearance of the application site, and patient's reaction.

b. *Electronic medical record (EMR):* Using an EMR such as SimChart for the Medical Office, use the correct radio buttons, drop-down menus, and free text fields to document the method of application (chemical cold or hot pack), location and duration of the application, appearance of the application site, and patient's reaction.

Chemical packs. **A,** Chemical cold pack; **B,** Chemical hot pack.

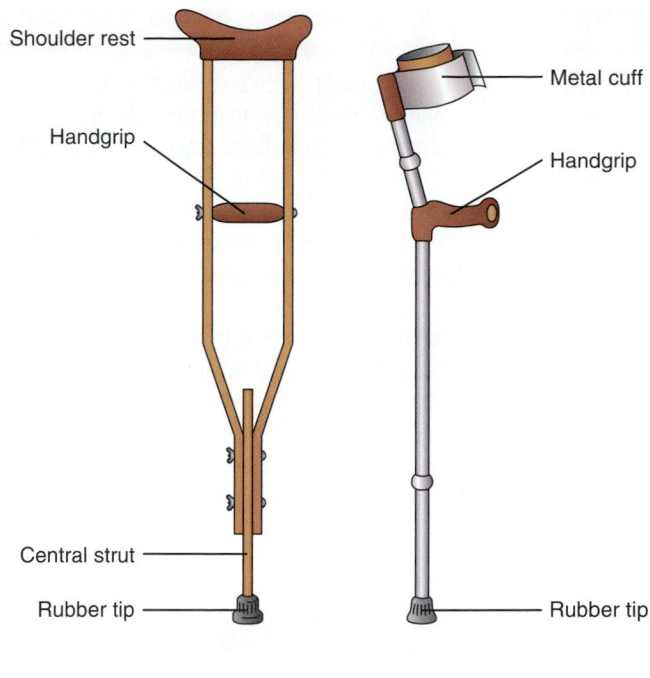

AXILLARY CRUTCH   **FOREARM CRUTCH**

Figure 22-2 Types of crutches.

AMBULATORY AIDS

Mechanical assistive devices are used by individuals who require aid in ambulation. The word **ambulation** means walking; patients who are **ambulatory** are able to walk as opposed to being confined to a wheelchair or a bed. Ambulatory aids include crutches, canes, and walkers. The device used depends on factors such as the type and severity of the disability, the amount of support required, and the patient's age and degree of muscular coordination. The ambulatory aid may be prescribed for a temporary condition, such as a fracture, a sprain to a lower extremity, and disability after orthopedic surgery. It also may be prescribed for a long-term condition, such as paralysis, deformity, and permanent weakness of the lower extremities.

CRUTCHES

Crutches are artificial supports that consist of wood or tubular aluminum. They are used for patients who require assistance in walking as a result of disease, injury, or birth defects of the lower extremities. Crutches function by removing weight from the legs and transferring it to the arms. The two main crutch types are the axillary crutch and the forearm crutch (Figure 22-2). The axillary crutch and the forearm crutch require rubber tips, which increase surface tension, to prevent the crutches from slipping on the floor.

The *axillary crutch* is used most frequently and is made of wood or tubular aluminum. This type of crutch has a shoulder rest and handgrips and extends from the ground almost to the patient's axilla.

The *forearm crutch*, also known as a *Lofstrand crutch*, consists of a single adjustable tube of aluminum that extends to the forearm. A metal cuff attached to the crutch fits securely around the patient's forearm, and a handgrip covered with rubber extends from the crutch for weight bearing. The metal cuff and the handgrip stabilize the patient's wrists to make walking safer and easier. One advantage of the forearm crutch is that the individual can release the handgrip, enabling use of the hand, while the metal cuff holds the crutch in place. Individuals who are paraplegic or have cerebral palsy use the forearm crutch most often.

Axillary Crutch Measurement

The patient must be measured for axillary crutches to ensure the correct crutch length and proper placement of the handgrip. Incorrectly fitted crutches increase the patient's risk of developing back pain, nerve damage, and injuries to the axillae and palms of the hands. Procedure 22-7 presents the correct way to measure a patient for axillary crutches.

If the crutches are too long, the shoulder rests exert pressure on the patient's axillae. This can injure the radial nerve in the brachial plexus, which eventually may lead to *crutch palsy*, a condition of muscular weakness in the forearm, wrist, and hand. In addition, crutches that are too long force the patient's shoulders forward, preventing the patient from pushing his or her body off the ground. Crutches that are too short force the patient to be bent over and uncomfortable, also making them awkward to use. If the handgrips are too low, pressure is put on the patient's axillae, whereas handgrips that are too high are awkward.

Wooden crutches are made with bolts and wing nuts, which allow proper adjustment of the length and handgrip level. Aluminum crutches consist of aluminum tubes. Spring-loaded pushbuttons on an inner tube "pop out" into holes on an outer tube to allow proper adjustment of the crutch length.

HIGHLIGHT on Ambulatory Aids

Many people who could benefit from ambulatory aids are not using them. The primary reason is that they do not know how to use them correctly, become discouraged, and quit using them.

Other types of aids available to assist individuals with physical disabilities include raised toilet seats, handlebars, carrying devices, tub seats, over-bed tables, and swivel cushions for assistance in getting into and out of cars.

If an individual needs help in learning to drive with a physical disability, the local bureau of vocational rehabilitation or the state motor vehicle department can provide information on qualified instruction available in the community.

Walking with an ambulatory aid is a physiologic stressor to the body because it requires more energy than normal walking.

Because of this, individuals need to rest frequently when using an ambulatory aid.

Many people need to have their crutches lengthened after they have had them for a while. This is because their posture improves as they gain confidence in walking with them. Children and teenagers who use crutches for a long time also need frequent adjustments as they grow.

A cane can provide security to the individual using it; however, it can be more trouble than it is worth if it is the incorrect size. It is estimated that two thirds of people who buy canes select one that is too long.

Some walkers are designed to fit over chairs and toilets, allowing the user additional support when rising or sitting. Folding walkers are available, and they are easy to store and transport. ∎

PATIENT TEACHING   Crutches

- Teach patients the guidelines for the proper use of crutches.
- Provide the patient with an exercise sheet that illustrates exercises to strengthen arm muscles before beginning crutch walking.
- Teach the patient the crutch gaits prescribed by the physician, and have the patient demonstrate the gaits before leaving the office.
- Provide the patient with a list of local vendors who provide crutch services, such as repairs and supplies (e.g., rubber tips, crutch pads).
- Provide the patient with printed educational materials on the use of crutches and crutch gaits. ∎

Crutch Guidelines

It is important that the patient receive specific guidelines to ensure safety while using crutches, to prevent injuries and falls. The medical assistant is responsible for instructing the patient in the following guidelines:

1. Wear well-fitting flat shoes with firm, nonskid soles to provide good traction and stability.
2. Use good posture to prevent strain on muscles and joints and to maintain proper body balance.
3. Support your weight with your hands on the handgrips and the axillary pads pressing against the sides of the rib cage. The body weight should not be supported by the axillae because pressure on the axillae may cause crutch palsy.
4. Look ahead when walking, rather than down at your feet.
5. Be aware of the surface on which you are walking. It should be clean, flat, dry, and well lighted. Throw rugs and objects serving as obstacles should temporarily be removed from your environment to prevent falls.

6. Keep the crutches about 4 to 6 inches out from the sides of your feet when walking to prevent obstruction of the pathway for the feet.
7. Take steps by moving the crutches forward a safe and comfortable distance, preferably 6 inches. When first learning to use the crutches, take small steps rather than large ones. Do not move forward more than 12 to 15 inches with each step. A greater distance might cause the crutches to slide forward and you to lose your balance.
8. Report tingling or numbness in the upper body to the physician. You might be using the crutches incorrectly, or they might be the wrong size for you.
9. Extra padding can be added to the shoulder rests of your crutches to make them more comfortable. If you do this, ensure that the extra padding does not press against your axillae, but rather against your lateral rib cage. The handgrips also can be padded for increased comfort.
10. To prevent slipping, keep the crutch tips dry to maintain their surface friction. If they become wet, dry them completely before use.
11. Inspect the crutch tips regularly. They should be securely attached. If the crutch tips are worn down, they should be replaced with tips of the proper size.
12. For wooden crutches, periodically check the wing nuts holding the central strut and handgrips in place to ensure that they are tight.

Crutch Gaits

The type of crutch gait used depends on the amount of weight the patient is able to support with one or both legs and the patient's physical condition and muscular coordination. The patient should learn a fast and a slow gait. The faster gait is used for making speed in open areas, and the slower one is used in crowded places. In addition, learning more than one gait reduces patient fatigue because a different combination of muscles is used for each gait. Procedure 22-8 provides guidelines and charts for use in instructing the patient on how to walk with crutches.

CANES

A cane is a lightweight, easily movable device made of wood or aluminum with a rubber tip and is used to help provide balance and support. Canes are generally used by patients who have weakness on one side of the body, such as patients with hemiparesis, joint disabilities, or defects of the neuromuscular system. The three main types of canes are the *standard cane,* the *tripod cane,* and the *quad cane* (Figure 22-3). The standard cane provides the least amount of support and is used by patients who require only slight assistance in walking. The tripod and quad canes have three and four legs, respectively, a bent shaft, and a T-shaped handle with grips. They are easier to hold and provide greater stability than a standard cane because of the wider base of support. In addition, multilegged canes are able to stand alone, which frees the arms when the patient is getting up from a chair. The disadvantage of a multilegged cane is that it is bulkier and more difficult to move.

A cane is held on the side of the body opposite the side that needs support. The cane length must be properly adjusted to ensure optimal stability. The cane handle should be approximately level with the greater trochanter, and the elbow should be flexed at a 25- to 30-degree angle. The patient should be instructed to stand erect and not lean on the cane to ensure good balance. Procedure 22-9 presents guidelines on instructing the patient on how to walk with a cane.

WALKERS

A walker is an ambulatory aid consisting of an aluminum frame with handgrips and four widely placed legs with rubber suction tips and one open side (Figure 22-4). A walker is light and easily movable. Walkers are available with wheels that facilitate movement of the walker. They are also available with a fold-up feature that allows them to be easily transported in a vehicle. For proper ambulation, the walker should extend from the ground to approximately the level of the patient's hip joint. Procedure 22-10 presents guidelines on instructing the patient on how to walk with a walker.

Walkers are used most often by geriatric patients with weakness or balance problems. Walkers also are used during the healing process for patients who have had knee or hip joint replacement surgery. These patients need more help with balance and walking than can be provided by crutches or a cane. Because of its wide base, a walker provides the patient with a great amount of stability and security. Disadvantages of a walker include a slow pace and difficulty in maneuvering the walker in a small room.

Figure 22-3 Examples of a quad cane *(left)* and a standard cane *(right).* (Courtesy 3M Health Care, St Paul, Minn.)

Figure 22-4 Walkers.

What Would You Do? | **What Would You *Not* Do?**

Case Study 2

Thaddeus Bernard calls the office. Thaddeus fractured the femur of his left leg 2 weeks ago in a skiing accident. The physician applied a long leg fiberglass cast, and Thaddeus was properly fitted with aluminum crutches. Thaddeus says that he is having some problems with his crutches. He is complaining of weakness in his forearms and hands and some tingling and numbness in his fingers. He also says that he has bruises under his arms. Thaddeus says that after he got home, his crutches didn't seem to fit right, so he readjusted them. Thaddeus is getting ready to return to college and wants to know the best way to carry his books while using crutches. ■

PROCEDURE 22-7   Measuring for Axillary Crutches

Outcome Measure an individual for axillary crutches

Equipment/Supplies

- Axillary crutches
- Goniometer

1. **Procedural Step.** Greet the patient and introduce yourself. Identify the patient and inform the patient that you will be measuring him or her for axillary crutches. Discuss the importance of properly fitted crutches with the patient.

Determining Crutch Length

For you to determine crutch length correctly, the patient must wear shoes while being measured. The measurement can be taken while the patient is standing.

2. **Procedural Step.** Ask the patient to stand erect.
3. **Procedural Step.** Position the crutches with the crutch tips at a distance of 2 inches (5 cm) in front of and 4 to 6 inches (15 cm) to the side of each foot. (The large dots in the figure represent crutch tips.)
4. **Procedural Step.** Adjust the crutch length so that the shoulder rests are approximately 1½ to 2 inches (about two finger widths) below the axillae.
   Wooden crutches. The length of the crutch is adjusted by removing the bolt and wing nut and sliding the central strut (support piece) at the bottom upward or downward as necessary to attain the proper length. The strut is secured by replacing the bolt and securely fastening the wing nut.
   Tubular aluminum crutches. The length of the crutch is adjusted by pressing the spring-loaded push button with your thumb and sliding the outer tube upward or downward as necessary to attain the proper length. The spring-loaded button on the inner tube should be allowed to "pop out" into the appropriate hole on the outer tube.

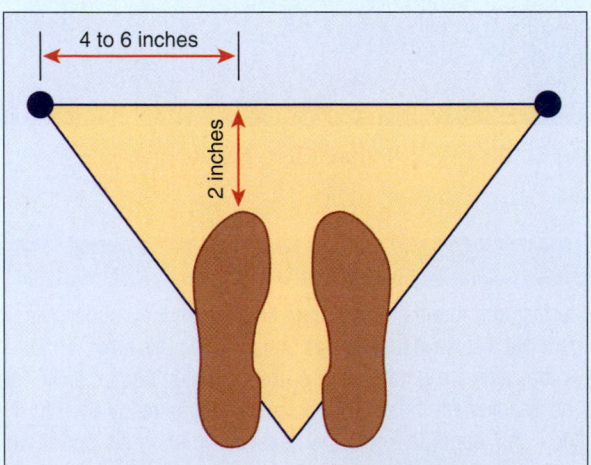

Position for measuring for crutches.

Handgrip Positioning

When the crutch length has been adjusted, correct placement of the handgrips must be determined.

5. **Procedural Step.** Ask the patient to stand erect with a crutch under each arm and to support his or her weight by the handgrips.
6. **Procedural Step.** Adjust the handgrips on the crutches so that the patient's elbow is flexed to an angle of approximately 30 degrees. The handgrip level is adjusted by removing the bolt and wing nut and sliding the handgrip upward or downward, as required. The handgrip is secured by replacing the bolt and tightly fastening the wing nut. The angle of elbow flexion can be verified by using a measuring device known as a *goniometer.* A goniometer is an instrument that measures the angle of a joint.
7. **Procedural Step.** Check the fit of the crutches. If the crutches are measured correctly, the medical assistant should be able to insert two fingers between the top of the crutches and the axillae when the patient is standing erect with the crutches under the arms.

Insert two fingers between the top of the crutch and the axilla.

8. **Procedural Step.** Chart the procedure in the patient's medical record.
   a. *Paper-based patient record:* Record the date and time and the axillary crutch measurement procedure.
   b. *Electronic medical record:* Using an EMR such as SimChart for the Medical Office, use the appropriate radio buttons, drop-down menus, and free text fields to document the axillary crutch measurement procedure.

PROCEDURE 22-8   Instructing a Patient in Crutch Gaits

Outcome Instruct a patient in the following crutch gaits: four-point, two-point, three-point, swing-to, and swing-through

Equipment/Supplies

- Axillary crutches

1. **Procedural Step.** Greet the patient and introduce yourself. Identify the patient and inform the patient that you will be instructing him or her in crutch gaits. Discuss the importance of the proper use of crutches with the patient.

2. **Procedural Step.** Instruct the patient in the tripod position as follows:
   a. Stand erect, and face straight ahead.
   b. Place the tips of the crutches 4 to 6 inches (15 cm) in front of the feet and 4 to 6 inches (10 to 15 cm) to the side of each foot. (The large dots in the figure represent crutch tips.)
   Principle: The tripod position is the basic crutch stance used before crutch walking. It provides a wide base of support and enhances stability and balance.

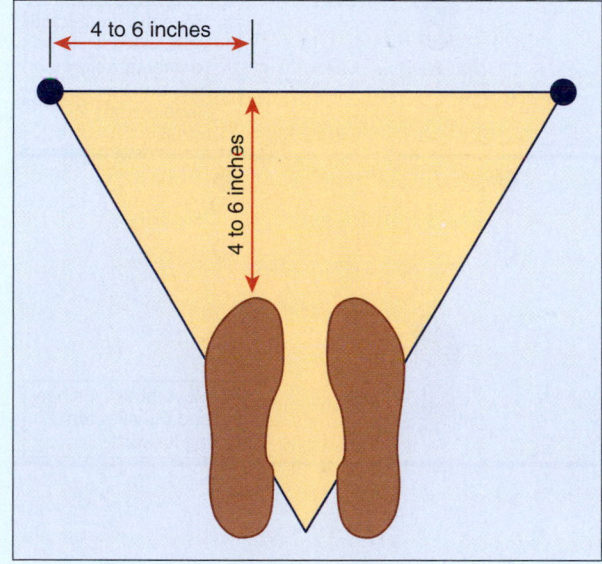

Tripod position.

3. **Procedural Step.** Instruct the patient in the following crutch gaits:

Four-Point Gait

The four-point gait is a basic and slow gait. To use this gait, the patient must be able to bear considerable weight on both legs. The four-point gait is the most stable and the safest of the crutch gaits because it provides at least three points of support at all times. It is used most often by patients who have leg muscle weakness or spasticity, poor muscular coordination or balance, or degenerative leg joint disease. Instruct the patient in the procedure for the four-point gait, following the steps in the accompanying figure.

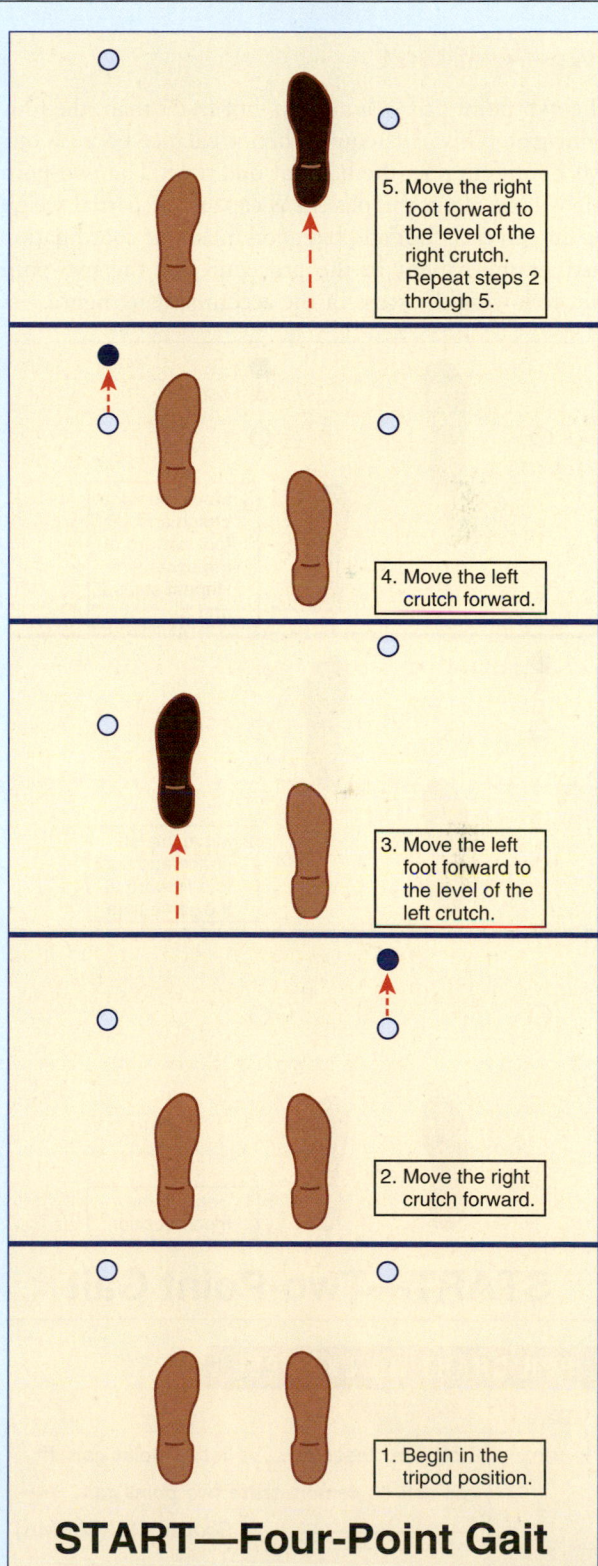

5. Move the right foot forward to the level of the right crutch. Repeat steps 2 through 5.

4. Move the left crutch forward.

3. Move the left foot forward to the level of the left crutch.

2. Move the right crutch forward.

1. Begin in the tripod position.

START—Four-Point Gait

Continued

PROCEDURE 22-8

PPR CHARTING EXAMPLE

Date	
12/15/XX	1:30 p.m. Instructed pt in four-point gait. Pt was able to demonstrate four-point gait. ——— ——————— M. Cooper, CMA (AAMA)

Two-Point Gait

The two-point gait is similar to, but faster than, the four-point gait. This gait requires better balance because only two points support the body at one time. The two-point gait is used when the patient is capable of partial weight bearing on each foot and has good muscular coordination. Instruct the patient in the procedure for the two-point gait, following the steps in the accompanying figure.

Three-Point Gait

The three-point gait is used by patients who cannot bear weight on one leg. The patient must be able to support his or her full weight on the unaffected leg. With this gait, the crutches and the unaffected leg alternately bear the patient's weight. This gait is used most often by amputees without a prosthesis, patients with musculoskeletal or soft tissue trauma to a lower extremity (e.g., fracture, sprain), patients with acute leg inflammation, and patients who have had recent leg surgery. To use this gait, the patient must have good muscular coordination and arm strength. Instruct the patient in the procedure for the three-point gait, following the steps in the accompanying figure.

START—Two-Point Gait

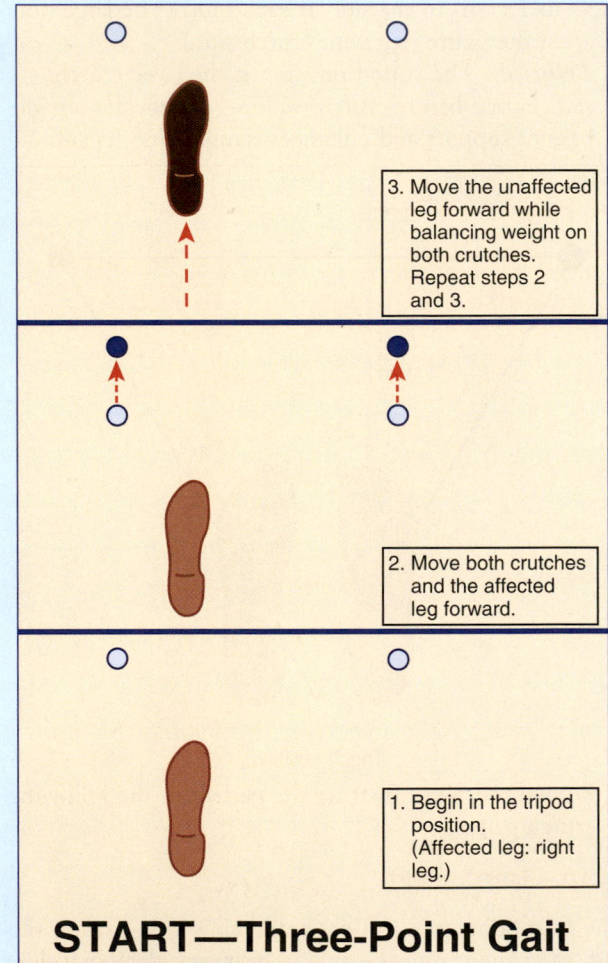

START—Three-Point Gait

PPR CHARTING EXAMPLE

Date	
12/16/XX	2:30 p.m. Instructed pt in two-point gait. Pt was able to demonstrate two-point gait. ——— ——————— M. Cooper, CMA (AAMA)

PPR CHARTING EXAMPLE

Date	
12/17/XX	2:30 p.m. Instructed pt in three-point gait. Pt was able to demonstrate three-point gait.——— ——————— M. Cooper, CMA (AAMA)

PROCEDURE 22-8   Instructing a Patient in Crutch Gaits—cont'd

Swing Gaits

The swing gaits include the swing-to gait and the swing-through gait and are used by patients with severe lower extremity disabilities, such as paralysis, and by patients who wear supporting braces on their legs.

Instruct the patient in the procedures for the swing-to and the swing-through crutch gaits, following the steps in the accompanying figures.

4. Procedural Step. Chart the procedure in the patient's medical record.

a. *Paper-based patient record:* Record the date and time and the type of instructions given to the patient. Document that the patient was able to properly demonstrate the crutch gaits (refer to the PPR charting example).

b. *Electronic medical record:* Using an EMR such as SimChart for the Medical Office, use the appropriate radio buttons, drop-down menus, and free text fields to document the type of instructions given to the patient. Document that the patient was able to properly demonstrate the crutch gaits.

PROCEDURE 22-8

3. Lift and swing the body to the crutches. Repeat steps 2 and 3.

2. Move both crutches forward together.

1. Begin in the tripod position.

START—Swing-To Gait

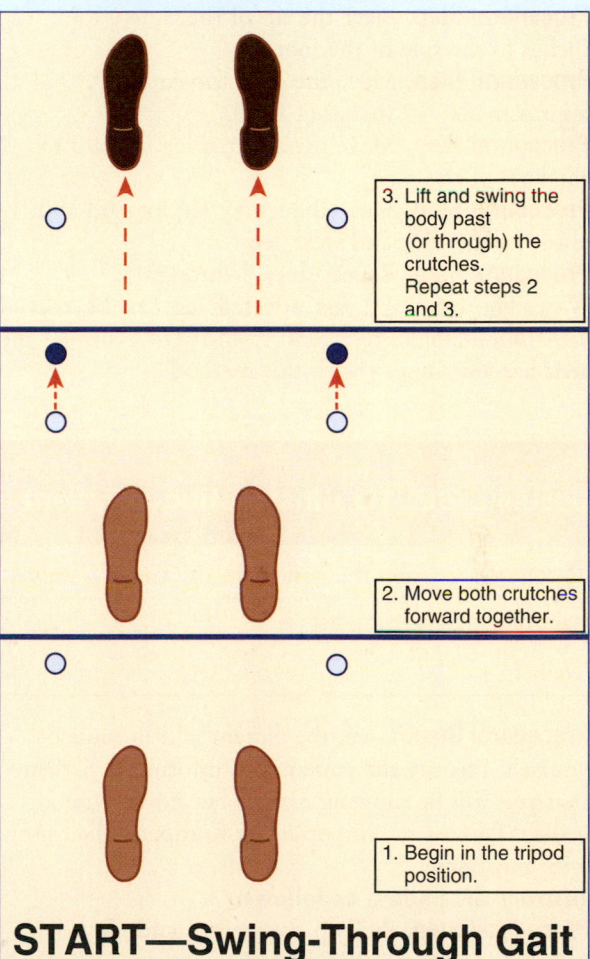

3. Lift and swing the body past (or through) the crutches. Repeat steps 2 and 3.

2. Move both crutches forward together.

1. Begin in the tripod position.

START—Swing-Through Gait

PPR CHARTING EXAMPLE

Date	
12/18/XX	3:30 p.m. Instructed pt in swing-to and swing-through gaits. Pt was able to demonstrate swing gaits.— M. Cooper, CMA (AAMA)

PROCEDURE 22-9 Instructing a Patient in Use of a Cane

Outcome Instruct the patient in the use of a cane

Equipment/Supplies

- Cane

1. **Procedural Step.** Greet the patient and introduce yourself. Identify the patient and inform the patient that you will be showing him or her how to use a cane. Discuss the importance of proper cane use with the patient.
   Instruct the patient as follows:
2. **Procedural Step.** Hold the cane on the strong side of the body (i.e., in the hand opposite the affected extremity).
3. **Procedural Step.** Place the tip of the cane 4 to 6 inches to the side of the foot.
4. **Procedural Step.** Move the cane forward approximately 12 inches (1 foot).
5. **Procedural Step.** Move the affected leg forward to the level of the cane.
6. **Procedural Step.** Move the strong leg forward and ahead of the cane and weak leg.
7. **Procedural Step.** Repeat steps 3 through 5.
   Note: The cane and the affected leg can be moved forward simultaneously (steps 3 and 4); however, the patient has less support with this method.

8. **Procedural Step.** Chart the procedure in the patient's medical record.
   a. *Paper-based patient record*: Record the date and time and the type of instructions given to the patient. Document that the patient was able demonstrate proper use of a cane (refer to the PPR charting example).
   b. *Electronic medical record*: Using an EMR such as SimChart for the Medical Office, use the appropriate radio buttons, drop-down menus, and free text fields to document the type of instructions given to the patient. Document that the patient was able demonstrate proper use of a cane.

PPR CHARTING EXAMPLE

Date	
12/20/XX	2:30 p.m. Instructed pt in the procedure for using a cane. Pt was able to demonstrate proper use of a cane. _____
	M. Cooper, CMA (AAMA)

PROCEDURE 22-10 Instructing a Patient in Use of a Walker

Outcome Instruct the patient in the use of a walker

Equipment/Supplies

- Walker

1. **Procedural Step.** Greet the patient and introduce yourself. Identify the patient and inform the patient that you will be showing him or her how to use a walker. Discuss the importance of proper walker use with the patient.
   Instruct the patient as follows:
2. **Procedural Step.** Pick up the walker, and move it forward approximately 6 inches.
3. **Procedural Step.** Move the right foot and then the left foot up to the walker.
4. **Procedural Step.** Repeat steps 1 and 2.
5. **Procedural Step.** Chart the procedure in the patient's medical record.
   a. *Paper-based patient record*: Record the date and time and the type of instructions given to the patient. Document that the patient was able

demonstrate proper use of a walker (refer to the PPR charting example).
   b. *Electronic medical record*: Using an EMR such as SimChart for the Medical Office, use the appropriate radio buttons, drop-down menus, and free text fields to document the type of instructions given to the patient. Document that the patient was able demonstrate proper use of a walker.

PPR CHARTING EXAMPLE

Date	
12/21/XX	9:30 a.m. Instructed pt in the procedure for using a walker. Pt was able to demonstrate proper use of a walker. _____
	M. Cooper, CMA (AAMA)

PROCEDURE 22-10

What Would You Do? What Would You *Not* Do? RESPONSES

Case Study 1
Page 470

What Did Marlyne Do?
- Empathized with Aaron for being in so much pain.
- Explained to Aaron that he should never sleep on a heating pad because the heat builds up and causes the type of burn he experienced.
- Explained to Aaron that it is best to apply heat for 15 to 30 minutes at a time with the pad set no higher than the medium setting. Told him the pad may not feel warm after his body gets used to it, but that it is still helping him. Told Aaron that the high setting could burn his skin.
- Told Aaron how to prevent low back pain by using good body mechanics, especially during lifting.

What Did Marlyne Not Do?
- Did not criticize Aaron for sleeping on the heating pad or turning the pad to the high setting.

Case Study 2
Page 479

What Did Marlyne Do?
- Listened carefully and empathetically to Thaddeus's problems with and concerns about his crutches.

- Explained to Thaddeus that the crutches were adjusted to fit him properly at the office and that he may have caused some problems by readjusting them.
- Scheduled an appointment for Thaddeus to come in that day so the physician could examine him and his crutches could be checked for proper length.
- Went over crutch guidelines and crutch gaits with Thaddeus again when he came to the office for his appointment.
- Told Thaddeus that he should use a backpack to carry his books to keep his hands free to move on his crutches. Stressed that he should keep his backpack as light as possible and keep the weight evenly distributed on his back (i.e., use both straps).

What Did Marlyne Not Do?
- Did not tell Thaddeus to readjust the crutches himself.
- Did not tell Thaddeus that he should have paid more attention when he was being instructed in crutch guidelines.

TERMINOLOGY REVIEW

Key Term	Word Parts	Definition
Ambulation		Walking or moving from one place to another.
Ambulatory		Able to walk as opposed to being confined to bed or a wheelchair.
Compress		A soft, moist, absorbent cloth that is folded in several layers and applied to a part of the body in the local application of heat or cold.
Edema		The retention of fluid in the tissues, resulting in swelling.
Erythema	*hem/o:* blood *erythr/o:* red	Reddening of the skin caused by dilation of superficial blood vessels in the skin.
Exudate		A discharge produced by the body's tissues.
Soak		The direct immersion of a body part in water or a medicated solution.
Sprain		Trauma to a joint that causes injury to the ligaments.
Strain		An overstretching of a muscle caused by trauma.
Suppuration		The process of pus formation.

ON THE WEB

For information on rehabilitation and disability:

National Rehabilitation Information Center (NARIC): www.naric.com

American Academy of Orthopaedic Surgeons: www.aaos.org

About.com: Orthopedics: orthopedics.about.com

American Physical Therapy Association: www.apta.org

American Chiropractic Association: www.acatoday.org

American Occupational Therapy Association: www.aota.org

National Stroke Association (NSA): www.stroke.org

Arthritis Foundation: www.arthritis.org

National Institute of Arthritis and Musculoskeletal and Skin Diseases: www.niams.nih.gov

American Academy of Physical Medicine and Rehabilitation: www.aapmr.org

The Gynecologic Examination and Prenatal Care

23

e Check out the Evolve site at http://evolve.elsevier.com/Bonewit/today/ to access additional interactive activities and exercises to help you study and prepare for success.

LEARNING OBJECTIVES | PROCEDURES

Gynecologic Examination
1. State the purpose of the gynecologic examination.
2. Identify the components of the gynecologic examination.

Breast Examination
3. Explain the purpose of a breast examination.

Instruct patient in the procedure for a breast self-examination.

Pelvic Examination
4. Explain the purpose of a pelvic examination.
5. List and describe the four parts of the pelvic examination.
6. State the purpose of a Pap test.
7. List the advantages and disadvantages of the liquid-based Pap test.
8. List and describe each category on a cytology request for a Pap test.

Prepare patient for a gynecologic examination.
Assist the physician with a gynecologic examination.
Complete a cytology request form.

Vaginal Infections
9. Identify the symptoms of each of the following:
   - Trichomoniasis
   - Candidiasis
   - Chlamydia
   - Gonorrhea
10. Explain how each of the above-listed infections is diagnosed.

Assist in the collection of a vaginal microbiologic specimen.

Prenatal Visits
11. Explain the purpose of each part of the prenatal record.
12. List and explain the purpose of each procedure included in the initial prenatal examination.
13. List and explain the purpose of each prenatal laboratory test.
14. Explain the purpose of return prenatal visits.
15. Explain the purpose of each of the following:
    - Multiple marker test
    - Ultrasound scan
    - Amniocentesis
    - Fetal heart rate monitoring

Calculate the expected date of delivery (EDD).

Complete a prenatal health history.
Assist with an initial prenatal examination.
Assist with a return prenatal examination.

CHAPTER OUTLINE

INTRODUCTION TO THE GYNECOLOGIC EXAMINATION AND
   PRENATAL CARE
GYNECOLOGIC EXAMINATION
Gynecology
Terms Related to Gynecology
Breast Examination

Pelvic Examination
Inspection of External Genitalia, Vagina, and Cervix
Pap Test
Bimanual Pelvic Examination
Rectal-Vaginal Examination

487

Vaginal Infections
Trichomoniasis
Candidiasis
Chlamydia
Gonorrhea
PRENATAL CARE
Obstetrics
Obstetric Terminology

Prenatal Visits
First Prenatal Visit
Prenatal Record
Initial Prenatal Examination
Return Prenatal Visits
Special Tests and Procedures
Medical Assisting Responsibilities

KEY TERMS

Gynecology
adnexal (ad-NEKS-al)
amenorrhea (AY-men-ah-REE-ah)
atypical (ay-TIP-ih-kul)
cervix (SER-viks)
colposcopy (kol-POS-koe-pee)
cytology (sy-TOL-oh-jee)
dysmenorrhea (DIS-men-ah-REE-ah)
dyspareunia (DIS-pah-ROO-nee-ah)
dysplasia (dis-PLAY-shah)
ectocervix (EK-toe-SER-viks)
endocervix (EN-doe-SER-viks)
external os (eks-TER-nal AHS)
gynecology (gie-nuh-KOL-oh-jee)
menopause (MEN-oh-paws)
menorrhagia (men-uh-RAY-jee-ah)
metrorrhagia (met-ro-RAY-jee-ah)
perimenopause
    (PEAR-ee-MEN-oh-paws)

perineum (pear-ih-NEE-um)
risk factor
vulva (VUL-va)
Obstetrics
abortion (ah-BOR-shun)
Braxton Hicks contractions (BRAK-stun
    HIKS con-TRAK-shuns)
dilation (die-LAY-shun) (of the cervix)
effacement (eh-FAYS-ment)
embryo (EM-bree-oh)
engagement
expected date of delivery (EDD)
fetal heart rate
fetal heart tones
fetus (FEE-tus)
fundus (FUN-dus)
gestation (jess-TAY-shun)
gestational (jess-TAY-shun-al) age
infant

multigravida (MUL-tee-GRAV-ih-duh)
multipara (mul-TIH-pear-uh)
nullipara (nul-IH-pear-uh)
obstetrics (ob-STEH-triks)
position
postpartum (poest-PAR-tum)
preeclampsia (PREE-ih-KLAMP-see-ah)
prenatal (pree-NAY-tul)
presentation
primigravida (PRIH-mih-GRAV-ih-duh)
primipara (prih-MIH-pear-uh)
puerperium (PYOO-ur-PEER-ee-um)
quickening
toxemia (tok-SEE-mee-uh)
trimester (try-MES-ter)

INTRODUCTION TO THE GYNECOLOGIC EXAMINATION AND PRENATAL CARE

The medical assistant should have knowledge of gynecology and obstetrics to assist in examinations and treatments in these specialties. Gynecologic examinations are frequently and routinely performed in the medical office. Prenatal care consists of a series of scheduled medical office visits for the promotion of the health of the mother and fetus during the pregnancy. Obtaining the patient's cooperation makes the gynecologic or prenatal examination proceed more smoothly and as a result makes the patient feel more comfortable. The medical assistant can help by explaining the purpose of the procedure to the patient. If the patient understands the beneficial results to be derived from the examination, she is more likely to participate as required. This chapter discusses the gynecologic examination and prenatal care and the procedures involved in both.

GYNECOLOGIC EXAMINATION
GYNECOLOGY

Gynecology is the branch of medicine that deals with diseases of the reproductive organs of women. The gynecologic examination is frequently and routinely performed in the medical office and typically includes a *breast examination* and a *pelvic examination*.

The purpose of the gynecologic examination is to assess the health of the female reproductive organs to detect early signs of disease, leading to early diagnosis and treatment. This examination may be part of a general physical examination, or it may be performed by itself. Although assisting with the gynecologic examination is a routine procedure for the medical assistant, the patient may not consider it a routine examination. To reduce apprehension or embarrassment, the medical assistant should fully explain the procedure to the patient and offer to answer any questions.

Terms Related to Gynecology

The medical assistant should have a thorough knowledge of the female reproductive system (refer to Chapter 16) and the following terms associated with the female reproductive system:

Amenorrhea Absence or cessation of the menstrual period. Amenorrhea occurs normally before puberty, during pregnancy, and after menopause.

Cervix The lower narrow end of the uterus that opens into the vagina.

Colposcopy Examination of the cervix using a colposcope (a lighted instrument with a magnifying lens).

Dysmenorrhea Pain associated with the menstrual period.

Dyspareunia Pain in the vagina or pelvis experienced by a woman during sexual intercourse.

Dysplasia The growth of abnormal cells. Dysplasia is a precancerous condition that may or may not develop into cancer.

Menopause The permanent cessation of menstruation, which usually occurs between the ages of 45 and 55 with an average age of 51.

Menorrhagia Excessive bleeding during a menstrual period, in the number of days, the amount of blood, or both. Also called *dysfunctional uterine bleeding* (DUB).

Metrorrhagia Bleeding between menstrual periods.

Perimenopause Before the onset of menopause, the phase during which a woman with regular periods changes to irregular cycles and increased periods of amenorrhea.

Perineum The external region between the vaginal orifice and the anus in a female and between the scrotum and the anus in a male.

Risk factor Anything that increases an individual's chance of developing a disease. Some risk factors (e.g., smoking) can be avoided, but others (e.g., age and family history) cannot.

BREAST EXAMINATION

The physician usually begins the gynecologic examination with the breast examination. The medical assistant is responsible for assisting the patient into the supine position. The physician inspects the breasts and nipples for swelling, dimpling, puckering, and change in skin texture. The nipples are checked for abnormalities such as bleeding and discharge. The breasts and axillary lymph nodes are palpated for lumps, hard knots, and thickening. The American Cancer Society (ACS) recommends that women in their 20s and 30s undergo a clinical breast examination by a physician every 3 years and then every year for women aged 40 and older. The ACS further recommends that women undergo an annual mammogram starting at age 40 and continuing for as long as they are in good health.

The patient should know how to examine her breasts at home for the presence of lumps and other changes with a breast self-examination (BSE). Most breast cancers are first discovered by women themselves. The American College of Obstetricians and Gynecologists recommends that women 20 years of age and older examine their breasts once every month. The ACS states that a BSE is an option for women starting in their 20s. The medical assistant may be responsible for instructing the patient in this procedure at the medical office (Procedure 23-1). If a lump or other change is discovered, the woman should schedule an appointment with her physician as soon as possible. Most breast lumps are not cancerous, but the physician must make that diagnosis.

Putting It All Into Practice

My name is Yin-Ling Wu, and I am a Registered Medical Assistant. I work with 10 physicians in a large clinic. My primary job responsibilities include documenting patient histories and complaints, taking vital signs, and assisting physicians with patient examinations and procedures.

One experience that has probably affected me more than any other occurred while I was working in obstetrics and gynecology. A full-term prenatal patient came in for a routine weekly appointment late one afternoon. By this stage of the pregnancy, you have seen the patients often enough to develop a more personal relationship. I was obtaining her vital signs and asking the routine questions when she said, "I haven't felt the baby move for 2 days." This immediately sent up a red flag, but I was careful to hide my concern until I was out of her room. The physician was unable to pick up any fetal heart tones, so she immediately did an ultrasound. It showed that the fetus had died. The patient was alone and extremely upset. I stayed with her until her family came.

Although little medical treatment was given during this time, I do believe that my medical assisting training and experience made a difference in my knowing what to do and say to help comfort the patient through this crisis. ■

What Would You Do? | What Would You *Not* Do?

Case Study 1

Carol Wooster, 42 years old, has come to the office for a gynecologic examination. She has not had a gynecologic examination in 10 years. Mrs. Wooster picked up a BSE brochure at a local health fair and performed a breast self-examination at home. She is now concerned because she found some unusual things. Her right breast is slightly larger than her left breast, her left nipple is pulled in, and she found some freckles on her right breast. Mrs. Wooster explains that she has not had a gynecologic examination in such a long time because her periods have been normal and regular. She also says that the physician will probably want her to have a mammogram, and she has heard that it hurts to have one. Mrs. Wooster is afraid that the physician will be annoyed with her for not having had a gynecologic examination sooner. ■

Answer questions that patients have about breast self-examination.

When should I examine my breasts?

Beginning at age 20, the American College of Obstetricians and Gynecologists recommends that you examine your breasts once a month according to your reproductive status as follows:

- *Regular periods:* Approximately 2 to 3 days after your menstrual period has ended. At this time, your breasts are least likely to be tender or swollen, and it will be easier to perform the examination.
- *No periods (because of menopause or hysterectomy):* Any day of the month is fine; however, it helps to choose a particular day, such as the first day of the month or an easy-to-remember date such as your birthday.
- *Hormone therapy:* If you are taking hormones, talk to your physician about when to examine your breasts.

Why is it important to examine my breasts every month?

The purpose of a breast self-examination is not just to find lumps, but also to notice when there are changes in your breasts. The best way to do this is to become as familiar as possible with your breasts. By examining your breasts once every month, you will learn what is normal for you, and it will be easier to notice changes.

What is considered normal?

Breast tissue normally feels a little lumpy and uneven. The left and right breasts may not be the same size; most women's breasts are slightly different in size. Many women have a normal thickening or ridge of firm tissue under the lower curve of the breast where it attaches to the chest wall. Throughout your life, changes also can occur in the size, shape, and feel of your breasts because of aging, weight changes, the menstrual cycle, pregnancy, breast feeding, and use of birth control pills or other hormones.

What should be reported to the physician?

Early breast cancer does not usually cause pain. When breast cancer first develops, there may be no symptoms at all. As the cancer grows, it can cause changes that should be reported to the physician. Contact your physician immediately if any of the following changes occurs:

- Any new lump, hard knot, or thickening in the breast or underarm area
- A change in the size or shape of the breast
- A puckering or dimpling of the skin of the breast or nipple
- A change in skin texture of the breast or nipple
- A nipple that becomes retracted (pulled in)
- A discharge or bleeding from the nipple ■

PELVIC EXAMINATION

The purpose of the pelvic examination is to assess the size, shape, and location of the reproductive organs and to detect the presence of disease. The pelvic examination consists of the following components:

- Inspection of the external genitalia, vagina, and cervix
- Collection of a specimen for a Pap test
- Bimanual pelvic examination
- Rectal-vaginal examination

For the pelvic examination, the patient is positioned in the lithotomy position. The patient lies on the table on her back, with her feet in the stirrups and her buttocks at the bottom edge of the table. The stirrups should be level with the examining table and pulled out approximately 1 foot from the edge of the table. The patient's knees should be bent and relaxed, and her thighs should be rotated outward as far as is comfortable. This position helps relax the vulva and perineum and facilitates insertion of the vaginal speculum. The patient should be properly draped to reduce exposure and to provide warmth. The lithotomy position is difficult to maintain, and the patient should not be placed in this position until the physician is ready to begin the examination.

The medical assistant can help the patient relax during the examination by telling her to breathe deeply, slowly, and evenly through the mouth. If the patient is relaxed, it is easier for the physician to insert the vaginal speculum and

to perform the bimanual pelvic examination; it also is more comfortable for the patient. It is recommended that the medical assistant remain in the room during the pelvic examination to provide legal protection for the physician, to reassure the patient, and to assist the physician. Procedure 23-2 outlines the medical assistant's role in assisting the physician with a gynecologic examination.

Inspection of External Genitalia, Vagina, and Cervix

The physician begins the pelvic examination with inspection of the external genitalia. The **vulva** is inspected for swelling, ulceration, and redness.

Next, the physician inserts a vaginal speculum into the vagina. Specula are available in two forms—plastic and metal. Plastic specula are used most commonly in the medical office; they are disposable and are designed to be used only once. Metal specula are reusable and must be sanitized and sterilized after each use. Vaginal specula come in three sizes—small, medium, and large. The physician determines the size required based on the physical and sexual maturity of the patient. The function of the speculum is to hold the walls of the vagina apart to allow visual inspection of the vagina and cervix (Figure 23-1).

A metal vaginal speculum is cold and should be warmed before use by placing it on a heating pad or by storing it in a warming drawer. A warmed speculum is more comfortable for the patient. It is important not to overheat the speculum, however; one that is too hot is just as uncomfortable

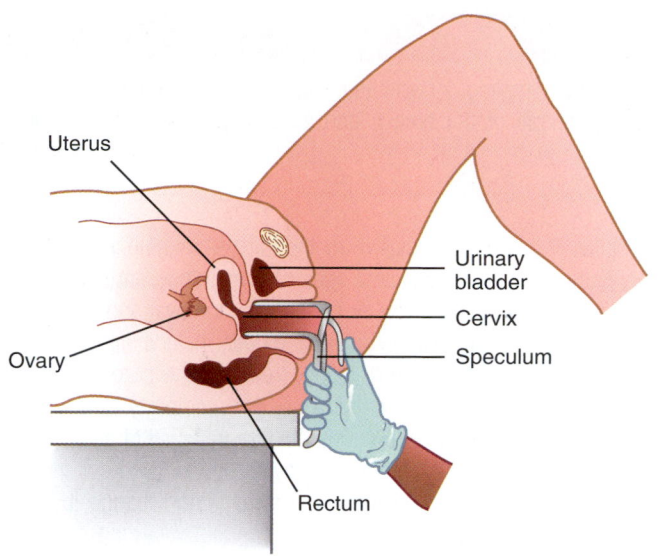

Figure 23-1 Insertion of the vaginal speculum for visualization of the vagina and cervix.

as one that is too cold. A disposable plastic speculum does not hold the cold and does not need to be warmed.

The physician inspects the vagina and cervix for color, lacerations, ulcerations, redness, nodules, and discharge. If an abnormal discharge is present, the physician obtains a specimen for laboratory evaluation. Examples of pathologic conditions that produce a discharge include vaginal infections such as *trichomoniasis, candidiasis, chlamydia,* and *gonorrhea,* which are discussed in detail later.

Pap Test

A Pap test is usually part of the pelvic examination. It is a simple and painless **cytology** evaluation named after its developer, Dr. George Papanicolaou (1883-1962). It is used for the early detection of cervical cancer. Almost all cancers of the cervix can be cured if detected early enough. The Pap test also is used to detect abnormal (**atypical**) cells of the cervix that might develop into cancer if not treated. In some cases the Pap test can detect cancer of the endometrium; however, it is less reliable in doing so.

HIGHLIGHT on Breast Cancer

Breast cancer is one of the most common types of cancer among American women. The American Cancer Society estimates that one of every eight women in the United States develops breast cancer at some point in her lifetime. Every year, more than 200,000 women learn they have breast cancer, and about 40,000 of them die from the disease. Most women (82%) diagnosed with breast cancer are older than 50 years, but breast cancer does occur in younger women.

Survival Rate

The 5-year survival rate for breast cancer that has spread to a distant site in the body (metastasized) is only 21%. The 5-year survival rate for small, localized tumors is 94%. If the cancer has spread to lymph nodes in the region of the breast, the 5-year survival rate is 73%. These encouraging statistics are the result of advances in the early detection of breast cancer and better treatment, including improved surgical procedures, radiation therapy, chemotherapy, hormonal therapy, and biologic therapy.

Recommendations for Early Detection

A three-point program is recommended for the early detection of breast cancer: (1) monthly breast self-examination, (2) periodic clinical breast examination by a physician, and (3) screening mammography.

Risk Factors

Breast cancer results from the abnormal growth of cells in breast tissue. It occurs more often in the left breast than in the right, and more often in the upper outer quadrant of the breast. The cause of abnormal growths in the breasts is unknown; therefore, every woman should consider herself at risk for breast cancer. Certain factors seem to place a woman at higher than normal risk for breast cancer, however, including the following:

- *Gender.* Women are much more likely than men to develop breast cancer.
- *Age.* The risk of breast cancer increases as women get older. Most women diagnosed with breast cancer are older than age 50.
- *Personal history.* Women with cancer in one breast have a greater chance of developing a new cancer in the other breast or in another part of the same breast.
- *Family history.* A woman's risk of developing breast cancer increases if her mother, sister, or daughter had breast cancer, especially at a young age.
- *Dense breast tissue.* Women with dense breast tissue (meaning they have more glandular tissue than fat tissue as seen on a mammogram) have a higher risk of developing breast cancer.
- *Breast biopsy.* Women who have had a breast biopsy that indicated certain types of benign breast disease (characterized by atypical hyperplasia) have an increased risk of developing breast cancer.
- *Breast cancer genes.* A woman who has inherited mutations in breast cancer genes (mutations of the *BRCA1* and *BRCA2* genes) from either parent is more likely to develop breast cancer.
- *Reproductive history.* Women who began menstruating at an early age (before age 12) or who went through menopause at a late age (after age 55) have a slightly increased risk of breast cancer.

Continued

HIGHLIGHT on Breast Cancer—cont'd

- *Childbearing.* Women who have never had a child or women who had their first child late (after age 30) have a slightly increased risk of developing breast cancer.
- *Hormone replacement therapy (HRT).* Studies indicate that the long-term use of estrogen and progesterone combination hormone replacement therapy for relief of menopausal symptoms increases the risk of breast cancer.
- *Radiation treatment.* Women who have had radiation of the chest before age 30 as treatment for another type of cancer (e.g., Hodgkin disease) have a significantly increased risk of developing breast cancer.
- *Race.* Caucasian women are diagnosed more frequently than Hispanic, Asian, or African American women.
- *Lifestyle factors.* Studies suggest that the use of alcohol (more than two drinks per day) increases the risk of breast cancer. Obesity, especially for women after menopause, also may increase the risk of breast cancer.

Warning Signs

The warning signs of possible breast cancer include a lump, hard knot, or thickening in the breast or armpit; a change in breast color or texture; dimpling or puckering; nipple discharge; changes in the size or shape of the breast; and an enlargement of the lymph nodes.

Diagnosis

A biopsy is the only conclusive method of determining whether a breast lump or suspicious area seen on a mammogram is benign or malignant. A biopsy involves the surgical removal and analysis of all or part of the lump. Biopsy methods include fine needle aspiration biopsy, core needle biopsy (removal of a core of tissue from the lump), vacuum-assisted biopsy (Mammotome), large core biopsy, and open surgical excisional biopsy (removal of all or part of the entire lump). The physician may recommend one or more of these procedures to evaluate a lump or other change in the breast.

Eighty percent of breast lumps are benign. A lump or suspicious area is often the result of a benign breast condition, such as normal hormonal changes, fibrocystic breast disease, or a fibroadenoma. ∎

Almost all cervical cancers are caused by the human papillomavirus (HPV). HPV is a common virus that can be transmitted from one individual to another during sexual intercourse. There are many strains of HPV, however, most of these strains do not pose a health risk. Certain strains of HPV are called *high-risk strains* because they can cause changes to a woman's cervix that can lead to cervical cancer over time.

Although HPV infection has the strongest link to the development of cervical cancer, there are other factors that place a woman at higher risk for cervical cancer. These include the following:

- Cigarette smoking
- Weakened immune system as a result of human immunodeficiency virus (HIV) infection, organ transplantation, chemotherapy, or long-term steroid use
- Having given birth to three or more children
- Use of oral contraceptives for more than 5 years
- Diethylstilbestrol (DES) exposure before birth

The American Cancer Society (ACS) recommends that women begin cervical cancer screening at 21 years of age with a Pap test. Screening (with a Pap test) should be performed every 3 years until 29 years of age. The ACS guidelines further state that beginning at age 30, the preferred method of screening is with a Pap test combined with an HPV test every 5 years until 65 years of age. The ACS guidelines state that another option for woman between the ages of 30 and 65 is to undergo screening every 3 years with just the Pap test. Women who are at high risk for cervical cancer or who have had abnormal Pap test results should be screened more often. The ACS recommends that women over the age of 65 who have had regular screening in the past 10 years discontinue cervical cancer screening as long as no serious precancerous conditions have been detected in the last 20 years.

Patient Instructions

The patient should be instructed to schedule her Pap test 10 to 20 days after the first day of her last menstrual period (LMP). This is because it is recommended that the Pap test not be collected during the patient's menstrual period. The patient should be told not to douche or insert tampons, medications, or contraceptive spermicides into the vagina for 2 days before having a Pap test. Douching and tampon insertion reduce the number of cells available for analysis, and vaginal medications and spermicides change the pH of the vagina, making the specimen nonrepresentative or invalid. The patient also should be told to abstain from sexual intercourse for 2 days before the Pap test. Recent sexual intercourse can produce inflammatory changes that can interfere with visualization of abnormal cells that may be present.

Specimen Collection

The outermost layer of the cervix consists of a thin, flat layer of cells, approximately 10 layers thick, known as *squamous epithelial cells.* With the speculum in place, the physician collects a sampling of these cells for evaluation by the laboratory. A scraping of epithelial cells is taken from the ectocervix and the endocervix. A scraping of cells also can be collected from the vagina; however, this is not usually done unless the physician has observed a lesion on the vaginal wall, or the maturation index is to be determined. The technique used by the physician to collect the epithelial cells is described next.

Vaginal Specimen

If a vaginal specimen is needed, it is collected first, before the cervical and endocervical specimens are obtained. The rounded end of the plastic spatula is used to collect the specimen. If a routine vaginal specimen is being obtained, it is collected from the vaginal pool in the posterior fornix of the vagina, which is located just below the cervix (Figure 23-2, A). If the physician is collecting a specimen from a lesion on the vaginal wall, a scraping of cells is taken from the area of the lesion. To obtain a specimen for determination of the maturation index (discussed later), the physician obtains the vaginal specimen from the upper one third of the lateral vaginal wall.

Cervical Specimen

The physician obtains the cervical specimen by placing the S-shaped end of the plastic spatula just inside the cervical canal at the **external os** and rotating the blade 360 degrees over the surface of the ectocervix at the squamocolumnar

junction, where cervical cancer is most often found (Figure 23-2, B). The ectocervix is the part of the cervix that projects into the vagina and is lined with stratified squamous epithelium.

Endocervical Specimen

The endocervix consists of the mucous membrane lining the endocervical canal. Collection of the endocervical specimen is accomplished by inserting an endocervical brush into the endocervical canal and rotating the brush (Figure 23-2, C). The endocervical brush is made up of soft bristles designed to be inserted into the canal without causing damage to it.

Preparation Methods

Two methods are used to prepare a specimen for a Pap test. The conventional method is the *direct smear* (Pap smear), and the newer method is the *liquid-based preparation.*

Direct Smear

With the direct smear method, a thin smear of each specimen is spread on a glass slide that has a frosted edge. The

Vaginal Specimen

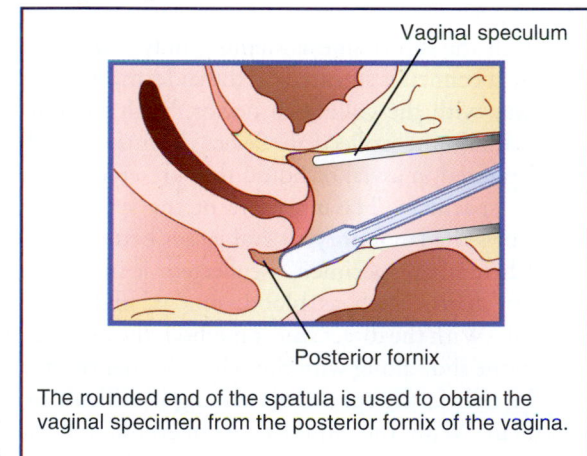

The rounded end of the spatula is used to obtain the vaginal specimen from the posterior fornix of the vagina.

A

Cervical Specimen

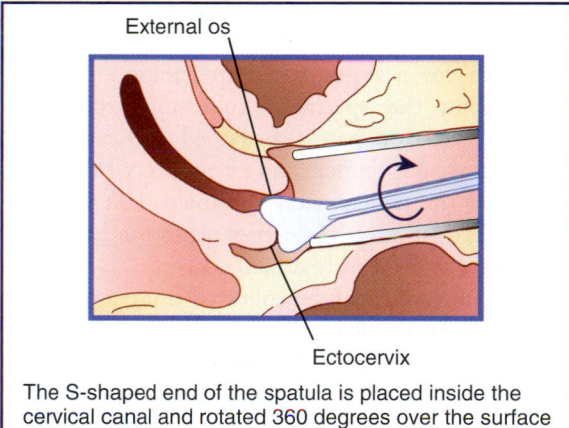

The S-shaped end of the spatula is placed inside the cervical canal and rotated 360 degrees over the surface of the cervix.

B

Endocervical Specimen

An endocervical brush is inserted into the endocervical canal and rotated to obtain a specimen.

C

Figure 23-2 Obtaining the Pap specimen.

medical assistant must label each slide on its frosted edge with a lead pencil according to the source of the specimen as follows: *V* (vaginal), *C* (cervical), or *E* (endocervical). Slides on which all three specimens can be placed also are available. These slides are divided into thirds and are prelabeled with *V, C,* and *E.*

The smears must be fixed immediately by flooding the slides with 95% ethyl alcohol or by lightly spraying the slides with a commercial cytology spray fixative. The slides must be fixed before they dry to avoid inaccurate results. The purposes of the fixative are to maintain the normal appearance of the cells; to protect the slides from contaminants in the air, such as dust and bacteria; and to attach the smear firmly to the slide. The cytology fixative must be allowed to dry thoroughly; the slides are then ready for transport to a laboratory for evaluation. To protect the slides during transport, they must be placed in a slide container designed especially for this purpose.

Liquid-Based Preparation

The most commonly used method to prepare the Pap specimen for evaluation is the liquid-based preparation method. Brand names include ThinPrep, and SurePath. Use of the liquid-based method improves the quality of the specimen, resulting in fewer slides that are unsatisfactory for evaluation. A better-quality specimen also reduces the occurrence of false-negative test results.

The specimen for a liquid-based preparation can be obtained by using the specimen collection technique described earlier. A plastic spatula (S-shaped end) is used to collect the ectocervical specimen, and an endocervical brush is used to collect the endocervical specimen. If a vaginal specimen is needed, it is collected first using the rounded end of the spatula as previously described.

The Pap specimen also can be collected using a broom, a collection device made of flexible plastic. The physician inserts the central bristles of the broom into the endocervical canal deep enough to allow the shorter bristles to contact the outside of the cervix fully. The broom is gently pushed and rotated in a clockwise direction (Figure 23-3). In this way, specimens from the ectocervix and the endocervix can be collected at the same time.

When the Pap specimen has been collected, the medical assistant is responsible for performing one of the following steps depending on the brand of liquid-based preparation being used:
- ThinPrep: Rinse the collection device in the vial of liquid preservative, and discard the collection device.
- SurePath: Remove the tip of the collection device, and deposit it in the vial of preservative. Discard the handle.

The preservative maintains the specimen and prevents it from drying out during transport to the laboratory. After it is received by the laboratory, the vial is placed in an automated slide preparation processor. The automated processor performs several important functions. First, it separates the cells from debris present in the specimen, and then it

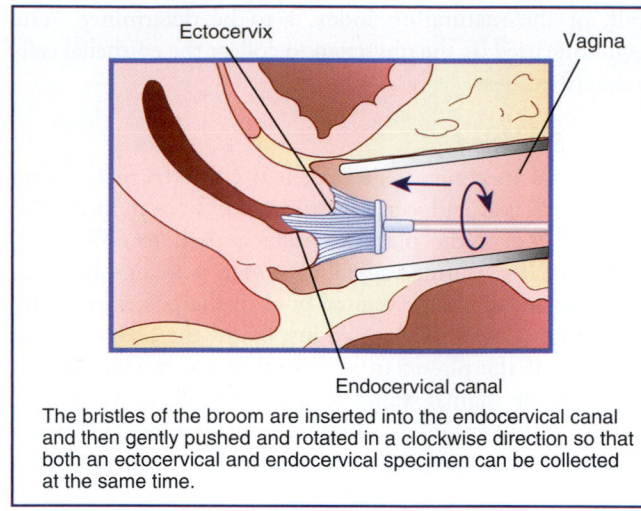

The bristles of the broom are inserted into the endocervical canal and then gently pushed and rotated in a clockwise direction so that both an ectocervical and endocervical specimen can be collected at the same time.

Figure 23-3 Collecting a Pap specimen using a broom.

disperses a representative cell sample onto a slide in a thin, uniform layer. The slide is next immersed in a fixative to maintain the normal appearance of the cells.

The ways in which the liquid-based method provides a better-quality specimen than the direct smear method are as follows:
- With the direct smear method, only a small portion of the specimen is smeared on the slide; most of it is thrown away with the collection device. With the liquid-based method, the collection device is rinsed or the tip is deposited in a vial of liquid that preserves all or most of the specimen. Having more of the specimen available allows the laboratory to evaluate it better.
- When a Pap specimen is collected, it includes unnecessary debris, such as blood, mucus, and inflammatory cells. With the direct smear method, the debris is smeared on the slide along with the cells. This debris may obscure the cells in the specimen, making it difficult to evaluate them. With the liquid-based method, the automated processor removes a large portion of the debris from the specimen and transfers the cells to a glass slide. This provides the cytotechnologist with a clear, unobstructed view of the epithelial cells.
- With the direct smear method the cells have a tendency to clump together when they are smeared on the slide, making them more difficult to evaluate. With the liquid-based method, the automated processor disperses the cells onto the slide in a thin, even layer. In this way, the cells are spread out, making it easier for the cytotechnologist to evaluate them.

Cytology Request

A cytology request must accompany all Pap specimens. Figure 23-4 is an example of hard copy cytology request form. They may also be computer-generated, but all of the same core information is necessary. The medical assistant is

GYN CYTOLOGY REQUISITION

THOMAS WOODSIDE, MD
501 MAIN ST
ST. LOUIS, MO 63146
(314) 555–0093

PATIENT INFO

| Patient's Name (Last) | (First) | (MI) | Date of Birth MO | DAY | YR | Collection Time AM PM | Collection Date MO | DAY | YR | Patient's ID # |

Patient's Address   Phone

City   State   ZIP

RESP. PARTY

Name of Responsible Party (if different from patient)

Address of Responsible Party   APT #

City   State   ZIP

INSURANCE

Patient's Relationship to Responsible Party   ☐ 1. Self   ☐ 2. Spouse   ☐ 3. Child   ☐ 4. Other

Insurance Comany Name	Plan	Carrier Code
Subscriber/Member #	Location	Group #
Insurance Address		Physician's Provider #
City	State	ZIP
Employer's Name or Number	Insured SSN	

Diagnosis/Signs/Symptoms in ICD-9 Format (Highest Specificity)

R E Q U I R E D

ICD-9 codes are the internationally accepted method of describing the clinical picture of the patient. All diagnoses should be provided by the ordering physician or his or her authorized designee. The following is a partial list of of common diagnoses in ICD-9 format. Most third party payers require an ICD-9 code to indicate the medical necessity of the test(s) and or profile(s) ordered. For a complete list of all ICD-9 codes, please refer to a current ICD-9 manual.

V76.2	Routine Cervical Pap Smear	616.0	Cervicitis	626.8	Abnormal Bleeding
V15.89	High Risk Cervical Screening	616.10	Vaginitis	627.1	Postmenopausal Bleeding
V22.2	Pregnancy	617.0	Endometriosis, Uterus	627.3	Atrophic Vaginitis
079.4	Human Papillomavirus	622.1	Dysplasia, Cervix	795.0	Abnormal Cervical Pap Smear
180.0	Malignant Neoplasm, Cervix	623.0	Dysplasia, Vagina		

COLLECTION METHOD

Liquid-Based Prep
192055 ☐ ThinPrep Pap Test
192039 ☐ ThinPrep Pap Test w/reflex to HPV Hybrid Capture when ASC-US or SIL
192047 ☐ ThinPrep Pap Test w/reflex to high-risk only HPV Hybrid Capture when ASC-US

Pap Smear
009100 ☐ 1 Slide   009191 ☐ 2 Slides

Pap Smear and Maturation Index
009209 ☐ 1 Slide   190074 ☐ 2 Slides

SOURCE OF SPECIMEN
☐ Cervical
☐ Endocervical
☐ Vaginal

Date LMP
___ / ___ / ___
Mo   Day   Year

COLLECTION TECHNIQUE
☐ Spatula
☐ Brush
☐ Broom
☐ Other _____

PATIENT HISTORY
☐ Pregnant   ☐ PMP Bleeding
☐ Lactating   ☐ Postpartum
☐ Oral Contraceptives   ☐ IUD
☐ Postmenopausal   ☐ Postcoital Bleeding
☐ Hormone Replacement Therapy   ☐ DES Exposure
☐ Previous Abnormal Pap Test
☐ Other _____

PREVIOUS TREATMENT   Date/Results
☐ None
☐ Colposcopy and Bx _____
☐ Cryosurgery _____
☐ LEEP _____
☐ Laser Vaporization _____
☐ Conization _____
☐ Hysterectomy _____
☐ Radiation _____
☐ Chemotherapy _____

Figure 23-4 Cytology request form.

responsible for completing the request, which includes the following categories.

General Information

General information includes the physician's name, address, and phone number and the patient's name, address, identification number, date of birth, and date of LMP. Insurance information also is required in this section for third-party billing.

Date and Time of Collection

The date and time of collection indicate to the laboratory the number of days that have passed since the collection, providing the laboratory with information regarding the freshness of the specimen.

Collection Method

Under the collection method category, the medical assistant must indicate whether the specimen is a direct smear (Pap smear) or a liquid-based preparation.

Source of the Specimen

The purpose of this category is to identify the origin of the specimen because it is impossible for the laboratory to obtain this information by looking at the specimen. The medical assistant checks one or more of the following boxes on the form: cervical, endocervical, or vaginal.

Collection Technique

The collection device or devices used to obtain the specimen must be indicated. The medical assistant checks one or more of the following boxes on the form: spatula, brush, or broom.

Patient History

Information on the present and past health status of the patient is specified under the patient history category. The medical assistant must check the following boxes that apply to the patient: pregnant, lactating, oral contraceptives, postmenopausal, hormone replacement therapy, postmenopausal bleeding, postpartum, intrauterine device (IUD), postcoital bleeding, DES exposure, and previous abnormal smear. This information assists the laboratory in evaluating the specimen.

Previous Treatment

Any previous treatment for a precancerous or cancerous condition of the cervix is indicated under this category. The medical assistant checks the appropriate box on the form if any of the following procedures have been performed on the patient: colposcopy and biopsy, cryosurgery, loop electrocautery excision procedure (LEEP), laser vaporization, conization, hysterectomy, radiation, and chemotherapy.

With use of an electronic health record, all of the above information is entered into an electronic requisition form using the appropriate radio buttons, drop-down menus, and free text fields..

Evaluation of the Pap Specimen

Before a Pap slide can be evaluated, it must be stained by a laboratory technician. Staining is performed on slides prepared by the direct smear method and the liquid-based method. The purpose of staining is to allow better viewing of the morphology of the epithelial cells. The slide is studied under a microscope for evidence of abnormalities by a specially trained technician, known as a *cytotechnologist*. When an abnormality is detected, it is reviewed by a *cytopathologist* (a physician specializing in pathology), who makes a final evaluation. The findings are recorded on a cytology report and returned to the medical office.

A more recent development in the evaluation of Pap slides is the use of automated cytology computer imaging devices. An abnormal slide may contain only a few abnormal cells among thousands of normal cells. Because of this, these abnormal cells may be missed during the evaluation by the cytotechnologist. A cytology computer imaging device is able to examine every cell on the slide and select and display cells that appear "most abnormal." The cytotechnologist can evaluate these cells further under a microscope. In this way, the cytotechnologist is able to focus his or her expertise and decision making on preselected areas of the slide.

Maturation Index

The maturation index must be performed on a sampling of cells taken from the upper third of the lateral vaginal wall. The *maturation index* refers to the percentage of parabasal, intermediate, and superficial cells present in the specimen. The maturation index provides the physician with an endocrine evaluation of the patient, which can assist in evaluating the cause of infertility, menopausal or postmenopausal bleeding, or amenorrhea and can help assess the results of treatment with hormones. If the physician orders a maturation index along with the Pap test, the medical assistant must indicate this on the cytology request by checking the box labeled *Maturation Index* (see Figure 23-4). Numerous factors affect the results of the maturation index; it is important to indicate on the cytology request the presence of abnormal bleeding; hormone treatment; or treatment with digitalis, corticosteroids, or thyroid medication.

Cytology Report

The Bethesda System (TBS) is the standard for reporting the results of a Pap test on the cytology report (Figure 23-5). The National Cancer Institute in Bethesda, Maryland, developed this system. It provides a detailed cytologic description (Table 23-1) rather than a numeric result (as with the previous class I through V system). For this reason, TBS is a more effective means of communicating the results of the Pap test to the physician.

Bimanual Pelvic Examination

After obtaining the specimen for the Pap test, the physician withdraws the speculum and performs a bimanual pelvic examination. The physician inserts the index and middle

GYN CYTOLOGY REPORT

RIVERVIEW MEDICAL LABORATORY
DEPARTMENT OF PATHOLOGY
2501 GRANT AVENUE
ST. LOUIS, MO 63146
(314) 555–3443

PATIENT: Heather Jones
PATIENT NO: 45876
DOB: 10/20/65
SUBMITTING: T. Woodside, MD

	SPECIMEN TYPE	
Date of Specimen: 7/01/XX		
Date Received: 7/02/XX	☒ ThinPrep	☐ Conventional Pap Smear
Date Reported: 7/06/XX		
Performed By: Richard McVay, Cytotechnologist	Checked By: Melissa Wagner, Pathologist	

SPECIMEN ADEQUACY	GENERAL CATEGORIZATION
☒ Satisfactory for Evaluation ☐ Unsatisfactory for Evaluation	☐ Negative for Intraepithelial Lesion or Malignancy (*see Interpretation/Result*) ☒ Epithelial Cell Abnormality (*see Interpretation/Result*) ☐ Other (*see Interpretation/Result*)

INTERPRETATION/RESULT

A. BENIGN CELLULAR CHANGES

☐ Infection:
- ☐ Trichomonas vaginalis
- ☐ Fungal organisms morphologically compatible w/ Candida species
- ☐ Cellular changes associated with herpes simplex virus
- ☐ Bacterial infection morphologically compatible with gardnerella
- ☐ Cytoplasmic inclusions suggestive of chlamydia

☐ Reactive changes
- ☐ Without inflammation
- ☐ With inflammation
- ☐ Atrophy with inflammation (atrophic vaginitis)
- ☐ Radiation effect
- ☐ Repair
- ☐ Hyperkeratosis
- ☐ Parakeratosis

B. EPITHELIAL CELL ABNORMALITIES

☒ Squamous Cell
- ☒ Atypical Squamous Cells of Undetermined Significance (ASC-US)
- ☐ Atypical Squamous Cells of Higher Risk (ASC-H)
- ☐ Low-Grade Squamous Intraepithelial Lesion (LSIL)
- ☐ High-Grade Squamous Intraepithelial Lesion (HSIL)
- ☐ Squamous Cell Carcinoma

☐ Glandular Cell
- ☐ Atypical Glandular Cells of Undetermined Significance (AGUS)
- ☐ Adenocarcinoma

Figure 23-5 Cytology report form (The Bethesda System).

Table 23-1 Pap Test Results

Test Result	Interpretation
Negative for intraepithelial lesion or malignancy	Epithelial cells were normal, and there were no precancerous or cancerous findings.
Atypical squamous cells of undetermined significance (ASC-US)	Cells are only slightly abnormal. Nature and cause of abnormality cannot be determined. These slightly altered cells usually return to normal on their own, resulting in negative results on subsequent Pap tests.
Atypical squamous cells of higher risk (ASC-H)	Minor abnormal changes in cells with unknown causes, but at risk of progressing to high-grade lesion (HSIL). Further testing is required to determine whether this is a minor condition or one that may progress to HSIL.
Low-grade squamous intraepithelial lesion (LSIL)	Abnormal cells that show definite minor changes but are unlikely to progress to cancer (general term for this is *mild dysplasia*). LSIL may be caused by HPV infection, but of a type that is not likely to lead to cervical cancer.
High-grade squamous intraepithelial lesion (HSIL)	Abnormal cell changes that have a higher likelihood of progressing to cancer. Although not cancerous yet, abnormal cells may become cancerous if treatment is not obtained (general term for this is *moderate-to-severe dysplasia*). HSIL is often caused by HPV infection of a type associated with cervical cancer.
Carcinoma	Usually means patient has cervical cancer. Most women with cervical cancer also test positive for HPV infection.

HPV, Human papillomavirus.

fingers of a lubricated gloved hand into the vagina. The fingers of the other hand are placed on the woman's lower abdomen. Between the two hands, the physician can palpate the size, shape, and position of the uterus and ovaries and can detect tenderness or lumps (Figure 23-6).

Rectal-Vaginal Examination

The last part of the pelvic examination is a rectal-vaginal examination. The physician inserts one gloved finger into the vagina and another gloved finger into the rectum to obtain information about the tone and alignment of the pelvic organs and the **adnexal** region (ovaries, fallopian tubes, and ligaments of the uterus). The presence of hemorrhoids, fistulas, and fissures also can be noted. During this examination, the physician may want to obtain some fecal material from the rectum to perform a fecal occult blood test (e.g., Hemoccult). This is typically performed on women beginning at 40 years of age. The medical assistant is responsible for assisting with the collection and testing the specimen for occult blood. This procedure (fecal occult blood testing) is presented in detail in Chapter 28.

Text continued on p. 504

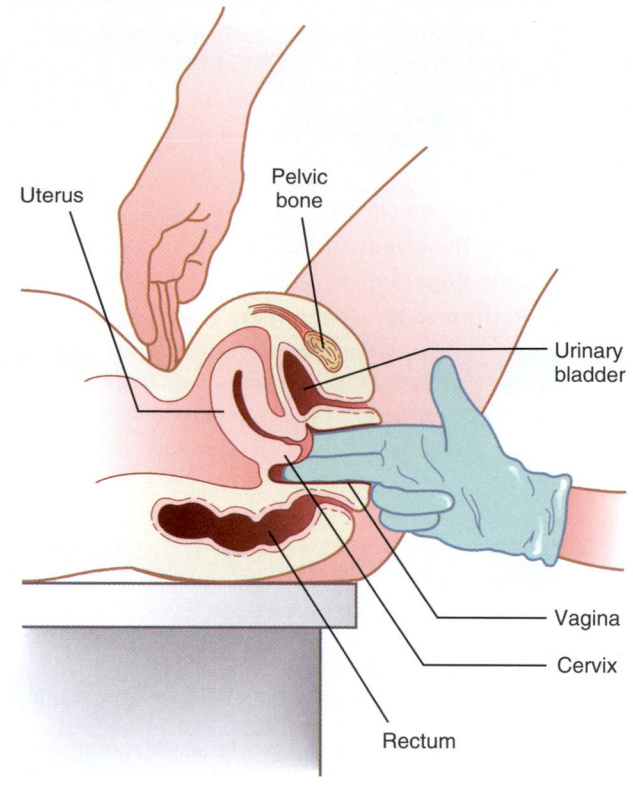

Figure 23-6 The bimanual pelvic examination.

PROCEDURE 23-1   Breast Self-Examination Instructions

Outcome Instruct a patient in the procedure for performing a breast self-examination

Equipment/Supplies

- Small pillow

1. **Procedural Step.** Greet the patient and introduce yourself. Identify the patient and inform the patient that you will be showing her how to perform a breast self-examination. Discuss with her the purpose of a breast self-examination and when to examine the breasts (see the box *Patient Teaching: Breast Self-Examination*).

2. **Procedural Step.** Explain to the patient that a complete breast self-examination should be performed in three ways—before a mirror, lying down, and in the shower.
   Principle. Using three methods results in a thorough examination, making it more likely that breast changes will be detected.
   Instruct the patient in the procedure for performing a breast self-examination as follows:

Before a Mirror

3. **Procedural Step.** Remove clothing from the waist up. Stand in front of a large mirror with your arms relaxed at your sides. Observe each breast for the following:
   a. Change in size or shape
   b. Swelling, puckering, or dimpling of the skin
   c. Change in skin texture
   d. Retraction of the nipple
   e. Changes in size or position of one nipple compared with the other
   Principle. Puckering and dimpling of the skin or retraction of the nipple may mean that a tumor is pulling the skin inward.

PROCEDURE 23-1   Breast Self-Examination Instructions—cont'd

4. Procedural Step. Slowly raise your arms over your head, and repeat the same inspection listed in Procedural Step 3.
Principle. When the arms are moved at the same time into the same positions, both breasts and nipples should react to the movement in the same way. A change in one breast (e.g., dimpling or puckering of the skin) and not the other should be reported to your physician.

Raise your arms over your head.

5. Procedural Step. Rest your palms on your hips and press down firmly to flex your chest muscles. Repeat the inspection in Procedural Step 3.
Principle. Flexing the chest muscles allows abnormalities to become more apparent.

Press down firmly to flex the chest muscles.

6. Procedural Step. Gently squeeze the nipple of each breast with your fingertips and look for a discharge.

Lying Down

7. Procedural Step. To examine the right breast, lie on your back and place a small pillow (or folded towel) under your right shoulder. Place your right hand behind your head.
Principle. The purpose of this step is to flatten the breast and distribute the breast tissue more evenly on the chest, making it easier to palpate the breast tissue.

8. Procedural Step. Extend your left hand with the fingers held flat. The pads of the middle three fingers of the left hand are used to perform the

examination. The finger pads include the top third of each finger. Do not use the tips of the fingers. Use small rotating motions (about the size of a dime) and continuous firm pressure with the finger pads.
Principle. The finger pads are more sensitive than the fingertips, making it easier to detect an abnormality.

Use the pads of the middle three fingers.

9. Procedural Step. Use one of the following patterns to move around the breast: circular, vertical strip, or wedge. Choose the pattern that is easiest for you. When you have chosen a pattern, use the same pattern each time you examine your breasts.

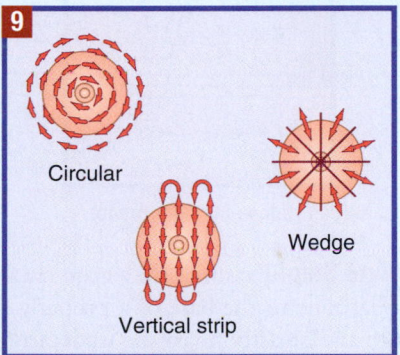

Circular

Wedge

Vertical strip

Use one of three patterns to examine the breasts.

Circular

a. Visualize the breast as a clock face.
b. Start at the outside top edge of the breast.
c. Proceed clockwise around the entire outer rim of the breast until your fingers return to the starting point.
d. Move in about 1 inch toward the nipple, and make the same circling motion again.
e. Move around the breast in smaller and smaller circles until you reach the nipple.

Vertical Strip

a. Mentally divide the breast into strips.
b. Start in the underarm area and slowly move your fingers downward until they are below the breast.
c. Move your fingers about 1 inch toward the middle, and slowly move back up.
d. Repeat until the entire breast has been examined.

Continued

PROCEDURE 23-1

Wedge

a. Mentally divide your breast into wedges, similar to the pieces of a pie.

b. Starting at the outer edge of the breast, move your fingers toward the nipple and back to the edge of the breast.

c. Check your entire breast, covering one small wedge-shaped section at a time.

Principle. Using a specific pattern ensures that the entire breast is examined.

10. Procedural Step. Holding the middle three fingers of your hand together with the thumb extended, use your finger pads and the pattern you selected to examine the right breast thoroughly. Press firmly enough to feel the different breast tissues. The breast should be palpated for lumps, hard knots, and thickening. Breast tissue normally feels a little lumpy and uneven.

Examine the right breast.

11. Procedural Step. Examine the entire chest area from your collarbone to the base of a properly fitted bra and from the breastbone to the underarm. Pay special attention to the area between the breast and the underarm, including the underarm itself. A ridge of firm tissue in the lower curve of the breast is normal. Continue the examination until every part of the breast has been examined, including the nipple.

Principle. An enlarged node in the armpit also can be a sign of breast cancer even if nothing can be felt in the breast.

12. Procedural Step. Repeat this procedure on the left breast. Place a small pillow (or folded towel) under the left shoulder, and place your left hand behind your head. Use the finger pads of the right hand to examine the left breast.

In the Shower

13. Procedural Step. Gently lather each breast.

Principle. Fingers glide easily over wet, soapy skin, making it easier to detect changes in the breast.

14. Procedural Step. Place your right hand behind your head. Extend your left hand with the fingers held flat. With the finger pads of the middle three fingers, use small rotating motions (about the size of a dime) and continuous firm pressure with the finger pads to examine the right breast. Use your preferred pattern (circular, vertical strip, or wedge) to palpate for lumps, hard knots, and thickening. Examine the area between the breast and the underarm, including the underarm itself.

Principle. The upright position makes it easier to examine the upper and outer portions of the breast.

15. Procedural Step. Repeat the procedure on the left breast. Place the left arm behind the head, and use the right fingers to examine the left breast.

Examine the breasts in the shower.

16. Procedural Step. Instruct the patient to report lumps and other changes to the physician immediately. Reassure the patient that most breast lumps are not cancerous, but the only way to know for sure is to see the physician as soon as possible.

17. Procedural Step. Chart the procedure in the patient's medical record.

a. *Paper-based patient record.* Record the date and time and the type of instructions given to the patient. If you gave a printed instruction sheet or educational brochure to the patient, document this as well (refer to the PPR charting example).

PPR CHARTING EXAMPLE	
Date	
9/7/XX	11:00 a.m. Instructions provided for a BSE. Pt given a BSE educational brochure.
	———————————— Y. Wu, RMA

b. *Electronic medical record (EMR):* Using an EMR such as SimChart for the Medical Office, document the type of instructions given to the patient using the appropriate radio buttons, drop-down menus, and free text fields. If you gave a printed instruction sheet or educational brochure to the patient, document this as well.

PROCEDURE 23-2   Assisting with a Gynecologic Examination

Outcome Assist with a gynecologic examination

The following procedure describes the medical assistant's role in assisting with a gynecologic examination consisting of breast and pelvic examinations, including a liquid-based Pap test and a fecal occult blood test.

Equipment/Supplies

- Disposable gloves
- Examining gown and drape
- Disposable vaginal speculum
- Vial with preservative (ThinPrep, SurePath)
- Plastic spatula and endocervical brush or cytology broom
- Water-based lubricant
- Gauze pads
- Fecal occult blood test
- Tissues
- Cytology request form
- Biohazard specimen transport bag

1. **Procedural Step.** Sanitize your hands.
2. **Procedural Step.** Assemble the equipment. Complete as much of the cytology request form as possible. Some information on the form, such as the last menstrual period (LMP), requires input from the patient and must be completed later.

Assemble equipment.

3. **Procedural Step.** Check the expiration date on the specimen vial. Label the vial with the date and the patient's name, date of birth, and identification number. The identification number is located on the cytology request form.
   Principle. If the vial is outdated, it should be discarded because it may lead to inaccurate test results.
4. **Procedural Step.** Greet the patient and introduce yourself.
5. **Procedural Step.** Escort the patient to the examining room and ask her to be seated. Identify the patient. Seat yourself so that you are facing the patient. Ask the patient whether she has any problems or concerns, and chart this information in the patient's medical record. Ask the patient the necessary questions to complete the rest of the cytology request form.

6. **Procedural Step.** Measure the patient's vital signs, height, and weight, and chart the results in the patient's medical record.
7. **Procedural Step.** Instruct and prepare the patient for the examination as follows:
   a. Ask the patient whether she needs to empty the bladder before the examination. If a urine specimen is needed, instruct the patient in the proper collection of the specimen.
   b. Provide the patient with a patient gown. Instruct the patient to remove all clothing and to put on the patient gown with the opening in front. If the patient is wearing socks, tell her she can keep them on. Offer assistance if you sense the patient may have trouble undressing.
   c. Tell the patient to have a seat on the examining table after she has put on the examining gown.
   d. Inform the patient that the physician will be with her soon, and leave the room to give her privacy.
   Principle. An empty bladder makes the examination easier and is more comfortable for the patient. Wearing socks helps keep the patient's feet warm during the examination.

Instruct and prepare the patient for the examination.

Continued

PROCEDURE 23-2

PROCEDURE 23-2 Assisting with a Gynecologic Examination—cont'd

8. Procedural Step. Make the medical record available for review by the physician. The medical office has a designated location where the record is placed, such as a small shelf mounted on the wall next to the outside of the examining room door or a chart holder on the outside of the examining room door. Position the medical record so that patient-identifiable information is not visible. If your office uses an EMR, you do not need to perform this step. With an EMR, the physician accesses the patient's record on the computer.

Principle: The physician will want to review the patient's measurements and urine test results documented by the medical assistant. HIPAA requires protection of a patient's health information.

9. Procedural Step. Check to make sure the patient is ready to be seen by the physician. Before entering a patient's room, always knock lightly on the door to let the patient know you are getting ready to enter the room. Inform the physician that the patient is ready. This may be done using a color-coded flagging system mounted on the wall next to the examining room.

10. Procedural Step. Assist the patient into a supine position, and properly drape her for the breast examination.

11. Procedural Step. Assist the patient into the lithotomy position for the pelvic examination.

12. Procedural Step. Prepare the vaginal speculum by thinly lubricating the blades of the speculum with a water-based lubricant. Never apply lubricant to the tip of the speculum.

Principle. Lubricating the vaginal speculum facilitates its insertion into the vagina.

13. Procedural Step. Prepare the light for the physician as follows:
   a. *Overhead examination lamp:* Adjust and focus the light for the physician.
   b. *Speculum-illumination system:* Snap the light source device into the light holder on the vaginal speculum and turn it on. The lighting system produces a beam of light that shines through the blades of the speculum for visualization of the vagina and cervix.

Principle. Visualization of the vagina and cervix requires direct light.

14. Procedural Step. Hand the vaginal speculum to the physician. Reassure the patient, and help her relax the abdominal muscles during the examination by telling her to breathe deeply, slowly, and evenly through the mouth.

Principle. If the patient is relaxed, the examination proceeds more smoothly and is more comfortable for her.

15. Procedural Step. Apply gloves, and assist with the collection of the Pap specimen as follows:

ThinPrep

Spatula and Brush Method

   a. Remove the cap from the ThinPrep vial, and hold it so that the physician can insert the spatula into the vial.
   b. Rinse the plastic spatula in the liquid preservative by vigorously swirling it around in the solution 10 times.

15. b.

Vigorously swirl the spatula in the preservative.

   c. Discard the spatula in a biohazard waste container.
   d. Hold the vial so that the physician can insert the endocervical brush into the vial.
   e. Rinse the brush in the liquid preservative by vigorously rotating it in the solution 10 times while pushing the brush against the vial wall. Swirl the brush in the solution to further release cellular material.
   f. Discard the brush in a biohazard waste container. Securely tighten the cap so that the torque line on the cap passes the torque line on the vial.

PROCEDURE 23-2 Assisting with a Gynecologic Examination—cont'd

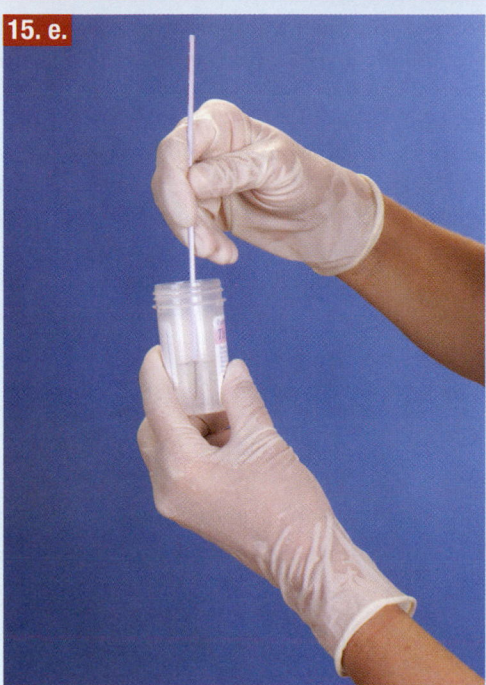

Rotate the brush in the preservative.

Broom Method

a. Remove the cap from the ThinPrep vial, and hold it so that the physician can insert the broom into the vial.

b. Rinse the broom in the liquid preservative by pushing the broom vigorously into the bottom of the vial 10 times. This motion forces the broom bristles apart, releasing cervical cells into the solution. Swirl the broom vigorously in the liquid preservative to further release cellular material.

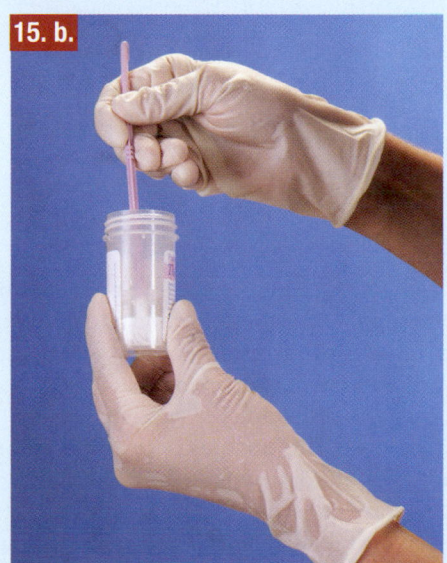

Push the broom vigorously into the bottom of the vial.

c. Discard the broom in a biohazard waste container. Tighten the cap so that the torque line on the cap passes the torque line on the vial.

SurePath

a. Remove the cap from the SurePath vial, and hold it so that the physician can insert the collection device into the vial.

b. Break off (spatula and brush method) or disconnect the tip (broom method) of the collection device from the handle.

c. Discard the handle of the collection device in a waste container.

d. Repeat these steps until the physician has collected all of the specimens needed for the Pap test.

e. Securely tighten the cap on the vial.

16. Procedural Step. Turn off the examining lamp or disconnect the light source from the vaginal speculum. Discard the disposable vaginal speculum in a biohazard waste container. Apply lubricant to a gauze square. Hold it out so that the physician can apply lubricant to his or her gloves to perform the bimanual and rectal-vaginal examinations. Assist with the collection of the fecal specimen for the fecal occult blood test.

Principle. Applying lubricant to a gauze square (rather than directly to the physician's gloved fingers) prevents the opening of the tube of lubricant from touching the physician's gloves and contaminating the contents of the tube.

Hold the gauze with the lubricant for the physician.

Continued

PROCEDURE 23-2 Assisting with a Gynecologic Examination—cont'd

17. Procedural Step. After the examination, assist the patient into a sitting position, and allow her the opportunity to rest for a moment. Offer the patient tissues to remove excess lubricant from the perineum. Assist the patient off the examining table. *Principle.* Some patients (especially geriatric) become dizzy after lying on the examining table and should be allowed to rest after sitting up.

18. Procedural Step. Instruct the patient to get dressed. Tell the patient how and when she will be notified of the Pap test results.

19. Procedural Step. Test the fecal occult blood specimen, and chart the results in the patient's medical record.

20. Procedural Step. Prepare the Pap specimen for transport to the laboratory. Place the vial in a biohazard specimen transport bag, and seal the bag. Insert the cytology requisition into the outside pocket of the bag, and tuck the top of the requisition under the flap. Place the bag in the appropriate location for pickup by the laboratory.

21. Procedural Step. Chart the transport of the Pap specimen to an outside laboratory in the patient's medical record.

22. Procedural Step. Clean the examining room.

PPR CHARTING EXAMPLE

Date	
9/7/XX	10:00 a.m. Hemoccult: negative.
	Instructions provided for BSE. ThinPrep
	Pap specimen to Medical Center Laboratory
	for cytology. ——————— Y. Wu, RMA

Insert the cytology request into the outside pocket.

VAGINAL INFECTIONS

The vagina provides a warm, moist environment, which tends to encourage the growth of various organisms that can result in a vaginal infection, or *vaginitis*. If an unusual vaginal discharge is present, suggesting a vaginal infection, a specimen is obtained to identify the invading organism. A sample of the vaginal discharge is collected at the medical office and is evaluated there or placed in an appropriate specimen container that is picked up by a laboratory courier and transported to an outside medical laboratory for evaluation.

The medical assistant is responsible for assembling the appropriate supplies for the collection and evaluation of the suspected invading organism. The medical assistant must label all specimens with the patient's name and date of birth, the date, and the source of the specimen. If the specimen is to be transported to an outside medical laboratory for evaluation, a laboratory request form must be completed. The request form indicates the source of the specimen, the physician's clinical diagnosis, and the laboratory test requested. The physician's clinical assessment of the patient's signs and symptoms, along with the results of the laboratory

Figure 23-7 *Trichomonas vaginalis* under a microscope. (Modified from Mahon C, Manuselis G: *Textbook of diagnostic microbiology,* ed 5, St Louis, 2015, Saunders.)

Wet Preparation

A small amount of the vaginal discharge is placed on the slide.

A drop of normal saline is added to the specimen.

A coverslip is placed over the specimen to protect it during examination under the microscope.

Figure 23-8 Preparing a wet preparation for the identification of *Trichomonas vaginalis.*

evaluation of the specimen, are used to diagnose the presence of a vaginal infection.

Medical assistants should protect themselves from infection with a pathogen while assisting with the collection and evaluation of the specimen by practicing good techniques of medical asepsis. Methods used to identify the invading organism and supplies required for the collection and evaluation of organisms that cause common vaginal infections are presented next.

Trichomoniasis

Trichomonas vaginalis, the causative agent of trichomoniasis ("trich"), is a pear-shaped protozoan with four flagella, which allow for the motility of the organism (Figure 23-7). Trichomoniasis is usually, but not always, spread through sexual intercourse. Symptoms of this infection include a profuse, frothy vaginal discharge that is usually yellowish green and has an unpleasant odor; itching and irritation of the vulva and vagina; dyspareunia; and dysuria. The cervix may exhibit small red spots, a condition known as "strawberry cervix."

Trichomonas may be identified at the medical office by a wet preparation, which involves using a sterile swab to place a small amount of the discharge on a microscope slide, adding a drop of isotonic saline to it, and placing a coverslip over the mixture to protect it (Figure 23-8). The slide is examined under the microscope and observed for the presence of the lashing movements of the flagella and the motility of the organism. If the physician prefers to have an outside laboratory evaluate the specimen, it must be placed in the appropriate specimen container and transported to the laboratory for evaluation.

Candidiasis

Candida albicans is a yeastlike fungus normally found in the intestinal tract and is a frequent contaminant of the vagina; however, it usually does not produce symptoms indicating a vaginal infection. Conditions such as pregnancy, diabetes

mellitus, and prolonged antibiotic therapy produce changes in the vagina that may precipitate a candidal infection of the vagina, commonly referred to as a "yeast infection." Symptoms of candidiasis include white patches on the mucous membrane of the vagina; a thick, odorless, cottage cheese–like discharge; vulval irritation; and dysuria. The discharge is extremely irritating and usually results in burning and intense itching.

Candida may be identified microscopically in the medical office by placing a specimen of the vaginal discharge on a slide using a sterile swab and adding a drop of a 10% solution of potassium hydroxide (KOH). The KOH dissolves cellular debris present in the smear and allows better visualization of yeast buds, spores, or hyphae (fungus filaments) indicating the presence of *C. albicans* (Figure 23-9). If the physician prefers to have an outside laboratory evaluate the specimen, it must be placed in the appropriate specimen container and transported to the laboratory.

Chlamydia

Chlamydia is caused by the bacterium *Chlamydia trachomatis.* Chlamydia is the most frequently reported and fastest spreading sexually transmitted disease in the United States, particularly among adolescent girls and young women. Because of this, the CDC recommends annual routine

Figure 23-9 *Candida albicans* under a microscope. The arrow is pointing to one of the yeast buds. (Modified from Mahon C, Manuselis G: *Textbook of diagnostic microbiology*, ed 5, St Louis, 2015, Saunders.)

screening for chlamydia of all sexually active females 25 years of age or younger.

Most women with chlamydia have no symptoms and are not aware of having the condition. Because of this, many women do not seek medical care until serious complications have occurred. After infection, chlamydia first attacks the cervix, resulting in cervicitis. If symptoms do occur, they may include one or more of the following: dysuria, itching and irritation of the genital area, and a yellowish, odorless vaginal discharge. These symptoms usually appear 1 to 3 weeks after the patient has been infected.

If not treated, chlamydia can spread further into the female reproductive tract and cause *pelvic inflammatory disease* (PID). The symptoms of PID include lower abdominal pain, fever, nausea and vomiting, dyspareunia, vaginal discharge, and bleeding between periods. Complications of PID are serious and include chronic pelvic pain, scarring of the fallopian tubes, ectopic pregnancy, and infertility.

Symptoms of a chlamydial infection in men include mild dysuria and a thin, watery discharge from the penis. Men are more likely to have symptoms than women; however, the symptoms may appear only early in the day and be so mild that they are ignored. If the infection is not treated, it can cause *epididymitis,* a painful condition of the testicles that could result in infertility.

Chlamydia is most frequently diagnosed using a nucleic acid amplification test (NAAT) or a nucleic acid hybridization test known as the *DNA probe test.* These tests are able to detect the presence of the genes (DNA) of *Chlamydia* bacteria. The physician uses a sterile swab to collect a specimen. The specimen is collected from the endocervical canal of a female patient and from the urethra of a male patient. Male patients should be instructed not to void for 1 hour before the collection of the specimen to prevent *Chlamydia* organisms from being washed out of the urethra. After collection, the specimen is placed in a tube containing a transport medium to preserve the specimen until it reaches the laboratory. See the box *Chlamydia and Gonorrhea Specimen*

Collection for detailed instructions on how to assist with the collection of a chlamydia specimen.

Gonorrhea

Gonorrhea is caused by the bacterium *Neisseria gonorrhoeae,* which is a gram-negative diplococcus. Gonorrhea is an infection of the genitourinary tract that is transmitted through sexual intercourse. Chlamydia often occurs in association with gonorrhea; approximately 25% to 40% of patients infected with gonorrhea also have chlamydia. The CDC recommends annual routine screening for gonorrhea in all sexually active women at risk for infection. Women younger than 25 years of age are at highest risk for a gonorrhea infection. Other risk factors include a previous gonorrhea infection, the presence of other STDs, and new or multiple sex partners.

Women who have contracted gonorrhea may have no symptoms or may exhibit dysuria and a yellow vaginal discharge. The symptoms of gonorrhea (if they occur) appear 2 to 10 days after infection and may be so mild that they are ignored. As the disease progresses, it can spread farther into the reproductive tract, resulting in PID. As mentioned previously, PID can lead to serious complications such as infertility.

Men who have contracted gonorrhea exhibit more symptoms than women, including dysuria and a whitish discharge from the penis, which may progress to a thick and creamy discharge. The burning and pain experienced during urination are often severe, which usually prompts an infected man to seek early treatment. If not treated, gonorrhea may cause epididymitis, which could lead to infertility.

The medical office most frequently uses a DNA probe test or a nucleic acid amplification test (NAAT) to diagnose gonorrhea. These tests detect the presence of the genes of the gonorrhea bacterium. The procedure for obtaining a specimen for the DNA probe test is outlined in the box *Chlamydia and Gonorrhea Specimen Collection.*

What Would You Do? What Would You *Not* Do?

Case Study 2

Dagny Fairchild comes to the office. She is 16 years old; her father is a lawyer and her mother is a chemical engineer. Her boyfriend was diagnosed 2 weeks ago with chlamydia. Dagny was hesitant to come in because she does not have any symptoms and her boyfriend always uses a condom. She is worried about her parents finding out that she is sexually active and what they will think if she has a sexually transmitted disease (STD). Dagny also is afraid and extremely embarrassed about what will be "done to her" to determine whether she has chlamydia. She tells Yin-Ling that she is thinking of leaving the office and not seeing the physician at all. (*Note:* Dagny lives in a state that allows minors to receive health care services without parental consent.) ∎

Chlamydia and Gonorrhea Specimen Collection

DNA-Based Detection Test

The procedure for collecting a specimen for the DNA test is outlined here. Chlamydia and gonorrhea tests can be performed on the same specimen.

1. The medical assistant assembles supplies needed to collect the specimen, including a vaginal speculum, clean disposable gloves, and the DNA probe collection kit. The collection kit includes cotton-tipped swabs and a tube of transport medium.
2. The transport tube must be labeled with the following information: patient's name, date of birth, and identification number; date and time of collection; and physician's name and telephone number.

**DNA-probe set-up
(Female patient)**

**DNA-probe set-up
(Male patient)**

3. The physician collects the specimen as follows:
   - *Female patient:* The physician inserts a vaginal speculum into the vagina. Using a cotton-tipped swab, the physician first removes excess mucus or discharge from the cervix. Next, the physician collects the specimen by inserting another cotton-tipped swab into the endocervical canal and rotating it for 15 to 30 seconds. This ensures a good sampling of the specimen.
   - *Male patient:* The patient must not urinate for 1 hour before the collection to prevent any urethral discharge from being washed away. The physician inserts a small-tipped cotton swab 2 to 4 cm into the penis. The swab is gently rotated for 2 to 3 seconds to dislodge cells and to ensure contact with all urethral surfaces.
4. The physician withdraws the swab.
5. The medical assistant should ensure that the transport medium is at the bottom of the tube. The medical assistant unscrews the cap and holds the tube for the physician.
6. The physician inserts the swab into the transport tube and breaks off the shaft of the swab at the score line.

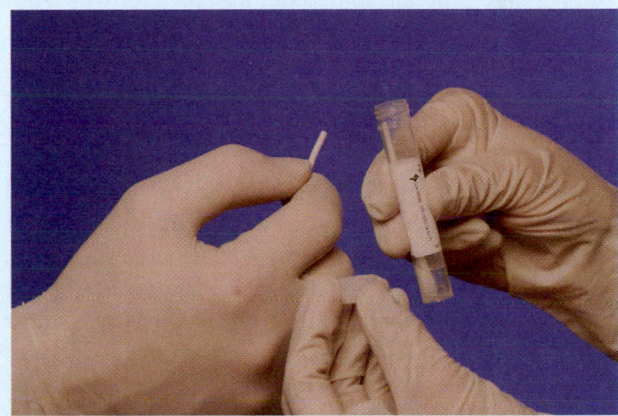

The physician inserts the swab into the tube and breaks off the shaft.

7. The medical assistant places the cap on the tube and twists it until it clicks into place. The tube is placed in a biohazard specimen transport bag along with the laboratory requisition for pickup by the laboratory.

Memories *from* Practicum

Yin-Ling Wu: During my practicum, I was assigned to an OB/GYN clinic. They had an ultrasound technician working there who ran all the scans on prenatal patients. The ultrasound scans I observed always looked like a big blob to me—I could never see anything.

One day, a patient whom one of the medical assistants knew really well came into the office. The patient agreed to let us all come in for her ultrasound. It was her first time getting an ultrasound. When the technician put the ultrasound probe on her abdomen, we could see the outline of the whole baby. You could even see a tiny arm and fingers, and it looked like the baby was waving. The look of joy and amazement on the mom's face was unforgettable. After that, I knew I was in the right profession. ■

PRENATAL CARE

OBSTETRICS

Obstetrics is the branch of medicine that deals with the supervision of women's health during pregnancy, childbirth, and the puerperium. **Prenatal** refers to the care of a pregnant woman before delivery of the infant. Prenatal care consists of a series of scheduled medical office visits for promotion of the health of the mother and fetus through prevention of disease and early detection, diagnosis, and treatment of problems common to pregnancy (e.g., anemia, urinary tract infection, and preeclampsia). Early detection of medical problems helps prevent serious complications in the mother and the fetus.

Obstetric Terminology

The medical assistant should know the common terms related to obstetrics, as follows:

Braxton Hicks contractions Intermittent and irregular painless uterine contractions that occur throughout pregnancy. They occur more frequently toward the end of pregnancy and are sometimes mistaken for true labor pains.

Dilation Stretching of the external os (of the cervix) from an opening of a few millimeters to an opening large enough to allow the passage of an infant (approximately 10 cm).

Effacement Thinning and shortening of the cervical canal from its normal length of 1 to 2 cm to a structure with paper-thin edges in which there is no canal at all. Effacement occurs late in pregnancy, during labor, or both. The purpose of effacement, along with dilation, is to permit the passage of the infant into the birth canal.

Embryo The child in utero from the time of conception through the first 8 weeks of development. (i.e., the first 2 months of development).

Engagement The entrance of the fetal head or the presenting part into the pelvic inlet.

Fetus The child in utero, from the third month after conception to birth; during the first 2 months of development, it is called an *embryo.*

Fundus The dome-shaped upper portion of the uterus between the fallopian tubes.

Gestation The period of intrauterine development from conception to birth; the period of pregnancy. The average pregnancy lasts about 280 days, or 40 weeks, from the date of conception to childbirth.

Gestational age The age of the fetus between conception and birth.

Infant A child from birth to 12 months old.

Multigravida A woman who has been pregnant more than once.

Multipara A woman who has completed two or more pregnancies to the age of viability regardless of whether they ended in live infants or stillbirths.

Nullipara A woman who has not carried a pregnancy to the point of fetal viability (20 weeks of gestation).

Position The relation of the presenting part of the fetus to the maternal pelvis.

Postpartum Occurring after childbirth.

Preeclampsia A major complication of pregnancy, the cause of which is unknown, characterized by increasing hypertension, albuminuria, and edema. If the condition is neglected or is not treated properly, preeclampsia may develop into eclampsia, which could cause maternal convulsions and coma. In general, preeclampsia occurs between the 20th week of pregnancy and the end of the first week postpartum.

Presentation Indication of the part of the fetus that is closest to the cervix and is delivered first. A cephalic presentation is a delivery in which the fetal head is presenting against the cervix. A breech presentation is a delivery in which the buttocks or feet are presented instead of the head.

Primigravida A woman who is pregnant for the first time.

Primipara A woman who has carried a pregnancy to fetal viability (20 weeks of gestation) for the first time regardless of whether the infant was stillborn or alive at birth.

Puerperium The period of time (usually 4 to 6 weeks) after delivery in which the uterus and the body systems are returning to normal.

Quickening The first movements of the fetus in utero as felt by the mother; usually occurs between 16 and 20 weeks of gestation and is felt consistently thereafter.

Toxemia A condition that can occur in pregnant women that includes preeclampsia and eclampsia. If preeclampsia goes undiagnosed or is not satisfactorily controlled, it could develop into eclampsia, which is characterized by convulsions and coma.

Trimester Three months, or one third, of the gestational period. The 9 months of pregnancy are divided into three trimesters, each consisting of 3 months. From conception to 3 months is the first trimester, from 4 to 6 months is the second trimester, and from 7 to 9 months is the third trimester.

PRENATAL VISITS

Medical office visits for prenatal and postpartum care of the pregnant woman can be grouped into three major categories as follows:
1. First prenatal visit
2. Return prenatal visits
3. 6 weeks postpartum visit

First Prenatal Visit

The first prenatal visit usually occurs after the woman has missed her second menstrual period; if problems exist, the woman is seen after missing her first menstrual period. Regardless of whether or not the patient is happy and excited about the pregnancy, the first visit is often a stressful experience for the patient. The medical assistant plays an important role in relaxing the patient and relieving her anxiety.

The first prenatal visit requires more time than subsequent prenatal visits; sufficient time should be scheduled to allow a complete and accurate initial assessment of the pregnant woman. The components of the first prenatal visit vary depending on the medical office, but they usually include the following:

- Completion of a prenatal record form.
- Initial prenatal examination, consisting of a complete physical examination. Of particular importance are the breast, abdominal, and pelvic examinations.
- Prenatal patient education.
- Laboratory tests.

Prenatal Record

The prenatal record provides information regarding the past and present health of the patient and serves as a database and flow sheet for subsequent prenatal visits. The prenatal record is essential in helping identify high-risk patients. The medical assistant is usually responsible for collecting a portion of the information required for the prenatal record. Many types of prenatal record forms are available (Figure 23-10). The specific form used in the medical office is based on the physician's preference and the method used for conducting the prenatal examination.

Obtaining and recording information in the prenatal record from one visit to the next provides an opportunity for the medical assistant to develop a rapport with the patient. It is also an excellent time to relay information to her regarding various aspects of the prenatal and postnatal periods, such as an explanation of the changes occurring in her body, the signs and symptoms of labor, nutrition of the infant (breast feeding and bottle feeding), and care of the newborn infant. The prenatal record form should be completed in a quiet setting that is free from distractions. This gives the patient the confidence to discuss areas of concern openly, which helps ensure a complete and accurate prenatal history.

Past Medical History

The past medical history focuses on conditions that could affect the health of the mother and fetus, such as diabetes, hypertension, heart disease, autoimmune disorders, kidney disease, liver disease, varicosities or phlebitis, alcohol and tobacco intake, drug addiction, Rh sensitization, pulmonary disease (e.g., tuberculosis, asthma), bleeding tendencies, surgeries, anesthetic complications, previous abnormal Pap test results, infertility problems, sexually transmitted diseases, and allergies. In addition, the medical assistant solicits information from the patient regarding immunizations and childhood diseases to provide the physician with the information needed to assess her antibody protection against such diseases.

Menstrual History

A menstrual history is obtained from the patient. It includes the date of onset of menstruation, the menstrual interval cycle, the duration, the amount of flow (recorded as small, moderate, or large), and any gynecologic disorders. The form also includes a space for the patient to indicate whether or not she was using a method of contraception when she became pregnant.

Obstetric History

A thorough obstetric history is a component of the prenatal record and provides the opportunity to obtain information from the patient related to previous pregnancies.

If a woman is a multigravida, information about each pregnancy is obtained, including the date of delivery, gestation in weeks, length of labor in hours, birth weight and sex of the newborn, type of delivery (vaginal or cesarean section), type of anesthesia, and any maternal or infant complications. The obstetric history assists in identifying areas that may need to be investigated further or monitored during the prenatal period. Women with previous complications, such as premature labor, gestational diabetes, or postpartum hemorrhaging, are at risk for having these problems again.

Present Pregnancy History

The present pregnancy history establishes a baseline for the present health status of the prenatal patient. In addition, the patient is queried regarding any warning signs that may be present and that may place the mother or fetus in jeopardy, such as persistent headaches, visual disturbances, abdominal pain, vaginal bleeding, or discharge. The patient also is asked whether she has experienced any of the early signs of pregnancy, such as nausea, vomiting, fatigue, and breast changes.

All prescribed or over-the-counter medications (including vitamin supplements and herbal products) the patient is taking must be recorded. Certain medications cross the placental barrier and could be harmful to the developing fetus. The patient should be instructed not to take any medications without first checking with the physician.

In the space provided under the present pregnancy history, the medical assistant needs to record the date of the first day of the patient's LMP. The LMP is used to calculate due date, or **expected date of delivery (EDD)**, by use of the Nägele rule: Add 7 days to the date of the LMP, subtract 3 months, and add 1 year (EDD = LMP + 7 days − 3 months + 1 year). For example, if the date of the patient's LMP was June 10, 2016, the EDD is March 17, 2017. The problem is set up as follows:

6	10	2016 (LMP)
−3	+7	+1 (applying Nägele rule)
3	17	2017 (delivery date)

With use of the Nägele rule, approximately 4% of patients deliver spontaneously on the EDD; most patients

PRENATAL HEALTH HISTORY

PATIENT INFORMATION

Date: _____   EDD: _____   Referred By: _____

Name: _____   Phone (home): _____
       LAST   FIRST   MIDDLE   Phone (work): _____

Address: _____   Emergency Contact: _____
                                                Phone: _____
         CITY   STATE   ZIP

Date of Birth: ___/___/___ Age: ___ Marital Status: _____

Occupation: _____

Education: ☐ High School   ☐ College   ☐ Post-graduate

PAST MEDICAL HISTORY

	O Neg / + Pos	DETAIL POSITIVE REMARKS INCLUDE DATE AND TREATMENT		O Neg / + Pos	DETAIL POSITIVE REMARKS INCLUDE DATE AND TREATMENT
1. DIABETES			16. D (Rh) SENSITIZED		
2. HYPERTENSION			17. PULMONARY (TB, ASTHMA)		
3. HEART DISEASE			18. RHEUMATIC FEVER		
4. AUTOIMMUNE DISORDER			19. BLEEDING TENDENCY		
5. KIDNEY DISEASE/UTI			20. GYN SURGERY		
6. NEUROLOGIC/EPILEPSY			21. OPERATIONS/HOSPITALIZATIONS (YEAR AND REASON)		
7. PSYCHIATRIC					
8. HEPATITIS/LIVER DISEASE					
9. VARICOSITIES/PHLEBITIS					
10. THYROID DYSFUNCTION			22. ANESTHETIC COMPLICATIONS		
11. TRAUMA/DOMESTIC VIOLENCE			23. HISTORY OF ABNORMAL PAP		
12. BLOOD TRANSFUSION			24. UTERINE ANOMALY/DES		

	AMT/DAY PREPREG.	AMT/DAY PREG.	# YEARS USE			
				25. INFERTILITY		
				26. SEXUALLY TRANSMITTED DISEASE		
13. TOBACCO						
14. ALCOHOL						
15. STREET DRUGS				27. OTHER		

IMMUNIZATIONS:

Mark an X next to those you have had.

☐ Influenza   ☐ Chickenpox

☐ Hepatitis B   ☐ Pneumococcal

☐ Hib   ☐ Tuberculin Test

☐ Polio   ☐ Tetanus Booster

☐ MMR

ALLERGIES:

List all allergies (foods, drugs, environment).   ☐ None

_____
_____
_____
_____
_____

MENSTRUAL HISTORY

Menarche: Age of Onset _____

Frequency: Q _____ Days

Duration: _____ Days

Amount of Flow: ☐ Small   ☐ Moderate   ☐ Large

GYN Disorders (List): _____
_____
_____

On contraceptive at conception? ☐ Yes ☐ No

Figure 23-10 Example of a prenatal record form.

deliver during the period extending from 7 days before to 7 days after the EDD.

Gestation calculators are commercially available that can be used to determine the delivery date by lining up an arrow and the date of the LMP, using a movable inner cardboard wheel (Figure 23-11). These calculators require less time to determine the EDD than use of the Nägele rule, and they provide information on the probable size (length and weight) of the fetus on any given date. The accuracy of gestation calculators is comparable with that of the Nägele rule. In addition, there are also many online gestational calculators, as well as a variety of apps for mobile devices. If the patient is unsure of the date of her LMP, the physician estimates the length of gestation by other methods, such as fundal height measurement and sonography.

Interval Prenatal History

The interval prenatal history also is included in the prenatal record form; its purpose is to update the record. During every return visit, essential data, including weight, blood pressure, urine testing results, fundal height measurement, and fetal heart rate (FHR), are collected and recorded in

OBSTETRIC HISTORY

G _____ (Total Pregnancies) T _____ (Term) P _____ (Preterm) A _____ (Abortions) L _____ (Living Children)

PREVIOUS PREGNANCIES:

DATE MONTH/ YEAR	WEEKS GEST.	LENGTH OF LABOR	BIRTH WEIGHT	SEX M/F	TYPE DELIVERY	ANES.	MATERNAL COMPLICATIONS	INFANT COMPLICATIONS

PRESENT PREGNANCY HISTORY

NAUSEA			ABDOMINAL PAIN	
VOMITING			URINARY COMPLAINTS	
FATIGUE			VAGINAL BLEEDING	
BREAST CHANGES			VAGINAL DISCHARGE	
INDIGESTION			PRURITIS	
CONSTIPATION			ACCIDENTS	
PERSISTENT HEADACHES			SURGERY	
DIZZINESS			X-RAYS	
VISUAL DISTURBANCE			RUBELLA EXPOSURE	
EDEMA (SPECIFY AREA)			OTHER VIRAL INFECTIONS	

LMP _____ / _____ / _____
    Mo   Day   Year

Amount of Flow: ☐ Small   ☐ Moderate   ☐ Large

CURRENT MEDICATIONS: (Include prescription, OTC, herbal, and vitamins). ☐ None

Medication _____   **Frequency** _____

INITIAL PHYSICAL EXAMINATION

DATE ____ / ____ / ____

1. HEENT	☐ NORMAL ☐ ABNORMAL	12. VULVA	☐ NORMAL	☐ CONDYLOMA	☐ LESIONS
2. FUNDI	☐ NORMAL ☐ ABNORMAL	13. VAGINA	☐ NORMAL	☐ INFLAMMATION	☐ DISCHARGE
3. TEETH	☐ NORMAL ☐ ABNORMAL	14. CERVIX	☐ NORMAL	☐ INFLAMMATION	☐ LESIONS
4. THYROID	☐ NORMAL ☐ ABNORMAL	15. UTERUS SIZE	_____ WEEKS		☐ FIBROIDS
5. BREASTS	☐ NORMAL ☐ ABNORMAL	16. ADNEXA	☐ NORMAL	☐ MASS	
6. LUNGS	☐ NORMAL ☐ ABNORMAL	17. RECTUM	☐ NORMAL	☐ ABNORMAL	
7. HEART	☐ NORMAL ☐ ABNORMAL	18. DIAGONAL CONJUGATE	☐ REACHED	☐ NO	_____ CM
8. ABDOMEN	☐ NORMAL ☐ ABNORMAL	19. SPINES	☐ AVERAGE	☐ PROMINENT	☐ BLUNT
9. EXTREMITIES	☐ NORMAL ☐ ABNORMAL	20. SACRUM	☐ CONCAVE	☐ STRAIGHT	☐ ANTERIOR
10. SKIN	☐ NORMAL ☐ ABNORMAL	21. SUBPUBIC ARCH	☐ NORMAL	☐ WIDE	☐ NARROW
11. LYMPH NODES	☐ NORMAL ☐ ABNORMAL	22. GYNECOID PELVIC TYPE	☐ YES	☐ NO	

COMMENTS (Number and explain abnormals): _____
_____
_____

EXAM BY _____

Figure 23-10, cont'd

Continued

this section. A general inquiry is made regarding the occurrence of additional signs of pregnancy, such as fetal movement or Braxton Hicks contractions, and how the patient is feeling and any concerns or symptoms since the last prenatal visit.

This information is recorded and assists the medical staff in planning, implementing, and evaluating individual needs. Particular attention is focused on risk factors, such as hypertension, thrombophlebitis, and uterine bleeding, which could influence the course of the pregnancy.

Initial Prenatal Examination

Purpose

The initial prenatal examination is of particular importance because it results in confirmation of the pregnancy and establishes a baseline for the woman's state of health. It includes a thorough gynecologic examination (breast and pelvic examinations) and a general physical examination of the other body systems, although the latter may be performed during a subsequent prenatal visit, depending on the medical office routine.

PATIENT'S NAME _____

INTERVAL PRENATAL HISTORY

Date 20___	Weeks Gestation	Height of Fundus (cm)	Weight	B/P	Urine Glucose	Urine Protein	FHT	Vaginal Examination	Presentation	Edema	Discharge	Bleeding	Contractions	Fetal Activity	NST	Next Appt.	Initials

PLANS/EDUCATION   (COUNSELED ☑)

☐ ANESTHESIA PLANS _____
☐ TOXOPLASMOSIS PRECAUTIONS (CATS/RAW MEAT) _____
☐ CHILDBIRTH CLASSES _____
☐ PHYSICAL/SEXUAL ACTIVITY _____
☐ LABOR SIGNS _____
☐ NUTRITION COUNSELING _____
☐ BREAST OR BOTTLE FEEDING _____
☐ NEWBORN CAR SEAT _____
☐ POSTPARTUM BIRTH CONTROL _____
☐ ENVIRONMENTAL/WORK HAZARDS _____

☐ TUBAL STERILIZATION _____
☐ VBAC COUNSELING _____
☐ CIRCUMCISION _____
☐ TRAVEL _____
☐ LIFESTYLE, TOBACCO, ALCOHOL _____

REQUESTS _____
_____

TUBAL STERILIZATION
CONSENT SIGNED   DATE ___/___/___   INITIALS _____

Figure 23-10, cont'd

Women often have little or no medical supervision during their childbearing years; the physical examination is of particular importance in establishing a baseline for the woman's general state of health and in identifying high-risk prenatal patients. Conditions such as obesity, hypertension, severe varicosities, and uterine size inappropriate for the due date can be diagnosed by the physician, and necessary treatment or monitoring can be instituted to help prevent complications.

Preparation of the Patient

When the patient arrives at the medical office and the prenatal record form has been completed, the medical assistant is responsible for taking and recording the patient's vital signs, height, and weight to provide a database for subsequent prenatal visits. The patient is asked to disrobe completely and put on an examining gown with the opening in front. The medical assistant must give complete and thorough instructions so the patient knows exactly what is expected. The patient should be asked whether she needs to empty her bladder because an empty bladder facilitates the examination and is more comfortable for her. If the office policy is such that a specimen is needed for urine testing at the initial prenatal visit, the patient will be required to void.

Special precautions should be taken in assisting the prenatal patient. The medical assistant should support the patient as she gets onto and off the scale and examining

LABORATORY		PATIENT'S NAME _____			
INITIAL LABS	**DATE**	**RESULTS**		**REVIEWED**	**COMMENTS**
BLOOD TYPE	/ /	A B AB O			
Rh FACTOR	/ /	☐ Pos ☐ Neg			
Rh ANTIBODY SCREEN	/ /	☐ Pos ☐ Neg			
HCT/HGB	/ /	_____% _____ g/dL			
RUBELLA ANTIBODY TITER	/ /	Immune Nonimmune			
VDRL	/ /	☐ NR ☐ R			
HBsAg (HEPATITIS B)	/ /	☐ Pos ☐ Neg			
HIV	/ /	☐ Pos ☐ Neg ☐ Declined			
URINE CULTURE/SCREEN	/ /				
PAP TEST	/ /	☐ Normal ☐ Abnormal			
CHLAMYDIA (DNA PROBE)	/ /	☐ Pos ☐ Neg			
GONORRHEA (DNA PROBE)	/ /	☐ Pos ☐ Neg			
7–20 WEEK LABS (WHEN INDICATED/ELECTED)	**DATE**	**RESULTS**		**REVIEWED**	**COMMENTS**
ULTRASOUND #1 (7–12 WEEKS)	/ /	EDD:			
ULTRASOUND #2 (18–20 WEEKS)	/ /	EFW:			
TRIPLE SCREEN (15–20 WEEKS)	/ /				
CVS	/ /				
AMNIOCENTESIS	/ /				
24–28 WEEK LABS (WHEN INDICATED)	**DATE**	**RESULTS**		**REVIEWED**	**COMMENTS**
HCT/HGB	/ /	_____ % _____ g/dL			
GCT (24–28 WKS)	/ /	1 Hour _____			
GTT (IF SCREEN ABNORMAL)	/ /	_____ FBS _____ 1 Hour _____ 2 Hour _____ 3 Hour			
D (Rh) ANTIBODY SCREEN	/ /				
D IMMUNE GLOBULIN (RhIG) GIVEN (28 WKS)	/ /	SIGNATURE			
32–36 WEEK LABS	**DATE**	**RESULTS**		**REVIEWED**	**COMMENTS**
HCT/HGB (32 WKS)	/ /	_____ % _____ g/dL			
ULTRASOUND #3 (34 WKS)	/ /	EFW:			
GROUP B STREP (35–37 WKS)	/ /	☐ Pos ☐ Neg			
ADDITIONAL LAB TESTS	**DATE**	**RESULTS**		**REVIEWED**	**COMMENTS**
	/ /				
	/ /				
	/ /				
	/ /				
	/ /				

Figure 23-10, cont'd

table to ensure her safety and comfort. This is especially important as the pregnancy progresses and the patient becomes more awkward and off balance.

The medical assistant is responsible for setting up the tray required for the examination. The setup includes the equipment and supplies required for the procedures to be performed. During the prenatal examination, the medical assistant is responsible for positioning the patient as required for each aspect of the examination and assisting the physician as necessary.

Patient Education

At the conclusion of the initial prenatal examination and after the patient is dressed, the physician talks with her regarding instructions on diet, weight gain, rest, sleep, employment, exercise, travel, sexual intercourse, dental care, smoking, alcohol, and drugs. Many offices have a prenatal guidebook designed especially for this purpose that is given to each patient to use as a reference. Some offices also use a series of teaching films that the patient views during the return prenatal visit while waiting to see the physician. The physician also prescribes a daily vitamin supplement to be taken during the prenatal period to ensure that the mother and fetus obtain an adequate supply of vitamins and minerals.

When the physician is finished talking with the patient, the medical assistant is responsible for scheduling the next prenatal visit and for ensuring that the patient understands the instructions for maintaining health and preventing disease during the pregnancy. The medical assistant should tell the patient to report the occurrence of any warning signs during the pregnancy (see the *Warning Signs During Pregnancy* box) and not to take any medications without first checking with the physician. The patient also should be encouraged to contact the medical office should any questions or problems arise.

Warning Signs During Pregnancy

Signs of Infection
- Fever
- Vaginal discharge
- Dysuria
- Increased frequency of urination
- Marked decrease in urinary output

Signs of Spontaneous Abortion
- Vaginal bleeding
- Persistent low back pain
- Abdominal pain and cramping

Signs of Preeclampsia
- Severe, persistent headache
- Dizziness
- Blurred vision
- Sudden swelling of hands, feet, or face

- Sudden rapid weight gain
- Abdominal pain

Signs of Placental or Fetal Problems
- Vaginal spotting or bleeding
- Abdominal pain and cramping
- Back pain
- Noticeable decrease in fetal activity
- No fetal movement

Signs of Preterm Labor
- Regular or frequent contractions (more than four to six per hour)
- Recurring low, dull backache
- Menstrual-like cramping
- Unusual pressure in the pelvis, low back, abdomen, or thighs

Figure 23-11 Gestation calculator. The last menstrual period is July 20, and the expected date of delivery is April 25.

Laboratory Tests

The physician orders many laboratory tests to assist in the assessment of the patient's state of health and to detect problems that may put the pregnancy at risk. Several tests, such as the Pap test and the chlamydia and gonorrhea tests, require the physician to collect the specimens at the medical office and have them transported by laboratory courier to an outside laboratory for evaluation. The specimen required for the prenatal blood tests (known as a *prenatal profile*) must be obtained through a venipuncture to provide a sufficient quantity of blood for the number of tests ordered.

The blood specimen is collected at the medical office or at an outside laboratory.

It is important to have these initial tests completed as soon as possible to provide the physician with the test results by the time of the next scheduled prenatal visit. Based on the results of the prenatal examination and the laboratory tests, the physician may order additional tests to assess the patient's condition. Certain tests and procedures, such as the glucose challenge test (GCT) and the group B *Streptococcus* (GBS) test, are scheduled later in the pregnancy. The prenatal laboratory tests that are usually performed on a pregnant woman are described next.

Urine Tests
Urinalysis

A complete urinalysis, including physical, chemical, and microscopic analyses of the urine, is performed; a clean-catch midstream urine specimen is typically required for the test. If bacteria are found in the urine specimen, the physician usually requests a urine culture and sensitivity test to determine the possible presence of a urinary tract infection. A pregnancy test also may be performed on the urine specimen, if ordered by the physician.

Swab Tests
Pap Test

A Pap test is done for the detection of abnormalities of cell growth to diagnose precancerous or cancerous conditions of the cervix. This test also can be used for hormonal assessment (maturation index) and to assist in the detection of vaginal infections.

Chlamydia and Gonorrhea

Specimens are taken from the endocervical canal and sent to the laboratory to rule out chlamydia and gonorrhea. Chlamydia can be passed from an infected woman to her infant during childbirth, resulting in conjunctivitis and pneumonia in the newborn. If a gonorrheal infection is present at the time of delivery, the *N. gonorrhoeae* organism could infect the infant's eyes during passage through the birth canal. This may result in *ophthalmia neonatorum,* which, if not treated, could lead to blindness. For this reason, most states require that pregnant women be tested for gonorrhea, and that the eyes of newborns be treated with antibiotic drops immediately after birth to kill any gonococcal bacteria that may be present. A patient who is diagnosed with chlamydia or gonorrhea requires immediate treatment with an appropriate antibiotic to prevent problems for herself and her child.

Trichomoniasis and Candidiasis

If an excessive irritating vaginal discharge is present, the physician obtains a specimen to rule out trichomoniasis and candidiasis. It is important to control candidiasis before delivery to prevent the development of thrush, a yeastlike infection of the infant's mucous membranes of the mouth or throat.

Group B *Streptococcus*

GBS is a common bacterium often found in the vagina and rectum of healthy women. Normally, one in four pregnant women carries GBS. GBS is not harmful to a pregnant woman, but it can cause life-threatening infections in the newborn. While passing through the birth canal, a newborn can become infected with the bacteria carried by the mother. When infected, the infant may develop an infection of the blood (septicemia), pneumonia, or meningitis.

To prevent GBS infection of the newborn, a pregnant woman is tested for the bacteria between 35 and 37 weeks of gestation. Using two swabs, the physician collects specimens from the vagina and the rectum. The specimen swabs are placed in a transport tube and sent to the laboratory to be cultured for GBS. If GBS is found, intravenous antibiotics are administered to the woman every 4 hours during labor until delivery. In most cases, this antibiotic administration prevents the newborn from becoming infected with GBS. In situations in which the newborn does become infected with GBS, antibiotics are administered immediately, and the infant is closely monitored.

Blood Tests

Complete Blood Count

The complete blood count (CBC) is a basic screening test used to assist in assessing the patient's state of health. It includes a hemoglobin, hematocrit, white blood cell count, red blood cell count, differential white blood cell count, platelet count, and red blood cell indices. Of particular importance with respect to the prenatal patient are the hemoglobin and hematocrit evaluations, which are described here.

Hemoglobin and Hematocrit

Low hemoglobin or hematocrit values are seen in cases of anemia. Prenatal patients have a tendency to develop anemia because there is an increased demand for and correlating increased production of red blood cells during

pregnancy; the physician carefully reviews the results of these tests. If the hemoglobin or hematocrit value is low, further hematologic evaluation is usually required. If necessary, therapy is instituted, which usually consists of an iron supplement and nutritional counseling. The hemoglobin and hematocrit values are checked again at approximately 32 weeks of gestation as a precaution against anemia before delivery.

What Would You Do?	**What Would You *Not* Do?**

Case Study 3

Johanna Kruger is 24 years old and pregnant with her first child. She is at the office for her first prenatal visit. She is quite upset. Her best friend just had her first baby, and the baby died 24 hours later from a group B *Streptococcus* (GBS) infection. Johanna is afraid that the same thing will happen to her baby. She wants to be tested for GBS as soon as possible. She has some antibiotics at home and is thinking of taking them. Johanna is worried because she has been experiencing some problems with her pregnancy. She is sick all day, her breasts hurt, and yesterday she had some spotting. Johanna is hesitant to tell all of this to the physician because he might think she worries too much. ■

Rh Factor and ABO Blood Type

Tests are performed to anticipate ABO blood type and Rh factor incompatibilities. If the patient is Rh-negative, the father's blood type also must be evaluated. If the father's blood type is Rh positive, the possibility of an Rh incompatibility exists. This situation warrants the performance of an Rh antibody titer test and repeat antibody titers throughout the pregnancy to determine whether the mother's antibody level is increasing. An increased Rh antibody level could be dangerous to the developing fetus. It can result in severe anemia, jaundice, brain damage, heart failure, and sometimes death of the fetus.

Glucose Challenge Test

A glucose challenge test (GCT) is performed between 24 and 28 weeks of gestation to screen for gestational diabetes mellitus (GDM). This test works by assessing the body's response to a measured glucose solution. The patient does not need to fast for this test, and no preparation is required other than arriving at the laboratory at the scheduled time. To perform the GCT, the patient is asked to drink 50 g of a glucose solution, and her glucose level is measured 1 hour later. A woman with a glucose level of less than 140 mg/dL does not have GDM and requires no further testing. If the glucose level is greater than 140 mg/dL, the test result is abnormal. Not all women with elevated results have diabetes, however, and further testing using the 3-hour oral glucose tolerance test (OGTT) must be performed before a final diagnosis can be made. (*Note:* Refer to Chapter 33 for information on the OGTT.)

Syphilis Test

The microorganism that causes syphilis, *Treponema pallidum,* is able to cross the placental barrier and infect the fetus; this could result in intrauterine death or could cause the fetus to be born with congenital syphilis. Infants with congenital syphilis are often born with deformities and may become blind, deaf, paralyzed, or insane. The tests most commonly employed to screen for the presence of syphilis are the Venereal Disease Research Laboratory (VDRL) test and the rapid plasma reagin (RPR) test. The test results are reported as nonreactive, weakly reactive, or reactive. Because these tests are screening tests, a weakly reactive or reactive test result warrants more specific testing to arrive at a diagnosis of syphilis. Examples of these tests are the fluorescent treponemal antibody absorption (FTA-ABS) test and the *T. pallidum* particle agglutination assay (TPPA) test.

A prenatal test for syphilis is mandated by most states and should be performed early in the pregnancy, before fetal damage occurs. A patient who has contracted syphilis requires treatment with an appropriate antibiotic.

Rubella Antibody Titer

The rubella antibody titer assesses the level of antibody against rubella (German measles) in the patient's blood and is used to determine whether the woman is immune to rubella. If the mother contracts rubella during pregnancy, serious congenital abnormalities can occur in the fetus. Patients who lack immunity should be immunized against rubella within 6 weeks of delivery.

Rh Antibody Titer (on Rh-Negative Blood Specimens)

An Rh antibody titer detects the quantity of circulating Rh antibodies against red blood cells. These antibodies can occur in a pregnant woman who is Rh negative and is carrying an Rh-positive fetus; an Rh antibody titer is performed on all Rh-negative blood specimens. Repeat antibody titer levels also are performed during the pregnancy to determine whether the woman's antibody level is increasing. As was previously indicated, an increased Rh antibody level could be dangerous to the developing fetus. As a preventive measure, Rh-negative women with the potential for having an Rh-positive infant and who test negative for Rh antibodies are given two injections of Rh immune globulin (RhoGAM). The RhoGAM prevents the formation of Rh antibodies in the mother, which avoids Rh incompatibility complications during the next pregnancy. The first injection is given at 28 weeks of gestation, and the second injection is administered within 72 hours of delivery.

Hepatitis B and Human Immunodeficiency Virus

The Centers for Disease Control and Prevention (CDC) recommends that pregnant women have the hepatitis B surface antigen (HBsAg) test to screen for hepatitis B virus. Women who have positive HBsAg test results have an increased risk of spontaneous abortion or preterm labor. In addition, the mother may transmit hepatitis B to the infant, particularly during delivery or in the first few days of life. This risk can be greatly reduced by administering hepatitis B immune globulin (HBIG) and the hepatitis B vaccine within 12 hours of birth to the newborns of women who have tested positive for hepatitis B.

Infants born to women who are HIV positive are at risk of developing the disease. If antiretroviral drugs are taken during pregnancy and the infant is delivered by cesarean section, the chance of transmitting HIV to the infant is reduced significantly. Because of this, the CDC recommends that testing for HIV be included in the routine panel of prenatal screening tests for all pregnant women and that separate written consent not be required. The CDC further recommends that the patient should be notified that HIV testing will be performed unless the patient declines the test. The CDC recommends that repeat HIV screening be performed in the third trimester in geographic areas that have elevated rates of HIV infection among pregnant women.

Return Prenatal Visits

Return prenatal visits provide the opportunity for a continuous assessment of the health of the mother and the fetus. During each visit, essential data are collected and recorded in the prenatal record, resulting in an updated record at each visit, as is discussed in this section. If signs or symptoms of a pathologic condition are present, the physician performs select aspects of the physical examination as necessary to diagnose and treat the condition. In addition, diagnostic and laboratory tests may be ordered to assist in diagnosis and treatment. The usual schedule of visits for prenatal care is as follows:
- 0 to 28 weeks of gestation: every 4 weeks
- 29 to 35 weeks: every 2 weeks
- 36 weeks until delivery: every week

A patient who exhibits complications is seen more frequently for closer monitoring.

The return prenatal visit also provides the opportunity for the physician and the medical assistant to lend support to the mother, to provide her with ongoing prenatal education to reduce apprehension and anxiety, and to ensure that the mother is well informed and prepared during her pregnancy, childbirth, and the postpartum period. The medical assistant plays an important role in prenatal education and should take the necessary time with each patient to provide appropriate information and to allow the patient to ask questions. Procedure 23-3 outlines the medical assistant's role in the return prenatal visit.

The patient is asked to provide a urine specimen during each return prenatal visit. The medical assistant is responsible for testing the specimen for glucose and protein using a reagent strip and for documenting results in the prenatal record. A positive reaction to glucose may indicate the development of gestational diabetes mellitus or a prediabetic condition, and a positive reaction to protein may indicate a urinary tract infection or preeclampsia. Further testing usually is needed to arrive at a final diagnosis and to institute treatment. Hypertension is the most common medical disorder of pregnancy and occurs in 10% to 12% of all pregnancies. Because of this, the medical assistant must make sure to obtain an accurate blood pressure measurement.

During the return visit, the physician performs one or more of the following procedures, depending on the stage of the pregnancy: (1) palpation of the woman's abdomen to

Figure 23-12 Measurement of fundal height. The physician places one end of a centimeter tape measure on the superior aspect of the symphysis pubis and measures to the top of the uterine fundus.

measure fundal height, (2) measurement of the fetal heart rate, and (3) a vaginal examination. These procedures are discussed in detail next.

Fundal Height Measurement

The pregnant uterus rises gradually into the abdominal cavity, and the fundus is palpable between 8 and 13 weeks of gestation. The first fundal height measurement, which is usually performed during the first prenatal visit, is used as a guideline for all subsequent measurements. The physician measures the fundal height by placing one end of a flexible, nonstretchable centimeter tape measure on the superior aspect of the symphysis pubis and measuring to the crest or top of the uterine fundus (Figure 23-12). The measurement is recorded on a flow chart in the patient's prenatal record. By 20 weeks the fundus reaches the lower border of the umbilicus, and by 36 to 37 weeks it reaches the tip of the sternum. During the first and second trimesters, measuring the fundal height provides a rough estimate of the duration of the pregnancy (Figure 23-13).

Because fetal weights vary considerably during the third trimester, it is difficult to use fundal height measurements as an estimate of the duration of the pregnancy in the last trimester.

In addition to assessing the duration of the pregnancy, the fundal height measurements permit variations from normal to become apparent and are used to assess whether fetal growth is progressing normally. Growth that is too rapid or too slow must be evaluated further by the physician as a possible indication of high-risk conditions, such as multiple pregnancies, polyhydramnios, ovarian tumor, and

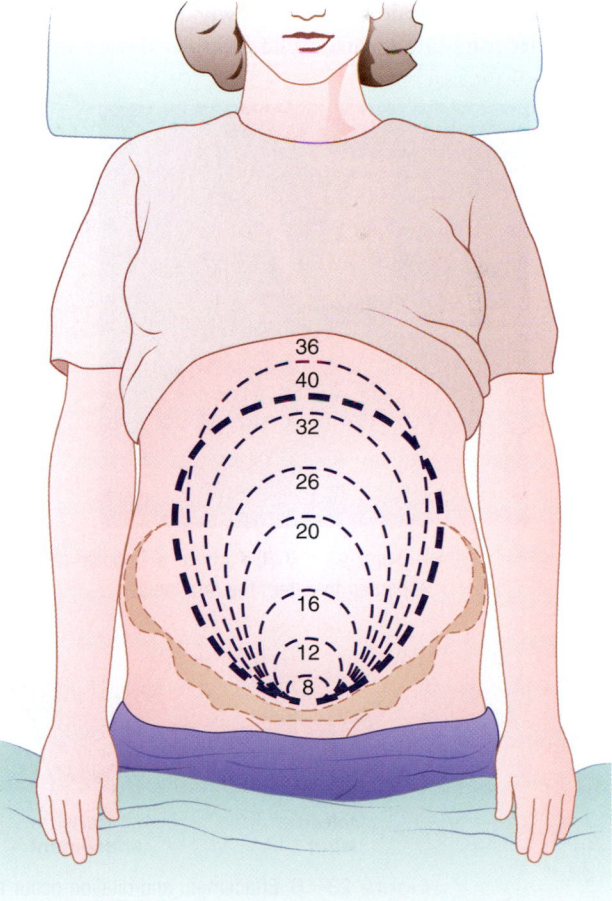

Figure 23-13 Fundal height showing gestational age in weeks.

intrauterine growth retardation; intrauterine death; or an error in estimating the fetal progress.

Fetal Heart Tones

The normal **fetal heart rate** is between 120 and 160 beats per minute with a regular rhythm. A very slow or rapid FHR usually indicates fetal distress. The term **fetal heart tones** refers to the heartbeat of the fetus as heard through the mother's abdominal wall. The fetal heart tones can be heard with a Doppler fetal pulse detector between 10 and 12 weeks of gestation. The Doppler fetal pulse detector converts ultrasonic waves into audible sounds of the fetal pulse.

The Doppler device consists of a main control unit and a probe (Figure 23-14, *A*). The probe head contains a transducer and electronic components, which generate the sound waves. The probe head is delicate and must be handled carefully, making sure not to drop or knock the head to prevent damaging it.

Because air is a poor conductor of sound, an ultrasound coupling gel must first be spread on the mother's abdomen in the area to be examined. The gel is usually applied by the medical assistant, and its purpose is to increase conductivity of the sound waves between the abdomen and the transducer.

The physician places the head of the probe into the gel on the mother's abdomen and slowly moves it until the fetal heart tones are located. The Doppler device amplifies

the fetal heart tones, and they are broadcast through a built-in loudspeaker in the main unit. A volume control provides adjustment of the sound level as required. (Fetal heart tones sound like the hoofbeats of a galloping horse, and when the probe is over the placenta, a windlike sound is heard.) The Doppler device also may have a liquid crystal diode (LCD) screen, which provides a digital display of the fetal pulse rate. Stereo headphones come with the Doppler device to allow private listening. The loudspeaker is muted when the headphones are connected (Figure 23-14, *B*).

After the procedure, the medical assistant should remove excess gel from the mother's abdomen with a paper towel. The probe head is cleaned using a damp cloth or a paper towel. The Doppler device should be properly stored in its carrying case to prevent it from becoming damaged.

Vaginal Examination

In the absence of vaginal bleeding, vaginal examinations may be performed at any time during the pregnancy; however, in a normal pregnancy, there is usually no need to perform a vaginal examination until the patient nears term. The vaginal examination is usually begun approximately 2 to 3 weeks from the EDD and is performed to confirm the presenting part and to determine the degree, if any, of cervical dilation and effacement. The purpose of dilation and effacement is to permit the passage of the infant from the uterus into the birth canal (Figure 23-15).

Figure 23-14 A, Parts of a Doppler device. **B,** The probe of the Doppler device is moved across the abdomen to detect the fetal pulse.

Figure 23-15 Effacement and dilation occur to permit the passage of the infant into the birth canal. The cervical canal shortens from its normal length of 1 to 2 cm to a structure with paper thin edges in which there is no canal at all. The cervix dilates from an opening a few millimeters wide to an opening large enough to allow the passage of the infant (approximately 10 cm).

Case Study 4

Wynita Lopez is at the office with her husband. She is 32 years old and 18 weeks pregnant. It took Wynita a long time—almost 6 years—to get pregnant. She is excited and happy about being pregnant but, at the same time, sad and confused. Her test results on her multiple marker test came back indicating the possibility that her baby has Down syndrome. A repeat test was done with the same results. Wynita just got finished having an ultrasound that showed a normal baby, but Wynita and her husband understand that the only way to know for sure is to have an amniocentesis. Wynita does not know what to do. She is afraid of having an amniocentesis because of the chance of miscarriage. She also knows her multiple marker test result could be a false positive. Wynita is unsure what her decision would be if the baby did have Down syndrome. Her husband is visibly distressed and wants Wynita to make all the decisions, saying he will be supportive of whatever she decides. Right now she wants as much information as she can get about all of this before she makes a decision. She feels "safer" being at the medical office and does not want to go home just yet. ■

Special Tests and Procedures

The pregnancy can be evaluated with one or more of the following special tests and procedures: multiple marker test, obstetric ultrasound scan, amniocentesis, and fetal heart rate monitoring. These are not considered routine procedures; however, they involve little or no risk to the mother or the fetus. Because some of these tests may be performed in the obstetric medical office, the medical assistant should have a general knowledge of these procedures.

Multiple Marker Test

The multiple marker test is a laboratory test available to pregnant women between 15 and 20 weeks of gestation. Its purpose is to screen for the presence of certain fetal abnormalities, which include neural tube defects, Down syndrome, trisomy 18, and ventral wall defect. Because the multiple marker test has a high incidence of false-positive test results, it is not a mandatory prenatal test; however, the American College of Obstetricians and Gynecologists believes that this test should be offered to all pregnant women regardless of maternal age.

The multiple marker test is a screening test. Abnormal test results always necessitate further testing, such as an ultrasound or amniocentesis, to determine whether a fetal abnormality actually exists.

Obstetric Ultrasound Scan

An obstetric ultrasound scan is a diagnostic imaging technique, similar to sonar, used to view the fetus in utero. It allows continuous viewing of the fetus and shows fetal movement. The physician or an ultrasound technologist performs the procedure. The primary purpose of an ultrasound scan is to evaluate the health of the fetus and to

Figure 23-16 Obstetric ultrasound scan.

determine gestational age. This is accomplished by viewing the image of the fetus and by taking various measurements of the image, such as crown-rump length; biparietal diameter, which is a side-to-side measurement of the fetal head; femur length; and abdominal circumference.

Obstetric ultrasound scanning uses high-frequency sound waves that are directed into the uterus through a transducer. When the sound waves reach the uterus, they "bounce" back to the transducer, similar to an echo. These reflected sound waves are converted into an image, or *sonogram* (Figure 23-16), which is displayed on a monitor screen. The monitor is usually positioned so the mother can observe the image on the screen if she wishes. Although an obstetric ultrasound scan can be performed at any time during the pregnancy, it is often performed at between 7 and 12 weeks of gestation and again at between 18 and 20 weeks. A third scan is sometimes done at around 34 weeks of gestation. Box 23-1 outlines this schedule and what can be assessed at these times.

Amniocentesis

Amniocentesis is a diagnostic procedure that can be performed between 15 and 18 weeks of gestation. Amniocentesis aids in prenatal diagnosis of certain genetically transmitted errors of metabolism, congenital abnormalities, and chromosomal disorders such as Down syndrome. It also is used to detect fetal jeopardy or distress and, later in the pregnancy, to assess fetal lung maturity. Amniocentesis also can determine whether the fetus is male or female.

To perform the procedure, the physician inserts a long, thin needle through the mother's abdomen and into the amniotic sac surrounding the fetus (Figure 23-17). An obstetric ultrasound scan is always performed in conjunction with amniocentesis so that the physician can view the position of the fetus, placenta, and amniotic fluid. This allows the physician to know the exact place to insert the needle. The physician withdraws a sample (about 1 tablespoon) of fluid, which contains fetal cells. The fluid is sent to a laboratory for study. It usually takes 1 to 3 weeks to evaluate the amniotic fluid and report the results.

BOX 23-1   Purpose of Obstetric Ultrasound Scanning

Between 7 and 12 Weeks

- To confirm pregnancy by detecting fetal heart motion
- To determine gestational age by taking measurements of the embryo and embryonic sac
- To detect an ectopic pregnancy

Twins.

Embryo at approximately 9 weeks of gestation. (From Greer IA, Cameron IT, Kitchener HC, Prentice A: *Mosby's color atlas and text of obstetrics and gynecology,* St Louis, 2001, Mosby.)

Between 18 and 20 Weeks

- To determine fetal growth, size, and weight by taking measurements of the fetus
- To detect the presence of multiple fetuses
- To examine the brain, spinal cord, heart, lungs, gastrointestinal tract, reproductive organs, kidneys, bladder, bowel, and extremities of the fetus
- To detect congenital abnormalities
- To determine the location of the placenta
- To determine the cause of bleeding or spotting

External female genitalia. *1,* Major labium; *2,* minor labium; *3,* vaginal cleft; *4,* thighs. (From Callen P: *Ultrasonography in obstetrics and gynecology,* ed 5, Philadelphia, 2008, Saunders.)

Erect fetal penis. *1,* Urethra; *2,* corpus cavernosum; *3,* shaft; *4,* glans; *5,* foreskin. (From Callen P: *Ultrasonography in obstetrics and gynecology,* ed 5, Philadelphia, 2008, Saunders.)

BOX 23-1   Purpose of Obstetric Ultrasound Scanning—cont'd

At 34 Weeks
- To evaluate fetal growth, size, and weight by taking measurements of the fetus
- To verify the location of the placenta
- To confirm fetal presentation in uncertain cases

Other Purposes
- To diagnose uterine and pelvic abnormalities during pregnancy
- To view the fetus, placenta, and amniotic fluid during tests such as amniocentesis and chorionic villus sampling
- To confirm intrauterine death

Amniocentesis being performed under ultrasound guidance. (From Greer IA, Cameron IT, Kitchener HC, Prentice A: *Mosby's color atlas and text of obstetrics and gynecology,* St. Louis, 2001, Mosby.)

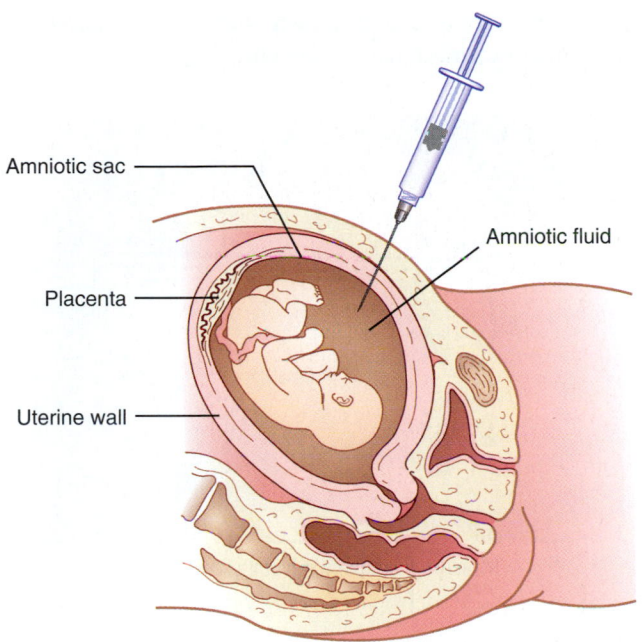

Figure 23-17 Amniocentesis.

Although the complication rate for amniocentesis is extremely low, the procedure is not risk free. There is a slight risk of bleeding, leakage of fluid, and infection of the amniotic fluid. There also is a slight possibility of miscarriage. Because of these risks, amniocentesis is offered only to women whose pregnancies are at risk for fetal abnormalities. This includes women who are 35 years old or older, women who have a child with a genetic or neural tube defect, women who have multiple marker test results, women who

have or whose partner has a chromosomal abnormality, and women who are carriers or whose partner is a carrier for a metabolic disease.

Fetal Heart Rate Monitoring
Fetal heart rate monitoring is performed later in the pregnancy to obtain information on the physical condition of the fetus. Specific conditions that may warrant this procedure are fetal growth that is not progressing well, decreased amniotic fluid, decreased fetal activity, elevation of the mother's blood pressure, gestational diabetes, and an overdue infant.

For this procedure an electronic microphone is strapped to the mother's abdomen to amplify the fetal heartbeat. A gel is usually applied under the microphone to make the sounds clearer. The fetal heartbeat is heard and displayed on a screen and printed on special paper.

MEDICAL ASSISTING RESPONSIBILITIES

The medical assistant has many important responsibilities in the return prenatal examination, which are outlined in Procedure 23-3. The medical assistant is responsible for assembling the equipment and supplies required for the examination, for obtaining information to update the prenatal record, for preparing the patient for the examination, and for assisting the physician during the examination. The physician depends on the medical assistant to have the urine test results and certain measurements, such as blood pressure and weight, completed and recorded in advance to allow him or her the opportunity to review these measurements before examining the patient.

PROCEDURE 23-3   Assisting with a Return Prenatal Examination

Outcome Assist with a return prenatal examination

Equipment/Supplies

- Urine specimen container
- Centimeter tape measure
- Doppler fetal pulse detector
- Ultrasound coupling gel
- Paper towel

- Disposable vaginal speculum
- Disposable gloves
- Water-based lubricant
- Gauze pads
- Examining gown and drape

1. Procedural Step. Sanitize your hands.

2. Procedural Step. Set up the tray for the prenatal examination. The equipment and supplies depend on the procedures to be included in the examination, which may include one or more of the following:
  a. Fundal height measurement
  b. Measurement of fetal heart tones
  c. Examination of the legs, feet, and face for edema and development of varicosities
  d. Taking a specimen for the diagnosis of a vaginal infection
  e. Vaginal examination

Set up the prenatal tray.

3. Procedural Step. Greet the patient and introduce yourself. Identify the patient and explain the procedure. Provide the patient with a urine specimen container, and ask her to obtain a urine specimen.
Principle. A urine specimen is needed to test for glucose and protein at each prenatal visit. In addition, an empty bladder makes the examination easier and is more comfortable for the patient.

4. Procedural Step. Escort the patient to the examining room, and ask her to be seated. Seat yourself so that you are facing the patient. Ask the patient whether she has experienced any problems since the last prenatal visit, and record information in the appropriate section in her prenatal record.

Principle. The physician investigates any unusual or abnormal signs or symptoms relayed by the patient.

5. Procedural Step. Measure the patient's blood pressure, and chart the results in the prenatal record. If the blood pressure is elevated, allow the patient to relax, and then measure the blood pressure again.
Principle. Taking the blood pressure again gives the opportunity to determine whether the elevation was caused by emotional excitement.

Measure the patient's blood pressure.

6. Procedural Step. Weigh the patient, and chart the results in the prenatal record.
Principle. Maternal weight gain or loss assists in assessing fetal development, as well as the mother's nutrition and state of health.

7. Procedural Step. Instruct and prepare the patient for the examination. Have her remove or pull up her outer clothing to expose the abdominal area. If the physician will be performing a vaginal examination, the patient also must remove her panties; otherwise, she may leave them on. Tell the patient to have a seat on the examining table when she is finished getting ready for the examination. Inform the patient that the physician will be with her soon, and leave the room to give her privacy.

8. Procedural Step. Using a reagent strip, test the urine specimen for glucose and protein, and chart

PROCEDURE 23-3   Assisting with a Return Prenatal Examination—cont'd

Weigh the patient.

the results in the prenatal record. *Note:* The urine specimen may be tested at any time before the physician examines the patient; however, a convenient time to test the specimen is while the patient is disrobing.

Principle. The prenatal patient's urine must be tested at every visit to assist in early detection and prevention of disease.

9. **Procedural Step.** Make the medical record available for review by the physician. The medical office has a designated location where the record is placed, such as a small shelf mounted on the wall next to the outside of the examining room door or in a chart holder on the outside of the examining room door. Position the medical record so that patient-identifiable information is not visible. If your office uses an EMR, you do not need to perform this step. With an EMR, they physician accesses the patient's record on the computer.

Principle. The physician will want to review the patient's chart and information documented by the medical assistant. HIPAA requires protection of a patient's health information.

10. **Procedural Step.** Check to make sure the patient is ready to be seen by the physician. Before entering a patient's room, always knock lightly on the door to let the patient know you are getting ready to enter the room. Inform the physician. This may be done using a color-coded flagging system mounted on the wall next to the examining room.

11. **Procedural Step.** Assist the patient into a supine position, and properly drape her. Provide support and reassurance to the patient to help her relax during the examination.

Principle. The patient should be properly draped so that she is warm and comfortable.

12. **Procedural Step.** Assist the physician as required for the prenatal examination, as follows:
   a. *Fundal height measurement:* Hand the physician the tape measure for determination of the fundal measurement.
   b. *Fetal heart tones:* Apply a liberal amount of coupling gel to the patient's abdomen. Turn on the Doppler fetal pulse detector and hand it to the physician. When the physician is finished, remove excess gel from the patient with a paper towel. Clean the probe head of the Doppler device with a damp cloth or a paper towel. Place the probe head back in its holder.

Apply a liberal amount of coupling gel.

   c. *Vaginal specimen:* Assist the patient into the lithotomy position if a specimen is to be taken for the detection of a vaginal infection. Assist with collection of the specimen as required.
   d. *Vaginal examination:* Assist the patient into the lithotomy position if a vaginal examination is to be performed.

Continued

PROCEDURE 23-3   Assisting with a Return Prenatal Examination—cont'd

13. Procedural Step. After the examination, assist the patient into a sitting position, and allow her the

Assist the patient off the examining table.

opportunity to rest for a moment. If a vaginal examination was performed, offer the patient tissues to remove excess lubricating jelly from the perineum. Assist her off the examining table to prevent falls. Instruct the patient to get dressed. Leave the room to provide the patient with privacy. *Principle.* The patient may become dizzy after being on the examining table and should be allowed to rest before getting off the table. The medical assistant must provide for the safety of the prenatal patient while she is getting off the examining table.

14. Procedural Step. Provide the prenatal patient teaching and further explanation of the physician's instructions as required to meet individual patient needs. Escort the patient to the reception area.

15. Procedural Step. Clean the examining room in preparation for the next patient, and, if necessary, prepare specimens for transport to an outside medical laboratory.

What Would You Do? What Would You *Not* Do? RESPONSES

Case Study 1
Page 489

What Did Yin-Ling Do?
❑ Reassured Mrs. Wooster that the physician is there to help her and stressed that he will be pleased that she has come to the office for an examination.
❑ Commended Mrs. Wooster on performing a breast self-examination at home and encouraged her to continue performing a BSE each month. Asked her whether she had any questions on how to perform a BSE.
❑ Told Mrs. Wooster that some breast changes are normal and others are not normal, and the only way to know for sure is to be examined by the physician.
❑ Told Mrs. Wooster that it is important to have a periodic gynecologic examination even if her periods are normal. Explained to her that some conditions can be present without symptoms. Took plenty of time with her so that she would feel comfortable coming back again in the future for a gynecologic examination. Gave Mrs. Wooster a patient information brochure on gynecologic examinations.
❑ Gave Mrs. Wooster a patient information brochure on mammograms and explained the mammogram procedure to reduce her apprehension. Explained that the procedure is not

painful, but there may be some minor discomfort. Provided her with some tips on reducing discomfort that may occur, such as avoiding caffeine several days before the procedure and having the office schedule the mammogram a week after her menstrual period.

What Did Yin-Ling Not Do?
❑ Did not criticize Mrs. Wooster for waiting so long to schedule a gynecologic examination.
❑ Did not tell Mrs. Wooster that there is no discomfort involved with a mammogram.

Case Study 2
Page 506

What Did Yin-Ling Do?
❑ Stressed to Dagny how important it is that she be seen by the physician. Explained that she could be infected with chlamydia and not know it because chlamydia often has no symptoms, especially in women.
❑ Explained to Dagny that state law allows her to be treated for a sexually transmitted disease without permission from her parents. Told her the law was created to encourage minors to seek treatment for sexually transmitted diseases.

What Would You Do? What Would You *Not* Do? RESPONSES—cont'd

❑ Commended Dagny on practicing safe sex. Relayed to her that if a condom is not used correctly, or if it tears, she might not be protected from getting a sexually transmitted disease. That is another reason she should be tested.

❑ Explained to Dagny what will occur during the examination and what the physician will be doing. Relayed techniques that Dagny could use to relax during the procedure.

What Did Yin-Ling Not Do?

❑ Did not tell Dagny everything would be all right and that she probably does not have chlamydia.

❑ Did not ask Dagny whether she knows how her boyfriend got chlamydia.

❑ Did not try to prevent Dagny from leaving if she still insists on doing so.

Case Study 3
Page 515

What Did Yin-Ling Do?

❑ Tried to calm Johanna by telling her that it is normal for her to be worried and concerned. Explained that the purpose of her prenatal visits is so that the physician can keep a close watch on her and detect any problems that might occur.

❑ Reassured Johanna that she does not need to be afraid to tell the physician any of her concerns because he is there to help her and her baby.

❑ Told Johanna that it is important not to take any medications during her pregnancy without first checking with the physician because some medications could be harmful to her baby.

❑ Told Johanna that her problems and concerns would be relayed to the physician and that he would want to talk to her about them. Explained that the physician also would talk with her about being tested for group B streptococcus.

What Did Yin-Ling Not Do?

❑ Did not tell Johanna that it was all right to take the antibiotics.

Case Study 4
Page 519

What Did Yin-Ling Do?

❑ Escorted Mr. and Mrs. Lopez to a private room in the office. Tried to relax them and told them that whatever they choose to do will be the right decision for them. Reassured them that they could stay at the office for as long as they wanted.

❑ Gave Mrs. Lopez the information she requested that was available at the office and provided her with a list of resources approved by the physician that she could contact for further information.

❑ Asked Mr. and Mrs. Lopez whether they had any more questions they wanted to ask the physician.

What Did Yin-Ling Not Do?

❑ Did not give Mr. and Mrs. Lopez advice on what they should do.

⟲ TERMINOLOGY REVIEW

Key Term	Word Parts	Definition
Abortion		The termination of the pregnancy before the fetus reaches the age of viability (20 weeks).
Adnexal		Adjacent.
Amenorrhea	*a-:* without *men/o:* menstruation *-orrhea:* flow, excessive discharge	The absence or cessation of the menstrual period. Amenorrhea occurs normally before puberty, during pregnancy, and after menopause.
Atypical	*a-:* without	Deviation from the normal.
Braxton Hicks contractions		Intermittent and irregular painless uterine contractions that occur throughout pregnancy. They occur more frequently toward the end of pregnancy and are sometimes mistaken for true labor pains.
Cervix		The lower narrow end of the uterus that opens into the vagina.
Colposcopy	*colp/o:* vagina *-scopy:* visual examination	Examination of the cervix using a colposcope (a lighted instrument with a magnifying lens).
Cytology	*cyt/o:* cell *-ology:* study of	The science that deals with the study of cells, including their origin, structure, function, and pathology.
Dilation (of the cervix)		The stretching of the external os from an opening a few millimeters wide to an opening large enough to allow the passage of an infant (approximately 10 cm).

Continued

↻ TERMINOLOGY REVIEW—cont'd

Key Term	Word Parts	Definition
Dysmenorrhea	*dys-:* difficult, painful, abnormal *men/o:* menstruation *-orrhea:* flow, excessive discharge	Pain associated with the menstrual period.
Dyspareunia	*dys-:* difficult, painful, abnormal	Pain in the vagina or pelvis experienced by a woman during sexual intercourse.
Dysplasia	*dys-:* difficult, painful, abnormal *plasia:* a growth	The growth of abnormal cells. Dysplasia is a precancerous condition that may or may not develop into cancer.
Ectocervix	*ecto-:* outside, outer	The part of the cervix that projects into the vagina and is lined with stratified squamous epithelium.
Effacement		The thinning and shortening of the cervical canal from its normal length of 1 to 2 cm to a structure with paper-thin edges in which there is no canal at all. Effacement occurs late in pregnancy, during labor, or both. The purpose of effacement along with dilation is to permit the passage of the infant into the birth canal.
Embryo		The child in utero from the time of conception through the first 8 weeks of development.
Endocervix	*endo-:* within	The mucous membrane lining the cervical canal.
Engagement		The entrance of the fetal head or the presenting part into the pelvic inlet.
Expected date of delivery (EDD)		Projected birth date of the infant.
External os		The opening of the cervical canal of the uterus into the vagina.
Fetal heart rate		The number of times per minute the fetal heart beats.
Fetal heart tones		The sounds of the heartbeat of the fetus heard through the mother's abdominal wall.
Fetus		The child in utero from the third month after conception to birth; during the first 2 months of development, it is called an *embryo.*
Fundus		The dome-shaped upper portion of the uterus between the fallopian tubes.
Gestation		The period of intrauterine development from conception to birth; the period of pregnancy. The average pregnancy lasts about 280 days, or 40 weeks, from the date of conception to childbirth.
Gestational age		The age of the fetus between conception and birth.
Gynecology	*gynec/o:* woman *-ology:* study of	The branch of medicine that deals with the diseases of reproductive organs of women.
Infant		A child from birth to 12 months of age.
Menopause	*men/o:* menstruation	The permanent cessation of menstruation, which usually occurs between the ages of 45 and 55.
Menorrhagia	*men/o:* menstruation *-orrhagia:* rapid flow of blood	Excessive bleeding during a menstrual period, in the number of days or the amount of blood or both. Also called *dysfunctional uterine bleeding (DUB).*
Metrorrhagia	*metr/o:* uterus *-orrhagia:* rapid flow of blood	Bleeding between menstrual periods.
Multigravida	*multi-:* many *gravid/o:* pregnancy	A woman who has been pregnant more than once.
Multipara	*multi-:* many *par/o:* bear, give birth to	A woman who has completed two or more pregnancies to the age of fetal viability regardless of whether they ended in live infants or stillbirths.
Nullipara	*nulli-:* none *par/o:* bear, give birth to	A woman who has not carried a pregnancy to the point of fetal viability (20 weeks of gestation).
Obstetrics		The branch of medicine concerned with the care of the woman during pregnancy, childbirth, and the postpartal period.
Perimenopause	*peri-:* surrounding *men/o:* menstruation	Before the onset of menopause, the phase during which the woman with regular periods changes to irregular cycles and increased periods of amenorrhea.

TERMINOLOGY REVIEW—cont'd

Key Term	Word Parts	Definition
Perineum		The external region between the vaginal orifice and the anus in a female and between the scrotum and the anus in a male.
Position		The relation of the presenting part of the fetus to the maternal pelvis.
Postpartum	*post-:* after *par/o:* bear, give birth to	Occurring after childbirth.
Preeclampsia		A major complication of pregnancy, the cause of which is unknown. Preeclampsia is characterized by increasing hypertension, albuminuria, and edema. If this condition is neglected or is not treated properly, it may develop into eclampsia, which could cause maternal convulsions and coma. Preeclampsia typically occurs between the 20th week of pregnancy and the end of the first week postpartum.
Prenatal	*pre-:* in front of, before *nat/o:* birth *-al:* pertaining to	Before birth.
Presentation		Indication of the part of the fetus that is closest to the cervix and is delivered first. A cephalic presentation is a delivery in which the fetal head is presenting against the cervix. A breech presentation is a delivery in which the buttocks or feet are presented instead of the head.
Primigravida	*prim/i:* first *gravid/o:* pregnancy	A woman who is pregnant for the first time.
Primipara	*prim/i:* first *par/o:* bear, give birth to	A woman who has carried a pregnancy to fetal viability (20 weeks of gestation) for the first time regardless of whether the infant was stillborn or alive at birth.
Puerperium		The period of time, usually 4 to 6 weeks after delivery, in which the uterus and the body systems are returning to normal.
Quickening		The first movements of the fetus in utero as felt by the mother, which usually occur between 16 and 20 weeks of gestation and are felt consistently thereafter.
Risk factor		Anything that increases an individual's chance of developing a disease. Some risk factors (e.g., smoking) can be avoided, but others cannot (e.g., age and family history).
Toxemia		A condition that can occur in pregnant women that includes preeclampsia and eclampsia. If preeclampsia goes undiagnosed or is not satisfactorily controlled, it could develop into eclampsia, characterized by convulsions and coma.
Trimester	*tri-:* three	Three months, or one third, of the gestational period of pregnancy.
Vulva		The region of the external female genital organs.

ON THE WEB

For information on sexually transmitted diseases:

National Institute of Allergy and Infectious Diseases: Sexually Transmitted Infections: http://www.niaid.nih.gov/topics/std/Pages/default.aspx

Centers for Disease Control and Prevention: Sexually Transmitted Diseases: www.cdc.gov/std

Planned Parenthood: www.plannedparenthood.org

Medline Plus Sexually Transmitted Diseases: www.nlm.nih.gov/medlineplus/sexuallytransmitteddiseases.html

WebMD Sexual Conditions: www.webmd.com/sexual-conditions

Your STD Help: yourstdhelp.com

Continued

ON THE WEB—cont'd

STD Support Website: herpes-coldsores.com/support/std.htm

American Social Health Association: www.ashastd.org

Herpes Information: www.gotherpes.com

HPV Information: www.gothpv.com

For information on women's health:

The Universe of Women's Health: www.obgyn.net

Women's Health: www.womenshealth.gov

CDC Women's Health: www.cdc.gov/women

Healthy Women: www.healthywomen.org

For information on contraceptives:

Planned Parenthood: www.plannedparenthood.org

Mayo Clinic Birth Control Options: www.mayoclinic.com/health/birth-control/MY01182

Ultimate Birth Control Links: www.ultimatebirthcontrol.com

Reproductive Health Online: reprolineplus.org

For information on menopause:

North American Menopause Society: www.menopause.org

Everything Menopause: www.everythingmenopause.com

Power Surge: www.power-surge.com

Project Aware: www.project-aware.org

Mayo Clinic Menopause Information: www.mayoclinic.com/health/menopause/DS00119

WebMD Menopause Health Center: www.webmd.com/menopause

Medline Plus Menopause: www.nlm.nih.gov/medlineplus/menopause.html

For information on pregnancy and childbirth:

Pregnancy and Childbirth: www.childbirth.org

Pregnancy and Childbirth: pregnancy.about.com

Childbirth Connection: www.childbirthconnection.org

Pregnancy: www.pregnancy.org

My Pregnancy Guide: www.mypregnancyguide.com

WebMD Health and Pregnancy: www.webmd.com/baby

StorkNet's Pregnancy Guide: www.pregnancyguideonline.com

What to Expect: www.whattoexpect.com

The American College of Obstetricians and Gynecologists: www.acog.com

American Baby: www.americanbaby.com

Baby Zone: www.babyzone.com

Baby Center: www.babycenter.com

Lamaze International: www.lamaze.org

LaLeche League International: www.llli.org

The Pediatric Examination

 Check out the Evolve site at http://evolve.elsevier.com/Bonewit/today/ to access additional interactive activities and exercises to help you study and prepare for success.

LEARNING OBJECTIVES

Pediatric Office Visits
1. List the components of the well-child visit.
2. State the usual schedule for well-child visits.
3. Explain the purpose of the sick-child visit.
4. List the procedures performed by the medical assistant during pediatric office visits.
5. Explain why it is important to develop a rapport with the pediatric patient.

Growth Measurements
6. State the importance of measuring the child's weight, height (or length), and head circumference during each office visit.
7. State the functions served by a growth chart.

Pediatric Blood Pressure Measurement
8. State the importance of measuring a child's blood pressure.
9. List the three factors that determine whether a child has hypertension.

Collection of a Urine Specimen
10. List the reasons for collecting a urine specimen from a child.

Pediatric Injections
11. State the range for the gauge and length of needles used for intramuscular and subcutaneous pediatric injections.
12. Explain the use of each of the following pediatric injection sites: vastus lateralis and deltoid.

Immunizations
13. Describe the schedule for immunization of infants and children recommended by the American Academy of Pediatrics.
14. State the information that must be provided to parents as required by the National Childhood Vaccine Injury Act.
15. List the information that must be recorded in the medical record after administering an immunization.

Newborn Screening Test
16. Explain the purpose of a newborn screening test.
17. List the symptoms of phenylketonuria.
18. State what occurs if phenylketonuria is left untreated.

PROCEDURES

Carry an infant using the following positions:
- Cradle
- Upright

Plot pediatric growth values on a growth chart.
Measure the weight and length of an infant.
Measure the head and chest circumference of an infant.

Measure the blood pressure of a child.

Collect a urine specimen using a pediatric urine collector.

Locate the following pediatric intramuscular injection sites:
- Vastus lateralis
- Deltoid

Administer an intramuscular injection to an infant.
Administer a subcutaneous injection to an infant.

Read and interpret a vaccine information statement.
Record information on an immunization administration record.

CHAPTER OUTLINE

INTRODUCTION TO THE PEDIATRIC EXAMINATION
PEDIATRIC OFFICE VISITS
DEVELOPING A RAPPORT
CARRYING THE INFANT
Cradle Position
Upright Position
GROWTH MEASUREMENTS
Weight
Length and Height
Head and Chest Circumference
Growth Charts
PEDIATRIC BLOOD PRESSURE MEASUREMENT

Special Guidelines for Children
Correct Cuff Size
Cooperation of the Child
Blood Pressure Classifications
COLLECTION OF A URINE SPECIMEN
PEDIATRIC INJECTIONS
Types of Needles
Pediatric Intramuscular Injection Sites
Pediatric Subcutaneous Injection Sites
IMMUNIZATIONS
National Childhood Vaccine Injury Act
NEWBORN SCREENING TEST

KEY TERMS

adolescent
immunity (ih-MYOO-nih-tee)
immunization (IM-yoo-nih-ZAY-shun)
infant
length

pediatrician (PEE-dee-uh-TRIH-shun)
pediatrics (pee-dee-AT-riks)
preschool (PREE-skool) child
school-age child
toddler (TOD-ler)

toxoid (TOKS-oid)
vaccine (vak-SEEN)
vertex (VER-teks)

INTRODUCTION TO THE PEDIATRIC EXAMINATION

Pediatrics is the branch of medicine that deals with the care and development of children and the diagnosis and treatment of diseases in children. A **pediatrician** is a physician who specializes in pediatrics. Many physicians in general practice accept pediatric patients. It is essential that the medical assistant develop the skills needed to assist the physician in the care and treatment of children.

PEDIATRIC OFFICE VISITS

There are two broad categories of pediatric patient office visits. The first is the *well-child visit* (also termed *health maintenance visit*), in which the physician progressively evaluates the growth and development of the child. A patient history and physical examination are performed during each well-child visit and are directed toward discovering any abnormal conditions commonly associated with the stage of development reached by the child. Table 24-1 provides an outline of normal development during infancy. The child also receives necessary immunizations during these visits.

Another important component of the well-child visit is *anticipatory guidance.* Anticipatory guidance is the process of providing parents with information to prepare them for anticipated developmental events and to assist them in promoting their children's well-being. Topics that are commonly included are safety, nutrition, sleep, play, exercise, development, and discipline.

The interval between well-child visits depends on the medical office, but it frequently follows this schedule after birth: 3 to 5 days, 1 month, 2 months, 4 months, 6 months, 9 months, 12 months, 15 months, 18 months, 24 months, 30 months, 3 years, 4 years, and once a year thereafter.

The second category of pediatric patient office visits is the *sick-child visit.* The child is exhibiting the signs and symptoms of disease, and the physician evaluates the patient's condition to arrive at a diagnosis and to prescribe treatment.

What Would You Do? What Would You *Not* Do?

Case Study 1

My-Lai Chang comes into the office with Christopher Chang, her 2-month-old son. Christopher is here for his 2-month well-child visit. Mrs. Chang is very distraught. She says that Christopher has episodes of nonstop crying every day that last 2 to 3 hours at a time. She is breast feeding Christopher and says that the crying is worse after he nurses. Although Mrs. Chang realizes that Christopher has colic, she feels guilty because it seems "her milk" is making it worse. She also is having problems with sore nipples and engorgement. She really wanted to breast feed Christopher, but she is thinking of stopping because it just seems too hard to do. Christopher measures in the 50th percentile for weight and length. Mrs. Chang is worried that he is not growing enough and thinks it is because she is not producing enough milk. ∎

Table 24-1 Milestones of Gross and Fine Motor Development in Infancy

Average Age (mo)	Gross Motor	Fine Motor
1	Turns head from side to side	Grasping reflex present
2	Holds head at 45-degree angle when prone	Holds rattle briefly
3	Begins rolling over	Grasps rattle or dangling objects
4	Slight head lag when pulled to sitting position	Brings objects to mouth
5	No head wobble when held in sitting position	Transfers objects from hand to hand
6	Sits without support	Manipulates and examines large objects with hands
7	Stands while holding on	Reaches for, grabs, and retains object
8	Pulls self to stand	Grasps objects with thumb and finger
9	Crawls backward	Begins to show hand preference
10	Creeps on hands and knees	Hits cup with spoon
11	Walks using furniture for support	Picks up small objects with thumb and forefinger (pincer grasp)
12	Stands alone easily	Puts three or more objects into container
12-16	Walks alone easily	Turns two or three pages in large cardboard book

From Leahy JM, Kizilay PE: *Foundations of nursing practice,* Philadelphia, 1998, Saunders.

During well-child and sick-child visits, the medical assistant performs many of the same procedures that have been presented in previous chapters (e.g., measurement of temperature, pulse, respiration, and blood pressure; measurement of weight and height; measurement of visual and hearing acuity; assisting with the physical examination). This chapter discusses procedures specifically related to the pediatric patient and variations in procedures previously presented.

DEVELOPING A RAPPORT

The medical assistant must establish a rapport with the pediatric patient. If the medical assistant gains the child's trust and confidence, the child is likely to cooperate during an examination or procedure. Interacting with children requires special techniques. The techniques employed depend on the age of the child. **Toddlers** (1 to 3 years old) and **preschool children** (3 to 6 years old) often respond well to making a game of the procedure. Explaining the purpose of an instrument (e.g., the stethoscope) to a **school-age child** (6 to 12 years old) and allowing him or her to hold the instrument or even to help during the procedure may overcome fears in that age group (Figure 24-1) **Adolescents** (12 to 18 years old) respond best by discussing the risks of a procedure and allowing them to have input in the decision making process.

The medical assistant should always explain the procedure to children who are able to understand. Each child must be approached at his or her level of understanding. To do this, the medical assistant should know what to expect from a child at a particular age, in terms of motor and social development. Each child has his or her own individual rate of development; the descriptions of normal development based on age are meant to serve as a guide only and may

have to be modified to meet individual needs. In addition, it is normal for an ill child to regress to an earlier level of behavior. Table 24-2 outlines techniques that can be used with various age groups to gain their cooperation during an examination or procedure.

CARRYING THE INFANT

An **infant** is a child from birth to 12 months old. The medical assistant needs to lift and carry the infant to perform various procedures, such as measurement of length and weight. The infant should be lifted and carried in a manner that is safe and comfortable. Proper positions include the cradle and upright positions.

CRADLE POSITION

The medical assistant slides one hand and forearm under the infant's back and grasps the infant's arm from behind. The thumb and fingers should encircle the infant's forearm. The infant's head, shoulders, and back are supported by the medical assistant's forearm. Next, the medical assistant slips the other hand and forearm up and under the infant's buttocks. The infant is cradled in the arm with his or her body resting against the medical assistant's chest (Figure 24-2).

UPRIGHT POSITION

The medical assistant slips one hand and forearm under the infant's head and shoulders. The fingers should be spread apart to support the infant's head and neck. The other hand and forearm are slipped under the infant's buttocks to help support the infant's weight. The infant should be allowed to rest against the medical assistant's chest with the cheek resting on the medical assistant's shoulder (Figure 24-3).

Figure 24-1 The medical assistant should develop a rapport with children to gain their trust and cooperation. Making a game of the procedure **(A)** and explaining the purpose of the stethoscope and allowing the child to hold it **(B)** help the child overcome fears.

Figure 24-2 Traci holds the infant in the cradle position.

Figure 24-3 Traci holds the infant in the upright position.

Table 24-2 Techniques for Interaction with Children

Technique	Infant (Birth-1 yr)	Toddler (1-3 yr)	Preschool (3-6 yr)	School Age (6-12 yr)	Adolescent (12-18 yr)
Avoid sudden motion and loud or abrupt noises	❤		❤		
Limit number of strangers in room	❤				
Use distractions, bright objects, rattles, and talking to gain cooperation	❤				
Physically restrain child if necessary to ensure safety	❤	❤	❤		
Allow physical contact with parent during procedure	❤	❤	❤		
Encourage parent to comfort child after procedure	❤	❤	❤		
Use play to explain procedure (e.g., dolls, puppets)		❤	❤		
Perform procedures quickly, if possible		❤	❤		
Use concrete terms, rather than abstract terms		❤	❤		
Avoid words that have more than one meaning (e.g., shot)		❤	❤		
Give child permission to cry, yell, or otherwise express pain verbally		❤	❤		
Praise child for cooperative behavior		❤	❤	❤	
Allow child to handle equipment, if possible			❤	❤	
Make sure child understands body part to be involved			❤	❤	
Try to describe how procedure will feel			❤	❤	
Tell child about any discomfort that may be felt, but don't dwell on it			❤	❤	
Stress benefits of anything child may find pleasurable afterward (e.g., stickers, feeling better)			❤	❤	
Give child choices when possible (e.g., arm to use)			❤	❤	
Suggest ways to maintain control (e.g., counting, deep breathing, relaxation)			❤	❤	
Use drawing and diagrams to illustrate parts of body that will be involved			❤	❤	
Encourage participation such as holding instrument during procedure			❤	❤	
Include child in decision-making process				❤	❤
Discuss risks of procedure					❤
Provide information about appearance changes that might result					❤
Give child educational brochures or have him or her view videos about procedure					❤
Ask parent to step out if child does not want parent in examining room					❤

GROWTH MEASUREMENTS

One of the best methods to evaluate the progress of a child is to measure his or her growth. The weight, height (or length), and head circumference (up to age 3 years) of a child should be measured during each office visit and plotted on a growth chart.

WEIGHT

A child's weight is often used to determine nutritional needs and the proper dosage of a medication to administer to the child. The medical assistant should exercise care in measuring weight. Infants are weighed in a recumbent position, as outlined in Procedure 24-1. Older children are weighed in a standing position, as presented in Chapter 20.

LENGTH AND HEIGHT

Another measure of a child's growth is **length,** or height (stature). Length is measured in children younger than 24 months. The recumbent length is a measurement from the **vertex** (top) of the head to the heel of the infant in a supine position, as outlined in Procedure 24-1. Two people are often needed to determine the length of an infant accurately. The parent's help can be requested; the medical assistant must provide the parent with thorough instructions on what is to be done. Older children have their height measured in a standing position (Figure 24-4), as presented in Chapter 20.

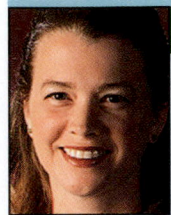

Putting It All Into Practice

My name is Traci Powell, and I am a Certified Medical Assistant. I work in the pediatrics department of a large multispecialty clinic. My job responsibilities are mostly clinical; however, I do assist in the front office when needed. I love working with the children and have enjoyed watching them grow over the years.

A co-worker and I recently organized a local AAMA (American Association of Medical Assistants) chapter. Our chapter provides AAMA continuing education units (CEUs). Our members attend state and national conventions every year, and they hold state and national leadership positions. It is my goal to see the medical assisting profession continue to grow and advance in the health care field.

It is interesting how your education, training, and experience all come together, especially in a crisis. Early one morning when I arrived at work, a mother was waiting with a small child who was approximately 2 years old. The child was dusky in color, panicky, and having trouble breathing. Apparently the child had gotten into some dry beans the previous night and had inhaled one into her lung. None of the physicians was in the building yet, and this child was in respiratory distress. We immediately called a Code Blue, put her on oxygen, and made arrangements for an ambulance to take her to Children's Hospital, where a surgeon was waiting. All went well, and she is a healthy little girl today.

Looking back, I am grateful for a good, solid medical assisting education; a PALS (Pediatric Advance Life Support) certification; and experience in working with children so that I was able to help that child through a life-threatening experience. I firmly believe that no matter how long a person has been in the medical field or what his or her profession is, continuing education is essential to stay current in the ever-changing health care field. ■

Figure 24-4 Measuring the height of a child.

head circumference growth chart. Measurement of head circumference is an important screening measure for microencephaly and macroencephaly.

At birth a newborn's head circumference is about 2 cm larger than his or her chest circumference. The chest grows at a faster rate than the cranium, and between 6 months and 2 years of age the measurements are about the same. After age 2 years, the chest circumference is greater than the head circumference. The measurement of the chest circumference is valuable in a comparison with the head circumference, but not by itself. The chest circumference is not typically measured on a routine basis; this measurement is done only when a heart or lung abnormality is suspected. Procedure 24-2 outlines the procedure for measuring the head and chest circumference of an infant.

GROWTH CHARTS

Growth charts should be part of every child's permanent record. The National Center for Health Statistics developed growth charts to assist physicians in determining whether the growth of a child is normal. The charts can be used to identify children with growth or nutritional abnormalities. The medical assistant may be responsible for plotting the child's measurements on a preprinted growth chart (Procedure 24-3). In offices with an electronic medical record, the growth percentiles are automatically calculated and plotted on a growth chart when the child's growth measurements are entered into the computer. This "electronic" growth

HEAD AND CHEST CIRCUMFERENCE

Infancy is a period of rapid brain growth. Because of this, the head circumference is an important measurement. The head circumference for a newborn ranges from 32 to 38 cm, or 12½ to 15 inches. A 10-cm (4-inch) increase in head circumference occurs within the first year of life.

The head circumference of children younger than 3 years should be routinely measured and plotted on a chart is maintained in the child's electronic medical record and can be printed out if needed.

Growth charts provide a means of comparing a child's weight and length (or height) with those of other children of the same age. For example, the medical assistant calculates the growth percentile of an 18-month-old boy and finds that he is in the 25th percentile for weight and the 80th percentile for length. This means that 75% of 18-month-old boys weigh more than he does, and 25% weigh less than he does. It also means that 20% of 18-month-old boys are taller, and 80% are shorter. Although comparing a child with other children of the same age is

one use of growth charts (particularly by parents), it is not the most important use.

The primary use of growth charts is to look at the child's growth pattern. If a child has always hovered around a certain percentile in height and weight, there is no need for concern. If a child is in the 20th percentile for weight but has always been in this percentile, he is likely growing normally. It would be more of a concern if the child had been in the 75th percentile and dropped to the 20th percentile. The physician investigates any significant change or rapid increase or decrease in a child's growth pattern.

HIGHLIGHT on Childhood Obesity

Statistics

An epidemic of childhood obesity is occurring in the United States; the incidence of obesity in children has doubled over the past 20 years. Approximately 32% of Americans younger than age 19 are overweight or obese, which equates to one of every three children. A child is considered overweight if his or her weight falls in the 85th to 95th percentile for age, gender, and height on the National Center for Health Statistics growth charts. When a child's weight exceeds the 95th percentile for age, gender, and height, he or she is considered obese.

Causes

The primary causes of childhood obesity are overeating and inadequate exercise. Other causes include hormonal and genetic problems, but these are much less likely, occurring in only 5% of obese children. The risk of obesity tends to be greater among children who have obese parents. After age 3, the likelihood that obesity will persist into adulthood increases as an obese child gets older. When an obese child reaches age 6, the probability is more than 50% that obesity will persist into adulthood. Of obese adolescents, 70% to 80% remain obese as adults.

Related Problems

Problems associated with childhood obesity include high blood pressure, type 2 diabetes, orthopedic problems caused by increased stress on weight-bearing joints, skin disorders such as dermatitis, sleep apnea, low self-esteem, social isolation, and feelings of rejection and depression. Some authorities believe that the social and psychological problems are the most significant consequences of childhood obesity.

Prevention

It is much easier to prevent childhood obesity than to treat it after it has occurred. Authorities believe that the primary focus should be on educating parents about the problems associated with childhood obesity and helping them employ preventive measures. Guidelines for preventing childhood obesity include the following:

- Provide a healthy diet, with 30% or fewer of the total calories consumed each day coming from fat.
- Encourage active play.
- Do not use food for reward, comfort, or bribes.
- Limit television, video, and computer time.
- Limit the amount of "junk" food kept in the home.
- Do not make the child eat when he or she is not hungry.
- Do not offer dessert as a reward for finishing a meal.
- Encourage the child to drink water instead of sweet beverages.
- Do not frequently eat at fast-food restaurants.

Treatment

The treatment of childhood obesity is difficult, and the success rate is not particularly high. Children seem to be most successful at losing weight and keeping it off when the entire family is involved. Parents should eat healthy meals and snacks with their children. The most successful diets are those that use ordinary foods in controlled portions, rather than diets that require the avoidance of specific foods. Parents also should spend time being active with their children. Activities should stress self-improvement rather than competition. ■

PROCEDURE 24-1   Measuring the Weight and Length of an Infant

Outcome Measure the weight and length of an infant

Equipment/Supplies

• Pediatric balance scale (table model)

1. **Procedural Step.** Sanitize your hands.
2. **Procedural Step.** Greet the infant's parent and introduce yourself. Identify the infant and explain the procedure to the parent. The weight of the infant is usually measured first. Depending on the medical office policy, ask the parent to perform one of the following:
   a. Remove the infant's clothing and put a dry diaper on the infant.
   b. Remove the infant's clothing, including the diaper.
   Principle. The infant should not be weighed with a wet diaper because it could increase the infant's weight considerably. Also, growth charts for infants and young children base their percentiles on the weight of the child without clothing.
3. **Procedural Step.** Unlock the pediatric scale, and place a clean paper protector on it. Check the balance scale for accuracy, making sure to compensate for the weight of the paper.
   Principle. The paper protector prevents cross-contamination and reduces the spread of disease from one patient to another.
4. **Procedural Step.** Gently place the infant on his or her back on the table of the scale. Place one hand slightly above the infant as a safety precaution.
5. **Procedural Step.** Balance the scale as follows:
   a. Move the lower weight to the notched groove that does not cause the indicator point to drop to the bottom of the calibration area. Ensure that the lower weight is seated firmly in its groove.
   b. Slowly slide the upper weight along its calibration bar by tapping it gently until the indicator point comes to rest at the center of the balance area.
   Principle. Not seating the lower weight firmly in its groove results in an inaccurate reading.

Balance the scale.

6. **Procedural Step.** Read the results while the infant is lying still. Jot down this value or make a mental note of it. (*Note:* The result on the pictured scale is 15 lb, 2 oz.)

Read the results in pounds and ounces.

7. **Procedural Step.** Return the balance to its resting position, and lock the scale.
8. **Procedural Step.** Place the vertex (top) of the infant's head against the headboard at the zero mark. Ask the parent to hold the infant's head in this position.

Properly position the infant.

9. **Procedural Step.** Straighten the infant's knees, and place the soles of his or her feet firmly against the upright footboard (to create a right angle).

PROCEDURE 24-1 Measuring the Weight and Length of an Infant—cont'd

10. **Procedural Step.** Read the infant's length in inches to the nearest ⅛ inch from the measure. Jot down this value or make a mental note of it. (*Note:* The result on this scale is 25½ inches.)

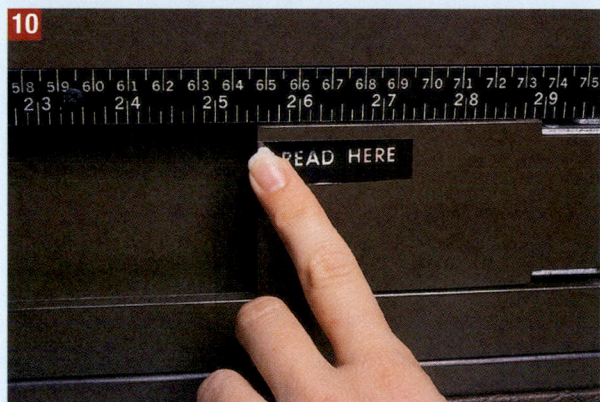
Read the length in inches.

11. **Procedural Step.** Gently remove the infant from the table, and hand him or her to the parent. Return the headboard and footboard to their resting positions.

12. **Procedural Step.** Sanitize your hands.
13. **Procedural Step.** Chart the results in the patient's medical record.
    a. *Paper-based patient record:* Record the date and time and the infant's weight and length measurements (refer to the PPR charting example).

PPR CHARTING EXAMPLE

Date	
8/10/XX	9:30 a.m. Wt. 15 lb 2 oz. Length 25 ½ in. ——
	—— T. Powell, CMA (AAMA)

    b. *Electronic medical record:* Document the infant's weight and length measurements using the appropriate radio buttons, drop-down menus, and free text fields. The electronic medical record will automatically calculate the child's growth percentiles and plot them on a growth chart once you enter the infant's weight and length measurements into the computer.

PROCEDURE 24-2 Measuring Head and Chest Circumference of an Infant

Outcome Measure the head and chest circumference of an infant

Equipment/Supplies
• Flexible nonstretch tape measure

Measurement of Head Circumference

1. **Procedural Step.** Sanitize your hands, and assemble the equipment.
2. **Procedural Step.** Position the infant. The infant should be placed on his or her back on the examining table. An alternative position is to have the parent hold the infant.
3. **Procedural Step.** Position the tape measure around the infant's head at the greatest circumference. This is usually accomplished by placing the tape slightly above the eyebrows and pinna of the ears and around the occipital prominence at the back of the skull.

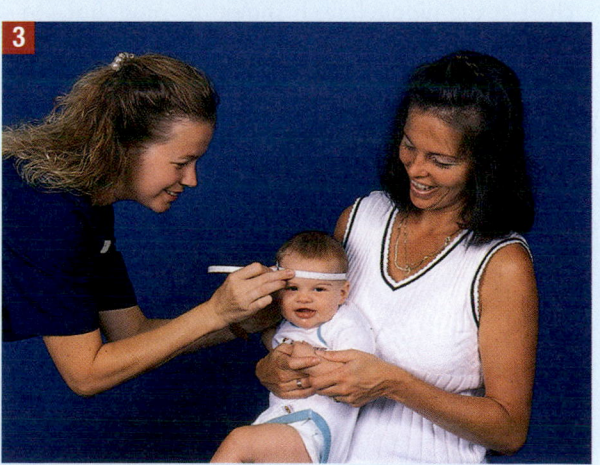
Position the tape measure around the infant's head.

Continued

PROCEDURE **24-2**   **Measuring Head and Chest Circumference of an Infant—cont'd**

4. Procedural Step. Read the results in centimeters (or inches) to the nearest 0.5 cm (or ¼ inch). Jot down this value or make a mental note of it. Sanitize your hands.

5. Procedural Step. Chart the results in the patient's medical record.

   a. *Paper-based patient record:* Record the date and time and the infant's head circumference measurement in centimeters (refer to the PPR charting example).

Encircle the tape around the infant's chest.

PPR CHARTING EXAMPLE

Date	
8/10/XX	10:00 a.m. Head circumference: 42.5 cm. ___
	——————————— T. Powell, CMA (AAMA)

   b. *Electronic medical record:* Document the infant's head circumference measurement using the appropriate radio buttons, drop-down menus, and free text fields. The electronic medical record will automatically calculate the child's head circumference percentile and plot it on a growth chart once you enter the infant's head circumference measurement into the computer.

Measurement of Chest Circumference

1. Procedural Step. Position the infant on his or her back on the examining table.

2. Procedural Step. Encircle the tape around the infant's chest at the nipple line. It should be snug, but not so tight that it leaves a mark.

3. Procedural Step. Read the results in centimeters (or inches) to the nearest 0.5 cm (or ¼ inch). Jot down this value or make a mental note of it. Sanitize your hands.

4. Procedural Step. Chart the results in the patient's medical record.

   a. *Paper-based patient record:* Record the date and time and the infant's chest circumference measurement in centimeters (refer to the PPR charting example).

PPR CHARTING EXAMPLE

Date	
8/15/XX	10:00 a.m. Chest circumference: 42 cm. ___
	——————————— T. Powell, CMA (AAMA)

   b. *Electronic medical record:* Document the infant's chest circumference measurement using the appropriate radio buttons, drop-down menus, and free text fields.

PROCEDURE 24-3   Calculating Growth Percentiles

Outcome Plot a pediatric growth value on a growth chart

Equipment/Supplies

- Pediatric growth chart

1. **Procedural Step.** Select the proper growth chart.
2. **Procedural Step.** Locate the child's age in the horizontal column at the bottom of the chart.
3. **Procedural Step.** Locate the growth value in the vertical column under the appropriate category (weight, length or stature, and head circumference).
4. **Procedural Step.** Draw an imaginary vertical line from the child's age mark and an imaginary horizontal line from the child's growth mark. Find the site at which the two lines intersect on the graph, and place a dot on this site.

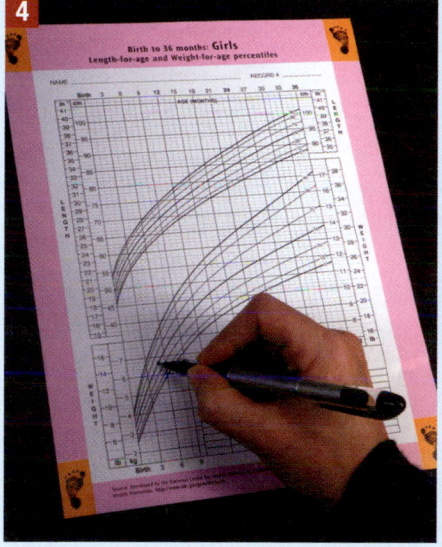

5. **Procedural Step.** To determine the percentile in which the child falls, follow the curved percentile line upward to read the value located on the right side of the chart. Interpolation is needed if the value does not fall exactly on a percentile line. (*Interpolation* means that you must estimate a percentile that falls between a larger and a smaller known percentile.)
6. **Procedural Step.** Chart the results in the patient's medical record. Include the date and time and each growth percentile. (Refer to the PPR charting example).

The weight (15 lb, 2 oz), length ($25\frac{1}{2}$ inches), and head circumference (42.5 cm) of the child in Procedures 24-1 and 24-2 have been plotted on a growth chart. This child is 5 months old. Locate these values on the appropriate growth chart to ensure you obtain the same percentiles.

In a medical office that uses an electronic medical record, the growth percentiles are automatically calculated when you enter the child's weight, length, and head circumference measurements into the computer. The growth percentiles are plotted and displayed on an electronic growth chart that is maintained as part of the child's electronic record.

PPR CHARTING EXAMPLE	
Date	
10/22/XX	10:30 a.m. Weight: 55%. Length: 70%. _____
	Head Circum: 67% —— T. Powell, CMA (AAMA)

Continued

PROCEDURE 24-3

PROCEDURE 24-3

Birth to 36 months: Girls
Length-for-age and Weight-for-age percentiles

NAME _____

RECORD # _____

AGE (MONTHS)

Birth 3 6 9 **12** 15 18 21 **24** 27 30 33 **36**

LENGTH

WEIGHT

Mother's Stature _____		Gestational		Comment
Father's Stature _____		Age: ____ Weeks		
Date	Age	Weight	Length	Head Circ.
	Birth			

95
90
75
50
25
10
5

Published May 30, 2000 (modified 4/20/01).
SOURCE Developed by the National Center for Health Statistics in collaboration with
the National Center for Chronic Disease Prevention and Health Promotion (2000).
http://www.cdc.gov/growthcharts

SAFER · HEALTHIER · PEOPLE™

PROCEDURE 24-3 Calculating Growth Percentiles—cont'd

Birth to 36 months: Boys
Length-for-age and Weight-for-age percentiles

NAME _____

RECORD# _____

| Mother's Stature _____ | Gestational |
| Father's Stature _____ | Age: _____ Weeks | Comment |

Date	Age	Weight	Length	Head Circ.
	Birth			

Published May 30, 2000 (modified 4/20/01).
SOURCE: Developed by the National Center for Health Statistics in collaboration with
the National Center for Chronic Disease Prevention and Health Promotion (2000).
http://www.cdc.gov/growthcharts

SAFER • HEALTHIER • PEOPLE™

PEDIATRIC BLOOD PRESSURE MEASUREMENT

The American Academy of Pediatrics recommends that all children 3 years old and older have their blood pressure measured annually. Measuring pediatric blood pressure helps to identify children at risk for developing hypertension as adults. High blood pressure in children can be caused by kidney disease and to a lesser degree by heart disease. When the condition is treated, the blood pressure usually returns to normal. Overweight children usually have higher blood pressure than children of normal weight. Losing weight through a prescribed diet and regular physical activity often reduces blood pressure in these children.

SPECIAL GUIDELINES FOR CHILDREN

The procedure for measuring blood pressure in children is the same as that for adults and is presented in Chapter 19. Some special pediatric guidelines must be taken into consideration.

CORRECT CUFF SIZE

The most important criterion in obtaining an accurate pediatric blood pressure measurement is selecting the correct cuff size. If the cuff is too small, the reading may be falsely high. If the cuff is too large, the reading may be falsely low. Blood pressure cuffs come in a variety of sizes and are measured in centimeters. The size of a cuff refers to its inner inflatable bladder, rather than its cloth cover. Table 24-3 lists the range of cuff sizes commercially available. The name of the cuff (e.g., child, adult) does not imply that it

is appropriate for that age. An 8-year-old overweight child may need an adult-sized cuff.

For an accurate blood pressure measurement, the bladder of the cuff should encircle 80% to 100% of the arm. The child's arm circumference should be assessed at the midpoint between the acromion process (shoulder) and the olecranon process (elbow). Figure 24-5 shows how to determine the correct pediatric cuff size.

COOPERATION OF THE CHILD

Another important factor to consider when taking pediatric blood pressure is preparing the child for the procedure. It is important to gain the child's cooperation and to ensure that the child is relaxed. Apprehension can cause the blood pressure to be falsely high. To reduce a child's anxiety level, carefully explain the procedure to the child, and, if appropriate, allow him or her to handle the equipment before measurement of the blood pressure. The blood pressure should be measured after the child has been sitting quietly for 3 to 5 minutes (Figure 24-6).

Table 24-3 Acceptable Bladder Dimensions for Arms of Different Sizes		
Cuff	Bladder Length (cm)	Arm Circumference Range at Midpoint (cm)
Newborn	6	Less than 6
Infant	15	6-15
Child	21	16-21
Small adult	24	22-26
Adult	30	27-34
Large adult	38	35-44
Adult thigh	42	45-52

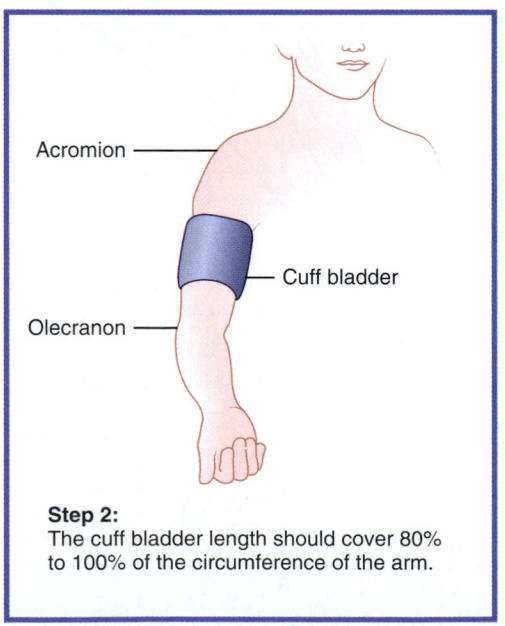

Step 1: The child's arm circumference should be assessed midpoint between the acromion process and the olecranon process.

Step 2: The cuff bladder length should cover 80% to 100% of the circumference of the arm.

Figure 24-5 Determination of proper blood pressure cuff size.

Figure 24-6 Traci measures the blood pressure of a pediatric patient.

BLOOD PRESSURE CLASSIFICATIONS

Blood pressure varies depending on the age of the child and his or her height and gender. The National High Blood Pressure Education Program (NHBPEP) prepared a set of tables that physicians use to determine whether a child's blood pressure is higher than the average among children of the same age and height. If a child has a blood pressure that is higher than 90% to 95% of most other children of the same age, height, and gender, the child may have high blood pressure.

The NHBPEP tables (one for boys and one for girls) allow precise classification of blood pressure according to body size, which avoids misclassifying children at the extreme ends of normal growth. A very tall child would not be mistakenly diagnosed as having hypertension, and hypertension would not be missed in a very short child. The NHBPEP tables used by physicians to assist in the diagnosis of hypertension in children can be found at the National Heart, Lung, and Blood Institute website.

Blood pressure varies throughout the day in children as a result of normal fluctuations in physical activity and emotional stress. If a child's blood pressure is elevated, two more readings must be taken at different visits before the physician can make a diagnosis of hypertension.

Memories *from* Practicum

Traci Powell: I still remember how difficult it was at times as a student. I had been out of high school for more than a year, so I had to get back into the routine of studying. I worried about whether I would do well, whether I would be able to find a good job, and whether I would like medical assisting. Adding to these concerns was the financial burden of putting myself through school. I took advantage of grants and a student loan. Throughout the last 6 months of my education, I also worked full-time as an aide on the midnight shift at a nursing home while attending school full-time during the day. As if that were not enough, my first child was well on her way into this world as I was finishing up the last quarter of my degree. There were so many times that I was tired, frustrated, and broke, but I kept pushing myself to do my best because I knew this was going to be my lifetime career, and I wanted to excel in my profession. My determination paid off. Today I have a great medical assisting position that I love, with an institution that is one of the best employers in the area. ■

COLLECTION OF A URINE SPECIMEN

A urinalysis may be performed on a pediatric patient for the following reasons: to screen for the presence of disease as part of a general physical examination, to assist in the diagnosis of a pathologic condition (e.g., urinary tract

What Would You Do? What Would You *Not* Do?

Case Study 2

Wanda Tilley comes to the office with her 10-year-old daughter, Courtney. Courtney has a skin condition on her legs that needs to be evaluated by the physician. Courtney has been obese since she was 4 years old. Mrs. Tilley also is obese and is not too concerned about Courtney's weight. She says that Courtney must have inherited her "fat gene," and there's not much that can be done about it. Courtney's favorite activities are playing video games and reading. She would like to join the community swim team, but she's too embarrassed for anyone to see her in a bathing suit. Courtney says the other kids are always making fun of her at school. She says that they call her "two-ton Tilley" and "double-roll," and they don't want to sit with her at lunch. Courtney wants her mom to home-school her because she's getting to the point where she can't take it anymore. She doesn't want the doctor to examine her because he'll see how fat she is and say bad things about it. ■

infection), or to evaluate the effectiveness of therapy. The collection of a urine specimen from a child who exhibits bladder control is performed using the technique outlined in Chapter 30. Collecting a urine specimen from an infant or young child who cannot urinate voluntarily involves the use of a pediatric urine collector. Pediatric urine collectors are designed to be used with both sexes. The urine collector consists of a clear plastic disposable bag containing a hypoallergenic pressure-sensitive adhesive around the opening of the bag. The adhesive firmly attaches the urine collector to the genitalia. Procedure 24-4 outlines the procedure for applying a pediatric urine collector.

PROCEDURE 24-4 Applying a Pediatric Urine Collector

Outcome Apply a pediatric urine collector

Equipment/Supplies

- Disposable gloves
- Personal antiseptic wipes
- Pediatric urine collector bag
- Urine specimen container and label
- Regular waste container

---

1. **Procedural Step.** Sanitize your hands.
2. **Procedural Step.** Assemble the equipment.
3. **Procedural Step.** Greet the infant's parent and introduce yourself. Identify the infant and explain the procedure to the parent.
4. **Procedural Step.** Apply gloves. Position the child. The child should be placed on his or her back with the legs spread apart. The medical assistant may need another individual to hold the child's legs apart.
   Principle. This position facilitates cleansing of the genitalia and permits proper application of the urine collector bag.
5. **Procedural Step.** Cleanse the child's genitalia.
   Female: Using a front-to-back motion (pubis to anus), cleanse each side of the meatus with a separate wipe. With a third wipe, cleanse directly down the middle (directly over the urinary meatus). Discard each wipe after cleansing. Allow the area to dry completely.
   Male: If the child is not circumcised, retract the foreskin of the penis. Cleanse the area around the meatus and the urethral opening (meatal orifice) in a manner similar to that used to cleanse the female patient. Use a separate wipe for each swipe. Cleanse the scrotum last, using a fresh wipe. Discard each wipe after cleansing. Allow the area to dry completely.
   Principle. The urinary meatus and surrounding area must be cleansed to prevent contaminants, such as baby powder, fecal material, and microorganisms, from entering the urine specimen, which could affect the test results. A front-to-back motion must be used to prevent drawing microorganisms from the anal area into the area being cleansed. The area must be completely dry to ensure an airtight adhesion of the collection bag to prevent leakage of urine.
6. **Procedural Step.** Remove the paper backing from the urine collector bag. This exposes the hypoallergenic adhesive surface around the opening of the bag. Firmly attach the bag in the following manner:
   Female: Stretch the perineum taut, and firmly place the bottom of the adhesive surface on the infant's perineum. Starting at the perineum and working upward, firmly press the adhesive surface to the skin surrounding the external genitalia, ensuring there is no puckering. The opening of the bag should be directly over the urinary meatus. The excess of the bag should be positioned toward the child's feet.
   Male: Position the bag so that the child's penis and scrotum are projected through the opening of the bag. Starting at the perineum and working upward, firmly press the adhesive surface to the skin surrounding the penis and scrotum, ensuring there is no puckering. The excess of the bag should be positioned toward the child's feet.
   Principle. The adhesive surface of the bag must be attached securely with no puckering to prevent leakage.

6 (1)

Remove paper backing from the urine collector bag.

PROCEDURE 24-4 Applying a Pediatric Urine Collector—cont'd

6 (2)

Firmly press the adhesive surface to the skin surrounding the external genitalia.

6 (3)

A, Male: The penis and scrotum are projected through the opening of the bag. **B, Female:** The opening of the bag should be directly over the urinary meatus.

7. **Procedural Step.** Loosely diaper the child. Check the urine collector bag every 15 minutes until a urine specimen is obtained.
Principle. The diaper helps hold the urine collector bag in place. The bag must be checked frequently. Once the infant has urinated, moisture from the urine may cause the adhesive surface to become loose and leak, especially with an active infant.

8. **Procedural Step.** When the child has voided, gently remove the urine collector bag by holding the bottom of the adhesive surface against the infant's skin and carefully peeling the bag off from the top to the bottom.
Principle. The bag must be removed gently because pulling the adhesive away too quickly may cause discomfort and irritation of the child's skin.

9. **Procedural Step.** Cleanse the genital area with a personal antiseptic wipe. Rediaper the child.

10. **Procedural Step.** Transfer the urine specimen into a urine specimen container, and tightly apply the lid. Label the container with the child's name and date of birth, the date, the time of collection, and the type of specimen (i.e., urine). Dispose of the collector bag in a regular waste container. (*Note:* The urine collector bag can be used as a urine container to transport the specimen to the laboratory. This is accomplished by folding the adhesive sponge ring in half along its vertical axis and pressing the adhesive surfaces firmly together to ensure a tight seal.)

11. **Procedural Step.** Based on the medical office routine, test the urine specimen or prepare it for transfer to an outside laboratory; be sure to include a completed laboratory request form. If the specimen cannot be tested or transferred immediately, preserve it by placing it in the refrigerator.
Principle. Changes occur in a urine specimen that is left sitting out at room temperature, which can lead to inaccurate test results.

12. **Procedural Step.** Remove the gloves, and sanitize your hands.

13. **Procedural Step.** Chart the procedure in the patient's medical record.
    a. *Paper-based patient record:* Record the date, the time of collection, and the type of specimen (i.e., urine). If the specimen is to be transported to an outside laboratory, indicate this information, including the laboratory tests ordered (refer to the PPR charting example).

Continued

PROCEDURE 24-4 Applying a Pediatric Urine Collector—cont'd

PPR CHARTING EXAMPLE

Date	
8/12/XX	10:15 a.m. Urine specimen collected for culture. Picked up by Medical Center Lab on 8/12/XX. ———— T. Powell, CMA (AAMA)

b. *Electronic medical record:* Document the type of specimen (i.e., urine) and the testing that was completed, using the appropriate radio buttons, drop-down menus, and free text fields. If the specimen is to be transported to an outside laboratory, document this information including the laboratory tests ordered.

PEDIATRIC INJECTIONS

Administering an injection to a child is an important responsibility. The experience a child has with early injections influences the child's attitude toward later ones. If the child is old enough to understand, the procedure should be explained. The medical assistant should be honest and should attempt to gain the child's trust and cooperation. The child should be told the truth about the injection—that it will hurt, but only for a short time. It also is advisable to explain that the medicine is being given to help him or her. Another person should be present to assist. The assistant can help position the child and can divert or restrain him or her if necessary. If the child struggles and fights excessively, the medical assistant should delay the injection and consult the physician.

The administration of injections is presented in Chapter 26. Before undertaking the study of pediatric injections, the medical assistant should review this chapter thoroughly, concentrating on the locations of injection sites and the procedures for preparing and administering injections. The same basic technique is used to administer an injection to an adult and a child. Variations in procedure are explained in the following section.

TYPES OF NEEDLES

The gauge and length of the needle used for intramuscular injections vary, depending on the consistency of the medication to be administered and the size of the child. Thick or oily preparations require a larger needle lumen, and the needle must be long enough to reach muscle tissue. A needle length ranging from ⅝ inch to 1 inch is typically used to administer an intramuscular injection to a child, and in general the gauge of the needle ranges from 22 to 25, depending on the viscosity (thickness) of the medication. The length of the needle used to administer a pediatric subcutaneous injection ranges from ½ inch to ⅝ inch, and the gauge of the needle ranges from 23 to 25.

PEDIATRIC INTRAMUSCULAR INJECTION SITES

Pediatric injection sites vary based on the age of the child. The specific site to be injected is stated in the package insert accompanying the medication. Until the child is walking, the gluteus muscle is small and not well developed and is covered with a thick layer of fat. An injection in the dorsogluteal site (Figure 24-7) may come dangerously close to the sciatic nerve. The danger is increased if the child is squirming or fighting. Because serious trauma can result from incorrect administration of an injection in this area, the dorsogluteal site should never be used as an injection site for an infant or young child.

The vastus lateralis muscle site is recommended for injections of infants and young children. It is located on the anterior surface of the midlateral thigh, away from major nerves and blood vessels, and it is large enough to accommodate the injected medication (Figure 24-8, *A*). To locate the vastus lateralis site in an infant or young child, divide

Figure 24-7 Dorsogluteal intramuscular injection site. (Courtesy Wyeth Laboratories, Philadelphia, Pa.)

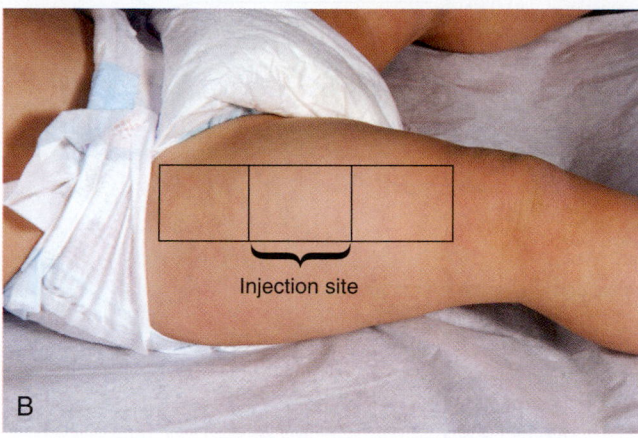

Figure 24-8 **A,** Vastus lateralis intramuscular injection site. **B,** Location of the vastus lateralis injection site in an infant. Divide the mid-anterior thigh into thirds. The injection is administered into the middle third of the thigh. (**A,** Courtesy Wyeth Laboratories, Philadelphia, Pa.)

the mid–anterior thigh into thirds. The injection is administered into the middle third of the thigh (Figure 24-8, *B*).

The length of the needle used depends on the overall size of the thigh. The needle should be long enough to penetrate the muscle belly for proper absorption to occur. A 1-inch needle is often used for a normal-sized infant or child; however, the length of the needle may need to be decreased (e.g., ⅝ inch) for newborns or preterm infants and increased (e.g., 1¼ inches) for overweight children. For administration of the injection, the infant is placed on his or her back. The thigh is grasped to compress the muscle tissue and to stabilize the extremity (Figure 24-9, *A*). The injection is administered as illustrated in Figure 24-9, *B*, by following the procedure outlined in Chapter 26.

The deltoid muscle is shallow and can accommodate only a small amount of medication. In addition, repeated injections at this site are painful. Because the deltoid site is so small in an infant, the deltoid site should not be used to administer an injection until a child is at least 18 months old. The length of the needle should be adjusted according to the amount of subcutaneous tissue over the injection site. For example, a ⅝-inch needle is often used for a normal-sized 4-year-old, but a 1-inch needle may be required for an obese child of the same age. For administration of the injection, the deltoid muscle mass should be grasped at the injection site and compressed between the thumb and fingers. The needle should be inserted pointing slightly upward toward the shoulder (Figure 24-10).

After the injection has been given, the medical assistant or the child's parent should hold the infant, provide comfort, and show approval so that the child associates something other than pain with this procedure.

PEDIATRIC SUBCUTANEOUS INJECTION SITES

A subcutaneous injection is made into the subcutaneous tissue, which consists of adipose (fat) tissue and is located

Figure 24-9 **A,** Compression of the vastus lateralis muscle. **B,** Intramuscular injection into the vastus lateralis injection site.

just under the skin. Subcutaneous tissue is located all over the body; however, certain sites are more commonly used because they are located where bones and blood vessels are not near the surface of the skin. The recommended subcutaneous site for an infant younger than 12 months of age is the anterior thigh. For a child 12 months of age or older,

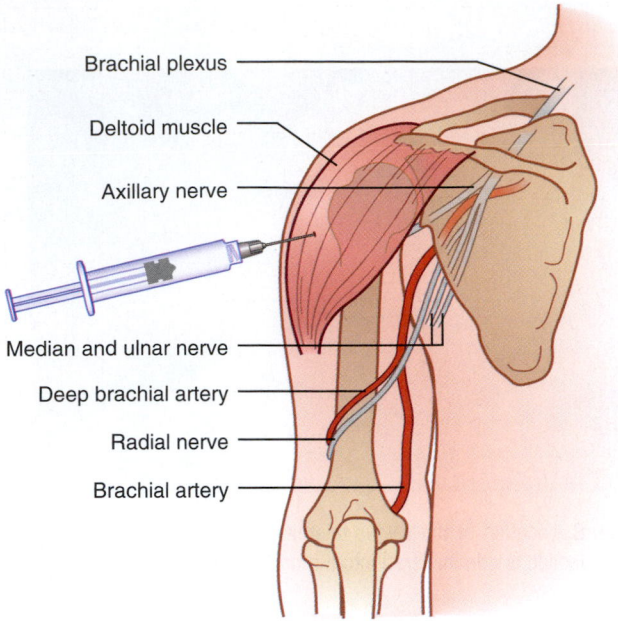

Brachial plexus
Deltoid muscle
Axillary nerve
Median and ulnar nerve
Deep brachial artery
Radial nerve
Brachial artery

Figure 24-10 Deltoid intramuscular injection site. (Courtesy Wyeth Laboratories, Philadelphia, Pa.)

the recommended subcutaneous site is the lateral part of the upper arm.

For administration of the injection, the area surrounding the injection site should be grasped and held in a cushion fashion and the needle should be inserted at a 45-degree angle. This ensures that the subcutaneous tissue and not muscle tissue is entered. The designated pediatric subcutaneous injection sites do not contain any large blood vessels. Because of this, the CDC recommends that aspiration of the syringe is not necessary before administration of a vaccine through the subcutaneous route. Studies show that not aspirating before administration of the vaccine reduces pain at the injection site. It is extremely important, however, that the medical assistant always review and follow the medication administration policies set forth at her or his medical office.

IMMUNIZATIONS

Immunity is the resistance of the body to the effects of harmful agents, such as pathogenic microorganisms and their toxins. The process of becoming immune or rendering an individual immune through the use of a **vaccine** or **toxoid** is known as active, artificial **immunization.** Immunizations build the body's defenses and protect an individual from attack by certain infectious diseases.

Immunizations should be administered to infants and young children during well-child visits according to an immunization schedule. The American Academy of Pediatrics recommends that the schedule outlined in Figure 24-11 be followed. This schedule is intended as a guide to be used with any modifications needed to meet the requirements of an individual or group.

The medical assistant should be familiar with every immunization that is given, including its use, common side effects, route of administration, dose, and method of storage. The drug manufacturer includes a package insert with each vaccine and toxoid that contains valuable information about the drug. Drug references, such as the *Physician's Desk Reference,* also can be used to locate information on immunizations. Immunizations administered to infants and children, along with brand names, routes of administration, and common minor problems, are listed in Table 24-4. Certain immunizations can be administered together in the same injection. A combined immunization is just as effective as the individual immunization and results in fewer injections for the infant or child. For example, diphtheria, tetanus, and pertussis (DTaP), hepatitis B, and polio (DTaP-HepB-IPV) immunizations can be combined together in the same injection. Table 24-5 provides a list of combined immunizations administered to infants and children, along with brand names and the routes of administration.

Parents should be provided with an immunization record card (Figure 24-12) at their infant's first well-child visit. They should be instructed to bring this card to every visit so that their child's immunizations can be recorded. Parents should be informed of the possible normal side effects of each immunization and given instructions on how to respond if they occur.

NATIONAL CHILDHOOD VACCINE INJURY ACT

The National Childhood Vaccine Injury Act (NCVIA), which became effective in 1988, requires that parents be provided with information about the benefits and risks of childhood immunizations. To help medical offices comply with these regulations, the Centers for Disease Control and Prevention developed a set of vaccine information statements (VISs). A VIS explains, in lay terminology, the benefits and risks of a vaccine. It also contains information about reporting an adverse reaction, the National Vaccine Injury Compensation Program, and how to get more information about childhood diseases and vaccines. See Figure 24-13 for a DTaP VIS.

The NCVIA requires that the appropriate and most current VIS be given to the child's parent or guardian each and every time before the child receives a dose of any immunization listed in Table 24-4. The medical assistant must give the parent or guardian enough time to read the VIS and an opportunity to ask questions before the immunization is administered. In addition, the medical assistant must chart the following information in the patient's medical record: the name and publication date of each VIS provided to the parent, and the date the VIS was given to the parent. The publication date of the VIS is located at the bottom left or right corner of the VIS. Vaccine information statements also are available for pneumococcal polysaccharide, shingles (herpes zoster), rabies, yellow fever, typhoid, Japanese encephalitis, anthrax, and smallpox. Their use is

Vaccine	Birth	1 mo	2 mos	4 mos	6 mos	9 mos	12 mos	15 mos	18 mos	19–23 mos	2-3 yrs	4-6 yrs	7-10 yrs	11-12 yrs	13–15 yrs	16–18 yrs
Hepatitis B[1] (HepB)	1st dose	←2nd dose→			←3rd dose→											
Rotavirus[2] (RV) RV1 (2-dose series); RV5 (3-dose series)			1st dose	2nd dose	See footnote 2											
Diphtheria, tetanus, & acellular pertussis[3] (DTaP: <7 yrs)			1st dose	2nd dose	3rd dose			←4th dose→				5th dose				
Tetanus, diphtheria, & acellular pertussis[4] (Tdap: ≥7 yrs)														(Tdap)		
Haemophilus influenzae type b[5] (Hib)			1st dose	2nd dose	See footnote 5		←3rd or 4th dose, See footnote 5→									
Pneumococcal conjugate[6] (PCV13)			1st dose	2nd dose	3rd dose		←4th dose→									
Pneumococcal polysaccharide[6] (PPSV23)																
Inactivated poliovirus[7] (IPV: <18 yrs)			1st dose	2nd dose	←3rd dose→							4th dose				
Influenza[8] (IIV; LAIV) 2 doses for some: See footnote 8					Annual vaccination (IIV only) 1 or 2 doses						Annual vaccination (LAIV or IIV) 1 or 2 doses		Annual vaccination (LAIV or IIV) 1 dose only			
Measles, mumps, rubella[9] (MMR)					See footnote 9		←1st dose→					2nd dose				
Varicella[10] (VAR)							←1st dose→					2nd dose				
Hepatitis A[11] (HepA)							←2-dose series, See footnote 11→									
Human papillomavirus[12] (HPV2: females only; HPV4: males and females)														(3-dose series)		
Meningococcal[13] (Hib-MenCY ≥ 6 weeks; MenACWY-D ≥9 mos; MenACWY-CRM ≥ 2 mos)					See footnote 13									1st dose		Booster

▢ (yellow) Range of recommended ages for all children	▢ (green) Range of recommended ages for catch-up immunization	▢ (purple) Range of recommended ages for certain high-risk groups	▢ (green/purple) Range of recommended ages during which catch-up is encouraged and for certain high-risk groups	▢ (white) Not routinely recommended

This schedule includes recommendations in effect as of January 1, 2015. Any dose not administered at the recommended age should be administered at a subsequent visit, when indicated and feasible. The use of a combination vaccine generally is preferred over separate injections of its equivalent component vaccines. Vaccination providers should consult the relevant Advisory Committee on Immunization Practices (ACIP) statement for detailed recommendations, available online at http://www.cdc.gov/vaccines/hcp/acip-recs/index.html. Clinically significant adverse events that follow vaccination should be reported to the Vaccine Adverse Event Reporting System (VAERS) online (http://www.vaers.hhs.gov) or by telephone (800-822-7967). Suspected cases of vaccine-preventable diseases should be reported to the state or local health department. Additional information, including precautions and contraindications for vaccination, is available from CDC online (http://www.cdc.gov/vaccines/recs/vac-admin/contraindications.htm) or by telephone (800-CDC-INFO [800-232-4636]).

This schedule is approved by the Advisory Committee on Immunization Practices (http://www.cdc.gov/vaccines/acip), the American Academy of Pediatrics (http://www.aap.org), the American Academy of Family Physicians (http://www.aafp.org), and the American College of Obstetricians and Gynecologists (http://www.acog.org).

(From Department of Health and Human Services, Centers for Disease Control and Prevention, United States, 2014. For the remainder of the footnotes to this immunization schedule, please see http://www.cdc.gov/vaccines/schedules/downloads/child/0-18yrs-schedule.pdf.)

Footnotes — Recommended immunization schedule for persons aged 0 through 18 years—United States, 2015

For further guidance on the use of the vaccines mentioned below, see: http://www.cdc.gov/vaccines/pubs/acip-list.htm.

1. **Hepatitis B (HepB) vaccine. (Minimum age: birth)**
   Routine vaccination:
   At birth
   • Administer monovalent HepB vaccine to all newborns before hospital discharge.
   • For infants born to hepatitis B surface antigen (HBsAg)–positive mothers, administer HepB vaccine and 0.5 mL of hepatitis B immune globulin (HBIG) within 12 hours of birth. These infants should be tested for HBsAg and antibody to HBsAg (anti-HBs) 1 to 2 months after completion of the HepB series, at age 9 through 18 months (preferably at the next well-child visit).
   • If mother's HBsAg status is unknown, within 12 hours of birth administer HepB vaccine to all infants regardless of birth weight. For infants weighing <2,000 grams, administer HBIG in addition to HepB within 12 hours of birth. Determine mother's HBsAg status as soon as possible and, if she is HBsAg-positive, also administer HBIG for infants weighing ≥2,000 grams (no later than age 1 week).
   Doses following the birth dose
   • The second dose should be administered at age 1 or 2 months. Monovalent HepB vaccine should be used for doses administered before age 6 weeks.
   • Infants who did not receive a birth dose should receive 3 doses of a HepB-containing vaccine on a schedule of 0, 1 to 2 months, and 6 months starting as soon as feasible. See Figure 2.
   • The minimum interval between dose 1 and dose 2 is 4 weeks and between dose 2 and 3 is 8 weeks. The final (third or fourth) dose in the HepB vaccine series should be administered no earlier than age 24 weeks, and at least 16 weeks after the first dose.
   • Administration of a total of 4 doses of HepB vaccine is recommended when a combination vaccine containing HepB is administered after the birth dose.
   Catch-up vaccination:
   • Unvaccinated persons should complete a 3-dose series.
   • A 2-dose series (doses separated by at least 4 months) of adult formulation Recombivax HB is licensed for use in children aged 11 through 15 years.
   • For other catch-up issues, see Figure 2.
2. **Rotavirus (RV) vaccines. (Minimum age: 6 weeks for both RV-1 [Rotarix] and RV-5 [RotaTeq]).**
   Routine vaccination:
   • Administer a series of RV vaccine to all infants as follows:
      1. If RV-1 is used, administer a 2-dose series at 2 and 4 months of age.
      2. If RV-5 is used, administer a 3-dose series at ages 2, 4, and 6 months.
      3. If any dose in series was RV-5 or vaccine product is unknown for any dose in the series, a total of 3 doses of RV vaccine should be administered.
   Catch-up vaccination:
   • The maximum age for the first dose in the series is 14 weeks, 6 days.
   • Vaccination should not be initiated for infants aged 15 weeks 0 days or older.
   • The maximum age for the final dose in the series is 8 months, 0 days.
   • If RV-1 (Rotarix) is administered for the first and second doses, a third dose is not indicated.
   • For other catch-up issues, see Figure 2.
3. **Diphtheria and tetanus toxoids and acellular pertussis (DTaP) vaccine. (Minimum age: 6 weeks)**
   Routine vaccination:

• Administer a 5-dose series of DTaP vaccine at ages 2, 4, 6, 15–18 months, and 4 through 6 years. The fourth dose may be administered as early as age 12 months, provided at least 6 months have elapsed since the third dose.
   Catch-up vaccination:
   • The fifth (booster) dose of DTaP vaccine is not necessary if the fourth dose was administered at age 4 years or older.
   • For other catch-up issues, see Figure 2.
4. **Tetanus and diphtheria toxoids and acellular pertussis (Tdap) vaccine. (Minimum age: 10 years for Boostrix, 11 years for Adacel).**
   Routine vaccination:
   • Administer 1 dose of Tdap vaccine to all adolescents aged 11 through 12 years.
   • Tdap can be administered regardless of the interval since the last tetanus and diphtheria toxoid-containing vaccine.
   • Administer one dose of Tdap vaccine to pregnant adolescents during each pregnancy (preferred during 27 through 36 weeks gestation) regardless of number of years from prior Td or Tdap vaccination.
   Catch-up vaccination:
   • Persons aged 7 through 10 years who are not fully immunized with the childhood DTaP vaccine series, should receive Tdap vaccine as the first dose in the catch-up series; if additional doses are needed, use Td vaccine. For these children, an adolescent Tdap vaccine should not be given.
   • Persons aged 11 through 18 years who have not received Tdap vaccine should receive a dose followed by tetanus and diphtheria toxoids (Td) booster doses every 10 years thereafter.
   • An inadvertent dose of DTaP vaccine administered to children aged 7 through 10 years can count as part of the catch-up series. This dose can count as the adolescent Tdap dose, or the child can later receive a Tdap booster dose at age 11–12 years.
   • For other catch-up issues, see Figure 2.
5. *Haemophilus influenzae* type b (Hib) conjugate vaccine. (Minimum age: 6 weeks)
   Routine vaccination:
   • Administer a Hib vaccine primary series and a booster dose to all infants. The primary series doses should be administered at 2, 4, and 6 months of age; however, if PRP-OMP (PedvaxHib or Comvax) is administered at 2 and 4 months of age, a dose at age 6 months is not indicated. One booster dose should be administered at age 12 through15 months.
   • Hiberix (PRP-T) should only be used for the booster (final) dose in children aged 12 months through 4 years, who have received at least 1 dose of Hib.
   Catch-up vaccination:
   • If dose 1 was administered at ages 12-14 months, administer booster (as final dose) at least 8 weeks after dose 1.
   • If the first 2 doses were PRP-OMP (PedvaxHIB or Comvax), and were administered at age 11 months or younger, the third (and final) dose should be administered at age 12 through 15 months and at least 8 weeks after the second dose.
   • If the first dose was administered at age 7 through 11 months, administer the second dose at least 4 weeks later and a final dose at age 12 through 15 months, regardless of Hib vaccine (PRP-T or PRP-OMP) used for first dose.
   • For unvaccinated children aged 15 months or older, administer only 1 dose.

Figure 24-11 Immunization schedule. (From Department of Health and Human Services, Centers for Disease Control and Prevention, United States, 2015.)

Table 24-4 Infant and Childhood Immunizations

Immunization (and Abbreviation)	Brand Names	Route of Administration	Common Minor Problems after Administration
Hep B (hepatitis B vaccine)	Engerix-B Recombivax HB	IM	Mild fever Soreness at injection site
DTaP (diphtheria and tetanus toxoids and acellular pertussis vaccine)	Acel-Imune Certiva Daptacel Infanrix Tripedia	IM	Fever, irritability, tiredness, poor appetite, and vomiting Redness or swelling at injection site Soreness or tenderness at injection site (occurs 1-3 days after the injection and occurs more often after the fourth or fifth dose in the series than after earlier doses)
Hib (*Haemophilus influenzae* type b vaccine)	ActHIB HibTITER PedvaxHIB	IM	Redness, swelling, and warmth at injection site; fever greater than 101°F (38.3°C) (occurs within 1 day after injection; may last 2 to 3 days)
IPV (inactivated polio vaccine)	IPOL	IM or SC	Soreness at the injection site
PCV (pneumococcal conjugate vaccine)	Prevnar	IM	Redness, swelling, and tenderness at the injection site; fever Irritability and drowsiness Loss of appetite
RV (rotavirus vaccine)	Rotarix RotaTeq	PO	Irritability, temporary diarrhea, and vomiting
MMR (measles, mumps, and rubella vaccines)	M-M-R II	SC	Fever, mild rash, swelling of glands in the cheeks or neck (occur 7-12 days after administration)
Var (varicella) (chickenpox vaccine)	Varivax	SC	Fever, mild rash Soreness or swelling at injection site
Hep A (hepatitis A vaccine)	Havrix Vaqta	IM	Soreness at the injection site Headache, loss of appetite, and tiredness (usually last 1-2 days)
MCV4 (meningococcal vaccine)	Menactra	IM	Pain and redness at injection site Fever (usually lasts 1-2 days)
HPV (human papillomavirus vaccine)	Gardasil Cervarix	IM	Pain, redness, swelling, or itching at injection site Fever
Influenza vaccine (injection)	Afluria Fluarix FluLaval FluShield Fluvirin Fluzone Fluzone Intradermal	IM ID	Soreness, redness, or swelling at the injection site, fever and malaise Hoarseness; sore, red, or itchy eyes Cough, fever, aches (occur soon after injection and usually last 1-2 days)
Influenza vaccine (nasal spray)	FluMist	IN	Runny nose, nasal congestion or cough Headache, muscle aches, abdominal pain, or occasional vomiting or diarrhea Fever; wheezing

ID, intradermal; *IM,* intramuscular; *IN,* intranasal; *PO,* oral; *SC,* subcutaneous.

Table 24-5 Infant and Childhood Combination Immunizations

Combined Immunization	Brand Name	Route of Administration
DTaP-HepB-IPV	Pediarix	IM
DTaP-Hib-IPV	Pentacel	IM
DTaP-IPV	Kinrix	IM
DTaP-Hib	TriHIBit	IM
Hib-HepB	Comvax	IM
MMRV	ProQuad	SC

See Table 24-4 for the common minor problems that may occur following administration of each individual immunization.
DTaP, Diphtheria, tetanus, and pertussis; *HepB,* hepatitis B; *Hib,* Haemophilus influenzae type b; *IM,* intramuscular; *IPV,* inactivated polio vaccine; *MMRV,* measles, mumps, rubella, varicella; *SC,* subcutaneous.

strongly encouraged by the NCVIA but is not required, because these vaccines are not administered to children on a routine basis.

The NCVIA also requires that the following information be recorded in each patient's medical record or on a permanent office log after administration of the vaccine: the date of administration of the vaccine, the manufacturer and lot number of the vaccine, the signature and title of the health care provider who administered the vaccine, and the name and address of the medical office where the vaccine was administered. Figure 24-14 shows an example of an immunization administrative record that is included in a patient's medical record.

IMMUNIZATION RECORD

Name _____

Birthdate _____

Immunization	DATE	DATE	DATE	DATE	DATE
Hep B (Hepatitis B)					
DTaP (Diphtheria, Tetanus, and Pertussis)					
Hib (*Haemophilius influenzae* Type b)					
IPV (Inactivated Polio Vaccine)					
PCV (Pneumococcal Conjugate Vaccine)					
RV (Rotavirus vaccine)					
MMR (Measles, Mumps, Rubella)					
Varicella (Chickenpox)					
Hep A (Hepatitis A)					
MCV4 (Meningococcal Vaccine)					
HPV (Human Papillomavirus)					
Influenza					
Tuberculin (Mantoux) RESULT					
Tetanus Booster					
Other					

Figure 24-12 Immunization record card.

DIPHTHERIA TETANUS & PERTUSSIS VACCINES

WHAT YOU NEED TO KNOW

1 | Why get vaccinated?

Diphtheria, tetanus, and pertussis are serious diseases caused by bacteria. Diphtheria and pertussis are spread from person to person. Tetanus enters the body through cuts or wounds.

DIPHTHERIA causes a thick covering in the back of the throat.
- It can lead to breathing problems, paralysis, heart failure, and even death.

TETANUS (Lockjaw) causes painful tightening of the muscles, usually all over the body.
- It can lead to "locking" of the jaw so the victim cannot open his mouth or swallow. Tetanus leads to death in up to 2 out of 10 cases.

PERTUSSIS (Whooping Cough) causes coughing spells so bad that it is hard for infants to eat, drink, or breathe. These spells can last for weeks.
- It can lead to pneumonia, seizures (jerking and staring spells), brain damage, and death.

Diphtheria, tetanus, and pertussis vaccine (DTaP) can help prevent these diseases. Most children who are vaccinated with DTaP will be protected throughout childhood. Many more children would get these diseases if we stopped vaccinating.

DTaP is a safer version of an older vaccine called DTP. DTP is no longer used in the United States.

2 | Who should get DTaP vaccine and when?

Children should get 5 doses of DTaP vaccine, one dose at each of the following ages:

2 months	15-18 months
4 months	4-6 years
6 months	

DTaP may be given at the same time as other vaccines.

3 | Some children should not get DTaP vaccine or should wait

- Children with minor illnesses, such as a cold, may be vaccinated. But children who are moderately or severely ill should usually wait until they recover before getting DTaP vaccine.

- Any child who had a life-threatening allergic reaction after a dose of DTaP should not get another dose.

- Any child who suffered a brain or nervous system disease within 7 days after a dose of DTaP should not get another dose.

- Talk with your doctor if your child:
  - had a seizure or collapsed after a dose of DTaP,
  - cried non-stop for 3 hours or more after a dose of DTaP,
  - had a fever over 105°F after a dose of DTaP.

Ask your health care provider for more information. Some of these children should not get another dose of pertussis vaccine, but may get a vaccine without pertussis, called **DT**.

4 | Older children and adults

DTaP is not licensed for adolescents, adults, or children 7 years of age and older.

But older people still need protection. A vaccine called **Tdap** is similar to DTaP. A single dose of Tdap is recommended for people 11 through 64 years of age. Another vaccine, called **Td**, protects against tetanus and diphtheria, but not pertussis. It is recommended every 10 years. There are separate Vaccine Information Statements for these vaccines.

Diphtheria/Tetanus/Pertussis	5/17/2007

Figure 24-13 Vaccine information statement for diphtheria, tetanus, and pertussis (DTaP). (Courtesy Centers for Disease Control and Prevention, Atlanta, Ga.)

5 | What are the risks from DTaP vaccine?

Getting diphtheria, tetanus, or pertussis disease is much riskier than getting DTaP vaccine.

However, a vaccine, like any medicine, is capable of causing serious problems, such as severe allergic reactions. The risk of DTaP vaccine causing serious harm, or death, is extremely small.

Mild Problems (Common)

- Fever (up to about 1 child in 4)
- Redness or swelling where the shot was given (up to about 1 child in 4)
- Soreness or tenderness where the shot was given (up to about 1 child in 4)

These problems occur more often after the 4th and 5th doses of the DTaP series than after earlier doses. Sometimes the 4th or 5th dose of DTaP vaccine is followed by swelling of the entire arm or leg in which the shot was given, lasting 1-7 days (up to about 1 child in 30).

Other mild problems include:

- Fussiness (up to about 1 child in 3)
- Tiredness or poor appetite (up to about 1 child in 10)
- Vomiting (up to about 1 child in 50)

These problems generally occur 1-3 days after the shot.

Moderate Problems (Uncommon)

- Seizure (jerking or staring) (about 1 child out of 14,000)
- Non-stop crying, for 3 hours or more (up to about 1 child out of 1,000)
- High fever, over 105°F (about 1 child out of 16,000)

Severe Problems (Very Rare)

- Serious allergic reaction (less than 1 out of a million doses)
- Several other severe problems have been reported after DTaP vaccine. These include:
  - Long-term seizures, coma, or lowered consciousness
  - Permanent brain damage.

  These are so rare it is hard to tell if they are caused by the vaccine.

Controlling fever is especially important for children who have had seizures, for any reason. It is also important if another family member has had seizures. You can reduce fever and pain by giving your child an *aspirin-free* pain reliever when the shot is given, and for the next 24 hours, following the package instructions.

6 | What if there is a moderate or severe reaction?

What should I look for?

Any unusual conditions, such as a serious allergic reaction, high fever or unusual behavior. Serious allergic reactions are extremely rare with any vaccine. If one were to occur, it would most likely be within a few minutes to a few hours after the shot. Signs can include difficulty breathing, hoarseness or wheezing, hives, paleness, weakness, a fast heart beat or dizziness. If a high fever or seizure were to occur, it would usually be within a week after the shot.

What should I do?

- **Call** a doctor, or get the person to a doctor right away.
- **Tell** your doctor what happened, the date and time it happened, and when the vaccination was given.
- **Ask** your doctor, nurse, or health department to report the reaction by filing a Vaccine Adverse Event Reporting System (VAERS) form.

  Or you can file this report through the VAERS web site at **www.vaers.hhs.gov**, or by calling **1-800-822-7967**. *VAERS does not provide medical advice*

7 | The National Vaccine Injury Compensation Program

In the rare event that you or your child has a serious reaction to a vaccine, a federal program has been created to help pay for the care of those who have been harmed.

For details about the National Vaccine Injury Compensation Program, call **1-800-338-2382** or visit the program's website at **www.hrsa.gov/vaccinecompensation.**

8 | How can I learn more?

- Ask your health care provider. They can give you the vaccine package insert or suggest other sources of information.

- Call your local or state health department's immunization program.

- Contact the Centers for Disease Control and Prevention (CDC):
  - Call **1-800-232-4636 (1-800-CDC-INFO)**
  - Visit the National Immunization Program's website at **www.cdc.gov/nip**

U.S. DEPARTMENT OF HEALTH & HUMAN SERVICES
Centers for Disease Control and Prevention

Vaccine Information Statement	
DTaP (5/17/07)	42 U.S.C. § 300aa-26

Figure 24-13, cont'd

IMMUNIZATION ADMINISTRATION RECORD

Name _____
(first)   (MI)   (last)

DOB _____

Physician _____

Address _____

_____

SITE ABBREVIATIONS:
RVL: Right vastus lateralis
LVL: Left vastus lateralis
RD: Right deltoid
LD: Left deltoid
PO: By mouth
IN: Intranasal

Vaccine	Type of Vaccine[1] (generic abbreviation)	Date Given (mo/day/yr)	Dose	Site	Vaccine		Vaccine Information Statement		Signature and Title of Vaccinator
					Lot #	Mfr.	Date on VIS	Date Given	
Hepatitis B[2] (e.g., HepB, Hib-HepB, DTaP-HepB-IPV) Give IM.									
Diphtheria, Tetanus, Pertussis[2] (e.g., DTaP, DTaP-Hib, DTaP-HepB-IPV, DT, DTaP-Hib-IPV, Tdap, DTaP-IPV, Td) Give IM.									
Haemophilus influenzae type b[2] (e.g., Hib, Hib-HepB, DTaP-Hib-IPV, DTaP-Hib) Give IM.									
Polio[2] (e.g., IPV, DTaP-HepB-IPV, DTaP-Hib-IPV, DTaP-IPV) Give IPV SC or IM. Give all others IM.									
Pneumococcal (e.g., PCV, conjugate; PPV, polysaccharide) Give PCV IM. Give PPV SC or IM.									
Rotovirus Give oral.									
Measles, Mumps, Rubella[5] (e.g., MMR, MMRV) Give SC.									
Varicella[5] (e.g., Var, MMRV) Give SC.									
Hepatitis A Give IM									
Meningococcal (e.g., MCV4, MPSV4) Give MCV4 IM and MPSV4 SC.									
Human papillomavirus (e.g., HPV) Give IM									
Influenza[5] (e.g., TIV, inactivated; LAIV, live attenuated) Give TIV IM. Give LAIV IN.									
Other									

1. Record the generic abbreviation for the type of vaccine given (e.g., DTaP-Hib, PCV), *not* the trade name.
2. For combination vaccines, fill in a row for each separate antigen in the combination.

Figure 24-14 Immunization administration record included in a patient's medical record. (Modified from Immunization Action Coalition, St Paul, Minn.)

NEWBORN SCREENING TEST

A newborn screening test is performed on an infant to screen for the presence of certain metabolic and endocrine diseases. The diseases that are screened for vary by state but typically include phenylketonuria (PKU), biotinidase deficiency, congenital adrenal hyperplasia, maple sugar urine disease, congenital hypothyroidism, galactosemia, homocystinuria, and sickle cell anemia. The most important of these is PKU, which is discussed in greater detail in the following paragraphs.

PKU is a congenital hereditary disease caused by a lack of the enzyme *phenylalanine hydroxylase*. This enzyme is needed to convert phenylalanine, an amino acid, into tyrosine, which is an amino acid needed for normal metabolic functioning. Without this enzyme, phenylalanine accumulates in the blood and, if the accumulation is left untreated, causes mental retardation and other abnormalities, such as tremors and poor muscle coordination. In most cases, on early detection a special low-phenylalanine diet and close periodic monitoring can prevent adverse effects. Normal development usually occurs if treatment is started before the child reaches 3 to 4 weeks of age. To promote the best development of cognitive abilities, most authorities recommend lifelong dietary restriction of phenylalanine. Although PKU is not a common condition (affecting 1 in every 12,000 births), early diagnosis and treatment lead to a better prognosis.

Phenylalanine can be detected in the blood of an affected infant only after the infant has been receiving breast or formula milk. Infants taking formula can be tested earlier than breast-fed infants because formula contains phenylalanine, whereas the "first breast milk," or colostrum, does not. The test results of breast-fed infants are usually invalid until the mother begins producing milk.

All states require by law that infants undergo newborn screening. The best time to perform the test is between 1 and 7 days after birth. In most states the newborn screening test is performed before the infant leaves the hospital. If the test has abnormal or invalid results, the infant needs to be retested. Most repeat tests are required because of invalid test results caused by the collection of an inadequate amount of the blood specimen. Newborn screening retesting is usually performed at a hospital laboratory but may sometimes be performed in the medical office.

The newborn screening test card (Figure 24-15) includes an information section that must be completed before the test is performed. The newborn screening test is performed

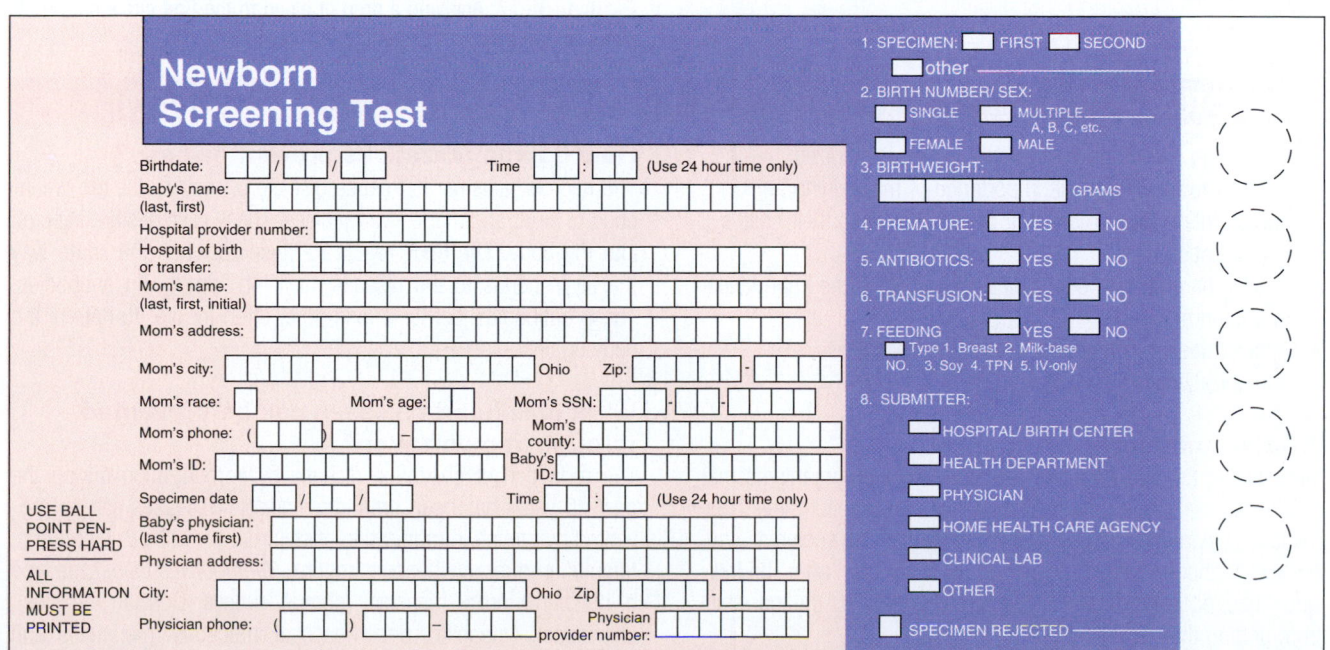

Figure 24-15 Newborn screening test card.

Medial curve ———————— ———————— Lateral curve

The shading indicates the appropriate area for making the puncture.

A

B

Figure 24-16 **A,** Heel puncture sites for a pediatric patient. **B,** Puncture of the medial posterior curve of the plantar surface of an infant's heel.

on capillary blood obtained from the fleshy part of the lateral or medial posterior curve of the plantar surface of the infant's heel (Figure 24-16). The blood specimen is placed on a special filter paper attached to the newborn screening test card (Figure 24-17) and is mailed to an outside laboratory for analysis. The results are ready in a few days. If one of the newborn screening test results is positive, further testing is performed.

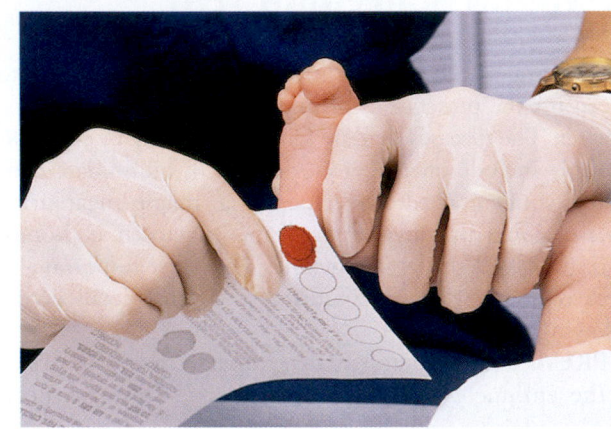

Figure 24-17 Applying a drop of blood to the first circle on the filter paper on the newborn screening test card.

PATIENT TEACHING Childhood Immunizations

- Encourage parents to have their children immunized.
- Emphasize to parents the importance of maintaining an immunization record card that documents all of their child's immunizations.
- Provide parents with educational materials on the importance of immunizations.
- Answer questions patients have about childhood immunizations.

What is immunity?

Immunity is the resistance of the body to microorganisms that cause disease. When an individual has an infection, the body responds by producing disease-fighting substances known as *antibodies*. Antibodies usually remain in the body even after the individual has recovered from the disease. This protects the individual from getting that disease again.

How do immunizations prevent disease?

The microorganisms that cause disease or their toxins are weakened or killed and made into vaccines. These vaccines are injected into the body. The body reacts to these vaccines the same way that it responds to the disease itself—by producing antibodies. These antibodies last for a long time, often for life, to defend the body against disease.

What childhood diseases can be prevented through immunization?

The reduction of childhood disease by immunization during the past 40 years has been dramatic. Fourteen diseases can be prevented by routine immunization of children: hepatitis B, diphtheria, tetanus, pertussis (whooping cough), *Haemophilus influenzae* type b infections, polio, measles, mumps, rubella (German measles), chickenpox (varicella), pneumococcal infections (meningitis and blood infections), hepatitis A, rotavirus, and influenza (flu). Except for tetanus, all these diseases are contagious. They can be spread from child to child and from one community to another. When children are not protected against them, serious outbreaks of disease can still occur.

Haven't most of these diseases been eliminated in the United States?

Although most of the vaccine-preventable diseases have been reduced to very low levels in the United States, this is not true worldwide. Some of these diseases are quite prevalent in other countries. An infected traveler can bring these diseases into the United States without knowing it. If Americans were not immunized, these diseases could quickly spread throughout the population and cause an epidemic. Only when a disease has been eradicated worldwide is it safe to stop vaccinating for that particular disease.

Do immunizations have side effects?

Vaccines are among the safest and most reliable medications available. Minor side effects may occur, however, after administration of an immunization. They do not last long and may include a slight fever and irritability; redness, swelling, and soreness at the injection site; and a mild rash. Rarely, the effects can be more serious; if any unusual symptoms occur after immunization, it is important to contact the physician immediately. Overall, the benefits of vaccines to prevent childhood diseases are greater than the possible risks for almost all children.

Are immunizations required by law?

Every state has laws requiring immunization against some or all of these diseases before children enter school. Children who get their immunizations benefit from the protection these immunizations provide; immunizations also contribute to the well-being of everyone by reducing the chance for disease to spread. School immunization requirements for each state can be found at the following websites: www.nnii.org/vaccineInfo/index.cfm#state and www.immunize.org/states. ■

What Would You Do? What Would You *Not* Do? RESPONSES

Case Study 1
Page 530

What Did Traci Do?
- Listened patiently to Mrs. Chang and allowed her to vent her frustrations.
- Reassured Mrs. Chang that her milk is very nutritious for Christopher. Gave her a brochure on breast feeding that included information on what to do for sore nipples and engorgement.
- Gave Mrs. Chang the names and phone numbers of community resources for nursing mothers.
- Told Mrs. Chang that Christopher's weight and length do not fall in the underweight category on his growth chart. Showed her Christopher's growth chart so that she could see that Christopher is progressing normally.

What Did Traci Not Do?
- Did not tell Mrs. Chang to cheer up because the colic would eventually go away on its own.
- Did not give a personal opinion on whether Mrs. Chang should breast feed or bottle feed her infant.

Case Study 2
Page 543

What Did Traci Do?
- Explained to Mrs. Tilley that childhood obesity has doubled in the past 20 years and has become a serious health concern.
- Told Mrs. Tilley that she could have a big impact on Courtney's life by preparing healthy meals and eating them with her and by becoming involved in activities with Courtney, such as taking walks.
- Spent some time talking with Courtney about her interests and complimented Courtney on her achievements.
- Encouraged Courtney to join the swim team. Told her that lots of people do not like to be seen in a bathing suit and encouraged her not to let that stand in her way of doing something she wants to do.
- Reassured Courtney that the doctor wants to help her and that he would never say anything bad about her weight.

What Did Traci Not Do?
- Did not agree with Mrs. Tilley that there is nothing that can be done about Courtney's weight problem.
- Did not tell Courtney that she needs to lose weight or she might develop serious health problems such as diabetes.

Case Study 3
Page 555

What Did Traci Do?
- Explained to Stacy that it is rare, but sometimes a child develops polio from getting the oral polio vaccine. Told her that this does not occur with the injectable polio vaccine.
- Explained to Stacy that chickenpox is usually a mild disease, but it can be serious, especially in young infants and adults.
- Explained to Stacy that most side effects from vaccines are mild and that complications from the diseases far outweigh the possible side effects.

Continued

What Would You Do? What Would You *Not* Do? RESPONSES—cont'd

- ❏ Told Stacy that these diseases have been reduced to very low levels in the United States, but they still occur in other countries. Explained that infected travelers can bring these diseases to the United States and infect individuals who are not immunized.
- ❏ Reminded Stacy that these immunizations are required for Matthew to start kindergarten.
- ❏ Talked with Matthew on his level about why he needs to be immunized.
- ❏ Told Matthew that they would play a game so that it wouldn't hurt as much. Taught him to hold up his finger and pretend that it was a birthday candle; when the injection was given, told him to keep blowing out the candle until he was told to stop.

- ❏ Told Matthew that he could choose a prize from the treasure chest after he had his immunizations.

What Did Traci **Not** *Do?*
- ❏ Did not ignore or minimize Stacy's concerns.
- ❏ Did not tell Stacy that the answers to all her questions are in the vaccine information sheets that she was just given.
- ❏ Did not tell Stacy it would be all right to skip Matthew's immunizations.
- ❏ Did not refer to the immunizations as "shots" when talking with Matthew.
- ❏ Did not tell Matthew that it would not hurt when he gets his immunizations.

TERMINOLOGY REVIEW

Key Term	Word Parts	Definition
Adolescent		An individual 12 to 18 years old.
Immunity		The resistance of the body to the effects of a harmful agent, such as a pathogenic microorganism and its toxins.
Immunization (active, artificial)		The process of becoming immune or of rendering an individual immune through the use of a vaccine or toxoid.
Infant		A child from birth to 12 months old.
Length (recumbent)		The measurement from the vertex of the head to the heel of the foot of a patient in a supine position.
Pediatrician	*pedi/a:* child	A physician who specializes in the care and development of children and the diagnosis and treatment of children's diseases.
Pediatrics	*pedi/a:* child	The branch of medicine that deals with the care and development of children and the diagnosis and treatment of children's diseases.
Preschool child	*pre-:* in front of; before	A child 3 to 6 years old.
School-age child		A child 6 to 12 years old.
Toddler		A child 1 to 3 years old.
Toxoid		A toxin (a poisonous substance produced by a bacterium) that has been treated by heat or chemicals to destroy its harmful properties. It is administered to an individual to prevent an infectious disease by stimulating the production of antibodies in that individual.
Vaccine		A suspension of attenuated (weakened) or killed microorganisms administered to an individual to prevent an infectious disease by stimulating the production of antibodies in that individual.
Vertex		The top of the head.

ON THE WEB

For information on child health:

KidsHealth: www.kidshealth.org

Baby Center: www.babycenter.com

The Child Health Site: www.thechildhealthsite.com

Healthy Children: www.healthychildren.org

Pediatric on Call: www.pediatriconcall.com

Kids Source Online: www.kidsource.com

American Academy of Pediatrics: www.aap.org

Child and Youth Health: www.cyh.com

Girls' Health: www.girlshealth.gov

For information on childhood conditions:

Attention-Deficit/Hyperactivity Disorder: www.add-adhd.org

Attention Deficit Disorder Association: www.add.org

Cerebral Palsy: www.about-cerebral-palsy.org

American Academy for Cerebral Palsy and Developmental Medicine: www.aacpdm.org

Child Abuse: www.preventchildabuse.org

American Professional Society on the Abuse of Children: www.apsac.org

Cystic Fibrosis: www.cysticfibrosis.com

Cystic Fibrosis Foundation: www.cff.org

Dental Health: Colgate World of Care: www.colgate.com

American Dental Association: www.ada.org

The Tooth Fairy Online: www.asis.com/toothfairy

Diabetes: American Diabetes Association: www.diabetes.org

Children with Diabetes: www.childrenwithdiabetes.com

Down Syndrome: downsyndrome.com

National Down Syndrome Society: www.ndss.org

Spina Bifida Association: www.spinabifidaassociation.org

National Sudden and Unexpected Infant/Child Death and Pregnancy Loss Resource Center: www.sidscenter.org

Influenza Information: www.cdc.gov/flu

SIDS Alliance: www.sidsalliance.org

For information on immunizations:

Immunization Action Coalition: www.immunize.org

Centers for Disease Control and Prevention: Vaccines and Immunizations: www.cdc.gov/vaccines

American Academy of Pediatrics Childhood Immunization Support Program: www2.aap.org/immunization

American Academy of Family Physicians: Recommendations for Immunizations: www.aafp.org

Vaccine Information: www.vaccineinformation.org

The Children's Hospital of Philadelphia Vaccine Education Center: www.chop.edu

Every Child by Two: www.ecbt.org

National Network for Immunization Information: www.immunizationinfo.org

Drug Information Online: www.drugs.com

25 Minor Office Surgery

ⓔ Check out the Evolve site at http://evolve.elsevier.com/Bonewit/today/ to access additional interactive activities and exercises to help you study and prepare for success.

LEARNING OBJECTIVES

Surgical Asepsis

1. State the characteristics of a minor surgical procedure.
2. Identify procedures that require the use of surgical asepsis.
3. Describe the medical assistant's responsibilities during a minor surgical procedure.
4. List the guidelines to follow to maintain surgical asepsis during a sterile procedure.
5. Identify and explain the use and care of instruments commonly used for minor office surgery.

Wound Healing

6. Explain the differences between a closed and an open wound, and give examples.
7. List and explain the three phases of the healing process.
8. List and describe the different types of wound drainage.
9. List the functions of a dressing.

Sutures

10. Explain the method used to measure the diameter of suturing material.
11. Describe the two types of sutures (absorbable and nonabsorbable), and give examples of their uses.
12. Categorize suturing needles according to type of point and shape.

Medical Office Surgical Procedures

13. Explain the purpose of and procedure for each of the following minor surgical operations: sebaceous cyst removal, incision and drainage of a localized infection, mole removal, needle biopsy, ingrown toenail removal, colposcopy, cervical punch biopsy, and cryosurgery.
14. Explain the principles underlying each step in the minor office surgery procedures.

PROCEDURES

Apply and remove sterile gloves.
Open a sterile package.
Add an article to a sterile field.
Pour a sterile solution.

Change a sterile dressing.

Remove sutures.
Remove surgical staples.
Apply and remove adhesive skin closures.
Set up a tray for each of the following minor surgical procedures:
- Suture insertion
- Sebaceous cyst removal
- Incision and drainage of a localized infection
- Mole removal
- Needle biopsy
- Ingrown toenail removal
- Colposcopy
- Cervical punch biopsy
- Cryosurgery

Assist the physician with minor office surgery.

LEARNING OBJECTIVES

Bandaging

15. State the functions of a bandage, and list the guidelines for applying a bandage.
16. Identify the common types of bandages used in the medical office.

PROCEDURES

Apply each of the following bandage turns:
- Circular
- Spiral
- Spiral-reverse
- Figure-eight
- Recurrent

CHAPTER OUTLINE

INTRODUCTION TO MINOR OFFICE SURGERY
SURGICAL ASEPSIS
INSTRUMENTS USED IN MINOR OFFICE SURGERY
Scalpels
Scissors
Forceps
Miscellaneous Instruments
Care of Surgical Instruments
COMMERCIALLY PREPARED STERILE PACKAGES
WOUNDS
Wound Healing
Phases of Wound Healing
Wound Drainage
STERILE DRESSING CHANGE
SUTURES
Types of Sutures
Suture Size and Packaging
Suture Needles
Insertion of Sutures
Suture Insertion Setup
Procedure: Suture Insertion
Suture Removal
Surgical Skin Staples
Adhesive Skin Closures
ASSISTING WITH MINOR OFFICE SURGERY
Tray Setup
Methods Used to Set up a Sterile Tray
Side Table
Skin Preparation
Shaving the Site
Cleansing the Site
Antiseptic Application

Local Anesthetic
Preparing the Anesthetic
Assisting the Physician
MEDICAL OFFICE SURGICAL PROCEDURES
Sebaceous Cyst Removal
Procedure: Sebaceous Cyst Removal
Postoperative Instructions: Sebaceous Cyst Removal
Surgical Incision and Drainage of Localized Infections
Procedure: Incision and Drainage
Postoperative Instructions: Incision and Drainage
Mole Removal
Procedure: Mole Shave Excision
Procedure: Surgical Mole Excision
Postoperative Instructions: Shave Excision and Surgical Excision
Laser Mole Surgery
Needle Biopsy
Procedure: Needle Biopsy
Postoperative Instructions: Needle Biopsy
Ingrown Toenail Removal
Procedure: Ingrown Toenail
Postoperative Instructions: Ingrown Toenail
Colposcopy
Procedure: Colposcopy
Cervical Punch Biopsy
Procedure: Cervical Punch Biopsy
Postoperative Instructions: Cervical Punch Biopsy
Cryosurgery
Cervical Cryosurgery
Procedure: Cervical Cryosurgery
Skin Lesions
BANDAGING
Guidelines for Application
Types of Bandages
Bandage Turns

KEY TERMS

abrasion (ah-BRAY-shun)
abscess (AB-sess)
absorbable suture (ab-SOR-ba-bul SOO-chur)
approximation (ah-PROKS-ih-MAY-shun)
bandage
biopsy (BYE-op-see)
capillary action (KAP-ill-air-ee AK-shun)

colposcope (KOL-poh-skope)
colposcopy (kol-POS-koh-pee)
contaminate (kon-TAM-in-ate)
contusion (kon-TOO-shun)
cryosurgery (KRY-oh-SURJ-er-ee)
exudate (EKS-oo-date)
fibroblast (FYE-broh-blast)
forceps (FORE-seps)

furuncle (FYOOR-un-kul)
hemostasis (hee-moe-STAY-sis)
incision (in-SIH-shun)
infection (in-FEK-shun)
infiltration (in-fill-TRAY-shun)
inflammation (in-flah-MAY-shun)
laceration (lass-ur-AY-shun)
ligate (LIH-gate)

local anesthetic (LOE-kul an-es-STET-ik)
Mayo (MAY-oe) tray
needle biopsy (NEE-dul BYE-op-see)
nonabsorbable suture (non-ab-SOR-ba-
    bul SOO-chur)
postoperative (post-OP-er-uh-tiv)
preoperative (pree-OP-er-uh-tiv)

puncture (PUNK-shur)
scalpel (SKAL-pul)
scissors
sebaceous cyst (suh-BAY-shus SIST)
serum (SEER-um)
sterile (STARE-ul)
surgery

surgical asepsis (SUR-jih-kul
    ay-SEP-sis)
sutures (SOO-churz)
swaged (SWAYJD) needle
wound

INTRODUCTION TO MINOR OFFICE SURGERY

The term **surgery** is defined as the branch of medicine that deals with operative and manual procedures for correction of deformities and defects, repair of injuries, and diagnosis and treatment of certain diseases. *Minor office surgery* (also known as *minor surgery*) refers to a surgical procedure that is restricted to the management of minor conditions and injuries that does not require the use of general anesthesia. Minor surgical procedures have the following characteristics:

- Are performed in an ambulatory health care facility, such as a physician's office or clinic
- Can be performed in a short period of time, usually in less than 1 hour
- Require a local anesthetic, a topical anesthetic, or no anesthetic
- Can be performed safely with a minimum of discomfort to the patient
- Do not, under normal circumstances, pose a major risk to life or to the function of an organ or body parts

Various types of minor surgical operations are performed in the medical office, such as insertion of sutures, sebaceous cyst removal, incision and drainage of infections, mole removal, needle biopsies, cervical biopsies, and ingrown toenail removal. The physician explains the nature of the surgical procedure and any risks to the patient and offers to answer questions. The medical assistant is responsible for **preoperative** instructions (e.g., explaining the patient preparation required for the procedure) and for obtaining the patient's signature on a written consent to treatment form, which grants the physician permission to perform the surgery (Figure 25-1).

Additional responsibilities of the medical assistant include preparing the treatment room, preparing the patient, preparing the minor surgery tray, assisting the physician during the procedure, administering **postoperative** care to the patient, and cleaning the treatment room after the procedure.

The treatment room must be spotlessly clean, and the medical assistant should ensure that the physician has adequate lighting for the procedure. The patient is positioned and draped according to the procedure to be performed. The skin is prepared as specified by the physician. Hair around the operative site is a contaminant and may need to be removed by shaving. The skin is cleansed, and an appropriate antiseptic is applied to the area to reduce the number of microorganisms present.

The medical assistant prepares the minor surgery tray using **sterile** technique. The specific instruments and supplies included in each setup vary, depending on the type of surgery to be performed and the physician's preference. The medical assistant must become familiar with the instruments and supplies required for each surgical procedure performed in the medical office.

During the minor surgery, the medical assistant is present to assist the physician as needed and to lend support to the patient. The medical assistant should become completely familiar with the assisting techniques (e.g., swabbing blood from the operative site) required for each surgical procedure performed in the medical office and should learn to anticipate the physician's needs to help the procedure go quickly and smoothly.

After the minor surgery, the medical assistant should remain with the patient as a safety precaution to prevent accidental falls and other injuries and to make sure the patient understands the postoperative instructions. The medical assistant removes and properly cares for all used instruments and supplies and cleans the treatment room in preparation for the next patient.

SURGICAL ASEPSIS

Surgical asepsis, also known as *sterile technique,* refers to practices that keep objects and areas sterile, or free from all living microorganisms and spores. Surgical asepsis protects the patient from pathogenic microorganisms that may enter the body and cause disease. It is always employed under the following circumstances: when caring for broken skin, such as open wounds and suture punctures; when a skin surface is being penetrated, as by a surgical incision for a mole removal or the administration of an injection (the needle must remain sterile); and when a body cavity is entered that is normally sterile, such as during the insertion of a urinary catheter. Sterility of instruments and supplies is achieved through the use of disposable sterile items or by sterilizing reusable articles.

A sterile object that touches any unsterile object is automatically considered contaminated and must not be used.

(attach label or complete blanks)

First name: _____ Last name: _____

Date of Birth: _____ Month _____ Day _____ Year

Account Number: _____

Procedure Consent Form

I, _____ , hereby consent to have

Dr. _____ perform _____ .

I have been fully informed of the following by my physician:

1. The nature of my condition.
2. The nature and purpose of the procedure.
3. An explanation of risks involved with the procedure.
4. Alternative treatments or procedures available.
5. The likely results of the procedure.
6. The risks involved with declining or delaying the procedure.

My physician has offered to answer all questions concerning the proposed procedure.

I am aware that the practice of medicine and surgery is not an exact science, and I acknowledge that no guarantees have been made to me about the results of the procedure.

Patient _____ Date _____
(or guardian and relationship)

Witnessed _____ Date _____

Figure 25-1 Consent to treatment form.

If the medical assistant is in doubt or has a question concerning the sterility of an article, he or she should consider it contaminated and replace it with a sterile article.

Sterility of the hands cannot be attained. Sanitizing the hands renders them medically aseptic and must be performed before and after every surgical procedure using proper technique (see Chapter 17). To prevent contamination of sterile articles, sterile gloves must be worn while picking up or transferring articles during a sterile procedure. Procedure 25-1 describes the procedure for applying and removing sterile gloves.

Specific guidelines must be observed during a sterile procedure to maintain surgical asepsis. See the accompanying box, *Guidelines for Surgical Asepsis*.

INSTRUMENTS USED IN MINOR OFFICE SURGERY

A variety of surgical instruments are used for minor office surgery. Most instruments are made of stainless steel and have either a bright, highly polished finish or a dull finish. The medical assistant should become familiar with the name, use, and proper care of all instruments used in the medical office. Surgical instruments are named according to one or more of the following: (1) function (e.g., splinter forceps); (2) design (e.g., mosquito hemostatic forceps); and (3) the individual who developed the instrument (e.g., Kelly hemostatic forceps). The parts of an instrument are illustrated in Figure 25-2; some common instruments are described here and are illustrated in Figure 25-3.

SCALPELS

A **scalpel** is a small straight surgical knife consisting of a handle and a thin, sharp steel blade. A scalpel is used to make surgical incisions and can divide tissue with the least possible trauma to surrounding structures. Both disposable and reusable scalpels are available. A disposable scalpel consists of a nonslip plastic handle and a permanently attached steel blade that is individually packaged to maintain sterility. Scalpels that are reusable consist of a reusable stainless steel handle to which a disposable steel blade is attached.

Guidelines for Surgical Asepsis

1. Take precautions to prevent sterile packages from becoming wet. Wet packages draw microorganisms into the package owing to the **capillary action** (the action that causes liquid to rise along a wick, a tube, or a gauze dressing) of the liquid, resulting in contamination of the sterile package. If a sterile package that has been prepared at the medical office becomes wet, it must be rewrapped and resterilized; if a disposable sterile package becomes wet, it must be discarded.

2. A 1-inch border around the sterile field is considered contaminated or unsterile because this area may have become contaminated while the sterile field was being set up.

3. Always face the sterile field. If you must turn your back to it or leave the room, a sterile towel must be placed over the sterile field.

4. Hold all sterile articles above waist level. Anything out of sight might become contaminated. The sterile articles also should be held in front of you and should not touch your uniform.

5. To avoid contamination, place all sterile items in the center, not around the edges, of the sterile field.

6. Be careful not to spill water or solutions on the sterile field. The area beneath the field is contaminated, and microorganisms are drawn up onto the field by the capillary action of the liquid, resulting in contamination of the field.

7. Do not talk, cough, or sneeze over a sterile field. Water vapor from the nose, mouth, and lungs is carried outward by the air and contaminates the sterile field.

8. Do not reach over a sterile field. Dust or lint from your clothing may fall onto it, or your unsterile clothing may accidentally touch it.

9. Do not pass soiled dressings over the sterile field.

10. Always acknowledge if you have contaminated the sterile field so that proper steps can be taken to regain sterility.

Figure 25-2 Parts of an instrument.

The blade comes individually packaged in a moisture-proof sterile package.

SCISSORS

Scissors are cutting instruments that have ring handles and straight (str) or curved (cvd) blades. Both blade tips may be sharp (s/s), both may be blunt (b/b), or one tip may be blunt and the other sharp (b/s). The two parts of a pair of scissors come together at a hinge joint known as a *box lock* (see Figure 25-2). The type of scissors employed depends on the intended use. The various types of scissors are listed and described next.

- *Operating scissors* have straight delicate blades with sharp cutting edges and are used to cut through tissue. They are available with sharp/sharp, blunt/blunt, or blunt/sharp blade tips.

- *Suture scissors* are used to remove sutures. The hook on the tip aids in getting under a suture, and the blunt end prevents puncturing of the tissues.

- *Bandage scissors* are inserted beneath a dressing or bandage to cut it for removal. The flat blunt prow can be inserted beneath a dressing without puncturing the skin.

- *Dissecting scissors* have thick beveled blades with a fine cutting edge used to divide or separate tissue rather than cut it. Dissecting scissors are available with straight or curved blades. Both blade tips of dissecting scissors are blunt.

FORCEPS

Forceps are instruments for grasping, squeezing, or holding tissue or an item such as sterile gauze. Some forceps have two prongs and a spring handle (e.g., thumb, tissue, splinter, dressing forceps) that provides the proper tension for grasping an object such as tissue, a foreign object, or sterile gauze. Some forceps have serrations (e.g., thumb and hemostatic forceps), which are sawlike teeth that grasp tissue and prevent it from slipping out of the jaws of the instrument. As is shown in Figure 25-3, some varieties have toothed clasps on the handle, known as *ratchets* (see Figure 25-2), to hold the tips securely together and lock them in place (e.g., Allis tissue forceps, hemostatic forceps). The ratchets are designed to allow locked closure of the instrument at two or more positions. The various types of forceps are listed and described next.

- *Thumb forceps* have serrated tips and are used to pick up tissue or to hold tissue between adjacent surfaces.

Scalpels

Operating Scissors (Straight) Blunt-Blunt

Operating Scissors Sharp-Sharp

Operating Scissors Sharp-Blunt

Littauer Suture Scissors Straight

Lister Bandage Scissors

Mayo Dissecting Scissors Curved

Mayo Dissecting Scissors Straight

Standard Thumb Forceps

Standard Tissue Forceps 1 × 2 Teeth

Plain Splinter Forceps

Adson Dressing Forceps

Allis Tissue Forceps

Figure 25-3 Instruments used in minor office surgery. (Courtesy Elmed, Addison, Ill.)

Halsted Mosquito
Hemostatic Forceps
Straight or Curved

Kelly Hemostatic
Forceps
Straight or Curved

Foerster
Sponge Forceps

Rochester-Pean
Hemostatic Forceps
Straight or Curved

Ochsner-Kocher Hemostatic
Forceps Straight or Curved
1 × 2 Teeth

Crile-Wood
Needle Holder

Sharp   Blunt

Volkmann Rake Retractor

Senn-Mueller Retractor

Figure 25-3, cont'd

- *Tissue forceps* have teeth, which are used to grasp tissue and prevent it from slipping. Tissue forceps are identified by the number of apposing teeth on each jaw (e.g., 1 × 2, 2 × 3, 3 × 4). Tissue forceps are sometimes referred to as "rat-toothed" forceps because the pointed projections resemble the teeth of a rat. The teeth should approximate tightly when the instrument is closed.
- *Splinter forceps* have sharp points that are useful in removing foreign objects, such as splinters, from the tissues.
- *Dressing forceps* are used in the application and removal of dressings. They are also used to hold or grasp sterile

gauze or sutures during a surgical procedure. Dressing forceps have blunt ends that contain coarse cross-striations used for grasping.

- *Hemostatic forceps* have serrated tips, ratchets, ring handles, and box locks and are available with straight or curved blades. Hemostats are used to clamp off blood vessels and to establish **hemostasis** until the vessels can be closed with sutures. The serrations on a hemostat prevent the blood vessel from slipping out of the jaws of the instrument. The ratchets keep the hemostat tightly shut and locked in place when it is closed. The ring handles allow for a secure grasp of the hemostat and also are used to select the desired ratchet position. The serrated blades should mesh together smoothly when the hemostat is closed; if they spring back open, the instrument is in need of repair. *Mosquito hemostatic forceps* have small, fine tips and are smaller and more delicate than standard Kelly hemostatic forceps. Mosquito hemostatic forceps are used to hold delicate tissue or to clamp off smaller blood vessels, whereas standard hemostatic forceps are used to grasp and compress larger blood vessels.
- *Sponge forceps* have ring handles, ratchets, box locks, and large serrated rings on the blade tips for holding sponges. A *sponge* is a porous, absorbent pad, such as a 4-inch gauze pad, used to absorb fluids, apply medication, or cleanse an area.

MISCELLANEOUS INSTRUMENTS

Various miscellaneous instruments used in the medical office are listed and described next.

- *Needle holders* have serrated tips, ring handles, ratchets, and box locks. A needle holder is used to firmly grasp a curved needle for insertion of the needle through the skin flaps of an incision. The serrated tips of a needle holder are designed to hold a curved needle securely without damaging it. A needle holder is sometimes referred to as a "driver" because it functions to "drive" the curved needle through the skin.
- *Retractors* are used to hold tissues aside to improve the exposure of the operative area.

CARE OF SURGICAL INSTRUMENTS

Surgical instruments are expensive, are delicate yet durable, and last for many years if handled and maintained properly. The care an instrument receives depends to a large degree on the parts making up the instrument (e.g., box lock, ratchet, cutting edge, serrations). The medical assistant works with instruments while setting up a sterile tray, performing certain procedures such as suture removal and sterile dressing change, and cleaning up after minor office surgery and during the sanitization and sterilization process. During each of these procedures, guidelines must be

followed to prolong the life span of each instrument and to ensure its proper functioning:

1. Always handle instruments carefully. Dropping an instrument on the floor or throwing an instrument into a basin could damage it.
2. Do not pile instruments in a heap because they become entangled and might be damaged when separated.
3. Keep sharp instruments separate from the rest of the instruments to prevent damaging or dulling the cutting edge. Also, keep delicate instruments, such as lensed instruments, separate to protect them from damage.
4. To prolong the proper functioning of the ratchet, keep instruments with a ratchet in an open position when not in use.
5. Rinse blood and body secretions off an instrument as soon as possible to prevent them from drying and hardening on the instrument.
6. When performing procedures that require surgical instruments, always use the instrument for the purpose for which it was designed. Substituting one type of instrument for another could damage it.
7. Sanitize and sterilize instruments using proper technique.

Putting It All Into Practice

My name is Trudy Browning, and I have worked as the office manager of an internal medicine office for the past 7 years. My job includes front and back office duties, including scheduling appointments, transcription, patient calls, patient workups, injections, electrocardiograms, and venipuncture. The most interesting part of my job is dealing with the many different personalities of the patients I come in contact with daily.

A patient who had not been to the clinic for a while came in one day. His graduation from college had been delayed because he had developed a pilonidal cyst that needed to be surgically removed. At onset, these cysts can be very painful and usually require daily cleaning and packing. From my experience with pilonidal cyst care, I knew that 1 to 2 months of treatment are usually required before full recovery is achieved.

The physician and I prepared for the initial treatment and noticed that the surgical site was very large and deep. We knew this treatment would take much longer than usual. Treatment was provided daily for 3 months. Subsequent treatments continued every other day for 2 months. Through our continuous contact, we became good friends with the patient.

Our patient graduated at the end of the spring quarter and moved out of state. He stays in contact with us and is still undergoing treatment. He made a difference in our lives because he always maintained a positive attitude and was very pleasant, making our job easier. We made a difference in his life through the good health care we provided and our continuing friendship. ∎

7. Procedural Step. Remove your thumb from the cuff and pull the glove on. Turn back the cuff.

Turn back the cuff.

8. Procedural Step. Turn back the cuff of the first glove by reaching under the cuff with the other gloved hand. Do not allow your sterile gloved hand to come in contact with the inside of the cuff. Adjust the gloves to a comfortable position. Inspect the gloves for tears.

Principle. The area under the folded cuff is sterile and may be touched by the sterile gloved hand. The inside of the cuff has previously been touched by your clean hands and is not sterile. If a tear is present, a new pair of gloves must be applied.

Removing Sterile Gloves

1. Procedural Step. With your gloved left hand, grasp the outside of the right glove 1 to 2 inches from the top. (*Note:* It does not matter which glove is removed first—you may start with the left glove if you prefer.)

Grasp the outside of the glove.

2. Procedural Step. Slowly pull the right glove off the hand. It turns inside out as it is removed from your hand.

3. Procedural Step. Pull the right glove free, and scrunch it into a ball with your gloved left hand.

Scrunch the glove into a ball.

4. Procedural Step. Place the index and middle fingers of the right hand on the inside of the left glove. Do not allow your clean hand to touch the outside of the glove.

Place the fingers on the inside of the glove.

5. Procedural Step. Pull the second glove off the left hand. It turns inside out as it is removed from your hand, enclosing the balled-up right glove. Discard both gloves in an appropriate waste container. If your gloves are visibly contaminated with blood or other potentially infectious materials, discard them in a biohazard waste container; otherwise, they can be discarded in a regular waste container.

PROCEDURE 25-1   Applying and Removing Sterile Gloves—cont'd

Pull the glove off the hand.

6. Procedural Step. Sanitize your hands thoroughly to remove any microorganisms that may have come in contact with your hands.

PROCEDURE 25-2   Opening a Sterile Package

Outcome Open a sterile package. A sterile package that has been wrapped according to the procedure for wrapping presented in Chapter 18 is opened using the procedure outlined here. The sterile package may be in the form of a commercially prepared disposable package (e.g., sterile dressing change) or a pack that has been assembled and sterilized at the medical office (e.g., sebaceous cyst removal pack); in both cases, the inside of the sterile wrapper serves as the sterile field.

Equipment/Supplies

- Sterile package

1. **Procedural Step.** Sanitize your hands.
2. **Procedural Step.** Assemble the equipment.
3. **Procedural Step.** Check the pack to make sure it is not wet, torn, or opened. These factors cause contamination of the sterile contents and the pack must not be used. If autoclave tape has been used to close the pack, check to make sure the tape has changed color.
   Principle. Autoclave tape indicates that the pack has been through the sterilization process, but it does not verify that the contents of the pack are sterile.

Check the sterilization indicator.

Continued

PROCEDURE 25-2

4. **Procedural Step.** Place the wrapped package on the table so that the top flap of the wrapper opens away from you. Always face the sterile field, and do not talk, laugh, cough, or sneeze over the field. These actions contaminate the sterile field.
5. **Procedural Step.** Loosen and remove the fastener on the wrapped package, and discard it in a waste container.
6. **Procedural Step.** Open the first flap away from the body. Handle only the outside of the wrapper. *Principle.* The medical assistant should open the sterile package so as not to reach over the sterile contents. Otherwise, dust or lint from unsterile clothing may fall on the contents of the package and cause contamination.

Open the left and right flaps.

8. **Procedural Step.** Open the flap closest to the body by lifting it toward you. Touch only the outside of the wrapper.

Open the first flap away from the body.

7. **Procedural Step.** Without crossing over the sterile field, open the left and right flaps.

Open the flap closest to the body.

9. **Procedural Step.** Adjust the sterile wrapper by the corners as needed to make sure it lies in proper position on the tray or table.
10. **Procedural Step.** Check the sterilization indicator on the inside of the pack to make sure it has changed appropriately. This indicates that the contents of the pack are sterile.

PROCEDURE 25-3   Pouring a Sterile Solution

Outcome Pour a sterile solution

Equipment/Supplies

- Sterile solution
- Sterile container
- Sterile towel

1. **Procedural Step.** Read the label of the solution to ensure that you have the correct solution.
2. **Procedural Step.** Check the expiration date on the solution. Do not use an outdated solution.
   Principle. Outdated solutions may produce undesirable effects and should be discarded.
3. **Procedural Step.** Check the solution label a second time to make sure you have the correct solution.
4. **Procedural Step.** Place the palm of your hand over the label. Remove the cap by touching only the outside, and place the cap on a flat surface with the open end up. Do not place the cap on the sterile field, as the outside of the cap is contaminated.
   Principle. Palming the label prevents the solution from dripping on the label and obscuring it. Handling the cap by the outside prevents contamination of the inside. Placing the cap with the open end up prevents contamination of the inside of the cap by an unsterile surface.
5. **Procedural Step.** Rinse the lip of the bottle (if it has been previously used) by pouring a small amount of solution into a separate container.
   Principle. Rinsing the lip washes away any microorganisms that may be on it.
6. **Procedural Step.** Pour the proper amount of solution into the sterile container at a height of approximately

6 inches. Do not allow the neck of the bottle to come in contact with the sterile container, and be careful not to splash solution onto the sterile field.
Principle. Pouring from a height of approximately 6 inches reduces splashing and prevents contamination of the sterile container with the outside of the (unsterile) bottle.

Pour the proper amount of solution.

7. **Procedural Step.** Replace the cap on the container without contaminating it. Check the label a third time to ensure that you have poured the correct solution.

---

so, the steps of surgical asepsis outlined in Procedure 25-3 should be followed.

WOUNDS

A **wound** is a break in the continuity of an external or internal surface caused by physical means. Wounds can be accidental or intentional (as when the physician makes an incision during a surgical operation). There are two basic types of wounds: closed and open.

A *closed wound* involves an injury to the underlying tissues of the body without a break in the skin surface or mucous membrane; an example is a contusion, or bruise. A **contusion** results when the tissues under the skin are injured and is often caused by a blunt object. Blood vessels rupture, allowing blood to seep into the tissues, which results in a bluish discoloration of the skin. After several days, the color of the contusion turns greenish yellow as a result of oxidation of blood pigments. Bruising commonly

occurs with injuries such as fractures, sprains, strains, and black eyes. *Open wounds* involve a break in the skin surface or mucous membrane that exposes the underlying tissues; examples include incisions, lacerations, punctures, and abrasions. Figure 25-5 illustrates specific wounds.

- An **incision** is a clean, smooth cut caused by a sharp instrument, such as a knife, razor, or piece of glass. Deep incisions are accompanied by profuse bleeding; in addition, damage to muscles, tendons, and nerves may occur.
- A **laceration** is a wound in which the tissues are torn apart, rather than cut, leaving ragged and irregular edges. Lacerations are caused by dull knives, large objects that have been driven into the skin, and heavy machinery. Deep lacerations result in profuse bleeding, and a scar often results from the jagged tearing of the tissues.
- A **puncture** is a wound made by a sharp-pointed object piercing the skin layers—for example, a nail, splinter, needle, wire, knife, bullet, or animal bite. A puncture wound has a very small external skin opening, and for

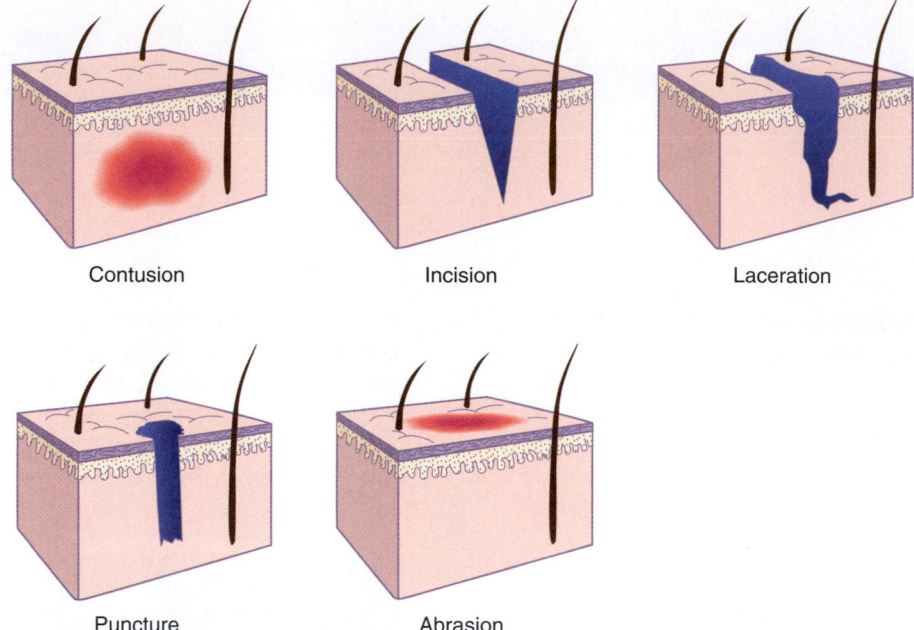

Figure 25-5 Types of wounds.

this reason bleeding is usually minor. A tetanus booster may be administered with this type of wound because the tetanus bacteria grow best in a warm anaerobic environment, such as the one in a puncture.

- An **abrasion** or scrape is a wound in which the outer layers of the skin are scraped or rubbed off, resulting in oozing of blood from ruptured capillaries. Abrasions are often caused by falling on gravel and floors (floor burn). These falls can result in skinned knees and elbows.

WOUND HEALING

The skin is a protective barrier for the body and is considered its first line of defense. When the surface of the skin has been broken, it is easy for microorganisms to enter and cause **infection.** The body has a natural healing process that works to destroy invading microorganisms and to restore the structure and function of damaged tissues, as is described next.

Phases of Wound Healing

Wound healing occurs in three phases, which are described here and illustrated in Figure 25-6.

Phase 1

Phase 1, also called the *inflammatory phase,* begins as soon as the body is injured. This phase lasts approximately 3 to 4 days. During this phase, a fibrin network forms, resulting in a blood clot that "plugs" up the opening of the wound and stops the flow of blood. The blood clot eventually becomes the scab. The inflammatory process also occurs during this phase. **Inflammation** is the protective response of the body to trauma, such as cuts and abrasions, and to the entrance of foreign matter, such as microorganisms. During inflammation, the blood supply to the wound increases, which brings white blood cells and nutrients to the site to assist in the healing

Phase 1: Inflammatory Phase

Phase 2: Granulation Phase

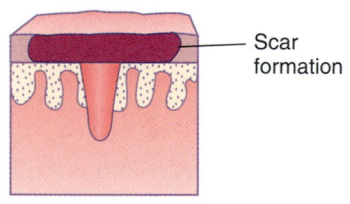

Phase 3: Maturation Phase

Figure 25-6 Phases of wound healing.

process. The four local signs of inflammation are redness, swelling, pain, and warmth. The purpose of inflammation is to destroy invading microorganisms and to remove damaged tissue debris from the area so that proper healing can occur.

Phase 2

Phase 2 is also called the *granulation phase* and typically lasts 4 to 20 days. During this phase, **fibroblasts** migrate to the wound and begin to synthesize collagen. Collagen is a white protein that provides strength to the wound. As the amount of collagen increases, the wound becomes stronger, and the chance that the wound will open decreases. There also is a growth of new capillaries during this phase to provide the damaged tissue with an abundant supply of blood. As the capillary network develops, the tissue becomes a translucent red color. This tissue is known as *granulation tissue.* Granulation tissue consists primarily of collagen and is fragile and shiny and bleeds easily.

Phase 3

Phase 3, also known as the *maturation phase,* begins as soon as granulation tissue forms and can last for 2 years. During this phase, collagen continues to be synthesized, and the granulation tissue eventually hardens to white scar tissue. Scar tissue is not true skin and does not contain nerves or have a blood supply.

The medical assistant should always inspect the wound when providing wound care. The wound should be observed for signs of inflammation and the amount of healing that has occurred. This information should be documented in the patient's record.

Wound Drainage

The medical term for drainage is **exudate.** An exudate is material, such as fluid and cells, that has escaped from blood vessels during the inflammatory process. The exudate is deposited in tissue or on tissue surfaces and is often present in a wound. When providing wound care, the medical assistant should always inspect the wound for drainage and document this information in the patient's record. There are three major types of exudates: serous, sanguineous, and purulent.

- *Serous exudate.* A serous exudate consists chiefly of **serum,** which is the clear portion of the blood. Serous drainage is clear and watery. An example of a serous exudate is the fluid in a blister from a burn.
- *Sanguineous exudate.* A sanguineous exudate is red and consists of red blood cells. This type of drainage results when capillaries are damaged, allowing the escape of red blood cells, and is frequently seen in open wounds. A bright-red sanguineous exudate indicates fresh bleeding, and a dark exudate indicates older bleeding.

- *Purulent exudate.* A purulent exudate contains pus, which consists of leukocytes, dead liquefied tissue debris, and dead and living bacteria. Purulent drainage is usually thick and has an unpleasant odor. It is white in color but may acquire tinges of pink, green, or yellow depending on the type of infecting organism. The process of pus formation is *suppuration.*

In addition to the exudates just described, mixed types of exudates are often observed in a wound. A *serosanguineous exudate* consists of clear and blood-tinged drainage and is commonly seen in surgical incisions. A *purosanguineous exudate* consists of pus and blood and is often seen in a new wound that is infected.

STERILE DRESSING CHANGE

Surgical asepsis must be maintained when one is caring for and applying a dry sterile dressing (abbreviated as *DSD*) to an open wound. The medical assistant must take care to prevent infection in clean wounds and to decrease infection in wounds already infected. The function of a sterile dressing is to protect the wound from contamination and trauma, to absorb drainage, and to restrict motion, which may interfere with proper wound healing. The size, type, and amount of dressing material used during a sterile dressing change depend on the size and location of the wound and the amount of drainage.

Sterile folded *gauze pads* are used in the medical office for a sterile dressing change. This type of dressing absorbs drainage, but the gauze has a tendency to stick to the wound when the drainage dries. Gauze pads come in a variety of sizes, including 4×4, 3×3, and 2×2; the 4×4 size is used most frequently.

Nonadherent pads also are used as a sterile dressing; they have one surface impregnated with agents that prevent the dressing from sticking to the wound. One brand of this type of material is Telfa pads. The nonadherent side, which is shiny, is placed next to the wound. Telfa dressings are often used to cover burned skin. Procedure 25-4 presents the procedure for changing a sterile dressing.

PROCEDURE 25-4

PROCEDURE 25-4   Changing a Sterile Dressing

Outcome   Change a sterile dressing

Equipment/Supplies

- Mayo stand
- Biohazard waste container

Side Table

- Clean disposable gloves
- Antiseptic swabs
- Sterile gloves
- Plastic waste bag
- Surgical tape
- Scissors

Sterile Field

- Sterile dressing
- Sterile thumb forceps

1. **Procedural Step.** Wash your hands with an antimicrobial soap.
2. **Procedural Step.** Assemble the equipment. Set up the nonsterile items on a side table or counter. Position the waterproof waste bag in a location convenient for disposal of contaminated items.

Prepare the side table.

3. **Procedural Step.** Greet the patient and introduce yourself. Identify the patient by full name and date of birth and explain the procedure. Instruct the patient not to move during the procedure. Adjust the light so that it is focused on the dressing.
4. **Procedural Step.** Apply clean gloves. Loosen the tape on the dressing, and pull it toward the wound. Carefully and gently remove the soiled dressing by pulling it upward. Do not touch the inside of the dressing that was next to the open wound. If the dressing is stuck to the wound, it can be loosened by moistening it with a normal saline solution. Place the soiled dressing in the waste bag without allowing the dressing to touch the outside of the bag.
   Principle. Gentle dressing removal avoids unnecessary stress on the wound. Touching the inside of the dressing can transfer an infected discharge to your gloves.

Remove the soiled dressing.

5. **Procedural Step.** Inspect the wound, and observe for the following: amount of healing; presence of inflammation; and presence of drainage, including the amount (scant, moderate, or profuse) and type of drainage.
   Principle. Drainage is classified as serous (containing serum), sanguineous (red and composed of blood), serosanguineous (containing serum and blood), or purulent (containing pus and appearing white with tinges of yellow, pink, or green, depending on the type of infecting microorganism). Purulent drainage is usually thick and has an unpleasant odor.
6. **Procedural Step.** Open the pouch containing the sterile antiseptic swabs, and place it in a convenient location or hold it in your nondominant hand.
7. **Procedural Step.** Using the antiseptic swabs, apply the antiseptic to the wound. Apply the antiseptic from the top to the bottom of the wound, working from the center to the outside of the wound. Use a new swab for each motion. Discard each contaminated swab in the waste bag after use.
   Principle. The purpose of the antiseptic is to decrease the number of microorganisms in the wound.

PROCEDURE 25-4 Changing a Sterile Dressing—cont'd

Apply an antiseptic to the wound.

8. Procedural Step. Remove the clean disposable gloves, and discard them in the waste bag without contaminating yourself. Sanitize your hands and prepare the sterile field using surgical asepsis. Items are either placed onto a sterile field or are contained in a prepackaged setup. Instruct the patient not to talk, laugh, sneeze, or cough over the sterile field. *Principle.* Microorganisms are carried in water vapor from the mouth, nose, and lungs and can be transferred onto the sterile field.

Prepare the sterile field.

9. Procedural Step. Open a package of sterile gloves, and apply them.

10. Procedural Step. Pick up the sterile dressing with your gloved hand or sterile forceps. Place the sterile dressing over the wound by lightly dropping it in place. Do not move the dressing once you have dropped it into place. Discard the gloves or forceps in the waste bag. *Principle.* Dropping the dressing over the wound and not moving it prevent the transfer of microorganisms from the skin to the center of the wound.

11. Procedural Step. Apply hypoallergenic adhesive tape to hold the dressing in place. The tape must be long enough to adhere to the skin, but not so long that it loosens when the patient moves. The strips of tape should be evenly spaced, with strips at each end of the dressing.

12. Procedural Step. Instruct the patient in wound care as follows:

a. Provide the patient with written wound care instructions (see the patient teaching box on wound care in this chapter).

b. Explain the wound care instructions, and ask the patient whether he or she has any questions. Tell the patient to keep the wound clean and dry and to contact the office if signs of infection occur such as excessive swelling, pain, or discharge.

c. Ask the patient to sign the instruction sheet on the appropriate line.

d. Witness the patient's signature by signing your name in the appropriate space on the form. Include today's date.

e. Before the patient leaves the medical office, make a copy of the instruction sheet. Give a signed copy of the wound care instructions to the patient.

f. File the instruction sheet.
Paper-based patient record: File the original instruction sheet in the patient's medical record.
Electronic medical record: Scan the instruction sheet into the patient's electronic record.

Principle. The filed copy protects the physician legally in the event that the patient fails to follow the instructions and causes further harm or damage to the wound.

Instruct the patient in wound care.

Continued

PROCEDURE 25-4

PROCEDURE 25-4   Changing a Sterile Dressing—cont'd

13. **Procedural Step.** Return the equipment. Tightly secure the bag containing the soiled dressing and contaminated articles, and dispose of it in a biohazard waste container.
    Principle. Contaminated items must be disposed of properly to prevent the spread of infection.
14. **Procedural Step.** Sanitize your hands.
15. **Procedural Step.** Chart the procedure in the patient's medical record.
    a. *Paper-based patient record:* Record the date and time, location of the dressing, condition of the wound, type and amount of drainage, care of the wound, and any problems the patient experienced with the wound. Also chart the instructions given to the patient on wound care (refer to the PPR charting example).

    b. *Electronic medical record:* Document the location of the dressing, condition of the wound, type and amount of drainage, care of the wound, and any problems the patient has experienced with the wound using the appropriate radio buttons, drop-down menus, and free text fields. Also, document the instructions given to the patient on wound care.

PPR CHARTING EXAMPLE

Date	
9/20/XX	10:30 a.m. Dressing changed Ⓛ ant forearm. Scant amt of serous drainage noted. Sl redness around incision line. Sutures intact and suture line in good approximation. Incision cleaned c̄ Betadine and DSD applied. No complaints of pain or discomfort. Explained wound care. Written instructions provided. Signed copy filed in chart. To return in 2 days for suture removal. ————————————— T. Browning, CMA (AAMA)

SUTURES

Insertion and removal of **sutures** are commonly performed in the medical office. Sutures may be required to close a surgical incision or to repair an accidental wound. They **approximate,** or bring together, the edges of the wound with surgical stitches and hold them in place until enough healing has taken place so that the wound can withstand ordinary stress and no longer needs support from the sutures. Sutures also protect the wound from further contamination and minimize the amount of scar formation. A **local anesthetic** is necessary to numb the area before the sutures are inserted.

TYPES OF SUTURES

Sutures are available in two types: absorbable and nonabsorbable. **Absorbable sutures** are made of a material that is gradually digested and absorbed by the body in a relatively short period of time. The amount of time can range from 7 days to several months, depending on the type of tissue being sutured and the size and type of absorbable suture being used.

Absorbable sutures consist of surgical gut (Surgigut) or synthetic materials, such as polyglycolic acid (Dexon), polyglactin 910 (Vicryl), polydioxanone (PDS II), polyglyconate (Maxon), and poliglecaprone (Monocryl), lactomer (Polysorb), and Caprosyn (Figure 25-7, *A*). Surgical gut is made

Figure 25-7 Swaged suture packets. **A,** Absorbable sutures. **B,** Nonabsorbable sutures.

from sheep or cow intestine. This type of suturing material is gradually digested by tissue enzymes and is absorbed by the body's tissues 7 to 21 days after insertion, depending on the kind of surgical gut employed. *Plain surgical gut* has a rapid absorption time, whereas *chromic surgical gut* is treated to slow down its rate of absorption in the tissues. Absorbable sutures frequently are used to suture subcutaneous tissue, fascia, intestines, bladder, and peritoneum and to **ligate,** or tie off, vessels. Because suturing of this type of tissue is typically done during surgery performed by the physician in the hospital with the patient under a general anesthetic, the medical office may not stock absorbable suture material.

Nonabsorbable sutures (Figure 25-7, *B*) are not absorbed by the body and may remain permanently in the body tissues and become encapsulated by fibrous tissue or may be removed (e.g., skin sutures). Nonabsorbable sutures are used to suture skin; this type of suture is used frequently in the medical office. Nonabsorbable sutures are made from materials that are not affected by tissue enzymes. These materials include silk (Sofsilk), nylon (Ethilon), polyester (Ti-Cron, Surgidac), polypropylene (Prolene, Surgipro), polybutester (Novafil and Vascufil), stainless steel, and surgical skin staples.

Memories *from* Practicum

Trudy Browning: I remember observing my first minor office surgery during my practicum. It was a sebaceous cyst removal. The cyst was located on the calf of the patient's left leg. I helped in setting up the surgical tray and prepared and draped the site. I tried to explain to the patient what was going to occur to prepare her for the procedure. I think the patient was calmer than I was. The physician entered the room with a medical assistant on hand. Although I was in the room primarily to observe, I helped the physician with his surgical gloves and in numbing the site. I watched the physician make the incision and cut out and remove a large cyst.

Everything was going smoothly until the physician started to suture the wound. I felt like someone had turned the heat up really high; the room seemed to get really hot. I started to feel dizzy. I smiled at the physician and excused myself. He just smiled back at me, and I left the room. I went outside the room and caught my breath. I regained my composure and reentered the room. The physician was still suturing the wound. As I watched him run the needle through the skin and pull the suture tight, it really got to me. I smiled and told the physician that I would wait outside until they were done. After the physician left the room, I went back to help clean up. I felt so stupid. Later that day, the physician looked at me and said, "Got a little warm in there, didn't it?" He just laughed and said that what I did was normal and not to worry about it. He made me feel better about myself. After that incident, I went in alone and helped him with cyst removals, and it didn't bother me at all. ∎

SUTURE SIZE AND PACKAGING

Sutures are measured by their gauge, which refers to the diameter of the suturing material. The sizes range from numbers below 0 (pronounced "aught") to numbers above 0. The diameter of the suture material increases with each number above 0 and decreases with each number below 0. If the size of a particular suture material ranges from 7-0 to 5, available sizes include 7-0, 6-0, 5-0, 4-0, 3-0, 2-0, 0, 1, 2, 3, 4, and 5. Size 7-0 sutures are very fine sutures, and size 5 sutures are very heavy sutures. Size 2-0 (00) sutures have a smaller diameter than size 0 sutures.

Nonabsorbable sutures with a smaller gauge (5-0 to 6-0) are used for suturing incisions in delicate tissue, such as the face and neck, whereas nonabsorbable heavy sutures are used for firmer tissue, such as the chest and abdomen. Finer sutures leave less scar formation and are used when cosmetic results are desired.

Sutures come in a box of individually packaged sutures (Figure 25-8, *A*). The box of sutures is stamped with an expiration date that must be checked each time a suture package is removed from the box. Each individual suture package consists of an outer peel-apart envelope and a sterile inner packet (Figure 25-8, *B*). Packages are labeled according to the type of suture material (e.g., surgical silk), the size (e.g., 4-0), the length of the suturing material (e.g., 18 inches), the date of manufacture, and the expiration date of the suture. The type and size of material used are based on the nature and location of the tissue being sutured and the physician's preference. To repair a laceration of the arm, the physician might use a 4-0 surgical silk suture. The physician informs the medical assistant of the type and size of sutures needed.

SUTURE NEEDLES

Needles used for suturing are made from stainless steel alloys and are categorized according to their type of point and their shape. A needle with a sharp point is a *cutting needle,* and one with a round point is a *noncutting needle.* Cutting needles (Figure 25-9, *A*) are used for firm tissues such as skin; the sharp point helps push the needle through the tissue. Noncutting or blunt needles are used to penetrate tissues that offer a small amount of resistance, such as the fascia, intestine, liver, spleen, kidneys, subcutaneous tissue, and muscle.

A suture needle may be curved or straight (see Figure 25-9, *A*). *Curved needles* permit the physician to dip in and out of the tissue. A needle holder must be used with a curved needle. A *straight needle* is used when the tissue can be displaced sufficiently to permit the needle to be pushed and pulled through the tissue. Straight needles do not require the use of a needle holder.

Some needles have an eye through which the suture material is inserted; however, most needles are **swaged** (Figure 25-9, *B*). *Swaged* means that the suture and needle are one continuous unit; the needle is permanently attached

Figure 25-8 A, Sutures come in a box of individually packaged sutures. **B,** Each individual suture package consists of an outer peel-apart envelope and a sterile inner packet.

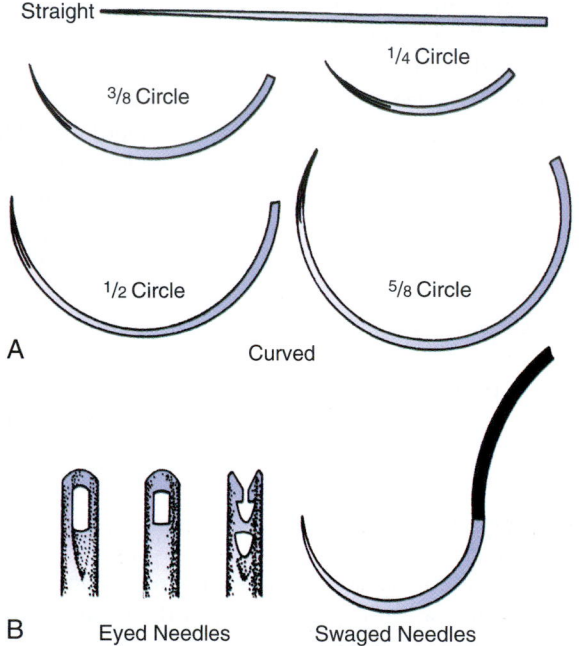

Figure 25-9 Common suture needles. **A,** Needles with a cutting point. **B,** Eyed needles and a swaged needle. (**B,** modified from Nealon TF Jr: *Fundamental skills in surgery,* ed 4, Philadelphia, 1994, Saunders.)

INSERTION OF SUTURES

The medical assistant may be responsible for preparing the suture tray and for assisting the physician during the insertion of the sutures. The physician designates the size and type of suture material and needle required. Because sutures, needles, and suture-needle combinations (swaged needles) are contained in peel-apart packages, they can be added to the sterile field by flipping them onto the sterile field or by placing them there with a sterile gloved hand (Figure 25-10).

Suture Insertion Setup

The items required for a suture insertion setup are listed next.

Items Placed to the Side of the Sterile Field

* Clean disposable gloves
* Antiseptic solution
* Surgical scrub brush
* Antiseptic swabs
* Sterile gloves
* Local anesthetic
* Antiseptic wipe to cleanse the vial
* Tetanus toxoid with needle and syringe

to the end of the suture. Swaged needles are used frequently because they offer several advantages over eyed needles. One advantage is that the suture material does not slip off the needle, as might occur with suture material threaded through the eye of a needle. Another advantage is that tissue trauma is reduced because a swaged needle has only a single strand of suture that must be pulled through the tissue compared with a double strand in an eyed needle. The swaged needle can be pulled through the tissue with less resulting trauma. Swaged suture packets are labeled to specify the gauge, type, and length of suture material, the type of needle point (cutting or noncutting), and the needle shape (curved or straight) (see Figure 25-7).

Suture insertion side table.

Flipping sutures onto the sterile field.

The physician removing the sutures with a sterile gloved hand.

Figure 25-10 Adding sutures to a sterile field.

Items Included on the Sterile Field

- Fenestrated drape
- Syringe and needle for drawing up the local anesthetic
- Hemostatic forceps
- Thumb forceps
- Tissue forceps
- Dissecting scissors
- Operating scissors
- Needle holder
- Suture
- Sterile 4 × 4 gauze

Suture insertion sterile field.

Procedure: Suture Insertion

Sutures are inserted as follows:
1. A local anesthetic is used to numb the area.
2. The physician inserts sutures to close a surgical incision or to repair an accidental wound.
3. A sterile dressing may be applied to the operative site.

Postoperative Instructions: Suture Insertion

Postoperative instructions include the following:
1. Keep the dressing clean and dry.
2. Contact the medical office if any signs of infection occur at the incision site, including excessive redness, swelling, discharge, or an increase in pain.
3. Notify the medical office if the sutures become loose or break.

Provide the patient with written instructions on wound care to refer to at home, and instruct the patient when to return for removal of the sutures.

SUTURE REMOVAL

When the wound has healed such that it no longer needs the support of nonabsorbable suture material, the sutures must be removed. The length of time the sutures remain in place depends on their location and the amount of healing that must occur. Some areas of the body, such as the head and neck, have a good blood supply; the sutures do not need to remain there as long as they do in other areas because this area heals more rapidly.

Sutures must always be left in place long enough for proper healing to occur. The physician determines the length of time, but in general, skin sutures inserted in the face and neck are removed in 3 to 5 days, and sutures inserted in other areas, such as the skin of the chest, arms, legs, hands, and feet, are removed in 7 to 14 days.

What Would You Do? **What Would You *Not* Do?**

Case Study 1

Kerry Ventura brings her 6-year-old son Cory to the medical office. Cory got a new bike for his birthday and just learned how to ride it without training wheels. While going around a corner, he lost his balance and fell and cut his left knee. The incision is about 1½ inches long. Cory is going to need sutures to approximate the wound. Mrs. Ventura is very upset and blames herself. She says that she should have been watching him more closely. Mrs. Ventura wants to know why Steri-Strips can't be used to close the incision. She says that it would be a lot less painful for Cory than having stitches. When asked to sign the consent to treatment form for Cory, Mrs. Ventura says she does not want to sign the form until her husband has a chance to read it. She says that right now he is in Japan for 2 weeks on a business trip. ■

Figure 25-11 Disposable skin stapler.

SURGICAL SKIN STAPLES

Surgical skin staples are often used to close wounds. Stapling is the fastest method of closure of long skin incisions. In addition, trauma to the tissue is reduced because the tissue does not have to be handled much when the staples are inserted. Surgical staples are stainless steel and are inserted into the skin using a special skin stapler. Skin staplers are available as reusable or disposable devices. The skin stapler holds a cartridge that contains a prescribed number and size of staples (Figure 25-11).

The physician inserts the staples by gently approximating the tissues with tissue forceps. The skin stapler is held over the site, and the staple is inserted into the skin. Skin stapling produces excellent cosmetic results, and the staples are easy to remove with a specially designed staple remover.

The medical assistant is frequently responsible for removing sutures and staples. This procedure should be done only after the physician has given a written or verbal order to the medical assistant. Procedure 25-5 presents the method used to remove sutures and skin staples.

ADHESIVE SKIN CLOSURES

Adhesive skin closures may be used for wound repair to approximate the edges of a laceration or incision. Skin

Figure 25-12 Adhesive skin closures in different sizes.

closures consist of sterile, hypoallergenic tape that is commercially available in a variety of widths and lengths and is strong enough to approximate a wound until healing occurs. Brand names for adhesive skin closures are Steri-Strip (3M Corporation, St Paul, Minn) and Proxi-Strip (Ethicon, Bridgewater, NJ) (Figure 25-12).

Adhesive skin closures may be used when not much tension exists on the skin edges. The strips of tape are applied transversely across the line of incision to approximate the skin edges. The advantages of adhesive skin closures are that they eliminate the need for sutures and a local anesthetic, they are easy to apply and remove, they have a lower incidence of wound infection compared with sutures, and they result in less scarring than sutures. The disadvantage of this method is that there is less precision in bringing the wound edges together compared with suturing the wound. In addition, adhesive skin closures cannot be used on certain areas of the body where the adhesive has difficulty adhering to the skin. This includes areas that harbor moisture (e.g., palms of the hands, soles of the feet,

axillae) and hairy areas of the body (e.g., scalp, a man's chest).

The medical assistant frequently is responsible for applying adhesive skin closures. Procedure 25-6 outlines this procedure. Approximately 5 to 10 days after application, the skin closures usually loosen and fall off on their own. If they require removal by the medical assistant, the method presented at the end of Procedure 25-6 should be followed.

Text continued on p. 590

PROCEDURE 25-5   Removing Sutures and Staples

Outcome Remove sutures and staples

Equipment/Supplies

- Antiseptic swabs
- Clean disposable gloves
- Sterile 4 × 4 gauze

- Surgical tape
- Mayo stand
- Biohazard waste container

For Suture Removal

- Suture removal kit, which includes the following:
  - Suture scissors

- Thumb forceps
- Sterile 4 × 4 gauze

For Staple Removal

- Staple removal kit, which includes the following:
  - Staple remover

- Sterile 4 × 4 gauze

---

1. **Procedural Step.** Wash your hands with an antimicrobial soap. Assemble the equipment.
   Principle. Washing the hands with an antimicrobial soap removes microorganisms from the hands and also deposits an antimicrobial film on your hands to discourage the growth of bacteria.

Staple removal setup.

2. **Procedural Step.** Greet the patient and introduce yourself. Identify the patient by full name and date of birth and explain the procedure.
3. **Procedural Step.** Position the patient as required to provide good access to the site. Adjust the light so that it is focused on the wound. Verify that the sutures (or staples) are intact and that the incision

Suture removal setup.

Continued

PROCEDURE 25-6 **Applying and Removing Adhesive Skin Closures**

Outcome Apply and remove adhesive skin closures

Equipment/Supplies

- Clean disposable gloves
- Sterile gloves
- Antiseptic solution
- Surgical scrub brush
- Antiseptic swabs
- Tincture of benzoin

- Sterile cotton-tipped applicator
- Adhesive skin closure strips
- Sterile 4 × 4 gauze pads
- Surgical tape
- Biohazard waster container

Application of Adhesive Skin Closures

1. **Procedural Step.** Wash your hands with an antimicrobial soap and assemble the equipment. Check the expiration date on the adhesive skin closures.

Assemble the equipment.

2. **Procedural Step.** Greet the patient and introduce yourself.
3. **Procedural Step.** Identify the patient by full name and date of birth and explain the procedure.
4. **Procedural Step.** Position the patient as required for application of the strips. Adjust the light so that it is focused on the wound. Apply clean gloves. Inspect the wound for signs of redness, swelling, and drainage. (*Note:* Document this information in the patient's record after completing the procedure.)
5. **Procedural Step.** Gently scrub the wound using an antiseptic solution (e.g., Betadine solution) and a sterile gauze pad or a surgical scrub brush. Clean at least 3 inches around the wound, removing all debris, skin oil, and exudates. Allow the skin to dry or pat dry with gauze pads. (*Note:* Change gloves as needed to maintain cleanliness.)

Clean the wound.

6. **Procedural Step.** Apply an antiseptic to the site using antiseptic swabs such as Betadine swabs. Apply the antiseptic from the top to the bottom of the wound, working from the center to the outside of the wound. Use a new swab for each motion. Allow the skin to dry completely.
Principle. The antiseptic decreases the number of microorganisms in the wound. The skin must be completely dry to ensure adhesion of the skin closures to the skin.

Apply an antiseptic to the wound.

7. Procedural Step. If dictated by the medical office policy, apply a thin coat of tincture of benzoin to the skin parallel to each side of the wound with a sterile cotton-tipped applicator. Do not allow the tincture of benzoin to touch the wound. Allow the skin to dry. Remove the gloves, and wash your hands with an antimicrobial soap.
Principle. Tincture of benzoin facilitates adhesion of the strips to the skin.

Apply tincture of benzoin.

8. Procedural Step. Open the plastic peel-apart package of strips using sterile technique as follows:
a. Grasp each flap of the package between the thumbs and bent index fingers. Pull the package apart.
b. Peel back the package until it is completely open.
c. Lay the opened package flat on a clean dry surface. The inside of the package serves as the sterile field.

9. Procedural Step. Apply sterile gloves. Fold the card of strips along its perforated tab, and tear off the tab, which exposes the ends of the strips, making them easier to grasp. Peel a strip of tape off the card at a 45-degree angle to the card.

Peel a strip of tape off the card.

10. Procedural Step. Check that the skin surface is dry. Position the first strip over the center of the wound as follows:
a. Secure one end of the strip of tape to the skin on one side of the wound by pressing down firmly on the tape.
b. Stretch the strip transversely across the line of the incision until the edges of the wound are approximated exactly. If necessary, use your gloved hand to assist in bringing the edges of the wound together.
c. Secure the strip on the skin on the other side of the wound by pressing down firmly on the tape.
Principle. Approximating the wound exactly facilitates good healing and minimizes scar formation.

Position the first strip over the center of the wound.

11. Procedural Step. Apply the second strip perpendicular to the wound on one side of the center strip. The space between the strips should be approximately ⅛ inch. Apply a third strip on the other side of the center strip at a ⅛-inch interval. Continue applying the strips at ⅛-inch intervals until the edges of the wound are approximated. If at any time the skin surfaces become moist with perspiration, blood, or serum, wipe the area dry with a sterile gauze pad before applying the next strip.
Principle. Applying the strips in this manner facilitates good approximation of the wound. Spacing the strips at ⅛-inch intervals allows proper drainage of the wound.

Continued

PROCEDURE 25-6   Applying and Removing Adhesive Skin Closures—cont'd

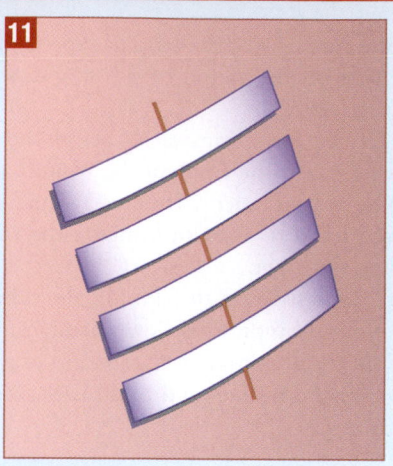

Apply the strips until the edges of the wound are approximated.

12. Procedural Step. Apply two closures approximately ½ inch from the ends of the strips and parallel to the wound (ladder fashion).
Principle. Applying a strip along each edge redistributes the tension and assists in holding the strips firmly in place.

Apply a strip along each edge.

13. Procedural Step. Apply a dry sterile dressing over the strips if indicated by the physician (see Procedure 25-4).
14. Procedural Step. Remove the gloves, and sanitize your hands.
15. Procedural Step. Instruct the patient in wound care as follows:
a. Provide the patient with written wound care instructions (see the patient teaching box on wound care in this chapter).

b. Explain the wound care instructions, and ask the patient whether he or she has any questions.
c. Ask the patient to sign the instruction sheet on the appropriate line.
d. Witness the patient's signature by signing your name in the appropriate space on the form. Include today's date.
e. Before the patient leaves the medical office, make a copy of the instruction sheet. Give a signed copy of the wound care instructions to the patient.
f. File the instruction sheet.

Ask the patient to sign the instruction sheet.

Paper-based patient record: File the original instruction sheet in the patient's medical record.
Electronic medical record: Scan the instruction sheet into the patient's electronic record.
Principle. An instruction sheet signed by the patient provides legal documentation that wound care instructions were provided to the patient in the event that the patient fails to follow the instructions and causes further harm or damage to the wound.
16. Procedural Step. Chart the procedure in the patient's medical record.
a. *Paper-based patient record:* Record the date and time, the appearance of the wound, the wound preparation, the number of strips applied, the location of the wound, the care of the wound, and the patient's reaction. Chart verbal and written instructions given to the patient concerning wound care (refer to the PPR charting example).

PROCEDURE 25-6 Applying and Removing Adhesive Skin Closures—cont'd

PPR CHARTING EXAMPLE

Date	
9/20/XX	10:30 a.m. Incision approx 5 cm long located on Ⓡ post forearm. Redness noted on edge of wound. Sl amt of serous drainage noted. Wound scrubbed c̄ Betadine sol and Betadine antiseptic applied. Applied Steri-Strips x4. Incision in good approximation. Applied DSD. Explained wound care. Written instructions provided. Signed copy filed in chart. To return in 5 days for removal of strips. _____
	_____ T. Browning, CMA (AAMA)

b. *Electronic medical record:* Document the appearance of the wound, wound preparation, the number of strips applied, the location of the wound, the care of the wound, and the patient's reaction using the appropriate radio buttons, drop-down menus, and free text fields. Also, document verbal and written instructions given to the patient concerning wound care.

Removal of Adhesive Skin Closures

Adhesive skin closures usually loosen and fall off on their own approximately 5 to 10 days after application. If they require removal, the procedure outlined here should be followed by the medical assistant.

1. **Procedural Step.** Sanitize your hands. Greet the patient and introduce yourself. Identify the patient by full name and date of birth and explain the procedure.
2. **Procedural Step.** Position the patient as required. Adjust the light so that it is focused on the wound. Check that the skin closures are intact and that the incision line is approximated and not gaping. Check that the incision line is not infected. If the incision line is not approximated, or if redness, swelling, or a discharge is present, do not remove the skin closures; notify the physician.
3. **Procedural Step.** Position a 4 × 4 gauze pad in a convenient location. Apply clean gloves.
4. **Procedural Step.** Remove the skin closures as follows:
   a. Gently grasp one end of a strip of tape with the dominant hand.
   b. Stabilize the skin with one finger of the nondominant hand.
   c. Slowly loosen and peel off one half of the strip of tape from the outside to the wound margin,

keeping the peeled-off section of the strip close to the skin surface and pulled back over itself. As you remove the strip from the skin, continue moving the finger as necessary to support the newly exposed skin. Always pull the strip toward the wound. Never pull the strip away from the wound because tension on the wound site could disrupt the healing process.
   d. Remove the other half of the strip of tape from the outside to the wound margin in the manner just described.
   e. When both halves of the strip are completely loosened, gently lift the strip up and away from the wound surface. Place the strip on a 4 × 4 gauze pad.
   f. Continue in this manner until all the skin closures have been removed.
5. **Procedural Step.** Cleanse the site with an antiseptic swab. Apply a dry sterile dressing if indicated by the physician (see Procedure 25-4).
6. **Procedural Step.** Dispose of the strips and gauze in a biohazard waste container. Remove the gloves, and sanitize your hands.
7. **Procedural Step.** Chart the procedure in the patient's medical record.
   a. *Paper-based patient record:* Record the date and time, the status of the skin closures, the number of skin closures removed, the location of the site, the care of the wound, and the patient's reaction. Chart any instructions given to the patient (refer to the PPR charting example).

PPR CHARTING EXAMPLE

Date	
9/25/XX	10:30 a.m. Skin closures intact and in good approximation. No signs of infection. Strips x 4 removed from Ⓡ post forearm. Incision line cleaned c̄ Betadine and DSD applied. Instructions provided on dressing care.
	_____ T. Browning, CMA (AAMA)

b. *Electronic medical record:* Document the status of the skin closures, the number of skin closures removed, the location of the site, the care of the wound, and the patient's reaction, using the appropriate radio buttons, drop-down menus, and free text fields. Also, document any instructions given to the patient.

Continued

ASSISTING WITH MINOR OFFICE SURGERY

TRAY SETUP

Assisting with minor office surgery requires a thorough knowledge of the instruments and supplies for each tray setup and the type of assistance required by the physician during the surgery. The medical assistant must be able to work quickly and efficiently and to anticipate the physician's needs.

The instruments and supplies for the surgery must be set on a sterile field. Many offices maintain index cards indicating the appropriate instruments and supplies for each minor office surgery tray setup. The card also may include information regarding the type of skin preparation, the position of the patient, the physician's glove size, the type of suture material, preoperative instructions, and postoperative instructions. In general, the index cards are kept in a file box and are filed alphabetically by the type of surgery. The medical assistant should pull the card before setting up for the minor office surgery and use it as a guide to ensure that all required articles are placed on the sterile field. The medical assistant may set up the sterile tray before or after preparing the patient's skin. The sterile tray setup must not become contaminated. If the medical assistant must turn away from the sterile tray or leave the room after setting up, a sterile towel must be placed over the tray to maintain sterility.

Methods Used to Set up a Sterile Tray

A common method used to set up a sterile tray is to use prepackaged sterile setups wrapped in disposable sterilization paper or muslin that are prepared by the medical office through autoclave sterilization (see Procedure 25-2). These setups are labeled according to use (e.g., suture pack, cyst removal pack) and contain most of the instruments and supplies required for the minor office surgery indicated on the label. The medical assistant opens the wrapped package on a flat surface, such as a **Mayo tray.** A Mayo tray is a broad, flat metal tray placed on a stand that can be used to hold sterile instruments and supplies; the inside of the wrapped package is sterile and serves as the sterile field. Several additional articles not contained in the prepackaged setup (e.g., an antiseptic, sterile 4 × 4 gauze pads, disposable syringes and needles, sutures) may need to be added to the sterile field when the package is opened. Items in peel-apart packages are added by flipping them onto the sterile field or by placing them on the field using a sterile gloved hand.

If an antiseptic solution is poured into a basin on the sterile field, this is performed according to Procedure 25-3.

Another method used to set up a sterile tray is to place all necessary articles on the sterile field by flipping them onto the sterile field from peel-apart packages. With this method, the sterile field is prepared by placing a sterile towel over a tray such as a Mayo tray or another flat surface. The sterile towel must be handled by the corners only so as not to contaminate it. It must not be fanned through the air,

but instead must be laid down gently and slowly to prevent airborne contamination.

Side Table

Some articles required for minor office surgery are not placed on the sterile field but are set on an adjacent table or counter. These articles, such as a surgical scrub brush, are not sterile and must not be placed on the sterile field. The local anesthetic, which is a sterile solution, is in a vial that is not sterile and must *not* be placed on the sterile field. The physician needs to apply gloves to perform the surgery. Although the gloves are sterile, the outside wrapper is not; the package of gloves must not be placed on the sterile field. In addition, it is easier for the physician to apply gloves from a side table or counter. To facilitate application of the gloves, the medical assistant opens the outside wrapper for the physician.

SKIN PREPARATION

The patient's skin must be prepared before the minor office surgery because the skin contains an abundance of microorganisms. If these microorganisms were to enter the body through the operative site, a wound infection could develop. It is impossible to sterilize skin because chemical agents required to kill all living microorganisms are too strong to be placed on the skin surfaces. The operative site and an area surrounding it must be cleaned and prepared in such a way as to remove as many microorganisms as possible to reduce the risk of surgical wound contamination.

Shaving the Site

Hair supports the growth of microorganisms, and the physician may want the medical assistant to shave the skin at and around the operative site. Shave preparation trays are commercially available and include several gauze sponges, a measured amount of antiseptic soap, a container for soapy water, and a disposable safety razor. The skin should be pulled taut as it is shaved, and the medical assistant must be careful to prevent nicks. When all the hair has been removed, the shaved area should be rinsed and dried thoroughly.

Cleansing the Site

The operative site must be cleaned with an antiseptic solution such as povidone-iodine (Betadine Surgical Scrub) or chlorhexidine gluconate (Hibiclens) (Figure 25-13). The medical assistant should scrub the operative area with a surgical scrub brush using a firm circular motion, moving from the inside outward. The area is rinsed using gauze pads saturated with water and is blotted dry with sterile gauze.

Antiseptic Application

When the patient's skin has been shaved (if required) and cleansed, an antiseptic is applied to the operative area, followed by the application of a sterile drape. The antiseptic decreases the number of microorganisms on the patient's skin; a common antiseptic is Betadine. A disposable sterile *fenestrated drape* (Figure 25-14) is the type of drape most

Figure 25-13 Cleansing solutions.

Figure 25-14 Fenestrated drape.

commonly used. It has an opening that is placed directly over the operative site. A fenestrated drape covers a wide area of skin around the operative area, leaving only the operative site exposed. This provides a sterile area around the operative site and decreases contamination of the patient's surgical wound.

LOCAL ANESTHETIC

Minor office surgeries often require the use of a local anesthetic; the local anesthetic most frequently used in the medical office is lidocaine hydrochloride (Xylocaine). The physician injects the local anesthetic into the tissue surrounding the operative site, a process termed **infiltration,** to produce a loss of sensation in that area and prevent the patient from feeling pain during the surgery. When first injected into the tissues, lidocaine causes the patient to experience a brief burning or stinging sensation at the injection site. The local anesthetic begins working in 5 to 15 minutes and has a duration of action of 1 to 3 hours, depending on the type of anesthetic.

Some physicians prefer to use a local anesthetic containing *epinephrine.* Epinephrine is a vasoconstrictor that prolongs the local effect of the anesthetic and decreases the rate of systemic absorption of the local anesthetic. It accomplishes this by constricting blood vessels at the operative site. The physician informs the medical assistant of the type, strength, and amount of local anesthetic needed for the minor office surgery. Xylocaine is available in 0.5%, 1%, 1.5%, and 2% solutions. The physician may order 1 mL of Xylocaine 2% with epinephrine to suture a laceration of the forearm.

Preparing the Anesthetic

The local anesthetic is drawn up into the syringe according to the procedure presented in Chapter 26. The vial must first be cleansed using an antiseptic wipe. The correct amount of anesthetic solution is withdrawn into the syringe. This may be performed by the medical assistant or the physician. The medical assistant withdraws the anesthetic into the syringe and hands it to the physician, who has not yet applied sterile gloves. The physician injects the anesthetic into the patient's tissues and then applies sterile gloves to begin the surgery.

The physician may prefer to draw the anesthetic solution into the syringe after he or she has applied sterile gloves. The medical assistant should first show the label of the vial to the physician and should then hold the vial securely while the physician withdraws the medication (Figure 25-15). The medical assistant must hold the vial because the outside of the vial is medically aseptic and cannot be touched by the physician's sterile gloved hand.

If the medical assistant prepares the anesthetic injection, the needle and syringe are not placed on the sterile field, but are assembled off to the side. If the physician withdraws the anesthetic, the needle and syringe are placed on the sterile field.

ASSISTING THE PHYSICIAN

The type of assistance required by the physician during minor office surgery is based on the type of surgery and the physician's preference. Some physicians want the medical assistant to apply sterile gloves and assist directly by handing instruments and supplies from the sterile field. An instrument should be handed to the physician in a firm, confident manner so that the instrument does not slip out of the physician's hand and drop on the floor. The instrument should be placed in the physician's hand in its functional position—that is, the position in which it is to be used (Figure 25-16). If the instrument is handed correctly, the physician should not have to reposition the instrument to use it.

The medical assistant is responsible for adding any instruments or supplies to the sterile field that the physician requires after the surgery has begun, such as another hemostat, additional 4 × 4 gauze pads, and sutures. This is usually accomplished by using peel-apart packages and either flipping the contents onto the sterile field or holding the

PROCEDURE 25-7   Assisting with Minor Office Surgery

Outcome Set up a surgical tray, and assist with minor office surgery

Equipment/Supplies

- Mayo stand
- Instruments and supplies for the type of surgery to be performed
- Biohazard waste container

Preparing the Tray

1. **Procedural Step.** Determine the type of minor office surgery to be performed. The physician instructs the medical assistant as to the type of surgery and provides any additional information needed to set up for the surgery, such as the type of local anesthetic and sutures to be used. If the medical office maintains a minor office surgery filing system, pull the file card that indicates the instruments and supplies required for the type of surgery to be performed.

2. **Procedural Step.** Prepare the examining room. Make sure the room is clean and well lighted.

3. **Procedural Step.** Sanitize your hands.

4. **Procedural Step.** Set up nonsterile articles on a side table or counter. If a specimen container is included in the setup, perform one of the following (based on the medical office policy):
   a. Attach a computer-generated bar code label to the specimen container *or*
   b. Clearly label the tubes and containers with the patient's name and date of birth, the date, your initials, and any other information required by the laboratory, such as the source of the specimen.

   Principle. Articles that are not sterile cannot be placed on the sterile field because they would contaminate it. Two unique identifiers should be used when labeling the specimen (e.g., patient's name and date of birth).

5. **Procedural Step.** Wash your hands with an antimicrobial soap and set up the minor office surgery tray on a clean, dry, flat surface, using the principles of surgical asepsis. The sterile tray can be set up as follows:
   Prepackaged setup
   a. Select the appropriate package from the supply shelf, and place it on a Mayo tray or other flat surface.
   b. Open the prepackaged setup using the inside of the wrapper as the sterile field. Check the sterilization indicator to make sure the contents of the pack are sterile.

Open the sterile pack using the inside of the wrapper as the sterile field.

   c. Add other articles to the sterile field that are needed for the surgery but not contained in the sterile package, such as 4 × 4 gauze, sutures, and a fenestrated drape. If sutures are required for the setup, make sure to check the expiration date of the sutures.

Transferring articles to a sterile field

   a. Pick up the folded sterile towel by two corner ends and allow it to unfold; make sure it does not touch an unsterile surface.
   b. Lay the sterile towel down gently and slowly over the Mayo tray, making sure it does not brush against an unsterile surface such as your uniform. Do not allow your arms to pass over the towel as you lay it down because this would result in contamination of the sterile field.

PROCEDURE 25-7   Assisting with Minor Office Surgery—cont'd

Lay the sterile towel down gently and slowly.

c. Transfer instruments and supplies to the sterile field from wrapped or peel-apart packages.
Principle. The principles of surgical asepsis must be followed to prevent contamination of the sterile field.

6. **Procedural Step.** Apply a sterile glove, and arrange the articles neatly on the sterile field. Do not allow one article to lie on top of another. Check that all the instruments and supplies required for the surgery are available on the sterile field.
Principle. Instruments and supplies can be located quickly and efficiently on a neat and orderly sterile field. Sterile gloves must be used to prevent contamination of the sterile articles.

Arrange the articles neatly on the sterile field.

7. **Procedural Step.** Cover the tray setup with a sterile towel by picking up the towel by two corner ends and placing it gently and slowly over the setup. Do not allow your arms to pass over the sterile field as you lay it down.
Principle. The towel prevents the sterile tray from becoming contaminated. The towel must be picked up by the corner ends to prevent contaminating it and should be moved slowly and not fanned through the air to prevent airborne contamination. Passing the arms over the sterile field results in contamination of the field.

Cover the tray setup with a sterile towel.

Preparing the Patient

8. **Procedural Step.** Greet the patient and introduce yourself. Identify the patient by full name and date of birth. Explain the procedure, and prepare the patient for the minor office surgery as follows:
a. Try to allay the patient's fear or anxiety.
b. Ask the patient whether he or she needs to void before the surgery.
c. Provide instructions to the patient about any clothing that must be removed and putting on an examination gown, if required. Enough clothing must be removed to expose the operative area completely and to avoid getting the antiseptic or blood on the patient's clothing.
d. Instruct the patient not to move during the procedure and not to talk, laugh, sneeze, or cough over the sterile field.
Principle. Minor office surgery is often a frightening experience for the patient, and reassurance should be offered to reduce apprehension. The amount of clothing that must be removed depends on the type of minor office surgery being performed. By moving, the patient may accidentally contaminate the sterile field or touch the operative site. Microorganisms are carried

Continued

in water vapor from the mouth, nose, and lungs and can be transferred onto the sterile field.

9. **Procedural Step.** Position the patient. The position is determined by the type of minor office surgery to be performed. The patient is positioned in such a way as to provide the best possible exposure and accessibility to the operative site. *Note:* If a difficult position must be maintained, such as the knee-chest position, the patient should not be positioned until the physician is ready to begin the minor office surgery.

10. **Procedural Step.** Adjust the light so that it is focused on the operative site.

11. **Procedural Step.** Prepare the patient's skin by performing the following:
    a. Apply clean disposable gloves.
    b. If hair is present, the skin at and around the operative site may need to be shaved. The skin should be pulled taut as it is shaved. The area is rinsed and dried thoroughly.
    c. Cleanse the patient's skin with an antiseptic solution and a surgical scrub brush using a firm, circular motion and moving from the inside outward. Do not return to an area just cleansed. The area is rinsed using gauze pads saturated with water and blotted dry with a sterile gauze pad.

Cleanse the patient's skin with an antiseptic solution.

    d. Apply an antiseptic to the site using antiseptic swabs such as Betadine. Allow the skin to dry. Alternatively, the physician may place a fenestrated drape over the operative site and then apply the antiseptic.
    e. Remove the gloves, and sanitize your hands.

12. **Procedural Step.** Verify that everything is prepared for the minor office surgery, and inform the physician that the patient is ready.

Assisting the Physician

13. **Procedural Step.** Assist the physician as required during the minor office surgery, following the principles of surgical asepsis. The physician drapes the patient, injects the local anesthetic, and performs the surgery. The responsibilities of the medical assistant may include the following:
    a. Uncover the sterile tray setup by picking up the sterile towel covering it. The towel should be picked up by two corner ends and removed slowly and gently without allowing the arms to pass over the sterile field.
    b. Open the outer glove wrapper for the physician to facilitate the application of sterile gloves.
    c. Withdraw the local anesthetic into a syringe and hand it to the physician, or hold the vial while the physician withdraws the local anesthetic. If lidocaine (Xylocaine) is used, the physician or medical assistant should inform the patient to expect a brief burning or stinging sensation as it is injected into the tissues.
    d. Adjust the light as needed by the physician for good visualization of the operative site.
    e. Restrain patients such as children.
    f. Relax and reassure the patient during the minor office surgery.
    g. Hand instruments and supplies to the physician. (Sterile gloves are required.)
    h. Keep the sterile field neat and orderly. (Sterile gloves are required.)
    i. Hold a basin in which the physician can deposit soiled instruments and supplies, such as hemostats and gauze sponges. (Clean gloves are required.)

Hold a basin for the physician to deposit soiled instruments.

PROCEDURE 25-7 Assisting with Minor Office Surgery—cont'd

j. Retract tissue from an area to allow the physician the best access to and visibility of the operative site. (Sterile gloves are required.)

k. Sponge blood from the operative site. (Sterile gloves are required.)

l. Add instruments and supplies to the sterile field as required by the physician.

m. Hold the specimen container to accept a tissue specimen received from the physician. (Clean gloves are required.) Do not touch the inside of the container because it is sterile. After the physician inserts the specimen, replace the container lid and close it tightly.

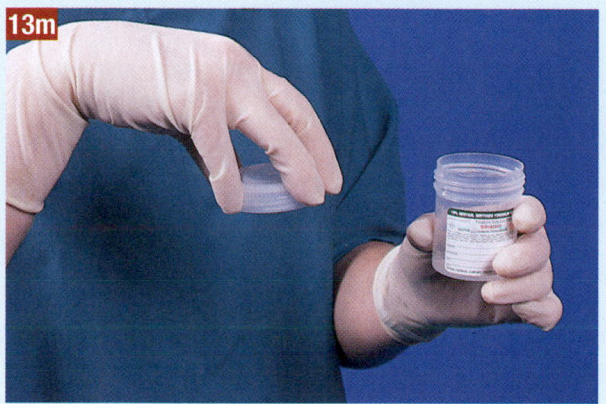

Hold the container to accept a tissue specimen.

n. After the physician has inserted a suture, cut the ends of the suture material approximately 1/8 inch above the knot of the suture. (Sterile gloves are required.)

14. **Procedural Step.** Apply a sterile dressing to the surgical wound, if ordered by the physician (see Procedure 25-4).

Principle. The sterile dressing protects the wound from contamination and injury and absorbs drainage.

15. **Procedural Step.** After the surgery, perform the following:

a. Stay with the patient as a safety precaution and to assist and instruct the patient.

b. Ensure that postoperative instructions regarding any type of medical care to be administered at home are understood. If the patient has a wound or if sutures have been inserted, he or she should be told to keep the area clean and dry and to report any signs of infection, such as excessive redness, swelling, discharge, or increased pain. Provide the patient with written wound care instructions (see the patient teaching box on wound care in this chapter). Ask the patient if he or she has any questions. Have the patient sign the instruction sheet. Witness the patient's signature. Before the patient leaves the office, make a copy of the instruction sheet. Give a copy to the patient.

c. File the instruction sheet.
Paper-based patient record: File the original instruction sheet in the patient's medical record.
Electronic medical record: Scan the instruction sheet into the patient's electronic record.

d. Relay information regarding the return visit for postoperative care, such as the removal of sutures or a dressing change.

e. Help the patient off the table to prevent falls.

f. Instruct the patient to get dressed, offering assistance if needed.

g. Any instructions or information given must be documented in the patient's medical record.

Principle. The patient (especially an elderly one) may become dizzy after the minor office surgery and may fall when getting off the examining table. The filed copy protects the physician legally, in the event that the patient fails to follow instructions and causes harm or damage to the operative site.

16. **Procedural Step.** If a specimen was collected, it must be transferred to the laboratory in a tightly closed, properly labeled specimen container. Prepare the specimen for transport. Complete a biopsy request form to accompany the specimen. Place the specimen container in a biohazard specimen bag and seal it. Insert the biopsy request in the outer pocket of the bag and tuck the requisition under the flap. Place the bag in the appropriate location for pickup by the laboratory.

17. **Procedural Step.** Chart specimen transport information in the patient's medical record.

a. *Paper-based patient record:* Record the date the specimen was picked up or sent to the laboratory and the name of the laboratory (refer to the PPR charting example).

PPR CHARTING EXAMPLE

Date	
9/25/XX	2:00 p.m. Applied DSD to (R) post forearm. Instructed patient on suture care. Written instructions provided. Signed copy filed in chart. To return in 5 days for removal of sutures. Sebaceous cyst specimen sent to Medical Center Laboratory for biopsy on 9/25/XX. —— T. Browning, CMA (AAMA)

Continued

PROCEDURE 25-7

PROCEDURE 25-7 for side margin

b. *Electronic medical record:* Document the date the specimen was picked up or sent to the laboratory, as well as the name of the laboratory, using the appropriate radio buttons, drop-down menus, and free text fields.

Principle. Recording information regarding transport of the specimen documents that the specimen was sent to the laboratory.

18. **Procedural Step.** Clean the examining room. Handle the instruments carefully so as not to damage them. Be especially careful with sharp instruments to prevent cutting yourself. Blood and body secretions should be rinsed off the instruments immediately to prevent them from drying and hardening. The instruments must be sanitized and sterilized when it is convenient to do so; follow the procedures presented in Chapter 18. Discard disposable articles contaminated with blood or other potentially infectious materials in a biohazard waste container.

Principle. Surgical instruments are expensive and must be handled carefully to prolong their life span. Hardened blood and secretions on an instrument are difficult to remove. Disposable articles must be discarded in an appropriate manner to prevent the spread of infection.

MEDICAL OFFICE SURGICAL PROCEDURES

The most common surgical procedures performed in the medical office are presented on the following pages. A discussion of the procedure and the items required for each tray setup are included. The medical assistant should take into account, however, that the instruments and supplies may vary slightly from those listed here, based on the physician's preference.

SEBACEOUS CYST REMOVAL

A **sebaceous cyst** (also known as an *epidermal cyst*) is a thin, closed sac or capsule located just under the surface of the skin. A sebaceous cyst forms when the outlet of a sebaceous (oil) gland becomes obstructed. The cyst contains *sebum,* which is made up of secretions from the sebaceous gland. The built-up secretion of sebum causes swelling, and the lining of the cyst consists of the stretched sebaceous gland. A sebaceous cyst is usually white or yellow in appearance and varies in size from less than ¼ inch (0.6 cm) in diameter to nearly 2 inches (5 cm) in diameter. It is usually a movable, dome-shaped mass with a smooth surface that is filled with a thick, fatty-white, cheesy material that has a foul odor. This type of cyst can occur anywhere on the body except on the palms of the hands and the soles of the feet—these areas do not contain sebaceous glands. Sebaceous cysts tend to occur most frequently on the scalp, face (Figure 25-18), ears, neck, back, and genital area.

A sebaceous cyst is usually slow-growing, painless, and nontender and may disappear on its own. A sebaceous cyst usually does not require surgical removal unless it becomes infected. An infected cyst is painful, tender, red, and swollen and may have a grayish-white, foul-smelling discharge. Because it is difficult to remove an infected sebaceous cyst, the physician usually drains the cyst and allows it to heal

Figure 25-18 Sebaceous cyst. (From Scully C: *Medical problems in dentistry,* ed 6, Norwalk, 2010, Churchill Livingstone.)

and then performs the cyst excision at a later time. Other reasons for removing a sebaceous cyst include cosmetic concerns and the need to reduce discomfort from a cyst that is located in a body area that is easily irritated, such as the armpit.

Surgical excision of a sebaceous cyst is a simple procedure that involves complete removal of the sac wall and its contents. Most sebaceous cysts are benign and are not usually biopsied unless they have an unusual appearance that may indicate a more serious problem. The side tray setup includes the items needed for a tissue biopsy (specimen container and laboratory request form); however, these items would not be placed on the tray if the physician determines that a biopsy of the sebaceous cyst is not warranted.

Procedure: Sebaceous Cyst Removal

A sebaceous cyst is removed as follows:
1. A local anesthetic is used to numb the area.
2. The physician makes an incision using either a single cut down the center or an oval cut on both sides of the cyst.

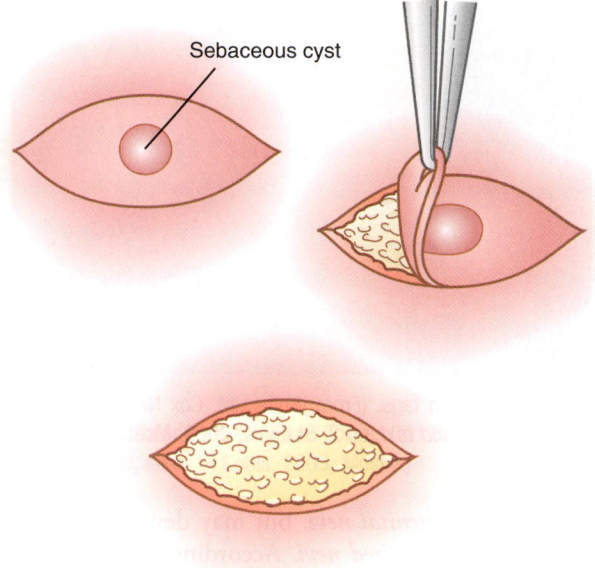

Figure 25-19 Sebaceous cyst removal. The physician makes an incision, removes the cyst, and sutures the surgical incision. (From Nealon TF Jr: *Fundamental skills in surgery,* ed 4, Philadelphia, 1994, Saunders.)

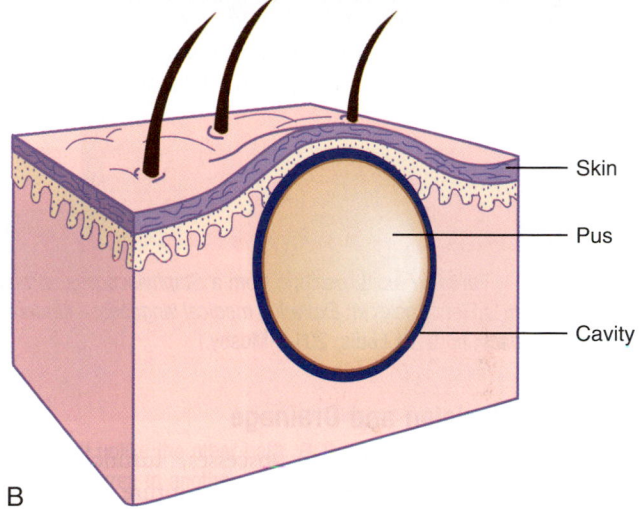

Figure 25-20 **A,** *Staphylococcus* skin abscess. **B,** An abscess is a collection of pus in a cavity surrounded by inflamed tissue. (**A,** From Braverman IM: *Skin signs of systemic disease,* ed 3, Philadelphia, 1998, Saunders. **B,** From Nealon TF Jr: *Fundamental skills in surgery,* ed 4, Philadelphia, 1994, Saunders.)

The physician then removes the cyst and sutures the surgical incision (Figure 25-19).

3. If the cyst is to be biopsied, it is placed in a specimen container with a preservative and sent to the laboratory for examination by a pathologist.
4. A sterile dressing is applied to the operative site.

Sebaceous cyst removal sterile field.

Postoperative Instructions: Sebaceous Cyst Removal

Postoperative instructions include the following:
1. Keep the dressing clean and dry.
2. Report any signs that the wound is infected, which include fever, increased pain, swelling, redness, warmth, and discharge.

3. Notify the medical office if the sutures become loose or break.

Provide the patient with written instructions on wound care to refer to at home, and instruct the patient when to return for removal of the sutures.

SURGICAL INCISION AND DRAINAGE OF LOCALIZED INFECTIONS

An **abscess** is a collection of pus in a cavity surrounded by inflamed tissue (Figure 25-20, *A*). It is caused by a pathogen that invades the tissues, usually via a break in the skin. An abscess serves as a defense mechanism of the body to keep an infection localized by walling off the microorganisms, preventing them from spreading through the body (Figure 25-20, *B*). A **furuncle,** also known as a *boil,* is a localized staphylococcal infection that originates deep within a hair follicle (Figure 25-21). Furuncles produce pain and itching. The skin initially becomes red and then turns white and necrotic over the top of the furuncle. Erythema and induration usually surround it.

examination. The primary goal of colposcopy is to prevent cervical cancer by detecting precancerous lesions early and treating them.

Blood cells make it more difficult for the physician to observe the cervix; therefore, a colposcopy is usually performed 1 week after the end of the menstrual period. To prepare for the procedure, the patient should be told not to douche; use tampons, vaginal medications, or spermicides;

or have intercourse for 24 hours before the examination. The lens of the colposcope is positioned approximately 12 inches (30 cm) from the opening of the vagina. The lens magnifies tissue, facilitating the inspection of cervical cells and the obtaining of a biopsy specimen. For a routine colposcopic examination, a magnification ranging from 6× to 15× is typically used. The colposcope may be placed on an adjustable stand or attached to the side of the examining table and swung out before use.

Procedure: Colposcopy

Colposcopy is performed as follows:
1. The patient is assisted into a lithotomy position and is prepared as for a pelvic examination.
2. The physician inserts a vaginal speculum into the vagina.
3. A long, cotton-tipped applicator moistened with saline is used to wipe the cervix to remove the mucous film that normally covers it. The saline also provides better visualization of the cervical epithelium because dry cervical epithelium is not transparent and does not allow satisfactory viewing of the vascular pattern of the cervix.
4. The colposcope is focused on the cervix, and the physician inspects the saline-moistened cervix.
5. The cervix is swabbed with acetic acid, using a long, cotton-tipped applicator. The acetic acid dissolves cervical mucus and other secretions. It also causes abnormal tissue to turn white, which allows easier visualization of abnormal areas of the cervix.
6. The cervical epithelium also may be stained with Lugol iodine solution using a long, cotton-tipped applicator. This provides another means to identify unhealthy epithelium. The healthy epithelium of the cervix contains glycogen, which is able to absorb the iodine, causing the epithelium to stain a dark brown color. Conversely, abnormal epithelium, such as would constitute a malignancy, does not contain glycogen and is unable to absorb the iodine.
7. If an abnormal area is observed, the physician obtains a cervical biopsy specimen using punch biopsy forceps, which is described next.

Figure 25-28 A colposcope. (From Apgar BS, Brotzman GL, Spitzer M: *Colposcopy: principles and practice—an integrated textbook and atlas*, Philadelphia, 2002, Saunders.)

Figure 25-29 **A,** Normal cervix. **B,** Abnormal cervix. (From Damjanov I: *Pathology for the health-related professions*, ed 4, St Louis, 2012, Saunders.)

CERVICAL PUNCH BIOPSY

A cervical biopsy is performed in combination with colposcopy to remove a cervical tissue specimen for examination by a pathologist. The purpose of the biopsy is to detect the presence of cervical dysplasia or cancer of the cervix. *Cervical dysplasia* is an abnormal growth of cells on the surface of the cervix that are precancerous. *Precancerous* means that abnormal cells have the potential to develop into cancer in the future. Cervical dysplasia can range from mild to moderate to severe. A cervical punch biopsy can also be used to diagnose polyps on the cervix and genital warts. Genital warts may indicate infection with human papillomavirus (HPV), which is a risk factor for developing cervical cancer. Performing a cervical punch biopsy helps the physician determine the type of abnormal tissue present on the cervix so that the physician can determine the best form of treatment for the patient's condition.

Cervical biopsies are most frequently performed after abnormal Pap test results. Although an abnormal Pap test result is a cause for concern, the majority of abnormal Pap test results are not caused by cervical cancer, but rather by a vaginal infection. To prevent inaccurate test results, the cervical biopsy is usually performed 1 week after the end of the menstrual period, when the cervix is the least vascular. To prepare for the procedure, the patient should be told not to douche; use tampons, vaginal medications, or spermicides; or have intercourse for 24 hours before the procedure to prevent inaccurate test results.

What Would You Do? What Would You *Not* Do?

Case Study 3

Sadira Wisal has been referred to the office by her family physician for a colposcopy. Her last Pap test results came back as abnormal, and a repeat Pap test 3 months later also had abnormal results. While having her vital signs taken, Sadira bursts into tears. She tearfully explains that she's afraid that she has cancer, and that no one at her regular physician's office told her what to expect from this procedure. Sadira does not understand why she has to have this procedure done, and she does not know what the physician will be doing during the procedure. She says that she feels stupid, but she does not even know what a cervix is. Sadira also worries that the procedure will affect her ability to have children. ■

Procedure: Cervical Punch Biopsy

A cervical punch biopsy is performed as follows:
1. The patient is positioned and draped in a lithotomy position. An anesthetic is not needed because the cervix has few pain receptors. The patient may experience no discomfort during the procedure or a certain amount of discomfort ranging from mild to moderate in intensity. Some patients experience mild cramping and pinching when the specimen is being removed from the cervix.
2. The physician inserts a vaginal speculum into the vagina for proper visualization of the cervix.
3. The cervix is wiped with saline and then swabbed with ascetic acid.
4. To assist in obtaining the specimen, the physician may stain the cervix with Lugol iodine solution.
5. The colposcope is focused on the cervix, and the physician inspects the cervix.
6. Using cervical biopsy punch forceps, the physician obtains several tissue specimens (Figure 25-30, *A*) from the abnormal cervical epithelium (Figure 25-30, *B*). The patient may feel a pinching sensation and mild cramps each time a specimen is removed from the cervix.
7. The specimen is placed in a container with a preservative and is sent to the laboratory for examination by a pathologist.
8. If bleeding occurs, the physician controls it with gauze packing, a hemostatic solution (e.g., Monsel solution), or electrocautery.
9. The patient is given a sanitary pad at the office after the procedure to absorb any discharge.

Postoperative Instructions: Cervical Punch Biopsy

Postoperative instructions include the following:
1. A minimum amount of cramping and bleeding may follow the procedure and last up to 1 week. Contact the medical office if the bleeding lasts longer than 2 weeks.
2. A thick, dark-colored vaginal discharge may occur after the procedure (if Monsel solution was used to control bleeding) and may last for several days.
3. Do not douche, use tampons, or have intercourse for 1 week after the procedure to allow proper healing of the cervix to take place.
4. Contact the medical office if any of the following occurs: bleeding that is heavier than normal menstrual bleeding, a foul-smelling vaginal discharge, fever, or lower abdominal pain.

Provide the patient with written instructions to refer to at home. An appointment is scheduled approximately 1 week after the procedure to make sure that healing is taking place and to discuss the biopsy results.

CRYOSURGERY

Cervical Cryosurgery

Cervical **cryosurgery,** also known as *cryotherapy,* uses freezing temperatures to treat certain gynecologic conditions. Cryosurgery is most often performed as a treatment for cervical dysplasia to destroy abnormal cervical cells that show changes that may lead to cancer. Cryosurgery is done only after a colposcopy confirms the presence of cervical dysplasia. Cryosurgery is also used for the treatment of chronic cervicitis, which is inflammation of the cervix.

Cervical cryosurgery can be performed without an anesthetic, although occasionally a mild analgesic is necessary immediately afterward. The cryosurgery unit consists of a long metal cryoprobe attached to a cooling-agent tank

A

B

Figure 25-30 Cervical punch biopsy. **A,** Obtaining a tissue specimen from the cervix using cervical biopsy punch forceps. **B,** Cervical biopsy punch forceps. (Courtesy Elmed, Addison, Ill.)

Figure 25-31 Cryosurgery unit. (From Zakus S: *Clinical skills for medical assistants,* ed 4, Philadelphia, 2001, Saunders.)

(Figure 25-31). The principal cooling agents are liquid nitrogen and compressed nitrogen gas. The cryoprobe is inserted into the vagina and placed firmly in contact with the abnormal area. The cooling agent flows through the cryoprobe, freezing the cervical tissue to −20° C. This causes the abnormal cells to die and slough off so that the

cervical covering can eventually be replaced with new, healthy epithelial tissue. Regeneration of cervical tissue occurs within approximately 4 to 6 weeks after the procedure. After cryosurgery, the patient will be required to have a Pap test every 3 to 6 months for a period of time determined by the physician.

Procedure: Cervical Cryosurgery

Cryosurgery is performed as follows:
1. The patient is draped and assisted into the lithotomy position.
2. The physician inserts a vaginal speculum for proper visualization of the cervix.
3. The cervix is swabbed with an acid-saline solution to remove mucus and other contaminants.
4. The metal cryoprobe is inserted into the vagina and placed firmly in contact with the affected area, and the cryosurgery unit is turned on.
5. The cooling agent flows through the cryoprobe and causes the metal probe to freeze and destroy superficial abnormal cervical tissue. The physician allows the cryoprobe to come in contact with the cervical area for approximately 3 minutes. During the procedure, the patient may experience some pain resembling menstrual cramping.
6. The cryoprobe is removed for 3 to 5 minutes to permit the cervical tissue to return to its normal temperature.

The freezing procedure is then repeated for an additional 3 minutes.

7. When the procedure has been completed, the medical assistant should assist the patient as necessary and observe her for signs of discomfort or vertigo.

8. The patient is given a sanitary pad at the office after the procedure to absorb any discharge.

Postoperative Instructions: Cervical Cryosurgery

Postoperative instructions include the following:

1. Normal activities can be resumed the day after the cryosurgery.

2. On the first postoperative day, a clear, watery vaginal discharge occurs, which lasts for 2 to 4 weeks. The discharge is caused by the shedding of the dead cervical tissue and gradually diminishes as the healing progresses.

3. Use sanitary pads (rather than tampons) to absorb the watery discharge.

4. Do not douche, use tampons, or have intercourse for 2 to 3 weeks after the procedure to allow proper healing of the cervix to take place.

5. Contact the medical office if any of the following occurs: bleeding that is heavier than normal menstrual bleeding, a foul-smelling vaginal discharge, fever, or lower abdominal pain.

Provide the patient with written instructions to refer to at home. The patient must schedule a return visit 6 weeks after the procedure to ensure that proper healing has occurred.

Skin Lesions

In the medical office, cryosurgery also may be used to remove benign skin lesions, such as common warts and skin tags. Only a small amount of cooling agent is required for skin lesions, so the cryosurgery unit is considerably smaller than the one described for cervical cryosurgery. Most physicians use liquid nitrogen contained in a small, pressurized, stainless steel canister with an attached probe. The physician applies the liquid nitrogen to the skin lesion until it turns white, which indicates that freezing of the tissue has occurred. During the procedure, the patient feels a slight burning or stinging sensation as the cooling agent is applied. After cryosurgery, a blister develops and dries to a scab in 1 week to 10 days and eventually sloughs off. The patient should be told to keep the area clean and dry until the scab has sloughed off. In some cases the treatment may not result in complete destruction of the lesion; two or more treatments may be required to remove the lesion.

BANDAGING

A **bandage** is a strip of woven material used to wrap or cover a part of the body. The function of the bandage may be to apply pressure to control bleeding, to protect a wound from contamination, to hold a dressing in place, or to protect, support, or immobilize an injured part of the body.

GUIDELINES FOR APPLICATION

The bandage should be applied so that it feels comfortable to the patient, and it must be fastened securely with metal clips or adhesive tape. Guidelines for applying a bandage are as follows:

1. Observe the principles of medical asepsis during the application of a bandage.

2. Ensure that the area to which a bandage is applied is clean and dry.

3. Do not apply a bandage directly over an open wound. To prevent contamination of the wound, first apply a sterile dressing and then the bandage. The bandage should extend at least 2 inches (5 cm) beyond the edge of the dressing.

4. To prevent irritation, do not allow the skin surfaces of two body parts (e.g., two fingers) to touch. In addition, the patient's perspiration provides a moist environment that encourages the growth of microorganisms. A piece of gauze should be inserted between the two body parts.

5. Ensure that joints and prominent parts of bones are padded to prevent the bandage from rubbing the skin and causing irritation.

6. Bandage the body part in its normal position with joints slightly flexed to avoid muscle strain.

7. Apply the bandage from the distal to the proximal part of the body to aid the venous return of blood to the heart.

8. As you apply the bandage, ask the patient whether it feels comfortable. The bandage should fit snugly enough that it does not fall off, but not so tightly that it impedes circulation.

9. If possible, leave the fingers and toes exposed when bandaging an extremity. This provides the opportunity to check them for signs of impairment in circulation. Signs indicating that the bandage is too tight include coldness, pallor, numbness, cyanosis of the nail beds, swelling, pain, and tingling sensations. If any of these signs occurs, loosen the bandage immediately.

10. If a bandage roll is dropped during the procedure, obtain a new bandage and begin again.

TYPES OF BANDAGES

Three basic types of bandages are used in the medical office. A *roller bandage* is a long strip of soft material wound on itself to form a roll. It ranges from $\frac{1}{2}$ inch to 6 inches (1.3 to 15.2 cm) wide and from 2 to 5 yards (1.83 to 4.57 m) long. The width used depends on the part being bandaged. Roller bandages usually are made of sterilized gauze. Gauze is porous and lightweight, molds easily to a body part, and is relatively inexpensive and easily disposed of. Because it is made of loosely woven cotton, however, it may slip and fray easily. *Kling gauze* is a special type of gauze that stretches; this allows it to cling, and as a result it molds and conforms better to the body part than does regular gauze.

Elastic bandages are made of woven cotton that contains elastic fibers. One brand name of elastic bandages is the Ace

↻ TERMINOLOGY REVIEW—cont'd

Key Term	Word Parts	Definition
Sterile		Free of all living microorganisms and bacterial spores.
Surgery		The branch of medicine that deals with operative and manual procedures for correction of deformities and defects, repair of injuries, and diagnosis and treatment of certain diseases.
Surgical asepsis	*a:* without or absence of -*sepsis:* infection	Practices that keep objects and areas sterile or free from microorganisms.
Sutures		Material used to approximate tissues with surgical stitches.
Swaged needle		A needle with suturing material permanently attached to its end.
Wound		A break in the continuity of an external or internal surface caused by physical means.

ON THE WEB

For information on surgery and emergency medicine:

American College of Surgeons: www.facs.org

Surgery: www.surgery.com

American Red Cross: www.redcross.org

Ethicon Incorporated: www.ethicon.com

Federal Emergency Management Agency: www.fema.gov

Administration of Medication and Intravenous Therapy

26

LEARNING OBJECTIVES

Introduction to the Administration of Medication

1. Explain the difference among administering, prescribing, and dispensing medication.
2. State the common routes for administering medication.
3. List and describe the six sections of the *Physicians' Desk Reference* (PDR).
4. List and describe the categories of information in a drug package insert.
5. Describe the Food and Drug Administration's responsibilities with respect to drugs.
6. List and define the four names of drugs.
7. Classify drugs according to preparation.
8. Classify drugs according to the action they have on the body.
9. List the guidelines for writing metric notations.
10. List and describe the five schedules for controlled drugs.
11. List and explain the parts of a prescription.
12. Describe the functions performed by an electronic medical record (EMR) prescription program.
13. Explain the purpose of a medication record.
14. Describe the factors that affect the action of drugs in the body.
15. List and describe the possible adverse effects of medication.
16. List the guidelines for preparing and administering medication.

Oral Administration

17. Explain why the oral route is most frequently used to administer medication.
18. State where the absorption of most oral medications occurs.

Parenteral Administration

19. State the advantages and disadvantages of the parenteral route of administration.
20. Identify the parts of a needle and syringe and explain their functions.
21. State the ranges of gauge and length of needles for each of the following injections: intradermal, subcutaneous, and intramuscular.
22. State the purpose of safety-engineered syringes.
23. Describe the dispensing units available for injectable medications.
24. State which tissue layers of the body are used for intradermal, subcutaneous, and intramuscular injections.
25. List the medications commonly administered through each of the following routes: intradermal, subcutaneous, and intramuscular.
26. Explain the reason for administering medication with the Z-track method.

PROCEDURES

Research a drug using the PDR.
Interpret a drug package insert.
Calculate drug dosage.
Complete a prescription form.
Complete a medication record form.

Prepare and administer oral medications.

Reconstitute a powdered drug for parenteral administration.
Withdraw medication from a vial.
Withdraw medication from an ampule.
Locate appropriate subcutaneous injection sites.
Administer a subcutaneous injection.
Locate each of the following intramuscular injection sites: dorsogluteal, deltoid, vastus lateralis, and ventrogluteal.
Administer an intramuscular injection.
Administer an injection using the Z-track method.
Administer an intradermal injection.

LEARNING OBJECTIVES

PROCEDURES

Tuberculin Testing

27. Explain the difference between active and latent tuberculosis.
28. Explain the purpose of tuberculin skin testing.
29. Identify the categories of individuals who should have a tuberculin test.
30. Explain the significance of a positive reaction to a tuberculin test.
31. List the diagnostic procedures that might be performed following a positive tuberculin test.
32. State the guidelines that should be followed when administering and reading a Mantoux tuberculin skin test.
33. State the advantages of the tuberculosis blood test.

Administer a Mantoux tuberculin skin test, and read the test results.
Complete a tuberculosis test record card.

Allergy Testing

34. Define an allergy, and name common allergens.
35. Explain what occurs during an allergic reaction.
36. List the guidelines for direct skin allergy testing.
37. State the purpose of each of the following types of allergy tests: patch testing, skin-prick testing, intradermal skin testing, and in vitro blood testing.

Perform allergy skin testing.

Intravenous Therapy

38. Explain the advantages of outpatient intravenous (IV) therapy.
39. Identify the role of the entry-level medical assistant in IV therapy.
40. State the indications for outpatient IV therapy.

CHAPTER OUTLINE

INTRODUCTION TO THE ADMINISTRATION OF MEDICATION
ADMINISTERING, PRESCRIBING, AND DISPENSING MEDICATION
LEGAL ASPECTS
ROUTES OF ADMINISTRATION
DRUG REFERENCES
FOOD AND DRUG ADMINISTRATION
DRUG NOMENCLATURE
CLASSIFICATION OF DRUGS BASED ON PREPARATION
Liquid Preparations
Solid Preparations
CLASSIFICATION OF DRUGS BASED ON ACTION
SYSTEMS OF MEASUREMENT FOR MEDICATION
Metric System
Household System
CONVERTING UNITS OF MEASUREMENT
CONTROLLED DRUGS
PRESCRIPTION
Parts of a Prescription
Generic Prescribing
Electronic Medical Record Prescription Program
MEDICATION RECORD
FACTORS AFFECTING DRUG ACTION
Therapeutic Effect
Age
Route of Administration
Size

Time of Administration
Tolerance
Undesirable Effects of Drugs
Adverse Reactions
Drug Interactions
Allergic Drug Reaction
Idiosyncratic Reaction
GUIDELINES FOR PREPARATION AND ADMINISTRATION OF MEDICATION
ORAL ADMINISTRATION
PARENTERAL ADMINISTRATION
Parts of a Needle and Syringe
Needle
Syringe
Safety-Engineered Syringes
Preparation of Parenteral Medication
Vials
Ampules
Prefilled Syringes
Storage
Reconstitution of Powdered Drugs
Subcutaneous Injections
Intramuscular Injections
Intramuscular Injection Sites
Z-Track Method
Intradermal Injections
TUBERCULIN SKIN TESTING
Tuberculosis
Purpose of Tuberculin Skin Testing
Tuberculin Skin Test Reactions

Mantoux Tuberculin Skin Test
Guidelines for Administering a Mantoux Tuberculin Skin Test
Guidelines for Reading Mantoux Tuberculin Skin Test Results
Two-Step Tuberculin Skin Test
Tuberculosis Blood Test
ALLERGY TESTING
Allergy
Allergic Reaction
Diagnosis and Treatment
Types of Allergy Tests

Direct Skin Testing
In Vitro Allergy Blood Testing
INTRAVENOUS THERAPY
Advantages of Outpatient Intravenous Therapy
Earlier Hospital Discharge
Avoidance of Hospitalization
Medical Office–Based Intravenous Therapy
Indications for Outpatient Intravenous Therapy
Scheduling the Intravenous Therapy
Medical Office Guidelines

KEY TERMS

adverse reaction (AD-vers ree-AK-shun)
allergen (AL-er-jen)
allergy (AL-er-jee)
ampule (AM-pyool)
anaphylactic reaction (an-uh-ful-AK-tik ree-AK-shun)
chemotherapy
controlled drug
conversion (kon-VER-shun)
cubic centimeter (KYOO-bik SEN-tih-mee-ter)
DEA number
dose
drug

enteral nutrition
gauge (GAYJ)
hemophilia
immune globulin
induration (in-dur-AY-shun)
infusion
inhalation (in-hal-AY-shun administration)
inscription (in-SKRIP-shun)
intradermal injection (in-tra-DER-mal in-JEK-shun)
intramuscular (in-tra-MUS-kyoo-lar) injection
intravenous (in-tra-VEE-nus) (IV) therapy

oral (OR-ul) administration
parenteral (par-EN-ter-al)
pharmacology (far-ma-KOL-oh-jee)
prescription
signatura (sig-na-CHUR-ah)
subcutaneous (sub-kyoo-TAY-nee-us) injection
sublingual (sub-LIN-gwal) administration
subscription (sub-SKRIP-shun)
superscription (soo-per-SKRIP-shun)
topical (TOP-ih-kul) administration
transfusion
vial (VIE-ul)
wheal (WEE-ul)

INTRODUCTION TO THE ADMINISTRATION OF MEDICATION

Pharmacology is the study of drugs and includes the preparation, use, and action of drugs in the body. A **drug** is a chemical that is used for the treatment, prevention, or diagnosis of disease. Most drugs are produced synthetically, but they also can be obtained from other sources, such as animals, plants, and minerals.

ADMINISTERING, PRESCRIBING, AND DISPENSING MEDICATION

Medication may be administered, prescribed, or dispensed in the medical office. Medication that is *administered* is actually given to a patient at the office. Medication is *prescribed* when a physician provides a patient with a handwritten or computer-generated prescription for a drug to be filled at a pharmacy. Prescriptions also can be sent electronically, telephoned, or faxed to the pharmacy by the physician, depending on the preference of the patient. *Dispensed* medication is given to a patient at the office to be taken at home; for example, the physician gives a patient drug samples to take home.

LEGAL ASPECTS

An important responsibility of the medical assistant is the administration of medication. (One should check the laws of the state to ensure that it is legally permissible for the medical assistant to administer medication.) The medical assistant should administer medication only under the direction of the physician. In all states, it is unlawful to administer medication in the medical office without the consent of the physician.

ROUTES OF ADMINISTRATION

Common routes of administration of medication are oral, sublingual, inhalation, buccal, rectal, vaginal, topical, intradermal, subcutaneous (subcut), intramuscular (IM), and intravenous (IV). The route of administration depends on the type of drug being given, the dosage form, the intended action, and the rapidity of response desired. The route by which medication is most commonly administered in the medical office is the parenteral route. **Parenteral** refers to sites outside the gastrointestinal tract; this term is most commonly used to refer to the administration of medication by injection.

SECTION 4: PRODUCT IDENTIFICATION GUIDE

This section provides a full-color (actual size) photograph of the tablets and capsules included in the PDR. The drugs are arranged alphabetically by manufacturer. A variety of other dosage forms are also illustrated, but are shown in less than actual size (e.g., inhalers, injectable drugs in vials). This section provides valuable assistance in identifying a drug.

SECTION 5: PRODUCT INFORMATION

This index makes up the main section of the PDR and contains product information on approximately 3000 drug products. The drugs are arranged alphabetically by manufacturer; under the manufacturer, the drugs are listed alphabetically by brand name. The information included in this section consists of the actual drug package inserts. The following information is included for each medication:

DESCRIPTION: This category consists of a general description of the drug and includes the following information: brand name (with pronunciation), generic name, drug category, dosage form (e.g., tablets, capsules), route of administration, chemical name and structural formula, and the inactive ingredients contained in the drug. This category also indicates if the product requires a prescription (Rx) or if it is available over-the-counter (OTC). The symbol C and a Roman numeral appearing next to the drug indicates that it is a scheduled drug and that a prescription written for this drug requires the physicians' DEA number.

CLINICAL PHARMACOLOGY: This category describes how the drug functions in the body to produce its therapeutic effect. Also included is an analysis of the absorption, distribution, metabolism, and excretion of the drug after it enters the body.

INDICATIONS AND USAGE: This category presents a list of the conditions that the drug has been formally approved to treat by the U.S. Food and Drug Administration (FDA).

CONTRAINDICATIONS: This category includes situations in which the drug should not be used because the risk of using the drug in these situations outweighs any possible benefit. Contraindications include administration of the drug to patients known to have a hypersensitivity (allergy) to it and use of the drug in patients who have a substantial risk of being harmed by it because of their particular age, sex, concurrent use of another drug, disease state, or condition (e.g., pregnancy).

WARNINGS: This category describes serious adverse reactions and potential safety hazards that may occasionally occur with the use of the drug and what should be done if they occur.

PRECAUTIONS: This category includes information regarding any special care that needs to be taken by the physician for the safe and effective use of the drug. Information typically presented in this category includes:

- **General Precautions:** Lists any disease states or situations that may require special consideration when the drug is being taken.
- **Information for Patients:** Includes information that should be relayed to the patient to ensure safe and effective use of the drug.
- **Laboratory Tests:** Indicates the laboratory tests that may be helpful in following the patient's response to the drug or in identifying possible adverse reactions to the drug.
- **Drug Interactions:** Lists any known interactions of this drug with other drugs that can affect the proper functioning of the drug.
- **Laboratory Test Interactions:** Includes any laboratory tests that may be affected when taking the medication.
- **Pregnancy:** Indicates the pregnancy category of the drug.

ADVERSE REACTIONS: This category describes the unintended and undesirable effects that may occur with the use of the drug. Some adverse reactions are harmless and therefore often tolerated by the patient in order to obtain the therapeutic effect of the drug. Other adverse reactions may be harmful to the patient and warrant discontinuing the medication.

OVERDOSAGE: This category describes symptoms associated with an overdosage of the drug, as well as the complications that can occur and the treatment to institute for an overdosage.

DOSAGE AND ADMINISTRATION: This category lists the recommended adult dosage, the usual dosage range of the drug, and the route of administration (e.g., by mouth, sublingual, IM). Also included is information about the intervals recommended between doses, the usual duration of treatment, and any modification of dosage needed for special groups such as children, the elderly, and patients with renal or hepatic disease.

HOW SUPPLIED: This category indicates the dosage forms that are available (e.g., 20-mg tablets), the units in which the dosage form is available (e.g., bottles of 100; 5-mL multiple-dose vial), information to help identify the dosage form (shape and color), and the handling and storage conditions for the drug.

Figure 26-1, cont'd

FOOD AND DRUG ADMINISTRATION

The U.S. Food and Drug Administration (FDA) is a federal agency in the Department of Health and Human Services. The FDA is responsible for determining whether new food products, drugs, vaccines, medical devices, cosmetics, and other products are safe before they are released for human use.

The FDA determines the safety and effectiveness of prescription and nonprescription (over-the-counter [OTC]) drugs. Pharmaceutical manufacturers are required to submit new drug applications to the FDA for review and approval before products can be released for human use.

The FDA also is responsible for determining whether a medication will be available with or without a prescription. Medications that require a prescription have been determined by the FDA to be safe and effective when used under the guidance of a physician. The label on a prescription medication container must bear the following symbol and word: *Rx only*.

Nonprescription medications are drugs that the FDA determines to be safe and effective for use without physician supervision. Nonprescription medications have a low incidence of adverse reactions when the consumer follows the directions and warnings on the label. Examples of nonprescription medications include mild pain relievers, topical antibiotics, topical corticosteroids, cold medications, and laxatives.

DRUG NOMENCLATURE

Each drug has four names: chemical, generic, official, and brand (also known as *trade*) names.

1. *Chemical name.* The chemical name provides a precise description of the drug's chemical composition; pharmaceutical manufacturers and pharmacists are most concerned with the chemical makeup of a drug.
2. *Generic name.* The generic name is assigned by the pharmaceutical manufacturer that develops the drug, before it receives official approval from the FDA. The generic name is often a shortened derivative of the chemical name.
3. *Official name.* The official name is the name under which the drug is listed in official publications, such as the *United States Pharmacopeia* (USP) and the *National Formulary* (NF). Official publications set specific standards to regulate the strength, purity, packaging, safety, labeling, and dosage form of each drug. The generic name is frequently used for the official name.
4. *Brand name.* The brand name is the name under which a pharmaceutical manufacturer markets a drug. Because a drug may be manufactured by more than one pharmaceutical company, it may have several brand names. The generic name of a common analgesic is acetaminophen; brand names for this drug include Tylenol, Tempra, Datril, Exdol, Panadol, and Liquiprin.

The medical assistant should be familiar with the generic and brand names of medications commonly prescribed and administered in the medical office.

What Would You Do? What Would You *Not* Do?

Case Study 1

Carol Okasinski, 56 years old, is a new patient. She was a patient of another physician in the community; however, his receptionist was often rude to her, and she decided not to go there anymore. Mrs. Okasinski is obese and has hypertension, type 2 diabetes, osteoarthritis in her hands and knees, and problems with depression. While filling in the health history form, she says she cannot fill in the names of the medications she is taking. She is on a lot of medications prescribed by her previous physician. She says she could not get the childproof pill containers open because of the arthritis in her hands, so she had her husband throw away the childproof containers and transfer each medication into an easy-to-open plastic container. She knows when to take her medications, but she does not know the names of them or why she is taking them. She has brought in a bag with all her medications in their plastic containers. ∎

CLASSIFICATION OF DRUGS BASED ON PREPARATION

Drugs are available in two basic forms: liquid and solid. A medication may be available in both these forms (liquid and solid), which permits it to be administered to different types of patients. A liquid preparation of an antibiotic is administered to young children, and the solid preparation (e.g., tablets) of the same medication is administered to older children and adults. The following list includes the common categories of drugs based on preparation.

LIQUID PREPARATIONS

Elixir A drug that is dissolved in a solution of alcohol and water. Elixirs are sweetened and flavored and are taken orally. *Example:* Dimetapp elixir.

Emulsion A mixture of fats or oils in water. *Example:* Durezol ophthalmic emulsion.

Liniment A drug combined with oil, soap, alcohol, or water. Liniments are applied externally, using friction, to produce a feeling of heat or warmth. *Example:* Heet liniment.

Lotion An aqueous preparation that contains suspended ingredients. Lotions are used to treat external skin conditions. They work to soothe, protect, and moisten the skin and to destroy harmful bacteria. *Example:* Caladryl lotion.

Solution A liquid preparation that contains one or more completely dissolved substances. The dissolved substance is known as the *solute,* and the liquid in which it is dissolved is known as the *solvent.* Most drugs administered parenterally (by injection) consist of solutions. *Example:* Depo-Provera injectable solution.

Spirit A drug combined with an alcoholic solution that is volatile (a substance that is volatile evaporates readily). *Example:* Aromatic spirit of ammonia.

Spray A fine stream of medicated vapor, usually used to treat nose and throat conditions. *Example:* Dristan nasal spray.

Suspension A drug that contains solid insoluble drug particles in a liquid; the preparation must be shaken before administration. *Example:* Amoxicillin oral suspension.

Suspension aerosol A pressurized form in which solid aerosol or liquid drug particles are suspended in a gas to be dispensed in a cloud or mist. *Example:* Proventil inhalation aerosol.

Syrup A drug dissolved in a solution of sugar, water, and sometimes a flavoring to disguise an unpleasant taste. *Example:* Robitussin cough syrup.

Tincture A drug dissolved in a solution of alcohol or alcohol and water. *Example:* Tincture of iodine.

SOLID PREPARATIONS

Tablet A powdered drug that has been pressed into a disc. Some tablets are scored—that is, they are marked with an indentation so that they can be broken into halves or quarters for proper dosage. *Example:* Tylenol tablets.

Chewable tablet A powdered drug that has been flavored and pressed into a disc. Chewable tablets are often used for antacids, antiflatulents, and children's medications. *Example:* Pepto-Bismol chewable tablets.

Sublingual tablet A powdered drug that has been pressed into a disc and is designed to dissolve under the tongue, which permits its rapid absorption into the bloodstream. *Example:* Nitroglycerin sublingual tablets (Nitrostat).

Enteric-coated tablet A tablet coated with a substance that prevents it from dissolving until it reaches the intestines. The coating protects the drug from being destroyed by gastric juices and prevents it from irritating the stomach lining. To prevent the active ingredients from being released prematurely in the stomach, enteric-coated tablets must not be crushed or chewed. *Example:* Ecotrin enteric-coated aspirin.

Capsule A drug contained in a gelatin capsule that is water-soluble and functions to prevent the patient from tasting the drug. *Example:* Benadryl capsules.

Sustained-release capsule A capsule that contains granules that dissolve at different rates to provide a gradual and continuous release of medication. This reduces the number of doses that must be administered. (Sustained-release medication also comes in other preparations, such as tablets and caplets.) *Example:* Sudafed 12-hour sustained-release capsules.

Caplet A drug contained in an oblong tablet with a smooth coating to make swallowing easier. *Example:* Advil caplets.

Lozenge A drug contained in a candy-like base. Lozenges are circular and are designed to dissolve on the tongue. *Example:* Chloraseptic throat lozenges.

Cream A drug combined in a base that is usually nongreasy, resulting in a semisolid preparation. Creams are applied externally to the skin. *Example:* Hydrocortisone topical cream.

Ointment A drug with an oil base, resulting in a semisolid preparation. Ointments are applied externally to the skin and are usually greasy. *Example:* Cortisporin topical ointment.

Suppository A drug mixed with a firm base, such as cocoa butter, that is designed to melt at body temperature. A suppository is shaped into a cylinder or a cone for easy insertion into a body cavity, such as the rectum or vagina. *Example:* Preparation H suppositories.

Transdermal patch A patch with an adhesive backing, which contains a drug, that is applied to the skin. The drug enters the circulation after being absorbed through the skin. *Example:* Nitroglycerin patches (Nitro-Dur).

CLASSIFICATION OF DRUGS BASED ON ACTION

Drugs also can be classified according to the action they have on the body. The medical assistant should know in which category a particular drug belongs and its primary uses and major therapeutic effects. Table 26-1 contains classifications based on action and examples of drugs that are commonly administered and prescribed in the medical office.

Text continued on p. 632

Table 26-1 Classification of Drugs Based on Action

Drug Category	Primary Use and Major Therapeutic Effects	COMMONLY PRESCRIBED DRUGS	
		Generic	Brand
Analgesics (opioid)	*Indications for Use:* Used to manage moderate to severe pain *Desired Effects:* Work by altering perception of and response to painful stimuli *Side Effects:* Sedation, pruritis, dizziness, nausea, vomiting, constipation, physical dependence, tolerance, respiratory depression.	codeine/acetaminophen (APAP) fentanyl hydrocodone/APAP hydrocodone/aspirin (ASA) hydrocodone/ibuprofen meperidine oxycodone oxycodone/APAP oxycodone/ASA propoxyphene propoxyphene N/APAP tramadol	▸Tylenol w/ Codeine (III) Actiq ▸Vicodin (III) Lortab/ASA (III) ▸Vicoprofen (III) Demerol (II) ▸OxyContin (II) ▸Percocet (II) Percodan (II) Darvon (IV) ▸Darvocet-N (IV) ▸Ultram
Analgesics (barbiturate)	*Indications for Use:* Used to manage moderate to severe pain of tension headaches *Desired Effects:* Work by relieving pain and relaxing muscle contractions *Side Effects:* Drowsiness, lightheadedness, dizziness, sedation, shortness of breath, naurea, vomiting, abdominal pain, intoxicated feeling	butalbital/APAP/caffeine butalbital/ASA/caffeine	▸Fioricet (III) Fiorinal (III)

Table 26-1 Classification of Drugs Based on Action—cont'd

Drug Category	Primary Use and Major Therapeutic Effects	COMMONLY PRESCRIBED DRUGS Generic	COMMONLY PRESCRIBED DRUGS Brand
Analgesics/ antipyretics	*Indications for Use:* Used to manage mild to moderate pain and to reduce fever *Desired Effects:* Work by relieving pain and reducing fever *Side Effects*: Nausea, dyspepsia, ulceration or bleeding, diarrhea, headache, dizziness.	acetaminophen aspirin	Tylenol* Bayer* Ecotrin*
Analgesics/ antipyretics		**Nonsteroidal Antiinflammatory Drugs (NSAIDs)** diclofenac ibuprofen naproxen	 Voltaren Advil* ▸Motrin* Aleve* ▸Anaprox ▸Naprosyn
Anesthetics (local)	*Indications for Use:* Used to produce local anesthesia through loss of feeling to a body part *Desired Effects:* Work by preventing initiation and conduction of normal nerve impulses in body part *Side Effects*: Mild bruising, swelling, or itching at the injection site.	lidocaine dibucaine	Xylocaine Nupercainal ointment*
Antacids	*Indications for Use:* Used to treat heartburn, hyperacidity, indigestion, and gastroesophageal reflux disease and to promote healing of ulcers *Desired Effects:* Work by neutralizing gastric acid to relieve gastric pain and irritation *Side Effects*: Nausea, constipation, diarrhea, headache, hyperacidity.	aluminum hydroxide/magnesium hydroxide calcium carbonate sodium bicarbonate/ASA	Maalox* Mylanta* Tums* Alka-Seltzer*
Anthelmintics	*Indications for Use:* Used to treat worm infections (pinworms, roundworms, hookworms) *Desired Effects*: Work by destroying worms *Side Effects*: Abdominal pain, diarrhea, headache, dizziness	mebendazole	Vermox
Anti-Alzheimer agents	*Indications for Use:* Used to treat mild to moderate dementia associated with Alzheimer disease *Desired Effects:* Work by elevating acetylcholine concentration in the cerebral cortex *Side Effects*: Headache, fatigue, dizziness, nausea, vomiting, diarrhea, loss of appetite, joint pain, insomnia	donepezil memantine rivastigmine	▸Aricept ▸Namenda Exelon
Antianemics	**Iron Supplements** *Indications for Use:* Used to prevent or cure iron-deficiency anemia *Desired Effects:* Work by increasing amount of iron in body *Side Effects*: Upset stomach, cramps, constipation, diarrhea, nausea, vomiting **Vitamin B$_{12}$ Injections** *Indications for Use:* Used to treat pernicious anemia *Desired Effects:* Work by increasing amount of vitamin B$_{12}$ in body *Side Effects*: Headache, dizziness, weakness, nausea, upset stomach, diarrhea, numbness or tingling, pain, swelling and redness at injection site, joint pain. **Folic Acid Supplements** *Indications for Use:* Used to promote normal fetal development *Desired Effects:* Work by stimulating production of red blood cells, white blood cells, and platelets *Side Effects*: Allergic reaction	ferrous sulfate iron dextran cyanocobalamin folic acid	Feosol* DexFerrum INFeD Cobex Cyanoject ▸Folvite

Table 26-1 Classification of Drugs Based on Action—cont'd

Drug Category	Primary Use and Major Therapeutic Effects	COMMONLY PRESCRIBED DRUGS	
		Generic	Brand
Antianginals	*Indications for Use:* Used to relieve or prevent angina attacks *Desired Effects:* Work by increasing blood supply to myocardial tissue *Side Effects:* Headache, dizziness, lightheadedness, fainting, fatigue	**Nitrates** isosorbide dinitrate isosorbide mononitrate nitroglycerin **Beta-Blockers** atenolol propranolol metoprolol **Calcium Channel Blockers** amlodipine bepridil diltiazem nifedipine verapamil	Sorbitrate ‣Imdur Nitro-Bid Nitro-Dur Nitrostat Tenormin Inderal ‣Toprol-XL ‣Norvasc Vascor Cardizem Dilacor XR Adalat Procardia XL ‣Calan Isoptin Verelan
Antianxiety agents	*Indications for Use:* Used to treat anxiety *Desired Effects:* Work at many levels in central nervous system to produce anxiolytic (anxiety-relieving) effect *Side Effects:* Drowsiness, lack of energy, clumsiness, slurred speech, confusion, disorientation, depression, dizziness, impaired thinking, memory loss	alprazolam buspirone chlordiazepoxide diazepam lorazepam	‣Xanax (IV) BuSpar Librium (IV) ‣Valium (IV) ‣Ativan (IV)
Anticholinergics	*Indications for Use:* Used preoperatively to decrease oral and respiratory secretions *Desired Effects:* Work by blocking effects of acetylcholine in autonomic nervous system *Side Effects:* Dry mouth and eyes, decreased sweating, blurred vision, constipation, flushing of the face, urinary retention	atropine	Atro-Pen
Anticoagulants	*Indications for Use:* Used to prevent and treat venous thrombosis, pulmonary embolism, and myocardial infarction by preventing clot extension and formation *Desired Effects:* Work by delaying or preventing blood coagulation *Side Effects:* Hemorrhaging, hematuria, bruising, bleeding gums, nosebleeds, bloody or black stools, menorrhagia	heparin enoxaparin warfarin	 ‣Lovenox ‣Coumadin
Anticonvulsants	*Indications for Use:* Used to prevent or relieve seizures *Desired Effects:* Work by decreasing incidence and severity of seizures *Side Effects:* Constipation, nausea, vomiting, dizziness, drowsiness	carbamazepine clonazepam divalproex gabapentin lamotrigine phenytoin pregabalin topiramate	Tegretol ‣Klonopin (IV) ‣Depakote ‣Neurontin ‣Lamictal ‣Dilantin ‣Lyrica ‣Topamax

Table 26-1 Classification of Drugs Based on Action—cont'd

Drug Category	Primary Use and Major Therapeutic Effects	COMMONLY PRESCRIBED DRUGS	
		Generic	Brand
Antidepressants	*Indications for Use:* Used to prevent, cure, or alleviate depression and to treat anxiety disorders (panic attacks) and obsessive-convulsive disorder *Desired Effects:* Work by inhibiting reuptake of neurotransmitters in the central nervous system *Side Effects:* Nausea, increased appetite, weight gain, loss of sexual desire, fatigue, drowsiness	**Selective Serotonin Reuptake Inhibitors (SSRIs)** citalopram escitalopram fluoxetine fluvoxamine paroxetine sertraline **Serotonin-Norepinephrine Reuptake Inhibitors (SNRIs)** desvenlafaxine duloxetine venlafaxine **Miscellaneous** amitriptyline bupropion mirtazapine nefazodone trazodone	 ▸Celexa ▸Lexapro ▸Prozac Luvox ▸Paxil ▸Zoloft Pristiq ▸Cymbalta ▸Effexor XR ▸Elavil ▸Wellbutrin SR ▸Remeron Serzone ▸Desyrel
Antidiabetics	**Oral Hypoglycemics** *Indications for Use:* Used to manage non–insulin-dependent type 2 diabetes mellitus *Desired Effects:* Work by stimulating release of insulin from pancreas and increasing sensitivity to insulin *Side Effects:* Headache, stomach upset, loss of appetite, nausea, diarrhea, vomiting, hypoglycemia	glimepiride glipizide glyburide metformin pioglitazone rosiglitazone	▸Amaryl ▸Glucotrol XL ▸Micronase ▸Glucophage ▸Actos ▸Avandia
Antidiabetics	**Insulins** *Indications for Use:* Used to manage diabetes mellitus *Desired Effects:* Work by reducing blood glucose levels *Side Effects:* Hypoglycemia, headache, weight gain, pain, redness and irritation at the injection site	regular insulin NPH insulin NPH/regular insulin insulin glargine insulin lispro	Humulin R* Novolin R* Humulin N* Novolin N* Humulin 70/30* Novolin 70/30* ▸Lantus Humalog
Antidiarrheals	*Indications for Use:* Used to control and relieve diarrhea *Desired Effects:* Work by inhibiting peristalsis, reducing fecal volume, and preventing loss of fluids and electrolytes *Side Effects:* Abdominal pain, constipation, dizziness, dry mouth, drowsiness	bismuth subsalicylate diphenoxylate/atropine kaolin/pectin loperamide	Pepto-Bismol* Lomotil (V) Kaopectate* Imodium*
Antidysrhythmics	*Indications for Use:* Used to control or prevent cardiac dysrhythmias *Desired Effects:* Work by decreasing myocardial excitability and slowing conduction velocity *Side Effects:* Dry mouth and throat, dizziness, diarrhea, loss of appetite, lightheadedness, blurred vision	metoprolol procainamide propranolol	▸Lopressor ▸Toprol-XL Pronestyl Inderal
Antiemetics	*Indications for Use:* Used to prevent or relieve nausea and vomiting *Desired Effects:* Work by depressing chemoreceptor trigger zone in central nervous system to inhibit nausea and vomiting *Side Effects:* Dry mouth, drowsiness, dysuria, dizziness, blurred vision	dronabinol ondansetron prochlorperazine promethazine meclizine	Marinol (III) Zofran Compazine ▸Phenergan Bonine*

Continued

Table 26-1 Classification of Drugs Based on Action—cont'd

Drug Category	Primary Use and Major Therapeutic Effects	Generic	Brand
Antiflatulents	*Indications for Use:* Used to relieve discomfort of excess gas and bloating in gastrointestinal tract *Desired Effects:* Work by causing coalescence of gas bubbles in intestinal tract *Side Effects:* Nausea, constipation, hypersensitivity reaction	simethicone	Gas-X* Mylanta Gas*
Antifungals	*Indications for Use:* Used to treat fungal infections *Desired Effects:* Work by killing or inhibiting growth of susceptible fungi *Side Effects:* Mild stomach pain, headache, dizziness, unusual or unpleasant taste in the mouth	amphotericin B clotrimazole fluconazole itraconazole ketoconazole miconazole nystatin terbinafine	Fungizone Gyne-Lotrimin* ▸Diflucan Sporanox Nizoral Monistat* Mycostatin* ▸Lamisil
Antigout agents	*Indications for Use:* Used to prevent attacks of gout *Desired Effects:* Work by inhibiting production of uric acid *Side Effects:* Skin rash, diarrhea, nausea, itching, drowsiness	allopurinol colchicine	▸Zyloprim Colchicine tablets
Antihistamines	*Indications for Use:* Used to relieve symptoms associated with allergies (increased sneezing; rhinorrhea; itchy eyes, nose, and throat) *Desired Effects:* Work by blocking effects of histamine at histamine receptor sites *Side Effects:* Dry mouth, drowsiness, dizziness, nausea, vomiting, blurred vision, urinary retention	brompheniramine cetirizine chlorpheniramine desloratadine diphenhydramine fexofenadine/pseudoephedrine levocetirizine loratadine promethazine	Dimetane* ▸Zyrtec* Chlor-Trimetron* Teldrin* ▸Clarinex Benadryl* ▸Allegra Xyzal ▸Claritin* ▸Phenergan
Antihypertensives	*Indications for Use:* Used to manage hypertension *Desired Effects:* Work by causing systemic vasodilation to reduce blood pressure *Side Effects:* Constipation, dehydration, dizziness, lightheadedness, drowsiness,	**Angiotensin-Converting Enzyme (ACE) Inhibitors** benazepril captopril enalapril lisinopril quinapril ramipril **Peripherally Acting Adrenergic Blockers** clonidine doxazosin prazosin **Angiotensin II Receptor Antagonists** candesartan irbesartan losartan olmesartan telmisartan valsartan **Beta-Blockers** atenolol carvedilol metoprolol propranolol sotalol	 Lotensin Capoten ▸Vasotec ▸Prinivil ▸Accupril ▸Altace ▸Catapres Cardura Minipress Atacand ▸Avapro ▸Cozaar ▸Benicar Micardis ▸Diovan ▸Tenormin ▸Coreg ▸Lopressor ▸Toprol-XL Inderal Betapace

COMMONLY PRESCRIBED DRUGS

Table 26-1 Classification of Drugs Based on Action—cont'd

Drug Category	Primary Use and Major Therapeutic Effects	COMMONLY PRESCRIBED DRUGS	
		Generic	Brand
		Calcium Channel Blockers	
		amlodipine	▸Norvasc
		diltiazem	▸Cardizem
		felodipine	Plendil
		Vasodilator	
		hydralazine	Apresoline
		Miscellaneous	
		amlodipine/atorvastatin	Caduet
		amlodipine/benazepril	▸Lotrel
		bisoprolol/hydrochlorothiazide	Ziac
		irbesartan/hydrochlorothiazide	▸Avalide
		losartan/hydrochlorothiazide	▸Hyzaar
		olmesartan/hydrochlorothiazide	▸Benicar HCT
		triamterene/hydrochlorothiazide	▸Maxzide
		valsartan/hydrochlorothiazide	Diovan HCT
Antiimpotence agents	*Indications for Use:* Used to treat erectile dysfunction *Desired Effects:* Work by promoting increased blood flow to penis *Side Effects*: Headache, flushing, indigestion, stuffy or runny nose, temporary vision changes	sildenafil tadalafil vardenafil	▸Viagra ▸Cialis Levitra
Antiinfectives	*Indications for Use:* Used to treat infections *Desired Effects:* Work by killing or inhibiting growth of bacteria *Side Effects*: Vomiting, diarrhea, allergic reaction, abdominal cramps, vaginal itching or discharge, white patches on the tongue	**Penicillins** amoxicillin amoxicillin/clavulanate ampicillin benzathine penicillin penicillin V procaine penicillin Macrolides azithromycin clarithromycin erythromycin	▸Amoxil ▸Trimox ▸Augmentin Omnipen Bicillin ▸Veetids Wycillin ▸Zithromax Biaxin Ery-Tab
		Cephalosporins cefaclor cefdinir cefprozil ceftriaxone cefuroxime cephalexin	 Ceclor ▸Omnicef ▸Cefzil Rocephin Ceftin ▸Keflex
		Fluoroquinolones ciprofloxacin levofloxacin moxifloxacin ofloxacin	 ▸Cipro ▸Levaquin Avelox Floxin
		Tetracyclines doxycycline minocycline tetracycline	 Doryx ▸Vibramycin Arestin Achromycin Sumycin
		Aminoglycosides gentamicin kanamycin neomycin tobramycin	 Garamycin Kantrex Neobiotic Nebcin

Continued

Table 26-1 Classification of Drugs Based on Action—cont'd

Drug Category	Primary Use and Major Therapeutic Effects	COMMONLY PRESCRIBED DRUGS	
		Generic	Brand
		Sulfonamides	
		sulfamethoxazole	Gantanol
		trimethoprim/sulfamethoxazole	‣Bactrim
		Miscellaneous	
		clindamycin	Cleocin
		chloramphenicol	Chloromycetin
		nitrofurantoin	‣Macrobid
			Macrodantin
		vancomycin	Vancocin
Antiinflammatories	*Indications for Use:* Used to relieve signs and symptoms of osteoarthritis and rheumatoid arthritis in adults *Desired Effects:* Work by decreasing pain and inflammation *Side Effects:* Vomiting, nausea, constipation, reduced appetite, headache, dizziness, rash, drowsiness	aspirin celecoxib etodolac ibuprofen indomethacin meloxicam nabumetone naproxen piroxicam valdecoxib	Bayer* Ecotrin* ‣Celebrex Lodine Advil* Motrin* Indocin ‣Mobic ‣Relafen Aleve* Anaprox Naprosyn Feldene Bextra
Antimanics	*Indications for Use:* Used to treat bipolar affective disorders *Desired Effects:* Work by altering cation transport in nerves and muscles *Side Effects:* Restlessness, mild tremor of hands, mild thirst, loss of appetite, stomach pain, flatulence, indigestion, weight gain or loss	lithium	Eskalith Eskalith CR
Antimigraine agents	*Indications for Use:* Used in acute treatment of migraine attacks *Desired Effects:* Work by causing vasoconstriction in large intracranial arteries *Side Effects:* Dizziness, flushing, nausea, vomiting, sore throat, tingling sensation, abdominal pain	sumatriptan	‣Imitrex
Antineoplastics	*Indications for Use:* Used to treat tumors *Desired Effects:* Work by preventing development, growth, or proliferation of malignant cells *Side Effects:* Nausea, vomiting, loss of appetite, diarrhea, hair loss, bone marrow depression	cyclophosphamide methotrexate	Cytoxan Mexate Folex
Anti-Parkinson agents	*Indications for Use:* Used to treat symptoms of Parkinson disease *Desired Effects:* Work by restoring balance between acetylcholine and dopamine in central nervous system *Side Effects:* Nausea, vomiting, sleepiness, dizziness, headache, low blood pressure	carbidopa/levodopa ropinirole	Sinemet Requip
Antiprotozoals	*Indications for Use:* Used to treat protozoal infections *Desired Effects:* Work by destroying protozoa *Side Effects:* Diarrhea, nausea, vomiting, stomach pain	metronidazole	Flagyl

Table 26-1 Classification of Drugs Based on Action—cont'd

Drug Category	Primary Use and Major Therapeutic Effects	COMMONLY PRESCRIBED DRUGS	
		Generic	Brand
Antipsychotics	Indications for Use: Used to treat psychotic disorders Desired Effects: Work by blocking dopamine and serotonin receptors in central nervous system Side Effects: Drowsiness, rapid heartbeat, dizziness, weight gain	haloperidol aripiprazole olanzapine risperidone quetiapine	Haldol ‣Abilify ‣Zyprexa ‣Risperdal ‣Seroquel
Antiretrovirals	Indications for Use: Used to manage human immunodeficiency virus (HIV) infections and to reduce maternal-fetal transmission of HIV Desired Effects: Work by inhibiting replication of retroviruses Side Effects: Nausea, diarrhea, loss of appetite, headache, fatigue, peripheral neuropathy, lipodystrophy	efavirenz emtricitabine lamivudine ritonavir tenofovir zidovudine	Sustiva Emtriva Epivir Norvir Viread Retrovir
Antispasmodics	Indications for Use: Used to control hypermotility in irritable bowel syndrome, spastic colitis, spastic bladder, and pylorospasm Desired Effects: Work by preventing or relieving spasms of gastrointestinal or genitourinary tract Side Effects: Flatulence, bloating, dizziness, heartburn, dry mouth, constipation,	dicyclomine hyoscyamine	Bentyl Levsin
Antituberculars	Indications for Use: Used to treat tuberculosis Desired Effects: Work by killing or inhibiting growth of mycobacteria Side Effects: Diarrhea, stomach pain, nausea, vomiting, loss of appetite, unusual tiredness or weakness	isoniazid rifampin	INH Rifadin
Antitussives	Indications for Use: Used in prevention or relief of coughs caused by minor viral upper respiratory infections or inhaled irritants Desired Effects: Work by suppressing cough reflex by direct effect on cough center in central nervous system Side Effects: Irritability, dizziness, drowsiness, nausea, vomiting	benzonatate chlorpheniramine/hydrocodone dextromethorphan guaifenesin/codeine	Tessalon Tussionex (III) Robitussin DM* Robitussin A-C (V)
Antiulcer agents	Indications for Use: Used to manage ulcers, gastroesophageal reflux disease, heartburn, indigestion, and gastric hyperacidity Desired Effects: Work by preventing accumulation of acid in stomach Side Effects: Headache, mild diarrhea, nausea, stomach pain, flatulence, constipation, dry mouth	**Proton Pump Inhibitors** esomeprazole lansoprazole omeprazole pantoprazole rabeprazole **H₂-Receptor Antagonists** cimetidine famotidine ranitidine	 ‣Nexium ‣Prevacid ‣Prilosec* ‣Protonix ‣AcipHex Tagamet* ‣Pepcid AC* ‣Zantac*
Antivirals	Indications for Use: Used to manage viral infections Desired Effects: Work by inhibiting viral replication Side Effects: Nausea, vomiting, dizziness, diarrhea, headache, insomnia	acyclovir famciclovir Valacyclovir oseltamivir	‣Zovirax Famvir ‣Valtrex Tamiflu
Bone resorption inhibitors	Indications for Use: Used to treat and prevent osteoporosis Desired Effects: Work by inhibiting reabsorption of bone Side Effects: Nausea, vomiting, stomach pain, diarrhea, headache, dizziness, pain the extremities, loss of voice	alendronate ibandronate raloxifene risedronate	‣Fosamax Boniva ‣Evista ‣Actonel

Continued

Table 26-1 Classification of Drugs Based on Action—cont'd

Drug Category	Primary Use and Major Therapeutic Effects	COMMONLY PRESCRIBED DRUGS	
		Generic	Brand
Bronchodilators	*Indications for Use:* Used to manage reversible airway obstruction caused by asthma or chronic obstructive pulmonary disease *Desired Effects:* Work by relaxing smooth muscle of respiratory tract resulting in bronchodilation *Side Effects:* Dry mouth, constipation, diarrhea, headache, heart palpitations, dizziness, trembling, nervousness, muscle aches or cramps	albuterol fluticasone/salmeterol formoterol ipratropium/albuterol levalbuterol montelukast salmeterol theophylline tiotropium	‣Proventil ‣ProAir HFA ‣Advair Diskus Foradil ‣Combivent Xopenex ‣Singulair Serevent Bronkodyl ‣Spiriva
Cardiac glycosides	*Indications for Use:* Used to treat congestive heart failure and cardiac arrhythmias *Desired Effects:* Work by increasing strength and force of myocardial contractions and slowing heart rate *Side Effects:* Cardiac arrhythmias, nausea, vomiting, diarrhea, loss of appetite, dizziness, weakness, headache, blurred vision, depression	digitoxin digoxin	Crystodigin ‣Digitek Lanoxicaps ‣Lanoxin
Central nervous system stimulants	*Indications for Use:* Used to treat narcolepsy and manage attention-deficit/hyperactivity disorder *Desired Effects:* Work by increasing level of catecholamines in central nervous system *Side Effects:* Loss of appetite, increased anxiety level, weight loss, dizziness, headache, irritability, facial tics, restlessness, panic attacks, insomnia, tachycardia	atomoxetine dextroamphetamine dextroamphetamine saccharate and sulfate lisdexamfetamine methylphenidate	‣Strattera Dexedrine (II) ‣Adderall (II) Vyvanse (II) ‣Ritalin (II) ‣Concerta (II)
Contraceptives (hormonal)	*Indications for Use:* Used to prevent pregnancy and to regulate menstrual cycle *Desired Effects:* Work by inhibiting ovulation *Side Effects:* Headache, dizziness, lightheadedness, stomach upset, bloating, nausea, weight gain, metrorrhagia, breast tenderness, mood changes	**Oral Contraceptives** ethinyl estradiol/drospirenone ethinyl estradiol/levonorgestrel ethinyl estradiol/norethindrone ethinyl estradiol/norgestimate **Injectable Contraceptives** medroxyprogesterone **Transdermal Contraceptives** ethinyl estradiol/norelgestromin **Vaginal Ring Contraceptives** ethinyl estradiol/etonogestrel	 ‣Yasmin Yaz Alesse Levien Kariva ‣Ortho-Novum ‣Loestrin Fe ‣Ortho Tri-Cyclen Tri-Sprintec ‣Depo-Provera ‣Ortho Evra NuvaRing
Corticosteroids	**Systemic Corticosteroids** *Indications for Use:* Used to treat inflammation, allergies, asthma, and autoimmune disorders and as replacement therapy in adrenal insufficiency *Desired Effects:* Work by suppressing inflammation and modifying normal immune response *Side Effects:* Increased appetite, weight gain, sudden mood swings, easy bruising, muscle weakness, blurred vision, increased growth of body hair, swollen face	cortisone fluticasone hydrocortisone methylprednisolone triamcinolone	Cortone ‣Flovent Cortef Medrol Depo-Medrol Aristocort

Table 26-1 Classification of Drugs Based on Action—cont'd

Drug Category	Primary Use and Major Therapeutic Effects	COMMONLY PRESCRIBED DRUGS	
		Generic	Brand
	Nasal Corticosteroids *Indications for Use:* Used to treat chronic nasal inflammatory conditions (e.g., allergic rhinitis) *Desired Effects:* Work by suppressing inflammation and reducing hypersecretions of respiratory tract *Side Effects:* Nosebleed, sinus pain, sore throat, burning, dryness or irritation inside the nose	fluticasone mometasone prednisone triamcinolone	‣Flonase ‣Nasonex ‣Deltasone ‣Sterapred ‣Nasacort
Decongestants	*Indications for Use:* Used to decrease nasal congestion *Desired Effects:* Work by producing vasoconstriction in respiratory tract mucosa *Side Effects:* Irritation of the lining of the nose, headache, nausea, dry mouth, nervousness, insomnia, dizziness	oxymetazoline phenylephrine pseudoephedrine	Afrin* Dristan* Neo-Synephrine* Sudafed*
Diuretics	*Indications for Use:* Used to manage hypertension, edema in congestive heart failure, and renal disease *Desired Effects:* Work by removing excess fluid from the body by increasing urine output *Side Effects:* Dry mouth, increased thirst, weakness, lethargy, drowsiness, muscle pain or cramps, confusion, oliguria, headache, dizziness	**Loop Diuretics** bumetanide furosemide **Thiazide Diuretics** chlorthalidone hydrochlorothiazide **Potassium-Sparing Diuretics** spironolactone triamterene	Bumex ‣Lasix Hygroton ‣Microzide Aldactone Dyrenium
Electrolyte replacements	*Indications for Use:* Used to treat or prevent electrolyte depletion *Desired Effects:* Work by replacing electrolytes in body *Side Effects:* Nausea, vomiting, diarrhea, flatulence, high blood pressure, arrhythmias	**Potassium Supplements** potassium chloride	‣K-Dur ‣Klor-Con
Emetics	*Indications for Use:* Used to treat poisoning *Desired Effects:* Work by inducing vomiting *Side Effects:* Diarrhea, lethargy, stomach cramps, prolonged vomiting	syrup of ipecac	
Expectorants	*Indications for Use:* Used to manage coughs by expelling mucus *Desired Effects:* Work by decreasing viscosity of bronchial secretions to promote clearance of mucus from respiratory tract *Side Effects:* Nausea, vomiting, stomach upset, dizziness, headache, drowsiness, diarrhea, constipation	guaifenesin	Robitussin* Mucinex* Naldecon*
Hormone replacements	*Indications for Use:* Used to treat moderate to severe vasomotor symptoms of menopause *Desired Effects:* Work by restoring hormonal balance *Side Effects:* Headache, nausea, vaginal discharge, fluid retention, weight gain, breast tenderness	conjugated estrogens conjugated estrogen/progesterone estradiol/norethindrone	‣Premarin ‣Prempro Activella

Continued

Table 26-1 Classification of Drugs Based on Action—cont'd

Drug Category	Primary Use and Major Therapeutic Effects	COMMONLY PRESCRIBED DRUGS	
		Generic	Brand
Immunizations	*Indications for Use:* Used to prevent (vaccine-preventable) diseases *Desired Effects:* Work by stimulating body to produce antibodies *Side Effects:* Pain, redness, tenderness and swelling at the injection site, fatigue, headache, nausea, dizziness, fever	diphtheria, tetanus toxoids, and acellular pertussis vaccine	Acel-Imune Certiva Daptacel Infanrix Tripedia
		Haemophilus b conjugate vaccine	ActHIB HibTITER
		hepatitis A vaccine	Havrix Vaqta
		hepatitis B vaccine	Engerix-B Recombivax HB
		human papillomavirus vaccine	Gardasil
		inactivated polio vaccine	IPOL
		influenza virus vaccine types A and B	Afluria FluShield Fluzone FluMist
		measles, mumps, and rubella vaccine	M-M-R II
		meningococcal conjugate vaccine	Menactra
		pneumococcal conjugate vaccine	Prevnar Pneumovax II
		rotavirus	Rotarix RotaShield
		rubella vaccine	Meruvax II
		varicella vaccine	Varivax
Immunosuppressants	*Indications for Use:* Used to treat severe rheumatoid arthritis and to prevent and treat rejection of transplanted organs *Desired Effects:* Work by inhibiting body's normal immune response *Side Effects:* Abdominal discomfort, swollen and painful gums, acne, increased hair growth, headache, diarrhea, nausea, flushing, cramps	cyclosporine methotrexate	Sandimmune Neoral Rheumatrex
Laxatives	*Indications for Use:* Used to relieve constipation *Desired Effects:* Work by promoting defecation of normal, soft stool *Side Effects:* Bloating, cramping, flatulence, diarrhea, nausea, dehydration	bisacodyl docusate phenolphthalein psyllium	Dulcolax* Colace* Phenolax* Metamucil*
Lipid-lowering agents	*Indications for Use:* Used to lower cholesterol to reduce risk of myocardial infarction and stroke *Desired Effects:* Work by inhibiting enzyme needed to synthesize cholesterol in body *Side Effects:* Headache, diarrhea, constipation, muscle aches and weakness, nausea, vomiting, stomach upset, bloating, cramping	atorvastatin ezetimibe ezetimibe/simvastatin fenofibrate fluvastatin gemfibrozil lovastatin pravastatin rosuvastatin simvastatin	▸Lipitor ▸Zetia ▸Vytorin ▸Tricor Lescol Lopid ▸Mevacor ▸Pravachol ▸Crestor ▸Zocor
Muscle relaxants (skeletal)	*Indications for Use:* Used to treat acute painful musculoskeletal conditions *Desired Effects:* Work by relaxing skeletal muscles *Side Effects:* Headache, drowsiness, dizziness, dry mouth, nausea, blurred vision, stomach upset	baclofen carisoprodol cyclobenzaprine metaxalone methocarbamol tizanidine	▸Lioresal ▸Soma ▸Flexeril Skelaxin Robaxin ▸Zanaflex

Table 26-1 Classification of Drugs Based on Action—cont'd

Drug Category	Primary Use and Major Therapeutic Effects	COMMONLY PRESCRIBED DRUGS	
		Generic	Brand
Ophthalmic antiinfectives	*Indications for Use:* Used to treat eye infections *Desired Effects:* Work by destroying bacteria *Side Effects:* Temporary blurred vision, tearing, eye redness, eye discomfort, allergic reaction	dexamethasone/tobramycin moxifloxacin polymyxin/bacitracin polymyxin/neomycin polymyxin/trimethoprim tobramycin	TobraDex Vigamox Polysporin Neosporin Polytrim Tobrex
Otic preparations	*Indications for Use:* Used to treat ear conditions		
	Analgesics *Desired Effects:* Work by relieving ear pain *Side Effects:* Allergic reaction	benzocaine	Auralgan
	Antiinfectives *Desired Effects:* Work by treating otitis externa *Side Effects:* Temporary stinging or burning in the ear, allergic reaction	neomycin/polymyxin/ hydrocortisone ofloxacin	Cortisporin Otic Floxin Otic
	Cerumenolytics *Desired Effects:* Work by softening cerumen *Side Effects:* Temporary decrease in hearing and feeling of fullness in the ear	carbamide peroxide	Debrox*
Platelet inhibitors	*Indications for Use:* Used to reduce incidence of myocardial infarction and stroke *Desired Effects:* Work by interfering with ability of platelets to adhere to each other *Side Effects:* Itching, eczema, rash, head or joint pain, bruising, diarrhea, stomach upset	clopidogrel salicylates	▸Plavix Aspirin*
Sedatives and hypnotics	*Indications for Use:* Used for short-term treatment of insomnia *Desired Effects:* Work by promoting sleep by central nervous system depression *Side Effects:* Burning or tingling in the extremities, change in appetite, constipation, diarrhea, dizziness, daytime drowsiness, loss of coordination, headache, mental slowing, stomach pain, unusual dreams	eszopiclone flurazepam hydroxyzine phenobarbital temazepam zolpidem	▸Lunesta (IV) Dalmane (IV) Atarax Vistaril Luminal (IV) ▸Restoril (IV) ▸Ambien (IV)
Smoking deterrents	*Indications for Use:* Used to manage nicotine withdrawal to cease cigarette smoking *Desired Effects:* Work by providing nicotine during controlled withdrawal from cigarette smoking *Side Effects:* Dry mouth, nausea, stomach pain, headache, dizziness, vision changes, sore throat, muscle pain	bupropion nicotine varenicline	Zyban Nicorette Gum* Nicotrol Inhaler Nicoderm Patch* Commit Lozenges* Chantix
Thrombolytic agents	*Indications for Use:* Used for acute management of coronary thrombosis (myocardial infarction) *Desired Effects:* Work by dissolving existing clots *Side Effects:* Bleeding, arrhythmias, dizziness, headache, shortness of breath, allergic reaction	alteplase anistreplase reteplase streptokinase	Activase Eminase Retavase Streptase
Thyroid preparations	**Thyroid Hormones** *Indications for Use:* Used as replacement or substitute therapy for diminished or absent thyroid functioning of many causes *Desired Effects:* Work by increasing basal metabolic rate *Side Effects:* Hair loss, fast or irregular heart rate, hot flashes, irritability, sweating, mood changes, insomnia, vomiting, diarrhea, appetite changes, weight changes	levothyroxine	▸Levoxyl ▸Synthroid

Continued

Table 26-1 Classification of Drugs Based on Action—cont'd

| Drug Category | Primary Use and Major Therapeutic Effects | COMMONLY PRESCRIBED DRUGS | |
		Generic	Brand
	Antithyroid Agents *Indications for Use:* Used to treat hyperthyroidism *Desired Effects:* Work by inhibiting thyroid hormone synthesis, reducing basal metabolic rate *Side Effects:* Headache, drowsiness, dizziness, nausea, vomiting, stomach upset, itching, muscle, joint or nerve pain, hair loss	methimazole	Tapazole
Urinary tract antispasmodics	*Indications for Use:* Used to treat overactive bladder function *Desired Effects:* Work by inhibiting bladder contractions *Side Effects:* Dry mouth, dry eyes, blurred vision, dizziness, drowsiness, constipation, diarrhea, stomach pain or upset, joint pain, headache	oxybutynin tolterodine	Ditropan ▸Detrol
Vasopressors	*Indications for Use:* Used to treat severe allergic reactions and cardiac arrest *Desired Effects:* Work by increasing blood pressure and cardiac output and by dilating bronchi *Side Effects:* Sweating, nausea, vomiting, pale skin, feeling short of breath, dizziness, weakness or tremors, headache, feeling nervous or anxious	epinephrine	Adrenalin EpiPen
Weight control agents	*Indications for Use:* Used to manage obesity		
	Appetite Suppressants *Desired Effects:* Work by suppressing appetite center in central nervous system *Side Effects:* Nausea, vomiting, diarrhea, upset stomach, headache, blurred vision, nervousness, insomnia, dizziness, fatigue, dry mouth	diethylpropion phentermine sibutramine orlistat	Tenuate (IV) Fastin (IV) Meridia (IV) Xenical
	Lipase Inhibitors *Desired Effects:* Work by inhibiting action of lipase to decrease absorption of dietary fats *Side Effects:* Oily or fatty stools, orange or brown colored oil in stool, flatulence with an oily discharge, loose stools, increased number of bowel movements, stomach pain, nausea, vomiting.		Alli*

▸Top-200 most prescribed drugs.
(II), Schedule II drug; *(III)*, Schedule III drug; *(IV)*, Schedule IV drug.
*Available OTC (over the counter).

SYSTEMS OF MEASUREMENT FOR MEDICATION

Two systems of measurement are used in the United States for prescribing, administering, and dispensing medication: the metric system and the household system. The metric system is the most common system used to measure medication because it provides a more exact measurement and is easier to use. The household system is not as accurate as the metric system for the measurement of medication and usually is used only when a patient takes liquid medication at home.

Systems of measurement have units of weight, volume, and length. *Weight* refers to the heaviness of an item, and *volume* refers to the amount of space occupied by a substance. *Length* is a unit of linear measurement of the distance from one point to another. Although length is not used to administer medication, it is used in other aspects of the medical office. The head circumference of infants is measured in centimeters (cm), a metric unit of linear measurement.

To prepare and administer medication properly and to avoid medication errors, the medical assistant must have a thorough knowledge of the specific units of measurement for these two systems and must be able to convert within each system and from one system to another. A basic discussion of the metricand household systems is presented next. A more thorough study of these systems, including conversion of units and dose calculation, is included in Chapter 26 of the Study Guide.

METRIC SYSTEM

The metric system was developed in France in the latter part of the 18th century in an effort to simplify measurement. Most European countries are required by law to use this system for the measurement of weight, volume, and length. Overall, the metric system is used for most scientific and medical measurements. Pharmaceutical companies use the metric system to measure and label medications.

The metric system employs a uniform decimal scale based on units of 10, making it very flexible and logical. The basic metric units of measurement are the gram, liter, and meter. The *gram* is a unit of weight used to measure solids, the *liter* is a unit of volume used to measure liquids, and the *meter* is a linear unit used to measure length or distance. The metric units used most often in the administration of medication in the medical office are the milligram, gram, milliliter, and cubic centimeter. Because a **cubic centimeter** (cc) is the amount of space occupied by 1 milliliter (mL), these two units can be used interchangeably (i.e., 1 mL = 1 cc).

Prefixes added to the words *gram, liter,* and *meter* designate smaller or larger units of measurement in the metric system. The same prefixes are used with all three units. For example, *milli-* is used as follows: *milli*gram, *milli*liter, and *milli*meter. A prefix changes the value of the basic unit of measurement by the same amount. The prefix *milli-* describes a unit that is $\frac{1}{1000}$ of the basic unit: 1 gram is equal to 1000 milligrams, 1 liter is equal to 1000 milliliters, and 1 meter is equal to 1000 millimeters. The box *Metric Notation Guidelines* lists the metric units of measurement and equivalent values in different units. Specific guidelines are used in the medical notation of metric units and doses, which also are presented in the box. To read prescriptions and medication orders, to document medication administration, and, most important, to avoid medication errors, the medical assistant must be familiar with and be able to follow these guidelines.

Metric Notation Guidelines

Follow these guidelines when using the metric notation of measurement and dosage.
1. The units of metric measurement are written using the following abbreviations.
   Weight
   microgram: mcg
   milligram: mg
   gram: g
   kilogram: kg
   Volume
   milliliter: mL
   liter: L
2. Do not use a period with the abbreviations for metric units because the period might be mistaken for another letter or symbol.
   Correct: mg
   mL
   Incorrect: mg.
   mL.
3. Place the numeral that expresses the quantity of the dose in front of the abbreviation. To make it easier to read, leave a (single) space between the quantity and the abbreviation.
   Correct: 5 mL
   Incorrect: mL 5
   5mL
4. Write a fraction of a dose as a decimal.
   Correct: 0.5 g
   Incorrect: ½ g

5. If the dose is a fraction of a unit, place a zero before the decimal point as a means of focusing on the fractional dose. This reduces the possibility of misreading the dose as a whole number.
   Correct: 0.5 g (this reduces the possibility of not seeing the decimal point and reading the dose as 5 grams)
   Incorrect: .5 g
6. Do not place a decimal point and a zero after a whole number. The decimal point may be overlooked, resulting in a 10-fold overdose error.
   Correct: 1 mL (this reduces the possibility of not seeing the decimal point and reading the dose as 10 mL)
   Incorrect: 1.0 mL

Metric System: Conversion of Equivalent Values
Weight
1000 micrograms = 1 milligram
1000 milligrams = 1 gram
1000 grams = 1 kilogram
Volume
1000 milliliters = 1 liter
1000 liters = 1 kiloliter
1 milliliter = 1 cubic centimeter

HOUSEHOLD SYSTEM

The household system is more complicated and less accurate for administering liquid medication than the metric system. Nevertheless, most individuals are familiar with this system because of its frequent use in the United States. This system of measurement may be the only one the patient can understand and safely use to take liquid medication at home. Most patients are more comfortable measuring medication in teaspoons than in milliliters. In addition, the patient is more likely to have household measuring devices on hand than to have metric measuring devices. If a precise measurement is needed, however, the metric system must be used, and the medical assistant should instruct the patient in the use of the metric measuring device.

Volume is the only household unit of measurement used to administer medication. The basic unit of liquid volume in the household system is the *drop (gtt)*, which is approximately equal to 0.6 mL in the metric system. These two units cannot be considered exact equivalents because the size of the drop varies based on temperature, the viscosity of the liquid, and the size of the dropper. The remaining units, in order of increasing volume, are *teaspoon, tablespoon, ounce (fluid ounce), cup,* and *glass.* Table 26-2 lists the units of liquid volume measurement in the household system and equivalent values in different units.

CONVERTING UNITS OF MEASUREMENT

Changing from one unit of measurement to another is known as **conversion.** Conversion is required when medication is ordered in a unit of measurement that differs from the medication's label. The dose quantity must be mathematically translated or converted to the unit of measurement of the medication on hand. If the physician orders 5 grams of an oral solid medication, and the medication label expresses the drug strength in milligrams, the medical assistant would need to convert the grams into milligrams to know how much medication to administer. Converting units of measurement can be classified into the following categories: (1) conversion of units within a measurement system, and (2) conversion of units from one measurement system to another.

Converting units within a measurement system allows a quantity to be expressed in two different but equal units of measurement within *one* system. An example of converting units of weight within the metric system is as follows: 1 gram is equal to 1000 milligrams. Converting from one measurement system to another allows a quantity written in one measurement system to be expressed in an equivalent unit of measurement in *another* system. An example of a conversion from the metric system to the household system is as follows: 5 milliliters (metric system) is equivalent to 1 teaspoon (household system).

Conversion requires the use of a conversion table to indicate the equivalent values of various units of measurement. Conversion tables of equivalent values are included in this chapter:

- Metric conversion—*Metric Notation Guidelines* box
- Household conversion—Table 26-2

Tables used to convert from one system to another consist of approximate rather than exact equivalents, and a 10% error usually occurs in making these conversions. Conversion tables used to convert from the household system to the metric system are presented in Table 26-3.

The medical assistant must be careful to avoid errors in interpolation when using conversion tables. The numbers on conversion tables are small and close together; it is easy to misread the chart from one column to the other. To reduce this possibility, a straightedge, such as a ruler, should be used when reading a conversion table.

Table 26-2 Household System: Conversion of Common Values	
Abbreviations	
drop	gtt
teaspoon	tsp
tablespoon	T
ounce	oz
cup	c
Volume	
60 gtt =	1 tsp
3 tsp =	1 T
6 tsp =	1 oz
2 T =	1 oz
6 oz =	1 teacup
8 oz =	1 glass

Table 26-3 Equivalences in Household and Metric Units (Volume)	
Household	**Metric**
1 gtt	= 0.06 mL
15 gtts	= 1 mL (1 cc)
1 tsp	= 5 (4) mL*
1 T	= 15 mL
2 T	= 30 mL
1 oz	= 30 mL
1 teacup	= 180 mL
1 glass	= 240 mL

*The American standard teaspoon is accepted as 5 mL; however, 4 mL can be used as the equivalent to provide a more accurate conversion.

CONTROLLED DRUGS

As a result of federal and state legislation, restrictions are placed on drugs that have potential for abuse. These drugs are known as **controlled drugs.** They are classified into five categories, called *schedules,* which are based on their abuse potential. Table 26-4 lists, describes, and provides examples of the schedules for controlled drugs.

To administer, prescribe, or dispense controlled drugs, the physician must register every 3 years with the Drug Enforcement Administration (DEA). The physician is assigned a registration number known as the **DEA number.** Every time a prescription for a controlled drug is written, the physician must put his or her DEA number in the appropriate space on the prescription blank.

PRESCRIPTION

A **prescription** is a physician's order authorizing the dispensing of a drug by a pharmacist. Prescriptions can be authorized by different forms, including handwritten and computer-generated prescriptions, or they can be telephoned, faxed, or sent electronically to a pharmacy.

Abbreviations and symbols are usually used to write a prescription. They also are used to document medication information in the patient's chart. Common abbreviations used in the medical office for writing prescriptions are included in Table 26-5.

The medical assistant should ensure that all prescription pads are kept in a safe place and out of reach of individuals who may want to obtain drugs illegally. The stock supply of prescription pads should be locked in a drawer.

Table 26-4 Classification of Controlled Drugs

Classification	Description and Prescription Regulations	EXAMPLES Generic	Brand
Schedule I	High potential for abuse Currently no accepted medical use in treatment in the United States There is a lack of accepted safety for use of the drug under medical supervision Use may lead to severe physical or psychological dependence May be used for research with appropriate limitations Not available for prescribing	GHB heroin LSD MDMA ("ecstasy") mescaline methaqualone (Quaalude) psilocybin	
Schedule II	High potential for abuse Currently accepted medical use in treatment in the United States or a currently accepted medical use with severe restrictions Abuse may lead to severe psychological or physical dependence Prescription must be in writing in indelible ink or typed Emergency telephone order permitted only for immediate amount needed to treat patient; written prescription must be provided to pharmacist within 7 days No refills allowed Manufacturer's label marked C-II	**Analgesics** cocaine codeine fentanyl hydrocodone combined with nonopioid analgesic hydromorphone meperidine methadone morphine oxycodone oxycodone/acetaminophen (APAP) oxycodone/aspirin (ASA) **Central Nervous System Stimulants** dextroamphetamine lisdexamfetamine methylphenidate methamphetamine **Sedatives/Hypnotics** amobarbital glutethimide pentobarbital secobarbital	 Duragesic Vicodin, Lortab, Lorcet, Tussionex, Vicoprofen Dilaudid Demerol Dolophine Roxanol OxyContin Percocet Percodan Adderall Vyvanse Ritalin, Concerta Desoxyn Amytal Doriden Nembutal Seconal

Continued

Table 26-4 Classification of Controlled Drugs—cont'd

Classification	Description and Prescription Regulations	EXAMPLES	
		Generic	**Brand**
Schedule III	Less potential for abuse than drugs in Schedules I and II Currently accepted medical use in treatment in the United States Abuse may lead to moderate or low physical dependence or high psychological dependence Telephone and fax orders permitted If authorized by physician, prescription can be refilled five times within 6 months from issue date Prescription expires 6 months from issue date Manufacturer's label marked C-III	**Anabolic Steroids** oxandrolone oxymetholone **Analgesics** buprenorphine butalbital compound codeine combined with nonopioid analgesic **Central Nervous System Stimulant** benzphetamine **Male Hormone** testosterone **Sedative/Hypnotic** butabarbital	Anavar Anapolon Buprenex Fioricet, Fiorinal Tylenol w/ Codeine, Empirin w/ Codeine Didrex Depotest, Delatestryl Butisol
Schedule IV	Lower potential for abuse than drugs in Schedule III Currently accepted medical use in treatment in the United States Abuse may lead to limited physical or psychological dependence Telephone and fax orders permitted If authorized by physician, prescription can be refilled five times within 6 months of issue date Prescription expires 6 months from issue date Manufacturer's label marked C-IV	**Analgesics** butorphanol pentazocine propoxyphene **Antianxiety Agents** alprazolam chlordiazepoxide diazepam halazepam lorazepam meprobamate oxazepam **Anticonvulsant** clonazepam **Central Nervous System Stimulants** modafinil pemoline **Sedatives/Hypnotics** chloral hydrate eszopiclone ethchlorvynol flurazepam midazolam phenobarbital temazepam triazolam zaleplon zolpidem **Weight Control Agents** diethylpropion phentermine sibutramine	Stadol Talwin Darvon, Darvocet-N Xanax Librium Valium Paxipam Ativan Equanil Serax Klonopin Provigil Cylert Noctec Lunesta Placidyl Dalmane Versed Luminal Restoril Halcion Sonata Ambien Tenuate Fastin Meridia

Table 26-4 Classification of Controlled Drugs—cont'd

Classification	Description and Prescription Regulations	EXAMPLES Generic	EXAMPLES Brand
Schedule V	Low potential for abuse Accepted medical use in United States Abuse may lead to limited physical or psychological dependence Telephone and fax orders permitted Prescribing policies determined by state and local regulations. In most states: • Number of refills determined by physician • Prescription expires 1 year from issue date • Some are available without prescription to patients older than 18 years of age (with proper identification) • Manufacturer's label marked C-V	Cough suppressants with small amounts of codeine Antidiarrheals containing paregoric diphenoxylate/atropine	Robitussin A-C, Cheracol syrup Parepectolin, Kapectolin PG Lomotil

Table 26-5 Common Abbreviations and Symbols Used in Medication Documentation

Abbreviation or Symbol	Meaning	Abbreviation or Symbol	Meaning
$\overline{aa}$	of each	OTC	over the counter
ac	before meals	oz	ounce
ad lib	as desired	$\overline{p}$	after
aq	water	pc	after meals
admin	administer, administration	Pt or pt	patient
AM or a.m.	morning	per	by
APAP	acetaminophen	PM or p.m.	evening
ASA	aspirin	po or PO	by mouth
bid	twice a day	prn	as needed
$\overline{c}$	with	qAM	every morning
cap(s)	capsule(s)	qh	every hour
DAW	dispense as written	q(2, 3, 4)h	every (2, 3, 4) hours
dil	dilute	qid	four times a day
g	gram	qs	of sufficient quantity
gtt(s)	drop(s)	Rx	prescription
h or hr	hour	$\overline{s}$	without
ID	intradermal	subcut	subcutaneous
IM	intramuscular	SL	sublingual
IV	intravenous	sol	solution
kg	kilogram	STAT	immediately
L	liter	T	tablespoon
liq	liquid	tab(s)	tablet(s)
mcg	microgram	tid	three times a day
med(s)	medication(s)	tsp	teaspoon
mg	milligram	#	number
min	minute	×	times
mL	milliliter	Ø	no, none
NPO	nothing by mouth		

Putting It All into Practice

My name is Theresa Cline, and I work for four physicians in a family practice medical office. I have worked there ever since I graduated from college with an associate's degree in medical assisting. One experience that I will never forget taught our entire office staff a valuable lesson. It involved a woman who came to our office because she had lacerated her wrist while using a butcher knife. After the wound was sutured, I gave her a tetanus injection because she was past due for one. Shortly thereafter, she became very nauseated and dizzy, and I made her lie down on the examining table. She asked me to get her a cold drink of water, and I left the room to do so. Apparently, while I was gone, she must have tried to sit up or turn over because she rolled off the table and struck the back of her head on the floor. She sustained a laceration to her scalp, which also had to be sutured. Owing to her persistent symptoms of severe nausea, vomiting, and headache, it was decided that she should be admitted to the hospital for neurologic observation and x-ray studies.

The vital lesson that this experience taught everyone in our office was that you must never leave a patient alone, not even for a minute to get something, if there is the slightest indication that he or she is not feeling perfectly fine. Another staff member should be called to obtain whatever is needed. From that point on, this has been our office policy and procedure. ■

PARTS OF A PRESCRIPTION

A prescription is a handwritten (Figure 26-2) or computer-generated document that includes directions to the pharmacist for filling the prescription and instructions to the patient for taking the medication. The prescription must include the following specific information:

- *Date.* A pharmacist cannot fill a prescription unless the date the prescription was issued is indicated on the prescription. The reason for this is that a prescription expires after a certain length of time. In most states, a prescription for a drug (with the exception of controlled drugs) expires 1 year from the date of issue. After this time, the prescription (or any refills left on the prescription) cannot be filled.
- *Physician's name, address, telephone number, and fax number.* This information is preprinted on prescription forms that are handwritten and automatically printed on forms that are computer generated. This information identifies the physician issuing the prescription and provides the necessary information should the pharmacist have a question and need to contact the medical office.
- *Patient's name and address.* This information is important for insurance billing and for properly dispensing the medication.
- *Patient's date of birth and age.* The patient's age is important to the pharmacist when he or she double-checks the physician's order to ensure that the proper dose is being

---

Larry Douglas, M.D.
11 West Union Street
Athens, OH 45701

Phone   740-555-8993   **FAX**   740-555-7222

Patient Name   Holly Roberts   **DOB**   10/1/XX

     Address   72 Hill St., Athens, OH 45701   **Age**   24

                                                Date   07/12/XX

R⎫ **Superscription**

    Inscription { Amoxil 250 mg

    Subscription { Disp: #30 (thirty)

    Signatura { Sig: Take 1 capsule 3 times a day for 10 days

☐ **Dispense as Written**

Refill   (NR)   1   2   3   4   5

                             Signature   *Larry Douglas, M.D.*

                             DEA # _____

Figure 26-2 Example of a handwritten prescription.

dispensed. The most common errors in dosage occur among children and the elderly, who may not require the standard dose of a drug because patients in these age groups metabolize drugs differently. Knowing the patient's age also allows the pharmacist to double-check that the drug is age appropriate for the patient. For example, ciprofloxacin (e.g., Cipro) should not be taken by children and adolescents because this antibiotic can damage cartilage in individuals younger than 18 years.

- *Superscription.* The **superscription** consists of the abbreviation *Rx*. This symbol comes from the Latin word *recipe* and means "take."
- *Inscription.* The **inscription** states the name of the drug and the dose (e.g., Amoxil 250 mg). Most drugs are available in various doses; it is important that the correct dose be prescribed. For example, Amoxil comes in the following doses: 125 mg, 250 mg, and 500 mg.
- *Subscription.* The **subscription** gives directions to the pharmacist. At present, it is usually used to designate the number of doses to be dispensed. To prevent a prescription from being altered illegally, it is recommended that numbers and letters be used to indicate the quantity to be dispensed (e.g., #30 [thirty]).
- *Signatura.* The **signatura** (abbreviated *Sig.*) comes from the Latin term *signa*, which means "write" or "label." The signatura indicates the information to be included on the medication label. It consists of directions to the patient for taking the medication. The name of the medication also is included on the label so that the patient can identify the medication.
- *Refill.* This part of the prescription indicates the number of times the prescription may be refilled.
- *Physician's signature.* A prescription cannot be filled unless it is signed by the physician.

- *DEA number.* The number assigned to the physician by the Drug Enforcement Administration must appear on the prescription for a controlled drug. See Table 26-4 for examples of controlled drugs.

GENERIC PRESCRIBING

Generic prescribing means that the physician writes the prescription using the generic rather than the brand name of the drug. Because many pharmaceutical manufacturers may produce the same generic drug and sell it under different brand names, price competition often results. If the physician prescribes a drug using its generic name, the pharmacist is permitted to fill it with the drug that offers the best savings to the patient. In addition, most states allow the pharmacist the option of filling the prescription with a chemically equivalent generic drug, even if the drug has been prescribed by brand name. If the physician wants the prescription to be filled with a specific brand of drug, instructions must be indicated on the prescription form, such as "Dispense as Written (DAW)," or words of a similar meaning (see Figure 26-2).

COMPLETING A PRESCRIPTION FORM

The physician is responsible for having accurate and pertinent information on the prescription form. If the physician so delegates, a prescription form can be completed by the medical assistant and signed by the physician. The physician must review the prescription thoroughly before signing it to ensure all of the information is correct. If the medical assistant is delegated this responsibility, he or she must carefully follow the important guidelines presented in the box *Guidelines for Completing a Prescription Form*.

Guidelines for Completing a Prescription Form

Using a Paper Form
- Work in a quiet, well lit area that is free of distractions.
- Use an indelible black ink pen to write on the form
- Print all information on the form
- Ensure that all information is spelled correctly.
- Review the metric notation guidelines presented in the box *Metric Notation Guidelines*. (Most prescriptions are written in metric units.)
- Always ask the physician if you have questions about the prescription.
- Complete all of the required information on the form; it includes the following:
  1. Patient's name, address, date of birth, and age
     - Clearly print all of this information on the form. Never leave the address, date of birth, and age categories blank.

2. Date
   - Indicate today's date on the prescription form.
3. Name of the medication
   - The physician may prescribe the medication using either the generic or the brand name.
   - Make sure to spell the name of the drug correctly. If you are unsure, use a drug reference to find the correct spelling of a drug.
4. Medication dosage
   - Never leave a decimal point "naked." If the dosage is a fraction of a unit, a zero must be placed before the decimal point as a means of focusing on the fractional dose. This reduces the possibility of misreading the dose as a whole number. *Example:* 0.5 mL (not .5 mL).

Continued

Guidelines for Completing a Prescription Form—cont'd

- Never place a decimal point and a zero after a whole number because the decimal point may be overlooked, resulting in a 10-fold overdose error. *Example:* 5 mg (not 5.0 mg).

5. Quantity to dispense
   - Use numbers and letters to indicate the quantity to be dispensed. *Example:* Disp: #30 (thirty).
   - Ensure that the quantity is correct. The number of prescribed pills should match the duration of treatment. *Example:* If the patient has been prescribed 3 tablets a day for 7 days, the quantity should be written as follows: Disp: #21 (twenty-one).

6. Directions for taking the medication
   - Clearly indicate the directions for taking the medication. Many authorities recommend writing the directions without abbreviations. *Example:* Sig: Take 1 capsule 3 times a day for 10 days.

7. Refills
   - Never leave this category blank.
   - If there are no refills, indicate this clearly on the form. The method for doing this is based on the setup of the preprinted form.
     Example: Refill: (NR) 1 2 3 4 5
     (on this form, the information is circled)
     Example: Refill: 0
     (on this form, the information is written in)

8. Dispense as written
   - If the physician does not allow a substitution (e.g., generic equivalent) for this medication, check this category.

9. DEA number
   - If the prescription is for a controlled drug, clearly indicate the physician's DEA number on the form.

10. Group practice
    - If there is more than one physician in the practice, circle (or check) the name of the physician

prescribing the medication. This avoids confusion if the pharmacist cannot read the physician's signature. *Example:*
   James Ortman, MD, Mark Rothstein, MD, Richard Bontrager, MD

- Give the prescription to the physician to review and sign.
- Document the prescription order in the patient's medication record if directed by the physician. Give the prescription to the patient. Provide the patient with guidelines for taking the medication (see patient teaching box on prescription medications).
- Ask the patient whether he or she has any questions about the medication.

Using an Electronic Medical Record

1. Access the patient's electronic medical record, verifying the date of birth.
2. Access the prescription screen and verify the autofilled information (i.e., date, patient name, date of birth, address, and age).
3. Select the correct medication from the drop-down menu.
4. Select the correct medication dose from the drop-down menu, or enter it in the free text field.
5. Enter the quantity to dispense.
6. Enter the directions for taking the medication, using the drop-down menu or the free text fields.
7. Enter the correct information in the Refills field. This field should not be left blank; there should be either a number indicated or "no refills."
8. If the physician has indicated that there should be no substitution for this medication, the "Dispense as Written" radio button should be selected.
9. Forward the prescription to the physician for review and his or her electronic signature.
10. Save the prescription in the patient's record, print a copy for the patient or send it electronically to the pharmacy, and update the patient's medication list.

PATIENT TEACHING   Prescription Medications

To avoid adverse reactions, teach patients the proper guidelines for taking prescription medication. These guidelines are as follows:

- *Know the names of all your prescription and nonprescription medications. Know the generic and brand names of each of your medications.* Nonprescription drugs are known as *over-the-counter (OTC) drugs;* they are drugs that can be purchased without a prescription. Vitamin supplements and herbal products are considered OTC drugs.
- *Know why you are taking each medication.* It is important to know the desired therapeutic outcome, dose, frequency and

time of administration, and common side effects of each medication, and guidelines ("do's and don't's") to follow when taking the medication. Never take your medication in the dark or without your reading glasses (if needed for close vision).

- *Take your medication exactly as prescribed, at the right times, and in the right amounts.* The medication may not work properly if it is not taken as directed. If the dose is too small, the drug may not produce its intended therapeutic effect; exceeding the recommended dose could result in a toxic effect. Make sure you know what to do if you are late in taking a dose or miss a dose of your medication. It is also important to know if any other medication or food interferes with your medication and should be avoided.

- *Inform the physician if new symptoms or adverse effects develop when you are taking the medication.* The physician may need to change your dose or prescribe a different medication. There are usually alternative medications that the physician can prescribe to treat your condition.

- *Take the medication for the prescribed duration of time, even after you begin to feel better.* If you do not complete the entire course of drug therapy, your condition may recur. Not taking all of a prescribed antibiotic may cause an infection to return, and it may be worse than the first infection.

- *Tell the physician if you decide not to take your medication.* Otherwise, the physician may think your medication is not working. Not taking a medication prescribed by the physician could be serious because this may allow your condition to worsen.

- *Do not take additional medications, including OTC medications, without checking with the physician.* All drugs, including OTC medications, are designed to have an effect on the body. Vitamin supplements and herbal products are considered OTC drugs. Some combinations of drugs cause serious reactions. In some cases, one drug cancels the effects of another and prevents it from working.

- *Never take a medication that was prescribed for someone else.* Physicians prescribe medication based on an individual's age, weight, sex, and condition. Taking a medication prescribed for someone else can have serious results.

- *Keep all medications in their original containers to avoid taking the wrong medication by mistake.* Store your medications in their original containers from the pharmacy. Basic information about your medication is on the original container. Medications that are not clearly marked may be taken inadvertently by the wrong person.

- *Store your medications in a safe place, away from the reach of children.* If you have young children, make sure your medication is dispensed in containers with child-resistant safety closures. After taking your medication, make sure that the cap of the container is closed tightly. Accidental drug poisoning in children is a common and preventable problem. Also, do not take your medication in front of young children because they may want to mimic your behavior.

- *Store medications in a cool, dry place or as stated on the label.* Do not store capsules or tablets in the bathroom or kitchen because heat or moisture may cause the medication to break down.

- *Properly discard unused portions of prescription medications and outdated OTC medications.* Unwanted medication may pose a risk to human health and the environment if disposed of improperly. Unused or expired medication should not be flushed down the toilet or drain unless the drug label or accompanying patient information specifically instructs you to do so.

Medications can be properly discarded as follows:

1. Community drug take-back program: Contact your city or county government's household trash and recycling service to determine if your community offers a drug take-back program. This type of program is considered the best option for disposing of medication and allows individuals in the community to bring unwanted medication to a central location for proper disposal.

2. Household disposal: If a take-back program is not available in your community, the following steps should be followed to dispose of unwanted medication:

   a. Remove the medication from its original container.

   b. Mix the medication with an undesirable substance, such as kitty litter or coffee grounds.

   c. Place the mixture in a disposable container such as a sealable plastic bag or an empty plastic container with a lid and discard it in the household trash.

   d. Remove personal information (including the prescription number) from an empty prescription medication container before discarding the container in the trash to protect the privacy of your personal health information. This can be accomplished by covering the information with a permanent marker or scratching it off. ∎

ELECTRONIC MEDICAL RECORD PRESCRIPTION PROGRAM

Electronic medical record (EMR) software includes a prescription program, which greatly reduces the amount of time needed to prescribe and refill medication. The prescription program generates and prints a prescription, which is then signed by the physician and given to the patient (Figure 26-3). The program can also transmit the prescription electronically to the patient's pharmacy. Both of these features eliminate the need for the pharmacist to decipher the physician's handwriting.

The EMR prescription program also has the capability to quickly refill a prescription and print a list of medications being taken by the patient. The patient can use this list to keep track of the medication he or she is taking (Figure 26-4).

MEDICATION RECORD

A medication record form (Figure 26-5) includes detailed information about each medication so that the physician

PRESCRIPTION: (Give to the pharmacist)	PRESCRIPTION: (Give to the pharmacist)
Huntington Clinic 701 Concord Ave Lexington, KY 48710 614-871-0033	Huntington Clinic 701 Concord Ave Lexington, KY 48710 614-871-0033
Doctor: John Blauser, MD	Doctor: John Blauser, MD
For: Danielle Travis Age: 28 DOB: 08/08/XX	For: Danielle Travis Age: 28 DOB: 08/08/XX
Date: 10/27/20XX	Date: 10/27/20XX
Address: 101 Coventry Lane Lexington, KY 48710	Address: 101 Coventry Lane Lexington, KY 48710
Rx: Amoxil (Generic - amoxicillin) (Dose/unit - 250 mg) (Form - Caps) (Disp - #30) (Frequency - One three times daily for 10 days) (Route - By mouth) (Refills-0).	Rx: Tylenol-3 (Generic - Acetaminophen/Codeine) (Dose/unit - 1 to 2) (Form - Tabs) (Disp - #15)(fifteen) (Frequency - Every 4 hours as needed for moderate to severe pain) (Route - By mouth) (Refills-0).
Dr: _____ *John Blauser, MD* _____	Dr: _____ *John Blauser, MD* _____

Figure 26-3 Example of a computer-generated prescription.

Huntington Clinic
701 Concord Ave
Lexington, KY 48710
614-871-0033

Patient: Clare Andrews
      352 Pinewood Dr.
      Lexington, KY 48710

Age/DOB: 12/25/1970
EMRN: 7016780

Medication List

Medication	Refills	Start
Abilify 15 mg tablet TAKE 1 TABLET DAILY	0	24Sep20XX
Acetaminophen-Codeine #3 300-30 mg tablet TAKE 1 TABLET EVERY 6 TO 8 HOURS AS NEEDED FOR PAIN	0	23Sep20XX
Clonazepam 1 mg tablet TAKE 1 TABLET EVERY 8 HOURS PRN	0	24Sep20XX
Etodolac CR 500 mg tablet extended release 24 hour 1-2 TABLETS PO ONCE DAILY WITH FOOD	0	21Sep20XX
Fish Oil 1000 mg capsule TAKE 1 CAPSULE DAILY	11	7Apr20XX
Flovent HFA 44 mcg/act aerosol INHALE 2 PUFFS TWICE DAILY	3	6Jan20XX
Fluticasone Propionate 50 mcg/act suspension USE 2 SPRAYS IN EACH NOSTRIL ONCE DAILY	3	9Sep20XX
Lamictal 200 mg tablet TAKE 2 TABLETS DAILY	0	24Sep20XX
Omeprazole 20 mg capsule delayed release TAKE 1 TABLET DAILY	11	24Sep20XX
Pamine 2.5 mg tablet TAKE 1 TABLET 3 TIMES DAILY	0	6Jan20XX
Proventil HFA 108 (90 base) mcg/act aerosol solution INHALE 1-2 PUFFS EVERY 4-6 HOURS AS NEEDED AND AS DIRECTED	3	21Jul20XX
Tramadol HCl 50 mg tablet TAKE 1 TABLET EVERY 6 HOURS	0	29Apr20XX
Voltaren 1% gel APPLY 2 GRAMS TOPICALLY 4 TIMES DAILY	6	24Sep20XX
WelChol 625 mg tablet TAKE 3 TABLETS TWICE DAILY WITH MEALS	11	29Apr20XX

Figure 26-4 Example of a computer-generated patient medication list.

MEDICATION RECORD								

Patient _John Walsh_
Birthdate _6/10/49_

ALLERGY
Ø

DATE	MEDICATION AND DOSAGE	FREQUENCY	RX	OTC	REFILLS			STOP
2/18/XX	Cipro 250 mg	⫶ q 12 h po x 10 days	X					2/28/XX
6/10/XX	Prevacid 15 mg	⫶ daily po	X					7/10/XX
6/10/XX	Lipitor 10 mg	⫶ daily po	X		1/6/XX			
6/10/XX	Prozac 20 mg	⫶ daily po	X		1/6/XX			
12/3/XX	Tobrex Ophthalmic Solution	1 drop q3h ® eye	X					12/10/XX
2/5/XX	Echinacea	⫶ daily po		X				
3/15/XX	Nitrostat 0.4 mg	⫶ prn pain SL Rep q 5 min prn pain, not to exceed 3 tabs	X					
3/15/XX	Inderal 40 mg	⫶ bid po	X					
3/15/XX	St Joseph ASA Enteric Coated 81 mg	⫶ daily po		X				

Figure 26-5 Example of a medication record.

can tell at a glance what medications and how much the patient is taking. Both prescription medications and OTC medications, including vitamin supplements and herbal products, must be recorded in the medication record.

The medication record is part of the patient's medical record. The medical assistant is often responsible for documenting medication information in the medication record. Care must be taken to ensure the information is correct and clearly stated.

In a paper-based patient record (PPR), the medical office may use a preprinted form to record the medication that a patient is taking. With an EMR, the medical assistant enters this information into a digital form on the screen of the monitor using free text entry, drop-down lists, and check-boxes.

A medication record typically includes the following information:

- Patient's name and date of birth
- Any drug allergies
- Date the medication was prescribed (for prescription medications) or date the patient started taking the medication (for OTC medications)
- Name and dose of the medication
- Frequency of administration of the medication
- Route of administration
- Prescription or OTC medication category
- Refills (prescription medication only)
- Date the patient stopped taking the medication

What Would You Do? What Would You *Not* Do?

Case Study 2

Linda Cardwell calls the medical office. Her daughter Rachel, 9 years old, was seen in the office 10 days ago. Rachel was diagnosed with strep throat, and the physician ordered Amoxil 250 mg tid × 7 days. Mrs. Cardwell says that after 3 days of taking the medication, Rachel was much better, so she stopped giving her the Amoxil because it was causing her to have diarrhea. Mrs. Cardwell says that her 12-year-old son started feeling achy all over and she gave him the Amoxil for 2 days, and it seemed to help. She also says that her husband started complaining of sinus problems, so she also gave him the Amoxil for 2 days. Mrs. Cardwell says that now Rachel's throat is hurting again, and she has a fever. She wants to know whether Rachel has developed another case of strep throat. Mrs. Cardwell says she does not know what to do because she does not have any Amoxil left to give Rachel. ■

FACTORS AFFECTING DRUG ACTION

THERAPEUTIC EFFECT

Each drug has an intended therapeutic effect—the reason the patient takes the medication. Certain factors affect the therapeutic action of drugs in the body, causing patients to respond differently to the same drug. Because of this, the drug therapy may need to be adjusted to meet these variations, which include the following.

Age

Children and the elderly tend to respond more strongly to drugs than young and middle-aged adults. The physician may calculate smaller doses for very young and geriatric patients.

Route of Administration

Medications administered by different routes are absorbed at different rates. Drugs administered orally are absorbed slowly because they must be digested first. Parenterally administered drugs are absorbed more quickly than orally administered drugs because they are injected directly into the body.

Size

A patient's body size has an effect on drug action. A thin individual may require a smaller quantity of a drug, and an obese individual may require more.

Time of Administration

A drug administered by the oral route is absorbed more rapidly when the stomach is empty than when it contains food. A drug may not produce the desired effect or may be absorbed too slowly if it is taken when food is present. Some drugs irritate the stomach's lining, however, and must be taken with food. The drug package insert or a drug reference should always be consulted to determine when a drug should be taken.

Tolerance

A patient taking a certain drug over a period of time may develop a tolerance to it. This means that the same dose of a drug no longer produces the desired effect after prolonged administration. The physician should be notified to determine whether a change of drug or dosage is needed.

UNDESIRABLE EFFECTS OF DRUGS

A drug may cause undesirable effects, which may occur immediately or may be delayed hours or even days after administration of the medication.

Adverse Reactions

Most drugs produce unintended and undesirable effects known as **adverse reactions.** Adverse reactions are secondary effects that occur along with the therapeutic effect of

Memories *from* **Practicum**

Theresa Cline: I can clearly remember the first time I gave an injection at my practicum site. I was worried that I would forget how to give an injection and look bad in front of my practicum supervisor and the patient. What made things worse is that the patient was a woman with very thin arms. I was giving her a flu shot, and I was so scared that the needle would hit her bone even though I was only using a 1-inch needle. When I walked into the room, my supervisor told the woman that I was a student and asked her if it was all right if I gave her the flu injection. The woman laughed and said, "Well, I guess so." That made me feel even more nervous. The patient then asked if it was my first shot. I told her "yes" and she said, "Just don't hurt me." When it came time to give the injection, everything that I had ever learned about injections came back to me. I gave the injection, and the woman told me I did a good job and that she didn't even feel it. That made me feel so good! My supervisor said, "If you can give a shot to her, you can give a shot to anyone." Every injection after that was a "piece of cake." I've learned just to take a deep breath before each difficult situation encountered in the office, and everything will work out. ■

the drug. Some adverse reactions, referred to as *side effects,* are harmless and are often tolerated by the patient to obtain the therapeutic effect of the drug. Most patients are willing to tolerate the dry mouth and drowsiness that may accompany an antihistamine to obtain its therapeutic effect. Other adverse reactions, such as a decrease in blood pressure or an allergic reaction, can be harmful to the patient and warrant discontinuing the medication.

Drug Interactions

When certain medications are used at the same time, drug interactions may produce undesirable effects. The medical assistant should inquire about other medications the patient is taking and record this information in the patient's chart for review by the physician.

Allergic Drug Reaction

The patient may exhibit an allergic reaction to a drug. The reaction is usually mild and takes the form of a rash, rhinitis, or pruritus. Occasionally, a patient has a severe allergic reaction that occurs suddenly and immediately. This is known as an **anaphylactic reaction.**

An anaphylactic reaction is the least common but the most serious type of allergic reaction. Symptoms begin with sneezing, urticaria (hives), itching, erythema, angioedema, and disorientation. Erythema is reddening of the skin caused by dilation of superficial blood vessels in the skin. Angioedema is a localized urticaria of the deeper tissues of the body. If not treated, the symptoms of anaphylaxis quickly increase in severity and progress to dyspnea, cyanosis, and shock. Blood pressure decreases, and the pulse becomes weak and thready. Convulsions, loss of consciousness, and death may occur if treatment is not initiated promptly.

To prevent an anaphylactic reaction to a drug or to reduce its danger, the medical assistant should stay with the patient after administration of the medication. The medical assistant should be especially alert for signs of an anaphylactic reaction after administering allergy skin tests or a penicillin or allergy injection. If a reaction occurs, the physician should be notified immediately so that he or she can begin treatment immediately. In general, treatment consists of one or more injections of epinephrine, depending on the severity of the reaction. Epinephrine goes to work immediately to reverse the life-threatening symptoms of anaphylaxis. When the patient's condition has been stabilized, he or she is usually given an injection of an antihistamine. The antihistamine takes longer to begin working but helps alleviate urticaria, itching, angioedema, and erythema. The medical assistant must ensure that an ample supply of epinephrine is on hand at all times. Many offices maintain emergency crash carts for this purpose.

Idiosyncratic Reaction

An idiosyncratic reaction is an abnormal or peculiar response to a drug that is unexplained and unpredictable. Elderly patients are most prone to idiosyncratic reactions to drugs and should be monitored closely when they are taking a new medication.

GUIDELINES FOR PREPARATION AND ADMINISTRATION OF MEDICATION

To prevent medication errors, the medical assistant should follow these guidelines when preparing and administering any drug:

1. Work in a quiet, well lit atmosphere that is free of distractions.
2. Always ask if you have a question about the medication order.
3. Know the drug to be given.
4. Select the proper drug. Check the label of the medication three times—as it is taken from its storage location, before preparing the medication, and after preparing the medication. Do not use a drug if the label is missing or is difficult to read.
5. Do not use a drug if the color has changed, if a precipitate has formed, or if it has an unusual odor.
6. Check the expiration date before preparing the drug for administration.
7. Prepare the proper dose of the drug. The term **dose** refers to the quantity of a drug to be administered at one time. Each medication has a dose range, or range of quantities of the drug that can produce therapeutic effects. It is important to administer the exact dose of the drug. A dose that is too small would not produce

a therapeutic effect, and a dose that is too large could be harmful or even fatal to the patient.

8. Correctly identify the patient so that the drug is administered to the intended patient. When medication is administered, the patient should be identified by his or her full name and date of birth.
9. Before administering the medication, check the patient's records or question the patient to ensure that he or she is not allergic to the medication.
10. If you are giving an injection, determine the appropriate route and site at which to administer the injection; the route and site are dictated by the type of injection being given. An allergy injection is given by the subcutaneous route, and an antibiotic injection is given by the intramuscular route. The site must be free from abrasions, lesions, bruises, and edema.
11. Use the proper technique to administer the medication.
12. Stay with the patient after administering the medication.
13. Document information properly in the patient's medical record immediately after administering the drug. If using a PPR, include the date and time, the name of the medication, the manufacturer and lot number (if required), the dose given, the route of administration, the site of administration, and any unusual observations or patient reactions. Sign the recording with your name and credentials. If you administer a medication that contains a fraction of a unit, place a 0 before the decimal point (e.g., 0.5 mg, not .5 mg) so that the dose is not misread as 5 mg. A decimal point and a zero should never be placed after a whole number. The decimal point may be overlooked and misread, resulting in a 10-fold overdose error (e.g., 20 mg, not 20.0 mg). If using an EMR, document the name of medication, the manufacturer and lot number (if required), the dose given, the route of administration, and any unusual observations or patient reactions using the appropriate radio buttons, drop-down menus, and free text fields.
14. Always follow the seven "rights" of preparing and administering medication in the medical office:
    Right patient
    Right medication
    Right dose
    Right route
    Right time
    Right technique
    Right documentation

ORAL ADMINISTRATION

The oral route is the most convenient and most used method of administering medication. **Oral administration** means that the drug is given by mouth in either a solid form (e.g., tablet, capsule) or a liquid form (e.g., suspension, syrup). Absorption of most oral medications occurs in the small intestine, although some may be absorbed in the mouth and stomach.

Many patients find it easier to swallow a tablet or a capsule with a glass of water. Water should not be offered after the patient has received a cough syrup, however, because the water would dilute the medication's beneficial effects. Unless the patient has a malabsorption problem or is unable to swallow, the oral route is considered the safest and most desirable route for administering medication. Procedure 26-1 outlines the procedure for the administration of oral medications.

PROCEDURE 26-1   Administering Oral Medication

Outcome Administer oral solid and liquid medications

Equipment/Supplies

- Medication ordered by the physician
- Medication order
- Medicine cup
- Medication tray

1. Procedural Step. Sanitize your hands.

2. Procedural Step. Assemble the equipment.

3. Procedural Step. Work in a quiet, well lit atmosphere.
Principle. Good lighting aids the medical assistant in reading the medication label.

4. Procedural Step. Select the correct medication from the shelf. Compare the medication with the physician's instructions and medication order. Check the drug label three times—while removing the medication from storage, while preparing the medication, and after preparing the medication. Check the expiration date.
Principle. If the medication is outdated, consult the physician because it may produce undesirable effects for which the medical assistant could be held responsible. To prevent a drug error, the medication should be carefully compared with the physician's instructions.

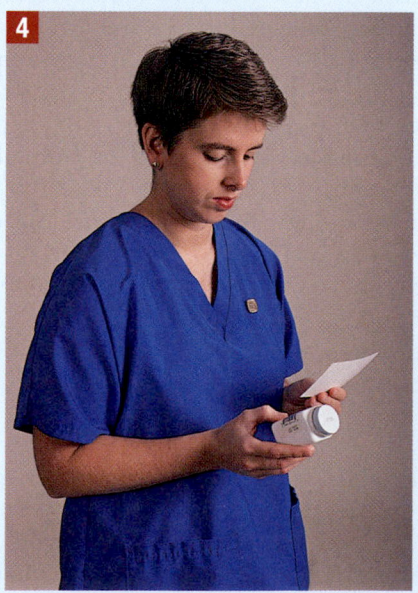

Compare the medication with the physician's instructions.

5. Procedural Step. Calculate the correct dose to be given, if necessary.

6. Procedural Step. Remove the bottle cap, touching the outside of the lid only.
Principle. Touching the inside of the lid contaminates it.

7. Procedural Step. Check the drug label again, and pour the medication.
Solid medications: Pour the correct number of capsules or tablets into the bottle cap. Transfer the medication to a medicine cup, being careful not to touch the inside of the cup.
Principle. Pouring the medication into the lid prevents contamination of the medication and lid.
Liquid medications: Place the lid of the bottle on a flat surface with the open end facing up. Palm the surface of the label.
With the opposite hand, place the thumbnail at the proper calibration on the medicine cup, and hold the cup at eye level. Pour the medication, and read the dose at the lowest level of the meniscus. (The meniscus is the curved surface of the liquid in a container. When a liquid is poured into a medicine cup, capillary action causes the liquid in contact with the cup to be drawn upward, resulting in a curved surface in the middle.)
Principle. Placing the bottle cap with the open end up prevents contamination of the inside of the cap. Palming the medication label prevents the medication from dripping on the label and obscuring it.

PROCEDURE 26-1   Administering Oral Medication—cont'd

Pour the correct number of capsules or tablets into the bottle cap.

Place the lid of the bottle on a flat surface with the open end facing up.

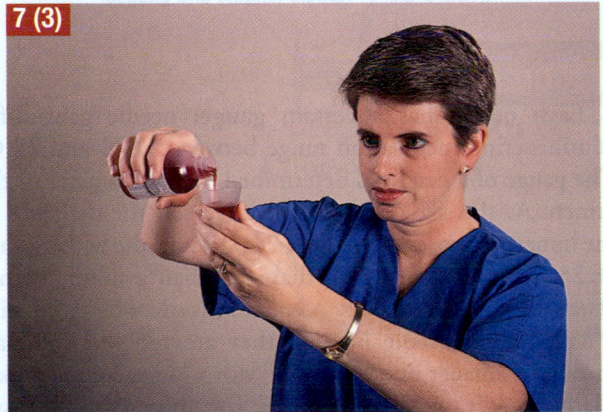

Hold the cup at eye level, and pour the medication.

8. **Procedural Step.** Replace the bottle cap, and check the drug label a third time to ensure it is the correct medication. Return the medication to its storage location.

9. **Procedural Step.** Greet the patient and introduce yourself. Identify the patient by full name and date of birth and explain the procedure. Explain the purpose of administering the medication.
Principle. It is crucial that no error be made in patient identity.

10. **Procedural Step.** Hand the medicine cup containing the medication to the patient, along with a glass of water. (If the medication is a cough syrup, do not offer water.)
Principle. Water helps the patient swallow the medication.

11. **Procedural Step.** Remain with the patient until the medication is swallowed. If the patient experiences any unusual reaction, notify the physician.

12. **Procedural Step.** Sanitize your hands.

13. **Procedural Step.** Chart the procedure in the patient's medical record.
   a. *Paper-based patient record:* Record the date and time, the name of the medication, the dose given, the route of administration, and any significant observations or patient reactions. The Latin abbreviation *po,* which means "by mouth," can be used to indicate the route of administration (refer to the PPR charting example).

PPR CHARTING EXAMPLE	
Date	
2/12/XX	9:30 a.m. Acetaminophen, 650 mg, po.
	———————— T. Cline, CMA (AAMA)

   b. *Electronic medical record:* Document the name of the medication, the dose given, the route of administration, and any significant observations or patient reactions, using the appropriate radio buttons, drop-down menus, and free text fields.

PARENTERAL ADMINISTRATION

The parenteral route of drug administration has several advantages. Medications given subcutaneously, intramuscularly, and intravenously are absorbed more rapidly and completely than medications given orally. In some cases, the parenteral route is the only way a drug can be given (e.g., insulin, most immunizations). If the patient is unconscious or has a gastric disturbance, such as nausea or vomiting, the parenteral route may be used to administer medication. If state laws permit, the medical assistant is usually responsible for administering subcutaneous, intramuscular, and medication, but rather for medical treatments, such as irrigating wounds and draining fluid from cysts.

SAFETY-ENGINEERED SYRINGES

OSHA stipulates requirements to reduce needlestick and other sharps injuries among health care workers. As was discussed in Chapter 17, employers are required to evaluate and implement commercially available safer medical devices that reduce occupational exposure to the lowest extent feasible.

Safer medical devices include safety-engineered syringes. *Safety-engineered syringes* incorporate a built-in safety feature to reduce the risk of a needlestick injury. Figure 26-10 illustrates types of safety-engineered syringes and the methods for using them.

Figure 26-10 Safety-engineered syringes.
A, Hinged-shield syringe.
1. After administering the injection, push the lever of the hinged shield forward.
2. Continue pushing until the needle tip is fully covered by the shield, then discard the syringe in a biohazard sharps container.
(Becton-Dickinson Safety Glide Syringe.)
B, Sliding-shield syringe.
1. After administering the injection, extend the sliding shield forward fully until a click is heard.
2. Lock the shield by twisting it in either direction until a click is heard. Discard the syringe in a biohazard sharps container.
(Monoject Safety Syringe.)

Figure 26-10, cont'd
C, Retractable needle.
1. Administer the injection by following the proper technique.
2. After administering the medication, continue depressing the plunger with the thumb. Use firm pressure past the point of initial resistance. This action delivers the full dose of medication to the patient and activates the needle retraction device, causing the needle to retract automatically from the patient's skin and into the barrel of the syringe.
3. Discard the syringe in a biohazard sharps container.
(Vanish Point Syringe.)

PREPARATION OF PARENTERAL MEDICATION

Medication used for injections is available in various types of dispensing units—vials, ampules, and prefilled syringes and cartridges.

Vials

A **vial** is a closed glass or plastic container with a rubber stopper; a soft metal or plastic cap protects the rubber stopper and must be removed the first time the medication is used. An injectable medication may be available in a single-dose vial, a multiple-dose vial, or both (Figure 26-11). A vial is labeled with specific information as illustrated in Figure 26-12.

Before the medication can be withdrawn, some vials require mixing (e.g., reconstituting a powdered drug, mixing a vial that separates on standing). Vials that require mixing should be rolled between the hands rather than shaken because shaking would cause the medication to foam, creating air bubbles that may enter the syringe when the medication is withdrawn.

To remove medication from a vial, an amount of air exactly equal to the amount of liquid to be removed is injected into the vial. The air should be inserted above the fluid level to avoid creating bubbles in the medication. If air is not injected first, a partial vacuum is created, and it is difficult to remove the medication. During the withdrawal of medication, the needle opening should be inserted below the fluid level to prevent the entrance of air bubbles. Air bubbles can be removed by tapping the barrel of the syringe with the fingertips. If the bubbles are allowed to remain, they take up space that the medication should occupy, which would prevent the patient from receiving the full dose of medication.

Ampules

An **ampule** is a small, sealed glass container that holds a single dose of medication (see Figure 26-11). An ampule has a constriction in the stem, known as the *neck,* which helps in opening it. Before opening, the medical assistant must ensure that there is no medication in the stem by tapping it lightly. A colored ring around the neck indicates where the ampule is prescored for easy opening. The ampule is opened by holding it firmly with gauze and breaking off the stem with a strong steady pressure.

A hazard with medication in ampules is the possibility of small glass particles getting into the ampule as the stem is broken off. When the medication is withdrawn into the syringe, the glass particles also might be withdrawn. To prevent this problem, a needle with a filter should be used that filters out small glass particles (Figure 26-13).

The needle opening is inserted into the base of the ampule below the fluid level to withdraw medication. To prevent contamination, the needle should not be permitted to touch the outside of the ampule. Air should never be injected into the ampule because it could force out some of the medication.

Prefilled Syringes

Some drugs come in *prefilled disposable syringes.* Using this type of dispensing unit does not require drawing up the medication. The name of the drug, the dose, and the expiration date are printed on the syringe (Figure 26-14).

STORAGE

The medical assistant should always read the drug package insert to determine the proper method for storing each parenteral medication because improper storage may alter the effectiveness of the medication.

RECONSTITUTION OF POWDERED DRUGS

Some parenteral medications are stable for only a short time in liquid form; these medications are prepared and stored in powdered form and require the addition of a liquid before administration. The process of adding a liquid to a powdered drug is known as *reconstitution.* The liquid used to reconstitute a powdered drug is known as the *diluent* and usually

Figure 26-11 The multiple-dose vial *(left)* and the single-dose vial *(middle)* consist of a closed glass container with a rubber stopper. The ampule *(right)* consists of a small, sealed glass container that holds a single dose of medication.

Figure 26-12 Information included on the label of a medication vial.

Figure 26-13 Filter needle used to withdraw medication from an ampule.

Figure 26-14 A prefilled disposable syringe of medication.

Figure 26-15 The measles, mumps, and rubella (MMR) vaccine is a parenteral medication that requires reconstitution before administration. The vial on the left contains the medication in powdered form, and the vial on the right contains the sterile diluent.

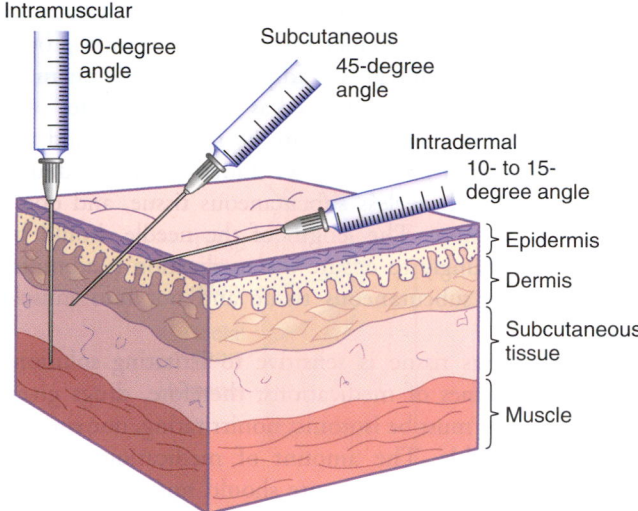

Figure 26-16 Angle of insertion for intradermal, subcutaneous, and intramuscular injections.

Figure 26-17 Common sites for subcutaneous injections. **A,** Upper outer arm. **B,** Lower abdomen. **C,** Upper outer thigh. **D,** Upper back. **E,** Flank region.

SUBCUTANEOUS INJECTIONS

A **subcutaneous injection** is made into the subcutaneous tissue, which consists of adipose (fat) tissue and is located just under the skin (Figure 26-16). Subcutaneous tissue is located all over the body; however, certain sites are more commonly used because they are located where bones and blood vessels are not near the surface of the skin. These sites include the upper lateral part of the arms, the anterior thigh, the upper back, and the abdomen (Figure 26-17). Absorption of medication from a subcutaneous injection occurs

consists of sterile water or normal saline. The powdered drug is contained in a single-dose or multiple-dose vial and is accompanied by specific instructions for reconstitution. An example of a parenteral medication that requires reconstitution is the measles, mumps, and rubella (MMR) immunization (Figure 26-15). The procedure for reconstituting powdered drugs is outlined in Procedure 26-3.

used to draw up the medication be removed from the syringe and replaced with a new sterile needle. This is because the point of the needle may not be as sharp after it has been inserted into rubber stopper of the medication vial. The medical assistant should follow the policy set forth by his or her medical office.)

Principle. The needle must remain sterile. The needle guard prevents the needle from becoming contaminated.

h. **Procedural Step.** Check the drug label for the third time, and return the medication to its proper storage location.

Withdrawing Medication From an Ampule

a. **Procedural Step.** Remove the needle (and needle guard) from the syringe, and attach a filter needle (and needle guard).

b. **Procedural Step.** Open the antiseptic wipe, and cleanse the neck of the ampule.
Principle. Cleansing the neck of the ampule removes dust and bacteria.

c. **Procedural Step.** Tap the stem of the ampule lightly to remove any medication in the neck of the ampule.

d. **Procedural Step.** Check the medication label a second time and place a piece of gauze around the neck of the ampule. Hold the base of the ampule between the first two fingers and the thumb of one hand. Hold the neck of the vial between the first two fingers and the thumb of the other hand. Apply a strong steady pressure with the thumbs, and break off the stem by snapping it quickly and firmly away from the body. Discard the stem and gauze in a biohazard sharps container.

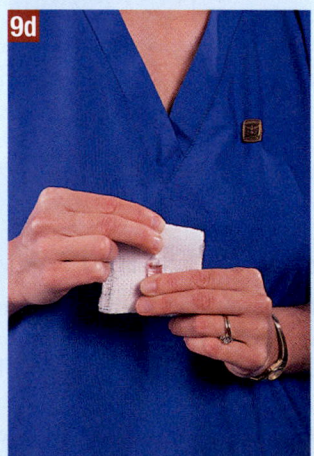

Snap the stem away from the body.

e. **Procedural Step.** Place the ampule on a flat surface. Remove the needle guard. Insert the filter needle opening below the fluid level.

Principle. The filter needle prevents glass particles from being withdrawn into the syringe.

f. **Procedural Step.** Withdraw the proper amount of medication by pulling back on the plunger. Keep the needle opening below the fluid level to prevent the entrance of air bubbles into the syringe. Tilt the ampule as needed to keep the needle opening immersed in the fluid.

Note: There is another method that can be used to remove medication from an ampule. Choose the method that is easiest for you. To perform this method, invert the ampule, making sure to keep the needle opening below the fluid level. Withdraw the proper amount of medication by pulling back on the plunger. Move the needle downward as necessary to keep the needle opening immersed in the fluid.

Principle. Air bubbles take up space the medication should occupy, resulting in an inaccurate measurement of medication.

Withdraw the medication.

g. **Procedural Step.** Remove the needle from the ampule, and replace the needle guard. Check the drug label for the third time, and dispose of the glass ampule in a biohazard sharps container.

h. **Procedural Step.** Remove the filter needle (and guard) from the syringe, and discard it in a biohazard sharps container. Reapply the needle (and guard) for administering the medication.

i. **Procedural Step.** If air bubbles are in the syringe, remove the needle guard, hold the syringe in a vertical position, and tap the barrel with the fingertips until the bubbles disappear. Remove the air at the top of the syringe by slowly pushing the plunger forward. If the syringe contains excess fluid, hold the syringe vertically over a sink with the needle tip up and slanted toward the sink. Slowly eject the excess fluid into the sink. Holding the syringe at eye level, check again to make sure you have drawn up the proper amount of medication. Replace the needle guard.

PROCEDURE **26-3**   Reconstituting Powdered Drugs

Outcome Reconstitute a powdered drug for parenteral administration

Equipment/Supplies

- Medication ordered by the physician
- Medication order
- Appropriate needle and syringe
- Antiseptic wipe
- Medication tray

1. **Procedural Step.** Follow steps 1 through 8 of Procedure 26-2.
2. **Procedural Step.** From the vial of the powdered drug, withdraw an amount of air equal to the amount of liquid to be injected into the vial. *Principle.* Removing air from the powdered drug vial allows room for injection of the diluent.
3. **Procedural Step.** Inject the air removed from the powdered drug vial into the vial of diluent. *Principle.* Air must be injected into the vial to prevent formation of a partial vacuum in the vial, which would make it difficult to remove the diluent.
4. **Procedural Step.** Invert the diluent vial, and withdraw the proper amount of liquid into the syringe. Remove air bubbles from the syringe. Holding the syringe at eye level, check again to make sure you have drawn up the proper amount of diluent. Carefully remove the needle from the vial.
5. **Procedural Step.** Insert the needle into the powdered drug vial, and inject the diluent into the vial. Remove the needle from the vial, and replace the needle guard.

Inject the diluent into the vial.

6. **Procedural Step.** Roll the vial between the hands to mix the powdered drug and liquid (unless indicated otherwise by the drug package insert). *Principle.* Shaking the vial may cause air bubbles to form.

Roll the vial between the hands.

7. **Procedural Step.** Label multiple-dose vials with the date of preparation and your initials.
8. **Procedural Step.** Administer the injection.
9. **Procedural Step.** Store multiple-dose vials as indicated by the manufacturer's instructions. Because reconstituted drugs are stable for a short time, carefully check the date of preparation on the multiple-dose vial before administering the medication again.

PROCEDURE 26-3

PROCEDURE 26-5   Administering an Intramuscular Injection—cont'd

Inject the medication slowly and steadily.

Apply gentle pressure to the injection site.

10. **Procedural Step.** Place a gauze pad gently over the injection site and remove the needle quickly, keeping it at the same angle as for insertion.
Principle. Withdrawing the needle quickly and at the same angle as for insertion reduces patient discomfort. Placing a gauze pad over the injection site helps prevent tissue movement as the needle is withdrawn, also reducing patient discomfort. Using a gauze pad prevents a stinging sensation from the alcohol.

11. **Procedural Step.** Apply gentle pressure to the injection site with a gauze pad. If you are using a safety syringe with a shield, activate the safety feature at this time by following the steps outlined in Figure 26-10.
Principle. Gentle pressure helps distribute the medication so that it is absorbed by the muscle tissue. Avoid vigorous massaging because this could damage underlying tissues.

12. **Procedural Step.** Properly dispose of the needle and syringe in a biohazard sharps container.
Principle. Proper disposal is required by the OSHA standard to prevent accidental needlestick injuries.

13. **Procedural Step.** Remove the gloves, and sanitize your hands.

14. **Procedural Step.** Chart the procedure in the patient's medical record.

a. *Paper-based patient record:* Record the date and time, the name of the medication, the manufacturer and lot number, the dose given, the route of administration, the injection site used, and any significant observations or patient reactions (refer to the PPR charting example).

PPR CHARTING EXAMPLE

Date	
2/20/XX	9:30 a.m. Rocephin (Hoffmann-LaRoche, Lot #: U6261). Admin 1 gram, IM, (L) dorsogluteal. Tolerated injection well.————————— T. Cline, CMA (AAMA)

b. *Electronic medical record:* Document the name of the medication, the manufacturer and lot number, the dose given, the route of administration, the injection site used, and any significant observations or patient reactions, using the appropriate radio buttons, drop-down menus, and free text fields.
Principle. The lot number indicates the batch in which the medication was made. Should a problem arise with that batch, the drug can be recalled, and individuals who received it can be identified.

15. **Procedural Step.** Stay with the patient to ensure he or she is not experiencing any unusual reactions. If the patient experiences an unusual reaction, notify the physician immediately.

PROCEDURE 26-6 Z-Track Intramuscular Injection Technique

Outcome Administer an intramuscular injection using the Z-track method

Equipment/Supplies

- Medication ordered by the physician
- Medication order
- Appropriate needle and syringe
- Antiseptic wipe
- Disposable gloves
- Biohazard sharps container

1. **Procedural Step.** Follow steps 1 through 5 of Procedure 26-5.
2. **Procedural Step.** Apply gloves, and remove the needle guard. With the nondominant hand, pull the skin away laterally from the injection site approximately 1 to 1½ inches.
3. **Procedural Step.** Insert the needle quickly and smoothly at a 90-degree angle.
4. **Procedural Step.** Aspirate for 5 to 10 seconds to determine whether the needle is in a blood vessel. If blood appears, withdraw the needle and discard the needle and syringe. Prepare another injection and begin again.
5. **Procedural Step.** Inject the medication slowly and steadily.
6. **Procedural Step.** After injecting the medication, wait 10 seconds before withdrawing the needle to allow initial absorption of the medication.
7. **Procedural Step.** Withdraw the needle quickly, keeping it at the same angle as for insertion.
8. **Procedural Step.** Release the traction on the skin to seal off the needle track; doing so prevents the medication from reaching the subcutaneous tissue and skin surface.
9. **Procedural Step.** Do not apply pressure to the site because this could cause the medication to seep out.
10. **Procedural Step.** If you are using a safety syringe with a shield, activate the safety feature at this time by following the steps outlined in Figure 26-10.
11. **Procedural Step.** Properly dispose of the needle and syringe in a biohazard sharps container.

12. **Procedural Step.** Remove your gloves, and sanitize your hands.
13. **Procedural Step.** Chart the procedure in the patient's medical record.
    a. *Paper-based patient record:* Record the date and time, the name of the medication, the manufacturer and lot number, the dose given, the route of administration, the injection site used, and any significant observations or patient reactions (refer to the PPR charting example).

PPR CHARTING EXAMPLE

Date	
2/20/XX	10:30 a.m. Iron dextran (Watson Pharmaceuticals, Lot #: 1445). Admin 100 mg, IM, Z-track into Ⓡ dorsogluteal. No complaints of discomfort. —————————————— T. Cline, CMA (AAMA)

    b. *Electronic medical record:* Document the name of the medication, the manufacturer and lot number, the dose given, the route of administration, the injection site used, and any significant observations or patient reactions using the appropriate radio buttons, drop-down menus, and free text fields.
14. **Procedural Step.** Stay with the patient to ensure he or she is not experiencing any unusual reactions. If the patient experiences an unusual reaction, notify the physician immediately.

PROCEDURE 26-6

TUBERCULIN SKIN TESTING

TUBERCULOSIS

Tuberculosis (TB) is an infectious bacterial disease that can occur in almost any part of the body but usually attacks the lungs. Tuberculosis affecting the lungs is known as *pulmonary tuberculosis,* whereas tuberculosis occurring in other parts of the body is known as *extrapulmonary tuberculosis* and is most apt to occur in the brain, spine, kidneys, bones, and joints. The name of the bacterium that causes tuberculosis is *Mycobacterium tuberculosis,* which is a rod-shaped bacterium. Shortly (within weeks) after infection, a small percentage of individuals infected with TB bacteria develop active pulmonary tuberculosis. In these individuals, the TB bacteria are able to overcome the body's defense system. This is most apt to occur in young children and individuals with a weakened immune system. The TB bacteria then begin to multiply and attack the body, resulting in the destruction of tissue.

Symptoms of active pulmonary tuberculosis include a chronic cough lasting 3 weeks or longer that produces a mucopurulent sputum, occasional hemoptysis (coughing up blood), and chest pain. Systemic symptoms include fatigue, loss of appetite, weakness, unexplained weight loss, chills, low-grade fever, and sweating at night. If active tuberculosis is left untreated, it can result in serious complications such as permanent lung damage and even death.

Most people (90%) infected with the TB bacterium do not develop the active disease because their body defenses protect them. Body defenses may be able to destroy the TB bacteria immediately after they enter the body and completely clear them from the body. If this is not possible, the TB bacteria are engulfed by white blood cells known as macrophages. The body then builds a fibrous wall of tissue around these macrophages (infected with TB bacteria) to encapsulate them. Some of the TB bacteria may remain alive inside the capsule in a dormant or inactive state. During this time, the individual experiences no symptoms and cannot spread the disease to others. Individuals are said to have a latent tuberculosis infection (LTBI), and the only sign indicating that they have been infected with tuberculosis is a positive reaction to a TB test.

Individuals with latent tuberculosis may go on to develop active tuberculosis. This occurs in approximately 10% of individuals with LTBI. About half of these individuals develop active tuberculosis within 2 years after the initial infection, and the other half develop tuberculosis many years, even decades, after having become infected. The TB bacteria break out of the capsule and cause the symptoms of active tuberculosis (described previously). The development of LTBI into active tuberculosis is most apt to occur when the body's immune system is weakened, such as during a serious illness, or in patients who have an immune disorder such as human immunodeficiency virus (HIV) infection. The difference between active tuberculosis and latent tuberculosis is outlined in Table 26-6.

PURPOSE OF TUBERCULIN SKIN TESTING

The purpose of tuberculin skin testing is to identify individuals who are infected with *M. tuberculosis.* Early identification of individuals with active infectious tuberculosis leads to early treatment and prevents the spread of tuberculosis.

A TST is recommended for individuals who are at higher risk for tuberculosis exposure or infection, or at higher risk for progressing from latent tuberculosis to active tuberculosis. Examples include individuals who have close day-to-day contact with someone with active tuberculosis, individuals who have immigrated from a country with a high incidence of TB, and individuals who work or reside in facilities or institutions with people who are at high risk for TB (e.g.,

Table 26-6 Differences Between Active and Latent Tuberculosis (TB)		
Characteristics	**Active TB**	**Latent TB**
Symptoms	Patient usually feels sick and has symptoms of TB such as cough, fever, and weight loss.	Patient feels fine and has no symptoms.
TB bacterial status	Active TB bacteria are present in the body.	TB bacteria are present in the body that are alive but inactive.
TB test results	Patient usually has a positive TST or QFT-G blood test result.	Patient usually has a positive TST or QFT-G blood test result.
Diagnostic tests	Patient may have an abnormal chest radiograph and a positive sputum test result.	Patient has a normal chest radiograph and a negative sputum test result.
Ability to infect others	Patient is infectious and may spread the disease to others.	Patient is not infectious and cannot spread the TB to others.
Treatment	Patient needs treatment for active TB.	Physician may consider treatment for latent TB to prevent active TB disease.

QFT-G, QuantiFERON-TB Gold; *TST,* tuberculin skin testing.

hospitals and other health care facilities, correctional facilities, and nursing homes). Tuberculin skin testing may also be required as a prerequisite for employment, college entrance, entrance into the military service, and so on. A positive reaction to a TST test occurs 2 to 10 weeks after an individual is infected with tuberculosis. Because of this, a patient recently infected with TB bacteria may show a false-negative TST result and should be retested 10 weeks later.

The medical assistant is responsible for administering the TST and for reading the test results. Although tuberculin skin testing is relatively easy to perform, the procedure must be followed exactly to ensure accurate results. A patient with a tuberculous infection may fail to react to the TST if it is not performed correctly.

TUBERCULIN SKIN TEST REACTIONS

The substance used in the TST is tuberculin, which consists of a purified protein derivative (PPD) extracted from a culture of *M. tuberculosis* (the causative agent of tuberculosis), to test for sensitivity to the TB organism. The tuberculin PPD solution contains no live tuberculosis organisms and is completely harmless, making it safe to administer to people of all ages.

When introduced into the skin of an individual with an active or latent case of tuberculosis, tuberculin causes localized thickening of the skin, resulting in induration. **Induration,** which indicates a positive reaction, is an abnormally raised hardened area with clearly defined margins caused by an accumulation of small, sensitized lymphocytes (a type of white blood cell) that occurs in the area in which the tuberculin was injected into the skin (Figure 26-22). TST reactions are based on the amount of induration present and are interpreted according to the manufacturer's instructions that accompany the test.

A positive reaction to a TST indicates the presence of a tuberculous infection; however, it does not differentiate between active and latent forms of the infection. Therefore, a positive reaction warrants additional diagnostic procedures before the physician can make a final diagnosis. Other procedures used to detect an active tuberculous infection include chest x-ray and microbiologic examination and culture of the patient's sputum for TB bacteria.

MANTOUX TUBERCULIN SKIN TEST

The Mantoux TST is the most common method used for tuberculin skin testing. In the past, the Tine TST was used to screen individuals for active or latent tuberculosis. The Tine TST uses a sterile plastic unit containing four tuberculin-impregnated tines for puncturing the skin. However, most authorities believe that the Mantoux TST is more specific and accurate than the Tine TST. Because of this, the Tine TST is rarely used anymore.

The Mantoux TST is named after Charles Mantoux, the French physician who developed the test. The Mantoux TST is administered through an intradermal injection using a tuberculin syringe with a capacity of 1.0 mL and a short (⅜ to ½ inch) needle with a gauge of 26 to 27. The standard injected dose is 0.1 mL of tuberculin PPD solution containing 5 TU (tuberculin units). Brand names for Mantoux tests include Tubersol and Aplisol. Once opened, a vial of tuberculin PPD solution expires after 30 days and must be discarded. This is because oxidation and degradation of tuberculin reduce its potency, which can lead to inaccurate test results. The medical assistant should write the expiration date on the vial on opening. Before withdrawing tuberculin from the vial, the medical assistant should check both the manufacturer's expiration date and the 30-day expiration date marked by the medical assistant on the vial.

It is important to properly store the tuberculin PPD solution because it can be adversely affected by exposure to light and heat. The vial should be stored in the dark as much as possible; exposure to bright light should be avoided because this can diminish the potency of the PPD solution. A vial that has been exposed to light for an extended period of time should be discarded. The vial must be stored in the refrigerator at a temperature between 35° F to 46° F (2° C to 8° C). The vial should be returned to its refrigerated storage area as soon as possible after the proper dose has been drawn up into a syringe.

It is important that the medical assistant draw up the proper amount of tuberculin PPD solution. Injecting too much of the solution might elicit a reaction not caused by a tuberculous infection, and injecting too little of the solution results in insufficient solution being injected into the skin to elicit a reaction. This will invalidate the test because if no reaction occurs, it cannot be accepted as a negative reaction.

The medical assistant must make sure to inject the tuberculin solution into the superficial skin layers to form a tense, pale, raised area known as a **wheal.** If the injection is made into the subcutaneous layer, a wheal will not form and the test will yield a false-negative result, whereas a too-shallow injection may cause leakage of the tuberculin solution onto

Figure 26-22 Positive tuberculin skin test result. (From Nairn R: *Immunology for medical students,* ed 2, Philadelphia, 2007, Mosby.)

the skin. In either case, the medical assistant must repeat the TST at a site at least 2 inches (5 cm) away.

The medical assistant should not apply pressure to the site after injecting the tuberculin PPD solution because the solution is not intended to be absorbed into the tissues. In addition, applying pressure may cause leakage of the solution through the needle puncture site. The wheal will disappear on its own within a few minutes and should not be covered with an adhesive bandage.

Guidelines for Administering a Mantoux Tuberculin Skin Test

1. Use the anterior forearm, approximately 4 inches (10 cm) below the bend in the elbow, as the site of administration of the test. Avoid the following areas because they make the test harder to perform and interfere with good visualization and palpation of test reactions:
   - Hairy areas of the skin
   - Areas with visible veins
   - Scar tissue
   - Red or swollen areas
   - Bruised areas
   - Areas with lesions, dermatitis, or other skin irritations
   - Muscle ridges
2. Cleanse the skin thoroughly with an antiseptic wipe and allow it to dry completely before administering the test.
3. Be sure to inject the tuberculin slowly into the superficial layers of the skin. If the injection is performed correctly, a wheal should appear that is approximately 6 to 10 mm ($\frac{3}{8}$ inch) in diameter. If blood appears at the puncture site once the TST has been administered, this is not significant and will not interfere with the test. The blood can be removed by gently blotting the area with a gauze pad, making sure not to apply pressure.
4. Once the TST has been administered, the results must be read within 48 to 72 hours.

Guidelines for Reading Mantoux Tuberculin Skin Test Results

1. The TST results must be read in good lighting within 48 to 72 hours.
2. Use both inspection and palpation to read the TST results. Induration may not always be visible and therefore must be assessed through palpation.
3. If induration is present, rub your fingertip lightly from the area of normal skin (without induration) to the indurated area to assess its size. The diameter of induration must be assessed and measured transversely to the long axis of the forearm (left to right, not up and down). Measure the widest diameter of induration in millimeters using a flexible millimeter ruler. (*Note:* If you have difficulty locating the edges of the induration, the following technique will help. Take a ballpoint pen and place the tip of it on normal skin adjacent to the induration at a 45-degree angle. Then push the pen toward the indurated area. The pen will make an ink line on the normal skin

Figure 26-23 Positive tuberculin skin test showing induration and erythema. Induration is the only criterion used to determine a positive reaction. (From Abbas AK, Lichtman AH, Pillai, S: *Basic immunology functions and disorders of the immune system,* ed 4, Philadelphia, 2014, Saunders.)

and then will stop at the edge of the induration. Repeat this technique on the opposite side of the induration.
4. The extent of induration present is the only criterion used to determine a positive TST reaction (Figure 26-23). If erythema is present without induration, the results are interpreted as negative.
5. Record all reactions in millimeters to the nearest millimeter. If no induration is present, the TST results should be recorded as 0 mm. Results should never be recorded as positive or negative.
6. The interpretation of the TST test results depends on the following:
   a. Measurement (in mm) of the induration
   b. The individual's risk of being infected with tuberculosis (e.g., close contact with an individual with active TB increases the risk of being infected)
   c. The individual's risk of progression to disease if infected (e.g., HIV-infected individuals are more apt to progress from LTBI to active TB)
7. Mantoux TST results are interpreted according to the guidelines presented in Table 26-7. The procedure for administering and reading a Mantoux TST is presented in Procedure 26-7.

TWO-STEP TUBERCULIN SKIN TEST

The two-step TST is recommended by the Centers for Disease Control and Prevention (CDC) for the initial baseline testing of adults who are required to undergo periodic tuberculin skin testing. For example, most health care workers are required to have an initial TST when hired and then a yearly TST thereafter. On employment, the initial TST should consist of a baseline two-step test.

To understand the purpose of a two-step TST, it is first necessary to understand what can sometimes occur in individuals who were infected with tuberculosis many years ago.

Table 26-7 Interpretation of the Tuberculin Mantoux Skin Test*

Interpretation of the Mantoux skin test results is based on the individual's risk of being infected with tuberculosis (TB) and the risk of progression to disease if infected. Individuals with impaired immunity are more likely to have a weaker response to a tuberculin skin test. Because of this, there are three cutoff points for identifying a positive reaction to a Mantoux test.

Positive Reaction

An induration of 5 mm or more is classified as positive in individuals with the following high-risk factors for developing TB:
1. Individuals infected with HIV
2. Individuals who have had recent close contact with individuals who have active TB
3. Individuals who have fibrotic changes on a chest radiograph consistent with previously healed TB
4. Individuals who have had organ transplants
5. Individuals on immunosuppressive drug therapy (e.g., prolonged high-dose corticosteroid therapy, TNF-alpha–antagonist drug therapy [Remicade, Enbrel, Humira])

Negative Reaction

An induration of 4 mm or less

Positive Reaction

An induration of 10 mm or more is classified as positive in individuals who do not meet the aforementioned criteria but who have other risk factors for TB, including the following:
1. Individuals who inject illegal drugs
2. Individuals with the following conditions that weaken the immune system: diabetes mellitus; chronic renal failure; body weight that is 10% or more below ideal body weight; silicosis; gastrectomy; jejunoileal bypass; certain hematologic disorders such as leukemias and lymphomas; carcinoma of the head, neck, or lungs
3. Residents and employees of the following high-risk congregate settings: hospitals and other health care facilities, correctional facilities, nursing homes, homeless shelters, drug rehabilitation centers, residential facilities for patients with AIDS
4. Recent immigrants from countries with a high incidence of TB (countries in Asia, Africa, the Caribbean, Latin America, and Eastern Europe and Russia)
5. Children younger than 4 years
6. Infants, children, and adolescents exposed to adults at high risk for developing TB
7. Mycobacteriology laboratory personnel

Negative Reaction

An induration of 9 mm or less

Positive Reaction

An induration of 15 mm or more is classified as positive in individuals at low risk for developing TB, including individuals with no known risk factors for TB

Negative Reaction

An induration of 14 mm or less

AIDS, Acquired immunodeficiency syndrome; *HIV*, human immunodeficiency virus; *TNF*, tumor necrosis factor.
*The cutoff point may sometimes vary from state to state from those presented in this table.

Over a period of years, the ability of the immune system of an individual with a previous TB infection to react to the tuberculin solution may gradually diminish. When a TST is administered to such an individual, the body does not react at all or only weakly reacts, resulting in a false-negative test result. For example, a 42-year-old individual who was infected with tuberculosis during childhood may have a negative test result to an initial TST.

Administering a TST to an individual with a previous TB infection causes stimulation or "boosting" of the patient's immune system that takes place over several days after administration of the test. Basically, the first test "jogs the memory" of the immune system to recognize and react to the tuberculin. If another TST is administered after the

first TST, there is often a strong reaction to the tuberculin, resulting in a positive test result. This boosted reaction is caused by an old TB infection and should not be interpreted as a newly acquired infection. Misinterpretation could result in an unnecessary investigation to identify the source of the infection and unnecessary treatment of individuals. Although the booster effect can occur in an individual in any age group, it is most apt to occur in older individuals who were infected with tuberculosis at a younger age.

To perform a two-step TST, the medical assistant administers the Mantoux TST and instructs the patient to return to have the test result read within 48 to 72 hours as outlined in Procedure 26-7. If the TST result is positive, the individual is considered infected with TB bacteria, and further

HIGHLIGHT on Allergens

House Dust

There are many components in house dust to which an individual may be allergic; the most significant of these is the house dust mite. Dust mites thrive in warm humid conditions and feed on scales shed from human skin; they are often found in mattresses, carpets, stuffed animals, and upholstered furniture. An individual who is allergic to house dust reacts to the waste products of these dust mites.

There is no shortage of food for the dust mite because one person sheds up to 1 gram of scales per day, which is enough to feed thousands of mites for months. *Dermatophagoides pteronyssinus* and *Dermatophagoides farinae* are the most common house dust mites and are present in varying numbers in virtually every home. Mites occur in greatest numbers in bedding, particularly in mattresses; there may be 5000 mites in each gram of dust from a mattress. Sufferers often notice that symptoms become much worse when the bedding is disturbed and allergenic material becomes airborne. Practices that eliminate dust also reduce the number of dust mites in a household.

Insect Stings

It is estimated that 1 of every 125 Americans is allergic to the venom from insect stings. Approximately 40 people in the United States die each year from a severe allergic reaction to insect venom. The incidence of deaths is low because most people know they need to obtain medical attention immediately if an allergic reaction begins.

Almost all insects whose venom can cause allergic reactions belong to the order Hymenoptera, which includes honeybees and bumblebees, wasps, yellow jackets, and hornets. When a honeybee stings, its stinger remains embedded in the victim's skin, causing the bee to die as it tries to tear itself away. Wasps, yellow jackets, and hornets are more aggressive than bees and can sting repeatedly. Hornets are the most aggressive of the group and may sting even when not provoked. Yellow jackets are close behind in aggressiveness, but wasps usually sting only if someone interferes with them near their nest.

If an insect sting does not cause an allergic reaction within 30 minutes, chances are excellent that no problem will occur. A normal reaction to an insect sting includes localized pain, redness, swelling, and itching lasting 1 to 2 days. Any generalized reaction not arising directly from the area of the sting is almost certain to be an anaphylactic reaction, which begins with such symptoms as sneezing, urticaria, itching, angioedema, erythema, and disorientation and progresses to difficulty in breathing, dizziness, faintness, and loss of consciousness. Medical care should be sought immediately because most fatalities occur within 2 hours after the sting. Because time is a factor, individuals who are known to have a severe allergy to insect stings are provided with an anaphylactic emergency treatment kit that contains epinephrine in a prefilled syringe and oral antihistamines. They can carry the kit with them so that treatment for a severe allergic reaction can be started as soon as possible.

Penicillin

Penicillin is a common cause of allergic drug reactions. Approximately 2% to 5% of individuals are allergic to penicillin. The reaction may be mild and completely overlooked or confused with the symptoms of the disease being treated with penicillin, or it can be more serious and take the form of severe dermatitis or an anaphylactic reaction. Death as a result of a severe anaphylactic reaction is rare, occurring in only 0.01% of patients being treated with penicillin.

Penicillin was discovered in 1929 by Sir Alexander Fleming, but it was not used as a therapeutic drug until 1940. By 1944, it was evident that some of the side effects of penicillin were allergic reactions; the first recorded death as a result of an anaphylactic reaction to penicillin occurred in 1945.

Oral administration of penicillin is safer than a penicillin injection because it has a lower frequency of severe allergic reactions. There have been only six reported deaths from oral administration of penicillin.

Approximately 95% of serious reactions occur within 1 hour after a penicillin injection. The best preventive measure is to keep the patient under direct observation for at least 30 minutes after administration of the injection. ∎

(Figure 26-27). The number of allergen extracts applied during one office visit usually ranges between 20 and 30. Pricking the skin deposits the allergens in the outer layers of the skin to allow each to react with the body tissues.

The following guidelines should be followed for skin-prick testing: The extracts should be placed on the skin in rows in a specific pattern. This, along with labeling the test sites with a felt-tipped pen, tracks the location of each extract. Only a single drop of extract should be placed on the skin; more than this amount may cause the extracts to diffuse and run together. A sterile needle should be passed through the drop, and the point should lightly lift the top layer of skin without causing bleeding. It is important to wipe the needle dry with a sterile swab between pricks to prevent one extract from mixing with the next, leading to inaccurate test results.

The maximum reaction is usually seen in 15 to 20 minutes. During this time, the test sites should be left uncovered, and the patient should be instructed not to touch them. These areas should not be wiped because this removes the allergen extract, resulting in false-negative results. The results are read (after 15 to 20 minutes) using a millimeter ruler.

An area of induration surrounded by redness and itching characterizes a positive reaction. Positive results are recorded by measuring the size of the induration in millimeters and converting it to a numeric scale based on the extent of the induration (see Table 26-8). Any redness should be ignored. See Figure 26-29 for an illustration of skin test results. If a negative or only a mild reaction occurs and the physician still suspects the presence of an allergy, the physician may order intradermal skin testing.

Intradermal Skin Testing

Intradermal skin testing is similar to skin-prick testing but is more sensitive. The number of skin tests performed during one office visit ranges from 5 to 30. Because there is a greater chance of adverse allergic reactions to intradermal skin testing, the physician often starts with skin-prick testing in individuals who are suspected of being highly allergic as determined by the medical history and results of the physical examination.

Intradermal skin testing involves the injection of a small amount (0.02 mL to 0.05 mL) of allergen extract into the superficial skin layers through the intradermal route of administration (see Figure 26-28). A tuberculin syringe is used to administer the test, and the allergen extract is injected until a wheal forms (see Procedure 26-7). After 15 to 20 minutes, the test sites are observed for reactions. Positive reactions are characterized by an area of induration surrounded by redness and itching. As with skin-prick testing, positive results are recorded by measuring the size of the induration in millimeters and converting it to a numeric scale based on the amount of induration present (Figure 26-29; see Table 26-8).

In Vitro Allergy Blood Testing

An in vitro allergy blood test measures the amount of IgE antibodies in the blood that respond to common allergens. Examples of in vitro blood tests include enzyme-linked immunosorbent assay (ELISA), the radioallergosorbent test (RAST), and ImmunoCAP. For an in vitro allergy blood test, a sample of the patient's blood is sent to an outside laboratory, where it is exposed to allergens suspected of causing an allergic reaction in that patient. A detection device is used to measure the level of IgE antibodies that respond to each allergen being tested, and the results are reported as a numeric value. An elevated level of IgE antibodies responding to an allergen indicates the patient is allergic to that allergen.

Figure 26-27 Skin-prick testing. Skin-prick testing involves the application of numerous allergen extracts to the skin, followed by the pricking of each with a sterile needle.

Figure 26-28 Intradermal skin testing. Intradermal testing involves the injection of a small amount of allergen extract into the superficial skin layers through the intradermal route of administration.

| NEG | ±1 | +1 | +2 | +3 | +4 |

Figure 26-29 Skin-prick and intradermal skin test results. (Copyright and courtesy Hollister-Stier, Spokane, Wash.)

Advantages of the in vitro blood test over direct skin testing are as follows: The results are not affected by medication (e.g., antihistamines); there is no danger of adverse allergic reactions because the test is performed in vitro, meaning outside the body; and in vitro blood testing can be performed on patients who have skin eruptions and are unable to undergo direct skin testing because of the lack of an intact skin surface area. In vitro blood testing is expensive, however, and does not provide immediate test results, which are available with direct skin testing. Blood testing is often used to test for allergies when it is not possible to perform skin testing. These situations include the following:

1. The physician does not want the patient to be taken off of a medication that interferes with skin test results.
2. The physician suspects that skin testing could result in an anaphylactic reaction in that patient.
3. The patient has a severe skin condition such as widespread dermatitis.
4. The skin testing may be difficult to perform, as in a child younger than 4 years.

PROCEDURE 26-7   Administering an Intradermal Injection

Outcome Administer an intradermal injection and read the test results

Equipment/Supplies

- Skin test solution ordered by the physician
- Medication order
- Appropriate needle and syringe
- Antiseptic wipe
- Sterile 2 × 2 gauze pad
- Disposable gloves
- Millimeter ruler
- Tuberculosis (TB) skin test record card
- Biohazard sharps container

1. **Procedural Step.** Sanitize your hands and prepare the injection (see Procedure 26-2).
2. **Procedural Step.** Greet the patient and introduce yourself. Identify the patient by full name and date of birth. Explain the procedure and purpose of the injection.
   Principle. It is crucial that no error be made in patient identity. Explain the purpose of the injection to reassure an apprehensive patient.
3. **Procedural Step.** Select an appropriate injection site. The anterior forearm and the middle of the back are recommended sites for an intradermal injection. If using the anterior forearm, position the arm on a firm surface with the palm facing upward.
   Principle. The entire area should be exposed to ensure a safe and comfortable injection.
4. **Procedural Step.** Prepare the injection site. Cleanse the area with an antiseptic wipe. Using a circular motion, start with the injection site and move outward. Do not touch the site after cleansing it.
   Principle. Using a circular motion will carry material away from the injection site. Touching the site after cleansing will contaminate it, and the cleansing process will need to be repeated.
5. **Procedural Step.** Allow the area to dry completely.
   Principle. If the area is not permitted to dry, the antiseptic may enter the tissue when the skin is pierced, resulting in irritation and patient discomfort. In addition, the antiseptic may cause a reaction that could be mistaken for a positive test response.
6. **Procedural Step.** Apply gloves, and remove the needle guard. With the nondominant hand, stretch the skin taut at the proposed site of administration. Insert the needle at a 10- to 15-degree angle (almost parallel to the skin), with the bevel upward. The needle should be inserted about ⅛ inch until the bevel of the needle just penetrates the skin. Slight resistance may be felt as the needle is inserted. No aspiration is needed.
   Principle. Gloves provide a barrier against bloodborne pathogens. Stretching the patient's skin taut will permit easier insertion of the needle. The needle should be inserted at an angle almost parallel to the skin, to ensure penetration within the dermal layer of the skin. The needle must be inserted with the bevel facing up to allow proper wheal formation. If the needle is inserted with the bevel facing down, the skin test solution will be absorbed into the underlying subcutaneous tissue, and a wheal will not form.

Insert the needle at a 10- to 15-degree angle with the bevel upward.

PROCEDURE **26-7**   **Administering an Intradermal Injection—cont'd**

7. Procedural Step. Release the stretched skin. Hold the syringe steady, and inject the skin test solution slowly and steadily by depressing the plunger until a firm, tense, pale wheal forms (approximately 6 to 10 mm in diameter). Expect to feel a certain amount of resistance as you inject the solution; this helps in indicating that the needle is properly located in the superficial skin layers rather than in the deeper subcutaneous tissue. If a wheal does not form, the test must be repeated at another site that is at least 2 inches (5 cm) from the first site. If you are using a retractable safety syringe, activate it at this time by following the steps outlined in Figure 26-10, *C*, and continue to Step 9.

Principle. Moving the syringe once the needle has entered the skin causes patient discomfort. Test results are considered reliable only if a wheal forms.

Inject the medication to form a wheal.

8. Procedural Step. Place a gauze pad gently over the injection site and remove the needle quickly and at the same angle as for insertion.

Principle. Withdrawing the needle quickly and at the angle of insertion reduces patient discomfort. The gauze pad placed over the injection site helps prevent tissue movement as the needle is withdrawn, also reducing patient discomfort.

9. Procedural Step. Do not apply pressure to the injection site. If blood appears at the injection site, blot the site lightly with a gauze pad. If you are using a safety syringe with a shield, activate the safety feature at this time by following the steps outlined in Figure 26-10.

Principle. Applying pressure may cause leakage of the testing solution through the needle puncture site, resulting in inaccurate test results.

10. Procedural Step. Properly dispose of the needle and syringe in a biohazard sharps container.

Principle. Proper disposal of the needle and syringe is required by the OSHA standard to prevent accidental needlestick injuries.

Properly dispose of the needle and syringe.

11. Procedural Step. Remove gloves and sanitize your hands.

12. Procedural Step. Stay with the patient to make sure that he or she is not experiencing any unusual reactions. The medical assistant should be especially careful and alert for any sign of a patient reaction when administering allergy skin tests. If the patient experiences an unusual reaction, notify the physician immediately.

13. Procedural Step. Perform one of the following, based on the type of skin test being administered.

Allergy Skin Tests

a. Read the test results within 20 to 30 minutes, using inspection and palpation at the site of the injection to assess the presence of and to determine the amount of induration. Interpret the skin test results according to the information outlined in Table 26-8.

b. Chart the procedure in the patient's medical record.

(1) *Paper-based patient record:* Record the date and time, the injection site used, the names of the skin tests, the skin test results, and any significant observations or patient reactions (refer to the PPR charting example).

Continued

Figure 26-30 Intravenous therapy. (From Potter PA, Perry AG: *Basic nursing: essentials for practice*, ed 7, St Louis, 2011, Mosby.)

Figure 26-31 Patient receiving intravenous therapy in an outpatient setting. (Photo by Margaret Hartshorn. Courtesy Arizona Arthritis Center [www.arthritis.arizona.edu].)

ADVANTAGES OF OUTPATIENT INTRAVENOUS THERAPY

Administration of IV therapy in an outpatient setting is growing in acceptance by patients and the medical community. IV therapy may be administered in an outpatient setting for a variety of reasons. which include the following:

- Administration of IV medication
- Replacement of fluids and electrolytes
- Administration of nutritional supplements
- Administration of blood products
- Emergency administration of IV medication and fluids

Outpatient IV therapy is more convenient for the patient and reduces medical costs through earlier discharge from the hospital or avoidance of hospitalization altogether.

Earlier Hospital Discharge

When a hospitalized patient is receiving IV therapy and requires continued therapy, it is not always necessary or cost-effective to keep the patient in the hospital. If the patient is medically stable, he or she may no longer need the careful observation and daily nursing care provided by a hospital. By receiving IV therapy in an outpatient setting, the patient can be discharged earlier. Most patients, particularly children, are more comfortable in their home environment, which often contributes to faster healing. An example of this is a hospitalized patient with an infection who still needs IV antibiotic therapy but no longer needs to be hospitalized and who receives the therapy at an infusion clinic.

Avoidance of Hospitalization

Outpatient IV therapy provides an alternative to patients with an acute or chronic illness that requires IV therapy. Patients who do not require hospitalization for their condition are able to obtain their IV therapy in an outpatient setting. This allows patients the option of being able to continue their daily routine without major interruptions and provides them with greater independence and control over their condition. An example of this is a patient with rheumatoid arthritis who needs IV infliximab (Remicade) therapy and receives that therapy at the rheumatology medical office.

MEDICAL OFFICE–BASED INTRAVENOUS THERAPY

Some medical offices provide outpatient IV therapy. Outpatient IV therapy may be provided in an oncology office for the administration of IV chemotherapy. **Chemotherapy** refers to the treatment of cancer using antineoplastic medications. With the advent of newer rheumatology medications that must be given intravenously, some rheumatology offices have started to provide this service. There are distinct advantages to medical office–based IV therapy. It allows the physician to provide closer monitoring of a patient's response to the IV therapy and any adverse reactions exhibited by the patient. These benefits have prompted more physicians to consider office-based IV therapy.

Based on the potential future growth of IV therapy in the medical office and the current growth of other IV outpatient settings, such as infusion clinics and the patient's home, there is a need for medical assistants to acquire some basic knowledge in IV therapy. The medical assistant is often responsible for scheduling IV therapy and providing the patient with IV therapy instructions and information, such as the length of time required for the therapy. In addition, patients may have questions that the medical assistant may need to answer (or refer to the proper individual for answering) regarding their outpatient IV therapy. The entry-level medical assistant should be familiar with the basic theory of outpatient IV therapy, which is presented here.

Advanced IV theory and initiating, maintaining, and discontinuing IV therapy are not entry-level medical assisting competencies and are not addressed in this text. Certain requirements must be met before the medical assistant can perform IV therapy in the medical office. The medical assistant first should check the laws of his or her state to determine whether it is legally permissible for the medical assistant to perform this procedure. The medical assistant must acquire the proper training (theory and skills) by completing a recognized IV therapy training program, including supervised clinical practice. Although the IV procedure can appear simple when performed by an expert, it is a difficult skill that requires considerable practice to perfect.

INDICATIONS FOR OUTPATIENT INTRAVENOUS THERAPY

Outpatient IV therapy has been shown to be a safe and effective alternative to inpatient IV therapy for the treatment of certain conditions. Before prescribing outpatient IV therapy, the physician assesses the need for the therapy by determining whether the following criteria are met: The patient's condition warrants the use of IV therapy, no alternative routes are feasible or appropriate to deliver the therapy, and the patient does not need to be hospitalized to receive the IV therapy. After determining the need for outpatient IV therapy, the physician prescribes the appropriate medication or fluid and treatment plan, orders laboratory tests to monitor the patient's progress, and assesses the patient after the IV therapy.

Scheduling the Intravenous Therapy

If the patient receives the IV therapy at an outpatient site other than the medical office (e.g., an infusion clinic), the medical assistant may be responsible for scheduling the necessary services and providing the patient with IV therapy instructions, such as the length of time required for the therapy, any dietary restrictions, whether to wear loose-fitting comfortable clothing, and whether someone needs to transport the patient to and from the appointment.

Medical Office Guidelines

Medical offices that provide IV therapy on-site usually set up a special room to deliver the therapy, which often includes a lounge chair to provide for patient comfort during the therapy. With office-based IV therapy, the entry-level medical assistant is responsible for scheduling the IV therapy and providing the patient with the IV therapy instructions listed previously. The medical office employs an IV practitioner, such as a nurse or a specially trained medical assistant, to initiate, maintain, and discontinue the IV therapy. This practitioner must be completely familiar with all aspects of the IV therapy, including indications and uses, actions, dose and rate of infusion, incompatibilities, contraindications and precautions, antidote, and adverse effects. During the IV therapy, the practitioner must monitor carefully the patient's response to the therapy and be alert for adverse or allergic reactions. After the therapy is completed, the IV practitioner provides the patient with follow-up instructions, such as information on normal side effects that may occur when the patient returns home and any adverse reactions that need to be reported to the medical office.

What Would You Do? What Would You *Not* Do? RESPONSES

Case Study 1
Page 619

What Did Theresa Do?
❑ Asked Mrs. Okasinski what pharmacy she uses. Called the pharmacy and ask them to fax a copy of her medications to the medical office. Used the information from the pharmacy and the Product Identification section of the PDR to identify Mrs. Okasinski's medications.
❑ Documented the medications in her medical record for the physician to review.
❑ Explained to Mrs. Okasinski that when she has her prescriptions filled, she should request nonchildproof containers so that she will be able to use the original containers, which have the name and prescription information on them. This will make it easier to tell her medications apart.
❑ After the physician was finished with Mrs. Okasinski, made a list of all the medications she would be taking based on the physician's orders. Went over each medication with Mrs. Okasinski, and gave her a copy of the medication list to keep as a reference.

What Did Theresa Not Do?
❑ Did not criticize Mrs. Okasinski for taking her medications out of their original containers.

Case Study 2
Page 643

What Did Theresa Do?
❑ Explained to Mrs. Cardwell that for the infection to be completely eliminated from Rachel's body, she needed to be given all of the medication.
❑ Stressed to Mrs. Cardwell that medication prescribed to one person should never be given to someone else because it might cause him or her to have a bad reaction.
❑ Explained to Mrs. Cardwell that if side effects of medication ever occur, it is important to call the medical office for information on what to do.
❑ Told Mrs. Cardwell that Rachel needs to be seen by the doctor again, and scheduled an appointment for her. Asked if any other family members needed an appointment with the doctor.

Continued

What Would You Do? | What Would You *Not* Do? | RESPONSES—cont'd

What Did Theresa **Not** *Do?*
- ❏ Did not tell Mrs. Cardwell that she should have known better than to give Rachel's antibiotic to the other family members.

Case Study 3
Page 656

What Did Theresa Do?
- ❏ Explained to Danielle that if the injection were given in her arm, it would not be absorbed very well and she might not get better.

- ❏ Explained to Danielle that injections are given to patients every day at the office and that Danielle does not need to be embarrassed.
- ❏ Told Danielle that she would be draped extra well and that it would only take a minute to give the injection.

What Did Theresa **Not** *Do?*
- ❏ Did not disregard Danielle's concerns.
- ❏ Did not give the injection in the deltoid.

↻ TERMINOLOGY REVIEW

Key Term	Word Parts	Definition
Adverse reaction		An unintended and undesirable effect produced by a drug.
Allergen		A substance that is capable of causing an allergic reaction.
Allergy		An abnormal hypersensitivity of the body to substances that are ordinarily harmless.
Ampule		A small sealed glass container that holds a single dose of medication.
Anaphylactic reaction		A serious allergic reaction that requires immediate treatment.
Chemotherapy	*chem/o-:* chemical *-therapy:* treatment	The use of chemicals to treat disease. The term *chemotherapy* is most often used to refer to the treatment of cancer using antineoplastic medications.
Controlled drug		A drug that has restrictions placed on it by the federal government because of its potential for abuse.
Conversion		Changing from one system of measurement to another.
Cubic centimeter		The amount of space occupied by 1 milliliter (1 mL = 1 cc).
DEA number		A registration number assigned to physicians by the Drug Enforcement Administration for prescribing or dispensing controlled drugs.
Dose		The quantity of a drug to be administered at one time.
Drug		A chemical used for the treatment, prevention, or diagnosis of disease.
Enteral nutrition	*enter/o:* intestines *-al:* pertaining to	The delivery of nutrients through a tube inserted into the gastrointestinal tract.
Gauge		The diameter of the lumen of a needle used to administer medication.
Hemophilia	*hem/o:* blood *-philia:* love	An inherited bleeding disorder caused by a deficiency of a clotting factor needed for proper coagulation of the blood.
Immune globulin		A blood product consisting of pooled human plasma containing antibodies.
Induration		An abnormally raised, hardened area of the skin with clearly defined margins.
Infusion		The administration of fluids, medications, or nutrients into a vein.
Inhalation administration		The administration of medication by way of air or other vapor being drawn into the lungs.
Inscription		The part of a prescription that indicates the name of the drug and the drug dosage.

↻ TERMINOLOGY REVIEW—cont'd

Key Term	Word Parts	Definition
Intradermal injection	*intra-:* within *derm/o:* skin *-al:* pertaining to	Introduction of medication into the dermal layer of the skin.
Intramuscular injection	*intra-:* within *muscul/o:* muscle *-ar:* pertaining to	Introduction of medication into the muscular layer of the body.
Intravenous (IV) therapy	*intra-:* within *ven/o:* vein *-ous:* pertaining to	The administration of a liquid agent directly into a patient's vein, where it is distributed throughout the body by way of the circulatory system.
Oral administration		Administration of medication by mouth.
Parenteral		Administration of medication by injection.
Pharmacology	*pharmac/o:* drugs *-ology:* study of	The study of drugs.
Prescription		A physician's order authorizing the dispensing of a drug by a pharmacist.
Signatura		The part of a prescription that indicates the information to print on the medication label.
Subcutaneous injection	*sub-:* under, below *cutane/o:* skin *-ous:* pertaining to	Introduction of medication beneath the skin, into the subcutaneous or fatty layer of the body.
Sublingual administration	*sub-:* under, below *lingu/o:* tongue *-al:* pertaining to	Administration of medication by placing it under the tongue, where it dissolves and is absorbed through the mucous membrane.
Subscription	*sub-:* under, below	The part of the prescription that gives directions to the pharmacist and usually designates the number of doses to be dispensed.
Superscription	*super-:* over, above	The part of a prescription consisting of the abbreviation (from the Latin word *recipe,* meaning "take").
Topical administration		Application of a drug to a particular spot, usually for a local action.
Transfusion	*trans-:* through, across	The administration of whole blood or blood products by the intravenous route.
Vial		A closed glass container with a rubber stopper that holds medication.
Wheal		A tense, pale, raised area of the skin.

ON THE WEB

For information on pharmacology:

Food and Drug Administration: www.fda.gov

Drug Enforcement Administration: www.justice.gov/dea

RxList: The Internet Drug Index: www.rxlist.com

Drug Topics: drugtopics.modemmedicine.com

Medline Plus: www.nlm.nih.gov/medlineplus

Health Square: www.healthcentral.com/medications

For information on alcohol and drug abuse:

Alcoholics Anonymous (AA): www.aa.org

National Institute on Alcohol Abuse and Alcoholism (NIAAA): www.niaaa.nih.gov

National Council on Alcoholism and Drug Dependence (NCADD): www.ncadd.org

National Institute on Drug Abuse: www.drugabuse.gov

Substance Abuse and Mental Health Services Administration: www.samhsa.gov

Partnership for a Drug Free America: www.drugfree.org

Institute for a Drug-Free Workplace: www.drugfreeworkplace.org

Al-Anon/Alateen: www.al-anon.alateen.org

Mothers Against Drunk Driving (MADD): www.madd.org

For information on tuberculosis:

American Lung Association: www.lung.org

American Thoracic Society: www.thoracic.org

National Center for TB Prevention: www.cdc.gov/nchstp

For information on allergies:

American Academy of Allergy, Asthma, and Immunology: www.aaaai.org

National Institute of Allergy and Infectious Diseases (NIAID): www.niaid.nih.gov

Asthma and Allergy Foundation of America: www.aafa.org

Cardiopulmonary Procedures

27

Check out the Evolve site at http://evolve.elsevier.com/Bonewit/today/ to access additional interactive activities and exercises to help you study and prepare for success.

LEARNING OBJECTIVES	PROCEDURES

Electrocardiography

1. State the purpose of electrocardiography.
2. Identify each of the following components of the ECG cycle:
   - P wave
   - QRS complex
   - T wave
   - PR segment
   - ST segment
   - PR interval
   - QT interval
   - Baseline following the T wave
3. State the purpose of the standardization mark.
4. State the functions of the electrodes, amplifier, and galvanometer.
5. List the 12 leads that are included in an ECG.
6. Describe the function served by each of the following:
   - Three-channel recording
   - Interpretive electrocardiography
   - Electronic medical record connectivity
   - Teletransmission
7. Identify each of the following types of artifact, and state its causes:
   - Muscle
   - Wandering baseline
   - 60-cycle interference
   - Interrupted baseline

Record a 12-lead, three-channel electrocardiogram (ECG).

Holter Monitor Electrocardiography

8. List the reasons for applying a Holter monitor.

Cardiac Dysrhythmias

9. List the three categories of cardiac dysrhythmias.
10. State examples of cardiac dysrhythmias.

Identify cardiac dysrhythmias on a 12-lead ECG.

Pulmonary Function Testing

11. List the different pulmonary function tests.
12. List indications for performing spirometry testing.
13. Describe patient preparation for spirometry.
14. Explain the purpose of postbronchodilator spirometry.

Peak Flow Measurement

15. Identify the symptoms of an asthma attack.
16. List examples of asthma triggers.
17. Explain the difference between long-term control and quick-relief asthma medications.
18. Describe the purpose of a peak flow meter.

Measure a patient's peak flow rate.

Home Oxygen Therapy
19. Explain why oxygen is needed by the body.
20. Describe what occurs when the body cannot maintain an adequate blood oxygen level.
21. Identify the conditions that may require home oxygen therapy.
22. List and describe the three common types of oxygen delivery systems.
23. List and describe the two types of devices used to administer home oxygen therapy.
24. Describe oxygen safety guidelines.

CHAPTER OUTLINE

INTRODUCTION TO ELECTROCARDIOGRAPHY
CARDIAC CYCLE
Waves
Baseline, Segments, and Intervals
Segments
Intervals
ELECTROCARDIOGRAPH PAPER
STANDARDIZATION OF THE ELECTROCARDIOGRAPH
ELECTROCARDIOGRAPH LEADS
Electrodes
Bipolar Leads
AUGMENTED LEADS
Chest Leads
PAPER SPEED
PATIENT PREPARATION
MAINTENANCE OF THE ELECTROCARDIOGRAPH
ELECTROCARDIOGRAPHIC CAPABILITIES
Three-Channel Recording Capability
Interpretive Electrocardiograph
Electronic Medical Record Connectivity
Teletransmission
ARTIFACTS
Muscle Artifact
Wandering Baseline Artifact
60-Cycle Interference Artifact
Interrupted Baseline Artifact
HOLTER MONITOR ELECTROCARDIOGRAPHY

Purpose
Digital Holter Monitor
Evaluating Results
CARDIAC DYSRHYTHMIAS
PULMONARY FUNCTION TESTS
Spirometry
Patient Preparation
Postbronchodilator Spirometry
PEAK FLOW MEASUREMENT
Asthma
Asthma Attack
Diagnosis and Treatment
Peak Flow Meter
Peak Flow Rate
Schedule of Use
Purpose of Peak Flow Measurements
Care and Maintenance
HOME OXYGEN THERAPY
Oxygen Delivery Systems
Compressed Oxygen Gas
Liquid Oxygen
Oxygen Concentrator
Oxygen Administration Devices
Nasal Cannula
Face Mask
Oxygen Safety Guidelines

KEY TERMS

amplitude (AM-pli-tood)
artifact (AR-tih-fakt)
atherosclerosis (ath-roe-skler-OH-sus)
baseline
cardiac cycle
dysrhythmia (dis-RITH-mee-ah)
ECG cycle
electrocardiogram
   (ee-LEK-troe-KAR-dee-oh-gram)

electrocardiograph
   (ee-LEK-troe-KAR-dee-oh-graf)
electrode (ee-LEK-trode)
electrolyte (ee-LEK-troe-lite)
flow rate
hypoxemia
hypoxia
interval (IN-ter-val)
ischemia (is-KEEM-ee-ah)

normal sinus rhythm
oxygen therapy
peak flow rate
segment
spirometer (spih-ROM-ih-ter)
spirometry (spih-ROM-ih-tree)
wheezing

INTRODUCTION TO ELECTROCARDIOGRAPHY

The **electrocardiograph** is an instrument used to record the electrical activity of the heart. The **electrocardiogram** (ECG) is the graphic representation of this activity. The ECG exhibits the amount of electrical activity produced by the heart and the time required for the impulse to travel through the heart.

Cardiovascular disorders can cause abnormal changes to occur on the ECG. Because of this, electrocardiography is used for the following purposes:

- To evaluate the following symptoms: chest pain, shortness of breath, dizziness, or heart palpitations
- To detect an abnormality in the heart's rate or rhythm (**dysrhythmia**)
- To detect the presence of impaired blood flow to the heart muscle known as myocardial ischemia. The term **ischemia** refers to a deficiency of blood in a body part usually caused by a blocked artery.
- To help diagnose damage to the heart caused by a myocardial infarction
- To determine the presence of hypertrophy (enlargement) of the heart
- To detect inflammation of the heart muscle (myocarditis) or the lining of the heart (pericarditis)
- To assess the effect on the heart of digitalis and other cardiac drugs
- To determine the presence of electrolyte disturbances
- To assess the progress of rheumatic fever
- To detect congenital heart defects
- Performed before surgery to assess cardiac risk during surgery
- As part of a complete physical examination

A 12-lead resting ECG cannot detect all cardiovascular disorders, nor can it always detect impending heart disease such as a myocardial infarction. An ECG is taken with the patient in a resting state and records only about 10 seconds of the heart's electrical activity. If a patient has a dysrhythmia that occurs intermittently, the abnormal heartbeat may not occur during this brief time period. A patient who experiences angina pectoris does not typically have symptoms while in a resting state, and an ECG run on such a patient may appear normal. Because of this, an ECG must be used in combination with the patient's symptoms, health history, physical examination, and other diagnostic and laboratory tests to obtain a complete assessment of cardiac functioning.

The medical assistant is frequently responsible for recording ECGs in the medical office. The medical assistant must acquire knowledge, and skill must be acquired in the following aspects of electrocardiography: preparation of the patient, operation of the electrocardiograph, identification and elimination of artifacts, and care and maintenance of the electrocardiograph.

Electrocardiographs are available in single-channel and three-channel recording formats. Because most medical

Figure 27-1 A three-channel electrocardiograph.

Putting It All Into Practice

My name is Janet Canterbury, and I work in the medical laboratory of an internal medicine office. I also run electrocardiograms, apply and remove Holter monitors, perform pulmonary function tests, and assist with cardiac stress testing.

One of my most rewarding experiences was when a young woman came into the office with severe chest pain. I immediately helped her back to an examining room. I ran an electrocardiogram, as ordered by the physician. After the physician read the electrocardiogram, he indicated the results did not look good and that the patient would have to be transported to the hospital. I went into the patient's room to comfort her. She asked me if she was going to have to go to the hospital. I replied, "Possibly." She immediately said, "No!" Then I began to explain to her how important it was to have more tests to make sure she would be alright. She finally agreed to go. After being taken to the hospital by an ambulance, she was later transferred to another hospital for a heart catheterization. A few weeks passed, and she came into the office. She hugged me and thanked me for possibly saving her life. It felt so good that I could help make a difference in a patient's life. ■

offices use a three-channel ECG, the information in this chapter focuses on the three-channel electrocardiograph (Figure 27-1).

CARDIAC CYCLE

The **cardiac cycle** represents one complete heartbeat. It consists of the contraction of the atria, the contraction of the ventricles, and the relaxation of the entire heart (as described previously). The electrocardiograph records the electrical activity that causes these events in the cardiac cycle. The **ECG cycle** is the graphic representation of the cardiac cycle (Figure 27-2).

Figure 27-2 Electrocardiogram (ECG) cycle.

WAVES

The normal ECG cycle consists of a P wave; the Q, R, and S waves (known as the *QRS complex*); and a T wave. The ECG cycle is recorded from left to right, beginning with the P wave.

P wave The P wave represents the electrical activity associated with the contraction of the atria, or *atrial depolarization.*

QRS complex The QRS complex represents the electrical activity associated with the contraction of the ventricles, or *ventricular depolarization,* and consists of the Q wave, the R wave, and the S wave. The ventricles are larger than the atria and therefore require a stronger electrical stimulus to depolarize the ventricles. That is why the R wave is taller than the P wave on the ECG graph cycle.

T wave The T wave represents the electrical recovery of the ventricles, or *ventricular repolarization.* The muscle cells are recovering in preparation for another impulse. (*Note:* Electrical recovery, known as *atrial repolarization,* follows the P wave. This repolarization occurs at the same time as ventricular depolarization [QRS complex]. Because of this, atrial repolarization is masked or hidden by the QRS complex and does not appear as a separate wave on the ECG cycle.)

U wave Occasionally a U wave follows a T wave. It is a small wave that is associated in some as yet undefined way with repolarization of the Purkinje fibers or repolarization of the papillary muscles of the heart.

BASELINE, SEGMENTS, AND INTERVALS

The flat, horizontal line that separates the various waves is known as the **baseline.** Following the U wave, the heart is at rest or *polarized.* Because no electrical activity is occurring in the heart during this time, the electrocardiograph does not have anything to record, which is why the baseline is flat.

The waves deflect either upward (positive deflection) or downward (negative deflection) from the baseline. The ECG cycle between the P wave and the T wave is divided into segments and intervals for the purpose of interpretation and analysis of the ECG by the physician. A **segment** is the portion of the ECG between two waves, and an **interval** is the length of a wave or the length of a wave with a segment.

Segments

PR segment The PR segment represents the time interval from the end of the atrial depolarization to the beginning of the ventricular depolarization. It is the time needed for the impulse to be delayed at the AV node and then travel through the bundle of His and Purkinje fibers to the ventricles.

ST segment The ST segment represents the time interval from the end of the ventricular depolarization to the beginning of repolarization of the ventricles.

Intervals

PR interval The PR interval represents the time interval from the beginning of the atrial depolarization to the beginning of the ventricular depolarization.

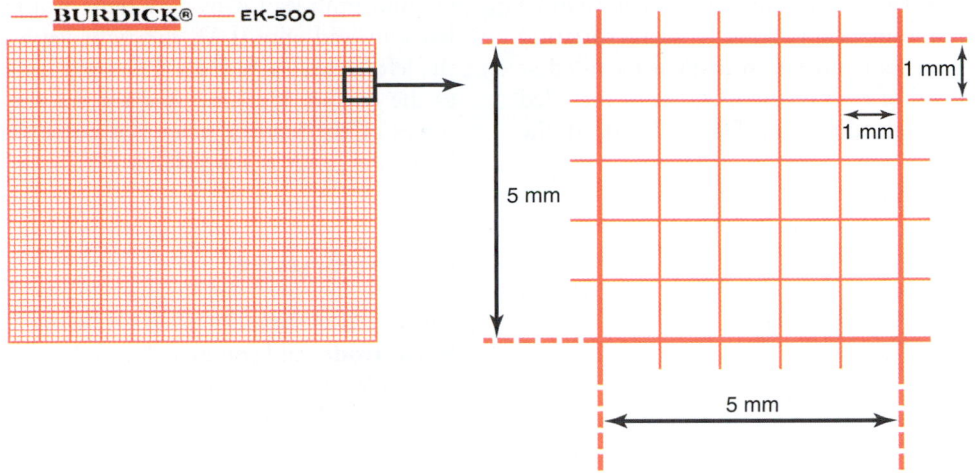

Figure 27-3 Diagram of electrocardiograph paper with a section enlarged to indicate the sizes of the large and small squares.

QT interval The QT interval is the time interval from the beginning of the ventricular depolarization to the end of repolarization of the ventricles.

Baseline The baseline after the T wave (or U wave, if present) represents the period when the entire heart returns to its resting, or polarized, state.

ELECTROCARDIOGRAPH PAPER

Electrocardiograph paper is divided into two sets of squares for the accurate and convenient manual measurement of the waves, intervals, and segments (Figure 27-3). Each small square is 1 mm high and 1 mm wide. Each large square (made up of 25 small squares) is 5 mm high and 5 mm wide. By manually measuring the various waves, intervals, and segments of the ECG graph cycle with ECG calipers or an ECG ruler, the physician is able to determine whether the electrical activity of the heart falls within normal limits. Heart disease can trigger abnormal changes in the ECG cycle, causing the results to fall outside of normal limits. For example, myocardial ischemia (often caused by coronary artery disease) can cause a depressed ST segment and an inverted T wave. A myocardial infarction can cause a larger than normal Q wave and an elevated ST segment.

Electrocardiograph paper contains a thermosensitive coating. A black or red graph is printed on top of this coating. The electrocardiograph uses a thermal print head to produce the ECG tracing. The print head has the ability to generate heat in a prescribed pattern. When the thermosensitive paper comes in contact with the heated print head, the coating turns black in the areas where it is heated, producing the ECG tracing. In addition to being heat sensitive, ECG paper is pressure sensitive and should be handled carefully to avoid making impressions that would interfere with proper reading of the ECG.

Normal Standard
Standardization mark is
10 mm high

Figure 27-4 Standardization mark.

STANDARDIZATION OF THE ELECTROCARDIOGRAPH

The electrocardiograph must be standardized, or calibrated, when an ECG is recorded. This is a quality control measure that ensures an accurate and reliable recording. It also means that an ECG run on one electrocardiograph compares in accuracy with a recording run on another machine. An ECG run on a properly calibrated electrocardiograph results in an accurate and reliable representation of the electrical activity of the patient's heart.

By international agreement, 1 millivolt (mV) of electricity should cause the stylus to move 10 mm high in **amplitude** (10 small squares). During the recording, the machine allows 1 mV to enter the electrocardiograph, which should result in an upward deflection of 10 mm. The marking that occurs on the ECG paper is known as a *standardization mark* (Figure 27-4). The width of the mark made by the machine is approximately 2 mm (two small squares). A three-channel electrocardiograph automatically records standardization marks on the ECG; a standardization mark is recorded at the beginning and end of each of the ECG strips included in the three-channel recording (see Figure 27-9). If the standardization mark is more or less than 10 mm in amplitude, the electrocardiograph must be adjusted; otherwise, the ECG recording may not be accurate. The manufacturer's operating manual must be consulted for proper adjustment information. An electrocardiograph must never be adjusted without use of the operating manual.

ELECTROCARDIOGRAPH LEADS

The standard ECG consists of 12 leads. A *lead* is a tracing of the electrical activity of the heart between two electrodes. Each lead provides an electrical "photograph" of the heart's activity from a different angle. Together, the 12 leads, or "photographs," facilitate a thorough interpretation of the heart's activity.

Ten lead wires are attached to the patient and are used to take the 12 electrical "photographs" of the heart. There are four limb lead wires: the right arm lead wire (RA), the left arm lead wire (LA), the right leg lead wire (RL), and the left leg lead wire (LL). The right leg lead wire is known as the *ground*. It is not used for the actual recording, but serves as an electrical reference point. There are six chest lead wires; each is abbreviated with a "V" and includes V_1, V_2, V_3, V_4, V_5, and V_6.

ELECTRODES

The electrical impulses given off by the heart are picked up by **electrodes** and conducted into the machine through lead wires. Electrodes are composed of a substance that is a good conductor of electricity. The electrical impulses given off by the heart are very small (0.0001 to 0.003 volt). To produce a readable ECG, they must be made larger, or amplified, by a device known as an *amplifier,* located within the electrocardiograph. The amplified voltages are changed into mechanical motion by the *galvanometer* and recorded on the electrocardiograph paper by a thermal print head (Figure 27-5).

Disposable electrodes are used to record a resting 12-lead ECG. The electrode contains a thin layer of a metallic

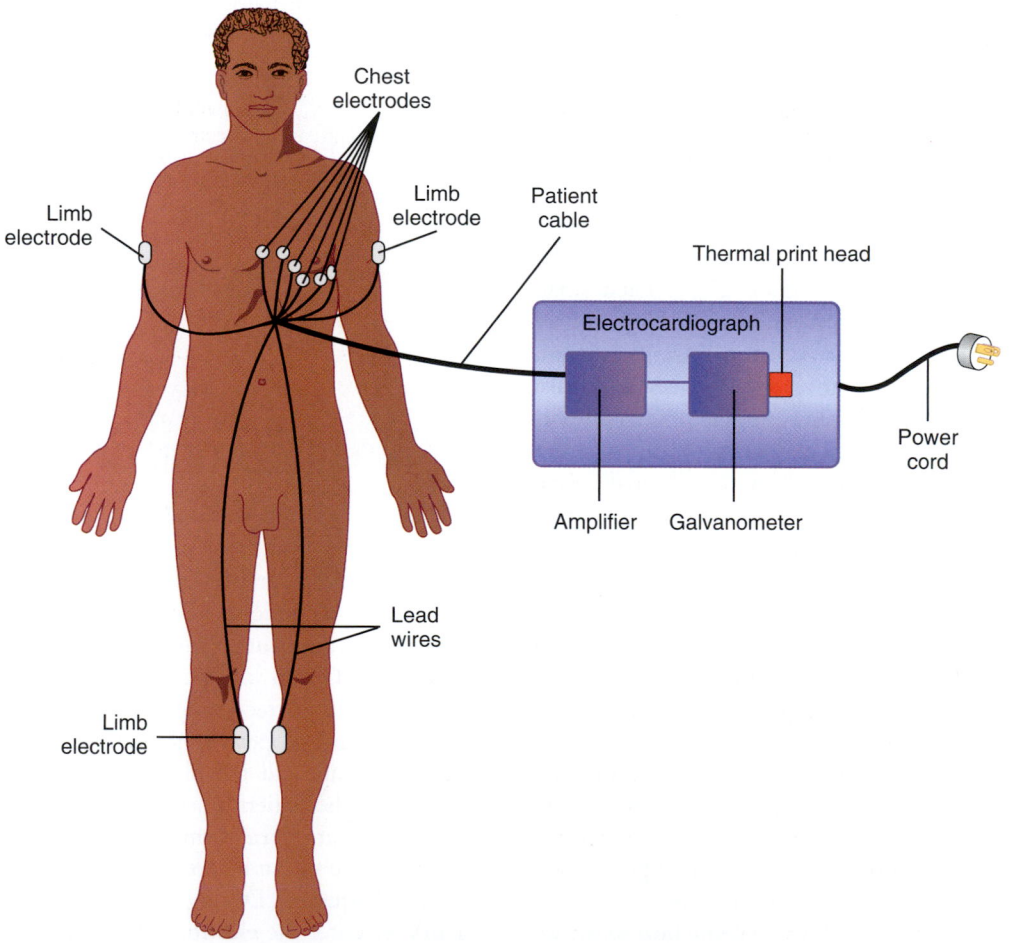

Figure 27-5 Diagram of the basic components of the electrocardiograph. The limb electrodes are attached to the fleshy parts of the limbs, and the lead wires are arranged to follow body contour. The patient cable is not dangling, and the power cord points away from the electrocardiograph.

Figure 27-6 Resting 12-lead electrocardiogram (ECG) electrodes. **A,** Disposable resting 12-lead electrode. **B,** The tab allows for attachment of the alligator clip. **C,** The back of the electrode contains an electrolyte gel combined with an adhesive. **D,** Disposable 12-lead electrodes are packaged in a foil-lined pouch and come on a card that contains 10 electrodes.

substance; this metallic substance is a good conductor of electricity. The electrode is square in shape and has a tab extending from one end (Figure 27-6, *A*). The tab allows for the firm attachment of an alligator clip (Figure 27-6, *B*).

The back of the electrode contains an electrolyte gel combined with an adhesive (Figure 27-6, *C*). An **electrolyte** is a substance that facilitates the transmission of the heart's electrical impulse. Skin is a poor conductor of electricity; therefore an electrolyte must be used when recording an ECG. The adhesive allows for firm adherence of the electrode to the patient's skin. There is no adhesive on the tab of the electrode, to allow for attachment of the alligator clip. The electrode is applied to the skin and held in place with its adhesive backing; it is thrown away after use.

Disposable 12-lead electrodes come on a card containing 10 electrodes (Figure 27-6, *D*). A foil-lined pouch is used to hold 10 cards of electrodes (or 100 electrodes per pouch). The foil-lined pouch preserves moisture to prevent the electrolyte from drying out.

Each electrode pouch (and the box containing the pouches) is stamped with an expiration date. The medical assistant must always check the expiration date of the electrodes before applying them. The electrolyte gel on

outdated electrodes may be dried out; a dried out electrolyte is unable to transmit a good ECG signal.

Electrodes are sensitive to environmental conditions and must be stored properly to prevent electrolyte drying. Electrodes should be stored in a cool area (less than 75° F or 24° C) away from sources of heat. When an electrode pouch is opened, the medical assistant should seal the pouch by folding over the end of it and then place the pouch (containing the remaining electrode cards) in a zipper-lock plastic bag to preserve moisture.

BIPOLAR LEADS

The first three leads of the 12-lead ECG are the bipolar leads; they are leads I, II, and III. The bipolar leads use two of the limb electrodes to record the heart's electrical activity. Lead I records the electric current traveling between the right arm and the left arm, lead II records the electric current traveling between the right arm and the left leg, and lead III records the electric current traveling between the left arm and the left leg (Figure 27-7).

Lead II shows the heart's rhythm more clearly than the other leads. Because of this, the physician often requests a

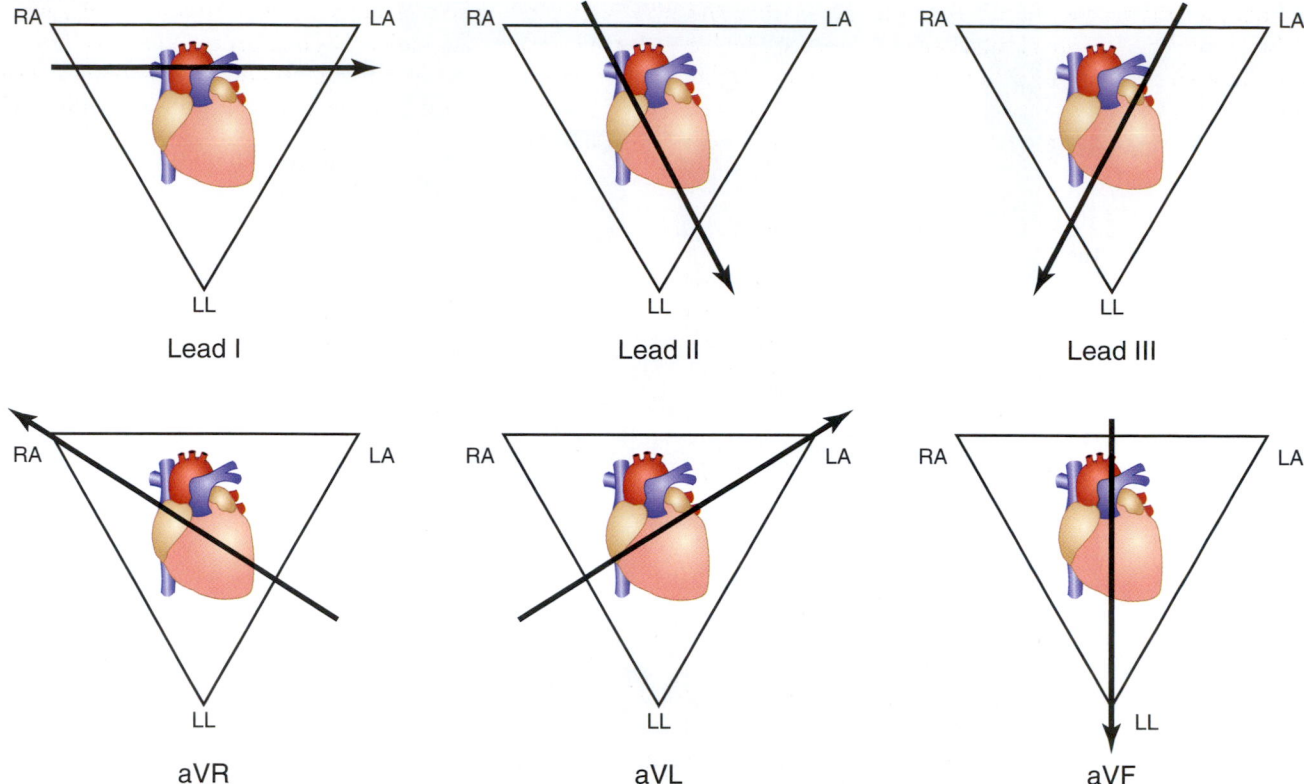

Figure 27-7 Diagram of the heart's voltage for leads I, II, III, aVR, aVL, and aVF.

rhythm strip, which is a longer recording (approximately 12 inches) of lead II (see Figure 27-9).

AUGMENTED LEADS

The next three leads are the augmented leads: aVR (augmented voltage—right arm), aVL (augmented voltage—left arm), and aVF (augmented voltage—left leg or foot). Lead aVR records the electric current traveling between the right arm electrode and a central point between the left arm and left leg. Lead aVL records the electric current traveling between the left arm electrode and a central point between the right arm and left leg. Lead aVF records the electric current traveling between the left leg electrode and a central point between the right and left arms. Leads I, II, III, aVR, aVL, and aVF provide an electrical "photograph" of the heart's activity from side to side and from the top to the bottom of the heart (see Figure 27-7).

CHEST LEADS

The last six leads are the chest, or precordial, leads(V_1, V_2, V_3, V_4, V_5, and V_6). These leads record the heart's voltage from front to back. The electric current traveling through the heart is recorded from a central point "inside" the heart to a point on the chest wall where the electrode is placed. These points correspond to the chest electrode placement sites. Figure 27-8 shows the proper location of the

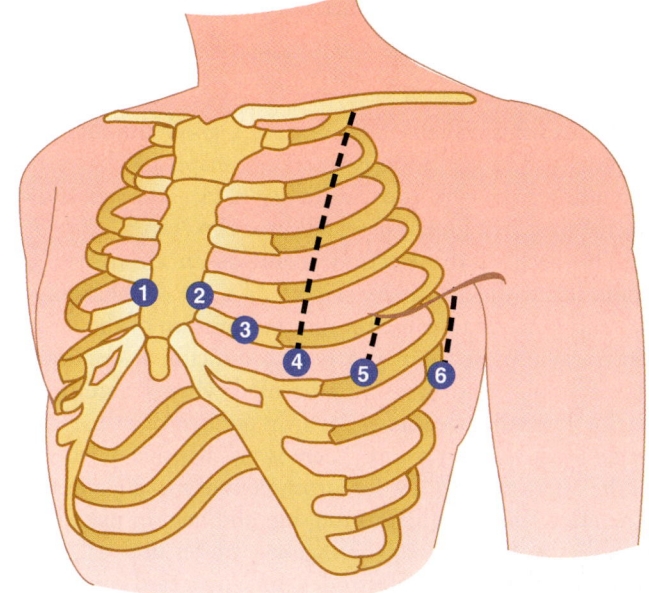

Figure 27-8 Recommended positions for electrocardiogram (ECG) chest electrodes:
1. V_1, fourth intercostal space at right margin of sternum
2. V_2, fourth intercostal space at left margin of sternum
3. V_3, midway between positions 2 and 4
4. V_4, fifth intercostal space at junction of left midclavicular line
5. V_5, at horizontal level of position 4 at left anterior axillary line
6. V_6, at horizontal level of position 4 at left midaxillary line

electrodes for the six chest leads. To ensure an accurate and reliable recording, the medical assistant must be able to locate these electrode placement sites accurately (by palpating the patient's chest). For example, if V_1 and V_2 are placed in the third intercostal spaces (instead of the fourth intercostal spaces), changes can occur to the P and T waves, which can falsely indicate heart disease. When first learning to locate the electrode sites for each chest lead, it helps to mark their locations on the patient's chest with a felt-tipped pen.

What Would You Do? | What Would You *Not* Do?

Case Study 1

Camilla Rossi is 22 years old and works at a Waffle House during the day and goes to business school at night. She comes to the office because she has been experiencing some heart problems. Over the past month, she has had three episodes of tachycardia, palpitations, trouble breathing, and profuse sweating. She is really scared that she has heart disease. Her grandfather just died from a heart attack, and she is afraid she will die next. The physician orders an ECG, but Camilla is reluctant to have the procedure. She is embarrassed about having to disrobe from the waist up, and she is worried that she will get shocked by all the wires coming out of the machine. She says that she does not have health insurance, and she does not know how she would pay for such a fancy test. She wants to know whether there is a less expensive way to find out what is wrong with her. ■

HIGHLIGHT on Cardiac Stress Testing

Description

A cardiac stress test (also known as an *exercise tolerance test* or *exercise electrocardiogram [ECG]*) is a diagnostic procedure used to evaluate the cardiovascular health of individuals with known heart disease and individuals at high risk for developing heart disease, particularly coronary artery disease (CAD). Cardiac stress testing is usually performed in a hospital under the direction of a cardiologist and a cardiac technician so that emergency equipment and trained personnel are available to deal with any unusual situations that might arise. (*Note:* A *nuclear cardiac stress test* is a type of stress test that employs the use of a radioactive material injected through an intravenous line and is described in Chapter 28.)

Purpose

The purpose of cardiac stress testing is as follows:
1. To evaluate symptoms of ischemic heart disease that cannot be assessed by a resting ECG. Ischemic heart disease occurs as a result of an inadequate blood supply to the myocardium, which is most commonly caused by atherosclerosis. **Atherosclerosis** is a condition in which fibrous plaques of fatty deposits and cholesterol build up on the inner walls of arteries. This causes narrowing and partial blockage of the lumen of these arteries, along with hardening of the arterial wall. Atherosclerosis in the coronary arteries is called *coronary artery disease.* During rest, the myocardium supplied by the partially blocked artery may receive an adequate blood supply. If the individual exercises, however, the artery may not be able to supply enough blood to the myocardium, resulting in myocardial ischemia. Myocardial ischemia can cause chest discomfort and certain abnormal changes on the ECG.
2. To assist in evaluating symptoms indicating the presence of cardiac dysrhythmias.
3. To assess the effectiveness of cardiac drug therapy.
4. To follow the course of rehabilitation after a myocardial infarction or a cardiac surgical procedure, such as a coronary bypass operation or a coronary stent placement.
5. To determine an individual's fitness level for a strenuous exercise program, such as jogging.

Patient Preparation

Patient preparation for a cardiac stress test includes the following:
1. Refrain from smoking for 4 hours before the test.
2. Avoid strenuous physical activities for 8 to 12 hours before the test.
3. Do not consume alcohol or food and beverages containing caffeine for 12 hours before the test. These substances may interfere with obtaining accurate results.
4. Do not eat or drink anything except water for 4 hours before the test. This reduces the likelihood of nausea that may accompany strenuous activity after a meal.
5. Certain cardiac medications may need to be discontinued 1 to 2 days before the test; this determination is made by the physician.
6. Wear loose, comfortable clothing and sports shoes suitable for exercising.

How the Test Works

- Cardiac stress testing involves the continuous electrocardiographic monitoring of an individual during physical exercise. During exercise, the body's need for oxygen places added demands or "stress" on the heart, making it work harder. A cardiac stress test evaluates the response of the heart to maximum or near-maximum exertion.
- A resting 12-lead ECG is usually performed before a cardiac stress test, and the results of the resting ECG are compared with the results of the cardiac stress test.

Continued

HIGHLIGHT on Cardiac Stress Testing—cont'd

- The stress test is accomplis   by having the patient use a treadmill while connected t   electrocardiograph machine through lead wires and elec   les (see illustration).
- The intensity of the physica   ertion starts with a slow warm-up walk on the tread   The speed and incline of the treadmill are gradually i   eased every 3 minutes until the patient's target heart ra   s reached. During this time the ECG is continuously displaye   n a computer screen. The patient's blood pressure, he   rate, and physical symptoms are also monitored during th   est.
- If the signs and symptoms   myocardial ischemia appear, the test is stopped. These s   otoms include severe dyspnea, chest discomfort or pain, pa   , weakness, and dizziness. The test is also stopped if tl   ECG shows abnormal changes, if a serious, irregular heartb   occurs, or if there is an abnormal change in blood r   sure.
- Once the exercising is comp   e, the patient's blood pressure, heart rate, and EC   re monitored until they return to normal.

Interpretation of Results

The patient's response to the c   ac stress test is used to determine normal or abnormal resul   A normal response is a gradual increase in the patient's bloc   pressure as physical exertion increases, whereas an abnorma   sponse is a sudden increase or decrease in the patient's blooc   essure. The ECG of a normal individual undergoing exercise e   bits a shortened PR interval and a compressed QRS complex. An abnormal tracing indicative of myocardial ischemia results in a depressed ST segment and an inverted T wave. An abnormal cardiac stress test result usually warrants further testing, such as coronary angiography, to assess the extent and severity of the heart disease. ∎

Cardiac treadmill stress test. (From deWit SC: Medical-surgical nursing: concepts and practice, St Louis, 2008, Saunders.)

PAPER SPEED

Normally, the ECG is record   with the paper moving at a speed of 25 mm/sec. Occasio   ly the ECG cycles are close together (e.g., when the he   beat is fast), making the recording difficult to read. Th   nedical assistant can change the paper speed to 50 mm/se   o spread out the cycles. To alert the physician to the char   the medical assistant must make a notation of it on the   ording.

PATIENT PREPARATION

Minimal preparation is requi   for an ECG. The medical assistant should instruct the p   ent in the following guidelines, which facilitate placeme   of the electrodes and ensure good adhesion of the electro   to the patient's skin.

1. Do not apply body lotion   l, or powder on the day of the test. This may make   nore difficult to apply the electrodes.
2. Wear comfortable clothing   d a shirt or blouse that can be removed easily.
3. Women should not wear   ll-length hosiery, such as pantyhose or tights.

MAINTENANCE OF THE ELECTROCARDIOGRAPH

Electrocardiographs require periodic maintenance. The casing of the electrocardiograph should be cleaned frequently with a soft cloth, slightly dampened with a mild detergent, to remove dust and dirt. Commercial solvents and abrasives should not be used because they can damage the finish of the casing.

The patient cables, lead wires, and power cord should be cleaned periodically with a cloth moistened with a disinfectant cleaner. The cables should never be immersed in the cleaning solution because this could damage them. Inspect the cables frequently for cracks or fraying, and replace them if needed. Check the metal tip of each lead wire for adhesive/electrolyte gel residue, which can interfere with the transmission of a good ECG signal from the electrode. Remove any residue with an alcohol wipe using pressure and friction.

The reusable alligator clips should be cleaned thoroughly with an alcohol wipe after patient use. Check the alligator clips periodically to make sure they fit snugly on the metal tip of each lead wire.

ELECTROCARDIOGRAPHIC CAPABILITIES

Electrocardiographs have a variety of capabilities that permit specific recording and transmittal options.

THREE-CHANNEL RECORDING CAPABILITY

Most medical offices use a three-channel electrocardiograph. An electrocardiograph with a three-channel recording capability can record the electrical activity of the heart through three leads simultaneously. This is in contrast to a single-channel electrocardiograph, which records only one lead at a time. The advantage of a three-channel electrocardiograph is that an ECG can be produced in less time than would be required if each lead were recorded separately.

The leads that are recorded simultaneously are leads I, II, and III; followed by aVR, aVL, and aVF; followed by V_1, V_2, and V_3; followed by V_4, V_5, and V_6. Each lead is automatically labeled by the electrocardiograph with its appropriate abbreviation.

Recording three leads at one time requires three-channel recording paper, which is designed in a standard 8½- × 11-inch format. This size printout fits easily into a paper-based medical record (PPR). Most three-channel electrocardiographs have a *copy capability* that quickly produces a duplicate copy of an ECG that has just been recorded. Some three-channel electrocardiographs have a memory storage capability in which a specified number of ECGs can be stored in the machine for later retrieval. This allows an ECG that has been misplaced to be retrieved from the electrocardiograph's memory and printed out again. Figure 27-9 is an example of a three-channel ECG recording that also includes a rhythm strip. Procedure 27-1 describes how to run a 12-lead three-channel ECG.

Figure 27-9 A three-channel electrocardiogram (ECG) with a rhythm strip.

INTERPRETIVE ELECTROCARDIOGRAPH

An electrocardiograph with interpretive capabilities has a built-in computer program that analyzes the recording as it is being run. Interpretive electrocardiographs provide immediate information on the heart's activity, leading to earlier diagnosis and treatment. Patient data are used in the interpretation of the ECG and must be entered into the electrocardiograph using a keyboard before running the recording. The data generally required are the patient's age, sex, height, weight, and medications, which are presented at the top of the recording. The computer analysis of the ECG is also printed at the top of the recording, along with the reason for each interpretation (Figure 27-10). The results are reviewed and interpreted further by the physician before a diagnosis is made and treatment is initiated.

ELECTRONIC MEDICAL RECORD CONNECTIVITY

Electronic medical record (EMR) connectivity allows the electrocardiograph to be linked with the office's computer system, either wirelessly or through a USB port. This enables a digital image of the recording to be sent from the electrocardiograph to the computer. EMR software can display the digital image of the ECG on the screen of the computer. The software also analyzes the ECG and displays this information along with the reason for each interpretation. If needed, a copy of the ECG report can be printed out on a regular sheet of paper using an inkjet or laser printer. The ECG report is reviewed and interpreted further by the physician before a diagnosis is made and treatment is initiated. The ECG report is then stored electronically in the patient's EMR.

Figure 27-10 An electrocardiogram (ECG) recording that has been analyzed by an interpretive electrocardiograph. The computer analysis is printed at the top of the recording, along with the reason for each interpretation.

TELETRANSMISSION

An ECG that has been recorded in a digital format can be transmitted electronically to an ECG data interpretation site. The recording is interpreted by a cardiologist (often along with a computer analysis) at the interpretation site, and the ECG recording and its interpretation are electronically transmitted to the sending office the same day.

ARTIFACTS

The medical assistant is responsible for producing a clear and concise ECG recording that can be read and interpreted by both a computer and the physician. Structures sometimes appear in the recording that are not natural and interfere with the normal appearance of the ECG cycles. They are known as **artifacts** and represent additional electrical activity that is picked up by the electrocardiograph. The presence of artifacts affects the quality of the recording, making it difficult to manually measure the ECG cycles. Artifacts can also sometimes cause a false-positive result on an ECG that is analyzed by a computer. The medical assistant should be able to identify artifacts and correct them. There are several types of artifacts; the most common are muscle, wandering baseline, and 60-cycle interference (also known as *AC artifacts*).

In some circumstances, as when individuals have trouble holding still or in buildings with older electrical systems, normal methods to eliminate muscle and 60-cycle interference artifacts may be unsuccessful. Electrocardiographs have an artifact filter that can reduce artifacts when all else fails. Because the artifact filter also affects the diagnostic accuracy of the ECG, it should be used as little as possible.

If the medical assistant is unable to correct an artifact, the physician should be consulted. It is possible that the machine is broken. If an electrocardiograph service technician has to be contacted, the medical assistant should have the following information available to aid the service technician in locating the problem:

1. What already has been done to locate and correct the problem
2. Leads in which the artifact occurs
3. A sample of the artifact recorded by the machine

MUSCLE ARTIFACT

A muscle artifact (Figure 27-11, *A*) can be identified by its fuzzy, irregular baseline. There are two types of muscle artifacts: those caused by involuntary muscle movement (somatic tremor) and those caused by voluntary muscle movement. Muscle artifacts may be caused by the following:

1. *An apprehensive patient.* To reduce the patient's apprehension and relax muscles, explain the procedure and reassure the patient that having an ECG recorded is a painless procedure.

2. *Patient discomfort.* Ensure that the table is wide enough to support the patient's arms and legs adequately. The patient can be made more comfortable by placing a pillow under his or her head. Check that the room temperature is comfortable for the patient. A temperature that is warm enough for the medical assistant may be too cold for the patient who has removed clothing. This could result in shivering, which also would produce a muscle artifact on the ECG.

3. *Patient movement.* The patient must be instructed to lie still and not talk during the recording.

4. *A physical condition.* Several nervous system disorders, such as Parkinson disease, prevent relaxation, and the patient trembles continually. For these individuals, it is difficult to obtain an ECG that is free of artifacts. The artifacts can be reduced, however, by asking the patient to place his or her hands under the buttocks with the palms facing downward.

WANDERING BASELINE ARTIFACT

A wandering baseline artifact (Figure 27-11, *B*) can be caused by the following:

1. *Loose electrodes.* The medical assistant should ensure that the electrodes are attached firmly to the patient's skin. A loose electrode results in poor transmission of the electrical impulse from the patient's skin to the electrode. If an electrode pulls loose, it can be reattached with hypoallergenic tape or replaced with a new electrode. The alligator clips should be attached firmly to the tabs of the electrodes. To prevent pulling of the lead wires on the electrodes, the patient cable should be well supported on the table or the patient's abdomen and should not be allowed to dangle. Pulling on the electrodes can cause the electrodes to pull away from the patient's skin.

2. *Dried-out electrolyte.* If the electrolyte gel on an electrode is dried out, the medical assistant must replace it with a new electrode. Always check the expiration date stamped on the electrode pouch (or box) to make sure the electrodes are within their expiration date.

3. *Body creams, oils, or lotions on the skin in the area where the electrode is applied.* Creams, oils, or lotions prevent good adhesion of the electrodes to the patient's skin. The medical assistant should remove these substances by rubbing with alcohol, using friction.

4. *Excessive movement of the chest wall during respiration.* The medical assistant should encourage the patient to relax and breathe more calmly, using the diaphragm rather than expanding the chest.

60-CYCLE INTERFERENCE ARTIFACT

A 60-cycle interference artifact (also known as an *AC artifact*) is caused by electrical interference. Electric current can "leak" or spread out from the power used by electrical appliances in the room in which the ECG is being run. This current may be picked up by the patient and carried into

60〜 .05-30Hz
10 mm/mv

E350i R

A

Muscle artifact

E350i Rev. 1.26 GR1 10.1

B

Wandering baseline

I   aVR   VI

C

60-cycle interference

D

Interrupted baseline

Figure 27-11 Examples of electrocardiogram (ECG) artifacts. (**D** from Long BW: *Radiography essentials for limited practice,* ed 4, St Louis, 2013, Saunders.)

the electrocardiograph, where it would show up on the ECG recording as a 60-cycle interference artifact. This type of artifact appears as small, straight, spiked lines that are consistent (Figure 27-11, *C*), causing the baseline to be thick and unreadable. A 60-cycle interference artifact can be caused by the following:

1. *Lead wires not following body contour.* Dangling lead wires can pick up electric current. Arrange the wires to follow body contour and to lie flat.
2. *Other electrical equipment in the room.* Lamps, autoclaves, electrically powered examining tables, or other electrical equipment that is plugged in may be leaking electric current. Unplug all nearby electrical equipment. (*Note:* Jewelry and watches do not interfere with the recording; therefore it is not necessary for the patient to remove these items unless they interfere with proper placement of the electrodes.)
3. *Wiring in the walls, ceilings, or floors.* Try moving the patient table away from the walls.

4. *Improper grounding of the electrocardiograph.* The machine is automatically grounded when it is plugged in. Check the three-pronged plug of the ECG machine to make sure the prongs are not loose or damaged. Ensure that the plug is securely in the wall outlet. The right leg electrode is not used for recording the leads, but it picks up electric current that has "leaked" onto the patient and carries it into the electrocardiograph. The electric current is carried away by the machine's grounding system.

INTERRUPTED BASELINE ARTIFACT

Occasionally, an interrupted baseline (Figure 27-11, *D*) occurs that may be caused by the metal tip of a lead wire becoming detached or by a frayed or broken patient cable. If the latter is the case, a new patient cable should be ordered from the manufacturer.

PROCEDURE 27-1 **Running a 12-Lead, Three-Channel Electrocardiogram**

Outcome Record a 12-lead electrocardiogram (ECG)

Equipment/Supplies

- Three-channel electrocardiograph
- Disposable electrodes
- ECG paper

1. **Procedural Step.** Work in a quiet, relaxing atmosphere away from sources of electrical interference.
2. **Procedural Step.** Sanitize your hands, and assemble the equipment. Check the expiration date of the electrodes. Greet the patient and introduce yourself. Identify the patient by full name and date of birth.
   Principle. The electrolyte gel on outdated electrodes may be dried out, which can cause artifacts on the ECG.
3. **Procedural Step.** Help the patient relax by explaining the procedure. Tell the patient that having an ECG recording is painless. Explain that he or she must lie still, breathe normally, and not talk while the ECG is being recorded so that an accurate ECG can be obtained.
   Principle. Explaining the procedure helps reassure apprehensive patients. The patient should be mentally and physically relaxed for an accurate ECG recording; an apprehensive or moving patient produces muscle artifacts. Heavy breathing or sighing can cause a wandering baseline artifact.
4. **Procedural Step.** Prepare the patient. Ask him or her to remove clothing from the waist up. The lower legs also must be uncovered. Provide a female patient with a gown, and instruct her to put it on

with the opening in front. Assist the patient into a supine position on the table. The table should support the arms and legs adequately so that they do not dangle. Properly drape the patient to prevent exposure and to provide warmth. A pillow can be used to support the patient's head.
   Principle. The chest, upper arms, and lower legs must be uncovered to allow proper placement of the electrodes. The patient should be kept warm, and the arms and legs should not be allowed to dangle; otherwise, muscle artifacts could result.
5. **Procedural Step.** Position the electrocardiograph so that the power cord points away from the patient and does not pass under the table. It is usually easier for the medical assistant to work on the left side of the patient.
   Principle. Proper positioning of the electrocardiograph reduces 60-cycle interference artifacts.
6. **Procedural Step.** Prepare the patient's skin for application of the disposable electrodes. If the patient has sweaty or oily skin or has used lotion, rub the area to which the electrode will be applied with alcohol, and allow it to dry. If the patient's chest is hairy, dry shave it at each electrode site before applying the electrode.

Continued

Principle. The patient's skin must be dry and free of oil and body hair so that the adhesive backing of the electrodes sticks to the patient's skin and stays on during the procedure.

7. **Procedural Step.** Remove a card containing 10 electrodes from its foil-lined pouch and reseal the pouch. Apply the limb electrodes. Firmly apply the adhesive backing of the electrodes to the fleshy part of each of the four limbs (upper arms and lower legs). The electrode tabs should point toward the center of the body. The tabs of the arm electrodes should point downward, and the tabs of the leg electrodes should point upward. The adhesive backing of the electrode allows it to adhere firmly to the patient's skin.

Principle. The pouch should be resealed to preserve moisture and prevent the electrolyte on the remaining electrodes from drying out. The electrodes must be firmly attached to permit good transmission of the electrical impulse from the patient's skin to the electrode. Loose electrodes can cause artifacts to occur on the recording, making it difficult to analyze the recording. The tabs of the electrodes should be positioned toward the center of the body to provide a more stable connection when the lead wire is attached to the electrode and to prevent the lead wires from pulling onto the electrodes and causing artifacts.

A, Apply the leg electrodes. **B,** Apply the arm electrodes.

8. **Procedural Step.** Apply the chest electrodes. Properly locate each electrode placement site using palpation, and apply the electrode with the tab pointing downward. Continue until all six of the chest electrodes have been applied.

Principle. Positioning the tabs of the electrodes downward prevents the lead wires from pulling and causing artifacts.

Apply the chest electrodes.

9. **Procedural Step.** Connect the lead wires to the electrodes. This is accomplished by inserting an alligator clip onto the metal tip of each lead wire. Next, firmly attach an alligator clip to the tab of each electrode. The ends of the lead wires are usually color-coded (e.g., red for the arms and green for the legs) and identified with abbreviations to help the medical assistant connect the proper lead to each electrode. Arrange the lead wires to follow body contour.

Principle. The lead wires must be attached correctly to ensure an accurate and reliable ECG. Arranging the lead wires to follow body contour reduces the possibility of 60-cycle interference artifacts.

Connect the lead wires to the electrodes.

PROCEDURE 27-1   **Running a 12-Lead, Three-Channel Electrocardiogram—cont'd**

10. **Procedural Step.** Plug the patient cable into the machine. The cable should be supported on the table or on the patient's abdomen to prevent pulling of the lead wires on the electrodes.
    Principle. Pulling of the lead wires on the electrodes can cause the electrodes to pull away from the skin, resulting in artifacts.

11. **Procedural Step.** Turn on the electrocardiograph. Enter patient data using the soft-touch keypad. Always use your fingertips to enter the data. Pencils and other sharp objects can damage the keyboard. As the data are entered, they are displayed on the liquid crystal diode (LCD) screen. Patient data to be entered typically include the patient's name, a patient identification number, age, sex, height, weight, and medications.

Enter patient data.

12. **Procedural Step.** Remind the patient to lie still, breathe normally, and not talk. Press the AUTO (automatic) button, and run the recording. The machine automatically inserts a standardization mark at the beginning of each ECG strip, followed by the recording of the 12-lead ECG in a three-channel format. Another standardization mark is inserted at the end of each ECG strip. (*Note:* With most three-channel electrocardiographs, the machine checks for a clear ECG signal after the AUTO button is pressed. If the signal is "noisy," this may indicate that an electrode does not have a good connection with the patient's skin. The machine usually indicates which electrode is causing the problem [e.g., "V₆ noisy"]. Apply firm pressure

to the electrode causing the problem. If this does not correct the problem, replace the electrode with a new one and/or place a piece of nonallergenic tape over the electrode.)

13. **Procedural Step.** After the ECG has been recorded:
    a. Check the printout to ensure that the standardization mark is 10 mm high. If it is more or less than 10 mm, adjust the standardization mark according to the manufacturer's instructions, and run another ECG.
    b. Check the direction of the R wave in lead I. If your patient's limb leads are attached correctly, the R wave on lead I should have a positive deflection. If it has a negative deflection, the limb leads are not attached correctly. Reattach the limb leads properly and run another recording.
    c. Observe the recording for artifacts. If an artifact is present, determine the cause of the artifact, correct the problem, and run another ECG.

Check the standardization mark.

14. **Procedural Step.** Inform the patient that you are finished and he or she can now talk or move. Turn the machine off. Disconnect the lead wires. Remove and discard the electrodes.

15. **Procedural Step.** Assist the patient in stepping down from the table.

16. **Procedural Step.** Sanitize your hands.

17. **Procedural Step.** Chart the procedure in the patient's medical record.
    a. *Paper-based patient record:* Record the date and time and the name of the procedure (12-lead ECG). Refer to the PPR charting example.

Continued

PROCEDURE 27-1

PPR CHARTING EXAMPLE

Date	
6/12/XX	10:30 a.m. Completed a 12-lead ECG.
	Recording to physician for review. ———
	——————— J. Canterbury, CMA (AAMA)

b. *Electronic medical record:* Document the procedure performed (12-lead ECG) using the appropriate radio buttons, drop-down menus, and free text fields.

18. **Procedural Step.** Place the recording in the appropriate place to be reviewed by the physician.

19. **Procedural Step.** Return all equipment to its proper storage place.

Figure 27-12 Digital Holter monitor.

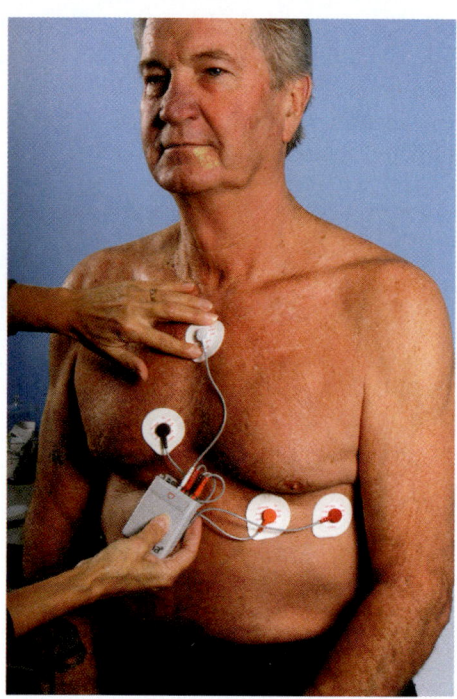

Figure 27-13 Digital Holter monitor. Electrical impulses given off by the heart are picked up by electrodes placed on the patient's chest.

HOLTER MONITOR ELECTROCARDIOGRAPHY

A Holter monitor is a portable ambulatory monitoring system for the continuous recording of the electrical activity of the heart for 24 hours or longer (Figure 27-12). The monitor is named for Dr. Norman Holter, an American biophysicist who invented this cardiac monitoring device. The original Holter monitor consisted of a large pack of equipment worn on the patient's back.

A Holter monitor is also known as an *ambulatory electrocardiographic monitor* (AEM). The purpose of a Holter monitor is to detect cardiac abnormalities that occur while the patient is engaged in his or her normal daily routine. Because of this, the Holter system is designed so that the patient is able to maintain his or her usual daily activities with minimal inconvenience while being monitored.

A Holter monitor is similar to a resting 12-lead ECG in that the electrical impulses given off by the heart are picked up by electrodes and transmitted through lead wires to a recording device (Figure 27-13). It is different from a resting 12-lead ECG in that only about 10 seconds of the heart's activity are recorded with a 12-lead ECG, whereas a Holter

monitor records the heartbeat continuously for an extended period of time. This allows the Holter monitor to pick up cardiac abnormalities that do not occur during the brief recording period of a resting 12-lead ECG.

PURPOSE

Holter monitor electrocardiography is an important noninvasive procedure used to diagnose cardiac rate, rhythm, and conduction abnormalities. Specifically, it is most frequently used for the following purposes:

- To assess the rate and rhythm of the heart during daily activities.
- To evaluate patients with unexplained chest pain, dizziness, or syncope (fainting).
- To discover intermittent cardiac dysrhythmias not picked up on a routine resting 12-lead ECG. A resting ECG

Figure 27-14 The digital Holter monitor is placed in a pouch hung around the patient's neck by a strap.

records only 40 to 50 heartbeats, whereas a Holter monitor records approximately 100,000 heartbeats in a 24-hour period.
- To detect myocardial ischemia.
- To assess the effectiveness of antidysrhythmic medications (e.g., digitalis, antianginal medications).
- To assess the effectiveness of a pacemaker.

DIGITAL HOLTER MONITOR

A digital Holter monitor is lightweight and battery powered. It uses either an external (removable) or an internal (non-removable) memory card to document the heart's activity (see Figure 27-12). The monitor can be clipped onto a belt around the patient's waist. It can also be held in a protective pouch that is hung around the patient's neck with a strap known as a *lanyard* (Figure 27-14). Digital monitors can continuously record the electrical activity of the heart for 24 hours, 48 hours, or 72 hours. Most physicians order a 24-hour recording, but they may occasionally order a 48- or 72-hour recording when the heart's activity needs to be recorded for a longer period of time. Throughout the monitoring period, the system continuously records the electrical activity of the heart and stores it on the memory card. The Holter monitor automatically stops recording after the monitoring period has been completed.

EVALUATING RESULTS

At the end of the monitoring period, the Holter monitor system is removed from the patient. The information on the memory card is then uploaded to a computer.

Specialized ECG software p orms calculations on the data and prepares an ECG sum ry report of the monitoring period, which is then di yed on the screen of the computer.

The computer-generated CG report summarizes information about the patient's rt rate and rhythm and any abnormalities that occurred ring the monitoring period. The report also includes s ted samples of the patient's cardiac activity, including tient event strips and any abnormal cardiac activity e ited by the patient, such as dysrhythmias. The results o e ECG summary report are reviewed and interpreted her by the physician. The ECG report can be printed t on regular sheets of paper with an inkjet or laser print nd stored in a PPR (patient-based paper record). It can o be stored electronically in the patient's EMR (electror medical record).

Memories *from* **Practicum**

Janet Canterbury: During my practicum, I was at an office w e electrocardiograms were one of the many cedures that were performed. For my first e trocardiogram, the patient was a man who a lot of hair on his chest, and I would need to shave the elec e placement sites on his chest. I was very nervous, but the cedure went well. When the electrocardiogram was run, he d me that I did a wonderful job and that it did not hurt at all t ve his chest shaved. I realized then that it was not so bad at all. That patient made me feel so good about what I do and lped me feel confident in the procedures I had ahead of me ■

CARDIAC DYSRHYTHMIAS

The normal ECG graph cy consists of a P wave, a QRS complex, and a T wave, wl t repeat in a regular pattern (see Figure 27-2). The term rmal sinus rhythm refers to an ECG that is within nor limits. This means that the waves, intervals, segments, l cardiac rate fall within the normal range. The normal h t rate ranges from 60 to 100 beats per minute. A rate slo than 60 beats per minute is *sinus bradycardia,* and a rate er than 100 beats per minute is *sinus tachycardia.*

Cardiac **dysrhythmia** is t term used to describe abnormal electrical activity in the rt causing an irregular heartbeat. Cardiac dysrhythmias be classified into one of the following categories: (1) a beats, (2) an abnormal rhythm, or (3) an abnorma eart rate. Cardiac dysrhythmias include atrial prematur ontraction, paroxysmal atrial tachycardia, atrial flutter, at fibrillation, premature ventricular contraction, ventricu tachycardia, and ventricular fibrillation.

PULMONARY FUNCTION TESTS

The purpose of a pulmonary function test (PFT) is to assess lung functioning, assisting in the detection and evaluation of pulmonary disease. Pulmonary function tests include spirometry, lung volumes, diffusion capacity, arterial blood gas studies, pulse oximetry, peak flow measurement, and cardiopulmonary exercise tests. The most frequently performed pulmonary function test is spirometry, which is described in the next section.

SPIROMETRY

Spirometry is a simple, noninvasive screening test that is often performed in the medical office. A computerized electronic instrument known as a **spirometer** is used to conduct the test (Figure 27-15). A spirometer measures how much air is pushed out of the lungs and how fast it is pushed out. The spirometry report is printed out as a table and graph. Spirometry is considered a screening test, and abnormal test results require that the patient undergo additional pulmonary function tests and possibly a computed tomography scan before a diagnosis can be made. Indications for performing spirometry include the following:

1. Patients who exhibit symptoms of lung dysfunction such as dyspnea
2. Individuals at high risk for lung disease because of smoking or exposure to environmental pollutants such as coal dust, asbestos, and exhaust fumes
3. Patients with lung disease, such as asthma, chronic bronchitis, and emphysema
4. Patients who are to undergo surgery (to assess probable lung performance during an operation)
5. Patients who need to be evaluated for lung disability or impairment for a compensation program (e.g., coal miners)

Figure 27-15 Spirometer.

Patient Preparation

Patient preparation is essential to obtain accurate test results. To prepare for the test, the patient should be instructed to do the following:

1. Do not eat a heavy meal for 8 hours before the test. (The patient must exert the diaphragm muscles, and a full stomach may interfere with this action.)
2. Stop smoking at least 8 hours before the test.
3. Do not take bronchodilators for 4 hours before the test.
4. Do not engage in strenuous activity for 4 hours before the test.
5. Wear loose, nonrestrictive clothing to keep the chest area as free as possible, which makes it easier to perform the breathing maneuver.

POSTBRONCHODILATOR SPIROMETRY

If the results of the spirometry test indicate a possible obstruction, the physician usually orders a postbronchodilator spirometry test. This test is performed by having the patient inhale a bronchodilator and running a spirometry test approximately 10 to 15 minutes later. The purpose of this test is to inform the physician as to how treatment would work in patients whose airways are obstructed.

What Would You Do? | **What Would You *Not* Do?**

Case Study 2

Joel Matthews, 48 years old, is at the office for a biannual checkup. Joel had a mild heart attack 2 years ago. Since then, he has completely changed his life. He's become a vegetarian and practices yoga every morning before going to work. After he gets home, he jogs 10 miles. He also lifts weights every other day and takes herbal vitamin supplements. Since his heart attack, he has lost 40 pounds and says that he has never felt better. The only thing he cannot seem to do is give up smoking. He started smoking when he was 17 years old and has cut back from two packs to one pack a day. He keeps trying to stop but says that he has been smoking so long that it might not be possible. Besides, with all the other healthy stuff he is doing, he thinks it probably cancels out the bad effects of the cigarettes. Joel is very concerned that if he does stop smoking, he will gain back all of the weight that it took him so long to lose. ■

PEAK FLOW MEASUREMENT
ASTHMA

Asthma is a chronic lung disease that affects the smaller bronchi and the bronchioles of the lungs.

Asthma can occur at any age but is more common in children and young adults. Asthma affects boys more

HIGHLIGHT on Smoking and Chronic Obstructive Pulmonary Disease (COPD)

COPD Defined

COPD is a chronic airway obstruction that results from emphysema or chronic bronchitis or a combination of these conditions. COPD is a chronic, debilitating, irreversible, and sometimes fatal disease.

More than 12 million Americans have been diagnosed with COPD; however, it is estimated that an additional 12 million Americans have the disease and remain undiagnosed. Smoking tobacco is the primary cause of COPD. In the United States, approximately 85% to 90% of deaths from COPD are caused by smoking. According to the American Lung Association, COPD is the fourth leading cause of death in the United States, behind heart disease, cancer, and stroke. COPD claims the lives of more than 120,000 Americans each year.

Emphysema

Emphysema is most often seen in older individuals with a long history of smoking. Emphysema due to smoking is caused by irreversible damage to the alveoli in the lungs from toxins present in cigarette smoke (see illustration). As alveoli continue to be damaged, the lungs are able to transfer less and less oxygen to the bloodstream. In addition, air becomes trapped in the damaged alveoli, making it difficult to remove during exhalation. Because of this, the primary symptom of emphysema is shortness of breath. Other symptoms include chronic cough, tiredness, and limited exercise tolerance. Close to 4 million people in the United States currently have been diagnosed with emphysema; of these, 2 million are women and 1.8 million are men. The reason is not yet understood, but only 10% to 15% of long-term smokers develop emphysema.

Emphysema caused by smoking. (From Little JW: Dental management of the medically compromised patient, ed 8, St Louis, 2013, Mosby.)

Chronic Bronchitis

Chronic bronchitis is an inflammation of the lining of the bronchiole tubes that causes swelling and excess production of mucus. Swelling and excess mucus narrow the bronchiole tubes and restrict airflow into and out of the lungs. Symptoms include chronic cough, shortness of breath, and coughing up of mucus. To be classified as chronic bronchitis, the symptoms must last 3 or more months out of the year for at least 2 years. As the disease progresses, the

lips and skin may exhibit cyanosis resulting from lack of oxygen in the blood. Chronic bronchitis is most often caused by long-term irritation of the bronchial tubes as a result of cigarette smoking; other causes include air pollution and exposure to dust or toxic gases in the workplace (e.g., coal mines). Chronic bronchitis often precedes or accompanies emphysema. It is estimated that 10 million Americans have chronic bronchitis. This condition affects individuals of all ages but has a higher incidence in individuals older than 45 years. Women are more than twice as likely to be diagnosed with chronic bronchitis as men.

Symptoms of COPD

Damage to the lungs caused by COPD occurs gradually over many years. In fact, more than 90% of patients who have COPD are over the age of 45 at the time of their diagnosis. Because there are no early symptoms, many people do not know they have COPD. By the time an individual experiences symptoms, it is usually a sign that irreversible lung damage has already occurred. The first symptoms of COPD include mild shortness of breath on exertion and occasional coughing. The disease slowly becomes more pronounced with severe episodes of dyspnea and coughing after even modest activity. As the disease progresses, the heart also can be affected and shortness of breath is present all the time, even while the patient is sitting quietly. At this point the individual's quality of life is greatly diminished. When the lungs and the heart are no longer able to deliver oxygen to the body's tissues, death occurs.

Treatment for COPD

The best treatment for COPD caused by smoking is for the patient to stop smoking. Continued smoking makes the COPD worse; quitting smoking slows the disease process. There are programs, support groups, nicotine replacement aids (e.g., nicotine patch, gum, lozenges, inhalers, nasal sprays), and prescription medications (e.g., Chantix, Zyban) to help individuals quit smoking. Other forms of treatment depend on the patient's condition and degree of lung impairment and may include the following:

1. Bronchodilators to relax and widen the bronchial tubes to increase airflow. They may be inhaled as aerosol sprays or taken orally.
2. Expectorants to thin the mucus so that it is easier to expel.
3. Antibiotics to treat infections that could interfere further with breathing and lung function.
4. Corticosteroids to reduce inflammation in the airways.
5. Breathing exercises to strengthen the muscles used to breathe.
6. Maintenance of overall good health habits, which include proper nutrition, adequate sleep, and regular exercise.
7. Oxygen therapy for patients with low blood oxygen to help with shortness of breath, allowing them to be more active.
8. Special measures including avoiding extremes of temperature (heat and cold), getting an annual influenza immunization, avoiding individuals with respiratory infection, and reducing exposure to air pollution.
9. Lung transplantation surgery is being performed on some patients who are in the later stages of COPD. ■

frequently before puberty and girls more frequently after puberty. In the United States, there are approximately 20 million individuals with asthma; of these, 6 million are children. Each year, more than 4000 deaths result from asthma.

Asthma is characterized by chronic inflammation of the small airways of the lungs and recurrent attacks of coughing, chest tightness, shortness of breath, and wheezing. **Wheezing** is a continuous, high-pitched, whistling, musical sound heard particularly during exhalation and sometimes during inhalation. In most patients, an asthma attack is followed by a symptom-free period. Asthma can be controlled by recognizing the warning signs and symptoms of an attack and treating them when they first occur. Failure to treat asthma can lead to serious complications, such as permanent lung damage.

Asthma Attack

Asthma attacks are highly individualized. Depending on the patient, asthma attacks vary in frequency and severity and may come on suddenly or gradually. An asthma attack may last for only 10 to 15 minutes or it may last for hours or even days.

In a normal individual, the airways to the lungs are fully open, allowing air to move easily into and out of the lungs. In a patient with asthma, the airways are always inflamed and hypersensitive to certain stimuli that do not affect the airways of normal individuals. These stimuli are known as *asthma triggers* because they can "trigger" an asthma attack.

Asthma triggers vary from one patient to another and may also vary from one season to the next. Examples of common allergens that may trigger an asthma attack include house dust, pollens, molds, animal danders, and cockroaches. Asthma attacks can also be triggered by environmental irritants, activities, or events, including air pollutants, tobacco smoke, chemical fumes (e.g., perfume, paint, gasoline), vigorous physical exercise, upper respiratory viral infections, exposure to cold, and emotional stress. It is sometimes difficult to determine what specific triggers cause a patient's asthma attacks.

When the inflamed airways of a patient with asthma are stimulated by a trigger, a series of reactions occur that affect the bronchial tubes. The bronchial tubes begin to constrict and swell, causing the patient to experience asthma

symptoms. Sometimes the symptoms are mild and go away, either on their own or with minimal treatment with medication. At other times, the symptoms become worse, leading to a full-blown asthma attack. During a severe asthma attack the bronchial tubes continue to constrict and swell and become clogged with mucus (Figure 27-16). This results in less air moving into and out of the lungs, which leads to a decrease in the amount of oxygen available to the body. The narrowed bronchial tubes and decreased oxygen supply cause the patient to experience coughing, chest tightness, shortness of breath, and wheezing. It is important to treat symptoms when they first begin to occur to prevent them from getting worse and causing a severe asthma attack, which may require emergency treatment.

Diagnosis and Treatment

The physician diagnoses asthma through a careful and detailed medical history. Of particular importance to the diagnosis of asthma are the patient's symptoms, family history of asthma, home and work environment, and living habits. The physician also performs a thorough physical examination to detect symptoms resulting from asthma, such as wheezing. When the medical history and physical examination have been completed, the physician usually orders laboratory and diagnostic tests, which may include pulmonary function tests (such as spirometry), allergy testing, and arterial blood gas studies.

Although asthma is a chronic disease with no cure, most patients with asthma are able to lead a normal life through proper management and treatment. The general treatment of asthma includes identifying and avoiding asthma triggers (if possible) and preventing and alleviating the symptoms through drug therapy. Two general categories of medication are prescribed for asthma: long-term–control medication and quick-relief medication.

Long-term–control medication helps relieve bronchial inflammation and prevents symptoms from occurring. Control medication helps the patient have fewer and milder asthma attacks and is typically taken every day. Corticosteroids are an example of a control medication; brand names include Flovent, Pulmicort, Asmanex, Qvar, and AeroBid. Other examples of long-term control medication include Singulair, Accolate, Serevent, Zyflo, and Advair.

A

B

Figure 27-16 A, Normal bronchial tube. **B,** Bronchial tube during an asthma attack.

Quick-relief medication (also called *rescue medication*) opens the airways quickly by dilating the bronchial tubes. It is taken when the patient is experiencing symptoms to prevent or control an asthma attack. Fast-acting bronchodilators are an example of quick-relief medication; brand names include Proventil, Ventolin, and Xopenex.

Many asthma medications are delivered through an *inhaler* (Figure 27-17), which allows the medication to go directly to the lungs. Quick-relief medications can be used in a breathing machine known as a *nebulizer* to treat an asthma attack at home. Other asthma medications are administered orally; however, they take longer to work because they first have to travel through the digestive and circulatory systems before reaching the lungs.

PEAK FLOW METER

A peak flow meter is a portable, handheld manual or digital device used to measure a breathing maneuver performed by the patient. *A manual peak flow meter* consists of a plastic tube with a sliding indicator that manually moves along a scale of numbers when the patient performs the breathing maneuver (Figure 27-18). A *digital peak flow meter* automatically measures the breathing maneuver and displays the measurement digitally on a screen (Figure 27-19). Because the manual meter is currently used most often, the remainder of this unit will focus on the manual peak flow meter.

A peak flow meter is used to measure how quickly air flows out of the lungs when the patient exhales forcefully. Peak flow meters are frequently used by patients with asthma and are recommended for patients with moderate to severe asthma. The measurements obtained from a peak flow meter are not as accurate as those obtained by spirometry; however, a peak flow meter can be used easily by a patient at home.

Peak flow measurements provide patients with important information such as when to take their medication and how

severe an asthma attack is. Several different brands of peak flow meters are available, and peak flow measurements may vary among brands. Because of this, a patient who purchases more than one meter should always buy the same brand to attain consistency among measurements.

Peak flow meters can be purchased over the counter and are available in two ranges: a low range and a full range. The *low-range meter* has a range from 0 to 300 and is used by young children and some older patients. The *full-range meter* has a range from 0 to 800 and is used by older children, teenagers, and adults (Figure 27-20). An adult has much larger bronchial tubes than a child and needs the wider range.

Figure 27-18 Manual peak flow meter.

Figure 27-19 Digital peak flow meter.

Figure 27-17 An inhaler is often used to deliver asthma medication to the bronchial tubes of the lungs. (From Potter PA: *Basic nursing: essentials for practice,* ed 7, St Louis, 2011, Mosby.)

Figure 27-25 Face mask.

Face Mask

A face mask consists of plastic and fits over the patient's nose and mouth. A face mask strap is then tightened around the patient's head to ensure a secure fit (Figure 27-25). Oxygen tubing is used to connect the face mask to the oxygen delivery system. A face mask is not used as frequently as a nasal cannula to administer oxygen because it is bulky and must be removed for eating or drinking and to communicate effectively.

A face mask is often used for patients who need a high flow of oxygen. It can deliver oxygen to the patient at a flow rate between 5 and 15 L/min. Wearing a nasal cannula for an extended period of time can cause irritation of the nose. Because of this, the patient might prefer to wear a nasal cannula during the day and a face mask at night to reduce the irritation that may occur from a nasal cannula. A face mask is also preferred by the patient if he or she has nasal congestion from a cold.

The face mask should be washed once or twice a week using liquid soap and water, then rinsed thoroughly and dried. The face mask should be replaced with a new one every 2 to 4 weeks, or sooner if it becomes cracked or discolored.

OXYGEN SAFETY GUIDELINES

Oxygen is a safe gas as long as it is used properly. Oxygen itself is not flammable, nor will it explode; however, it greatly increases the combustion rate of a fire. If something catches fire, oxygen will make the flame hotter and cause it to burn faster and more vigorously. The result is that a fire involving oxygen can appear explosive-like.

1. Store oxygen in a clean, dry, well-ventilated room. If kept in a closed area such as a closet, the small amount of oxygen gas that is continually vented from these units can accumulate in a confined space and become a fire hazard.
2. Compressed oxygen cylinders and liquid oxygen tanks must remain upright at all times. Secure oxygen cylinders and tanks to a fixed object, or place in a stand.
3. Never smoke while using oxygen. Do not allow smoking in the room where the oxygen is kept. Post "No Smoking: Oxygen in Use" signs where oxygen is kept.
4. Keep the oxygen supply at least 6 to 8 feet away from open flames such as gas stoves, lighted fireplaces, and candles.
5. Keep the oxygen supply at least 6 to 8 feet away from intense heat such as radiators, furnaces, and space heaters.
6. Keep the oxygen supply away from flammable products such as cleaning fluid, paint thinner, and aerosol sprays.
7. Do not lubricate oxygen equipment with oil or grease, because these substances are flammable.
8. Be sure to have functioning smoke detectors in the home.
9. Buy a fire extinguisher, and be familiar with how to use it.

What Would You Do? What Would You *Not* Do? RESPONSES

Case Study 1
Page 695

What Did Janet Do?
- ❏ Tried to reduce Camilla's fears by talking with her calmly and quietly.
- ❏ Explained to Camilla that an ECG is the best screening test available to check for heart problems.
- ❏ Reassured Camilla that she would be draped during the procedure and that she would be exposed as little as possible.
- ❏ Told Camilla that the wires may look a little scary, but there is no chance of being shocked by them. Explained that she won't feel anything when the test is being run.

- ❏ Told Camilla that she could talk with the billing clerk about setting up a payment plan for the test. Provided her with information about community resources that might help her pay for the test.

What Did Janet Not Do?
- ❏ Did not tell Camilla that she was too young to have heart problems.
- ❏ Did not tell Camilla that she needed to act more mature about being tested.

Case Study 2
Page 706

What Would You Do? What Would You *Not* Do? RESPONSES—cont'd

What Did Janet Do?

❑ Commended Joel on his weight loss and positive lifestyle changes.

❑ Shared a positive story with Joel about a patient who stopped smoking and did not gain weight.

❑ Asked Joel whether he would like any of the latest information on smoking cessation.

What Did Janet Not Do?

❑ Did not agree that Joel's positive lifestyle changes would counteract the bad effects of smoking.

❑ Did not lecture Joel on the dangers of smoking, because if he has been smoking since age 17 and has been trying to quit, he already knows what they are.

TERMINOLOGY REVIEW

Key Term	Word Parts	Definition
Amplitude		Refers to amount, extent, size, abundance, or fullness.
Artifact		Additional electrical activity picked up by the electrocardiograph that interferes with the normal appearance of the ECG cycles.
Atherosclerosis	*ather/o:* yellowish, fatty plaque *-sclerosis:* hardening of	Buildup of fibrous plaques of fatty deposits and cholesterol on the inner walls of an artery that causes narrowing, obstruction, and hardening of the artery.
Baseline		The flat horizontal line that separates the various waves of the ECG cycle.
Cardiac cycle	*cardi/o:* heart	One complete heartbeat.
Dysrhythmia	*dys-:* difficult, painful, abnormal *rhythm:* rhythm *-ia:* condition of diseased or abnormal state	An irregular heart rate or rhythm; also termed *arrhythmia.*
ECG cycle		The graphic representation of a heartbeat.
Electrocardiogram (ECG)	*electr/o:* electrical, electrical activity *cardi/o:* heart *-gram:* record of	The graphic representation of the electrical activity of the heart.
Electrocardiograph	*electr/o:* electrical, electrical activity *cardi/o:* heart *-graph:* instrument used to record	The instrument used to record the electrical activity of the heart.
Electrode	*electr/o:* electrical, electrical activity	A conductor of electricity, which is used to promote contact between the body and the electrocardiograph.
Electrolyte	*electr/o:* electrical, electrical activity	A chemical substance that promotes conduction of an electric current.
Flow rate		The number of liters of oxygen per minute that come out of an oxygen delivery system.
Hypoxemia	*hypo-:* below, deficient *ox/i:* oxygen *-emia:* blood condition	A decrease in the oxygen saturation of the blood.
Hypoxia	*hypo-:* below, deficient *ox/i:* oxygen *-ia:* condition of diseased or abnormal state	A reduction in the oxygen supply to the tissues of the body.
Interval		The length of a wave or the length of a wave with a segment.
Ischemia	*isch/o:* deficiency, blockage *-emia:* blood condition	Deficiency of blood in a body part.
Normal sinus rhythm		Refers to an ECG that is within normal limits.
Oxygen therapy		The administration of supplemental oxygen at concentrations greater than room air to treat or prevent hypoxemia.

Continued

↻ TERMINOLOGY REVIEW—cont'd

Key Term	Word Parts	Definition
Peak flow rate		The maximum volume of air that can be exhaled when the patient blows into a peak flow meter as forcefully and as rapidly as possible.
Segment		The portion of the ECG between two waves.
Spirometer	*spir/o:* breathe, breathing	An instrument for measuring air taken into and expelled from the lungs.
	-meter: instrument used to measure	
Spirometry	*spir/o:* breathe, breathing	Measurement of an individual's breathing capacity by means of a spirometer.
	-metry: measurement	
Wheezing		A continuous, high-pitched whistling musical sound heard particularly during exhalation and sometimes during inhalation.

ON THE WEB

For information on heart disease:

American Heart Association: www.americanheart.org

National Heart, Lung, and Blood Institute: www.nhlbi.nih.gov

American Association of Cardiovascular and Pulmonary Rehabilitation: www.aacvpr.org

My Heart Central: www.healthcentral.com/heart-disease

Health Communities: www.healthcommunities.com/health-topics/heart-health.shtml

Cardiology Channel: www.cardiosource.org/acc

American College of Cardiology: www.acc.org

The National Coalition for Women with Heart Disease: www.womenheart.org

For information on lung disease:

American Lung Association: www.lung.org

Pulmonary Channel: www.healthcommunities.com/health-topics/lung-conditions.shtml

Lung Cancer Online: www.lungcanceronline.org

American Association for Respiratory Care: www.aarc.org

Emphysema: emphysema.org

For information on smoking cessation:

Quit Net: www.quitnet.com

Smoking Cessation: www.smoking-cessation.org

National Center for Tobacco-free Kids: www.tobaccofreekids.org

Why Quit.com: www.whyquit.com

Quit Smoking Now: www.smokefree.gov

The Quit Smoking Company: www.quitsmoking.com

Specialty Examinations and Procedures: Colon Procedures, Male Reproductive Health, and Radiology and Diagnostic Imaging

 Check out the Evolve site at http://evolve.elsevier.com/Bonewit/today/ to access additional interactive activities and exercises to help you study and prepare for success.

LEARNING OBJECTIVES	PROCEDURES
Fecal Occult Blood Testing	
1. Explain the purpose of a fecal occult blood test.	Instruct a patient in the preparation and procedure for a fecal occult blood test (guaiac slide test).
2. Describe the patient preparation for fecal occult blood testing (guaiac slide method).	Develop a fecal occult blood test.
3. Explain the purpose of each type of preparation for fecal occult blood testing (guaiac slide method).	
Sigmoidoscopy	
4. Explain the purpose of a digital rectal examination before a sigmoidoscopic examination.	Instruct a patient in the preparation required for a sigmoidoscopy.
5. Explain the purpose of a sigmoidoscopy.	Assist the physician with sigmoidoscopy.
6. Describe the patient preparation for a sigmoidoscopy.	
Colonoscopy	
7. Explain the purpose of a colonoscopy.	Instruct a patient in the preparation required for a colonoscopy.
8. List the conditions that can be detected and assessed during a colonoscopy.	
9. Describe the patient preparation for a colonoscopy.	
Male Reproductive Health	
10. List the symptoms of prostate cancer.	Assist the physician with a digital rectal examination.
11. Explain the purpose of the digital rectal examination (DRE).	Instruct a patient in the preparation for a PSA test.
12. Explain the purpose of the prostate-specific antigen (PSA) test.	
13. State the risk factors for testicular cancer.	Teach a patient how to perform a testicular self-examination (TSE).
14. Describe the TSE schedule.	

Radiology

15. State the function of radiographs in medicine.
16. Explain the importance of proper patient preparation for a radiographic examination.
17. Explain the function of a contrast medium.
18. Describe the purpose of a fluoroscope.
19. Explain the purpose of each of the following types of radiographic examinations:
    - Mammography
    - Bone density scan
    - Upper gastrointestinal radiography
    - Lower gastrointestinal radiography
    - Intravenous pyelography

Instruct a patient in the proper preparation necessary for each of the following types of radiographic examinations:
- Mammography
  - Bone density scan
  - Upper gastrointestinal radiography
  - Lower gastrointestinal radiography
- Intravenous pyelography

Diagnostic Imaging

20. Explain the purpose of each of the following diagnostic imaging procedures:
    - Ultrasonography
    - Computed tomography
    - Magnetic resonance imaging
    - Nuclear medicine
21. Explain how nuclear medicine is used to produce an image of a body part or organ.
22. State the guidelines that may be required for nuclear medicine.

Instruct a patient on the purpose and advance preparation for each of the following diagnostic imaging procedures:
- Ultrasonography
  - Computed tomography
  - Magnetic resonance imaging
- Nuclear medicine

Digital Radiology

23. Explain the advantages of digital radiology.

CHAPTER OUTLINE

COLON PROCEDURES
Introduction to Colon Procedures
Blood in the Stool
Fecal Occult Blood Test
Guaiac Slide Test
Quality Control
Other Types of Stool Tests
Fecal Immunochemical Test
Fecal DNA Test
Sigmoidoscopy
Purpose
Patient Preparation for Sigmoidoscopy
Digital Rectal Examination
Sigmoidoscope
Colonoscopy
Purpose
Patient Preparation for Colonoscopy
Procedure
MALE REPRODUCTIVE HEALTH
Introduction to Male Reproductive Health
Prostate Cancer
Prostate Cancer Screening
Digital Rectal Examination
Prostate-Specific Antigen Test
Recommendations for Prostate Screening

Testicular Self-Examination
RADIOLOGY AND DIAGNOSTIC IMAGING
Introduction to Radiology
Contrast Media
Fluoroscopy
Positioning the Patient
Specific Radiographic Examinations
Mammography
Bone Density Scan
Gastrointestinal Series
Intravenous Pyelography
Other Types of Radiographs
Introduction to Diagnostic Imaging
Ultrasonography
Patient Preparation
Computed Tomography
Patient Preparation
Magnetic Resonance Imaging
Patient Preparation
Nuclear Medicine
Bone Scans
Nuclear Cardiac Stress Test
Guidelines
Digital Radiology

Colon Procedures

INTRODUCTION TO COLON PROCEDURES

Colon procedures are performed in the medical office or clinic and include the fecal occult blood test (FOBT), sigmoidoscopy, and sometimes colonoscopy, which are presented in this chapter. The FOBT is a screening test used to detect blood in the stool for the early detection of colorectal cancer. Stool specimens must be collected by the patient at home. Some patients initially may be reluctant to comply with the FOBT patient preparation requirements and collection of the stool specimens. The medical assistant can help by explaining the purpose of the test to the patient. If the patient understands the benefits to be derived from the test, he or she is more likely to participate as required.

Medical assistants are often responsible for explaining to a patient the preparation required for sigmoidoscopy and colonoscopy. The medical assistant should make sure the patient thoroughly understands the instructions. If the patient does not prepare properly, the procedure must be cancelled, which requires the patient to go through the preparation procedure again. The medical assistant assists the physician during a sigmoidoscopy, and he or she should have a thorough knowledge of the responsibilities accompanying this procedure.

BLOOD IN THE STOOL

Blood in the stool can indicate a number of gastrointestinal (GI) conditions, including hemorrhoids, diverticulitis, polyps, colitis, upper GI ulcers, and colorectal cancer. Some of these conditions (e.g., hemorrhoids) produce visible red blood on the outside of the stool, making it easy to detect. Blood entering the stool in an amount of 50 mL or more from conditions affecting the upper GI tract (e.g., peptic ulcers) causes the stool to exhibit **melena**, meaning it is

black and tarlike. The dark color is a result of oxidation of the iron in the blood (heme) by intestinal and bacterial enzymes. If a minute quantity of blood is present, however, it is not possible to detect it with the unaided eye. This hidden, or nonvisible, blood is termed **occult blood**, and its presence can be determined by testing the stool for blood.

Colorectal cancer is one of the most common forms of cancer in individuals older than the age of 50 years (see *Highlight on Colorectal Cancer*). During the early asymptomatic stages, almost all lesions (e.g., benign and malignant tumors) of the colon and rectum bleed a small amount on an intermittent basis, and this is usually in the form of occult blood. Discovery of occult blood in the stool does not mean that a patient has colorectal cancer. It does, however, warrant further diagnostic procedures, such as a colonoscopy, to determine if colorectal cancer is present. Early diagnosis and treatment of colorectal cancer increase the patient's survival rate. In most cases, when more pronounced symptoms of colorectal cancer start to appear (e.g., visible bleeding from the rectum, a change in bowel habits, abdominal pain), the cancer has reached an advanced stage.

FECAL OCCULT BLOOD TEST
GUAIAC SLIDE TEST

Routine screening of stool specimens for occult blood is frequently performed in the medical office. The guaiac slide test is a chemical test used to screen for fecal occult blood and is discussed in detail in this chapter. This test is commercially available with the brand names of Hemoccult, ColoScreen, and Seracult (Figure 28-1).

Fecal blood loss greater than 5 mL per day results in a positive reaction on a guaiac slide test. Individuals normally may lose up to 3 mL per day of blood in the feces owing to minor insignificant abrasions of the nasopharynx and GI tract, such as from brushing the teeth. To allow for normal blood loss, the guaiac slide test does not show a positive reaction until the blood in the stool reaches a level of 5 mL (or more) per day.

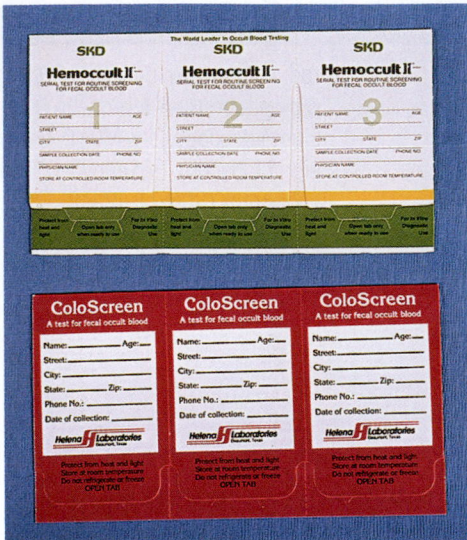

Figure 28-1 Examples of fecal occult blood testing kits. Hemoccult *(top)* and ColoScreen *(bottom)*.

The guaiac slide test is a simple and inexpensive method to screen for the presence of fecal occult blood; however, care must be taken to reduce the occurrence of false-positive and false-negative test results. This test is designed to assess the presence of blood in stool specimens collected from three bowel movements on three different days. The purpose of using three specimens is to provide for the detection of blood from GI lesions that exhibit intermittent bleeding, meaning they do not bleed every day. The patient must collect the three specimens at home and return the prepared slides to the medical office for developing. The medical assistant is responsible for providing the patient with instructions on patient preparation and collection and proper care and storage of the slides until they are returned to the medical office.

Purpose

The primary use of the guaiac slide test is to screen for the presence of occult blood caused by colorectal cancer. Other conditions that can cause blood in the stool include the following:
- Hemorrhoids
- Anal fissures
- Colorectal polyps
- Diverticulitis
- Peptic ulcers
- Ulcerative colitis
- Gastroesophageal reflux disease (GERD)
- Crohn disease

A positive test result on the guaiac slide test indicates only the presence of blood in the stool; the source and cause of the bleeding must still be determined. This means that additional diagnostic procedures must be performed before the physician can make a final diagnosis. These procedures may include colonoscopy, sigmoidoscopy, a double-contrast barium enema radiographic study, computed tomography

(CT) colonography, and a newer procedure known as *capsule endoscopy,* which uses a tiny wireless camera (that the patient swallows as a pill) to take photographs of the digestive tract.

Patient Preparation

Patient preparation for a guaiac slide test plays an important role in ensuring accurate test results. The patient must follow a special diet beginning 3 days before the test and must continue the diet until all three slides have been prepared. The patient is placed on a high-fiber, meat-free diet. Meat contains animal blood, which could lead to a false-positive test result. A high-fiber diet is used because it encourages bleeding from lesions that may bleed only occasionally. In addition, fiber adds bulk, which promotes bowel elimination and ensures adequate specimen collection.

Certain medications irritate the GI tract, which may result in a small amount of bleeding and thus could cause

Putting It All Into Practice

My name is Megan Baer, and I work in a large clinic that includes the specialties of family practice, gastroenterology, allergies, and dermatology. I am the clinical supervisor and oversee all of the clinical medical assistants and our "in-house" laboratory. I work closely with all physicians to meet the growing needs of the clinic.

Working with a gastroenterologist has been interesting and educational. When preparing a patient for a sigmoidoscopy, you must help the patient feel relaxed. This is an embarrassing situation for the patient, so you need to make him or her feel as comfortable as possible and maintain the patient's privacy and modesty. During the procedure, I talk to patients about the weather, their pets, and other interests to make them feel more relaxed and comfortable. This can help take their mind off the procedure.

One day I was assisting with a sigmoidoscopic examination, and a few minutes into the procedure the look on the physician's face told me something was wrong. When the examination was finished, the physician and I left the room and went back to his office. He informed me that what he saw on his examination was colorectal cancer, and at this stage not much could be done for the patient. The worst thing a physician has to do is give unpleasant news to a patient and see the look on the patient's face. Going into the room of a patient who has just received life-threatening information is something you don't forget. All you can do is be sympathetic and understanding and be a good listener. You have to be strong and not show your emotions even though your heart is breaking for the patient and the family. Always let patients know you are there for them.

Being with a patient who receives bad news about his or her health can make you think about your own life and how it affects not only you, but also your family and friends. I often think of how I would feel about receiving such news. I try to put myself in the patient's place and to be sincere and understanding and willing to lend an ear. ■

Table 28-1	Patient Preparation for the Fecal Occult Guaiac Slide Test: Dietary and Medication Guidelines
	Beginning 3 days before obtaining the first stool specimen, the patient should follow certain diet and medication modifications. These modifications should be followed until all three slides have been prepared.
Meats	Eat no red or rare meat (beef and lamb) or liver. Small amounts of well cooked pork, poultry, and fish are permitted. Red meat contains animal blood, which could cause a false-positive test result.
Vegetables	Eat moderate amounts of raw and cooked vegetables. Especially advised are lettuce, spinach, corn, and celery. Do not consume horseradish, turnips, broccoli, cauliflower, and radishes. These foods contain peroxidase, which sometimes can cause a false-positive test result.
Fruits	Eat moderate amounts of apples, bananas, oranges, peaches, pears, and plums. Avoid vitamin C in excess of 250 mg a day from citrus fruits and juices. Do not consume melons, because they contain peroxidase.
Miscellaneous high-fiber foods	Eat moderate amounts of whole-wheat bread, bran cereal, and popcorn. Foods high in fiber provide roughage to promote bowel elimination and encourage bleeding from "silent" lesions that bleed only occasionally.
Medications	Do not take medications or vitamin supplements that contain iron or vitamin C in excess of 250 mg for 3 days before and during the collection period. In addition, based on your medication therapy, the physician may stipulate additional medication restrictions. Certain medications cause irritation of the gastrointestinal tract, which may result in a small amount of bleeding. Nonsteroidal antiinflammatory drugs (NSAIDs) and more than one adult aspirin a day should be avoided for at least 7 days before and continuing through the test period. Examples of NSAIDs include ibuprofen (Advil, Motrin) and naproxen (Aleve). Acetaminophen (Tylenol) can be taken as needed.
Special guidelines	Inform the physician, and do not consume any of the food items listed previously, if you know from past experience that they cause you severe gastrointestinal discomfort or serious diarrhea. Ensure that the diet modifications have been followed for 3 days before collecting the first stool specimen. Do not initiate the test during a menstrual period or in the first 3 days after a menstrual period. The test should not be conducted when blood is visible in the stool or urine, such as from bleeding from hemorrhoids or a urinary tract infection. These conditions would result in false-positive test results. Store the slides with the flaps in a closed position at room temperature, and protect them from heat, sunlight, and fluorescent light. The slides must also be stored away from volatile chemicals such as ammonia, bleach, and other household cleaners. Improper storage can result in deterioration of the active reagents on the slides, leading to inaccurate test results.

a false-positive result on the guaiac slide test. Medications that should be avoided include ibuprofen (Motrin, Advil), naproxen (Aleve), and more than one adult aspirin per day. In addition, an iron supplement may cause a false-positive result, and a vitamin C supplement (greater than 250 mg per day) can cause a false-negative result. All of these substances should be discontinued before testing. Table 28-1 lists the specific patient preparation requirements for fecal occult blood testing using the guaiac slide test.

QUALITY CONTROL

Quality control methods must be employed with the guaiac slide test to ensure reliable and valid results. It is important to properly store the box containing the guaiac slides and developing solution. Adverse storage conditions can result in deterioration of the developing solution and the active reagents impregnated on the filter paper of the slides, leading to inaccurate test results. The box must be stored at a room temperature between 59°F (15°C) and 86°F (30°C). The contents of the box must be protected from heat, sunlight, and strong fluorescent light. In addition, the box should not be stored in close proximity to volatile chemicals such as ammonia, bleach, bromine, iodine, and disinfectant cleaners. If stored properly, the slides and developer will remain effective until the expiration date that is stamped on the side of the

box, each slide itself, and the container of developing solution.

A quality control procedure must be performed *after* the patient's test samples have been developed, read, and interpreted. This ensures that the test results are accurate and valid. The Hemoccult slide test contains an on-slide performance monitor that consists of positive and negative monitor areas. This monitor is located on the developing side of the filter paper under the back flap of the cardboard slide. The positive monitor area contains a control chemical that has been impregnated into the filter paper during the manufacturing process.

The medical assistant should apply 1 drop of the developing solution between the positive and negative performance monitor areas on each of the three slides. The results must be read within 10 seconds after application of the developer. If the slides and developer are functioning properly, the positive area turns blue, whereas the negative area shows no color change. Failure of the expected control results to occur indicates an error, and the test results are not considered valid; possible causes include the use of outdated slides or developing solution; an error in technique; and subjection of the slides to heat, sunlight, strong fluorescent light, or volatile chemicals. Procedure 28-1 outlines the medical assistant's responsibilities related to fecal occult blood testing using the Hemoccult guaiac slide test. Procedure 28-2 describes the development of a Hemoccult slide test.

What Would You Do? | What Would You *Not* Do?

Case Study 1

Beatrice Bernard is 52 years old and has come to the office for a physical examination. The physician wants Mrs. Bernard to perform a Hemoccult test. After being told the purpose of the test and how to prepare for it, Mrs. Bernard expresses some concerns. She does not like the idea of what she has to do to perform the test because it does not seem sanitary to her. She also thinks it will be a lot of work to prepare for the test. She has red meat for dinner at least four times a week, and she does not understand why she has to eliminate it from her meals. She says she takes a baby aspirin every day for "heart health" and would prefer not to stop taking it. Mrs. Bernard says that she has always taken very good care of herself, and she has never had problems with her colon. She also says no history of colon cancer has been reported in her family. Mrs. Bernard is too embarrassed to talk about this topic with the physician. She says she may just throw the test away when she gets home. ■

HIGHLIGHT on Colorectal Cancer

Incidence

Colorectal cancer is used to describe both cancer of the colon and cancer of the rectum. Based on what area is affected, these cancers are often referred to separately as *colon cancer* (see illustration) and *rectal cancer.* Colorectal cancer is the third leading cause of cancer-related deaths in the United States for both men and women. According to the American Cancer Society, every year approximately 150,000 people are diagnosed with colorectal cancer, and approximately 50,000 people die every year from this disease. As the U.S. population of baby boomers ages, these numbers may increase.

Colon cancer. (From Forbes CD: *Color atlas and text of clinical medicine,* ed 3, Philadelphia, 2003, Mosby.)

Risk Factors

The following factors increase the risk of developing colorectal cancer:

- Age: The risk of colorectal cancer increases significantly after 50 years of age and reaches a peak from ages 60 to 75 years. More than 90% of individuals diagnosed with colorectal cancer are older than 50 years.
- Colorectal polyps: A colorectal *polyp* is a grapelike growth that protrudes from the inner lining (mucosa) of the colon or rectum (see Figure 28-7). Individuals with large polyps or numerous polyps are particularly at risk for colorectal cancer. Most cases of colorectal cancer arise from *adenomatous* polyps that gradually become malignant over many years. Colorectal polyps are fairly common in individuals older than 50 years. Approximately 1 in 20 colorectal polyps can become cancerous if not removed.
- Personal history of colorectal cancer: Individuals who have been diagnosed previously with colorectal cancer are at higher risk for developing it in other parts of the colon and rectum, even if it was completely removed.
- History of inflammatory bowel disease of long duration, such as ulcerative colitis and Crohn disease.
- Strong family history of colorectal cancer.
- Known family history of hereditary colorectal cancer syndromes such as familial adenomatous polyposis (FAP) or hereditary nonpolyposis colon cancer (HNPCC).
- Other factors that have been associated with a higher incidence of colorectal cancer include smoking; heavy alcohol consumption; obesity; a diet high in fat, red meat, and processed meats (e.g., hot dogs, luncheon meats); low intake of fresh fruits and vegetables; and physical inactivity.

Symptoms

No or very few symptoms occur during the early stages of colorectal cancer. If colorectal cancer is detected and treated while the patient is still asymptomatic, the patient has a 90% chance of 5-year survival. By comparison, the 5-year survival rate for patients in whom colorectal cancer is diagnosed after symptoms appear is only 40%, and the 5-year survival rate when the cancer has spread to distant organs (metastasized) such as the liver or lungs is only 11%.

Symptoms that occur when colorectal cancer is more developed include the following:

- Bleeding from the rectum
- Blood in the stool
- A change in the shape of the stool (e.g., stools that are narrower than usual)
- A change in bowel habits (e.g., diarrhea, constipation)
- General abdominal discomfort (e.g., aches, pains, cramps)
- Unexplained weight loss
- Constant fatigue

HIGHLIGHT on Colorectal Cancer—cont'd

Recommendations for Early Detection

For the early prevention and detection of colorectal cancer, the American Cancer Society recommends that all adults 50 years old and older who are at average risk for colorectal cancer be screened using one of the following screening tests. Tests that detect both polyps and cancer are preferred over tests that detect only cancer. Individuals with risk factors for colorectal cancer should be screened at an earlier age and with greater frequency. For example, an individual who has a family history of colorectal cancer should begin colorectal cancer screening at 40 years of age.

Tests that detect both polyps and cancer include the following:

- Sigmoidoscopy: every 5 years*
- Colonoscopy: every 10 years
- Double-contrast barium enema: every 5 years*

- Computed tomography (CT) colonography (virtual colonoscopy): every 5 years*

Tests that detect only cancer include these:
- Fecal occult blood test: every year*
- Fecal immunochemical test: every year*
- Fecal DNA test: interval uncertain*

Cause

The cause of colorectal cancer is unknown, but studies have shown a higher incidence of this disease in countries such as the United States, in which populations have a diet that is high in meat and animal fat and low in fiber. This finding is supported by the fact that in countries such as Japan, in which the diet is high in fiber and low in fat, the incidence of colorectal cancer is much lower. ∎

*Colonoscopy should be performed if test results are positive.

PROCEDURE 28-1   Fecal Occult Blood Testing: Guaiac Slide Test

Outcome Instruct a patient in specimen collection for a Hemoccult guaiac slide test

Equipment/Supplies

- Hemoccult slide testing kit

1. Procedural Step. Obtain a Hemoccult testing kit. Check the expiration date on the slides.
Principle. Outdated slides can lead to inaccurate test results.

Check the expiration date.

2. Procedural Step. Greet the patient and introduce yourself. Identify the patient and explain the purpose of the test. Tell the patient that the test should not be conducted during a menstrual period or when hemorrhoids are bleeding or a urinary tract infection is present.

Principle. Bleeding from other (identifiable) sources causes a false-positive test result.

3. Procedural Step. Instruct the patient in proper preparation for the test. See the box *Highlight on Colorectal Cancer* for the specific guidelines the patient should follow. Tell the patient to begin the diet modifications 3 days before collecting the first stool specimen. Encourage the patient to adhere to the diet modifications.
Principle. The diet modifications may discourage patient compliance. The medical assistant should reinforce the importance of adhering to the diet requirements. Improper patient preparation can lead to inaccurate test results.

4. Procedural Step. Provide the patient with the Hemoccult testing kit. The kit consists of three identical cardboard slides attached to one another; each slide contains two squares, labeled "A" and "B." Three wooden applicator sticks and written instructions also are included in the testing kit.
Principle. Three slides are provided so that three stool specimens can be collected. The two squares in each slide (A and B) contain filter paper impregnated with guaiac, a chemical necessary for detection of blood in the stool.

Continued

PROCEDURE 28-1   Fecal Occult Blood Testing: Guaiac Slide Test—cont'd

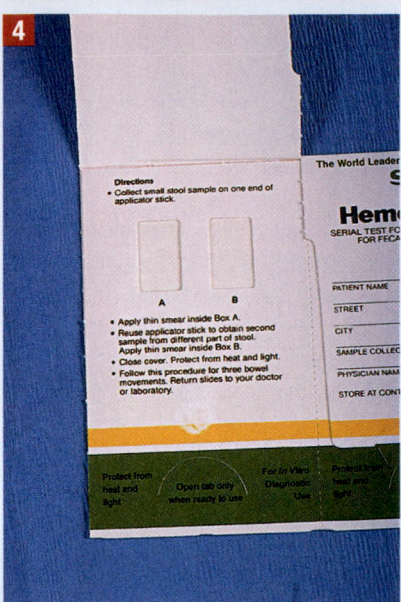

Each slide contains two squares labeled "A" and "B."

5. Procedural Step. Instruct the patient regarding completion of the information required on the front flap of each card. This includes the patient's name, address, phone number, and age and the date of the specimen collection. A ballpoint pen should be used to write this information.

Instruct the patient on how to complete the information section on the slides.

6. Procedural Step. Provide instructions on proper care and storage of the slides. Make it clear that the slides must be stored (with the flaps in a closed position) at room temperature and protected from heat, sunlight, strong fluorescent light, and volatile chemicals.
Principle. Adverse storage conditions can result in deterioration of the active reagents impregnated on the filter paper, leading to inaccurate test results.

7. Procedural Step. Instruct the patient on initiation of the test by telling him or her to begin the diet modifications and then to collect a stool specimen from the first bowel movement after the 3-day preparatory period.

8. Procedural Step. Instruct the patient on proper collection of the stool specimen:
   a. Fill in the sample collection date on the front flap of the first cardboard slide.
   b. Use a clean, dry container to collect the stool sample. The sample must be collected before it comes in contact with toilet bowl water. Allow the stool to fall into the collection container.
   c. Use one of the wooden applicators to obtain a specimen from one part of the stool sample.
   d. Open the front flap of the first cardboard slide (located on the left in the series of three).
   e. Spread a very thin smear of the specimen over the filter paper in the square labeled "A."
   f. Using the same wooden applicator, obtain another specimen from a different area of the stool.
   g. Spread a thin smear of the specimen over the filter paper in the square labeled "B."
   h. Close the front flap of the cardboard slide.
   i. Discard the wooden applicator in a waste container. Do not flush it down the toilet.
   j. Place the slides in a regular paper envelope to air-dry overnight.
Principle. Two squares are included in each slide to allow specimen collection from different parts of the stool because occult blood is not always uniformly distributed throughout the stool. Thick specimens prevent adequate light penetration through the filter paper, making it difficult to interpret the test results.

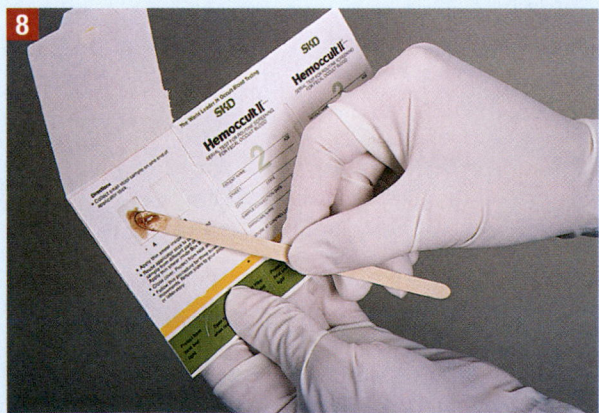

Spread a thin smear of the specimen over the filter paper.

PROCEDURE 28-1   Fecal Occult Blood Testing: Guaiac Slide Test—cont'd

9. **Procedural Step.** Instruct the patient to continue the testing period on 3 different days until all three specimens have been obtained as follows.
   a. Repeat Procedural Step 8 after the second bowel movement the next day. If you do not have a bowel movement on the next day, then collect the specimen on the following day. The specimens should be collected on 3 different days. Use the cardboard slide located in the middle of the series of three.
   b. Repeat Procedural Step 8 after the third bowel movement, using the cardboard slide located to the right in the series of three.
   c. Allow the completed slides to air-dry overnight in the paper envelope.

10. **Procedural Step.** Instruct the patient to place the cardboard slides in the envelope lined with foil, seal carefully, and return them as soon as possible to the medical office. Emphasize to the patient that only the foil-lined envelope can be used to mail the slides; a standard envelope cannot be used. Inform the patient that the slides must be returned no later than 14 days after the first specimen is collected.
   Principle. Standard paper envelopes are not approved by U.S. postal regulations for mailing fecal occult blood testing slides. Slides should not be developed after 14 days, because the test results may not be accurate.

11. **Procedural Step.** Give the patient an opportunity to ask questions; ensure that the patient understands the instructions for patient preparation and collection of the stool specimen and for storage of the slides.
    Principle. Improper patient preparation and poor collection technique can lead to inaccurate test results.

12. **Procedural Step.** Document in the patient's medical record.
    a. *Paper-based patient record:* Record the date and documentation that the Hemoccult test and instructions were given to the patient (refer to the PPR charting example).]

PPR CHARTING EXAMPLE

Date	
9/08/XX	9:00 a.m. Pt provided with a Hemoccult test and instructions for the procedure. ————————— M. Baer, CMA (AAMA)

   b. *Electronic medical record:* Document that the Hemoccult test and instructions were given to the patient using the appropriate radio buttons, drop-down menus, and free text fields.

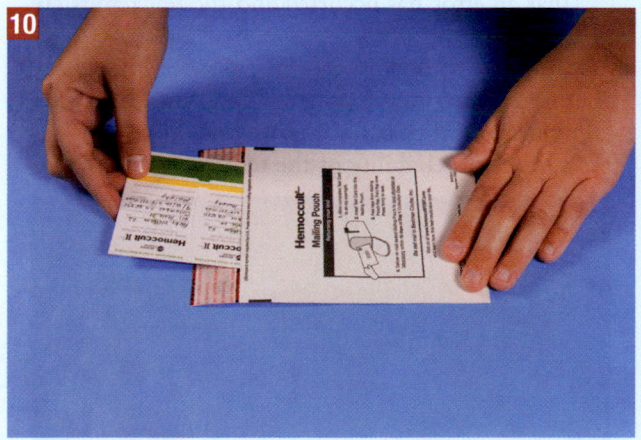

Place the cardboard slides in the envelope.

Figure 28-4 Flexible fiberoptic sigmoidoscope.

Figure 28-5 Collection of a specimen during a sigmoidoscopy.

laboratory. Removal of a precancerous polyp prevents it from developing into colon cancer in the future (see *Highlight on Colorectal Cancer*).

The medical assistant must prepare the patient for the procedure and assist the physician during the sigmoidoscopy. These responsibilities include the following:

- Determine whether the patient has prepared properly for the sigmoidoscopy
- Ask the patient whether he or she needs to void before the procedure
- Position and drape the patient in Sims position
- Reassure the patient and help him or her to relax
- Lubricate the physician's gloved index finger for the digital examination
- Lubricate the distal end of the sigmoidoscope before the physician inserts it (Figure 28-6)

Figure 28-6 The distal end of the sigmoidoscope must be lubricated before insertion.

- Assist with suction equipment
- Assist with the collection of a biopsy specimen by holding the specimen container to accept the specimen
- Assist the patient after the examination
- Prepare the biopsy specimen for transport to the laboratory
- Clean the examining room
- Sanitize and disinfect the sigmoidoscope

COLONOSCOPY

A **colonoscopy** is the visual examination of the mucosa of the rectum and the entire length of the colon (sigmoid colon, descending colon, transverse colon, and ascending colon) using a flexible fiberoptic **colonoscope**. A colonoscope is basically a sigmoidoscope but with a longer insertion tube. The colonoscope has a video camera attached to the distal end of the flexible insertion tube. The camera transmits images of the colon to a video screen for viewing by the physician (see Figure 28-3).

Before a patient undergoes a colonoscopy, the physician explains the nature of the procedure and any risks to the patient and offers to answer questions. The medical assistant may be responsible for obtaining the patient's signature on a written consent to treatment form, which grants the physician permission to perform the procedure.

PURPOSE

Colonoscopy is often performed after a positive FOBT result to determine the source and cause of the bleeding. It is also performed to evaluate patient symptoms related to the colon such as lower abdominal pain. Colonoscopy is considered the "gold standard" for assessing abnormalities of the colon. Conditions that can be detected and assessed during a colonoscopy include the following:

- Lesions of the colon or rectum (e.g., benign or malignant growths)
- Colorectal polyps (Figure 28-7)
- Hemorrhoids
- Fissures
- Infection and inflammation

Figure 28-7 Colon polyp. (From Lewis S: *Medical-surgical nursing,* ed 8, St Louis, 2011, Mosby.)

Colonoscopy is particularly valuable for the early detection of symptomatic and asymptomatic colorectal cancer. Early detection of colorectal cancer leads to early diagnosis and treatment, which increase the chance of survival for patients with this disease.

PATIENT PREPARATION FOR COLONOSCOPY

A colonoscopy is usually performed in a hospital on an outpatient basis or in a large medical clinic. The rectum and the entire colon must be flushed out completely so that the colon is empty and free of fecal material; this is known as a *full bowel prep.* This is one of the most important parts of the colonoscopy. Fecal material can interfere with good visualization of the wall of the colon, making it difficult for the physician to detect abnormalities.

The medical assistant may be responsible for providing the patient with instructions on preparing the colon. The patient should be encouraged to follow the instructions exactly. If the patient does not prepare properly, the colonoscopy is usually cancelled and must be rescheduled, which requires the patient to go through the bowel preparation procedure again. The patient preparation instructions may vary from one facility to another. General patient preparation recommendations for a colonoscopy are outlined in Table 28-3, along with patient instructions for after the procedure.

PROCEDURE

A sedative is administered intravenously before the colonoscopy. The sedative causes the patient to become relaxed, sleepy, and less aware of what is taking place. Some patients do not remember the procedure at all afterward.

The procedure itself is similar to a sigmoidoscopy. The patient is placed on his or her left side in Sims position. The physician performs a digital rectal examination (DRE) before inserting the colonoscope. The colonoscope is advanced all the way through the entire colon (approximately 4 to 5 feet) until it reaches the cecum. Air is inserted into the colon to distend it for better visualization. Suction is used to remove secretions such as mucus, blood, and liquid feces that interfere with proper visualization. The physician then slowly withdraws the colonoscope while carefully observing the mucosa of the colon for abnormalities.

If the physician discovers an abnormal lesion, a long thin instrument is passed through the lumen of the insertion tube to remove a specimen for biopsy. In addition, if a suspicious-looking polyp is discovered, the physician may remove it (polypectomy) or take a biopsy sample of it for analysis by the laboratory. Removal of a precancerous polyp prevents it from developing into colon cancer in the future.

After the procedure the patient may experience some bloating, abdominal cramping, and flatulence. If a polyp has been removed or if a biopsy has been performed, the patient may exhibit traces of blood in the stool for 1 to 2 days.

Table 28-3 Patient Preparation for Colonoscopy

It is important to follow the patient preparation requirements as carefully as possible to ensure accurate results. The following preparation is required for a colonoscopy.	
Beginning 5 days before the procedure	Discontinue taking iron, aspirin, and aspirin products. Iron can alter the color of the wall of the colon, and aspirin may cause bleeding if a polyp is removed from the colon.
Beginning 2 days before the procedure	Discontinue taking nonsteroidal antiinflammatory drugs such as ibuprofen and naproxen to minimize the risk of bleeding if a polyp is removed.
Medication restrictions	The physician will advise you of any other medication restrictions that need to be followed.
Beginning 1 day before the procedure and continuing until your examination is completed	a. Do not consume any solid food or milk products. b. Consume only gelatin (Jell-O) or popsicles (except purple or red, which could be mistaken for blood in the colon). c. Drink only clear liquids (water, apple juice, sport drinks [e.g., Gatorade], soft drinks, clear broth). Do not drink alcohol. d. Coffee or tea is permitted with no milk or cream.
Bowel preparation	Take a laxative on the afternoon (between 2 PM and 4 PM) before the procedure. The laxative is often in a powdered form (e.g., Colyte) and comes in a package that is attached to a plastic gallon container. Read the package instructions for preparing the laxative solution. The gallon container is filled with drinking water and mixed with the powdered laxative. After preparing the laxative solution, store it in the refrigerator. Most patients find it easier to drink the solution if it is chilled. a. Begin the bowel preparation by drinking one 8-ounce glass of the liquid laxative solution every 10 to 15 minutes until 2 quarts (eight 8-ounce glasses) have been consumed. It is best to drink the solution quickly rather than slowly sipping it. b. After drinking the first few glasses, you may experience nausea and a bloated feeling. This is temporary and will disappear once you start having bowel movements. If this occurs, you can slow down the drinking process or stop for 30 minutes and then resume drinking the solution every 15 minutes. c. Your first bowel movement should occur approximately 1 hour after you begin drinking the solution. You will need to have a bowel movement about 10 to 15 times. If your bowel movement is clear to pale yellow in color after drinking the first 2 quarts of the solution, you can stop drinking the solution. If your stool is not clear, continue drinking the solution every 15 minutes until your bowel movement is clear.
After midnight on the night before the examination	a. Do not eat or drink anything, including water. b. If medications need to be taken (as approved by the physician), take them with only a sip of water.
Transportation	Arrange to have someone drive you home after the procedure. You will be sedated during the procedure and cannot drive yourself, nor can you use public transportation.
After the procedure	You may experience some bloating, abdominal cramping, and flatulence. If you had a polyp removed or a biopsy specimen taken, it is normal to experience traces of blood in the stool for 1 to 2 days. Contact the office if you experience significant rectal bleeding, faintness, dizziness, shortness of breath, or heart palpitations.

Male Reproductive Health

INTRODUCTION TO MALE REPRODUCTIVE HEALTH

Two important areas related to male reproductive health are prostate screening and testicular self-examination (TSE). Preventive examinations and tests can assist in the detection of prostate and testicular cancers. Both of these areas are described in the following section.

PROSTATE CANCER

According to the American Cancer Society (ACS), prostate cancer is the second most common cause of cancer deaths in men, lung cancer being the most common. Every year,

approximately 200,000 men are diagnosed with prostate cancer, and approximately 27,000 die from this disease. The incidence of prostate cancer increases after age 50. Prostate cancer is found more often in African American men and men with a family history of prostate cancer.

The prostate gland surrounds the urethra and is located just below the bladder and in front of the rectum (Figure 28-8). It is approximately the size and shape of a walnut, and its function is to secrete fluid that transports sperm.

In the early stages, prostate cancer often causes no symptoms. Symptoms that occur when the cancer is more developed include the following:
- Difficulty in urinating
- Weak or interrupted urinary flow
- Pain or burning during urination
- Frequent urination, especially at night
- Blood in the urine
- Pain in the lower back, pelvis, or upper thighs

PROSTATE CANCER SCREENING

The primary screening tests for prostate cancer are the DRE and the prostate-specific antigen (PSA) test.

DIGITAL RECTAL EXAMINATION

The DRE is a quick and simple procedure that causes only momentary discomfort. During the examination the physician inserts a lubricated gloved finger into the patient's rectum. Because the prostate gland is located in front of the rectum, the physician is able to palpate the surface of the prostate gland through the rectal wall (see Figure 28-8). The physician palpates the gland to determine whether it is enlarged or has an abnormal consistency. Normally the prostate gland should feel soft, whereas malignant tissue is firm or hard. The sensitivity of the DRE is limited, however, because the physician can palpate only the posterior and lateral aspects of the prostate gland.

PROSTATE-SPECIFIC ANTIGEN TEST

The PSA test is a screening test that measures the amount of PSA in the blood. PSA is a protein normally produced by the cells of the membrane that covers the prostate gland. The normal range for PSA is 0 to 4 ng/mL of blood. The PSA level may become elevated in men who have a benign or malignant growth in the prostate. A PSA level of 4 to 10 ng/mL is considered slightly elevated; levels between 10 and 20 ng/mL are considered moderately elevated; and a value greater than 20 ng/mL is considered highly elevated. The higher the PSA level, the more likely that cancer is present. Other conditions (other than prostate cancer) that can cause an elevated PSA level include benign prostatic hyperplasia (BPH) and prostatitis.

The PSA level may normally increase after vigorous exercise, such as jogging or biking. The medical assistant should instruct the patient to engage in only normal activity for 2 days before having blood drawn for a PSA test. The patient also should be instructed not to have sexual intercourse for 2 days before the test because it can change the PSA level.

If the DRE is abnormal and/or the PSA test result is elevated, further testing may be performed to determine whether prostate cancer is present. To make this assessment, one or more of the following tests may be performed: transrectal ultrasound (TRUS), biopsy of the prostate gland, bone scan, and CT scan.

RECOMMENDATIONS FOR PROSTATE SCREENING

Screening refers to the process of testing an individual to detect a disease when that individual is not yet experiencing symptoms. For certain types of cancer (e.g., colorectal cancer, cervical cancer), screening allows the cancer to be discovered early, when it is more treatable, which increases the patient's survival rate.

The DRE and PSA screening tests for prostate cancer have certain limitations. Abnormal results from both of these tests do not necessarily indicate that cancer is present. In addition, normal results from these tests do not mean that cancer is *not* present. An elevated PSA test may lead to a biopsy and the detection of cancer in an individual, which can pose a dilemma. Many prostate cancers are slow growing and do not result in the death of an individual, particularly if the man is older or in poor health. Because it is sometimes difficult to determine the aggressiveness of the cancer, these individuals may still be treated with surgery or radiation, which can seriously affect a man's quality of life.

The ACS believes that available evidence does not currently support routine testing for prostate cancer. The ACS recommends that health care providers discuss the potential benefits and limitations of prostate screening with men older than 50 years. After this discussion, the PSA test and the DRE should be offered annually to men 50 years and older who are at average risk for prostate cancer and have

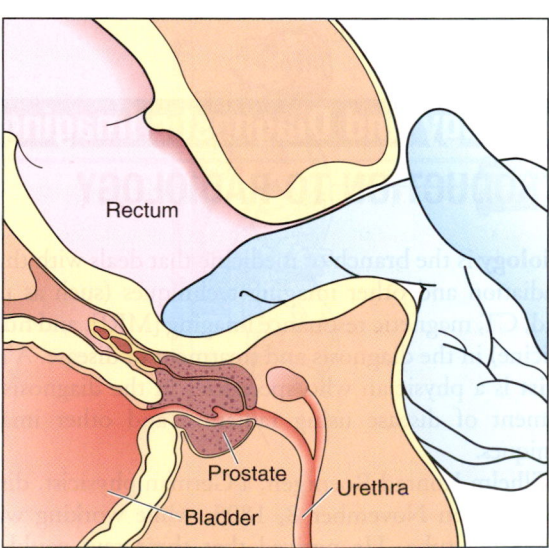

Figure 28-8 Digital rectal examination.

What Would You Do? | What Would You *Not* Do?

Case Study 2

Peter Bota, a 62-year-old retired Caucasian male, came to the medical office 1 week ago for a physical examination. The physician performed a digital rectal examination (DRE) but did not palpate anything abnormal. At that visit, Mr. Bota's blood was drawn for a prostate-specific antigen (PSA) test, and the results came back as slightly elevated (8 ng/mL). Mr. Bota has returned to the office and is waiting to talk with the physician about his test results and possible follow-up testing. Mr. Bota is extremely worried that he has cancer and wants to know the symptoms of prostate cancer. He also wants to know whether he did anything to cause prostate cancer. He says he does not smoke and drinks very little and that he walks his dog twice a day for exercise. ∎

bone mass. A score below −2.5 is defined as *osteoporosis.* The T-score is used to estimate the patient's risk of developing a fracture. The *Z-score* is derived by comparing the patient's measurements with an established database of normal individuals of the same age, gender, and ethnic group as the patient. An unusually high or low Z-score may indicate the need for further testing.

PATIENT TEACHING | Mammography

Answer questions that patients may have about mammography.

What is the purpose of mammography?

Mammography is a safe, low-dose radiographic examination used to screen for abnormal changes in the breasts. Mammography allows the physician to detect small lumps in the breast long before they can be felt. Although most breast lumps are not cancerous, breast cancer can be removed at an early stage when detected early, which usually results in treatment that is less deforming and has a much higher survival rate.

Who should have a mammogram?

The American Cancer Society recommends that women 40 years old and older have an annual mammogram because the risk of breast cancer increases after this age. Women with a family history of or other risk factors for breast cancer should follow the advice of the physician regarding mammography; age guidelines do not apply because these women undergo examination on a more frequent basis.

What occurs during the mammography procedure?

During mammography the breast is positioned on a special machine and is flattened with a compression paddle. Breast compression may be uncomfortable for some women. The discomfort can be reduced with avoidance of caffeine several days before the procedure and by scheduling the mammography the week after a menstrual period, when the breasts are less tender. Each breast is radiographed from above and from the side. A radiologist studies the resulting mammogram to detect any abnormalities. The results are reported to the physician.

Does mammography take the place of breast self-examination?

Mammography is not a substitute for breast self-examination. Women should continue to examine their breasts once a month and undergo a periodic breast examination by a physician. Most breast lumps are detected by women themselves.

- Encourage the patient to have a mammogram according to the schedule recommended by the American Cancer Society.
- Instruct the patient in the procedure for a breast self-examination.
- Provide the patient with educational materials on breast self-examination and mammography. ■

GASTROINTESTINAL SERIES

Upper Gastrointestinal Radiography

An upper GI study (UGI) is an examination of the upper digestive tract using fluoroscopy and radiography. The examination is helpful in the diagnosis of disorders of the esophagus, stomach, duodenum, and small intestine (e.g., GERD, hiatal hernia, peptic ulcer, benign and malignant tumors). The procedure may be ordered when the patient reports difficulty in swallowing, vomiting, abdominal pain, gastric reflux (burping up food [GERD]), severe indigestion, and blood in the stool.

Proper patient preparation is important for this procedure. The patient's stomach must be empty at the beginning of the study so that food does not obscure the radiographic image. To prepare for the examination, the patient must eat a light evening meal and then not eat or drink anything, including water and medications, after midnight on the day before the examination. Food and fluid in the GI tract have a degree of density and could cause confusing shadows on the radiograph.

The stomach varies little in density from the structures around it, and to make it show up on a radiograph a contrast medium must be used. The patient drinks a suspension of barium mixed with water and flavoring, which resembles a milkshake and has a chalky taste. Before drinking the barium, the patient may be asked to drink a carbonated beverage that consists of baking soda granules. This solution puts air into the stomach, causing it to expand. The combination of air and barium allows the radiologist to view the stomach in greater detail.

As the patient swallows the barium mixture, the radiologist observes its passage down the esophagus and into the stomach and duodenum with fluoroscopy. The barium coats the lining of the GI tract, making it visible on the screen of the fluoroscope. Radiographs are taken periodically during the examination to allow a detailed study of the upper GI tract and to obtain a permanent record. The patient's position is changed at various times so that the upper digestive tract can be visualized from different profiles. If the radiologist wants to observe the passage of barium through the small and large intestines, the patient must wait at the facility and return to the radiology examination room several times for additional radiographs. After the procedure, the radiologist prepares an upper GI report of the findings, which is sent to the patient's physician.

The medical assistant should explain to the patient that the barium suspension will appear in the stool for 1 to 3 days after the procedure and will cause the stool to have a whitish color. The barium mixture may cause constipation and the need for a laxative. To help prevent constipation, the patient should be instructed to increase fiber and fluid intake for several days after the procedure.

Lower Gastrointestinal Radiography

A lower GI study involves filling the colon with a barium sulfate mixture with a catheter (tube) inserted into the

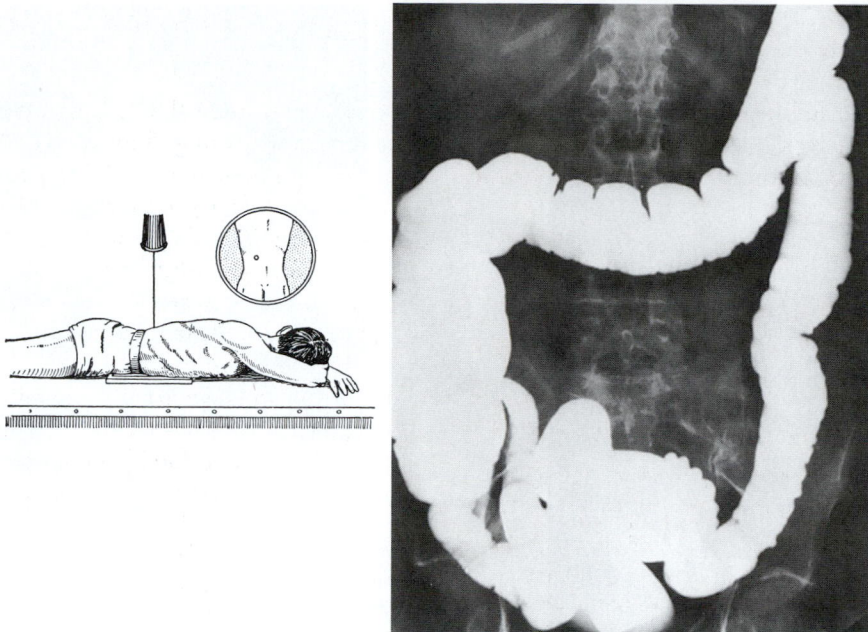

Figure 28-14 Lower gastrointestinal tract. Colon is distended with barium. Positioning of patient and radiograph. (From Meschan I: Synopsis of radiologic anatomy with computed tomography, Philadelphia, 1980, Saunders.)

rectum through the anus. Because of this, the procedure is sometimes called a *barium enema.* The examination uses fluoroscopy and radiography to observe and obtain permanent pictures of the colon and rectum (Figure 28-14). A lower GI study assists in diagnosis of disorders of the colon, such as polyps, cancerous tumors, and diverticulosis, and the extent of inflammatory bowel disease (e.g., ulcerative colitis, Crohn disease). The colon must be thoroughly cleansed in advance to remove gas and fecal material. Gas has a certain degree of density and shows up as confusing shadows on the radiograph. If fecal material appears on the film, the image of the colon is obscured.

Instructions for cleansing the colon may vary from one medical office to another, but in general the patient is instructed to consume only clear liquids the day before the examination, such as water, plain coffee and tea, clear broth, and strained fruit juice. A laxative should be taken on the day before the scheduled examination; an enema also may be necessary. An **enema** is an injection of fluid into the rectum to aid in the elimination of feces from the colon. The patient should not drink anything (except water) after midnight on the day before the examination. On the morning of the examination, the patient may be required to perform a warm water cleansing enema until the returns are clear.

The patient should report at the scheduled time and is instructed to relax on his or her side while the rectal catheter is inserted. As the barium enters the colon, the radiologist watches it on the fluoroscopic screen and periodically takes radiographs. The patient has a sensation of fullness and the urge to defecate as the barium enters the colon. The catheter usually has a balloon on the tip of it to prevent the barium

from coming back out. The patient is moved into various positions to allow the barium to fill the colon completely and to enable better visualization of the colon. The patient is allowed to evacuate the barium, and another radiograph is taken to finish the radiographic examination. After the procedure, the radiologist prepares a lower GI report of the findings, which is sent to the patient's physician.

A *double-contrast barium enema radiographic study* is similar to a lower GI study; however (in addition to the barium), it also employs the use of air that is inserted into the colon through the same catheter as the barium. The air distends the wall of the colon and allows the radiologist to view the colon in greater detail, making it easier to detect polyps and small cancerous tumors.

INTRAVENOUS PYELOGRAPHY

An intravenous pyelogram (IVP) is a radiograph of the kidneys, ureters, and bladder (Figure 28-15). An IVP is used to assist in the diagnosis of kidney stones, blockage or narrowing of the urinary tract, and growths within or near the urinary system.

The patient should consume only clear liquids starting at 4:00 PM the day before the examination. The evening before the examination, the patient must take a laxative such as magnesium citrate and/or Dulcolax tablets to remove gas and fecal material from the intestines. Removal of gas and fecal material permits proper visualization of the urinary tract. Starting at midnight the day before the examination, the patient should not eat, drink, smoke, or chew gum. Unless the patient is allergic to iodine, a contrast medium consisting of iodine is used and is administered

Figure 28-15 Intravenous pyelogram obtained 15 minutes after intravenous injection of a suitable contrast agent. (From Meschan I: Synopsis of radiologic anatomy with computed tomography, Philadelphia, 1980, Saunders.)

Figure 28-16 Three-dimensional (3-D) ultrasound examination of a third-trimester fetus. (From Leonard PC: Building a medical vocabulary: with Spanish translations, ed 9, St Louis, 2015, Saunders.)

Myelogram: Radiograph of the spinal column after injection of a radiopaque contrast medium.

Retrograde pyelogram: Radiograph of the kidneys and urinary tract after injection of radiopaque contrast medium directly into the ureter through a ureteral catheter. The dye flows to the kidneys through the ureters.

INTRODUCTION TO DIAGNOSTIC IMAGING

Diagnostic imaging procedures are performed frequently because they allow for the visualization of internal body structures in great detail. The most common diagnostic imaging procedures are **ultrasonography**, CT, MRI, and nuclear medicine scans. Diagnostic imaging procedures are usually performed in a hospital or a large clinic. The medical assistant, however, may need to relay information to a patient scheduled for such a procedure, including what to expect during the procedure and any patient preparation that may be required. The medical assistant should have a basic knowledge of diagnostic imaging procedures and the preparation necessary for each.

ULTRASONOGRAPHY

Ultrasonography, also called *ultrasound,* is the oldest of the diagnostic imaging procedures. Ultrasound uses high-frequency sound waves for the study of soft tissue structures. Recent advances have been made in technology in ultrasound. These include 3D ultrasound, in which sound waves are formatted into 3D images (Figure 28-16). Four-dimensional (4D) ultrasound is another new technology that consists of 3D ultrasound, but in motion.

intravenously to the patient. As the iodine enters the bloodstream, the patient may feel warm and flushed and have a metallic or salty taste in the mouth. This reaction is normal and lasts for only a few minutes. If the patient is allergic to iodine, a different type of contrast medium must be used. After the procedure the radiologist prepares an IVP report of the findings, which is sent to the patient's physician.

OTHER TYPES OF RADIOGRAPHS

Other types of radiographs that the medical assistant may encounter include the following:

Angiocardiogram: Radiograph of the heart in which valves and vessels are examined with radiography and fluoroscopy after introduction of a radiopaque contrast medium.

Bronchogram: Radiograph of the lungs after introduction of a radiopaque contrast medium.

Cerebral angiogram: Radiograph of the major arteries of the brain after injection of a radiopaque contrast medium.

Chest radiograph: Radiograph of the chest that does not use a contrast medium.

Cholangiogram: Radiograph of the bile ducts after administration of a radiopaque contrast medium.

Coronary angiogram: Radiograph of the coronary arteries after injection of a radiopaque contrast medium.

Cystogram: Radiograph of the urinary bladder after injection of a radiopaque contrast medium.

Hysterosalpingogram: Radiograph of the uterus and fallopian tubes after injection of a radiopaque contrast medium.

Ultrasound is frequently used in the diagnosis of conditions of the abdominal and pelvic organs, particularly the liver, gallbladder, spleen, pancreas, kidneys, uterus, ovaries, and abdominal aorta. Some examples of conditions that can be detected using ultrasound include breast cysts, gallstones, and kidney stones.

An ultrasound examination of the heart is called an **echocardiogram** and is used to determine the size, shape, and position of the heart and the movement of the heart valves and chambers. Ultrasonography is also used for guiding a needle or other device during a minimally invasive procedure such as amniocentesis, a needle biopsy, cortisone injection into a joint, and needle aspiration of fluid in a joint.

Ultrasonography offers many advantages as a diagnostic imaging procedure. It shows movement, allows continuous viewing of a structure, uses sound waves rather than radiation, and is less expensive than other imaging procedures. Ultrasound does have some minor limitations. Because sound waves are unable to penetrate bone and air- or gas-filled cavities such as the lungs, stomach, and intestines, ultrasound cannot be used in the evaluation of these structures. In addition, ultrasound may be difficult to use with obese patients because adipose tissue can interfere with sound wave transmission.

Before an ultrasound examination, a warm ultrasound gel must first be spread on the area to be examined. The purpose of the gel is to increase conductivity of the sound waves between the skin and the transducer. During the ultrasound examination, the examiner places a probe containing a transducer firmly on the patient's skin and moves it over the body areas to be examined. The transducer generates sound waves that are directed into the patient's tissues. The sound waves are reflected back to the transducer, similar to an echo. These sound waves are then transmitted to the ultrasound machine through a cable, where a computer converts them into an image. The size, shape, and consistency of the image are displayed on a video display screen; this image is known as a **sonogram** (Figure 28-17). The patient is often permitted to view the sonogram on the screen of the monitor as the procedure is performed. Selected images can be permanently recorded on paper, film, videotape, or a computerized storage medium. A radiologist reviews and interprets the images and prepares an ultrasound report that is sent to the patient's physician.

Although ultrasound is commonly used for a wide variety of noninvasive imaging procedures, individuals are most familiar with its use in obstetrics. Obstetric ultrasound is most frequently used to determine the gestational age of a fetus and to confirm the due date; to detect congenital abnormalities, ectopic pregnancy, and multiple pregnancy; and to determine the fetus's position and size late in pregnancy. If the fetus is old enough and is positioned correctly, it also may be possible to determine its gender. Because the ultrasound machine is a compact unit, most obstetricians perform this procedure in their medical offices. Ultrasound is also used by gynecologists to evaluate and treat infertility problems.

Doppler ultrasound is a special application of ultrasound. It measures the direction and speed of blood as it flows through blood vessels, such as major arteries and veins in the abdomen, arms, legs, and neck. Doppler ultrasound images can assist the physician in diagnosing blood flow blockages, narrowing of blood vessels as a result of atherosclerosis, and congenital malformations.

PATIENT PREPARATION

The medical assistant should tell the patient what to expect during an ultrasound examination and instruct the patient in the preparation required for the procedure, as follows:

1. Ultrasound is a safe and painless procedure that takes approximately 15 to 45 minutes to complete, depending on the body part examined.
2. The patient may need to prepare for the procedure, depending on the part of the body examined. An ultrasound of the gallbladder, liver, spleen, and pancreas necessitates that the patient fast for 8 to 12 hours. For an obstetric ultrasound, the patient needs to have a full

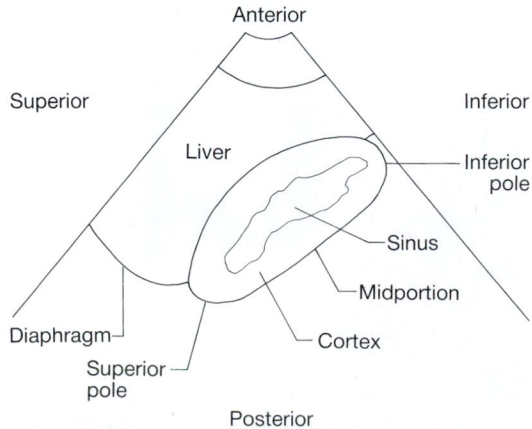

Figure 28-17 Sonogram of the right kidney. (From Tempkin BB: *Ultrasound scanning: principles and protocols,* ed 4, St Louis, 2015, Saunders.)

bladder. The patient should be instructed to consume approximately 32 ounces of fluid about 1 hour before the procedure.

3. The patient must remain still when requested during the procedure because movement can interfere with accurate results. In addition, the patient may be asked to change positions so that the organs can be seen at different angles.

COMPUTED TOMOGRAPHY

Computed tomography (also known as a *CT* scan) is an advanced radiographic examination that uses only a minimal amount of radiation. It produces a series of cross-sectional images of a body part, permitting the imaging of structures that cannot be visualized with conventional radiographic procedures. A CT scan allows the radiologist to view the bones and organs of the head and body in fine detail and has been used most successfully in diagnostic studies of the brain, abdomen, and pelvis. CT scans are used primarily to detect and evaluate tumors and other abnormalities and to monitor the effects of surgery, radiation therapy, or chemotherapy on tumors.

The scan is conducted by a skilled diagnostic imaging technician. The patient is positioned on a special motorized table (Figure 28-18). From an adjoining room, the technician mechanically moves the table into a doughnut-shaped device known as the *CT scanner* until the part of the body to be examined is inside the tubular opening of the scanner.

During the scan, two examinations are often performed. The first examination is a plain scan, and the second is a repeat scan after a contrast medium has been injected through a vein in the arm. The contrast medium makes possible a sharper image of internal structures of the body. The x-ray tube within the CT scanner rotates around the patient, taking multiple radiographic images in a rapid sequence at different angles. The series of radiographs is processed with a computer to produce cross-sectional

images of a body part similar to the slices of bread in a loaf. These images are permanently recorded on film or stored digitally on electronic media for evaluation by a radiologist (Figure 28-19). The radiologist reviews and interprets the images and prepares a CT report, which is sent to the patient's physician.

PATIENT PREPARATION

The medical assistant should tell the patient what to expect during the CT scan and should instruct the patient on the preparation required for the procedure, as follows:

1. Before the procedure the patient must remove all radiopaque objects, such as dentures, eyeglasses, and jewelry, because they interfere with a clear image of the body part examined.
2. If a contrast medium is to be used, the patient may need to fast for several hours before the procedure. It is important to ask the patient whether he or she is allergic to radiographic contrast media to avoid an adverse reaction.
3. The patient should lie motionless and breathe normally during the procedure. When a radiograph is being taken, the patient is usually asked to hold his or her breath so that the radiograph is not blurred. The patient hears mechanical clicking and whirring sounds from the scanner as pictures are taken.
4. Depending on the body part being examined, the procedure takes from 10 minutes to an hour to complete.

MAGNETIC RESONANCE IMAGING

MRI is used for imaging tissues of high fat and water content that cannot be seen with other radiologic techniques. MRI assists in the diagnosis of intracranial and spinal lesions and cardiovascular and soft tissue abnormalities, such as herniated discs and joint diseases. MRI allows the examiner to see through bone and view fluid-filled soft tissue in great detail.

MRI is a safe and painless procedure in which a strong magnetic field and ordinary radio waves produce computer-processed images of internal body structures. Because MRI does not involve radiation, the U.S. Food and Drug Administration has classified the MRI machine as a low-risk device.

The patient lies on a table inside the bore of the cylindric MRI machine while a diagnostic imaging technician in an adjoining room monitors the procedure (Figure 28-20). Because of the enclosed space, some patients may have difficulty with claustrophobia. The physician may order a sedative for these patients. Open MRI machines are less confining than traditional MRI machines; however, they are a newer technology and may not be available at some facilities.

The high-resolution, 3D images that are obtained with MRI are permanently recorded on film or stored digitally on electronic media for evaluation by a radiologist. The

Figure 28-18 Positioning patient for computed tomography (CT) scan. (From Kowalczyk N, Donnett K: *Integrated patient care for the imaging professional,* St Louis, 1996, Mosby.)

Figure 28-19 The computed tomography (CT) scanner takes multiple cross-sectional radiographic images. The images shown here are cross-sectional pictures of the head used to evaluate the orbits and sinuses. (From Snopek A: *Fundamentals of special radiographic procedures,* ed 4, Philadelphia, 1999, Saunders.)

Figure 28-20 Magnetic resonance imaging (MRI). The patient lies on a table inside the bore of the cylindrical MRI machine while MRI technicians in an adjoining room monitor the procedure. (From Frank E, Long B, Smith B, eds: Merrill's atlas of radiographic positions and radiologic procedures, vol 3, ed 12, 2012, Mosby.)

radiologist reviews and interprets the images and prepares an MRI report, which is sent to the patient's physician.

PATIENT PREPARATION

The medical assistant should tell the patient what to expect during the MRI and instruct the patient in the preparation required for the procedure, as follows:

1. MRI is a safe and painless procedure with a usual completion time between 20 minutes and 1½ hours.
2. No special preparation is necessary for the MRI examination. The patient may eat or drink before the examination and take any prescribed medication. The patient should wear loose, comfortable clothing, such as a jogging suit, for the procedure.
3. Because the procedure involves a strong magnet, the patient should remove any metal or magnetic-sensitive

objects, such as hairpins, eyeglasses, hearing aids, watches, rings, and credit cards. Avoid wearing cosmetics, as certain types of cosmetic preparations contain small amounts of metal. Individuals with a pacemaker or inner ear implant may not be able to undergo an MRI.

4. A contrast medium may be used for the procedure. It improves the resolution of the image by increasing the brightness in various parts of the body.

5. The patient must remain completely still for 15- to 20-minute intervals during the procedure. The patient hears a metallic clacking sound like a muffled drumbeat during the procedure. Earplugs or headphones are available for use if the patient desires.

What Would You Do? What Would You *Not* Do?

Case Study 3

Michael Wendl is an 18-year-old high school varsity football player. For the past 3 months, he has had pain and swelling in his left shoulder. The physician schedules a magnetic resonance imaging (MRI) scan to assist in determining the cause of the problem. Michael has had several radiographs over the past 2 years and is worried about the radiation exposure to his body. He wants to know how much radiation will be involved with the procedure. Michael has problems with claustrophobia and wants to know whether he can play a game on his iPhone during the procedure to distract him. He also wants to know whether he is allowed to eat anything before the procedure. ■

Memories *from* Practicum

Megan Baer: My first practicum was terrifying, but at the same time I was overwhelmed with excitement. I remember worrying about how I was going to remember all my clinical and administrative skills. I was worried that I would hurt someone or forget to do something important.

One day a patient came into our office upset and crying. The examination rooms were full, so I took her into our staff lounge. I sat her down, fixed her a cup of coffee, and asked her if I could help. She told me that her son had drowned 2 years ago on that day, her mother had cancer, and her husband had passed away 8 months previously. I listened to everything she had to say, and I comforted her until the physician was ready to see her. She walked over to me, hugged me, and said my smile and people skills were the best treatment for her depression that she had ever had. Her telling me that made me feel good about my career choice, and it made me realize how fulfilling it was. It did not take me long to realize that all the hands-on skills that I had learned in the classroom were not forgotten. I also realized that a smile and listening to people are just as important as my skills. ■

NUCLEAR MEDICINE

Nuclear medicine is an advanced diagnostic imaging procedure in which a tiny bit of radioactive material is introduced into the patient. The radiation is introduced into the body by a diagnostic imaging technician intravenously, by ingestion, or by inhalation. The technologist positions the patient on a scanning table that works in association with a specialized piece of equipment known as a *gamma camera.* The gamma camera is positioned above or below the scanning table and is able to detect the radiation being given off by the body part that has been targeted by the radiation. This is accomplished through the use of scintillation crystals. These crystals convert the radiation being given off by the body into light. This light is converted into electrical impulses, which are interpreted by a computer program contained within the gamma camera. The resulting information is displayed as still images or functional animations of body parts and organs. Because it can show the actual function of organs, nuclear medicine provides more detailed information for certain conditions than is provided by other diagnostic imaging examinations (e.g., CT scan, MRI).

The radioactive material used in nuclear medicine is known as a *radiopharmaceutical* (or radionuclide). Examples of commonly used radiopharmaceuticals include technetium-99m, iodine-123 and iodine-131, and thallium-201. Most radiopharmaceuticals are chemically bound to a complex known as a *tracer.* A tracer is designed to be attracted to specific areas of the body or, in some cases, to types of diseased tissue.

The most common nuclear medicine procedures include bone scans and nuclear cardiac stress tests, which are described in more detail in the next section. Other types of nuclear medicine procedures that may be performed include gallbladder procedures, thyroid studies, brain scans, lung scans, and liver procedures.

BONE SCANS

Bone scans are performed to detect small fractures (e.g., stress fractures) or lesions that may not be visible on other diagnostic imaging examinations. When a bone scan is performed, the patient is injected with a radiopharmaceutical. The patient must then wait at the facility for a predetermined period of time, based on the area being examined. The purpose of the waiting period is to allow the radiopharmaceutical to be absorbed sufficiently so that an accurate diagnosis can be made. The gamma camera detects the radiation given off by the small fracture, and it shows up as a "hot" spot on the nuclear images (Figure 28-21). The radiologist reviews the nuclear images and prepares a bone scan report, which is sent to the patient's physician.

Figure 28-21 Bone scan of the foot. *Arrows* show the hot spot that indicates a stress fracture. (From Donatelli RA: *Sports-specific rehabilitation,* St Louis, 2007, Churchill Livingstone.)

NUCLEAR CARDIAC STRESS TEST

A nuclear cardiac stress test is a diagnostic procedure used to evaluate the cardiovascular health of individuals with known heart disease or individuals at high risk for developing heart disease, particularly coronary artery disease (CAD). Although a nuclear stress test is more time-consuming and expensive to perform than a simple stress test (described in Chapter 27), it provides more accuracy in diagnosing CAD.

The radiopharmaceutical used for a nuclear stress test is usually technetium (99mTc) sestamibi (trade name is Cardiolite), which is administered intravenously and targets the heart. Nuclear images included in the stress test are taken by the gamma camera during two phases: a *resting phase* and a *stress phase* (which is a functional study). The resting phase is performed with the heart beating at a normal rate, whereas the stress phase is performed immediately after the patient exercises at his or her maximal (target) heart rate. The two sets of nuclear images—the resting images and the images taken under cardiac stress—are then compared with each other. These images assist the radiologist in determining which parts of the heart are healthy and functioning normally. The images also identify areas of the heart that exhibit decreased blood flow during exercise, meaning that a portion of the heart muscle is not receiving enough oxygen. A decreased oxygen supply to a portion of the heart is known as *cardiac ischemia* and is typically a result of the presence of CAD. The radiologist reviews and interprets the images and prepares a nuclear cardiac stress test report, which is sent to the patient's physician.

A PET (positron emission tomography) scan is a special type of nuclear imaging procedure. PET uses a special camera and computer to construct a 3D image of the area being scanned. This procedure is particularly useful in diagnosing conditions of the brain and heart, such as brain cancer and heart disease.

GUIDELINES

Specific guidelines that may be required for nuclear medicine examinations are as follows:

1. Depending on the type of nuclear medicine examination being performed, the patient may be required to be in a fasting state or to abstain from consuming certain foods or substances such as caffeine for a period of time. The medical assistant should check with the facility performing the examination so that proper dietary instructions can be relayed to the patient.

2. Nuclear medicine examinations are time-consuming because most examinations require multiple scans. The interval between scans is determined by the part being examined and the type of equipment and radiopharmaceutical being used. There may be a delay between administration of the radiopharmaceutical and when the patient is actually placed on the scanning table. Follow-up images that may be acquired later the same day or in some cases the following morning also may be needed. Because of this, the medical assistant must inform the patient of the amount of time required for the examination so that arrangements can be made with work and home schedules if needed.

3. Because most nuclear medicine examinations require that the patient lie still on a table for a prolonged time, the patient should be advised to wear comfortable clothing to the examination. If a nuclear medicine examination requires exercise as a component of the test, the patient should be instructed to wear appropriate exercise clothing, including athletic shoes.

DIGITAL RADIOLOGY

Modern advances in digital imaging technology have made inroads in the field of radiology. The result is the transformation of film-based radiology into a system of computer-displayed and stored digital images. To assist in understanding digital radiology, this transformation can be compared with the replacement of film cameras with digital cameras.

Figure 28-22 Digital image of a chest radiograph. (From Buck CJ: Electronic health record booster kit for the medical office, St Louis, 2009, Saunders.)

Images can be taken and viewed immediately and then sent electronically to a network of computers.

Digital radiology allows for increased efficiency and cost savings and better patient care. Higher-quality images and the ability to transfer these digital images electronically are two important benefits that affect the patient directly. As a result of this digital revolution, the medical assistant may be required to use the medical office computer to access, display (Figure 28-22), and permanently save images taken by the facilities providing digital imaging services.

What Would You Do? What Would You *Not* Do? RESPONSES

Case Study 1
Page 724

What Did Megan Do?
❏ Relayed to Mrs. Bernard that this is not the most fun test to perform, but that if colon cancer is detected early, the cure rate is very high.
❏ Explained to Mrs. Bernard that colon cancer increases after age 50, and that an individual can develop colon cancer without a family history of it.
❏ Told Mrs. Bernard that during the early stages of colon cancer no symptoms occur, so it is possible to feel fine but still have a problem.
❏ Explained to Mrs. Bernard in greater detail the reason for not eating red meat or taking aspirin during the testing period.
❏ Told Mrs. Bernard that disposable gloves can be given to her to take home to wear when she collects the specimens.
❏ Explained to Mrs. Bernard that the physician talks with patients every day about these types of things, and it is important to talk with him about all aspects of her health so that she receives the best care possible.

❏ Told Mrs. Bernard that the office will call her in 3 days to see whether she has any questions or is having any problems with the test.

What Did Megan Not Do?
❏ Told Mrs. Bernard that she is getting older and needs to be more concerned about performing health screening tests.

Case Study 2
Page 735

What Did Megan Do?
❏ Listened patiently and try to reassure and calm Mr. Bota. Told him that physicians do not yet know what causes prostate cancer.
❏ Explained that the PSA test is a screening test and that he should not jump to conclusions about the results.
❏ Told Mr. Bota that the physician will talk with him about his test results in a short while.
❏ Commended Mr. Bota on his healthy lifestyle habits and encouraged him to continue with them.

What Would You Do? What Would You *Not* Do? RESPONSES—cont'd

❑ Gave Mr. Bota some brochures on male reproductive health to read while he waited to be seen by the physician.

What Did Megan *Not* Do?
❑ Told Mr. Bota that there is nothing to worry about.

Case Study 3
Page 746

What Did Megan Do?
❑ Explained to Michael that MRI does not use radiation, so he would not be exposed to any radiation during the procedure.
❑ Told Michael that he would not be able to play a game on his iPhone during the procedure. Explained that MRI works with

a strong magnet that might damage the iPhone, and use of the iPhone also could interfere with a good image of the shoulder. Told Michael that he would need to lie still during the procedure.
❑ Told Michael the physician would be informed of his problem with claustrophobia. Explained that the physician may want to give him something to help him relax during the procedure.
❑ Told Michael that it is fine to eat before the procedure.

What Did Megan *Not* Do?
❑ Overlooked or minimized Michael's concern about claustrophobia.

TERMINOLOGY REVIEW

Key Term	Word Parts	Definition
Biopsy	*bi/o:* life *-opsy:* to view	The surgical removal and examination of tissue from the living body. Biopsies usually are performed to determine whether a tumor is benign or malignant.
Colonoscope	*colon/o:* colon *-scope:* instrument used for visual examination	An endoscope that is specially designed for passage through the anus to permit visualization of the rectum and the entire length of the colon.
Colonoscopy	*colon/o:* colon *-scopy:* visual examination	The visualization of the rectum and the entire colon using a colonoscope.
Contrast medium		A substance used to make a particular structure visible on a radiograph.
Echocardiogram	*ech/o:* sound *cardi/o:* heart *-gram:* record	An ultrasound examination of the heart.
Endoscope	*endo-:* within *-scope:* instrument used for visual examination	An instrument that consists of a tube and an optical system that is used for direct visual inspection of organs or cavities.
Enema		An injection of fluid into the rectum to aid in the elimination of feces from the colon.
Fluoroscope	*fluor/o:* fluorescence *-scope:* instrument used for visual examination	An instrument used to view internal organs and structures directly.
Fluoroscopy	*fluor/o:* fluorescence *-scopy:* visual examination	Examination of a patient with a fluoroscope.
Insufflate		To blow a powder, vapor, or gas (e.g., air) into a body cavity.
Melena		The darkening of the stool caused by the presence of blood in an amount of 50 mL or more.
Occult blood		Blood in such a small amount that it is not detectable by the unaided eye.
Peroxidase	*-oxia:* oxygen *-ase:* enzyme	As it pertains to the guaiac slide test, a substance that is able to transfer oxygen from hydrogen peroxide to oxidize guaiac, causing the guaiac to turn blue.
Radiograph	*radi/o:* radiation *-graph:* instrument used to record, x-ray film	A permanent record of a picture of an internal body organ or structure produced on radiographic film.
Radiography	*radi/o:* radiation *-graphy:* process of recording, x-ray filming	The taking of permanent records (radiographs) of internal body organs and structures by passing x-rays through the body to act on a specially sensitized film.

Continued

↻ TERMINOLOGY REVIEW—cont'd

Key Term	Word Parts	Definition
Radiologist	*radi/o:* radiation *-ologist:* one who studies and practices (specialist)	A physician who specializes in the diagnosis and treatment of disease using radiation and other imaging techniques.
Radiology	*radi/o:* radiation *-ology:* study of	The branch of medicine that deals with the use of radiation and other imaging techniques (such as ultrasound, computed tomography [CT], magnetic resonance imaging [MRI], and nuclear medicine) in the diagnosis and treatment of disease.
Radiolucent	*radi/o:* radiation *-lucent:* transparent	Describing a structure that permits the passage of x-rays.
Radiopaque	*radi/o:* radiation *-opaque:* opaque	Describing a structure that obstructs the passage of x-rays.
Sigmoidoscope	*sigmoid/o:* sigmoid (colon) *-scope:* instrument used for visual examination	An endoscope that is specially designed for passage through the anus to permit visualization of the rectum and sigmoid colon.
Sigmoidoscopy	*sigmoid/o:* sigmoid (colon) *-scopy:* visual examination	The visual examination of the rectum and sigmoid colon with use of a sigmoidoscope.
Sonogram	*son/o:* sound *-gram:* record	The record obtained with ultrasonography.
Ultrasonography	*ultra-:* beyond, excess *sono-:* sound *-graphy:* process of recording	The use of high-frequency sound waves to produce an image of an organ or tissue.

ON THE WEB

For information on colorectal cancer:

American Cancer Society: www.cancer.org

National Cancer Institute: www.cancer.gov

Prevent Cancer Foundation: www.preventcancer.org

Colon Cancer Alliance: www.ccalliance.org

Health Communities: www.healthcommunities.com/heath-topics/cancer.shtml

For information on prostate cancer:

Prostate Health: www.prostatehealth.com

Prostate Information: www.prostateinfo.com

Prostate.com: www.prostate.com

Prostate Cancer Foundation: www.pef.org

Prostatitis Foundation: www.prostatitis.org

Male Health: www.malehealthcenter.com

For information on radiography and diagnostic imaging:

American College of Radiology: www.acr.org

Whole Brain Atlas: www.med.harvard.edu/AANLIB/home.html

Radiology Information: www.radiologyinfo.org

Diagnostic Imaging: www.diagnosticimaging.com

ON THE WEB—cont'd

For information on breast cancer:

American Cancer Society: www.cancer.org

CDC Breast Cancer: www.cdc.gov/cancer

Cancer Treatment Centers of American: www.cancercenter.com

Breast Cancer org: www.breastcancer.org

National Breast Cancer Foundation: www.nationalbreastcancer.org

Breast Cancer.Net: www.breastcancer.net

Breast Cancer Basics: breastcancer.about.com

Introduction to the Clinical Laboratory

LEARNING OBJECTIVES

Clinical Laboratory

1. Explain the general purpose of a laboratory test.
2. Identify and define the eight categories of a laboratory test on the basis of function. List examples of tests included under each category.
3. List and explain specific uses of laboratory test results.
4. List and describe the components of the physician's office laboratory (POL).
5. List the information included in a laboratory directory.
6. Identify the purpose of a laboratory request form. List and explain the function of each type of information included on the form.
7. Identify the use of each of the following profiles, and list the tests included in each:
   • Comprehensive metabolic profile
   • Electrolyte profile
   • Hepatic function profile
   • Hepatitis profile
   • Lipid profile
   • Prenatal profile
   • Renal function profile
   • Rheumatoid profile
   • Thyroid function profile
8. Identify the purpose of the laboratory report form, and list the information included on it.
9. Describe the advantages of using a computer to send and receive laboratory documents.
10. Explain how an EMR program can be used to prepare a flow sheet for tests performed on a routine basis.

Collecting, Transporting, and Handling Specimens

11. Explain the purpose of advance patient preparation for the collection of a laboratory specimen.
12. List examples of specimens.
13. Identify and explain the guidelines that should be followed during specimen collection.
14. Explain why specimens must be handled and stored properly.
15. Identify the proper handling and storage techniques for each of the following specimens: blood, urine, microbiologic specimen, and stool specimen.

Laboratory Testing in the Medical Office

16. Describe the following CLIA test categories: waived, moderately complex, and highly complex.
17. List and describe the information included in a product insert that accompanies a CLIA-waived testing kit.
18. List the advantages of an automated blood analyzer.
19. Explain the purpose of quality control in the laboratory, and list quality control methods that should be employed when a CLIA-waived laboratory test is performed.
20. List the laboratory safety guidelines that should be followed in the medical office to prevent accidents.

PROCEDURES

Operate an emergency eyewash station.
Use a laboratory directory.

Complete a laboratory request form.
Read a laboratory report.
Operate an emergency eyewash station.
Inspect and test an emergency eyewash station.
Instruct a patient on the preparation necessary for a laboratory test that requires fasting.

Maintain laboratory test results using flow sheets.

Collect a specimen.
Handle and store a specimen.

Perform a CLIA-waived laboratory test by following the manufacturer's instructions.
Perform quality control procedures when conducting a CLIA-waived laboratory test.
Practice laboratory safety.

CHAPTER OUTLINE

INTRODUCTION TO THE CLINICAL LABORATORY
LABORATORY TESTS
PURPOSE OF LABORATORY TESTING
TYPES OF CLINICAL LABORATORIES
Physician's Office Laboratory
Components of the POL
Physical Structure
Refrigerator
Safety Measures
Room Temperature and Lighting
Maintenance
Outside Laboratories
Laboratory Directory
Collection and Testing Categories
LABORATORY REQUESTS
Purpose
Parts of Laboratory Request Form
LABORATORY REPORTS
LABORATORY DOCUMENTS AND THE EMR
PATIENT PREPARATION AND INSTRUCTIONS
Fasting
Medication Restrictions
COLLECTING, HANDLING, AND TRANSPORTING SPECIMENS
Guidelines for Specimen Collection

CLINICAL LABORATORY IMPROVEMENT AMENDMENTS
Purpose of CLIA 1988
Categories of Laboratory Testing
1. Waived Tests
2. Moderate-Complexity Tests
3. High-Complexity Tests
Requirements for Moderate-Complexity and High-Complexity Testing
CLIA-WAIVED LABORATORY TESTING
CLIA-Waived Testing Kits
CLIA-Waived Automated Analyzers
QUALITY CONTROL
1. Storage and Handling of Test Systems
2. Stability of Testing Components
3. Calibration
4. Controls
5. Collecting and Handling Specimens
6. Testing the Specimen
7. Interpreting and Reading Test Results
CATEGORIES OF TEST RESULTS
Qualitative Test Results
Quantitative Test Results
RECORDING TEST RESULTS
LABORATORY SAFETY

KEY TERMS

analyte
calibration
clinical diagnosis
control
fasting
homeostasis (hoe-mee-oh-STAY-sis)
in vivo (in-VEE-voe)
laboratory test

nonwaived test
plasma (PLAZ-ma)
product insert
profile
qualitative test
quality control
quantitative test
reagent

reference range
routine test
serum (SERE-um)
specimen (SPES-i-men)
test system
waived test

INTRODUCTION TO THE CLINICAL LABORATORY

Clinical laboratory test results are often used along with a thorough health history and physical examination to obtain essential data needed by the physician for the accurate diagnosis and management of a patient's condition. Clinical **laboratory tests** provide objective and quantitative information regarding the status of body conditions and functions. When the body is healthy, its systems function normally, and a state of equilibrium of the internal environment is said to exist; this is termed **homeostasis.** When the body is in a state of homeostasis, the physical and chemical

characteristics of body substances (e.g., fluids, secretions, excretions) are within an acceptable range known as the **reference range.**

When a pathologic condition exists, biologic changes occur within the body, altering the normal physiology or functioning of the body and resulting in an imbalance. These changes cause the patient to experience symptoms of that particular pathologic condition. Iron-deficiency anemia usually causes the patient to experience weakness, fatigue, pallor, irritability, and in some cases shortness of breath on exertion. In addition, these changes in the body's biologic processes may cause an alteration in the characteristics of body substances, such as an alteration in the chemical content of the blood or urine, an alteration in the antibody level, or an alteration in cell counts or cellular morphology.

Physical and chemical alterations of body substances become evident through abnormal values or results on laboratory tests—in other words, values outside the accepted reference range or limit for that particular test. Just as certain pathologic conditions cause specific symptoms to occur, certain pathologic conditions cause values outside of the reference range to occur for specific laboratory tests. Iron-deficiency anemia causes an alteration in normal red blood cell morphology and a decreased hemoglobin level.

An important realization is that a value outside of the reference range for a particular test may be seen with more than one pathologic condition. A decrease in the hemoglobin level is found with hyperthyroidism, cirrhosis of the liver, and autoimmune diseases. In this regard, the physician cannot rely solely on laboratory test results to make a diagnosis, but rather must rely also on the combination of data obtained from the health history, the physical examination, and diagnostic and laboratory test results.

LABORATORY TESTS

A **laboratory test** is defined as the clinical analysis and study of materials, fluids, or tissues obtained from patients to assist in the diagnosis and treatment of disease. Laboratory tests can be classified by function into one of the following categories: hematology, clinical chemistry, immunology and blood banking, urinalysis, microbiology, parasitology, cytology, and histology. Use of these classifications makes it easier to refer to laboratory tests.

The number of laboratory tests ordered for a patient varies depending on the physician's clinical findings. A clinical diagnosis of streptococcal sore throat usually requires only a strep test for confirmation. Many diseases cause more than one alteration in the physical and chemical characteristics of body substances, however, and a series of laboratory tests is often necessary to establish the pattern of abnormalities characteristic of a particular disease.

The medical assistant should realize that not all pathologic conditions necessitate the use of laboratory test results for arrival at a diagnosis; the information obtained from the patient's clinical signs and symptoms can be sufficient for a diagnosis of some conditions. In these instances, the physician is so certain of the clinical diagnosis that therapy can be instituted without laboratory confirmation. Most physicians diagnose acute purulent otitis media with the information obtained from patient symptoms (earache, fever, feeling of fullness in the ear) and from an otoscopic examination of the tympanic membrane (the tympanic membrane is red and bulging). Information obtained through the clinical signs and symptoms is sufficiently specific to otitis media to allow the physician to make a diagnosis and to prescribe treatment.

The medical assistant must acquire knowledge and skill in basic clinical laboratory methods and techniques. It is important that the medical assistant have knowledge of the laboratory tests that are performed most often, including the purpose of these tests, the reference range for each test, any advance patient preparation or special instructions, and any substances that might interfere with accurate test results, such as food or medication.

The medical assistant frequently works with this information when instructing a patient in advance preparation for a laboratory test; collecting, handling, and storing specimens; performing laboratory tests; and receiving and filing laboratory reports. It is essential that the medical assistant understand the value of laboratory tests and alert the physician to any abnormal results as soon as the test has been performed or the laboratory report has been received.

This chapter serves as an introduction to the clinical laboratory by providing an overview of methods and general guidelines to follow and by focusing on the relationship between the medical office and an outside laboratory. Specific information for collection, handling, storing, and testing of biologic specimens is presented in subsequent chapters.

PURPOSE OF LABORATORY TESTING

The most frequent use of laboratory test results is to assist in the diagnosis of a patient's condition. Laboratory test results also have many other significant medical uses. A summary of the purpose and function of laboratory testing follows.

1. *To assist in the diagnosis of pathologic conditions.* Laboratory tests are most frequently ordered by the physician to assist in the diagnosis of pathologic conditions. Along with the health history and the physical examination, laboratory test results provide the physician with essential data needed to arrive at a diagnosis and prescribe treatment. After obtaining the health history and performing the physical examination, the physician may order laboratory tests for these reasons:
   - *To confirm a clinical diagnosis.* A **clinical diagnosis** is defined as a tentative diagnosis of a patient's condition obtained through the evaluation of the health history and the physical examination, without the benefit of laboratory or diagnostic tests. The patient's signs and symptoms may provide a strong clinical diagnosis of a particular condition, and the physician may order laboratory tests simply to confirm that diagnosis. For example, the patient may have the typical signs and symptoms of diabetes mellitus, which would provide the physician with a fairly certain clinical diagnosis. In this instance, an oral glucose tolerance test (OGTT) may be ordered to confirm the diagnosis and to institute therapy.
   - *To assist in the differential diagnosis of a patient's condition.* Two or more diseases may have similar signs and symptoms; the physician orders laboratory tests to assist in the differential diagnosis of the patient's

condition. A diagnosis of streptococcal sore throat must be made with a laboratory test to differentiate it from other pathologic conditions with similar signs and symptoms, such as pharyngitis.

- *To obtain information regarding a patient's condition* when not enough concrete evidence exists to support a clinical diagnosis. The patient sometimes may have vague signs and symptoms, and laboratory tests are ordered to obtain information on what may be causing the patient's problem. For example, the patient may have nonspecific abdominal pain, and the physical examination may not yield enough information to support a clinical diagnosis. In this case, the physician may order a series of laboratory and diagnostic tests to assist in pinpointing the cause of the patient's problems.

2. *To evaluate the patient's progress and to regulate treatment.* When a diagnosis has been made, laboratory testing may be performed to evaluate the patient's progress and to regulate treatment. On the basis of the laboratory results, the therapy may need to be adjusted or further treatment prescribed. A patient undergoing iron therapy for iron-deficiency anemia should have a complete blood count (CBC) performed every month to assess the response to treatment and to ensure that the condition is improving. Another example is a patient who has had a cardiac valve replaced and is taking warfarin (Coumadin), an anticoagulant used to inhibit blood clotting. The patient must have a prothrombin time test at regular intervals to assess the clotting ability of the blood. On the basis of the test results, the medication may need to be adjusted to ensure the dosage is at a safe level. A patient with diabetes who measures his or her blood glucose level each day to regulate insulin dosage provides another example of laboratory tests used to regulate treatment.

3. *To establish a baseline level.* On the basis of such factors as age, gender, race, and geographic location, individuals have different normal levels within the established reference range for a particular test. In this respect, laboratory tests also can serve to establish each patient's baseline level with which future results can be compared. A patient who is going to receive warfarin (Coumadin) therapy should have a blood specimen drawn for a prothrombin time test before administration of this anticoagulant. The results serve as a baseline recording for that particular patient against which future prothrombin time test results can be compared.

4. *To prevent or reduce the severity of disease.* Laboratory tests also can help to prevent or reduce the severity of disease through early detection of abnormal findings. Certain conditions, such as high cholesterol, anemia, and diabetes, are relatively common disorders and sometimes may exist without symptoms in a patient, especially early in the development of the disease. Laboratory tests known as **routine tests** are performed on a routine basis on apparently healthy patients (usually as part of a general physical examination) to assist in the early detection of disease. These tests are relatively easy to perform and present a minimal hazard to the patient. The most commonly used routine tests are urinalysis, CBC, and routine blood chemistries.

5. *To comply with state laws.* Another reason for a laboratory test is its requirement by state law. The statutes of most states require a gonorrhea and syphilis test to be performed on pregnant women. The purpose of these tests is to protect the mother and fetus from harm by screening for the presence of these sexually transmitted diseases.

TYPES OF CLINICAL LABORATORIES

The medical office may use an outside laboratory for testing, or the office may contain its own laboratory, known as a *physician's office laboratory* (POL), in which the medical assistant performs various tests. Most medical offices use a combination of the two to fulfill the physician's need for test results.

PHYSICIAN'S OFFICE LABORATORY

In general, laboratory tests that are Clinical Laboratories Improvement Amendments (CLIA) waived and commonly required, such as glucose determination and urinalysis, are performed in the POL (Figure 29-1). CLIA consists of regulations developed in 1988 by the federal government to improve the quality of laboratory testing in the United States. A **waived test** is a laboratory test that has been determined by CLIA to be a simple procedure that is easy to perform and has a low risk of erroneous test results. CLIA regulations are described in greater detail later in this chapter.

Most physicians consider it too expensive in terms of equipment, supplies, and medical laboratory personnel to

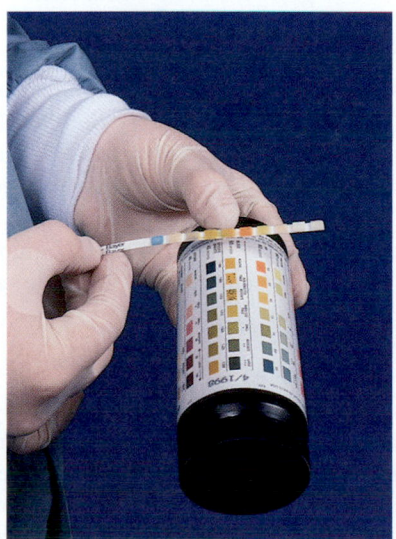

Figure 29-1 Urinalysis is frequently performed in a physician's office laboratory (POL).

perform laboratory tests that are any more complex than waived tests in the medical office. These tests are usually performed at an outside laboratory. Outside laboratories use highly sophisticated automated equipment to perform the tests, providing the medical offices with fast and reliable test results.

COMPONENTS OF THE POL

Physical Structure

The physical structure of the POL should meet certain requirements to provide a safe and effective working environment for performing laboratory tests and storing laboratory equipment and supplies. The POL should be a separate room or work area in the medical office. Laboratory work counters should be large enough to provide ample space for testing specimens. Cabinets should be available for storing equipment and supplies. The medical assistant should check the supply inventory periodically and reorder supplies as needed.

Refrigerator

A refrigerator should be available in the POL for storing specimens that require refrigeration, such as blood tubes and urine awaiting pickup by a courier from an outside laboratory. In addition, certain testing components, such as controls and testing reagents, may require refrigeration. The temperature of the refrigerator must be maintained at 36° F (2° C) to 46° F (8° C) to retard alterations in the physical and chemical compositions of specimens and to prevent deterioration of testing components that require refrigeration. The temperature of the refrigerator should be checked at least once each day and recorded on a refrigerator temperature log sheet. As specified by the Occupational Safety and Health Administration (OSHA) Standard, food must not be stored in the laboratory refrigerator, and a warning label must be attached to the refrigerator to alert employees to the presence of potentially infectious materials.

Safety Measures

Safety measures are an important component of the POL. Laboratory testing involves the collection and handling of specimens that may contain pathogens. In addition, many of the laboratory tests performed in the medical office involve the use of hazardous chemical reagents. It is important that safety measures in the form of equipment, supplies, and emergency devices be available and readily accessible in the POL.

Equipment and Supplies

Equipment and supplies necessary to comply with the OSHA Standard should be readily accessible in the POL. These supplies include handwashing facilities, alcohol-based hand rubs, gloves, safety goggles and masks, safety-engineered syringes and needles, and biohazard sharps containers and biohazard trash bags. Refer to Chapter 17 to review the OSHA Bloodborne Pathogens Standard.

Figure 29-2 Emergency eyewash station.

Labels: Activation paddle; Nozzle cover; Nozzle head; Eyewash bowl

Emergency Eyewash Station

It is recommended that an emergency eyewash station be located in the POL in the event of an accidental exposure incident to the eyes. An *emergency eyewash station* (Figure 29-2) is a device that is used to flush the eyes with tepid water (between 60° F and 100° F) when dust, irritants, other potentially infectious materials (OPIMs), or hazardous chemicals enter the eye. The eyewash station flushes both eyes simultaneously with water at a velocity low enough not to injure the eyes of the user. Once activated, the eyewash station remains operational without requiring the use of the user's hands until it is manually turned off.

The eyewash station should be easily accessible and located within a 10 second walking distance (approximately 55 feet) of the hazard. The first 10 to 15 seconds after exposure of the eye to a hazardous substance are critical, especially if a corrosive chemical is involved. A delay in treatment could result in permanent damage to the eye.

Procedure for Inspecting and Activating an Eyewash Station

It is important that the medical assistant inspect and activate the eyewash station each week to ensure that it is operating properly and to flush out the water supply lines. A more detailed inspection and activation should be performed on an annual basis by a qualified eyewash service technician. The procedure for performing a weekly eyewash check is outlined below:

1. Make sure the access route to the eyewash station is well-lit and free of obstructions.
2. Make sure the eyewash station is well-lit and the area around the eyewash station is free of clutter to avoid unnecessary delay in activating the eyewash station.
3. Make sure the protective nozzle covers are in place and in good condition. The covers protect the nozzle heads from airborne contaminants.

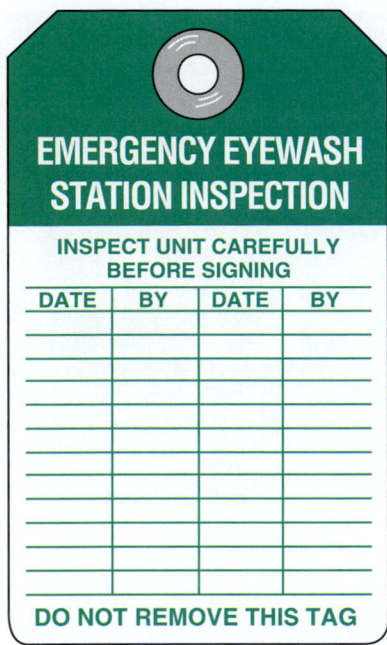

Figure 29-3 Emergency Eyewash Station Inspection Tag.

Figure 29-4 The eyelids must be held apart with the thumbs and forefingers to keep the eyes open.

4. Make sure the eyewash bowl is clean and free of debris.
5. Activate the eyewash device using the activation lever or paddle. The water flow from the nozzles should occur in one second or less following activation of the eyewash.
6. Make sure the protective nozzle covers come off automatically when the eyewash device is activated.
7. Activate the eyewash station for at least three minutes to flush out sediment, debris, or bacteria from the water supply lines.
8. Make sure the water flows continuously (once activated) without the use of the hands.
9. Make sure that the nozzle heads are not clogged and that water flows equally from both nozzle heads.
10. Return the activation lever or paddle to its resting position to turn off the flow of water.
11. Clean, disinfect, rinse, and completely dry the eyewash device including the nozzle heads and protective covers.
12. Replace the nozzle covers on the nozzle heads.
13. Report any problems to the appropriate personnel.
14. Document the inspection date and your initials on either an eyewash inspection log sheet or an eyewash inspection tag that is attached to the device (Figure 29-3).

Procedure for Operating an Emergency Eyewash Station

The medical assistant should be trained in the proper operation of the eyewash station at his or her medical office. A general procedure for the operation of an eyewash station is outlined below.

1. Immediately proceed to the emergency eyewash station after the eye(s) come in contact with a hazardous substance. Ask for assistance, if needed.
2. Activate the eyewash station using the activation lever or paddle. The protective covers will come off of the nozzle heads automatically and water will begin to flow out of the nozzles.
3. Hold both eyelids apart with your thumbs and forefingers to keep the eyes open (Figure 29-4). Most individuals respond to foreign substances in the eyes by closing their eyes tightly, therefore it is important to forcibly hold the eyes open.
4. Direct the flow of water at an angle to the eyes from the outside edge of the lower eye towards the inside of the eyes. Do not aim the water directly onto the eyes to prevent injury to the cornea.
5. If necessary, remove contact lenses to prevent the hazardous substance from becoming trapped under the lens. In most cases however, contact lenses are flushed out of the eyes by the water flow and do not need to be removed manually.
6. Continue to hold the eyelids apart and gently roll your eyeballs from left to right and up and down to make sure the water is reaching all areas of the eye.
7. Continue flushing for a full 15 minutes.
8. Return the activation lever or paddle to its resting position to turn off the flow of water.
9. Seek medical attention to determine if further treatment is required.
10. Clean, disinfect, rinse, and completely dry the eyewash device.

Room Temperature and Lighting

The temperature of the room should be maintained within a range that is conducive to performing laboratory tests and storing testing materials that require room temperature storage. Temperatures outside of this range can cause deterioration of testing materials, such as controls and testing reagents. Some automated analyzers are able to operate only within a specific temperature range. When a specimen is tested, a chemical reaction occurs between the specimen and the testing reagents to produce the test results. With some analyzers, the chemical reaction can occur only within a certain temperature range. If the temperature is outside of the required range, the analyzer cannot perform the test, resulting in an error message that appears on the screen of the analyzer. The temperature range required for the storage of testing materials and for performing tests is stated in the instructions accompanying them. It is usually a room temperature that falls between 59° F (15° C) and 86° F (30° C).

Adequate lighting is essential to assist in the proper collection, handling, and testing of specimens. Good lighting is also needed for the proper interpretation of test results that use a visual color comparison method to determine test results, such as the dipstick method of urinalysis.

Maintenance

The medical assistant is responsible for making sure the POL is clean and free of clutter. Biohazard sharps containers and trash bags should be replaced as needed. A disinfectant should be readily available for disinfecting the laboratory work counters each day. The medical assistant should know how to care for each piece of laboratory equipment; this information is indicated in the operating manual that accompanies the equipment.

OUTSIDE LABORATORIES

Outside laboratories include hospital and privately owned independent laboratories, which employ individuals specifically trained in clinical laboratory techniques and methods such as medical laboratory technologists and technicians. Because the medical assistant usually works closely with an outside laboratory, a basic knowledge of the relationship between the medical office and the outside laboratory (as described in this section) is important. If the specimen is collected at the medical office, the laboratory usually provides the medical office with the supplies and forms necessary to collect the specimen and prepare it for transport to the laboratory. The medical assistant is responsible for checking these supplies periodically and for reordering them from the laboratory as needed.

LABORATORY DIRECTORY

The outside laboratory provides the medical office with a laboratory directory (Figure 29-5), which serves as a valuable reference source for the proper collection and handling of specimens for transport to the outside laboratory. The laboratory may also maintain a website that includes a test menu of the specimen collection and handling requirements for each test performed by that laboratory. This allows the medical assistant to access this information easily and quickly using one or more of the following: a search box, an alphabetical index, or drop-down lists. If, after referring to the laboratory directory (or laboratory website), the

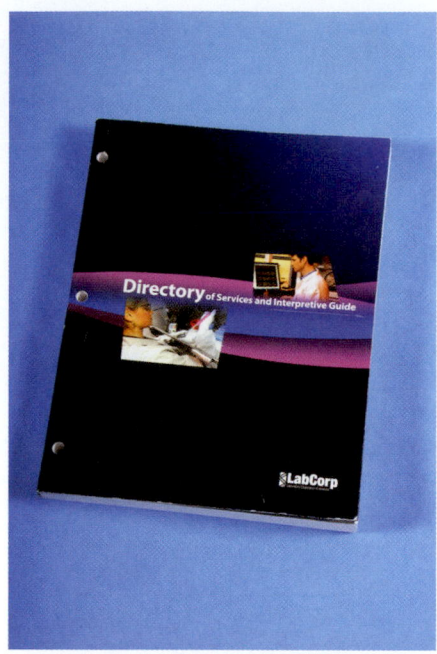

Figure 29-5 Laboratory directory.

medical assistant has a question regarding any aspect of the collection and handling of the specimen that is not clear, the laboratory should be contacted before he or she proceeds.

Laboratory directories vary in organization, depending on the laboratory. The following information is typically included in the directory for each test performed by the laboratory:
- Name and CPT code of the test
- Reference range
- Amount and type of specimen required
- Supplies necessary for collection of the specimen (e.g., blood tubes)
- Techniques to be used for collection of the specimen
- Special instructions
- Patient preparation
- Proper handling and storage of the specimen
- Instructions for transporting the specimen
- Causes for rejection of the specimen by the laboratory
- Uses and limitations of the test
- Methodology used to perform the test

Table 29-1 is a (modified) table of representative tests included in a laboratory directory to provide an overall understanding of the information included in a laboratory directory. The information presented in this modified directory includes all of the categories listed previously with the exception of the following: special instructions, instructions for transporting the specimen, uses and limitations of the test, and methodology used to perform the test. (*Note:* Refer to Figure 29-10 for an example of a laboratory test exactly as it is presented in a laboratory directory.)

Table 29-1 Representative Tests from a (Modified) Laboratory Directory

This table presents a modified table of representative tests included in a laboratory directory to provide you with an overall understanding of the components of a laboratory directory. The components presented in this modified directory include the name and CPT code of the test, reference range, amount and type of specimen required, supplies necessary for the collection of the specimen, techniques to use for collection of the specimen, patient preparation, proper handling and storage of the specimen, and causes for rejection of the specimen. This modified table does *not* include special instructions, instructions for transporting the specimen, uses and limitations of the test, and methodology used to perform the test. (*Note:* Refer to Figure 29-9 for an example of a laboratory test exactly as it is presented in a laboratory directory.)

Test and CPT Code	Specimen Requirements	Reference Range
ALT (alanine aminotransferase) CPT Code: 84460	2 mL serum in SST or transfer tube. Centrifuge and separate serum within 45 minutes after collection Refrigerate or store at RT.	45 U/L or less
AST (aspartate aminotransferase) CPT Code: 84450	2 mL serum in SST or transfer tube Centrifuge and separate serum from cells within 45 minutes after collection. Refrigerate or store at RT.	40 U/L or less
Bilirubin, total CPT Code: 82247	2 mL serum in SST or transfer tube. Centrifuge and separate serum from cells within 45 minutes after collection. Refrigerate. Protect from light.	0.1-1.2 mg/dL
Blood group (ABO) and Rh Type CPT Codes: 86900, 86901	5-mL lavender-top tube. A separate lavender-top tube is required for this test. Refrigerate or store at RT.	
BUN (blood urea nitrogen) CPT Code: 84520	2 mL serum in SST or transfer tube. Centrifuge and separate serum within 45 minutes after collection. Refrigerate serum.	7-25 mg/dL
Calcium, serum CPT Code: 82310	2 mL serum in SST or transfer tube. Centrifuge and separate serum from cells within 45 minutes after collection. Refrigerate or store at RT.	0-6 months: 8.9-11 mg/dL 7 months–adult: 8.5-10.6 mg/dL
CBC with differential CPT Code: 85025	5-mL lavender-top tube. Gently invert tube 8-10 times immediately after drawing. Refrigerate or store at RT.	Values given with report
CK (creatine kinase) CPT Code: 82550	3 mL serum in SST or transfer tube. Avoid exercise before venipuncture. Centrifuge and separate serum from cells within 45 minutes after collection. Refrigerate or store at RT.	Male: 17-148 U/L Female: 10-70 U/L
CRP (C-reactive protein) CPT Code: 86140	1 mL serum in SST or transfer tube. Avoid hemolysis. Centrifuge and separate serum from cells within 45 minutes after collection. Refrigerate or store at RT.	0.0-4.9 mg/L
Glucose, plasma CPT Code: 82947	5-mL gray-top tube. Patient should have fasted for 12 to 14 hours. Gently invert tube 8-10 times immediately after drawing. Refrigerate or store at RT.	65-99 mg/dL
LD (lactic acid dehydrogenase) CPT Code: 83615	3 mL serum in SST or transfer tube. Hemolysis invalidates results. Centrifuge and separate serum from cells within 45 minutes after collection. Refrigerate or store at RT.	100-250 IU/L
PT/INR (prothrombin time) CPT Code: 85610	5-mL light blue–top tube. Gently invert tube 3-4 times immediately after drawing. Clotting and hemolysis invalidate results. Store at RT.	PT/INR: 0.8-1.2 Patients on anticoagulant therapy: PT/INR: 2.0-3.0

Continued

Table 29-1 Representative Tests from a (Modified) Laboratory Directory—cont'd		
RPR (rapid plasma reagin) CPT Code: 86592	1 mL serum in SST or transfer tube. Centrifuge and separate serum from cells within 45 minutes after collection. Refrigerate.	Nonreactive
Sedimentation rate CPT Code: 85652	5-mL lavender-top tube. Gently invert tube 8-10 times immediately after drawing. Refrigerate.	Male: 0-15 mm/hr Over 50 years: 0-20 mm/hr Female: 0-20 mm/hr Over 50 years: 0-30 mm/hr
Triiodothyronine (T$_3$) CPT Code: 84480	1 mL serum in SST or transfer tube. Centrifuge and separate serum from cells within 45 minutes after collection. Refrigerate.	83-200 mg/dL
Thyroxine (T$_4$) CPT Code: 84436	2 mL serum in SST or transfer tube. Centrifuge and separate serum from cells within 45 minutes after collection. Refrigerate.	4.5-12.0 µg/dL
Triglycerides CPT Code: 84478	2 mL serum in SST or transfer tube. Patient should have fasted for 12-14 hr. Centrifuge and separate serum from cells within 45 minutes after collection. Refrigerate or store at RT.	Less than 150 mg/dL
Urinalysis, routine CPT Code: 81003	Random sample in urine transport tube. First morning specimen preferred (10 mL). Refrigerate.	Values given with report

INR, International normalized ratio; *RT,* room temperature; *SST,* serum separator tube.

COLLECTION AND TESTING CATEGORIES

Collection and testing of a specimen can be categorized as follows:

1. The specimen is collected and tested at the medical office.
2. The specimen is collected at the medical office and transferred to an outside laboratory for testing.
3. The patient is given a laboratory request to have the specimen collected and tested at an outside laboratory.

The medical assistant's responsibilities depend on which of these methods is used in the medical office. For example, a specimen collected at the medical office and transferred to an outside laboratory for testing involves a series of individual steps different from the steps followed when it is collected and tested at the medical office. The following clinical laboratory methods are presented in the remainder of this chapter to provide the student with the information needed to function competently in all three modes just described:

1. Completing laboratory request forms and reviewing laboratory reports
2. Informing the patient of any necessary advance preparation or special instructions
3. Collecting, handling, and transporting specimens
4. Performing CLIA-waived tests in the medical office
5. Practicing quality control and laboratory safety

LABORATORY REQUESTS
PURPOSE

A laboratory request is a printed form that contains a list of the most frequently ordered laboratory tests (Figure 29-6). A laboratory request is required when the specimen is collected at the medical office and transferred to an outside laboratory for testing, or when the specimen is to be collected and tested at an outside laboratory, in which case the request is given to the patient at the medical office to take to the laboratory. The request provides the outside laboratory with essential information necessary for accurate testing, reporting of results, and billing. Organizational formats for the request forms vary, depending on the laboratory. In general, most outside laboratories find it more convenient and economical to provide the medical office with one form for designating all tests, with the possible exception of the Pap test, in which case a separate form, known as a *cytology request,* is provided.

PARTS OF LABORATORY REQUEST FORM

The request form can be completed manually by the medical assistant by writing in all information required, or it may be completed on a computer screen by entering the information using a keyboard. Specific information that is required on the laboratory request form follows.

LABORATORY REQUISITION
Biomedical Laboratories, Inc.
100 Main Street
Athens, Georgia 45760

☐ Fax Send additional copy of report to:
☐ Call Client Number/Physician's Name   Phone/Fax number ( )
☐ Mail Physician's Address   City, State, Zip

Patient's Name (Last)	(First)	(MI)	Sex	Date of Birth MO|DAY|YEAR	Collection Time : AM PM	Fasting YES NO	Collection Date MO|DAY|YEAR

NPI/UPIN	Physician's ID #	Patient's SS #	Patient's ID #	Urine hrs/vol hrs____ vol____

PATIENT / RESP. PARTY

Physician's Name (Last, First)	Physician's Signature	Patient's Address	Phone
Medicare # (Include prefix/suffix)	☐ Primary ☐ Secondary	City	State ZIP
Medicaid # State	Physician's Provider #	Name of Responsible Party (if different from patient)	
Diagnosis/Signs/Symptoms in ICD-9 Format (Highest Specificity) **REQUIRED**		Address of Responsible Party (if different from patient) APT #	
		City State ZIP	

INSURANCE

Patient's Relationship to Responsible Party: ☐ 1–Self ☐ 2–Spouse ☐ 3–Child ☐ 4–Other

Performance Lab ☐   Carrier   Group #   Employee #   Mem

Insurance Company Name	Plan	Carrier Code
Subscriber/Member #	Location	Group #
Insurance Address	Physician's Provider #	
City	State ZIP	
Employer's Name or Number	Insured SS # (If not patient)	Worker's Comp ☐ Yes ☐ No

I hereby authorize the release of medical information related to the service subscribed herein and authorize payment directed to LabCorp.
X_____ Patient's Signature   Date

MEDICARE ADVANCE BENEFICIARY NOTICE
I have read the ABN on the reverse. If Medicare denies payment, I agree to pay for the identified test(s).
X_____ Patient's Signature   Date

NOTE: WHEN ORDERING TESTS FOR WHICH MEDICARE OR MEDICAID REIMBURSEMENT WILL BE SOUGHT, PHYSICIANS SHOULD ONLY ORDER TESTS THAT ARE MEDICALLY NECESSARY FOR THE DIAGNOSIS OR TREATMENT OF THE PATIENT. COMPONENTS OF THE ORGAN OR DISEASE PANELS/COMBINATIONS PRINTED BELOW ARE SHOWN ON THE REVERSE SIDE AND MAY ALSO BE ORDERED INDIVIDUALLY BELOW. COMPONENTS MAY BE BILLED SEPARATELY PER CARRIER POLICY.

PROFILES (See reverse for components)

80049	Basic Metabolic Profile	SST
80054	Comp Metabolic Profile	SST
80051	Electrolyte Profile	SST
80058	Hepatic Profile	SST
80059	Hepatitis Profile	SST
80061	Lipid Profile	SST
80091	Thyroid Profile	SST
80055	Prenatal Profile	RED LAV
80072	Rheumatoid Profile	SST

HEMATOLOGY

85025	CBC w Diff	LAV
85027	CBC w/o Diff	LAV
85014	Hematocrit	LAV
85018	Hemoglobin	LAV
85595	Platelet Count	LAV
85041	RBC Count	LAV
85048	WBC Count	LAV
85007	WBC Differential	LAV
89190	Nasal Smear, Eosin	Nasal Smear
85060	Pathologist Consult–Peripheral Smear	LAV

ALPHABETICAL/COMBINATION TESTS

86900 86901	ABO and Rh	LAV
82040	Albumin	SST
84075	Alkaline Phosphatase	SST
84460	ALT (SGPT)	SST
82150	Amylase, Serum	SST
86038	Antinuclear Antibodies	SST
84450	AST (SGOT)	SST
82607 82746	B₁₂ and Folate	SST
82250	Bilirubin, Total	SST

ALPHABETICAL TESTS CON'T

84520	BUN	SST
82310	Calcium	SST
80156	Carbamazepine (Tegretol®)	SER
82378	CEA	SST
82465	Cholesterol, Total	SST
82565	Creatinine	SST
80162	Digoxin	SER
82670	Estradiol	SST
82720	Ferritin, Serum	SST
82985	Fructosamine	SST
83001	FSH	SST
83001 83002	FSH and LH	SST
82977	GGT	SST
82947	Glucose, Plasma	GRY
82947	Glucose, Serum	SST
82950	Glucose, 2-hr. PP	SST
83036	Glycohemoglobin, Total	LAV
84703	hCG, Beta Subunit, Qual	SST
84702	hCG, Beta Subunit, Quant	SST
83718	HDL Cholesterol	SST
86677	Helicobacter pylori, IgG	SST
86706	Hep B Surface Antibody	SST
87340	Hep B Surface Antigen	SST
86803	Hep C Antibody	SST
83036	Hemoglobin A₁C	LAV
86701	HIV Antibodies	SST
83540	Iron, Total	SST
83540 83550	Iron and IBC	SST
83615	LDH	SST

ALPHABETICAL TESTS CON'T

83002	LH	SST
83690	Lipase	SER
80178	Lithium (Eskalith®)	SER
83735	Magnesium, Serum	SST
80184	Phenobarbital (Luminal®)	SER
80185	Phenytoin (Dilantin®)	SER
84132	Potassium	SST
84146	Prolactin, Serum	SST
84153	Prostate-Specific Antigen	SST
84066	Prostatic Acid Phos	SST
84155	Protein, Total	SST
85610	Prothrombin Time (PT)	BLU
85610 85730	PT and PTT Activated	BLU
85730	PTT Activated	BLU
86431	Rheumatoid Arthritis Factor	SST
86592	RPR	SST
86762	Rubella Antibodies, IgG	SST
85651	Sed Rate	LAV
84295	Sodium	SST
84403	Testosterone	SST
80198	Theophylline	SER
84436	Thyroxine (T₄)	SST
84478	Triglycerides	SST
84480	Triiodothyronine (T₃)	SST
84443	TSH, High Sensitivity	SST
84550	Uric Acid	SST
81003	Urinalysis Microscopic on Positives	URN
81001	Urinalysis with Microscopic	URN
80164	Valproic Acid (Depakene®)	SER

MICROBIOLOGY See Reverse Side

☐ ENDOCERVICAL ☐ THROAT ☐ URINE
☐ STOOL ☐ URETHRAL INDICATE SOURCE

87070	Aerobic Bacterial Culture	Bact Trnspt
87490 87590	Chlamydia/GC DNA Probe w/ Confirmation on Positives	Probe Trnspt
87490 87590	Chlamydia/GC DNA Probe Without Confirmation	Probe Trnspt
87490	Chlamydia DNA Probe	Probe Trnspt
87081	Genital, Beta-Hemolytic Strep Cult, Group B	Bact Trnspt
87070	Genital Culture, Routine	Bact Trnspt
87070	Lower Respiratory Culture	Steril Trnspt
87590	N. gonorrhoeae DNA Probe	Probe Trnspt
87015	Ova and Parasites	O & P Kit
87081 X2 87045	Stool Culture	Fecal Trnspt
87081	Throat, Beta-Hemolytic Strep Cult, Group A	Bact Trnspt
87060	Upper Respiratory Culture, Routine	Bact Trnspt
87086	Urine Culture, Routine	Urn Cul Trnspt

Clinical Information/Comments

OTHER TESTS/INDIVIDUAL COMPONENTS
TEST #   TEST NAMES

LAB USE ONLY

	STAT	VENIPUNCTURE	TRAVEL	NON LABCORP	VERBAL ORDER	CHART ORDER	HANDWRITTEN	24 HR TUV	PST/PSC #
	☐ 998074	☐ 998085	☐ 998096	☐ 998239	☐ 998250	☐ 998261	☐ 998272	☐ 998283	

CONTAINERS RECEIVED

SST SPUN	USST UNSPUN	SER SERUM TRNSPT	FRZ FRZ TRNS	RED RED	LAV LAVENDER	SLD SLIDE	BLU LT. BLUE	GRY GREY	GRN GREEN	RYB RYL BLU	YEL ACD	PLS PLASMA	URN URINE	24U 24 HR URINE	TA-U TART. ACID	FL FLUID	OT OTHER	BACT TRNSP	O & P KIT	PROBE TRNSP	URN CULT TRNSP	STERIL TRNSP	FECAL TRNSP	VIRAL TRNSP

300-0384

Figure 29-6 Laboratory request form.

1. *Physician's name and address.* The physician's name and address should be clearly indicated on the laboratory request form to facilitate the reporting of test results to the physician. Laboratory request forms are usually prenumbered with the physician's account number, which assists in identification, reporting, and billing of laboratory tests.

2. *Patient's name and address.* The patient's name and address must be documented on the form as requested by the laboratory; for example, the laboratory may want the patient's name designated with the last name first, middle initial, and then first name. The patient's address is needed for billing purposes and must include the city, state, and zip code.

3. *Patient's age and gender.* The reference ranges for some tests vary depending on the patient's age and gender. The reference range for hemoglobin concentration varies according to gender (12 to 16 g/dL for a woman; 14 to 18 g/dL for a man).

4. *Date and time of collection of the specimen.* The date of the specimen collection indicates to the laboratory the number of days that have passed since the collection, providing the laboratory with information regarding the freshness of the specimen. A time lapse that is too long between collection and testing of a specimen may affect the accuracy of some test results. The time of collection is significant with respect to certain laboratory tests. The reference range for serum cortisol varies depending on whether the specimen is collected in the morning or in the afternoon.

5. *Laboratory tests desired.* The tests desired by the physician are usually indicated by marking a box adjacent to those tests (and their corresponding CPT codes), as illustrated in Figure 29-5. A space designated as "additional tests" or "other tests" is provided on the laboratory request form for specifying the CPT code of a test that is desired but not listed on the request form. As previously indicated, the laboratory request form includes only the tests most frequently ordered. The laboratory directory contains a complete listing of all tests performed by the laboratory.

6. *Profiles.* Laboratory tests termed *profiles* may be ordered by the physician. A **profile** (also known as a *panel*) consists of an array of laboratory tests that have been determined to be the most sensitive and specific means of identifying a disease state or evaluating a particular organ or organ system. The profiles performed by an outside laboratory and the tests included in each are listed in the laboratory directory. A profile may be specific in nature—that is, all tests included relate to a specific organ of the body or a particular disease state. A specific profile is usually ordered when the physician does not have a definite clinical diagnosis but has a good idea of the patient's condition or what organ or organs are involved in the patient's condition. The physician orders a profile of the condition or organ in question. An example of a profile used to identify a

disease state is the rheumatoid profile, which is used to assist in the diagnosis of rheumatoid arthritis. An example of a profile used to evaluate an organ is the hepatic function profile, which is used to assess liver function and to assist in the diagnosis of a pathologic condition that affects the liver.

A profile also may be general in nature. A general metabolic profile contains numerous routine laboratory tests and is used primarily in a routine health screen of a patient. General metabolic profiles are used to detect any changes in the body's biologic processes that may be present, although the patient may not have had any symptoms to indicate that these changes have occurred. General metabolic profiles also are used when the patient's symptoms are so vague that the physician does not have enough concrete evidence to support a clinical diagnosis of a specific organ or disease state. An example of a general profile is the comprehensive metabolic profile; refer to Table 29-2 for a list of the tests included in this profile.

The medical assistant should have knowledge of the names of common profiles and the tests usually contained in each, which are listed in Table 29-2. The tests contained in each profile may vary slightly from one laboratory to another.

7. *Source of the specimen.* Certain tests require that the source of the specimen (e.g., throat, wound, ear, eye, urine, vagina) be recorded on the laboratory request form. This is done for identification of the origin of the specimen for the laboratory, because this information is not available by looking at the specimen. In many instances, the source dictates the test method used by the laboratory to evaluate the specimen for the presence of a possible pathogen. The test method used to detect the presence of *Streptococcus* in a specimen obtained from the throat would be different from that used to detect *Candida albicans* in a vaginal specimen.

8. *Physician's clinical diagnosis (in International Classification of Diseases [ICD] format).* The clinical diagnosis assists the laboratory in correlating clinical laboratory data with the needs of the physician. In some instances, further testing is performed by the laboratory if one test method proves inconclusive with respect to providing the physician with the information necessary to confirm or reject the clinical diagnosis. Another function of the clinical diagnosis is to assure laboratory personnel that the test results are within the framework of the diagnosis. When the results of a test disagree with the physician's clinical diagnosis, the laboratory repeats the test on the same or another specimen. The clinical diagnosis also alerts laboratory personnel to the possibility of the presence of a potentially dangerous pathogen, such as the hepatitis virus. In addition, this information is necessary for third-party billing by the laboratory. If the laboratory bills an insurance company for these tests, the ICD code for the clinical diagnosis needs to be on the insurance form. The processing of insurance forms

Table 29-2 Laboratory Profiles

Profile	Tests Included	Use
Comprehensive metabolic profile	Albumin ALP ALT AST Bilirubin (total) BUN Calcium Carbon dioxide Chloride Creatinine Glucose Inorganic phosphorus Potassium Protein (total) Sodium Triglycerides	General health screen that provides information on kidneys, liver, acid-base balance, blood glucose level, and blood proteins. Used to evaluate organ function and to check for conditions such as diabetes, liver disease, and kidney disease. Routinely ordered as part of blood workup for physical examination or medical examination (particularly when patient's symptoms are vague). Abnormal test results are usually followed up with more specific tests before a diagnosis is made.
Electrolyte profile	Carbon dioxide Chloride Potassium Sodium	Screen for electrolyte or acid-base imbalance and to monitor effect of treatment on disease or condition that causes electrolyte imbalance. This profile also is used to evaluate patient taking medication that can cause electrolyte imbalance.
Hepatic profile	Albumin ALP ALT AST Bilirubin (direct) Bilirubin (total) Protein (total)	Detection of pathologic conditions affecting the liver. This test is often ordered when symptoms indicating a liver condition occur, such as jaundice, dark urine, light-colored bowel movements, or pain or swelling in the abdomen. This profile may be ordered when an individual has been exposed to hepatitis, has a family history of liver disease, has excessive alcohol consumption, or is taking medication that can result in liver damage.
Hepatitis profile	Hepatitis A antibody, IgM Hepatitis B core antibody, total Hepatitis B surface antigen Hepatitis C antibody	Detection of viral hepatitis.
Lipid profile	Total cholesterol LDL cholesterol HDL cholesterol Triglycerides VLDL cholesterol (calculation) Total cholesterol/HDL Ratio (calculation)	Determination of risk of coronary artery disease.
Prenatal profile	ABO grouping and Rh typing CBC w/diff and w/plt Hepatitis B surface antigen Red cell antibody screen Rubella antibody screen Syphilis serology (RPR)	Establish baseline recordings and screenings of prenatal patients for disease or potential problems.
Renal function profile	Albumin BUN Calcium Carbon dioxide Chloride Creatinine Glucose Phosphorus Potassium Sodium	Detection of kidney problems. This profile shows how well the kidneys are functioning to remove excess fluid and waste. When a problem is detected, diagnostic imaging tests may be used for further evaluation and diagnosis.

Continued

Table 29-2 Laboratory Profiles—cont'd

Profile	Tests Included	Use
Rheumatoid profile	ANA CRP Rheumatoid factor Sedimentation rate Streptolysin O Uric acid	Assists in diagnosis of rheumatoid arthritis and helps distinguish it from other forms of arthritis and conditions with similar symptoms. This profile also is used to evaluate severity of rheumatoid arthritis, to monitor the condition and its complications, and to assess response to treatment.
Thyroid function profile	FTI Thyroxine (T_4) Triiodothyronine (T_3) Uptake	Detection of conditions affecting the thyroid gland.

ALP, Alkaline phosphatase; *ALT,* alanine aminotransferase; *ANA,* antinuclear antibody; *AST,* aspartate aminotransferase; *BUN,* blood urea nitrogen; *CBC,* complete blood count; *CRP,* C-reactive protein; *FTI,* free thyroxine index; *HDL,* high-density lipoprotein; *IgM,* immunoglobulin M; *LDL,* low-density lipoprotein; *VLDL,* very-low-density lipoprotein; *w/diff,* with differential; *w/plt,* with platelet count.

is facilitated by having the information at hand and not having to contact the medical office to obtain it.

9. *Medications.* Certain medications may interfere with the accuracy and validity of test results. The laboratory should be notified on the request form of any medications taken by the patient.

10. *STAT.* Sometimes the physician wants the laboratory test results reported as soon as possible. In this case, "STAT" should be clearly indicated in bold letters (or the appropriate STAT box checked) on the laboratory request form. Requests that are marked STAT are performed as soon as possible after receipt by the laboratory, and the results are telephoned or faxed to the physician as soon as they are available.

After the specimen has been collected, the completed request form must be placed with the specimen for transport to the outside laboratory. The medical assistant should realize the significance of this simple but important step. Numerous possible tests can be performed on one particular specimen, and without the request form the laboratory does not have the information it needs to carry out the physician's orders, causing delays in completing the tests and reporting results.

Putting It All Into Practice

My name is Korey McGrew, and I am employed by a group of physicians in a family practice medical office. Some of my duties include showing patients to examining rooms, taking vital signs, administering medications, transcription, filing, and many other duties that medical assistants perform. I have found that being a medical assistant has been challenging and rewarding, and I wish you the best of luck in reaching your goals.

When I first started working as a practicing medical assistant, I had a challenging venipuncture experience. The patient was a kind and personable 64-year-old man with hardening of the arteries. I tried to obtain the blood specimen from his arm but was not successful. The patient was calm and was not bothered at all by the unsuccessful stick. He said that it was hard to draw blood on him and to go ahead and try again. I decided to try taking blood from a vein on the back of his hand with a butterfly setup. To my relief, I obtained the blood specimen. I think that I was more nervous about this experience than the patient was. It is important to remain calm on the outside around patients even if you are nervous on the inside. ∎

What Would You Do? What Would You *Not* Do?

Case Study 1
Three days ago, Hildy McNicle was given a laboratory requisition at the medical office to have blood drawn and tested at an outside medical laboratory. Hildy calls the medical office and says she is a little confused. She called the laboratory for her test results, and they would not give them to her. They told her to call the medical office. She does not understand this because her blood was collected and tested at the laboratory, and it would seem logical to her that they would give her the test results, especially because she is paying the laboratory to perform the tests. The test results have come back with abnormal values, and the physician is at a medical convention and will not return until tomorrow. ∎

LABORATORY REPORTS

Laboratory report forms are used to relay the results of laboratory tests to the physician (Figure 29-7). The report is usually generated by a computer. It may consist of a preprinted form with the test results printed in the appropriate spaces on the form by a computer (as illustrated in Figure 29-7), or the entire report may be generated by the computer (Figure 29-8) and may be transmitted electronically. The report includes the following information:

1. Name, address, and telephone number of the laboratory
2. Physician's name and address

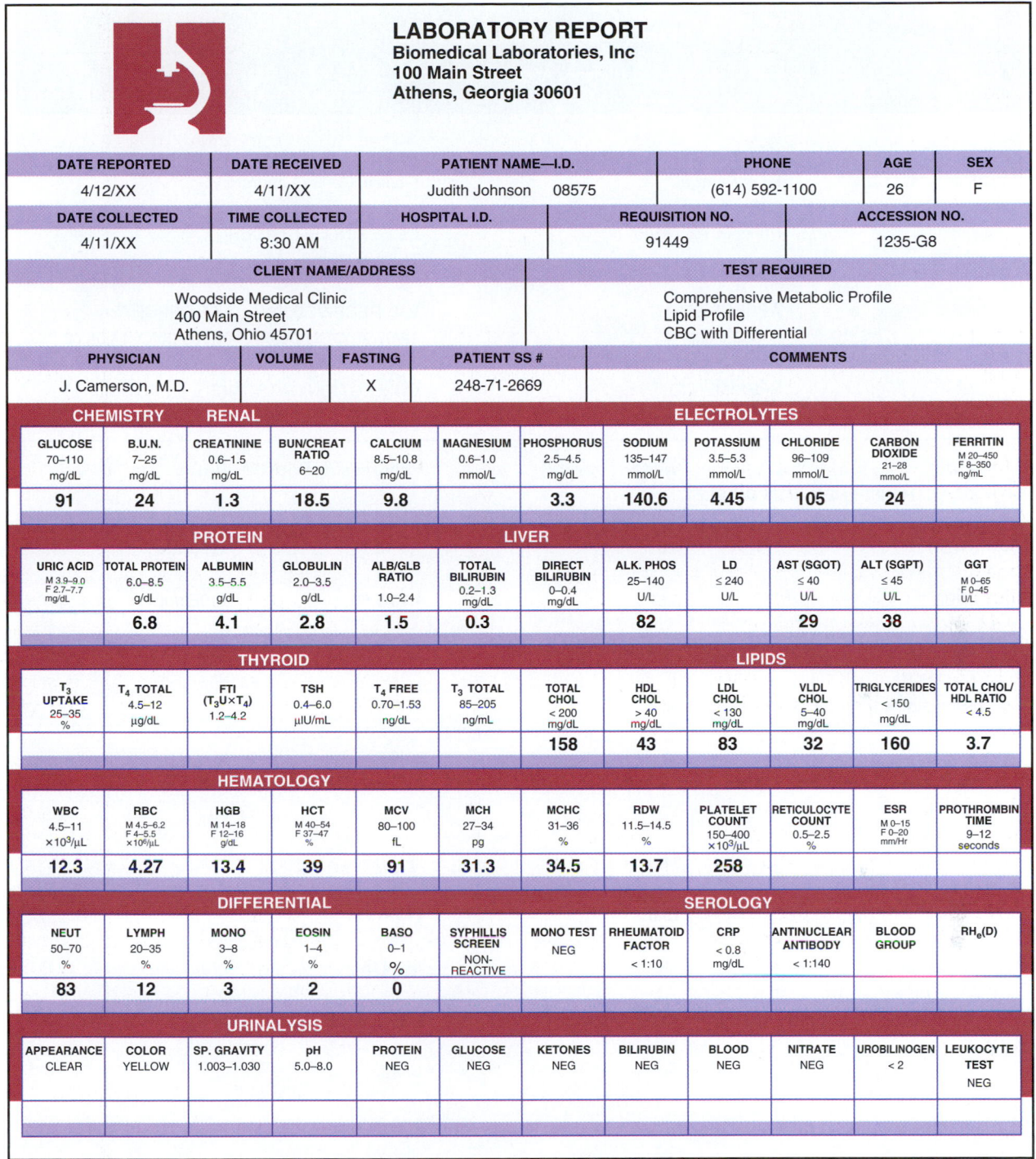

Figure 29-7 Laboratory report form.

3. Patient's name, age, and gender
4. Patient accession number
5. Date the specimen was received by the laboratory
6. Date the results were reported by the laboratory
7. Names of the tests performed
8. Results of the tests
9. Reference range for each test performed

A patient accession number or laboratory number is assigned to each specimen received by the laboratory. Its purpose is to provide positive identification of each

specimen within the laboratory and to allow easy access to the patient's laboratory records should a test result need to be located again. If the physician desires to have the laboratory test repeated, the accession number listed on the original report form must be included on the laboratory request form.

The **reference range** is also commonly referred to as a *reference interval* and a *reference value*. A reference range is defined as a certain established and acceptable parameter within which the laboratory test results of a healthy

Family Practice Health Care Center
3477 Arrowhead Ave
Phoenix, Arizona 78351
(942) 871-3746

ID#	SEX	PATIENT DEMOGRAPHICS	RESULTS PROVIDED BY
3368	F	Leah Percival	Medical Center Laboratory
		2973 Flint Dr.	
DOB		Phoenix, AZ 78366	**ORDERING PROVIDER**
4/28/78			Thomas Murphy, MD

AGE	ACCESSION #	LAB RECEIVED ON	LAB REPORTED ON
34	3380837630	12/07/20XX 11:00:53	12/05/20XX 14:08:00

LAB ID	SPECIMEN ID	COLLECTION DATE/TIME	FASTING
4739	30180906	12/04/20XX 2:53:00	NO

NAME	VALUE	REFERENCE RANGE	UNITS	FLAG
CBC WITH DIFFERENTIAL/PLATELET				
-WBC	4.6	4.0-10.5	x10e3/uL	
-RBC	3.57	4.10-5.60	x10E3/uL	L
-Hemoglobin	11.2	12.5-17.0	g/dL	L
-Hematocrit	32.9	36.0-50.0	%	L
-MCV	92	80-98	fL	
-MCH	31.4	27.0-34.0	pg	
-MCHC	34.0	32.0-36.0	g/dL	
-RDW	15.6	11.7-15.0	%	H
-Platelets	308	140-415	x10E3/uL	
-Neutrophils	73	40-74	%	
-Lymphs	14	14-46	%	
-Monocytes	11	4-13	%	
-Eos	1	0-7	%	
-Basos	1	0-3	%	
-Neutrophils (Absolute)	3.4	1.8-7.8	x10E3/uL	
-Lymphs (Absolute)	0.6	0.7-4.5	x10E3/uL	L

Figure 29-8 Computer-generated laboratory report.

individual are expected to fall. The reference range is used to interpret laboratory test results for a particular patient. A range, rather than a single value, is necessary for laboratory test results because of individual differences within a general population caused by factors such as age, gender, race, and geographic location. In addition, no test can be so accurate that a single value is possible. The reference range for each test varies slightly from one laboratory to another, depending on the test method, equipment, and reagents used to perform the test. Because of this, it is essential that the medical assistant compare the test results with reference ranges supplied by the laboratory performing the test rather than with a reference source such as a medical laboratory textbook.

Laboratory reports are delivered to the medical office by one or more of the following methods: faxed, mailed, hand-delivered by a laboratory courier, or sent electronically from the laboratory computer to the medical office computer. Abnormal results that pose a threat to the patient's health and laboratory reports marked STAT are telephoned or faxed to the medical office as soon as the tests have been completed, and a complete written report follows immediately thereafter. The laboratory usually supplies the medical office with telephone reporting pads to transcribe results from the telephone report to reduce errors.

The medical assistant may be responsible for reviewing laboratory reports as they are received. The medical assistant should compare the patient's test results with the reference ranges supplied by the laboratory and notify the physician of any abnormal test results. Most laboratory computer systems automatically flag and highlight abnormal results on the laboratory report. The physician carefully reviews each laboratory report received by the office, and the data obtained are correlated with information obtained from the health history and physical examination. The physician indicates that he or she is finished with the report usually by placing his or her signature on it. The medical assistant is then responsible for filing the laboratory report in the patient's chart, according to the medical office policy.

LABORATORY DOCUMENTS AND THE EMR

Many medical offices communicate with outside laboratories electronically using a computer system that interfaces with the computer system in the outside laboratory. This provides distinct advantages for the medical office using an electronic medical record (EMR). Laboratory requisition forms can be completed on a request form displayed on the computer screen using fill-in boxes, drop-down lists, and check-boxes. Depending on the medical office policy, the form can then be transmitted electronically to the medical laboratory or printed out and placed with the specimen for transport to the laboratory.

Once the patient's tests have been completed, the laboratory test results are sent electronically to the medical office. The laboratory report is placed in the physician's "electronic review box" for his or her review and electronic signature. Abnormal values are often highlighted on the report as shown in Figure 29-8. If a critical result appears on the laboratory report, an urgent message is e-mailed to the physician. After the physician reviews the laboratory report and places his or her electronic signature on the report, the report is electronically filed in the patient's EMR.

Other advantages of the laboratory component of an EMR include the ability to quickly view laboratory results in chronological order. In addition, results of a laboratory test performed on a routine basis (e.g., glucose testing, cholesterol testing) can be accessed by the computer and plotted on a flow sheet (Figure 29-9). This permits an abnormal trend to be identified early, so that appropriate action can be taken.

If an EMR medical office is not networked through computers with an outside laboratory, the laboratory reports received by the office must be scanned into the computer and electronically filed in the patient's EMR. A scanned report has some limitations. The computer can display the report, but the data on the report cannot be accessed or manipulated. Because of this, laboratory data cannot be used for many of the functions previously described. For example, the data on a scanned report cannot be accessed and incorporated into a flow sheet for trend analysis.

PATIENT PREPARATION AND INSTRUCTIONS

Factors such as food consumption, medication, activity, and time of day affect the laboratory results of certain tests. For some laboratory tests, advance patient preparation is necessary to obtain a high-quality specimen suitable for testing, which leads to accurate results and assists the physician in accurate diagnosis and treatment. The quality of laboratory test results can be only as good as the quality of the specimen obtained from the patient. A specimen obtained from a patient who has not prepared properly may invalidate the test results and necessitate calling the patient back to collect the specimen again.

The medical assistant is usually responsible for instructing the patient about the nature of the laboratory test and any advance preparation that might be necessary. A complete and thorough explanation of the information should be relayed clearly to the patient. The patient should be informed of the name of the test, how to prepare for the test, how the test is performed, and how and when to expect the test results. The medical assistant should make sure to explain the reason for the advance preparation, so the patient will be more likely to comply with the preparation necessary. It should be emphasized to the patient that the preparation is essential to obtain accurate

Figure 29-9 Cholesterol flow sheet generated by a computer. (Modified from Buck CJ: Electronic health record booster kit for the medical office, St Louis, 2009, Saunders.)

test results and to avoid having to collect the specimen again.

After the instructions have been explained, the medical assistant needs to verify that the patient completely understands them and should offer to answer any questions. It also is advisable to provide the patient with a written information sheet (Figure 29-10) to serve as a reference, should the patient forget some of the information after leaving the medical office. Some specimen collections may require that the patient remain at the collection site for a specified time; an example of this is the OGTT, which requires several hours for the collection of multiple, timed specimens. The patient should be told in advance of the time requirement, so that any necessary arrangements can be made with an employer or babysitter.

Sometimes the patient collects the specimen at home. The medical assistant is responsible for explaining detailed instructions to the patient on proper techniques for collection of the specimen. For example, if a first-voided morning urine specimen is necessary for the laboratory test, the medical assistant needs to provide the patient with the appropriate specimen container and to instruct the patient on proper collection, handling, and storage of the specimen until it reaches the medical office.

The specific type of preparation necessary for a particular test depends on the test ordered and the method used to run it. If the medical office uses an outside laboratory, the patient preparation necessary for each test can be found in the laboratory directory. If the test is performed in the medical office, the medical assistant should consult the manufacturer's instructions that accompany the test to obtain specific information regarding patient preparation. Advance patient

What Would You Do? | **What Would You *Not* Do?**

Case Study 2

Hans Volkman is leaving the medical office after being seen by the physician. The physician gave him a laboratory requisition for a complete blood count and a lipid profile. Hans notices that the clinical diagnosis on the form indicates iron-deficiency anemia and wants to know why the physician did not prescribe any medication for him if he thought he had anemia. Hans says that he told the physician his father had a heart attack at age 53 years and asked whether he would order a cholesterol test. He says the physician must have forgotten because the test was not marked on the laboratory form. Hans has been instructed to fast for the laboratory tests. He says that he stops every morning at the Coffee Cup restaurant and has coffee with cream and sugar, orange juice, and two doughnuts. He would like to know whether he could just have the coffee with cream and sugar before the tests. Hans says he has a hard time functioning in the morning without coffee. ■

preparation usually consists of fasting, diet modification (e.g., low-fat diet), or medication restrictions.

FASTING

Some blood specimens require the patient to fast before collection. The composition of blood is altered by the consumption of food because digested food is absorbed into the circulatory system, changing the results of certain laboratory tests. Food intake causes blood glucose and triglyceride laboratory tests to yield falsely high results. Any

ORAL GLUCOSE TOLERANCE TEST

PATIENT INFORMATION SHEET

General Information

Your physician has requested that you have an oral glucose tolerance test (OGTT). This test is performed to see how well your body processes glucose (sugar). Glucose is the primary source of energy for your body. The OGTT is primarily used to assist in diagnosis of diabetes. Your test is scheduled in the early morning because you will need to perform an overnight fast. The test generally lasts for a period of 3 hours.

Patient Preparation

It is very important that you prepare properly to ensure accurate test results. Patient preparation for this test includes the following:

1. For 3 days prior to the test you should consume a high-carbohydrate diet consisting of at least 150 grams of carbohydrate per day. Foods that are high in carbohydrate include bread, pasta, cereal, potatoes, rice, and crackers.
2. Do NOT drink or eat anything except water for 12 to 14 hours before the test.
3. Your physician will discuss what medications (if any) to discontinue before the test.

Testing Procedure

When you arrive at the testing facility, your blood will be drawn. You will then be given a glucose (sugar) solution to drink. Some people have a brief period of nausea after consuming the glucose solution. Your blood will be collected at intervals over a period of several hours.

During the testing procedure, you may experience some normal side effects such as weakness, a feeling of faintness, or perspiration. They are caused by a decrease in your body's glucose level as insulin is secreted in response to the glucose solution. These side effects are temporary and will only last for a short period of time. To ensure accurate test results, you need to adhere to the following during the testing procedure:

1. Sit quietly and do not leave the testing facility.
2. Do not eat or drink anything except water.
3. Do not smoke or chew gum during the procedure.

Following the Procedure

After the procedure you can eat and drink as usual and resume your normal activities. An appointment will be scheduled for you to discuss the test results with your physician.

Figure 29-10 Oral glucose tolerance test patient instruction sheet.

individual test (e.g., fasting blood glucose [FBG], OGTT) or profile including these tests (e.g., comprehensive metabolic profile, lipid profile) requires the patient to fast before the specimen is collected.

Fasting involves abstaining from food and fluids (except water) for a specified amount of time before the collection of the specimen (usually 12 to 14 hours). Fasting specimens are usually collected in the morning to allow food from the previous evening meal to be completely digested and absorbed. In addition, collection of the specimen in the morning causes the least amount of inconvenience to the patient in terms of abstaining from food and fluid.

The medical assistant must give detailed instructions to the patient, ensuring that the patient understands that fasting includes abstaining from food and fluid. The patient should be told, however, that it is permissible—in fact, advisable—to drink water because dehydration caused by water abstinence can alter certain test results.

The medical assistant should indicate a specific time to the patient for initiation of the fast. If the specimen is to be collected in the morning, the patient should be instructed to begin fasting at 6:00 PM on the previous evening. The patient also must be told the time to report for collection of the specimen.

MEDICATION RESTRICTIONS

Many medications affect the physical and chemical characteristics of body substances; medications taken by the patient may lead to inaccurate test results. Antibiotic therapy administered before collection of a throat specimen for strep testing may cause a falsely negative test result. The physician may ask the patient to avoid taking medication for a period of time before the collection of the specimen if discontinuing the medication would not cause any health threat or serious discomfort to the patient. Because medication is more likely to interfere with test results on urine than on blood, the patient is asked to discontinue medication 48 to 72 hours before the collection of a urine specimen and 4 to 24 hours before the collection of a blood specimen.

If the patient cannot be taken off medication, this information should be recorded on the laboratory request form for specimens transported to an outside laboratory for testing. This alerts the laboratory personnel to the presence of the medication. If the medication taken by the patient interferes with the method normally used to perform the test, the laboratory may be able to use an alternative method to obtain valid results. If the test is being performed in the medical office, the medical assistant should consult the manufacturer's instructions that accompany the test for the names of medications that interfere with test results.

The physician determines the need for a patient to discontinue medication before specimen collection. The medical assistant is responsible for ensuring that the patient understands any instructions regarding restrictions on medication and for recording medications the patient is taking on the laboratory request form.

What Would You Do? What Would You *Not* Do?

Case Study 3

Kathleen O'Leary is scheduled for a follow-up appointment today at the office. She was seen last week with fatigue, shortness of breath, weight loss, increased urination, and blurred vision. Kathleen was given a laboratory requisition to have blood drawn at an outside medical laboratory. The physician ordered a complete blood count with differential and a comprehensive metabolic profile. When the charts are prepared for the day, Kathleen's laboratory results are not in her chart. Kathleen is contacted by phone; she says she knows she should have gone to the laboratory to have her blood drawn, but she is afraid of needles and panics at the sight of blood. She says that the last time she had her blood drawn she started feeling hot and lightheaded and had to lie down on a table and was embarrassed. Kathleen says she also is worried the laboratory results might show something is wrong with her. She is thinking of not coming for her appointment today and hopes that she starts feeling better on her own. ■

COLLECTING, HANDLING, AND TRANSPORTING SPECIMENS

Clinical laboratory tests are performed on specimens obtained from the body. A **specimen** is a small sample or part taken from the body to represent the nature of the whole. Most laboratory tests are performed on specimens that are easily obtained from the body, such as blood, urine, feces, sputum, cervical and vaginal scrapings of cells, and secretions or discharge from various parts of the body (e.g., nose, throat, wound, ear, eye, vagina, urethra), for microbiologic analysis. Other examples of specimens analyzed in the laboratory but more difficult to obtain from the body include gastric juices, cerebrospinal fluid, pleural fluid, peritoneal fluid, synovial fluid, and tissue specimens for biopsy. The source of the specimen may not be indicative of the pathologic condition in question; for example, triiodothyronine and thyroxine tests are performed on blood serum but are used to detect a condition that affects the thyroid gland.

The medical assistant is responsible for the collection of most specimens obtained from patients in the medical office; of these, blood and urine constitute the largest percentage of specimens collected. Certain specimens, such as a sample of vaginal or urethral discharge, cerebrospinal fluid, or a tissue specimen, must be collected by the physician; in these cases, the medical assistant assists with the collection.

The most important goal of specimen collection and handling is to provide the laboratory with a sample that is as biologically representative as possible of the body substance collected. If the specimen is collected or handled improperly, the **in vivo** characteristics of the specimen may be adversely affected, which may cause inaccurate and unreliable test results; this may interfere with the accurate diagnosis and treatment of the patient's condition.

GUIDELINES FOR SPECIMEN COLLECTION

Specific guidelines that should be used regarding specimen collection and handling follow. Review and follow the OSHA Bloodborne Pathogens Standards during specimen collection (see Chapter 17).

1. *Review the requirements for collection and handling of the specimen,* which include the collection supplies necessary, the type of specimen to be collected (e.g., **serum, plasma,** whole blood, clotted blood, urine), the amount necessary for laboratory analysis, the techniques to follow to collect the specimen, and proper handling and storage of the specimen. The medical assistant must refer to the appropriate reference source to determine the collection and handling requirements for each test ordered by the physician. If the specimen is transported to an outside laboratory, this information is indicated in the laboratory directory. Figure 29-11 shows an example of the collection and handling requirements for a triglycerides test exactly as presented in a laboratory directory. The collection and handling requirements necessary for specimens tested in the medical office are listed in the manufacturer's instructions that accompany the test system. A **test system** is defined as a setup that includes all of the test components required to perform a laboratory test such as testing devices, controls, and testing reagents.

Triglycerides	
CPT code:	84478
Type of specimen:	Serum
Amount:	2 mL
Collection supplies:	SST or transfer tube
Collection techniques:	Let stand for 30 minutes. Separate serum from cells within 45 minutes of collection.
Patient preparation:	Patient should fast for 12 to 14 hours prior to collection.
Handling and storage:	Refrigerate or store at room temperature. Stable at room temperature for up to 7 days.
Causes for rejection:	Nonfasting specimen, improper labeling of tube
Reference range:	Desirable: Less than 150 mg/dL
	Borderline high: 150-199 mg/dL
	High: 200-499 mg/dL
	Very high: 500 mg/dL or greater

Use:

Measurement of triglyceride levels assists with the diagnosis and treatment of diabetes mellitus, nephrosis, liver obstruction, and pancreatitis. In association with HDL cholesterol and total cholesterol, a triglyceride determination assists in the assessment of the risk for developing coronary artery disease. Elevated levels may occur with liver disease, nephritic syndrome, hypothyroidism, increased alcohol consumption, poorly controlled diabetes, and pancreatitis.

Limitations:

- Women on estrogens (high estrogen contraceptives can increase blood triglyceride levels).
- An increase in the triglyceride level may occur during pregnancy.

Methodology:

Enzymatic

Figure 29-11 Collection and handling requirements for a triglyceride test from a laboratory directory.

2. *Assemble the equipment and supplies.* Use only the appropriate specimen containers as specified by the laboratory directory or manufacturer's instructions accompanying a test system. Substituting containers may not yield the proper type of specimen required or may affect the test results, as shown by the following examples. If serum is required and a tube containing an anticoagulant is used (instead of a tube without an anticoagulant), the blood separates into plasma and cells, rather than serum and cells, and the wrong type of blood specimen is obtained, which necessitates obtaining another specimen from the patient. Collection of a microbiologic specimen that may contain anaerobic pathogens with supplies meant for aerobic pathogens results in death of the anaerobic pathogen.

The specimen container should be sterile to prevent contamination of the specimen. Many specimens, especially microbiologic ones, are adversely affected by contaminants, such as extraneous microorganisms, which may affect the accuracy of the test results.

The medical assistant should check each container before use to ensure it is not broken, chipped, cracked, or otherwise damaged. Damaged containers are unsuitable for specimen collection and should be discarded. Some containers such as blood tubes have an expiration date (Figure 29-12). The medical assistant should make sure to check the expiration date on these containers to avoid using an outdated container.

3. *Label each specimen container.* The medical assistant should label each tube and specimen container.

Figure 29-12 Blood tube showing expiration date.

Figure 29-13 A, Computerized bar code label. **B,** Hand-labeled blood tube.

An unlabeled specimen is a cause for rejection of the specimen by an outside laboratory. Two *unique identifiers* should be used to label the specimen. A unique identifier is information that clearly identifies a specific patient, such as the patient's name and date of birth. A specimen can be labeled by attaching a computerized bar code label to the specimen (Figure 29-13, *A*). Laboratory instruments that do the testing are able to read the bar codes and automatically record results on a laboratory report for a particular patient using the demographic

information supplied by the bar code. A specimen can also be labeled by handwriting the information on the label, which should include the patient's name and date of birth, the date and time of collection, the medical assistant's initials, and any other information required by the laboratory, such as the source of the specimen (Figure 29-13, *B*). The information should be printed legibly, and the medical assistant should be certain that the information is accurate to avoid a mix-up of specimens. The medical assistant must also complete a laboratory request form to accompany the specimen, as described earlier in this chapter. (*Note:* The medical assistant should follow the medical office policy as to when the tubes should be labeled. Some offices prefer that the tubes be labeled *before* the specimen is drawn; other offices want the tubes to be labeled *after* the specimen has been drawn.)

4. *Identify the patient.* Proper patient identification is essential to avoid collecting a specimen from the wrong patient by mistake. After greeting the patient, the medical assistant should ask the patient to state his or her full name and date of birth. This information should be compared with the demographic data indicated in the patient's chart. The patient should *not* be asked whether he or she is a certain patient. For example, the patient should not be asked, "Are you Brad Thompson?" The patient may not hear the medical assistant correctly or may not be paying attention and may answer in the affirmative even if he is not that patient. A specimen that is not identified correctly could lead to an inaccurate patient diagnosis and the wrong treatment.

5. *Determine whether the patient has prepared properly.* If the patient was required to prepare before the specimen was collected, determine whether this was done properly. Improper preparation may lead to inaccurate test results. If a test that requires fasting, such as an FBG, is performed on a nonfasting specimen, the results are altered; in this case, they are falsely high. If the patient has not prepared properly, inform the physician; the physician may want the patient to prepare properly and return, or the physician may tell the medical assistant to go ahead with the collection but to alert the laboratory to the situation by marking the information on the laboratory request. In the example just given, "nonfasting specimen" would be written on the request form.

6. *Explain the procedure.* An explanation of the collection procedure helps relax and reassure the patient and gains the patient's confidence and cooperation, especially the first time the patient has a specimen collected.

7. *Collection of the specimen* involves a set of specific techniques for each type of specimen obtained. The information in this section is presented in general terms. Specific procedures for the collection of biologic specimens are included in this text in Chapters 30 through 34 (Urinalysis, Phlebotomy, Hematology, Blood Chemistry and Immunology, and Medical Microbiology).

Specimen collection involves a combination of medical and surgical aseptic techniques. Certain parts of the

Figure 29-14 Medical and surgical asepsis must be used when collecting a specimen.

collection materials, such as needles, swabs, and the insides of specimen containers, must remain sterile. If a culture medium is used during collection of a microbiologic specimen, the medical assistant must ensure that the lid of the container is removed only when the specimen is placed on the culture medium. Unnecessary removal of the lid results in contamination of the culture medium with extraneous microorganisms, which interferes with accurate test results. During the collection and handling of the specimen, the medical assistant must be careful to use medical and surgical asepsis to prevent contamination of the specimen, the patient, or himself or herself (Figure 29-14).

The medical assistant must collect the specimen using proper technique. The proper type of specimen must be collected as designated in the laboratory directory or by the instructions that accompany the test system. The collection procedure should be followed exactly to ensure a high-quality and reliable specimen. For example, collection of a random urine specimen when a clean-catch midstream specimen is required may affect the accuracy of the test results.

The medical assistant must be sure to collect the amount of specimen necessary for the test, which varies depending on the type of test being performed and the number of laboratory tests ordered on the specimen. If the medical assistant fails to collect the specified amount of a specimen that is being transported to an outside laboratory, the laboratory may not be able to perform the test, and the laboratory request is returned marked "quantity not sufficient" (QNS). This situation warrants calling the patient back for collection of another specimen.

8. *Process the specimen.* The specimen may need to be processed after collection. For example, when collecting a serum specimen using a serum separator tube (SST), the medical assistant must allow the tube to stand for 45 minutes and then centrifuge the specimen to separate the serum from the cells (with a gel barrier), as shown in Figure 29-15.

9. *Properly handle and store the specimen* to preserve its in vivo physical and chemical characteristics. Some

Figure 29-15 Serum specimen in a serum separator tube (SST) that has been centrifuged.

specimens, such as microbiologic specimens, are more sensitive to environmental influences and must be handled with special care. Whenever possible, laboratory tests are best performed on fresh specimens (for most specimens, within 1 hour after collection) because they yield the most reliable test results. When this is not possible, the specimen must be stored; storage may be required until it can be tested at the medical office or picked up by a laboratory courier from an outside laboratory. If the specimen is being picked up by a laboratory courier, the OSHA standard requires that it be placed in a biohazard specimen bag (Figure 29-16) to protect the courier from the possibility of an exposure incident. General guidelines for handling and storing biologic specimens most frequently collected in the medical office are presented in Table 29-3.

CLINICAL LABORATORY IMPROVEMENT AMENDMENTS
PURPOSE OF CLIA 1988

In 1988, Congress passed the Clinical Laboratory Improvement Amendments (CLIA 1988), which established standards for improving the quality of laboratory testing in the United States. CLIA 1988 consists of federal regulations governing all facilities that perform laboratory tests for health assessment or for the diagnosis, prevention, or treatment of disease. CLIA 1988 included facilities not previously covered under federal legislation, such as medical offices, health departments, and nursing homes. The Centers for Medicare and Medicaid Services (CMS) is a

Figure 29-19 Digital readout of results on an automated analyzer.

Figure 29-20 Clinical Laboratories Improvement Amendments (CLIA)–waived automated analyzers. Blood cholesterol analyzer *(left)* and hemoglobin analyzer *(right)*.

The ease of operating automated systems should not lead to a false sense of security because these systems have limitations that must be recognized—the most critical one being the failure of the equipment. One of the most important aspects of use of an automated system is the ability to recognize signs that indicate the system is malfunctioning, because malfunctioning may lead to inaccurate test results.

The manufacturer of each automated system provides an operating manual (and sometimes an instructional video) with the instrument that includes information needed to collect and handle the specimen, perform quality control procedures, and test the specimen. In addition, the manufacturer typically has personnel available for on-site training and service. It is important that the medical assistant become completely familiar with all aspects of the automated systems used to perform laboratory tests in his or her medical office. Quality control procedures are of particular importance to ensure that the analyzer is functioning properly and that the test results are reliable and accurate. Additional information on quality control procedures is presented later in this section.

When an automated analyzer is purchased, the testing components (e.g., controls, testing reagents) are usually purchased separately. The medical assistant is responsible for checking the supplies periodically and reordering them as needed. Each testing component comes with a product insert, which indicates the proper storage and stability requirements. Most testing components are stored at room temperature. If a testing component needs to be stored in the refrigerator, it must be allowed to come to room temperature before it is used. Unopened controls are stable until the expiration date marked on the container. Once opened, some controls are stable only for a certain period of time (e.g., 30 days). For these controls, the medical assistant

must write the date the control was opened *and* the date it should be discarded (expiration date) on the label of the control.

Some examples of brand names of CLIA-waived automated analyzers (Figure 29-20) include Cholestech LDX (Cholestech, Hayward, Calif), STAT-Site Hemoglobin Meter (Stanbio Laboratory, Boerne, Tex), CoaguChek system and Accu-Chek (Roche Diagnostics, Branchburg, NJ), A1C Now (Bayer Corporation, Morrisville, NJ),and Clinitek urine analyzer (Siemens Corporation, New York, NY).

QUALITY CONTROL

The ultimate goal in the clinical laboratory is to ensure that the laboratory test accurately measures what it is supposed to measure; this involves practicing and maintaining a quality control program. **Quality control** (QC) may be defined as the application of methods and means to ensure that test results are reliable and valid, and errors that may interfere with obtaining accurate test results are detected and eliminated. Practicing quality control methods ensures that test results represent the true status of the patient's condition and body functions and provide the physician with reliable information for making a diagnosis and prescribing treatment.

Quality control is an ongoing process that encompasses every aspect of patient preparation and specimen collection, handling, transport, and testing. The quality control methods that should be used to obtain precision and accuracy when using a CLIA-waived test system are presented here.

1. STORAGE AND HANDLING OF TEST SYSTEMS

a. Store the test system according to the manufacturer's instructions. Improper storage can cause deterioration of the testing components. Most test systems need to be stored at room temperature in a cool, dry area away from sources of heat and sunlight. Some testing components (e.g., controls, testing reagents) may need to be stored in the refrigerator.

b. Allow time for refrigerated testing components to reach room temperature before using them. It usually takes 15 to 30 minutes for a testing component to reach room temperature.

c. Controls often need to be shaken gently to mix them.

d. Do not transfer testing components from one testing kit to another.

e. Make sure environmental conditions are appropriate for running the test as specified in the manufacturer's instructions.

2. STABILITY OF TESTING COMPONENTS

a. Check the expiration date of each component in the test system before using it. Do not use a test component if it is past its expiration date.

b. Unopened controls are stable until the expiration date marked on the container. Once opened, some controls are stable only for a certain period of time (e.g., 30 days). For these controls, the date the control is opened *and* the date it should be discarded (expiration date) must be written on the label of the control after it has been opened. An opened control is stable until it reaches the expiration date stamped on the container or the expiration date indicated by the medical assistant on the container, whichever comes first.

c. Discard outdated testing components as soon as they reach their expiration dates.

3. CALIBRATION

Calibration is a mechanism used to check the precision and accuracy of a test system, such as an automated analyzer, to determine if the system is providing accurate results. A calibration check detects errors caused by laboratory equipment that is not working properly. Calibration is typically performed using a calibration device, often called a *standard*. The calibration device may come in the form of a calibration strip or cassette. The device is inserted into the analyzer (Figure 29-21, *A*), and the calibration results are displayed on the liquid crystal diode (LCD) screen of the analyzer or printed out by the analyzer. The calibration results are then compared with the expected results provided in the product insert or on the calibration device (Figure 29-21, *B*). Calibration guidelines include the following:

a. Perform the calibration procedure by following the manufacturer's instructions. Instructions include information on the type of calibration device to use, how to perform the calibration procedure, and what action should be taken if the procedure does not perform as expected.

b. Document calibration results in a quality control log. This is a CLIA recommendation (not a requirement) for CLIA-waived test systems.

c. If the calibration procedure does not perform as expected, patient testing should not be conducted until the problem has been identified and resolved.

d. The frequency of performing a calibration check is indicated in the manufacturer's instructions. At a minimum,

Figure 29-21 A, Calibrating an automated analyzer with a calibration device. **B,** Calibration results are compared with expected results on the calibration device.

a calibration check should be performed when a new lot number of testing reagents is put into use.

4. CONTROLS

A **control** is a solution that is used to monitor a test system to ensure the reliability and accuracy of test results. Controls come with a product insert, which lists the expected ranges for control results. There are two categories of controls: *external controls* and *internal controls.*

Internal controls: An internal control is built into some test systems (Figure 29-22). It evaluates whether certain aspects of the testing procedure are working properly. An internal control is performed at the same time that the testing procedure is performed. It checks for one or more of the following: whether a sufficient amount of the specimen was added, whether a sufficient amount of testing reagent was added, and whether the testing reagent migrated through the test device properly. If the internal control does not perform as expected, the test result is invalid and the specimen must be retested.

External controls: External controls are used to determine if the testing reagents are performing properly and to detect any errors in technique of the individual performing the test. External controls consist of commercially available solutions with known values. They may be included with the test system or may need to be purchased separately. In general, two levels of controls must be performed on a test system. A *low-level control* (also known as a *Level 1 control*) produces results that fall below the reference range for the test; a *high-level control* (also known as a *Level 2 control*) produces results that fall above the reference range for the test (Figure 29-23). The control procedure is performed in a manner similar to the procedure for performing the test on a specimen collected from a patient. Instead of adding the patient specimen to the testing device, however, the control is added to it. Control results are compared with expected results provided in the product insert. Failure of a control to produce expected results may be caused by

deterioration of testing components after improper storage or use of components past their expiration date, improper environmental testing conditions, or errors in technique used to perform the procedure. External control guidelines include the following:

a. Perform control procedures by following the instructions in the product insert. These instructions include information on how to perform the control procedure and what action should be taken if the controls do not perform as expected.

b. Document control results in a quality control log (Figure 29-24). This is a CLIA recommendation (not a requirement) for CLIA-waived test systems.

c. If the controls do not perform as expected, patient testing should not be conducted until the problem is identified and resolved. Factors that can cause abnormal control results include outdated controls or testing reagents, improper storage of testing components, and an error in the technique used to perform the procedure.

d. The frequency of performing external controls is indicated in the product insert. At a minimum, they should be performed on each new lot number of testing reagents and thereafter on a regular basis, such as monthly.

5. COLLECTING AND HANDLING SPECIMENS

a. Use the appropriate collection devices to collect the specimen. Do not substitute other devices.

b. Follow the manufacturer's instructions exactly for collecting and handling the specimen.

Negative   Positive

Figure 29-22 Internal control. The blue line next to the letter *C* indicates that the internal control has reacted as expected.

Figure 29-23 External controls. Low or level 1 control *(left)* and high or level 2 control *(right)*.

QUALITY CONTROL LOG

BLOOD GLUCOSE TEST

Name of meter: *Accu-Check Advantage*

Controls

TEST STRIPS:

Lot number: _____ *522677* _____

Exp date: _____ *4/30/20XX* _____

Code number _____ *635* _____

LOW LEVEL CONTROL:

Lot number _____ *63330* _____

Exp date _____ *11/29/20XX* _____

Expected range: _____ *18 – 64* _____

HIGH LEVEL CONTROL:

Lot number _____ *63330* _____

Exp date _____ *11/29/20XX* _____

Expected range: _____ *270 – 324* _____

Date	Low level control	Accept	Reject	High level control	Accept	Reject	Technician
9/20/XX	61	X		315	X		K. Mcgrew, CMA (AAMA)
9/21/XX	53	X		310	X		K. Mcgrew, CMA (AAMA)
9/22/XX	50	X		302	X		K. Mcgrew, CMA (AAMA)
9/23/XX	48	X		300	X		K. Mcgrew, CMA (AAMA)
9/24/XX	51	X		305	X		K. Mcgrew, CMA (AAMA)

Figure 29-24 Quality control log sheet for blood glucose testing.

c. If a specimen (e.g., urine) cannot be tested immediately, information is provided in the manufacturer's instructions on proper storage of the specimen until it can be tested.

6. TESTING THE SPECIMEN

a. If more than one patient is being tested at a time, label each testing device with the patient's name to prevent mix-up of specimens.

b. Follow the procedure in the manufacturer's instructions *exactly* for testing the specimen. Specific requirements may include the following:
   • Adding the proper amounts of reagents
   • Adding reagents in the proper order
   • Adhering to proper time intervals for various steps in the procedure
   • Reading results within the proper time frame

7. INTERPRETING AND READING TEST RESULTS

Testing kits often rely on a color change for the interpretation of test results. The color change is compared with a color chart or a color diagram (Figure 29-25) included with the testing kit. Test results derived from an automated analyzer do not need to be interpreted and are printed out or displayed on the LCD screen of the analyzer. The following guidelines should be followed when test results from a testing kit are interpreted:

Figure 29-25 Color diagram used to interpret test results.

a. Interpret the results according to instructions outlined in the product insert that accompanies the testing kit.
b. Test results are usually interpreted as positive, negative, or invalid. Invalid results may be caused by an improperly collected specimen or an error in technique in performing the testing procedure.
c. If a test result is invalid, retest a new sample with new testing materials. If the second test result is invalid, contact the manufacturer.

CATEGORIES OF TEST RESULTS

Laboratory test results are categorized as qualitative or quantitative.

QUALITATIVE TEST RESULTS

Qualitative test results indicate whether or not a substance is present in the specimen being tested; they also provide an approximate indication of the amount of substance present. Interpretation of qualitative results usually involves the use of a color comparison chart or a color diagram. Results are recorded in terms of 1+, 2+, or 3+; trace, small, moderate, or large; negative or positive; or reactive or nonreactive. Testing kits usually provide qualitative test results.

QUANTITATIVE TEST RESULTS

Quantitative test results indicate the exact amount of a chemical substance that is present in the body; results are reported in measurable units (e.g., mg/dL). No interpretation is required to read quantitative results. Automated analyzers provide quantitative test results, with the results being printed out or displayed on the LCD screen of the analyzer.

RECORDING TEST RESULTS

The medical assistant is responsible for recording laboratory test results. Careful recording is essential to avoid errors, which could affect the patient's diagnosis. It is usually unnecessary to chart results from laboratory reports returned from outside laboratories because the report itself is filed in the patient's record. In case of a STAT request or critical findings, the test results may be telephoned to the medical office, requiring the medical assistant to record results on a report form.

Results of laboratory tests performed by the medical assistant in the POL should be charted in the medical record and must include the date and time, name of the test, and test results. Quantitative test results should be recorded using the units of measurement of the test system (e.g., mg/dL). Qualitative test results should be recorded using words or abbreviations (e.g., positive, negative) and not symbols (e.g., +, −), because symbols can be accidentally changed or misinterpreted. The office may also maintain a log of the tests performed in the POL, which includes the patient's name, date and time, name of the test, the test results, and the name and credentials of the individual performing the test (Figure 29-26).

LABORATORY SAFETY

Laboratory safety is an important aspect of clinical laboratory testing in the medical office. As previously discussed, many of the laboratory tests performed in the medical office involve the use of hazardous chemical reagents, the handling of specimens that may contain pathogens, and the use of laboratory equipment. Practicing good technique in testing laboratory specimens and recognizing potential hazards help to reduce accidents in the laboratory. Some areas specifically related to laboratory safety in the medical office are described here.

The medical assistant should handle all chemical reagents carefully by adhering to the following instructions:
1. Review the SDS before using a laboratory chemical reagent to become familiar with its hazards, and measure to take to prevent injury and illness when handling the chemical reagent.
2. Ensure that all reagent containers are clearly and properly labeled.
3. If a label is loose, reattach it immediately.
4. Recap reagent containers immediately after use to prevent spills.

Laboratory specimens should be collected and handled carefully as follows:
1. Follow the OSHA Bloodborne Pathogens Standard in collecting and handling laboratory specimens.
2. Wash hands immediately if some of the material contained in the specimen is accidentally touched.
3. Avoid hand-to-mouth contact, such as eating, drinking, or applying makeup, while working with specimens.

	QUALITY CONTROL LOG			
	BLOOD GLUCOSE TEST			

ACCU-CHECK TEST STRIPS

Lot number: _____522677_____

Exp date: _____4/30/20XX_____

Code number _____635_____

Date	Patient name	Patinet ID	Glucose results (in mg/dL0)	Technician
9/20/XX	Thomas Jeffers	1341	98	K. Mcgrew, CMA (AAMA)
9/20/XX	Diana Woods	3744	74	K. Mcgrew, CMA (AAMA)
9/21/XX	Lauren Campbell	6497	115	K. Mcgrew, CMA (AAMA)
9/21/XX	Jason Coates	5310	78	K. Mcgrew, CMA (AAMA)
9/21/XX	Chloe Pearson	2333	85	K. Mcgrew, CMA (AAMA)
9/22/XX	Kathleen Dobson	1466	65	K. Mcgrew, CMA (AAMA)
9/22/XX	Larry Wilson	5399	102	K. Mcgrew, CMA (AAMA)
9/23/XX	Samantha Byran	2512	92	K. Mcgrew, CMA (AAMA)
9/24/XX	Abbey Paulson	1788	88	K. Mcgrew, CMA (AAMA)
9/24/XX	Michael Williams	3903	105	K. Mcgrew, CMA (AAMA)

Figure 29-26 Patient log of laboratory tests.

4. Immediately clean up any specimen spilled on the work-table, and cleanse the table with a disinfectant.
5. Properly dispose of all contaminated needles, syringes, specimen containers, and infectious waste used in specimen collection and testing.
6. Cover any break in the skin, such as a cut or scratch, with a bandage.
7. Ensure that all specimen containers are tightly capped to prevent leakage.
8. Do not store food in refrigerators where testing supplies or specimens are stored.
9. Handle all laboratory equipment and supplies properly and with care, as indicated by the manufacturer. For example, wait until the centrifuge comes to a complete stop before opening it.

Careful handling and storing of glassware to prevent breakage should be performed as follows:

1. Carefully arrange glassware in storage cabinets to prevent breakage.
2. Carefully remove glassware from storage cabinets.
3. If glassware does break, dispose of it in a puncture-resistant container to protect trash handlers from the shards.

30 Urinalysis

Check out the Evolve site at http://evolve.elsevier.com/Bonewit/today/ to access additional interactive activities and exercises to help you study and prepare for success.

LEARNING OBJECTIVES

Urinary System
1. List conditions that may cause polyuria and oliguria.
2. Define the terms used to describe symptoms of the urinary system.

Collection of Urine
3. Explain why a first-voided morning specimen is often preferred for urinalysis.
4. Explain the purpose of collecting a clean-catch midstream specimen.
5. Explain the purpose of a 24-hour urine collection.
6. List changes that may occur if urine is allowed to remain standing for longer than 1 hour.

Analysis of Urine
7. List factors that may cause urine to have an unusual color or become cloudy.
8. Identify the various tests that are included in the physical and chemical examination of urine.
9. List the structures that may be found in a microscopic examination of urine.

Urine Pregnancy Testing
10. Explain the basis for urine pregnancy tests.
11. List the guidelines that must be followed in a urine pregnancy test to ensure accurate test results.

PROCEDURES

Instruct a patient in the procedure for collecting a clean-catch midstream urine specimen.

Assess the color and appearance of a urine specimen. Perform a chemical assessment of a urine specimen. Prepare a urine specimen for microscopic analysis by the physician.

Perform a urine pregnancy test.

CHAPTER OUTLINE

COMPOSITION OF URINE
Terms Related to the Urinary System
COLLECTION OF URINE
Guidelines for Urine Collection
Urine Specimen Collection Methods
Random Specimen
First-Voided Morning Specimen
Clean-Catch Midstream Specimen
Twenty-Four–Hour Urine Specimen
ANALYSIS OF URINE
Physical Examination of Urine
Color
Appearance
Odor
Specific Gravity
Chemical Examination of Urine
Urine Testing Kits
pH

Glucose
Protein
Ketone
Bilirubin
Urobilinogen
Blood
Nitrite
Leukocytes
Reagent Strips
Guidelines for Reagent Strip Urine Testing
Quality Control Testing
Urine Analyzer
Microscopic Examination of Urine
Red Blood Cells
White Blood Cells
Epithelial Cells
Casts
Crystals

Miscellaneous Structures
URINE PREGNANCY TESTING
Human Chorionic Gonadotropin

Immunoassays
Guidelines for Urine Pregnancy Testing
SERUM PREGNANCY TEST

KEY TERMS

anuria (ah-NOOR-ee-ah)
bilirubinuria (bill-ih-roo-bin-YUR-ee-ah)
bladder catheterization
diuresis (di-ah-REE-sis)
dysuria (dis-YUR-ee-ah)
frequency
glycosuria (glie-koe-SOO-ree-ah)
hematuria (hem-ah-TOOR-ee-ah)
ketonuria (kee-toe-NOO-ree-ah)
ketosis (kee-TOE-sis)

micturition (mik-tur-ISH-un)
nephron (NEF-ron)
nocturia (nok-TOOR-ee-ah)
nocturnal enuresis (nok-TOOR-nal
  en-YUR-ee-sas)
oliguria (oh-lig-YUR-ee-ah)
pH (PEE-AYCH)
polyuria (pol-ee-YUR-ee-ah)
proteinuria (proe-teen-YUR-ee-ah)
pyuria (pi-YUR-ee-ah)

renal threshold (REE-nul-THRESH-hold)
retention
specific gravity
supernatant (soo-per-NAY-tent)
suprapubic aspiration
urgency
urinalysis (yur-in-AL-ih-sis)
urinary incontinence
void (VOYD)

COMPOSITION OF URINE

A physiologic change in the body caused by disease can create a disturbance in one or more of the functions of the kidney. Detection of such a disturbance can be made with the examination of urine and other body fluids such as blood.

Urine is composed of 95% water and 5% organic and inorganic waste products. Organic waste products consist of urea, uric acid, ammonia, and creatinine. Urea is present in the greatest amounts and is derived from the breakdown of proteins. Inorganic waste products include chloride, sodium, potassium, calcium, magnesium, phosphate, and sulfate.

A normal adult excretes approximately 750 to 2000 mL of urine per day. This amount varies according to the amount of fluid consumed and the amount of fluid lost through other means, such as perspiration, feces, and water vapor from the lungs. An excessive increase in urine output is known as **polyuria,** with the urine volume exceeding 2000 mL in 24 hours. Polyuria may be caused by the excessive intake of fluids or the intake of fluids that contain caffeine (e.g., coffee, tea, cola), which is a mild diuretic. Certain drugs, such as diuretics, and the pathologic conditions of diabetes mellitus, diabetes insipidus, and renal disease also may result in polyuria. Decreased or scanty urine output is known as **oliguria.** In the case of oliguria, the urine volume is less than 400 mL in 24 hours. Oliguria may occur with decreased fluid intake, dehydration, profuse perspiration, vomiting, diarrhea, or kidney disease. The normal act of voiding urine is known as **micturition.**

TERMS RELATED TO THE URINARY SYSTEM

The medical assistant should have a thorough knowledge of the following terms used to describe symptoms associated with the urinary system:

Anuria Failure of the kidneys to produce urine
Diuresis Secretion and passage of large amounts of urine
Dysuria Difficult or painful urination
Frequency The condition of having to urinate often
Hematuria Blood present in the urine
Nocturia Excessive (voluntary) urination during the night
Nocturnal enuresis Inability of an individual to control urination at night during sleep (bedwetting)
Oliguria Decreased output of urine
Polyuria Increased output of urine
Pyuria Pus present in the urine
Retention The inability to empty the bladder. The urine is being produced normally but is not being voided
Urgency The immediate need to urinate
Urinary incontinence The inability to retain urine

COLLECTION OF URINE

The advantages of urine testing are that urine is readily available and obtaining it does not require an invasive procedure or the use of special equipment. For accurate test results, however, the medical assistant must adhere to proper urine collection procedures to obtain the proper specimen as ordered by the physician.

GUIDELINES FOR URINE COLLECTION

The guidelines listed should be followed in collection of a urine specimen:
1. The medical assistant must obtain an adequate volume of urine as necessary for the type of test (usually 30 to 50 mL of urine).
2. Each specimen must be labeled properly with the patient's name and date of birth, the date and time of collection, and the type of specimen (i.e., urine) to avoid any mix-ups in specimens.

3. Any medication the patient is taking should be documented on the laboratory requisition and in the patient's medical record, because some medications may interfere with the accuracy of the test results.

4. If possible, the collection of a urine specimen should be avoided in women during menstruation and for several days thereafter because the specimen may become contaminated with blood. This results in a false-positive test result for blood in the urine.

5. The medical assistant should take into consideration that voiding may be difficult for patients under stress and anxiety. In these instances, understanding and patience should be conveyed to the patient.

6. A urine specimen may be difficult to obtain from a child, even with the assistance of a parent. In this case, the physician should be informed because another collection method may be used, such as a urine collection bag, suprapubic aspiration, or catheterization of the patient.

URINE SPECIMEN COLLECTION METHODS

The type of test to be performed often dictates the method used to collect the urine specimen. A first-voided morning specimen is recommended for pregnancy testing, and a clean-catch midstream specimen is necessary for identification of the presence of a urinary tract infection (UTI).

Most offices use disposable plastic urine specimen containers. These containers are available in different sizes and come with lids to prevent spillage and to reduce bacterial and other types of contamination.

What Would You Do?	**What Would You *Not* Do?**

Case Study 1
Yusuke Urameshi is at the office with fever and chills, urinary frequency, and painful and difficult urination. The physician suspects that Mr. Urameshi has prostatitis and orders a clean-catch urine specimen for a complete urinalysis, including a microscopic examination of the sediment. Mr. Urameshi tries to collect the specimen but is able to collect only 5 mL of urine. He says that he is worried about what is wrong with him and he thinks his nervousness is making it hard to get a specimen. Mr. Urameshi says that it is probably just as well because he did not understand how to cleanse himself, and he is not sure that he did it right. ∎

Random Specimen

Urine testing in the medical office is often performed on freshly voided, random specimens. The medical assistant instructs the patient to **void** into a clean, dry, wide-mouthed container, and the urine is tested immediately at the medical office.

First-Voided Morning Specimen

In many cases a first-voided morning specimen may be desired for testing because it contains the greatest concentration of dissolved substances, and a small amount of an abnormal substance that is present would be more easily detected. The patient should be instructed to collect the first specimen of the morning after rising and to preserve the specimen by refrigerating it until it is brought to the medical office. It is important to provide the patient with a specimen container to prevent the patient's use of a container from home that might harbor contaminants and affect the test results.

Clean-Catch Midstream Specimen

The urinary bladder and most of the urethra are normally free of microorganisms, whereas the distal urethra and the urinary meatus normally harbor microorganisms. If the urine is being cultured and examined for bacteria, a clean-catch midstream specimen is necessary to prevent contamination of the specimen with these normally present microorganisms. Only microorganisms that may be causing the patient's condition are desired in the urine specimen. A clean-catch midstream collection may be ordered for the detection of a UTI and the evaluation of the effectiveness of drug therapy in a patient undergoing treatment for such an infection.

The purpose of the clean-catch midstream collection is the removal of microorganisms from the urinary meatus and the distal urethra. This is accomplished by instructing the patient to thoroughly cleanse the area surrounding the meatus and to void a small amount of urine into the toilet, which flushes out microorganisms in the distal urethra. The urine specimen is collected in a sterile container using medically aseptic techniques. A properly collected specimen reduces the possibility of having to do a bladder catheterization or a suprapubic aspiration of the bladder. **Bladder catheterization** involves the passing of a sterile tube (the catheter) through the urethra and into the bladder to remove urine. **Suprapubic aspiration** involves the passing of a sterile needle through the abdominal wall into the bladder to remove urine. Both of these procedures must be performed using sterile technique.

Guidelines
Guidelines that should be followed when collecting a clean-catch midstream specimen are as follows:

1. A clean-catch midstream specimen is collected by the patient at the medical office. The medical assistant must provide complete instructions for collection of this specimen. Failure to instruct the patient adequately may necessitate a return to the medical office for the collection of another specimen because of bacterial contamination. Patient instructions for obtaining a clean-catch midstream specimen are presented in Procedure 30-1.

2. The medical assistant must label the container with the patient's name and date of birth, the date, the time of collection, and the type of specimen (clean-catch midstream specimen).

3. For reliable test results, the specimen should be tested immediately and should not be allowed to stand. If this

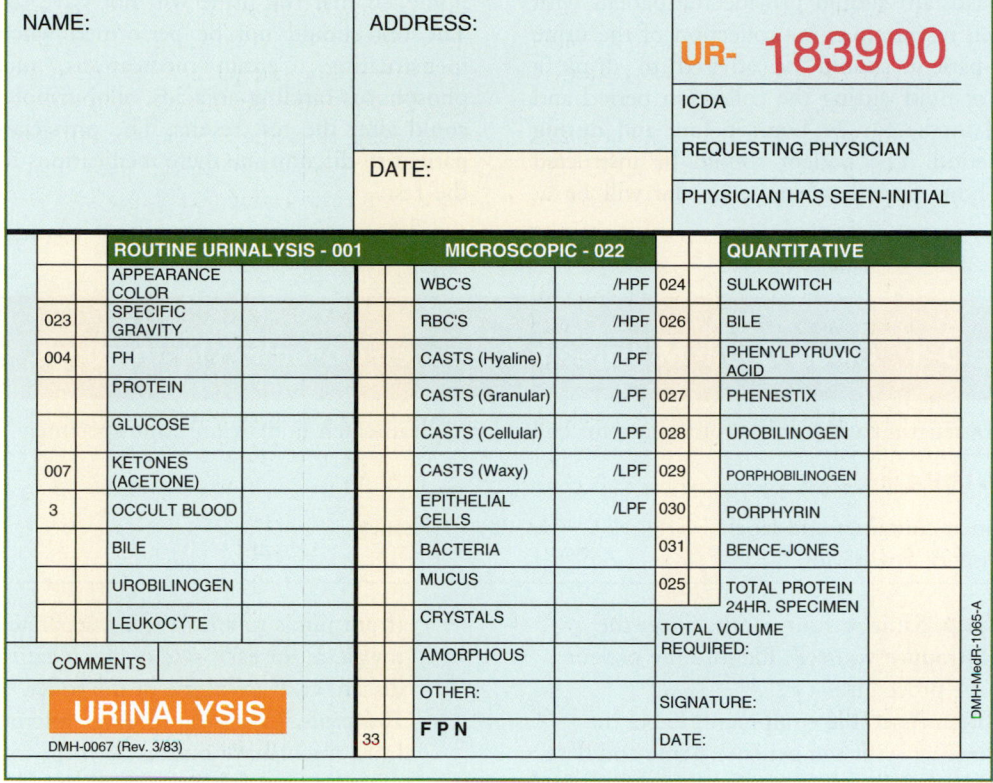

NAME:			ADDRESS:			UR- 183900	
						ICDA	
			DATE:			REQUESTING PHYSICIAN	
						PHYSICIAN HAS SEEN-INITIAL	

		ROUTINE URINALYSIS - 001				MICROSCOPIC - 022				QUANTITATIVE	
		APPEARANCE COLOR				WBC'S	/HPF	024		SULKOWITCH	
	023	SPECIFIC GRAVITY				RBC'S	/HPF	026		BILE	
	004	PH				CASTS (Hyaline)	/LPF			PHENYLPYRUVIC ACID	
		PROTEIN				CASTS (Granular)	/LPF	027		PHENESTIX	
		GLUCOSE				CASTS (Cellular)	/LPF	028		UROBILINOGEN	
	007	KETONES (ACETONE)				CASTS (Waxy)	/LPF	029		PORPHOBILINOGEN	
	3	OCCULT BLOOD				EPITHELIAL CELLS	/LPF	030		PORPHYRIN	
		BILE				BACTERIA		031		BENCE-JONES	
		UROBILINOGEN				MUCUS		025		TOTAL PROTEIN 24HR. SPECIMEN	
		LEUKOCYTE				CRYSTALS			TOTAL VOLUME REQUIRED:		
	COMMENTS					AMORPHOUS					
	URINALYSIS					OTHER:			SIGNATURE:		
	DMH-0067 (Rev. 3/83)			33		**F P N**			DATE:		

DMH-MedR-1065-A

Figure 30-1 Urinalysis laboratory request form.

is not possible, the specimen should be refrigerated, or a preservative should be added.

4. If the specimen is to be tested at an outside laboratory, completion of a laboratory requisition to accompany it is necessary. A urinalysis laboratory request form is shown in Figure 30-1.

5. The procedure is completed by sanitizing the hands and recording the procedure in the patient's chart. The information to be charted for specimens tested at the medical office includes the date and time, the type of specimen collected, and the laboratory test results. If the specimen is being transported to an outside laboratory for testing, record the date and time, the type of specimen collected, and the date the specimen was transported to the laboratory.

TWENTY-FOUR–HOUR URINE SPECIMEN

A 24-hour urine specimen is used for quantitative measurement of specific urinary components. With collection of urine over a 24-hour period, greater accuracy of measurement exists than with a random specimen. This is because body metabolism, exercise, and hydration can affect the excretion rate of substances in the urine. In addition, at certain times during a 24-hour period, increased excretion of substances (e.g., electrolytes, hormones, proteins, urobilinogen) is seen, and at other times decreased excretion is seen. Examples of substances measured in a 24-hour

specimen include calcium, cortisol, lead, potassium, protein, and urea nitrogen. A 24-hour specimen is often used in the diagnosis of the cause of kidney stone formation and in the control and prevention of new stone formation. It may also be used to perform a creatinine clearance test, which provides the physician with information on kidney function.

A large wide-mouthed container (3000 mL) is used to store the urine collected over the 24-hour period. To prevent changes in the quality of the urine specimen, the specimen must be kept refrigerated or placed in an ice chest. Some containers also contain a chemical preservative (in the form of crystals, tablets, or a liquid) to assist in maintaining the quality of the specimen. Examples of urine preservatives include hydrochloric acid, boric acid, acetic acid, and toluene. A hazardous chemical warning label should be attached to a specimen container with a preservative, and the patient should be instructed not to discard or touch the preservative in the container.

The patient is also provided with a container in which to collect each urine specimen. A female patient may be given a urine "hat," which is placed over the commode under the toilet seat; a male patient is often provided with a collection cup. After collection, the urine is poured into the large specimen container. This method makes collection easier and safer for the patient. If the patient voids urine directly into a specimen container that holds a preservative, the preservative could splash onto the patient's skin, resulting in a chemical burn.

The medical assistant should provide the patient with verbal and written instructions for collection of the urine specimen. The patient should be advised to drink a normal amount of fluid during the collection period and to avoid alcohol intake for 24 hours before and during the collection period. The patient should be instructed to choose a 24-hour period when he or she will be at home, so that the urine will not have to be transported. The test should not be performed when the patient is menstruating. Certain medications, such as thiazides, phosphorus-binding antacids, allopurinol, and vitamin C, could alter the test results. The physician may want the patient to discontinue these medications for 1 week before the test.

PROCEDURE 30-1   Clean-Catch Midstream Specimen Collection Instructions

Outcome Instruct a patient in the procedure for collecting a clean-catch midstream urine specimen

Equipment/Supplies

- Sterile specimen container and label
- Personal antiseptic towelettes
- Tissues

1. **Procedural Step.** Sanitize your hands. Greet the patient and introduce yourself. Identify the patient and explain the procedure.
2. **Procedural Step.** Assemble equipment. Label the specimen container with the patient's name and date of birth, the date, the type of specimen (clean-catch midstream), and your initials.

Assemble the equipment.

3. **Procedural Step.** Instruct a female patient on collection of the specimen as follows:
   a. Wash the hands, open the package of towelettes, and place them on their wrapper.
   b. Remove the lid from the specimen container and place it on a paper towel with the opening of the lid facing upward. Do not touch the inside of the lid or the inside of the specimen container.
   c. Pull undergarments down and sit on the toilet. Expose the urinary meatus by spreading apart the labia with one hand.
   d. Cleanse each side of the urinary meatus with an antiseptic towelette using a front-to-back motion

(from pubis to anus). Use a separate antiseptic towelette for each side of the meatus. After use, discard each towelette in the toilet.
   Principle. Cleansing removes microorganisms from the urinary meatus. A front-to-back motion must be used for cleansing to avoid drawing microorganisms from the anal region into the area that is being cleansed.
   e. Cleanse directly across the meatus (front to back) with a third antiseptic towelette. Discard the towelette.
   f. Continue to hold the labia apart, and void a small amount of urine into the toilet.
   Principle. Voiding a small amount flushes microorganisms out of the distal urethra.
   g. Without stopping the urine flow, collect the next amount of urine by voiding into the sterile container. Do not touch the inside of the container. Fill the specimen container about half full with urine.
   Principle. Touching the inside of the container contaminates it with microorganisms that normally reside on the skin.
   h. Void the last amount of urine into the toilet. This means that the first and last portions of the urine flow are not included in the specimen. Replace the lid of the specimen container.
   i. Wipe the area dry with a tissue, and discard it in the toilet. Flush the toilet and wash the hands.
4. **Procedural Step.** Instruct a male patient as follows:
   a. Wash the hands, open the towelettes, remove the lid from the specimen container, and remove undergarments.
   b. Stand in front of the toilet. Retract the foreskin of the penis (if uncircumcised).
   c. Cleanse the area around the meatus (glans penis) and the urethral opening (meatal orifice) by

PROCEDURE 30-1   Clean-Catch Midstream Specimen Collection Instructions—cont'd

wiping each side of the meatus with a separate antiseptic towelette.

d. Cleanse directly across the meatus with a third antiseptic towelette. After use, discard each towelette in the toilet.

e. Void a small amount of urine into the toilet.

f. Collect the next amount of urine by voiding into the sterile container without touching the inside of the container with the hands or penis. Fill the container about half full with urine.

g. Void the last amount of urine into the toilet and replace the lid on the container.

h. Wipe the area dry with a tissue, and discard it in the toilet. Flush the toilet and wash the hands.

5. Procedural Step. Provide the patient with instructions about what to do with the specimen after it has been collected (e.g., placing it in a designated area, directly handing it to the medical assistant).

6. Procedural Step. Test the specimen at the office or prepare the specimen for transport to an outside laboratory for testing. If the specimen is to be transported to an outside laboratory, do the following:

a. Place the specimen container in a biohazard specimen bag.

b. Place the laboratory request in the outside pocket of the specimen bag.

c. Properly preserve the specimen while awaiting pickup by a laboratory courier by placing it in a refrigerator.

7. Procedural Step. Chart the procedure in the patient's medical record.

a. *Paper-based patient record:* Record the date and time and the type of specimen collected (clean-catch midstream collection). Chart either the test results or the date the specimen was transported to the laboratory. Refer to the PPR charting example.

PPR CHARTING EXAMPLE

Date	
3/24/XX	10:15 a.m. Clean-catch midstream collected
	by pt. Sent to Medical Center Laboratory for
	C & S on 3/24/XX. —L. Proffitt, CMA (AAMA)

b. *Electronic medical record:* Document the type of specimen collected (clean-catch specimen, midstream collection) and the test results or the date the specimen was transported to the laboratory using the appropriate radio buttons, drop-down menus, and free text fields.

ANALYSIS OF URINE

Urinalysis is the analysis of urine and is the laboratory test most commonly performed in the medical office because a urine specimen is readily obtainable and can be easily tested. Urinalysis consists of *physical, chemical,* and *microscopic examinations.* Deviation from normal in any of the three areas assists the physician in the diagnosis and treatment of pathologic conditions, not only of the urinary system, but also of other body systems. Urinalysis may be performed as a screening measure as part of a general physical examination or to assist in the diagnosis of a pathologic condition. It also may assist in the evaluation of effectiveness of therapy after treatment has been initiated for a pathologic condition.

Urinalysis should be performed on a fresh or preserved specimen. If a specimen cannot be examined within 1 hour of voiding, it should be preserved at once in the refrigerator in a closed container and later returned to room temperature and mixed before testing. Chemical additives also are used to preserve urine specimens but usually are used only with specimens that require prolonged storage, such as specimens that must be shipped a long distance, because the chemical preservative sometimes interferes with the chemicals used to perform the urine test.

If the urine is allowed to stand at room temperature for longer than 1 hour, some of the following changes may occur:

1. Bacteria in the environment that get into the urine specimen work on the urea present in the urine, converting it to ammonia. Because ammonia is alkaline, an acid urine becomes alkaline, increasing the pH. In addition, an alkaline pH may result in a false-positive result on the protein test.

2. Bacteria multiply rapidly in the urine, resulting in a cloudy specimen and an increase in the nitrite.

3. If glucose is present in the specimen, it decreases in amount because microorganisms use the glucose as a source of food.

4. If any red or white blood cells are present, they may break down.

5. Casts decompose after several hours.

PHYSICAL EXAMINATION OF URINE

The physical examination of urine includes determination of the color, appearance, and specific gravity. The color and appearance of the urine specimen may be evaluated during preparation for another testing procedure, such as chemical testing of the urine, or before centrifugation of the specimen in preparation for microscopic analysis. For an accurate

HIGHLIGHT on Drug Testing in the Workplace

Statistics

Statistics suggest that the problem of drug abuse is growing in the workplace. On any one day, 8.9 to 16 million employees are estimated to be working under the influence of drugs. The effects of on-the-job drug use extend into every segment of the population and touch every business and industry. The Occupational Safety and Health Administration (OSHA) estimates that 65% of all work-related accidents can be traced to substance abuse. The Metropolitan Insurance Company states that drug abuse costs industry $81 billion annually because of accidents, turnover, absenteeism, lowered productivity, theft, and higher health care costs.

Testing Programs

Because of these economic and safety factors, businesses across the United States are adopting a less permissive attitude toward drug use and are beginning compulsory drug testing in the workplace. Approximately one third of U.S. employers have implemented drug-testing programs in the workplace. These employers include utility companies, transportation operations, sports associations, and governmental agencies. Currently, many companies test blue-collar and white-collar employees for drug use. Companies with drug-testing programs report a significant reduction in employee accidents, fewer sick days, and healthier employees.

A comprehensive drug-testing program includes the detection of drug use in the workplace, policies to discourage further abuse, and the referral of employees for treatment and rehabilitation. Drug testing may be performed for one or more of the following purposes: (1) preemployment drug screening, (2) testing for probable cause after unexplained behavior or an incident (e.g., an accident on the job), and (3) random sample testing of the workforce to detect use of controlled substances by employees on the job.

Testing Methods

Blood testing is the best means for determining precise information concerning the amount of drug used and when the drug was taken. Blood tests are costly, however, and are time-consuming to perform. Urine drug testing offers the next best alternative; it is noninvasive and technically easier and cheaper to perform. Current urine screening tests target the most common drugs of abuse: amphetamines, barbiturates, benzodiazepines, cocaine, marijuana, opiates, phencyclidine (PCP), methaqualone, and methadone.

Chain of Custody

The usual procedure for urine drug testing involves screening the specimen and confirming positive results with more specific urine tests. The specimen may be collected at the workplace, at the medical office, or at an outside laboratory. To help ensure reliable and valid drug-testing results, a security system or "chain of custody" must be followed in the collection and handling of the specimen. This typically includes ensuring the identification of the individual undergoing drug testing, taking precautions to avoid falsification of or tampering with specimens, properly labeling the urine specimen, sealing the sample in the specimen container after collection, and immediately sending it to the laboratory for analysis or refrigerating it at once for any delay in transport. Urine drug-testing kits are available for testing the specimen in the medical office. These kits provide immediate results and take only a few minutes to perform.

Disadvantages

The main disadvantage of urine drug testing is that a positive test result indicates only the presence of a drug in the urine; it does not provide any information regarding when the drug was taken. Drugs that are detected in the urine may or may not still be present in the blood, where they can affect an individual's behavior and impair performance. A positive urine test result does not reveal whether an individual is impaired by drugs. In addition, the initial urine screening tests are sometimes unreliable; unless positive results are confirmed with a more specific test, an individual may be unjustly accused of drug use. These factors and the violation of an individual's right to privacy are the main areas of dispute for individuals who oppose drug testing in the workplace.

Intervention

Companies with drug-testing programs have various options when results are positive, such as recommendations for drug treatment programs or disciplinary action. Many companies have established in-house employee assistance programs that include counseling and drug withdrawal therapy for employees who desire help. Most companies prefer to help current employees with rehabilitation instead of discharging them and hiring and training new employees. Studies show a 35% to 60% recovery rate for employees enrolled in drug treatment programs. ■

change has occurred, or if the *tested* strip gives off a color that does not match the shades on the color chart. Light, heat, and moisture can alter the effectiveness of the strips; care must be taken to store the test materials in a cool, dry area. Most test materials are packaged in light-resistant containers to protect them from light. The test materials must never be transferred from their original container to another because the other container may harbor traces of moisture, dirt, or chemicals that could affect the test results.

pH

The **pH** is the unit that indicates the acidity or alkalinity of a solution. The pH scale ranges from 0.0 to 14.0. The lower the number, the greater the acidity; the higher the number, the greater the alkalinity. A pH reading of 7.0 is neutral; a reading below 7.0 indicates acidity; and a reading above 7.0 indicates alkalinity.

The kidneys help regulate the acid-base balance of the body. For an accurate pH reading of the urine, the measurement should be performed on freshly voided urine. If the urine is allowed to remain standing, it becomes more alkaline as urea is converted to ammonia by bacterial action.

Although the pH of urine can normally range from 4.6 to 8.0, the pH of a freshly voided specimen of a patient on a normal diet is usually acidic and has a pH reading of about 6.0. An abnormally high pH reading on a fresh specimen (i.e., alkaline urine) may indicate a bacterial infection of the urinary tract.

Glucose

Normally, no glucose should be detectable in the urine. Glucose in the blood is filtered through the nephrons and is reabsorbed into the body. If the glucose concentration in the blood becomes too high, the kidney is unable to reabsorb all of it back into the blood, the renal threshold is exceeded, and glucose is spilled into the urine—a condition known as **glycosuria.** (The **renal threshold** is the concentration at which a substance in the blood that is not normally excreted by the kidney begins to appear in the urine.) The renal threshold for glucose is typically 160 to 180 mg/dL (100 mL of blood), but this number may vary among individuals. Diabetes mellitus is the most common cause of glycosuria. Some individuals have a low renal threshold, and glucose may appear in their urine after the consumption of a large quantity of foods containing sugar. This condition is known as *alimentary glycosuria.*

Protein

The presence of protein in the urine is known as **proteinuria.** Protein in the urine usually indicates a pathologic condition if found in several samples over time. A temporary increase in urine protein may be caused by stress or strenuous exercise. Some of the conditions that may cause proteinuria include glomerular filtration problems, renal disease, and bacterial infection of the urinary tract. If proteinuria occurs, the physician usually requests an examination of the sediment to determine, through visual observation, what is causing protein to be in the urine.

Ketone

Three types of ketone bodies exist: beta-hydroxybutyric acid, acetoacetic acid, and acetone. *Ketones* are the normal products of fat metabolism and can be used by muscle tissue as a source of energy. When more than normal amounts of fat are metabolized by the body, the muscles cannot handle all of the ketones that result. Large amounts of ketone accumulate in the tissues and body fluids; this condition is known as **ketosis.** The body rids itself of these excess ketones by excreting them in the urine. **Ketonuria** is the term that refers to the presence of ketone bodies in the urine. Conditions that may lead to ketonuria include uncontrolled diabetes mellitus, starvation, and a diet composed almost entirely of fat.

Bilirubin

The average life span of a red blood cell is 120 days. When a red blood cell breaks down, one of the substances released from the breakdown of hemoglobin is a vivid yellow pigment known as *bilirubin.* Normally, bilirubin is transported to the liver and excreted into the bile, and it eventually leaves the body through the intestines in the feces. Certain liver conditions, such as gallstones, hepatitis, and cirrhosis, may result in the presence of bilirubin in the urine, or **bilirubinuria.** The urine becomes yellow-brown or greenish, and a yellow foam appears when the urine is shaken.

Urobilinogen

Normally, bilirubin is excreted by the liver into the intestinal tract. Bacteria present in the intestines convert it to urobilinogen. Approximately 50% of the urobilinogen is reabsorbed into the body for reexcretion by the liver. Small amounts may appear in the urine, but most of the urobilinogen is excreted in the feces. An increase in the production of bilirubin increases the amount of urobilinogen excreted in the urine. Conditions such as excessive hemolysis of red blood cells, infectious hepatitis, cirrhosis, congestive heart failure, and infectious mononucleosis may increase the level of urobilinogen in the urine.

Blood

Blood is considered an abnormal constituent of urine, unless it is present as a contaminant during menstruation. The condition in which blood is found in the urine is termed *hematuria.* Hematuria may be the result of injury or disorders such as cystitis, tumors of the bladder, urethritis, kidney stones, and certain kidney disorders.

Nitrite

Nitrite in the urine indicates the presence of a pathogen in the (normally sterile) urinary tract, which results in a UTI. The pathogen possesses the ability to convert nitrate, which normally occurs in the urine, to nitrite, which is normally absent. The nitrite test must be performed with urine that has been in the bladder for at least 4 to 6 hours to ensure that bacteria have converted nitrate to nitrite. Therefore, use of a first-voided morning specimen is recommended. The test should *not* be performed on specimens that have been left standing out because a false-positive result may occur from bacterial contamination from the environment. The nitrite test is a screening test and is usually followed by a quantitative culture and identification of the invading pathogen.

Leukocytes

The presence of leukocytes in the urine is known as *leukocyturia* and accompanies inflammation of the kidneys and the lower urinary tract. Examples of specific conditions include acute and chronic pyelonephritis, cystitis, and urethritis. Reagent strips are available that contain a reagent area that permits the chemical detection of intact and lysed leukocytes in the urine. The advantage of detecting lysed leukocytes is that these cells cannot be observed during a microscopic examination of urine sediment and would otherwise remain undetected. The recommended urine specimen, particularly for women, is a clean-catch midstream collection to prevent contamination of the specimen with leukocytes from vaginal secretions leading to false-positive test results.

REAGENT STRIPS

In the medical office, reagent strips are the most commonly used diagnostic urine testing kit. Reagent strips consist of disposable plastic strips on which separate reagent areas are affixed for testing specific chemical constituents that may be present in the urine during pathologic conditions. The results provide the physician with information to assist in diagnosis of the following:

- Conditions affecting kidney function (e.g., kidney stones)
- Urinary tract infections
- Conditions affecting carbohydrate metabolism (e.g., diabetes mellitus)
- Conditions affecting liver function (e.g., hepatitis)

Test results also provide the physician with information related to the status of the patient's acid-base balance and urine concentration. Reagent strips are considered qualitative tests, and a positive result usually necessitates further testing. The number and type of reagent areas included on the reagent strip depend on the particular brand of reagent strips. Multistix 10 SG (Bayer Corporation, Tarrytown, NY) contains 10 reagent areas for testing pH, protein, glucose, ketone, bilirubin, blood, urobilinogen, nitrite, specific gravity, and leukocytes. The reagent strip urine testing procedure presented in this chapter (Procedure 30-2) is specifically for Multistix 10 SG; however, this procedure can be followed for the chemical testing of urine with most reagent strips. In all instances, the medical assistant should read the manufacturer's instructions before performing the test.

Guidelines for Reagent Strip Urine Testing

Testing urine with reagent strips is a relatively easy procedure to perform. Specific guidelines must be followed, however, to obtain accurate test results.

1. *Type of specimen.* The best results are obtained with a freshly voided and thoroughly mixed urine specimen. If the medical assistant is unable to test the specimen within 1 hour of voiding, the specimen should be refrigerated immediately and then allowed to return to room temperature before testing.
2. *Type of collection.* Most reagent strips are designed to be used with a random specimen collection; however, clean-catch midstream and first-voided morning specimens are suggested for specific tests. The nitrite test results are optimized with a first-voided morning specimen, whereas a clean-catch midstream collection is recommended for the leukocyte test.
3. *Specimen container.* The specimen container used must be thoroughly clean and free from any detergent or disinfectant residue because cleansing agents contain

oxidants that react with the chemicals on the reagent strip, leading to inaccurate test results. The container should be large enough to allow for complete immersion of all reagent strip areas.
4. *Time intervals.* Read the test results at the exact time intervals specified on the color chart. Do not read any test results after 2 minutes.
5. *Interpretation of results.* Of particular importance is the comparison of the reagent strip with the color chart. The reagent strip must be compared with the color chart in good lighting to obtain a good visual match of the color reactions with the color chart provided with the test kit.
6. *Storage of reagent strips.* The reagents on the strips are sensitive to light, heat, and moisture, and the bottle containing the strips must be stored in a cool, dry area away from direct sunlight, with the cap tightly closed to maintain reactivity of the reagent. The bottle may contain a desiccant that should not be removed because its purpose is to promote dryness by absorbing moisture. The bottle of reagent strips must be stored at a temperature between 59° F (15° C) and 86° F (30° C). The strips should not be stored in the refrigerator or freezer. A tan-to-brown discoloration or darkening on the reagent areas indicates deterioration of the chemical reagent strips, in which case the strips should not be used because the test results would be inaccurate.

Quality Control Testing

Quality control testing should be used in a chemical examination of urine with a reagent strip. Quality control testing ensures the reliability of test results by (1) determining whether the reagent strips are reacting properly, and (2) confirming that the test is being properly performed and accurately interpreted.

To check the reliability of Multistix reagent strips, the Chek-Stix control (Bayer Corporation) should be used. Each Chek-Stix control consists of a firm plastic strip to which are affixed synthetic ingredients (Figure 30-4). The

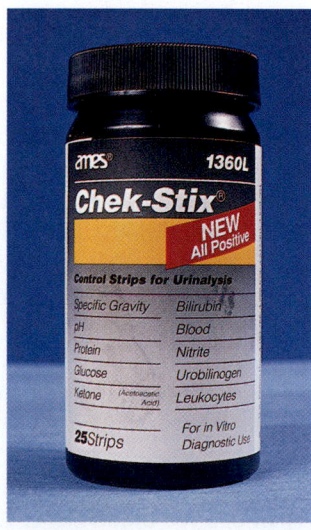

Figure 30-4 Chek-Stix control strips.

control strip is reconstituted by immersing it in distilled water for 30 minutes, which allows the ingredients on the strip to dissolve in the water. After reconstitution, the resulting solution is tested in the same manner as a urine specimen. The values to be expected are outlined in the product insert that accompanies the control strips. The results of the control test should be recorded in a quality control log. If the expected values are not obtained, the cause of the problem must be determined and corrected. Factors that can cause a problem include outdated reagent strips, improper storage of the strips, and an error in testing technique. The quality control test should be performed when each bottle of strips is opened for the first time or when a question of reliability arises regarding the testing strips.

Urine Analyzer

Urine analyzers are used to perform an automatic chemical examination of urine with reagent strips. They offer the advantage of the ability to perform the chemical analysis quickly and to interpret results automatically. These analyzers are used most often in medical offices that perform moderate-volume to large-volume urine testing.

The Clinitek Analyzer (Bayer Corporation) is an example of a urine analyzer that automatically reads Multistix SG and other (Bayer) urinalysis reagent strips (Figure 30-5, *A*). The results are printed out, and abnormal results are flagged to call attention to them (Figure 30-5, *B*). Different models are available; some can be used to perform a color and appearance analysis and a microscopic examination of the urine.

A

```
ID:  Erika Seager
     11-16-XX     5:37 PM

CLARITY:  Clear
COLOR: YELLOW

MULTISTIX 10 SG

GLU    NEGATIVE
BIL    NEGATIVE
KET    NEGATIVE
SG     1.025
BLO*   TRACE-LYSED
pH     5.5
PRO    NEGATIVE
URO    0.2 E.U./dL
NIT    NEGATIVE
LEU    NEGATIVE
```

B

Figure 30-5 A, Clinitek Urine Analyzer. **B,** Clinitek printout.

PROCEDURE 30-2

PROCEDURE 30-2 Chemical Testing of Urine With the Multistix 10 SG Reagent Strip

Outcome Perform a chemical assessment of a urine specimen

Equipment/Supplies

- Disposable gloves
- Multistix 10 SG reagent strips
- Urine container
- Timer
- Laboratory report form

1. **Procedural Step.** Perform the quality control testing procedure if using a new bottle of testing strips.
   Principle. Performing the quality control procedure ensures the reliability of test results.
2. **Procedural Step.** Obtain a freshly voided urine specimen from the patient with a clean container. The specimen should be uncentrifuged and at room temperature.
   Principle. The best results are obtained with a freshly voided specimen. The container should be clean because contaminants could affect the results. Uncentrifuged specimens ensure a homogeneous sample.
3. **Procedural Step.** Sanitize your hands.

4. **Procedural Step.** Assemble the equipment. Check the expiration date of the reagent strips.
   Principle. Outdated reagent strips may lead to inaccurate test results.
5. **Procedural Step.** Apply gloves. Remove a reagent strip from its plastic container, and recap the container immediately. Do not touch the test areas with your fingers or lay the strip on the table. It is permissible, however, to lay the reagent strip on a clean, dry paper towel.
   Principle. Recapping the container is necessary to prevent exposing the strips to environmental moisture, light, and heat, which cause altered reagent reactivity. Contamination of test areas by the hands or table surface may affect the accuracy of test results.

Continued

PROCEDURE 30-2   Chemical Testing of Urine With the Multistix 10 SG Reagent Strip—cont'd

6. Procedural Step. Thoroughly mix the urine specimen and remove the lid from the container. Using the dominant hand, completely immerse the reagent strip in the urine specimen, and remove it immediately. While removing, run the edge of the strip against the rim of the urine container to remove excess urine.

Principle. The strip should be completely immersed to ensure that all test areas are moistened for accurate test results. Prolonged immersion of the reagent strip and failure to remove excess urine may cause the reagents to dissolve and leach onto adjacent test areas, affecting the accuracy of the test results.

Completely immerse the reagent strip in the urine.

Run the edge of the strip against the urine container.

7. Procedural Step. With the nondominant hand, start the timer, pick up the reagent strip container, and rotate it to the color chart. Hold the reagent strip in a horizontal position and place it as close as possible to the corresponding color blocks on the color chart. Do not lay the strip directly on the color chart because this will result in soiling of the chart by the urine. Read the results carefully and at the exact reading times, starting with the shortest time specified on the color chart and as indicated here:

Glucose: 30 seconds	pH: 60 seconds
Bilirubin: 30 seconds	Protein: 60 seconds
Ketone: 40 seconds	Urobilinogen: 60 seconds
Specific gravity: 45 seconds	Nitrite: 60 seconds
Blood: 60 seconds	Leukocytes, 2 minutes

Principle. Holding the strip in a horizontal position avoids soiling your gloves with urine and prevents reagents from running over into adjacent testing areas, causing inaccurate test results. The strip must be read at the proper time interval to avoid dissolving out reagents, leading to inaccurate test results.

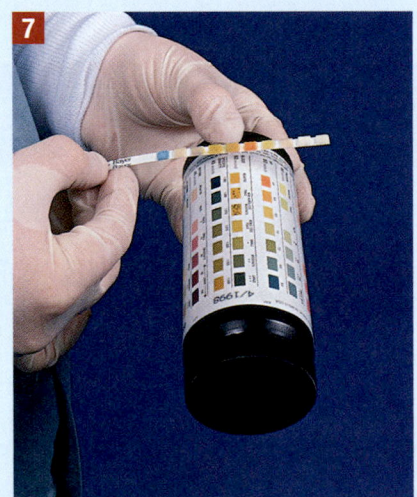

Hold the strip horizontally and read the results.

8. Procedural Step. Dispose of the strip in a regular waste container.

9. Procedural Step. Remove gloves, and sanitize your hands.

10. Procedural Step. Chart the results in the patient's medical record. The results should be charted by following the interpretation guide provided above each color block on the color chart.

a. *Paper-based patient record:* Most offices use a preprinted reporting form to make it easier to

PROCEDURE 30-2 Chemical Testing of Urine With the Multistix 10 SG Reagent Strip—cont'd

record results. The recording should include the date and time, the brand name of the test used (Multistix 10 SG), and the results (refer to the PPR charting example).

b. *Electronic medical record:* Document the brand name of the test used (Multistix 10 SG) and the results using the appropriate radio buttons, drop-down menus, and free text fields.

(Multistix Color Chart modified and printed by permission of Siemens Medical Solutions Diagnostics, Tarrytown, NY.)

MICROSCOPIC EXAMINATION OF URINE

Urine sediment is the solid material contained in the urine. A microscopic examination of the urine sediment performed by the physician helps clarify results of the physical and chemical examinations. A first-voided morning specimen is typically preferred because it is more concentrated and contains more dissolved substances; small amounts of abnormal substances are more likely to be detected. Use of a fresh specimen is important because changes occur in a specimen left standing out, as was previously discussed. These changes affect the reliability of the test results. The medical assistant is responsible for preparing the urine specimen for microscopic examination by the physician, as presented in Procedure 30-3.

Red Blood Cells

Red blood cells appear as round, colorless, biconcave discs that are highly refractile (Table 30-1). The presence of 0 to 5 per high-power field (HPF) is considered normal. More than this number may indicate bleeding somewhere along the urinary tract. Table 30-1 lists the possible causes of an abnormal number of red blood cells in the urine. Concentrated urine causes the red blood cells to become shrunken or *crenated,* whereas dilute urine causes them to swell and become rounded, which may cause them to hemolyze. If the red blood cells have hemolyzed, they cannot be seen under the microscope. The presence of blood in the urine still can be identified, however, with a reagent strip, such as Multistix, which is designed to detect free hemoglobin.

White Blood Cells

White blood cells are round and granular and have a nucleus (see Table 30-1). They are approximately 1.5 times as large as red blood cells. The presence of 0 to 8 per HPF is considered normal. More than this amount may indicate inflammation of the genitourinary tract. Table 30-1 lists the possible causes of an abnormal number of white blood cells in the urine.

Epithelial Cells

Most structures that make up the urinary system are composed of several layers of epithelial cells. The outer layer is constantly sloughed off and replaced by the cells underneath it. *Squamous epithelial cells* are large, clear, flat cells with an irregular shape. They contain a small nucleus and come from the urethra, bladder, and vagina. Squamous epithelial cells are normally present in small amounts in the urine. *Renal epithelial cells* are round and contain a large nucleus. They come from the deeper layers of the urinary tract, and their presence in the urine is considered abnormal. Table 30-1 lists the types of epithelial cells and possible causes of the presence of abnormal amounts in the urine.

Casts

Casts are cylindric structures formed in the lumen of the tubules that make up the nephron. Materials in the tubules harden, are flushed out, and appear in the urine in the form of casts. Various types of casts may be present in the urine. In general, their presence indicates a diseased condition.

Casts are named according to what they contain. *Hyaline casts* are pale, colorless cylinders with rounded edges that vary in size (see Table 30-1). *Granular casts* are hyaline casts that contain granules and are described as "coarsely granular" or "finely granular," depending on the size of the granules. *Fatty casts* are hyaline casts that contain fat droplets. *Waxy casts* are light yellow and have serrated edges; their name is derived from the fact that they appear to be made of wax. *Cellular casts* contain organized structures and are named according to what they contain. Examples include red blood cell casts, which are hyaline casts containing red blood cells; white blood cell casts, which are hyaline casts containing white blood cells; epithelial casts, which are hyaline casts containing epithelial cells; and bacterial casts, which are hyaline casts containing bacteria.

Crystals

A variety of crystals may be found in the urine. The type and number vary with the pH of the urine. Abnormal crystals include leucine, tyrosine, cystine, and cholesterol. Crystals that commonly appear in acid urine include amorphous urates, uric acid, and calcium oxalate (see Table 30-1). Crystals that commonly appear in alkaline urine include amorphous phosphate, triple phosphate, calcium phosphate, and ammonium urate crystals.

Miscellaneous Structures

Mucous threads are normally present in small amounts in the urine. They appear as long, wavy, threadlike structures with pointed ends.

Bacteria should not normally exist in the urinary tract. The presence of more than a few bacteria may indicate either contamination of the specimen during collection or a UTI. Bacteria are small structures that may be rod-shaped or round.

Yeast cells are smooth, refractile bodies with an oval shape. A distinguishing feature of yeast cells is small buds that project from the cells involved with reproduction. Yeast cells in the urine of female patients are usually a vaginal contaminant caused by the yeast *Candida albicans* and produce the

Memories *from* Practicum

Linda Proffitt: My main problem as a student on practicum was that I was a little shy. I learned that when your patient is relaxed, he or she is more likely to give you additional and important information about what is wrong. If your patient tenses up during a procedure, this can cause pain for the patient and make the procedure more difficult. When I started to make myself talk more to the patients and staff, things went more smoothly. ■

vaginal infection known as *candidiasis*. They also may be present in the urine of patients with diabetes mellitus.

Parasites may be present in the urine sediment as a contaminant from fecal or vaginal material. *Trichomonas vaginalis* is a parasite that causes trichomoniasis vaginitis.

Spermatozoa may be present in the urine of a man or woman after intercourse. The spermatozoa have round heads and long, slender, hairlike tails.

Table 30-1 lists the miscellaneous structures that may be present in the urine and the significance when found.

PATIENT TEACHING | **Urinary Tract Infections (UTIs)**

Answer questions that patients may have about UTIs.

What is a UTI?
Urinary tract infection (UTI) is a general term for the presence of bacteria in any portion of the urinary tract. UTIs, particularly those involving the bladder (cystitis) and urethra (urethritis), are common and treatable. A UTI is usually treated with an antibiotic. Use of all of the antibiotic for the full number of days prescribed by the physician is important, even if the symptoms disappear. If the medication is stopped too soon, the infection may recur and may be more difficult to treat than the original infection.

What are the symptoms of a UTI?
The symptoms of a simple UTI (cystitis) commonly include the frequent need to urinate, urgency (meaning the immediate need to urinate), a burning sensation during urination, and sometimes blood in the urine. Symptoms of a more complicated UTI involving the kidneys (pyelonephritis) include the aforementioned symptoms as well as lower abdominal discomfort, low back pain, fever, cloudy or foul-smelling urine, and blood in the urine.

Why do women have UTIs more frequently than men?
Women are more prone than men to the type of UTI called *cystitis* because the urethra of a woman is much shorter than that of a man, which makes travel up the urethra and into the bladder easier for bacteria. The most common source of infection is bacteria (*Escherichia coli*). E. coli organisms are normally found in the large intestine but can travel from the anal area to the urinary bladder, often as the result of poor hygienic practices. Cystitis occurs if E. coli organisms are able to overcome the body's natural defenses when the bacteria reach the urinary bladder and set up an infection.

What can women do to prevent a UTI?
Women prone to development of UTIs should practice the following prevention measures:
- Practice good hygienic measures by always cleaning the genital area from front to back after a bowel movement.
- Avoid possible irritants, such as bubble baths, perfumed soaps, feminine hygiene sprays, and the use of strong powders and bleaches for washing underclothes.
- Avoid clothing that traps moisture and encourages the growth of microorganisms, such as tight, constricting clothing; nylon panties; and pantyhose.
- Avoid activities that can contribute to irritation of the urinary meatus, such as prolonged bicycling, motorcycling, horseback riding, and travel that involves prolonged sitting.
- Urinate as soon as possible when you feel the urge. Holding urine in the bladder gives the bacteria more time to grow, which can cause a more severe infection. The more often you urinate, the more quickly the bacteria are removed from the bladder.
- Seek prompt treatment if you experience any of the symptoms of a UTI.

Encourage the patient with a UTI to drink plenty of water to help flush the bacteria out of the urinary tract.

Emphasize to the patient the importance of taking all of the antibiotic for the duration of time prescribed by the physician.

Emphasize the importance of practicing preventive measures to prevent the occurrence of UTIs.

Provide the patient with educational materials on UTIs. ∎

Table 30-1 Structures in Urine Sediment

Structure	Possible Causes	Microscopic Appearance
Red blood cells	Inflammatory diseases Acute glomerulonephritis Pyelonephritis Hypertension Renal infarction Trauma Stones Tumor Bleeding diseases Use of anticoagulants	 Red blood cells

Continued

Table 30-1 Structures in Urine Sediment—cont'd

Structure	Possible Causes	Microscopic Appearance
White blood cells	Pyelonephritis Cystitis Urethritis Prostatitis Transplant rejection (manifested by lymphocytes in urine) Tissue injury accompanied by severe inflammation (manifested by monocytes in urine) Inflammation, immune mechanisms, and other host defense mechanisms (manifested by histiocytes in urine)	 White blood cells
Squamous epithelial cells	Vaginal contamination	 Squamous epithelial cells
Renal tubular epithelial cells	Acute tubular necrosis Glomerulonephritis Acute infection Renal toxicity Viral infection	 Renal tubular epithelial cells
Hyaline casts	Normal urine Strenuous exercise Acute glomerulonephritis Acute pyelonephritis Malignant hypertension Chronic renal disease	 Hyaline cast*
Amorphous urate	Nonpathologic	 Amorphous urate crystals*
Uric acid	Usually nonpathologic; in large numbers, may indicate gout	 Uric acid crystals*

Table 30-1 Structures in Urine Sediment—cont'd

Structure	Possible Causes	Microscopic Appearance
Calcium oxalate	Usually nonpathologic; may be associated with stone formation	 Calcium oxalate crystals†
Bacteria	More than 100,000 bacteria per mL indicates urinary tract infection 10,000-100,000 bacteria per mL indicates that tests should be repeated Less than 10,000 bacteria per mL may signify urine in which any bacteria are urethral organisms or the result of contamination Bacteria accompanied by white blood cells or white blood cell or mixed casts may indicate acute pyelonephritis	 Bacteria (small rod structures)*
Yeast	May indicate contamination by yeasts from skin or hair May indicate diabetes mellitus or urinary tract infection *Candida albicans* may occur in patients with diabetes mellitus or in the contaminated urine of female patients with candidal vaginitis	 *C. albicans* (yeast)*
Parasites and parasitic ova	Usually indicate fecal or vaginal contamination and should be reported *Trichomonas* may be found in patients with urethritis and in contaminated urine of women with *Trichomonas* vaginitis Pinworm is a common contaminant and should be reported	 *Trichomonas* (parasite)*
Spermatozoa	Nonpathologic	 Spermatozoa*

PROCEDURE 30-3

Table 30-1 Structures in Urine Sediment—cont'd

Structure	Possible Causes	Microscopic Appearance
Urinary artifacts Hair (a) Pollen grains Bubbles Oil droplets Fibers (b) Powder (c) Dust Mucous threads (d) Glass particles	Nonpathologic May result from improper urine collection, improper slide preparation, or outside contamination	

(a) Hair†

(b) Fiber*

(c) Powder*

(d) Mucous threads‡

*Photomicrographs courtesy Bayer Corporation, Diagnostics Division, Elkhart, Ind.
†Photomicrograph from Lehman CA: *Saunders manual of clinical laboratory science,* Philadelphia, 1998, Saunders.
‡Photomicrograph from Stepp CA, Woods M: *Laboratory procedures for medical office personnel,* Philadelphia, 1998, Saunders.
Text courtesy Boehringer Mannheim Diagnostics, Indianapolis, Ind.

PROCEDURE 30-3   Prepare a Urine Specimen for Microscopic Examination: Kova Method

Outcome   Prepare a urine specimen for microscopic analysis by the physician

Equipment/Supplies

- Disposable gloves
- Urine specimen (first-voided morning specimen)
- Kova urine centrifuge tube
- Kova cap
- Kova pipet
- Kova slide
- Kova stain
- Test tube rack
- Urine centrifuge
- Mechanical stage microscope

PROCEDURE 30-3   Prepare a Urine Specimen for Microscopic Examination: Kova Method—cont'd

1. Procedural Step. Sanitize the hands, and assemble the equipment.

Assemble the equipment.

2. Procedural Step. Apply gloves. Mix the urine specimen with the Kova pipet.
Principle. The specimen must be well mixed to ensure accurate test results.

3. Procedural Step. Pour the urine specimen into the urine centrifuge tube. Fill it to the 12-mL graduation mark, and cap the tube.

Pour the specimen into the urine tube.

4. Procedural Step. Centrifuge the tube for 5 minutes at approximately 1500 revolutions per minute (rpm).
Principle. Centrifuging the specimen causes the solid elements in the urine to settle to the bottom of the tube.

Centrifuge the specimen.

5. Procedural Step. Remove the urine tube from the centrifuge; do not disturb or dislodge the sediment.

6. Procedural Step. Remove the cap. Insert the Kova pipet into the urine tube, and push it to the bottom of the tube until it seats firmly. Ensure that the clip on the bulb is hooked over the outside edge of the tube.

Insert the pipet until it seats firmly.

Continued

PROCEDURE 30-3

PROCEDURE 30-3   Prepare a Urine Specimen for Microscopic Examination: Kova Method—cont'd

7. Procedural Step. Decant the specimen by inverting the tube and pouring off the **supernatant** fluid. Approximately 1 mL of sediment is retained in the bottom of the tube.

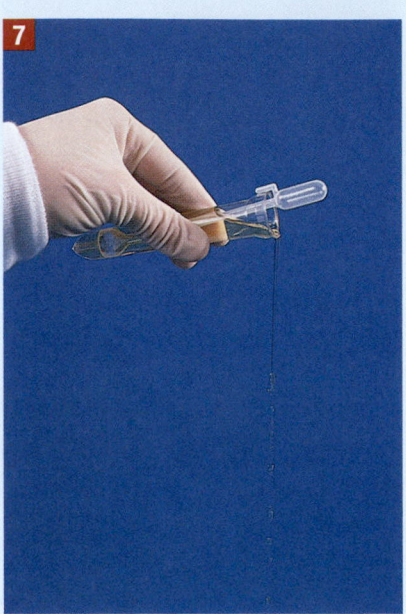

Pour the supernatant fluid.

8. Procedural Step. Remove the pipet from the tube. Add 1 drop of Kova stain to the tube. Place the pipet back in the tube, and mix the sediment and stain together vigorously with the pipet. Ensure that the sediment and the stain are well mixed. Place the urine tube in a test tube rack.
Principle. Kova stain improves the detail of the sediment for better visualization of structures under the microscope.

Mix the sediment and stain.

9. Procedural Step. Transfer a sample of the sediment to the Kova slide as follows:
a. Place the Kova slide on a flat surface with the open "envelope" areas facing upward.
b. Squeeze the bulb of the pipet to draw a sample of the sediment into the tip of the pipet.
c. Place the tip of the pipet so that it just touches the notched corner edge of the slide.
d. Gently squeeze the bulb to allow the specimen to fill the well. Do not overfill or underfill the well.
e. Place the pipet in the urine tube.

Fill the well with the specimen.

10. Procedural Step. Allow the specimen to sit for 1 minute to permit the sediment to settle in the well. *Principle.* Allowing the sediment to settle prevents structures from moving when the slide is viewed under the microscope.

11. Procedural Step. Place the slide on the stage of the microscope. Focus the specimen for the physician under the microscope by following the procedure presented in Procedure 34-1: Using the Microscope.

Focus the specimen for the physician.

PROCEDURE 30-3 Prepare a Urine Specimen for Microscopic Examination: Kova Method—cont'd

12. **Procedural Step.** When the physician is finished examining the urine sediment, remove the slide from the stage.
13. **Procedural Step.** Dispose of the plastic slide and pipet in a regular waste container. Rinse the remaining urine down the sink. Cap the empty plastic urine tube, and dispose of it in a regular waste container.
14. **Procedural Step.** Remove gloves, and sanitize your hands.

LAB REPORT

Date	Time	Name
3/18/XX	10:00 a.m.	Tanya Howe

MICROSCOPIC

WBCs	20 /HPF
RBCs	3 /HPF
CASTS (Hyaline)	0 /LPF
CASTS (Granular)	0 /LPF
CASTS (Cellular)	0 /LPF
CASTS (Waxy)	0 /LPF
EPITHELIAL CELLS	0 /LPF
BACTERIA	Freq
MUCUS	Occ
CRYSTALS	0 WBCs

_____ T. Bach, MD

URINE PREGNANCY TESTING

The diagnosis of pregnancy can be accomplished several ways. By the eighth week after fertilization, pregnancy can be confirmed with the medical history and physical examination. The physician may desire an earlier diagnosis, however, with a pregnancy test to initiate early prenatal care. A pregnancy test also may be necessary before certain medications are ordered or procedures are performed that may cause injury to a fetus.

In the medical office, immunologic tests are often used for pregnancy testing. These tests are performed on a concentrated urine specimen and rely on the presence of a hormone known as *human chorionic gonadotropin* (HCG) for a positive reaction.

HUMAN CHORIONIC GONADOTROPIN

HCG is produced by the developing fertilized egg, and small amounts of it are secreted into the urine and blood. Immediately after conception and implantation of the fertilized egg, the plasma level of HCG increases rapidly and can be used to detect pregnancy with a serum pregnancy test as early as 6 days before the first missed menstrual period. The highest plasma levels of HCG occur at about 8 weeks after conception. After this time, the production of HCG declines and remains at a lower level for the duration of the pregnancy. Within 72 hours of delivery, HCG disappears entirely from the plasma. As a result, pregnancy tests are more sensitive during the first trimester and may show a negative reaction when the level of HCG begins to decline during the second and third trimesters.

IMMUNOASSAYS

Immunoassays are used in the medical office for the detection of pregnancy. These tests are convenient to perform and provide immediate test results. Positive and negative reactions are evidenced by a specific visible reaction that is observed and interpreted by the individual performing the test.

Immunoassays are commercially available in testing kits that contain the required reagents and supplies to perform the test. Each kit can be used to perform a specific number of tests, ranging from 25 to 50. The instructions in the product insert accompanying the testing kit should be followed exactly to prevent inaccurate test results. When performed correctly, most urine pregnancy tests are 99% accurate with low occurrences of false-positive test results.

Immunoassays provide for the rapid, qualitative detection of HCG in a urine specimen; brand names include QuickVue One-Step HCG Urine Test (Quidel, San Diego, Calif), OSOM HCG Urine Test (Genzyme Diagnostics, Cambridge, Mass), and ICON HCG Pregnancy Test (Beckman Coulter, Brea, CA). Early prediction pregnancy tests may be able to detect pregnancy as early as 2 to 3 days before a first missed menstrual period. Urine pregnancy tests performed this early, however, may show a false-negative result and should be repeated later to confirm the results. Accurate results are much more probable if the urine is tested 1 week after a missed period.

Immunoassays take approximately 5 minutes to perform, and the test results are easily observed as a color change. Specific instructions for interpreting the test results are included in the product insert. The procedure for performing an immunoassay with QuickVue HCG Urine Test (Quidel) is outlined in Procedure 30-4.

GUIDELINES FOR URINE PREGNANCY TESTING

Specific guidelines must be followed in a urine pregnancy test to ensure accurate test results:

1. Use clean, preferably disposable, urine containers to collect the specimen. Traces of detergent in the specimen container may cause inaccurate test results.

2. The preferred specimen for a urine pregnancy test is a first-voided morning specimen because it contains the highest concentration of HCG; however, a random urine specimen can also be used. If the urine specimen cannot be tested immediately after voiding, it should be preserved in the refrigerator. A patient who collects the specimen at home should be given instructions on preserving the specimen.

3. The specific gravity of the urine specimen should be determined before the test is performed. A specific gravity of less than 1.007 is considered too dilute for pregnancy testing because it may lead to a false-negative test result.

4. The urine specimen should be at room temperature before the procedure is performed.

5. The urine pregnancy testing kit should be stored according to the information in the product insert. Most testing kits are stored at a room temperature between 59° F (15° C) and 86° F (30° C) and away from direct sunlight.

6. Testing kits past their expiration dates should not be used.

7. If more than one patient is being tested at a time, label each testing device with the patient's name to prevent a mix-up of specimens.

8. Most urine pregnancy testing kits include a built-in internal control to evaluate whether certain aspects of the testing procedure are working properly. The internal control is performed at the same time that the testing procedure is performed. The urine pregnancy internal control determines whether a sufficient amount of the specimen was added to the testing cassette and if the correct procedural technique was followed. If the internal control does not perform as expected, the test result is invalid and the specimen must be retested. It is recommended that the internal control be documented in a quality control log for the first pregnancy test run each day.

9. It is recommended that a positive and a negative external control be performed with each new lot of shipment of urine pregnancy testing kits, and then monthly thereafter. External controls are used to determine if the testing reagents are performing properly and to detect any errors in technique of the individual performing the test. External controls consist of commercially available solutions and may be included with the test system or may need to be purchased separately. The control procedure is performed in a similar manner to the procedure for performing the test on a specimen collected from a patient. Instead of adding the patient specimen to the testing device, however, the control is added to it. The positive control should produce a positive result, and the negative control should produce a negative result. The results should be documented in a quality control log (Figure 30-6). Failure of an external control to produce expected results may be caused by the following: deterioration of testing components as a result of improper storage, improper environmental testing conditions, or errors in technique used to perform the procedure.

10. Conditions other than a normal pregnancy that can result in a positive result include ectopic pregnancy and molar pregnancy.

What Would You Do? What Would You *Not* Do?

Case Study 3

Rita Lavelle is 8½ months pregnant and is at the clinic for a prenatal appointment. Lately, she has been having difficulty obtaining a urine specimen at the medical office because of her enlarged abdomen. At her last appointment, the office provided her with a urine specimen container so that she could obtain her specimen more easily at home. Rita brings in a first-voided urine specimen in a glass jar. She says her dog chewed up the specimen container from the office, so she used an empty peanut butter jar. The urine testing results from her specimen show that her glucose level is normal, but her protein level is 4+. Until this time, her urine test results all have been normal. Rita is concerned about her baby. She says that she was cleaning her bathroom cabinet yesterday and came across a pregnancy test; just for the fun of it, she decided to run the test. The results were negative, and now she is worried that something is wrong. Rita says that she has not been sleeping as well at night and that she has noticed more Braxton-Hicks contractions, but the baby has been kicking and moving as usual. ■

SERUM PREGNANCY TEST

The radioimmunoassay (RIA) for HCG is a quantitative test used to detect HCG in the serum of the blood. This test can detect pregnancy earlier and with greater accuracy than a urine pregnancy test. A serum pregnancy test can usually detect pregnancy at approximately the eighth day after fertilization, which is 6 days before the first missed menstrual period. This test uses a radioisotope technique and is capable

QUALITY CONTROL LOG

URINE PREGNANCY TEST

	Date	Name of test	Control lot #	Control expiration date	External positive control	External negative control	Technician
1	3/25 20XX	Quick Vue One Step HCG	140400	3/16/XX	+	−	*L. Proffit CMA (AAMA)*
2	4/22 20XX	Quick Vue One Step HCG	140400	3/16/XX	+	−	*L. Proffit CMA (AAMA)*
3	5/27 20XX	Quick Vue One Step HCG	140400	3/16/XX	+	−	*L. Proffit CMA (AAMA)*
4							
5							
6							
7							
8							
9							
10							

Figure 30-6 Quality control log for urine pregnancy testing.

of detecting minute amounts of HCG in the blood. This test is usually used to diagnose abnormalities, such as ectopic pregnancy; to follow the course of early pregnancy when abnormalities of embryonic development are suspected; and to provide an early diagnosis of pregnancy in individuals at high risk, such as patients with diabetes.

PROCEDURE 30-4   Performing a Urine Pregnancy Test

Outcome Perform a urine pregnancy test

Equipment/Supplies

- Disposable gloves
- Urine pregnancy testing kit (QuickVue HCG Urine Test by Quidel)
- Urine specimen (first-voided morning specimen)

1. Procedural Step. Sanitize the hands, and assemble the equipment. Check the expiration date on the urine pregnancy testing kit. It should not be used if the expiration date has passed. When a new testing kit is opened (and thereafter on a monthly basis), external positive and negative controls should be performed according to the instructions in the product insert accompanying the controls. Document the control results in a quality control log. If the controls do not perform as expected, patient testing should not be conducted until the problem has been identified and resolved.

Principle. An expired pregnancy test may produce inaccurate test results. Running positive and negative external controls ensures that the test results are valid and reliable. Factors that can cause abnormal control results include outdated controls or testing reagents, improper storage of testing components, and an error in the technique used to perform the procedure.

Continued

PROCEDURE 30-4   Performing a Urine Pregnancy Test—cont'd

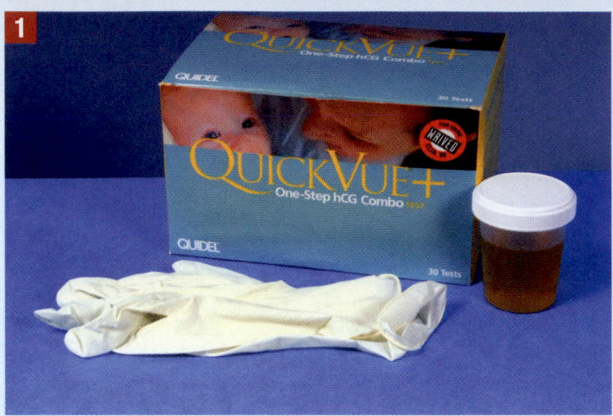

Assemble the equipment.

2. **Procedural Step.** Apply gloves. Rotate the urine specimen cup to mix the urine. Inspect the foil pouch containing the cassette. If it is torn or punctured, discard the test and obtain another one from the testing kit. Remove the test cassette from its foil pouch, and place it on a clean, dry, level surface. *Principle.* The foil pouch should not be opened until it is time to perform the test.

3. **Procedural Step.** Add 3 drops of urine to the round sample well on the test cassette with a disposable pipet supplied with the kit. The test cassette should not be handled or moved again until the test is ready for interpretation. Dispose of the pipet in a regular waste container.

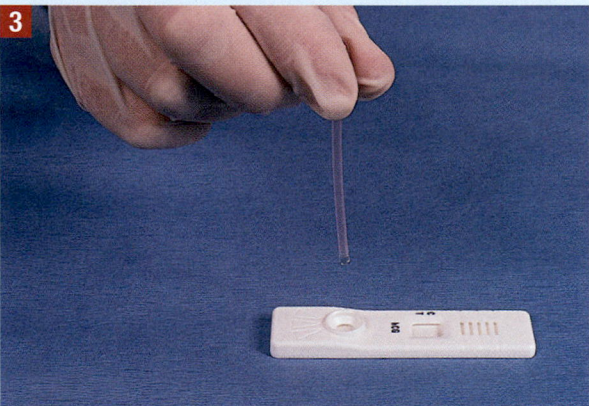

Add 3 drops of urine to the test well.

4. **Procedural Step.** Wait 3 minutes, and read the results by observing the test result window.
5. **Procedural Step.** Interpret the test results as follows:
Negative: The appearance of the blue procedural control line next to the letter *C* only and no pink to purple test line next to the letter *T* in the test

result window. In addition, the background of the test window should be clear and not interfere with the ability to read the test results. (*Note:* If the test result is negative and pregnancy is suspected, another specimen should be collected and tested 48 to 72 hours later.)
Positive: The appearance of any pink to purple line next to the letter *T* along with a blue procedural control line next to the letter *C* in the test result window. In addition, the background of the test window should be clear and should not interfere with the ability to read test results.
Invalid result: If no blue procedural control line appears within 3 minutes, or if the background of the test window interferes with reading the results, the test result is invalid, and the specimen must be retested with a new cassette.
Principle. The blue procedural control line is a positive internal quality control indicator designating that a sufficient urine sample was added to the cassette well and that the test is working properly. A background in the test window that is clear and does not interfere with reading the test results is a negative internal quality control indicator and also indicates that the test is working properly.

Negative   Positive
Interpret the results.

6. **Procedural Step.** Dispose of the test cassette in a regular waste container. Remove gloves, and sanitize your hands.
7. **Procedural Step.** Chart the results in the patient's medical record.
   a. *Paper-based patient record:* Record the date and time of the patient's last menstrual period (LMP), the name of the test, and the results recorded as either positive or negative (refer to the PPR charting example).

PROCEDURE 30-4 Performing a Urine Pregnancy Test—cont'd

PPR CHARTING EXAMPLE

Date	
3/25/XX	10:30 a.m. LMP: 2/20/XX.
	QuickVue preg test: Positive. _____
	_____ L. Proffitt, CMA (AAMA)

b. *Electronic medical record:* Document the patient's last menstrual period (LMP), the name of the test, and the results recorded as either positive or negative using the appropriate radio buttons, drop-down menus, and free text fields.

What Would You Do? What Would You *Not* Do? RESPONSES

Case Study 1
Page 788

What Did Linda Do?
❏ Took some time to try to calm and relax Mr. Urameshi. Reassured him that the physician would do everything he could to make Mr. Urameshi better.
❏ Offered Mr. Urameshi something to drink and told him it might help him obtain a specimen.
❏ Went over the directions again with Mr. Urameshi.
❏ Asked Mr. Urameshi if he would try again to obtain a specimen.

What Did Linda Not *Do?*
❏ Did not tell Mr. Urameshi that he was not trying hard enough.

Case Study 2
Page 793

What Did Linda Do?
❏ Asked Nora whether she takes all of the antibiotic she is prescribed when she has a UTI.
❏ Explained to Nora in terms she can understand why women seem to be more prone to development of UTIs.
❏ Explained to Nora what she could do to help prevent UTIs. Gave her a patient education brochure on UTIs to take home.
❏ Told Nora that the physician is not legally or ethically permitted to call in a prescription for her without seeing her. Also explained that it is in the best interests of her health care to be seen by the physician.

What Did Linda Not *Do?*
❏ Did not tell Nora that she could not test her urine at home.

Case Study 3
Page 808

What Did Linda Do?
❏ Told Rita that some peanut butter residue might have been left in the jar she used and might have affected the test results. Asked her to try to collect another specimen at the office so that the urine could be tested again.
❏ Told Rita that if something happens to the specimen container again, she should come to the office and get another one.
❏ Told Rita that several things could have caused her pregnancy test result to be negative. Explained to her that the test could have been outdated or not stored properly. Also explained that as a pregnancy gets farther along, less of the hormone that causes the test to be positive is secreted, so negative test results at the end of a pregnancy are not unusual.
❏ Reassured Rita that many women have trouble sleeping during the last month of pregnancy and that it is normal to have more Braxton-Hicks contractions as she gets closer to delivery.
❏ Told Rita that Linda would inform the physician of her symptoms so that he could discuss them in more detail with her.

What Did Linda Not *Do?*
❏ Did not criticize Rita for collecting her specimen in a peanut butter jar.
❏ Did not ignore or minimize Rita's concerns.

PROCEDURE 30-4

↻ TERMINOLOGY REVIEW

Key Term	Word Parts	Definition
Anuria	*an-:* without, absence of *ur/o:* urine *-ia:* condition of disease or abnormal state	Failure of the kidneys to produce urine.
Bilirubinuria	*bilirubino/o:* bilirubin *ur/o-:* urine *-ia:* condition of disease or abnormal state	The presence of bilirubin in the urine.
Bladder catheterization		The passing of a sterile catheter through the urethra and into the bladder to remove urine.
Diuresis		Secretion and passage of large amounts of urine.
Dysuria	*dys-:* difficult, labored, painful *ur/o:* urine *-ia:* condition of disease or abnormal state	Difficult or painful urination.
Frequency		The condition of having to urinate often.
Glycosuria	*glyc/o:* sugar *ur/o:* urine *-ia:* condition of disease or abnormal state	The presence of glucose in the urine.
Hematuria	*hemato/o:* blood *ur/o:* urine *-ia:* condition of disease or abnormal state	Blood present in the urine.
Ketonuria	*keton/o:* ketone *ur/o:* urine *-ia:* condition of disease or abnormal state	The presence of ketone bodies in the urine.
Ketosis	*keton/o:* ketone *-osis:* abnormal condition	An accumulation of large amounts of ketone bodies in the tissues and body fluids.
Micturition		The act of voiding urine.
Nephron		The functional unit of the kidney.
Nocturia	*noct/i:* night *ur/o:* urine *-ia:* condition of disease or abnormal state	Excessive (voluntary) urination during the night.
Nocturnal enuresis		Inability of an individual to control urination at night during sleep (bedwetting).
Oliguria	*olig/o:* scanty, few *ur/o:* urine *-ia:* condition of disease or abnormal state	Decreased or scanty output of urine.
pH		The unit that describes the acidity or alkalinity of a solution.
Polyuria	*poly-:* many *ur/o:* urine *-ia:* condition of disease or abnormal state	Increased output of urine.
Proteinuria	*protein-:* protein *ur/o:* urine *-ia:* condition of disease or abnormal state	The presence of protein in the urine.
Pyuria	*py/o:* pus *ur/o:* urine *-ia:* condition of disease or abnormal state	The presence of pus in the urine.
Renal threshold		The concentration at which a substance in the blood that is not normally excreted by the kidneys begins to appear in the urine.
Retention		The inability to empty the bladder. The urine is being produced normally but is not being voided.
Specific gravity		The weight of a substance compared with the weight of an equal volume of a substance known as the standard. In urinalysis, the *specific gravity* refers to the measurement of the amount of dissolved substances present in the urine compared with the same amount of distilled water.

TERMINOLOGY REVIEW—cont'd

Key Term	Word Parts	Definition
Supernatant	*super:* over, above	The clear liquid that remains at the top after a precipitate has settled.
Suprapubic aspiration	*supra-:* above *pub/o:* pubis *-ic:* pertaining to	The passing of a sterile needle through the abdominal wall into the bladder to remove urine.
Urgency		The immediate need to urinate.
Urinalysis	*urin/o:* urine	The physical, chemical, and microscopic analyses of urine.
Urinary incontinence		The inability to retain urine.
Void		To empty the bladder.

ON THE WEB

For information on kidney disease:

National Kidney Foundation: www.kidney.org

National Institute of Diabetes and Digestive and Kidney Diseases: www2.niddk.nih.gov

For information on drug abuse:

National Institute on Drug Abuse: www.drugabuse.gov

American Council for Drug Education: www.acde.org

Research Institute on Addictions: www.ria.buffalo.edu

Alcohol and Drug Abuse: www.alcoholanddrugabuse.com

DARE: www.dare.com

Coalition Against Drug Abuse: drugabuse.com

31 Phlebotomy

Check out the Evolve site at http://evolve.elsevier.com/Bonewit/today/ to access additional interactive activities and exercises to help you study and prepare for success.

LEARNING OBJECTIVES

Venipuncture

1. List and describe the general guidelines that should be followed when performing a venipuncture.
2. Explain how each of the following blood specimens is obtained:
   - Clotted blood
   - Serum
   - Whole blood
   - Plasma
3. List the layers into which the blood separates when an anticoagulant is added to the specimen.
4. List the layers into which the blood separates when an anticoagulant is not added to the specimen.
5. List the OSHA safety precautions that must be followed during venipuncture and when separating serum or plasma from whole blood.
6. State the additive content of each of the following vacuum tubes, and list the types of blood specimens that can be obtained from each: red, lavender, gray, light blue, green, royal blue.
7. Identify and explain the order of draw for the vacuum tube and butterfly methods of venipuncture.
8. List and describe the guidelines for use of evacuated tubes.
9. Identify possible problems during a venipuncture.
10. List four ways to prevent a blood specimen from becoming hemolyzed.
11. Explain how the serum separator tube functions in the collection of a serum specimen.

Skin Puncture

12. Explain when a skin puncture would be preferred over a venipuncture.
13. Describe each of the following skin puncture devices: disposable semiautomatic lancet and reusable semiautomatic lancet.
14. List and describe the guidelines for performing a finger puncture.

PROCEDURES

Perform a venipuncture using the vacuum tube method.
Perform a venipuncture using the butterfly method.

Obtain a capillary blood specimen using a disposable semiautomatic lancet.
Obtain a capillary blood specimen using a reusable semiautomatic lancet.

CHAPTER OUTLINE

INTRODUCTION TO PHLEBOTOMY
VENIPUNCTURE
General Guidelines for Venipuncture
Patient Preparation for Venipuncture
Review Collection and Handling Requirements
Identification of the Patient
Assemble the Equipment and Supplies
Reassuring the Patient
Patient Position for Venipuncture

Application of the Tourniquet
Guidelines for Applying the Tourniquet
Types of Tourniquets
Site Selection for Venipuncture
Guidelines for Site Selection
Alternative Venipuncture Sites
Types of Blood Specimens
OSHA Safety Precautions
VACUUM TUBE METHOD OF VENIPUNCTURE

Needle
Safety-Engineered Venipuncture Devices
Plastic Holder
Evacuated Tubes
Additive Content of Evacuated Tubes
Order of Draw for Multiple Tubes
Evacuated Tube Guidelines
BUTTERFLY METHOD OF VENIPUNCTURE
Guidelines for the Butterfly Method
PROBLEMS ENCOUNTERED WITH VENIPUNCTURE
Failure to Obtain Blood
Inappropriate Puncture Sites
Scarred and Sclerosed Veins
Rolling Veins
Collapsing Veins
Premature Needle Withdrawal
Hematoma

Hemolysis
Fainting
OBTAINING A SERUM SPECIMEN
Serum
Tube Selection
Preparation of the Specimen
Removal of Serum
Serum Separator Tubes
SKIN PUNCTURE
PUNCTURE SITES
SKIN PUNCTURE DEVICES
Disposable Semiautomatic Lancet
Reusable Semiautomatic Lancet
MICROCOLLECTION DEVICES
Capillary Tubes
Microcollection Tubes
GUIDELINES FOR PERFORMING A FINGER PUNCTURE

KEY TERMS

antecubital space (an-tih-KYOO-bih-tul SPAYS)
anticoagulant (an-tih-koe-AG-yoo-lent)
buffy coat
evacuated tube
hematoma (hee-mah-TOE-mah)

hemoconcentration (hee-moe-kon-sen-TRAY-shun)
hemolysis (hee-MOL-ih-sis)
osteochondritis (OS-tee-oh-kon-DRY-tis)
osteomyelitis (OS-tee-oh-mie-LIE-tis)
phlebotomist (fleh-BOT-oe-mist)

phlebotomy (fleh-BOT-oe-mee)
plasma
serum
venipuncture (VEN-ih-punk-chur)
venous reflux (VEEN-us-REE-fluks)
venous stasis (VEEN-us-STAE-sis)

INTRODUCTION TO PHLEBOTOMY

The purpose of phlebotomy is to collect a blood specimen for laboratory analysis. The word *phlebotomy* is derived from the Greek words for "vein" (*phlebos*) and "incision" (*otomy*) and literally means "making an incision into a vein." As used in the clinical laboratory sciences, **phlebotomy** is defined in general as the collection of blood. An individual who collects a blood sample is a **phlebotomist**.

Some blood specimens are tested in the medical office, and others are picked up and taken to an outside laboratory for testing. The latter specimens need to be placed in a biohazard specimen bag along with a laboratory request (Figure 31-1) so that laboratory personnel know what type of test the physician desires. The medical assistant may be responsible for completing the laboratory request form either on the computer or manually. The request form includes the physician's name and address; the patient's name, address, age, and gender; the date and time of collection of the specimen; the International Classification of Diseases (ICD) code of the clinical diagnosis; and a mark next to the type of test or tests to be performed.

Phlebotomy encompasses three major areas of blood collection:

- Arterial puncture
- Venipuncture
- Skin puncture

An arterial puncture is typically performed in a hospital to assess the oxygen level, carbon dioxide level, and acid-base balance of arterial blood; medical assistants do not perform arterial punctures. In the medical office, medical assistants perform venipunctures and skin punctures. This chapter focuses on these two ways to obtain blood.

VENIPUNCTURE

Venipuncture means the puncturing of a vein for the removal of a venous blood sample. In the medical office, a venipuncture is performed when a large blood specimen is needed for testing. Venipuncture is usually performed in the medical office using the following methods:

- Vacuum tube method
- Butterfly method

The vacuum tube method is the fastest and most convenient method and is used most often. This method relies on the use of an **evacuated tube**, which is a closed glass or plastic tube that contains a vacuum. The butterfly method is used for difficult draws, such as when a vein is small or

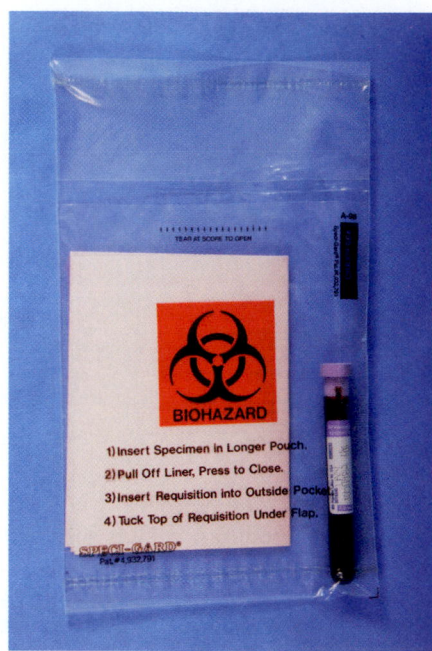

Figure 31-1 Specimen in a biohazard specimen bag along with the laboratory request form.

sclerosed (hardened). This chapter presents the theory and procedure for both of these methods.

GENERAL GUIDELINES FOR VENIPUNCTURE

General guidelines that are common to both methods of venipuncture include verifying any advance preparation, reviewing specimen collection and handling requirements, identifying the patient, reassuring the patient, assembling equipment and supplies, positioning the patient, applying the tourniquet, selecting a site for the venipuncture, obtaining the type of blood specimen required, and following the Occupational Safety and Health Administration (OSHA) Bloodborne Pathogens Standard.

PATIENT PREPARATION FOR VENIPUNCTURE

The patient should be given instructions an appropriate number of days before the specimen collection on any advance preparation that is required. Although most tests require no preparation, some tests require fasting or the avoidance of certain medications. *Fasting* involves abstaining from food or fluids (except water) for a specified amount of time before the collection of a specimen. If the medical assistant is unsure whether a laboratory test requires advance patient preparation, an appropriate reference source should be consulted. If the specimen is being tested at an outside laboratory, references consist of a laboratory directory and the laboratory's technical support staff. If the specimen is being tested at the medical office, references include the manufacturer's operating manual and/or product inserts included with blood analyzers and testing kits.

When a laboratory test requires advance preparation, before performing the venipuncture verify that the patient has prepared properly. If the patient has not properly prepared, do not collect the specimen unless directed otherwise by the physician. If the venipuncture is to be rescheduled, carefully review the preparation requirements with the patient.

REVIEW COLLECTION AND HANDLING REQUIREMENTS

The medical assistant must review the requirements for collecting and handling the blood specimen. These include the collection supplies necessary, the type of specimen to be collected (e.g., **serum**, **plasma**, whole blood, clotted blood), the amount necessary for laboratory analysis, the techniques to follow to collect the specimen, and the proper handling and storage of the specimen. The medical assistant must refer to the appropriate reference source to determine the collection and handling requirements for each test ordered by the physician. If the specimen is transported to an outside laboratory, this information is indicated in the laboratory directory. Figure 31-2 shows an example of the collection and handling requirements for a complete blood count (CBC) as it is presented in a laboratory directory. The collection and handling requirements necessary for specimens tested in the medical office are listed in the manufacturer's instructions that accompany the test system.

IDENTIFICATION OF THE PATIENT

It cannot be emphasized enough how important it is to identify the patient using two forms of identification (e.g., name and date of birth) before performing a venipuncture. Proper patient identification is essential to avoid collecting a specimen from the wrong patient by mistake. After greeting the patient, the medical assistant should ask the patient to state his or her full name and date of birth. This information should be compared with the demographic data indicated in the patient's medical record. The patient should *not* be asked whether he or she is a certain patient. For example, the patient should not be asked, "Are you Brad Thompson?" The patient may not hear the medical assistant correctly or may not be paying attention and may answer in the affirmative even if he is not that patient. Instead, ask the patient for his or her name and date of birth. If the patient is not properly identified, this in turn could lead to incorrect labeling of the specimen. A specimen that is not identified correctly could lead to an inaccurate patient diagnosis and the wrong treatment.

ASSEMBLE THE EQUIPMENT AND SUPPLIES

Use only the appropriate blood tubes as specified by the laboratory directory or manufacturer's instructions accompanying a test system. Substituting blood tubes may not

CBC (with differential and platelet count)

CPT Code: 85025

Tests included: WBC, RBC, hemoglobin, hematocrit, platelet count, differential, and red blood cell indices (MCV, MCH, MCHC, and RDW). If abnormal cells are observed on a manual differential or if the automated differential results meet specific flagging criteria, a full manual differential will be performed.

Type of specimen: Whole blood

Amount: 7 mL

Collection supplies: 7-mL lavender (EDTA) stoppered tube

Collection techniques: Red-stoppered and SST tubes should be collected before the lavender-stoppered tube. Completely fill tube to the exhaustion of the vacuum to ensure a proper blood to anticoagulant ratio. Gently invert tube 8-10 times immediately after drawing to mix the anticoagulant with the blood.

Patient preparation: None

Handling and storage: Store at room temperature for up to 24 hours following collection. Store in refrigerator for up to 48 hours following collection.

Causes for rejection: Hemolyzed or clotted specimen, under-filled tube, improper labeling of tube. Specimen collected in any tube other than an EDTA (lavender-stoppered) tube or a specimen that is more than 48 hours old.

Reference range: Values given with report

Use:
The CBC is used as a screening test to assess the overall health of an individual and to detect a wide range of hematologic conditions such as anemia, leukemia, and inflammatory processes. The CBC is also used to assist in managing medication and chemotherapeutic decisions.

Limitations:
- A manual differential can identify cells that may be misidentified by an automated analyzer
- Red blood cell indices are not a substitute for the direct examination of a blood smear

Methodology: Automated cell counter and microscopy

Figure 31-2 Collection and handling requirements for a complete blood count (CBC) from a laboratory directory.

yield the proper type of specimen required or may affect the test results, as shown by the following examples. If serum is required and a tube containing an anticoagulant is used (instead of a tube without an anticoagulant), the blood separates into plasma and cells, rather than serum and cells, and the wrong type of blood specimen is obtained, which necessitates obtaining another specimen from the patient.

The medical assistant should check each blood tube before use to ensure that it is not broken, chipped, cracked, or otherwise damaged. Damaged blood tubes are unsuitable for specimen collection and should be discarded. Blood tubes have an expiration date (Figure 31-3). The medical

assistant should make sure to check the expiration date on the tube to avoid using an outdated blood tube.

The medical assistant must be sure to label each blood tube. An unlabeled specimen is a cause for rejection of the specimen by an outside laboratory. Two *unique identifiers* should be used to label the specimen. A unique identifier is information that clearly identifies a specific patient, such as the patient's name and date of birth. A specimen can be labeled by attaching a computerized bar code label to the specimen (Figure 31-4, *A*). The bar code label includes (at least) two unique patient identifiers. A specimen can also be labeled by handwriting the information on the label, which should include the patient's name and date of birth (two unique identifiers), the date and time of collection, the medical assistant's initials, and any other information required by the laboratory (Figure 31-4, *B*). The information should be printed legibly, and the medical assistant should be certain that the information is accurate to avoid a mix-up of specimens. The medical assistant must also complete a laboratory request form to accompany the blood specimen. (*Note:* The medical assistant should follow the medical office policy as to when the tubes should be labeled. Some offices prefer the tubes be labeled *before* the specimen is drawn; other offices want the tubes to be labeled right *after* the specimen has been obtained.)

REASSURING THE PATIENT

Venipuncture is often a frightening experience for the patient. For many patients, the anticipation of the procedure is worse than the actual drawing of the blood. The medical assistant should take time to explain the procedure to the patient in an unhurried and confident manner. This helps to alleviate the patient's fears, which relaxes the patient's veins. Relaxed veins make venipuncture easier to perform and result in less pain for the patient.

Figure 31-3 Blood tube showing expiration date.

Instruct the patient to remain still during the procedure. Explain to the patient that a small amount of pain is associated with a venipuncture, but it is brief. Never tell the patient that the venipuncture will not hurt. Just before inserting the needle, tell the patient that he or she will "feel a small stick." This prevents startling the patient, which could cause the patient to move. Movement causes pain for the patient, and it may damage the venipuncture site.

PATIENT POSITION FOR VENIPUNCTURE

The patient position for venipuncture is especially important to the successful collection of a blood specimen. Proper positioning allows easy access to the vein and is more comfortable for the patient. The patient position depends on the vein to be used. The most common site for venipuncture is the **antecubital space**, and the information presented next refers to this site.

The patient should be seated comfortably in a chair. The arm should be extended downward to form a straight line from the shoulder to the wrist with the palm facing up; the arm should not bend at the elbow. The arm should be well supported on the armrest by a rolled towel or by having the patient place the fist of the other hand under the elbow (Figure 31-5).

A venipuncture should never be performed with the patient sitting on a stool or standing. The patient may faint and injure himself or herself. If the patient appears nervous or has fainted in the past from a venipuncture, it is best to place the patient in a semireclining position (semi-Fowler position) on the examining table. A pillow or a cushion should be placed under the patient's arm to support the arm in a straight line from the shoulder to the wrist.

Although unusual, it is possible for blood to flow from the evacuated tube back into the patient's vein during the procedure. This condition is known as **venous reflux**. Venous reflux could cause the patient to have an adverse reaction to a tube additive, particularly if the additive in the tube is ethylenediaminetetraacetic acid (EDTA). Venous

Figure 31-4 **A,** Computerized bar code label. **B,** Hand-labeled blood tube.

Figure 31-5 Patient position for obtaining a blood specimen from the antecubital veins.

reflux can occur only if the contents of the evacuated tube are in contact with the tube stopper while the specimen is being drawn. Venous reflux is prevented by keeping the patient's arm in a downward position so that the evacuated tube remains below the venipuncture site and fills from the bottom up.

APPLICATION OF THE TOURNIQUET

An important step in the venipuncture procedure is the application of the tourniquet. The tourniquet makes the patient's veins stand out so that they are easier to palpate. The tourniquet acts as a "dam" that causes the venous blood to slow down and pool in the veins in front of the tourniquet. This pooling of blood makes the veins more prominent so that they are more visible and can be palpated.

When applying a tourniquet, it is important to obtain the correct tourniquet tension. The tourniquet should be applied with enough tension to slow the venous flow without affecting the arterial flow. A tourniquet that is too tight obstructs both venous blood flow and arterial flow, which may result in a specimen that produces inaccurate test results. A tourniquet that is too loose fails to cause the veins to stand out enough to be palpated. A correctly applied tourniquet should fit snugly and not pinch the patient's skin.

Guidelines for Applying the Tourniquet

The following guidelines help to ensure successful application of the tourniquet:

1. Do not apply the tourniquet over sores or burned skin.
2. Place the tourniquet 3 to 4 inches above the bend in the elbow. This allows adequate room for cleansing the site and performing the venipuncture without the tourniquet getting in the way.
3. Apply the tourniquet so it is snug, but not so tight that it pinches the patient's skin or is otherwise painful to the patient.
4. When applying the tourniquet, ask the patient to clench his or her fist. This pushes blood from the lower arm

Putting It All Into Practice

My name is Dori Glover, and I work in a very busy, fast-paced family practice office for two physicians. I love my job. The physicians are great, with very different styles; the pace is fast; and the time flies by. I am constantly challenged, learning new things, meeting and helping people, and being a part of a team that works well together.

While performing a venipuncture for a routine blood chemistry profile (a procedure I have performed many times), I accidentally stuck myself after collecting the specimen. I could see the blood inside my glove, and I could see the patient's blood clinging to the point of the needle—my heart sank. I activated the safety shield and placed the needle and holder in the sharps container and tried to keep my cool and not alarm the patient. I mentally assessed the patient. He was an older man from a rural community, but I know you cannot always judge a book by its cover.

I excused myself and immediately proceeded to wash my hands thoroughly with soap and water and rinse, rinse, rinse! I then notified the physician. The physician questioned the patient regarding operations he had had in the previous year. He had undergone bypass surgery and had received 2 units of blood. Although blood is effectively screened, I thought about that one-in-a-zillion chance that it could have been contaminated. Thankfully, I had received the hepatitis B immunization series, but there was still concern regarding hepatitis C and, of course, HIV.

The patient was gracious and complied with our request to be tested for hepatitis and HIV. The physician and I discussed the situation, and we determined the risk to be low, but he nonetheless offered me the option of getting the HIV postexposure prophylactic treatment. This treatment is very toxic and is not something you want to receive needlessly. I declined and proceeded to wait in agony for the patient's test results. The word *relief* hardly describes how I felt when the patient's laboratory results came back negative!

This incident confirmed the importance of getting the hepatitis B immunization and paying attention to good technique when performing procedures involving blood. ∎

into the veins and makes them easier to palpate. You can ask the patient to clench and unclench the fist a few times; however, vigorous pumping should be avoided because it could lead to hemoconcentration, which could produce inaccurate test results.

5. Never leave the tourniquet on for longer than 1 minute because this would be uncomfortable for the patient. In addition, prolonged application of the tourniquet causes the venous blood to stagnate, or pool in one place too long—a condition known as **venous stasis**. When venous stasis occurs, the plasma portion of the blood filters into the tissues, causing hemoconcentration. **Hemoconcentration** is an increase in the concentration of nonfilterable blood components in the blood vessels, such as red blood cells, enzymes, iron, and calcium, as a result of a decrease in the fluid content of the blood. This

can result in inaccurate results for a variety of laboratory tests.

6. You should remove the tourniquet as soon as a good blood flow is established; however, this may not be practical when you are first learning the venipuncture procedure. Removing the tourniquet may cause the needle to move such that no more blood can be obtained, and the blood has to be redrawn. When you are learning the venipuncture procedure, it is better to wait until just before the needle is removed to remove the tourniquet.

7. *Always* remove the tourniquet before removing the needle from the patient's arm. If the needle is removed first, the pressure of the tourniquet causes blood to be forced out of the puncture site and into the surrounding tissue, resulting in a hematoma. A **hematoma** is defined as a swelling or mass of coagulated blood caused by a break in a blood vessel.

8. After use, wipe a tourniquet thoroughly with a disinfectant such as alcohol. Disposable tourniquets are available that are thrown away after one use.

Types of Tourniquets

The most common tourniquets are the *rubber* tourniquet and the *Velcro-closure* tourniquet. The type of tourniquet used is a matter of individual preference.

Rubber Tourniquet

The rubber tourniquet consists of a flat, soft band of rubber approximately 1 inch (2.5 cm) wide and 15 to 18 inches (38 to 45 cm) long. Rubber tourniquets are commercially available in latex or nonlatex rubber. They offer the advantage of being easily removable with one hand. The technique for applying a rubber tourniquet is described next and is illustrated in Figure 31-6.

Procedure: Rubber Tourniquet

1. Hold each end of the tourniquet with one hand. Position the tourniquet 3 to 4 inches (7.5 to 10 cm) above the bend in the elbow, making sure that the tourniquet lies flat against the patient's skin. Pull the ends away from each other to create tension (see Figure 31-6, *A*).

2. Bring the ends of the tourniquet toward each other and cross one over the other at the point of your grasp, with enough tension that the tourniquet is snug but is not pinching the patient's skin (see Figure 31-6, *B*).

3. Tuck a portion of the top length into the bottom length, forming a loop between the tourniquet and the patient's arm. This allows for a one-handed release of the tourniquet when pulled on one end. Make sure the flaps are directed upward so that they do not dangle into the working area (see Figure 31-6, *C*).

Velcro-Closure Tourniquet

The Velcro-closure tourniquet consists of a band of rubber or elastic material with Velcro attached at the ends. This type of tourniquet is easier to apply and is more comfortable for the patient than the rubber tourniquet. The disadvantage of the Velcro-closure tourniquet is that it is more difficult to remove with one hand than the rubber tourniquet. In addition, this type of tourniquet may not fit around the arms of extremely obese patients. The technique for applying a Velcro-closure tourniquet is described next and is illustrated in Figure 31-7.

Figure 31-6 Application of a rubber tourniquet. **A,** Create tension by pulling the ends of the tourniquet away from each other. **B,** With tension, cross one flap over the other at the point of your grasp. **C,** Form a loop by tucking a portion of the top length into the bottom length.

Figure 31-7 Application of a Velcro-closure tourniquet.

Procedure: Velcro-Closure Tourniquet

1. Hold each end of the tourniquet with one hand. Position the tourniquet 3 to 4 inches (7.5 to 10 cm) above the bend in the elbow.
2. Wrap the tourniquet around the arm, and secure it with the Velcro fastener. The tourniquet should be applied with enough tension that it is snug but is not pinching the patient's skin.

SITE SELECTION FOR VENIPUNCTURE

For most patients, the best site to use is the veins in the antecubital space (Figure 31-8). If the patient has large, visible antecubital veins, drawing blood is easy. If the patient has small veins or veins that cannot be palpated, obtaining a blood specimen can be quite a challenge, even for the most experienced medical assistant.

The antecubital space is the surface of the arm in front of the elbow. The antecubital veins typically have a wide lumen and are close to the surface of the skin, which makes them easily accessible. In addition, these veins typically have thick walls, making them less likely to collapse. Using the antecubital space spares the patient unnecessary pain because the skin is less sensitive there than at other sites, such as the back of the hand. The medical assistant should not be misled by the presence in some patients of many small, very blue "spidery" veins that lie close to the surface of the skin. These veins are not suitable for performing a venipuncture. The antecubital veins lie beneath these veins.

The best vein to use in the antecubital space is the *median cubital*. The median cubital is a prominent vein in the middle of the antecubital space and does not roll (see Figure 31-8). At times, however, the median cubital vein cannot be used—for example, when it lies deep in the

Figure 31-8 Antecubital veins.

tissues and cannot be palpated or is scarred from repeated venipunctures.

The *cephalic* and *basilic* veins are located on opposite sides of the antecubital space and provide an alternative site when the median cubital vein is unavailable. The cephalic vein is located on the thumb side of the antecubital space, and the basilic vein is located on the little finger side of the antecubital space. The disadvantage of these "side" veins is that they tend to roll or move away from the needle, escaping puncture. To prevent rolling, firm pressure should be applied below and to the side of the vein to stabilize it as the needle is inserted.

The brachial artery also is located in the antecubital space, but it lies deeper in the tissues. This is the artery that is used to measure blood pressure. Before performing a venipuncture, palpate for the presence of this artery. In contrast to a vein, an artery pulsates, is more elastic, and has a thicker wall than a vein. If the brachial artery is inadvertently punctured, the patient feels more than the usual amount of pain, and the blood is bright red and comes out in pulsing movements. If this situation occurs, the tourniquet should be removed and then the needle. Pressure with a gauze pad should be applied for 4 to 5 minutes.

Guidelines for Site Selection

Specific guidelines should be followed to facilitate the selection of a good vein:

1. Ensure that the lighting is adequate. Good lighting facilitates inspection of the veins.

2. Ensure that the veins "stand out" as much as possible. Before locating a venipuncture site, always apply the tourniquet, and have the patient make a fist. This combination makes the veins more prominent.

3. Examine the antecubital veins of both arms. The best site to perform a venipuncture varies with each individual. The patient may have larger veins in one arm than in the other. It is advisable to ask the patient whether he or she has had a venipuncture before. Most adults have had previous venipunctures and know which of their veins are best to use and which should be avoided. Listen to and evaluate information offered by the patient.

4. Use inspection and particularly palpation to select a vein. A vein does not have to be seen to be a good selection. If you cannot see a vein, palpation alone can be used to locate it. A vein feels like an elastic tube that "gives" under the pressure of the fingertips.

5. Always palpate for the median cubital vein (middle vein) first. It usually is bigger, is anchored better, bruises less, and poses the smallest risk of injuring underlying structures (e.g., nerves and arteries) than the other veins. Because of this, if the patient's median cubital vein cannot be seen but still can be palpated, it should be used as the first choice when selecting a vein. If the median cubital vein is good in both arms, select the one that appears the fullest. The cephalic vein located on the thumb side is the next best vein choice because it does not roll and bruise as easily as the basilic vein. The basilic vein, located on the little finger side of the antecubital space, is the least desirable venipuncture site in the antecubital space. Branches of the median nerve may lie close to this vein in some individuals. In addition, the basilic vein lies in close proximity to the brachial artery. Both of these conditions pose a risk of injury to underlying structures when blood is drawn from the basilic vein.

6. Thoroughly assess the patient's veins. To assess a vein as a possible site for venipuncture, place one or two fingertips (index and middle fingers) over it and press lightly, then release pressure. Do not use your thumb to palpate the vein because it is not as sensitive as the index finger. To be suitable for a venipuncture, the vein should feel round, firm, elastic, and engorged. When you depress and release an engorged vein, it should spring back in a rounded, filled state.

7. Determine the size, depth, and direction of the vein. When a suitable vein has been located, it should be palpated thoroughly and carefully to determine the direction of the vein and to estimate the size and depth of the vein. Palpate and trace the path of the vein several times by rolling your index finger back and forth over the vein to determine its size. Inspect and palpate the vein for problems. Some veins that appear suitable at first sight feel small, hard, bumpy, or flat when palpated.

8. Map the location of the site. After locating an acceptable vein, mentally "map" the location of the puncture site on the patient's arm with "skin marks." This

technique is particularly helpful if the vein cannot be seen, but only palpated. The puncture site may be located on or next to a skin mark, such as a freckle, a small wrinkle, or a pigmented area.

9. Do not leave the tourniquet on for longer than 1 minute. When first learning the venipuncture procedure, you may need to perform numerous assessments of the patient's arms to locate the best vein. After each assessment, remove the tourniquet for approximately 2 minutes to allow normal circulation of the blood to occur. This prevents patient discomfort and hemoconcentration, which can lead to inaccurate results for a variety of laboratory tests.

10. If a good vein cannot be found, the following techniques can be employed to make the veins more prominent:
   - Remove the tourniquet, and have the patient dangle the arm over the side of the chair for 1 to 2 minutes.
   - Tap the vein site sharply a few times with your index finger and second finger.
   - Gently massage the arm from the wrist to the elbow.
   - Apply a warm, moist washcloth to the area for 5 minutes.

ALTERNATIVE VENIPUNCTURE SITES

If it is impossible to locate a suitable vein in the antecubital space, alternative sites are available, including the inner forearm, the wrist area above the thumb, and the back of the hand (Figure 31-9). These alternative veins are smaller and have thinner walls than the antecubital veins and should be used for venipuncture only when all possibilities for obtaining the blood specimen at the antecubital site have been considered. If the medical assistant is able to palpate a small vein in the antecubital space, it may be possible to obtain blood there using the butterfly method of venipuncture.

The hand veins, in particular, should be used only as a last resort. The veins of the hand have a tendency to roll because they are not supported by much tissue and are close to the surface of the skin. This makes them more difficult to stick. In addition, an abundant supply of nerves is present in the hands, which makes this procedure more uncomfortable for the patient. Hand veins tend to have thin walls, which makes them more susceptible to collapsing, bruising, and phlebitis. In some patients, however, especially the obese and the elderly, the hand veins may be the only accessible site.

TYPES OF BLOOD SPECIMENS

The type of blood specimen required depends on the type of test to be performed. Serum is required for most blood chemistry studies, whereas whole blood is required for a CBC. The various types of blood specimens that the medical assistant would be required to obtain through the venipuncture procedure are as follows:

1. *Clotted blood.* Clotted blood is obtained from a tube that does not contain an anticoagulant. A tube without an anticoagulant causes the blood cells to clot.

Figure 31-9 Alternative venipuncture sites: the inner forearm, the wrist area above the thumb, and the back of the hand.

2. *Serum.* Serum is obtained from clotted blood by allowing the specimen to stand and then centrifuging it. Centrifuging a blood specimen that does not contain an anticoagulant causes the blood to separate into the following layers (Figure 31-10, *A*):
   - Top layer—serum
   - Bottom layer—clotted blood cells
3. *Whole blood.* Whole blood is obtained by using a tube that contains an **anticoagulant**. An anticoagulant is a substance that inhibits blood clotting. It is important to mix the anticoagulant with the blood by gently inverting the tube back and forth 8 to 10 times after collection.
4. *Plasma.* Plasma is obtained from whole blood that has been centrifuged. Centrifuging a blood specimen that contains an anticoagulant causes the blood to separate into the following layers (Figure 31-10, *B*):
   - Top layer—plasma
   - Middle layer—**buffy coat** (contains white blood cells and platelets)
   - Bottom layer—red blood cells

OSHA SAFETY PRECAUTIONS

The OSHA Bloodborne Pathogens Standard presented in Chapter 17 must be carefully followed during the venipuncture procedure to avoid exposure to bloodborne pathogens. The following OSHA requirements apply specifically to the

Figure 31-10 Layers into which the blood separates when there is no anticoagulant (**A**) and when an anticoagulant is present (**B**).

---

venipuncture procedure and to separation of serum from whole blood (see later):

1. Wear gloves when it is reasonably anticipated that you will have hand contact with blood.
2. Avoid hand-to-mouth contact, such as eating, drinking, or applying makeup, while working with blood specimens.
3. Wear a face shield or mask in combination with an eye protection device whenever splashes, spray, splatter, or droplets of blood may be generated.
4. Perform all procedures involving blood in a manner so as to minimize splashing, spraying, splattering, and generating droplets of blood.
5. Bandage cuts and other lesions on the hands before gloving.
6. Sanitize hands as soon as possible after removing gloves.
7. If your hands or other skin surfaces come in contact with blood, wash the area as soon as possible with soap and water.
8. If your mucous membranes (e.g., eyes, nose, mouth) come in contact with blood, flush them with water as soon as possible.
9. Do not bend, break, or shear contaminated venipuncture needles.
10. Do not recap a contaminated venipuncture needle.
11. Locate the sharps container as close as possible to the area of use. Immediately after use, place the contaminated venipuncture needle (and plastic holder) in the biohazard sharps container.
12. Place blood specimens in containers that prevent leakage during collection, handling, processing, storage, transport, and shipping.
13. Handle all laboratory equipment and supplies properly and with care as indicated by the manufacturer. For example, wait until the centrifuge comes to a complete stop before opening it.
14. Do not store food in refrigerators where testing supplies or specimens are stored.
15. If you are exposed to blood, report the incident immediately to your physician-employer.

What Would You Do? What Would You Not Do?

Case Study 1

Angela Castillo is 21 years old and comes to the office at 9:00 AM to have her blood drawn for a CBC and a thyroid profile. She has brought a friend along with her. Angela seems nervous, and her voice is shaking. She says this is the first venipuncture she has ever had. Angela asks whether her friend can stay with her to give her moral support while her blood is being drawn. Angela says that the blood has to be taken out of her left arm. She says she is right-handed and has a softball game this evening. When the veins of Angela's left arm are examined, a suitable vein cannot be located; however, she has a good median cubital vein in her right arm. Angela then wants to know whether the blood could be drawn from her left hand like they do on hospital television shows. ■

VACUUM TUBE METHOD OF VENIPUNCTURE

The vacuum tube method is frequently used to collect venous blood specimens. This method is considered ideal for collecting blood from normal healthy antecubital veins that are adequate in size to withstand the pressure of the vacuum in the evacuated tube. Procedure 31-1 outlines the venipuncture vacuum tube method. The vacuum tube system consists of a collection needle, a plastic holder, and an evacuated tube (Figure 31-11). One commercially available vacuum tube system is the Vacutainer System (Becton Dickinson, Franklin Lakes, NJ).

NEEDLE

The needle used with the vacuum tube method consists of a double-pointed stainless steel needle with a threaded hub near its center (Figure 31-12). The needle is coated with silicon, enabling it to penetrate the skin smoothly. The threaded hub of the needle screws into the plastic holder. Vacuum tube needles are packaged in sealed twist-apart plastic containers. The needle gauge and length are printed on the paper seal on the container (see Figure 31-12). A needle should not be used if the seal has been broken.

The double-pointed needle consists of an anterior needle and a posterior needle. The *anterior needle* is longer and has a beveled point designed to facilitate entry into the skin and the vein. The *posterior needle* is shorter, and its purpose is to pierce the rubber stopper of the evacuated tube. The posterior needle has a rubber sleeve that functions as a valve. Pushing the tube stopper of an evacuated tube onto the posterior needle compresses this rubber sleeve and exposes

Figure 31-11 Vacuum tube system.

Needle gauge and size

Plastic color-coded container

Anterior needle

Threaded hub

Posterior needle covered by the rubber sleeve

Figure 31-12 Vacuum tube needle in its container showing the gauge and size of the needle. The gauge of this needle is 21 G, and the size is 1 inch.

the opening of the needle, allowing blood to enter the tube. When a tube is removed, the sleeve slides back over the needle opening and stops the flow of blood.

Vacuum tube needles are available in sizes 20 G to 22 G, with 21-G needles used most often for routine venipuncture. A 22-G needle is recommended for children and adults with smaller veins, and a 20-G needle is sometimes used when a large-volume tube is used to collect a blood specimen. Manufacturers often color-code the needle guard and hub of venipuncture needles by gauge for easier identification—for example, Becton Dickinson uses the following color-coding system: yellow for 20-G needles, green for 21-G needles (see Figure 31-12), and black for 22-G needles. Vacuum tube needles come in two lengths: 1 inch and 1½ inches. The length used is based on individual preference; most medical assistants prefer the 1-inch needle for routine venipunctures. A 1-inch needle is less intimidating to the patient and tends to offer greater control because it allows the medical assistant to rest the fourth and fifth fingers on the patient's arm for stability. A 1½-inch needle allows more room for stabilizing the vein.

SAFETY-ENGINEERED VENIPUNCTURE DEVICES

OSHA stipulates requirements to reduce needlestick and other sharps injuries among health care workers. As discussed in Chapter 17, employers are required to evaluate and implement commercially available safer medical devices that reduce occupational exposure to the lowest extent feasible.

Safer medical devices include safety-engineered venipuncture devices. These devices incorporate a built-in safety

feature to reduce the risk of a needlestick injury. Figure 31-13 illustrates a safety-engineered venipuncture device and the method for using it.

PLASTIC HOLDER

The plastic holder consists of a plastic cylinder with two openings. The small opening is used to secure the double-pointed needle, and the large opening is used to hold the evacuated tube. The large opening has a plastic extension known as the *flange*. The flange assists in the insertion and removal of evacuated tubes and prevents the plastic holder from rolling when it is placed on a flat surface.

The plastic holder has an indentation about ½ inch from the hub of the needle. This marks the point at which the posterior needle starts to enter the rubber stopper of the tube. If a tube stopper is inserted past this point before the vein is entered, the tube fills with air, which prevents blood from entering the tube.

EVACUATED TUBES

Evacuated tubes consist of a glass or plastic tube with either a rubber stopper or a *Hemogard closure* stopper. The tube contains a premeasured vacuum that creates suction to pull the blood specimen into the tube. Evacuated tubes use a color-coded stopper system for ease in identifying the additive (or no additive) content of the tube. The additive content of evacuated tubes is described in the next section and is illustrated in Figures 31-14 and 31-15. A tube additive must not alter the blood components or affect the laboratory test to be performed.

The color of the tube stopper used depends on the type of test to be performed. The medical assistant must determine the correct color of the stopper to use for each collection. The color-coded stoppered tubes must not be substituted for one another because inaccurate test results could occur. If a CBC has been ordered by the physician, a lavender-stoppered tube must be used, and a tube with a different-colored stopper cannot be substituted for it.

Evacuated tubes are available in varying capacities that range from 2 mL to 10 mL (see Figure 31-14). The capacity of the tube used depends on the amount of the specimen required for the test. If the medical assistant is working with an outside laboratory, information on the amount of specimen required for a laboratory test and the stopper color of the tube required is indicated in the laboratory directory. If the test is being performed in the medical office, this information is indicated in the instructions accompanying the blood analyzer or testing kit.

Information regarding additive content, expiration date, and tube capacity is on the label of each package of evacuated tubes (Figure 31-16). In addition, evacuated tubes have a label affixed to them indicating the additive content, expiration date, and tube capacity, as well as a fill indicator to indicate when the vacuum has been exhausted and the tube is full.

Figure 31-13 Safety-engineered venipuncture device. **A,** Perform the venipuncture with the shield in a downward position. **B,** After performing the venipuncture, push the shield forward. **C,** Continue pushing until the needle tip is fully covered by the shield. Discard the needle and holder in a biohazard sharps container.

Figure 31-14 Vacutainer evacuated tubes. The stoppers of the evacuated tubes are color-coded for ease in identifying the additive content. The tubes with lavender, light blue, green, gray, and royal blue stoppers contain an anticoagulant and are used to obtain whole blood or plasma. The red-stoppered tube contains no additive and is used to obtain clotted blood or serum.

Gray: Sodium fluoride/potassium oxalate

Red: No anticoagulant

Lavender: EDTA

Gold: Serum separator tube

Figure 31-15 Hemogard tubes.

Figure 31-16 Evacuated tube package label.

A Hemogard closure stopper consists of a special rubber stopper and a plastic closure that overhangs the outside of the tube. Together, these components act as a single unit to reduce the likelihood of coming in contact with the contents of the tube. After collecting a blood specimen, the medical assistant may need to gain access to the blood in the tube for testing it or for further processing, such as in separating serum from whole blood. A conventional rubber stopper–evacuated tube "pops" as the top is removed, which may result in splattering of blood. The design of the Hemogard stopper works to prevent splattering of blood when the top is removed. The color coding of Hemogard closure stoppers is similar to that of rubber-stoppered tubes (see Figure 31-15).

Additive Content of Evacuated Tubes

Evacuated tubes use a color-coded system for ease in identifying the additive content of each type of tube (see Figures 31-14 and 31-15). The most frequently used evacuated tubes in the medical office are classified here according to the color of the stopper and the additive content:

1. *Red.* Red-stoppered tubes do not contain an anticoagulant and are used to obtain clotted blood or serum. Serum is required for serologic tests and most blood chemistries.

2. *Red/gray-speckled tube (often called a "tiger top" tube).* The tube has a gold stopper if Hemogard tubes are used. These tubes are used to obtain serum. These tubes do not contain an anticoagulant; however, they do contain an additive known as a *clot activator.* A clot activator consists of a substance that makes the red blood cells in the tube clot more quickly to yield serum. Red/gray- and gold-stoppered tubes also contain a gel that separates the cells from the serum when the tube is centrifuged. A tube with a clot activator must be inverted five times after the blood has been drawn to mix the clot activator with the blood specimen.

3. *Lavender.* Lavender-stoppered tubes contain the anticoagulant EDTA and are used to obtain whole blood or plasma. The most common use is to collect a blood specimen for a CBC.

4. *Light blue.* Light blue–stoppered tubes contain the anticoagulant sodium citrate and are used to obtain whole blood or plasma; the most common use is for coagulation tests, such as prothrombin time.

5. *Green.* Green-stoppered tubes contain the anticoagulant heparin and are commonly used to collect blood specimens to perform blood gas determinations and pH assays.

6. *Gray.* Gray-stoppered tubes contain sodium fluoride (a preservative) and potassium oxalate (an anticoagulant) and are used to obtain whole blood or plasma; the most common use is to collect blood specimens to perform blood alcohol and drug tests or an oral glucose tolerance test (OGTT).

7. *Royal blue.* Royal blue–stoppered tubes contain either EDTA or no additive at all. These tubes are made of a specially refined glass and rubber stopper and are used for the detection of trace elements, such as lead, zinc, arsenic, and copper, which are contracted through occupational or environmental exposure.

ORDER OF DRAW FOR MULTIPLE TUBES

When the vacuum tube system is used and when multiple tubes of blood are to be drawn, the following order of draw (Table 31-1) is recommended by the *Clinical and Laboratory Standards Institute (CLSI):*

1. *Blood culture tube:* Yellow-stoppered glass tube that contains the anticoagulant sodium polyanethol sulfonate

Table 31-1 Order of Draw for Collection of Multiple Evacuated Tubes

Order of Draw by Color of Stopper	Additive or Anticoagulant	Number of Inversions After Collection
Yellow	Sterile blood culture tube that contains SPS (sodium polyanethol sulfonate)	8 to 10 inversions
Light blue	Sodium citrate	3 to 4 inversions
Red	Glass: no additive / Plastic: clot activator	No inversions / 5 inversions
Red and gray	Serum separator gel and clot activator	5 inversions
Gold		
Green	Heparin	
Light green and gray	Plasma separator gel and lithium heparin	8 to 10 inversions
Light green		
Lavender	EDTA	8 to 10 inversions
Royal blue	EDTA No additive	8 to 10 inversions No inversions
Gray	Sodium fluoride, potassium oxalate	8 to 10 inversions

(SPS), which is used for blood cultures and other tests that require sterile specimens.

Rationale: To prevent contamination of the specimen by other tubes, which may lead to inaccurate test results.

2. *Coagulation tube:* Light blue–stoppered tube for coagulation tests.

Rationale: To prevent additives from other tubes from getting into the tube.

Note: The tubing of the butterfly setup contains 0.3 to 0.5 mL of air. If a light blue–stoppered tube is the first or only tube to be drawn, a 5-mL red-stoppered tube must be drawn first and discarded. This is because some of the tube's vacuum is exhausted by the air in the tubing (rather than blood), resulting in underfilling of the tube. If the light blue–stoppered tube is filled first, the underfilled tube results in an incorrect anticoagulant-to-blood ratio. An incorrect ratio when performing a coagulation test leads to inaccurate coagulation test results. It is also important to completely fill coagulation tubes to the exhaustion of the vacuum; failure to do so leads to erroneous coagulation test results.

3. *Serum tubes:* Tubes with or without a clot activator, and tubes with or without a gel barrier (e.g., red-stoppered tube; red/gray- or gold-stoppered tubes)

Rationale: To prevent contamination of serum tubes by tubes with an anticoagulant.

4. *Anticoagulant tubes* in this order of stopper color: green, lavender, royal blue (tube that contains EDTA), and gray

Rationale: To prevent cross-contamination among different types of anticoagulants, which may lead to inaccurate test results.

EVACUATED TUBE GUIDELINES

Certain guidelines should be followed when using evacuated tubes, as follows:

1. Select the proper evacuated tubes according to the tests to be performed and the amount of specimen required.
2. Check to ensure that the tube is not cracked. A cracked tube no longer has a vacuum.

Figure 31-17 Information included on a laboratory specimen bar code label.

3. Check the expiration date on each tube. Outdated tubes may no longer contain a vacuum, and as a result they would not be able to draw blood into the tube.

4. Make sure each tube is properly labeled. Proper labeling avoids mixing up specimens. Advances in specimen identification include the use of computer bar codes to identify specimens. Laboratory instruments that do the testing are able to read the bar codes and automatically record results onto the laboratory report form for a particular patient using the identification number supplied by the bar code. Along with the bar code, additional printed information is included on a bar code label (Figure 31-17). It is important to attach the correct bar code label to the blood tube. Inspect the label for printed information indicating the color of the stopper of the tube (e.g., LV for lavender) or type of tube (e.g., SST for serum separator tube) to which the label must be attached. For example, the bar code label illustrated in Figure 31-17 must be placed on a lavender (LV) tube for a specimen that is being collected to perform a CBC.

5. Before using tubes that contain powdered additives (e.g., gray-stoppered tube), gently tap the tube just below the stopper so that all of the additive is dislodged from the stopper. If an additive remains trapped in the stopper, erroneous test results may occur.

6. Take precautions to avoid premature loss of the tube's vacuum. Premature loss of vacuum can occur from the following:
   • Dropping the tube
   • Pushing the posterior needle through the tube stopper before puncturing the vein
   • Partially pulling the needle out of the vein after penetrating the patient's vein

7. Use a continuous, steady motion to make the puncture. Performing the puncture with a slow, timid motion or a rapid, jabbing motion is painful for the patient. In addition, a rapid motion could cause the needle to go completely through the vein, resulting in failure to obtain blood and possibly a hematoma.

8. When multiple tubes are to be drawn, follow the proper *order of draw*. This prevents contamination of nonadditive tubes by additive tubes and cross-contamination among different types of additive tubes, which could lead to inaccurate test results.

9. Fill evacuated tubes until the vacuum is exhausted, as evidenced by cessation of blood flow into the tube. The tube is almost but not quite full when the vacuum is exhausted. If the evacuated tube is removed before the vacuum is exhausted, a rush of air enters the tube, damaging the red blood cells. A tube that contains an anticoagulant must be filled completely to ensure the proper ratio of anticoagulant to the blood specimen.

10. Remove the last tube from the plastic holder before removing the needle from the patient's vein. This prevents blood from dripping out of the tip of the needle after it has been withdrawn from the patient's skin.

11. Mix tubes that contain a clot activator or an anticoagulant immediately after drawing by gently inverting them. Gentle inversion provides adequate mixing without causing **hemolysis**, or breakdown of blood cells. One inversion consists of one complete turn of the wrist (180 degrees) and then back again. Tubes with a clot activator should be inverted five times, and tubes with an anticoagulant (with the exception of sodium citrate tubes) should be inverted 8 to 10 times. Tubes containing sodium citrate (light-blue stopper) should be gently inverted three or four times (see Table 31-1). Inadequate mixing or not mixing tubes with an anticoagulant immediately after drawing the specimen may result in clotting of the blood, leading to inaccurate test results.

12. After the venipuncture, the top of the stopper may contain residual blood. Take precautions by following the OSHA Standard when handling these tubes.

PROCEDURE 31-1   Venipuncture—Vacuum Tube Method

Outcome Perform a venipuncture using the vacuum tube method

Equipment/Supplies

- Disposable gloves
- Tourniquet
- Antiseptic wipe
- Double-pointed needle with a safety shield
- Plastic holder
- Evacuated tubes with labels

- Sterile 2 × 2 gauze pad
- Adhesive bandage
- Biohazard sharps container
- Biohazard specimen bag
- Laboratory request form

1. **Procedural Step.** Review the requirements for collecting and handling the blood specimen as ordered by the physician. Sanitize your hands.

2. **Procedural Step.** Greet the patient and introduce yourself. Identify the patient by asking the patient to state his or her full name and date of birth. Compare this information with the demographic data in the patient's medical record.
   Principle. It is important to confirm that you have the correct patient to avoid collecting a specimen from the wrong patient.

3. **Procedural Step.** If the patient was required to prepare for the test (e.g., fasting, medication restriction), determine whether he or she has prepared properly. If the patient has not followed the patient preparation requirements, notify the physician for instructions on handling this situation.
   Principle. The patient must prepare properly so the medical assistant can obtain a high-quality specimen that will yield accurate test results.

4. **Procedural Step.** Assemble the equipment. Select the proper evacuated tubes for the tests to be performed. Check the expiration date on the tubes. Label each tube using one of the following methods: (a) attaching a computer bar code label to each tube to be drawn and labeling it with your initials, or (b) manually labeling each tube with the patient's name and date of birth, the date, and your initials. If the specimen is to be tested at an outside laboratory, complete a laboratory request form. (*Note:* Follow the medical office policy as to when the tubes should be labeled. Some offices prefer that tubes be labeled *before* the specimen is drawn; other offices want the tubes to be labeled right *after* the specimen has been drawn.)
   Principle. Outdated tubes may no longer contain a vacuum, and as a result they may not be able to draw blood into the tube. Proper labeling of blood specimens avoids a mix-up of specimens.

Assemble the equipment.

5. **Procedural Step.** Prepare the vacuum tube system. Remove the cap from the posterior needle using a twisting and pulling motion. Insert the posterior needle into the small opening on the plastic holder. Screw the plastic holder onto the Luer adapter, and tighten it securely.
   Principle. An unsecured needle can fall out of its plastic holder.

PROCEDURE 31-1 Venipuncture—Vacuum Tube Method—cont'd

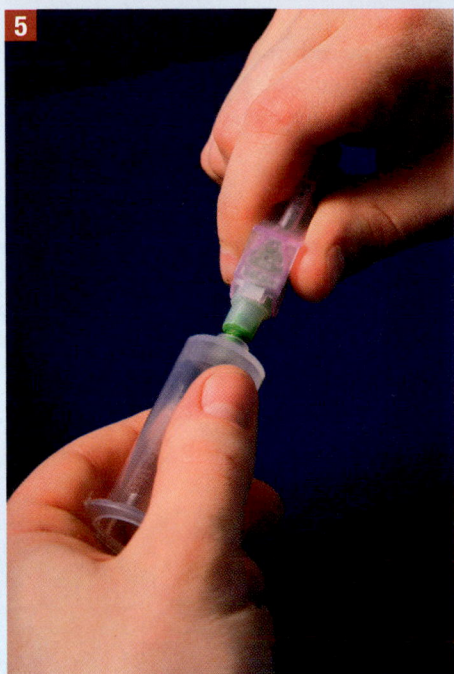

Insert the posterior needle into the plastic holder.

Apply the tourniquet.

6. **Procedural Step.** Open the sterile gauze packet, and lay it flat to allow the gauze pad to rest on the inside of its wrapper. Position the evacuated tubes in the correct order of draw. If the evacuated tube contains a powdered additive, tap the tube just below the stopper to release any additive adhering to the stopper.
   Principle. If an additive remains trapped in the stopper, erroneous test results may occur.

7. **Procedural Step.** Place the first tube loosely in the plastic holder.

8. **Procedural Step.** Explain the procedure to the patient, and reassure the patient. Perform a preliminary assessment of both arms to determine the best vein to use. It also is helpful to ask the patient which arm has been used in the past to obtain blood.
   Principle. Venipuncture is often a frightening experience for the patient, and reassurance should be offered to reduce apprehension.

9. **Procedural Step.** Apply the tourniquet. Position the tourniquet 3 to 4 inches above the bend in the elbow. The tourniquet should be snug but not tight. Ask the patient to clench the fist of the arm to which the tourniquet has been applied.
   Principle. The combined effect of the pressure of the tourniquet and the clenched fist should cause the antecubital veins to stand out so that accurate selection of a puncture site can be made.

10. **Procedural Step.** With a tourniquet in place, thoroughly assess the veins of first one arm and then the other to determine the best vein to use.

11. **Procedural Step.** Position the patient's arm. The arm with the vein selected for the venipuncture should be extended and placed in a straight line from the shoulder to the wrist with the antecubital veins facing anteriorly. The arm should be supported on the armrest by a rolled towel or by having the patient place the fist of the other hand under the elbow.
    Principle. This position allows easy access to the antecubital veins.

12. **Procedural Step.** Thoroughly palpate the selected vein. Gently palpate the vein with the fingertips to determine the direction of the vein and to estimate its size and depth. Never leave the tourniquet on an arm for longer than 1 minute at a time. (*Note:* If you need to perform several assessments to locate the best vein, the tourniquet must be removed and reapplied after a 2-minute waiting period.)
    Principle. Leaving the tourniquet on for longer than 1 minute is uncomfortable for the patient and may alter the test results.

Continued

PROCEDURE 31-1

PROCEDURE 31-1

PROCEDURE 31-1   Venipuncture—Vacuum Tube Method—cont'd

Palpate the vein.

13. **Procedural Step.** Remove the tourniquet and cleanse the site with an antiseptic wipe. Cleansing should be done in a circular motion, starting from the inside and moving away from the puncture site. Allow the site to air-dry; after cleansing, do not touch the area, wipe the area with gauze, or fan the area with your hand. Place the remaining supplies within comfortable reach of your nondominant hand.

    Principle. Using a circular motion helps carry foreign particles away from the puncture site. The site must be allowed to air-dry to allow the alcohol enough time to destroy microorganisms on the patient's skin. Residual alcohol entering the blood specimen can cause hemolysis, leading to inaccurate test results. In addition, residual alcohol causes the patient to experience a stinging sensation when the puncture is made. Touching or fanning the area causes contamination of the puncture site, and the cleansing process must be repeated. Items used during the procedure should be positioned so that you do not have to reach over the patient and possibly move the needle, resulting in pain, injury, or both.

14. **Procedural Step.** Reapply the tourniquet. Apply gloves. Rotate the needle's safety shield backward toward the holder (refer to Figure 31-13, *A*). Remove the cap from the needle using a twisting and pulling motion. Hold the vacuum tube system by placing the thumb of the dominant hand on top

of the plastic holder and the pads of the first three fingers underneath the holder and evacuated tube. The needle should be positioned with the bevel facing up. Position the evacuated tube so that the label is facing down.

Principle. Gloves provide a barrier against bloodborne pathogens. Positioning the needle with the bevel up allows easier entry into the skin and the vein, resulting in less pain for the patient. With the label facing down, you would be able to observe the blood as it fills the tube, which allows you to know when the tube is full.

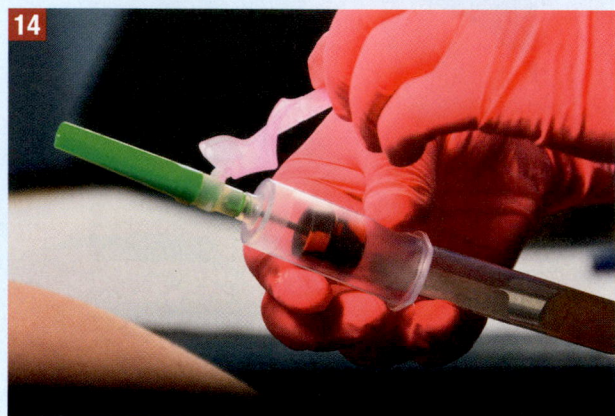

Rotate the safety shield backward.

15. **Procedural Step.** Anchor the vein. Grasp the patient's arm with the nondominant hand. Your thumb should be placed 1 to 2 inches below and to the side of the puncture site. Using your thumb, draw the skin taut over the vein in the direction of the patient's hand.

    Principle. The thumb helps hold the skin taut for easier entry and helps stabilize the vein to be punctured. Placing the thumb to the side keeps it out of the way of the vacuum tube setup, so that you can maintain a 15-degree angle when entering the vein.

16. **Procedural Step.** Position the needle at a 15-degree angle to the arm. Rest the backs of the fingers on the patient's forearm. Ensure that the needle points in the same direction as the vein to be entered. The needle should be positioned so that it enters the vein approximately ⅛ inch below the place where the vein is to be entered.

    Principle. An angle of less than 15 degrees may cause the needle to enter above the vein, preventing puncture. An angle of more than 15 degrees may cause the needle to go through the vein by puncturing the posterior wall. This could result in a hematoma.

PROCEDURE 31-1 Venipuncture—Vacuum Tube Method—cont'd

Position the needle.

17. Procedural Step. Tell the patient that he or she will "feel a small stick," and with one continuous steady motion, enter the skin and then the vein. You will feel a sensation of resistance followed by a "release" as the vein is entered. When the "release" is felt, you have entered the vein and should not advance the needle any farther.
Principle. Using one continuous steady motion helps to prevent tissue damage.

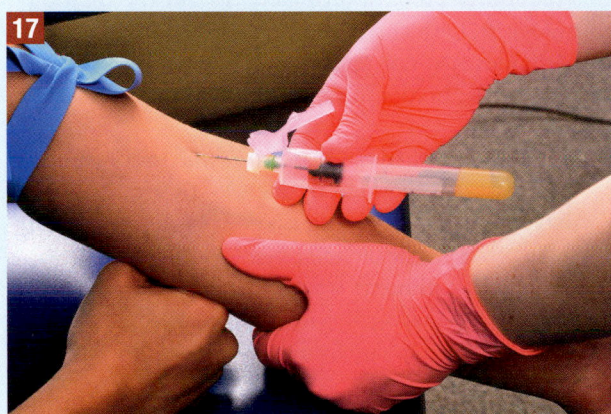

Make the puncture.

18. Procedural Step. Stabilize the vacuum tube setup by firmly grasping the holder between the thumb and the underlying fingers to prevent the needle from moving. Do *not* change hands during the procedure.
Principle. Stabilizing the holder helps prevent the needle from moving when a tube is inserted or removed. Changing hands may cause the needle to move, which is painful for the patient.

19. Procedural Step. With the nondominant hand, place the first two fingers on the underside of the flange on the plastic holder, and with the thumb, slowly push the tube forward to the end of the holder. This allows the posterior needle to puncture

the rubber stopper. Blood begins flowing into the tube if the (anterior) needle is in a vein.
Principle. Not using the flange may cause the needle to advance forward and go completely through the vein, resulting in failure to obtain blood; internal bleeding also may occur, resulting in a hematoma.

20. Procedural Step. Allow the evacuated tube to fill to the exhaustion of the vacuum, as indicated by cessation of the blood flow into the tube. The suction of the evacuated tube automatically draws the blood into the tube.
Principle. If the evacuated tube is removed before the vacuum is exhausted, a rush of air enters the tube, damaging the red blood cells. Also, a tube containing an additive, such as an anticoagulant, must be filled completely to ensure accurate test results.

Remove the tube from the holder.

21. Procedural Step. Remove the tube from the holder by grasping the tube with the fingers, placing the thumb or index finger against the flange, and pulling the tube off the posterior needle. Do not change the position of the needle in the vein. If the tube contains a clot activator, gently invert the tube back and forth five times before laying it down. If the tube contains an anticoagulant, gently invert the tube 8 to 10 times.
Principle. The rubber sheath covers the point of the needle, stopping the flow of blood until the next tube is inserted. Not using the flange to remove the tube can cause the needle to come out of the vein prematurely, resulting in blood being forced out of the puncture site. A tube containing an anticoagulant must be inverted immediately to prevent the blood from clotting. Careful mixing of the blood with a clot activator or an anticoagulant prevents hemolysis.

Continued

PROCEDURE 31-1

PROCEDURE 31-1   Venipuncture—Vacuum Tube Method—cont'd

Invert the tube 8 to 10 times.

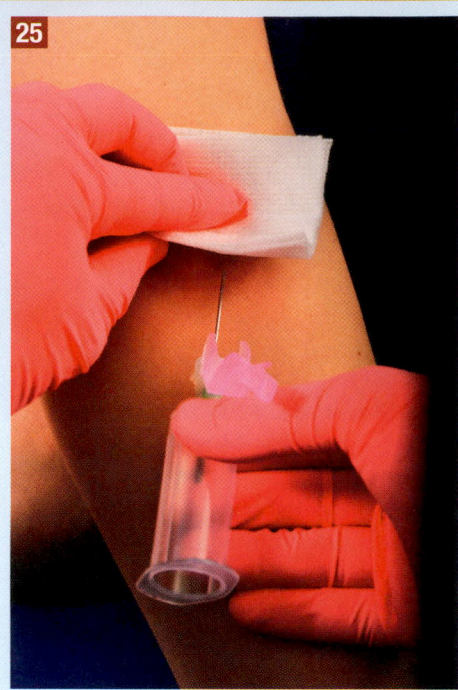

Withdraw the needle.

22. Procedural Step. Using the flange, carefully insert the next tube into the holder. Continue in this manner until the last tube has been filled.

23. Procedural Step. Remove the tension from the tourniquet by pulling upward on one of the flaps of the tourniquet. Ask the patient to unclench the fist.
Principle. The tourniquet tension must be removed before the needle. Otherwise, the pressure on the vein from the tourniquet could cause internal and external bleeding around the puncture site.

24. Procedural Step. Remove the last tube from the holder. Immediately invert the tube back and forth five times if it contains a clot activator and 8 to 10 times if it contains an anticoagulant.
Principle. Removing the last tube prevents blood from dripping out of the tip of the needle after it has been removed from the patient's arm.

25. Procedural Step. Place a sterile gauze pad slightly above the puncture site, and carefully withdraw the needle at the same angle as for penetration. Immediately move the gauze over the puncture site, and apply firm pressure. (Do not apply any pressure to the puncture site until the needle has been completely removed.) Push the safety shield forward with your thumb until you hear an audible click, which indicates the shield has locked into place. Do not push the shield forward by pressing it against a hard surface. (See Figure 31-13, *B, C.*)
Principle. Placing the gauze pad above the puncture helps prevent tissue movement as the needle is withdrawn and reduces patient discomfort. Careful withdrawal prevents further tissue damage.

26. Procedural Step. Immediately discard the plastic holder and attached needle in a biohazard sharps container. Do not remove the needle from the holder; the holder must be discarded and not reused.
Principle. Immediate disposal of the needle and holder unit is required by the OSHA Standard to prevent a needlestick injury; even though the safety shield encases the anterior needle, a needlestick injury can still occur from the posterior needle, which is covered only with a rubber sleeve. Plastic holders are often contaminated with blood and must not be reused.

27. Procedural Step. Continue to apply pressure with the gauze pad. Cooperative patients can be asked to assist by applying pressure with the gauze pad for 1 to 2 minutes. The arm can be elevated to facilitate clot formation. Do not allow the patient to bend the arm at the elbow because this increases blood loss from the puncture site.
Principle. Applying pressure reduces the leakage of blood from the puncture site externally or internally. Internal leakage of blood into the tissues could result in a hematoma.

28. Procedural Step. Stay with the patient until the bleeding has stopped. Remove the gauze, and inspect the puncture site to ensure that the opening is sealed with a clot. Apply an adhesive bandage to the puncture site. As an alternative, the gauze pad can be folded into quarters and taped on the puncture site to be used as a pressure bandage. Instruct the patient not to pick up anything heavy for about an hour. (*Note:* If swelling or discoloration occurs, apply an ice pack to the site after bandaging it.)

Principle. Lifting a heavy object causes pressure on the puncture site, which could result in bleeding.

29. Procedural Step. Place the tubes in an upright position in a test tube rack. Remove the gloves, and sanitize your hands.

30. Procedural Step. Chart the procedure in the patient's medical record.
   a. *Paper-based patient record:* Record the date and time, which arm and vein were used, unusual patient reaction, and your initials (refer to the PPR charting example).
   b. *Electronic medical record:* Document which arm and vein were used, as well as any unusual patient reactions, using the appropriate radio buttons, drop-down menus, and free text fields.

31. Procedural Step. If needed, process the specimen (e.g., centrifuging the specimen to separate serum from the cells). Test the specimen or prepare the specimen for transport to an outside laboratory for

testing according to the medical office policy. If the specimen is to be transported to an outside laboratory, do the following:
   a. Place the specimen tube in a biohazard specimen bag.
   b. Place the laboratory request in the outside pocket of the specimen bag.
   c. Properly handle and store the specimen while awaiting pickup by a laboratory courier.
   d. Chart the date the specimen was transported to the laboratory in the patient's medical record.

Principle. The biohazard bag protects the laboratory courier from the possibility of an exposure incident. The outside laboratory must have the completed request form to know which laboratory tests have been ordered by the physician. The specimen must be handled and stored properly to maintain the in vivo characteristics of the specimen.

PPR CHARTING EXAMPLE

Date	
4/5/XX	9:00 a.m. Venous blood specimen collected from ⓛ arm. Picked up by Medical Center Laboratory on 4/5/XX. ———————————————— ——————————— D. Glover, CMA (AAMA)

BUTTERFLY METHOD OF VENIPUNCTURE

The butterfly method of venipuncture is also called the *winged infusion method.* This is because a winged infusion set is used to perform the procedure. The term *butterfly* is derived from the plastic "wings" located between the needle and the tubing of the winged infusion set (Figure 31-18).

The butterfly method is used to collect blood from patients who are difficult to stick by conventional methods because it provides better control when making the puncture, and less pressure is exerted on the vein wall from the evacuated tube. The butterfly method is recommended for adults with small antecubital veins and children, who typically also have small antecubital veins. The butterfly method also is used when the antecubital veins are unavailable and veins in the forearm, wrist area, or back of the hand are used, as may occur with elderly and obese patients. These alternative veins are usually smaller and sometimes have a thin wall (e.g., hand veins), making them more likely to collapse with the vacuum tube method of venipuncture.

With the vacuum tube method, the "sucking action" exerted on the vein when the pressure in the vacuum is released causes the vein to collapse, blocking the flow of blood into the tube. The butterfly method results in less pressure on the vein wall because the pressure exerted by the evacuated tube must travel through a length of tubing before reaching the vein. Because the pressure against the vein wall is minimized, the vein is less likely to collapse with the butterfly method. Procedure 31-2 describes the venipuncture procedure with the butterfly method.

The gauge of the winged infusion needle used to collect a blood specimen ranges from 21 G to 23 G, and the length of the needle ranges from $\frac{1}{2}$ to $\frac{3}{4}$ inch. The needle is short and sharp, making it easier to stick difficult veins. For extremely small veins, a 23-G needle should be used to prevent rupture of the vein by a larger needle. In this case, it is preferable to use smaller-volume tubes (e.g., 2-mL evacuated tubes) because large evacuated tubes may put too much vacuum pressure on the vein, causing it to collapse. Manufacturers often color-code the wings of the infusion setup by gauge for easier identification—for example, Becton Dickinson uses the following color coding system:

Luer adapter

A

B

Hub adapter

Figure 31-18 Winged infusion set. **A,** Luer adapter with evacuated tube. **B,** Hub adapter with syringe.

A

B

Figure 31-19 Butterfly safety needle. The safety needle has a shield that covers the contaminated needle after it has been withdrawn from the patient's vein. **A,** The medical assistant has covered one half of the needle with the shield. **B,** The needle is completely covered with the shield.

green for 21-G needles and light blue for 23-G needles (see Figure 31-18).

The winged infusion needle is attached to a 7- or 12-inch length of tubing and a *Luer adapter,* which is attached to a (posterior) needle with a rubber sleeve. A plastic holder is screwed onto the Luer adapter, which allows it to be used with evacuated tubes (see Figure 31-18, *A*). Winged infusion sets also are available with a hub adapter that allows them to be used with a syringe (see Figure 31-18, *B*). Safety needles are available with a shield that covers the contaminated needle after it has been withdrawn from the patient's vein (Figure 31-19).

GUIDELINES FOR THE BUTTERFLY METHOD

Certain guidelines should be followed when performing the butterfly method of venipuncture, as follows:
1. Position the patient according to the site selected for the venipuncture as follows:
   - *Antecubital, wrist, and forearm veins.* Position the arm in a straight line from the shoulder to the wrist as described for the vacuum tube method of venipuncture.
   - *Hand veins.* Position the patient's hand on the armrest, and ask the patient to make a loose fist or to grasp a rolled towel. This combination causes the hand veins to stand out so that accurate selection of a puncture site can be made. Locate a suitable vein between the knuckles and the wrist bones. Hand veins are usually visible and easy to locate.
2. Position the tourniquet according to the venipuncture site as follows: If the veins of the forearm or wrist are used, apply the tourniquet to the forearm, approximately 3 inches above the puncture site. For hand veins, position the tourniquet on the arm just above the wrist bone (Figure 31-20).

3. Grasp the needle by compressing the plastic wings together. Insert the needle with the bevel facing up at a 15-degree angle to the skin. When the vein has been entered, decrease the angle to 5 degrees.
4. After decreasing the needle angle to 5 degrees, slowly thread the needle inside the vein an additional $\frac{1}{4}$ inch. This anchors or seats the needle in the center of the vein and allows the medical assistant to use both hands to change tubes.
5. To prevent venous reflux, keep the evacuated tube and holder in a downward position as in the vacuum tube venipuncture procedure. This technique ensures that the blood fills from the bottom up and not near the rubber stopper.
6. When multiple tubes are to be drawn, follow the proper order of draw. The order of draw for the butterfly method is identical to that for the vacuum tube method (previously presented). Following this order of draw prevents contamination of nonadditive tubes and cross-contamination of additive tubes.

A. Forearm site   B. Wrist site   C. Hand

Figure 31-20 Application of the tourniquet for alternative venipuncture sites.

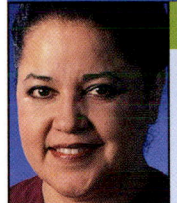

Memories *from* Practicum

Dori Glover: One of the most terrifying things for me as a student was learning venipuncture. Even though I would practice during classroom laboratory hours and felt comfortable with it, it still scared me to know I would have to draw on a real person one day. When the day arrived to draw on my laboratory partner, I became sick to my stomach. In the end, we both got through it just fine and walked away without hurting each other. I spent days trying to prepare myself for that first experience, but after it was over, I felt more confident and relaxed that I could do this. At my practicum site, I was able to perform several venipunctures a day, which raised my confidence level. Today venipuncture is my favorite responsibility of all. I would draw blood all day if I could. I know I could even draw with my eyes closed, but never would, of course! ∎

What Would You Do? What Would You *Not* Do?

Case Study 3

Maud Gabriel is at the office complaining of persistent headaches and abdominal pain over the past 3 months. The physician gives Mrs. Gabriel a laboratory requisition to have her blood drawn and tested at an outside laboratory. Mrs. Gabriel says that her daughter who lives with her works as a phlebotomist at the local hospital. Mrs. Gabriel wants to know whether her daughter can draw her blood at home and then drop it off at the laboratory. She says that the last time she had her blood drawn, they had to stick her two times and then she got a big bruise on her arm afterward. She says the laboratory technician kept digging around in her arm to find the vein and that it was quite painful. ∎

PROCEDURE 31-2 Venipuncture—Butterfly Method

Outcome Perform a venipuncture using the butterfly method

Equipment/Supplies

- Disposable gloves
- Tourniquet
- Antiseptic wipe
- Winged infusion set with a Luer adapter and safety shield
- Plastic holder

- Evacuated tubes with labels
- Sterile 2 × 2 gauze pad
- Adhesive bandage
- Biohazard sharps container
- Biohazard specimen bag
- Laboratory request form

Continued

PROCEDURE 31-2 Venipuncture—Butterfly Method—cont'd

1. **Procedural Step.** Review the requirements for collecting and handling the blood specimen as ordered by the physician. Sanitize your hands.

2. **Procedural Step.** Greet the patient and introduce yourself. Identify the patient by asking the patient to state his or her full name and date of birth. Compare this information with the demographic data in the patient's medical record. If the patient was required to prepare for the test (e.g., fasting, medication restriction), determine whether he or she has prepared properly. If the patient has not followed the patient preparation requirements, notify the physician for instructions on handling this situation.
   Principle. It is important to confirm that you have the correct patient to avoid collecting a specimen from the wrong patient. The patient must prepare properly for the medical assistant to obtain a high-quality specimen that will lead to accurate test results.

3. **Procedural Step.** Assemble the equipment. Select the proper evacuated tubes for the tests to be performed. Check the expiration date on the tubes. Label each tube using one of the following methods: (a) attaching a computer bar code label to each tube and labeling it with your initials, or (b) manually labeling each tube with the patient's name and date of birth, the date, and your initials. If the specimen is to be tested at an outside laboratory, complete a laboratory request form. (*Note:* Follow the medical office policy as to when the tubes should be labeled. Some offices prefer that tubes be labeled *before* the specimen is drawn; other offices want the tubes to be labeled right *after* the specimen has been drawn.)
   Principle. Outdated tubes may no longer contain a vacuum, and as a result they may not be able to draw blood into the tube. Proper labeling of blood specimens avoids the mix-up of specimens.

Assemble the equipment.

4. **Procedural Step.** Prepare the winged infusion set. Remove the winged infusion set from its package. Extend the tubing to its full length, and stretch it slightly to prevent it from recoiling. Insert the posterior needle into the small opening on the plastic holder. Screw the plastic holder onto the Luer adapter, and tighten it securely.
   Principle. Extending the tubing straightens it to permit a free flow of blood in the tubing. An unsecured needle can fall out of its plastic holder.

Screw the plastic holder onto the Luer adapter.

5. **Procedural Step.** Open the sterile gauze packet, and lay it flat to allow the gauze pad to rest on the inside of its wrapper. Position the evacuated tubes in the correct order of draw. If the evacuated tube contains a powdered additive, tap the tube just below the stopper to release any additive adhering to the stopper.
   Principle. If an additive remains trapped in the stopper, erroneous test results may occur.

6. **Procedural Step.** Place the first tube loosely in the plastic holder with the label facing down.
   Principle. With the label facing down, you can observe the blood as it fills the tube, which allows you to know when the tube is full.

7. **Procedural Step.** Explain the procedure to the patient, and reassure the patient. Perform a preliminary assessment of both arms to determine the best vein to use. It also is helpful to ask the patient which arm has been used in the past to obtain blood.
   Principle. Venipuncture is often a frightening experience for the patient, and reassurance should be offered to reduce apprehension.

8. **Procedural Step.** Apply the tourniquet. Position the tourniquet 3 to 4 inches above the bend in the elbow. The tourniquet should be snug but not tight.

Ask the patient to clench the fist of the arm to which the tourniquet has been applied.
Principle. The combined effect of the pressure of the tourniquet and the clenched fist should cause the antecubital veins to stand out so that accurate selection of a puncture site can be made.

9. **Procedural Step.** With a tourniquet in place, thoroughly assess the veins of first one arm and then the other to determine the best vein to use.

10. **Procedural Step.** Position the patient's arm. The arm with the vein selected for the venipuncture should be extended and placed in a straight line from the shoulder to the wrist with the antecubital veins facing anteriorly. The arm should be supported on the armrest by a rolled towel or by having the patient place the fist of the other hand under the elbow.
Principle. This position allows easy access to the antecubital veins.

11. **Procedural Step.** Thoroughly palpate the selected vein. Gently palpate the vein with the fingertips to determine the direction of the vein and to estimate its size and depth. Never leave the tourniquet on an arm for longer than 1 minute at a time. (*Note:* If you need to perform several assessments to locate the best vein, the tourniquet must be removed and reapplied after a 2-minute waiting period.)
Principle. Leaving the tourniquet on for longer than 1 minute is uncomfortable for the patient and may alter the test results.

12. **Procedural Step.** Remove the tourniquet and cleanse the site with an antiseptic. Cleansing should be done in a circular motion, starting from the inside and moving away from the puncture site. Allow the site to air-dry; after cleansing, do not touch the area, wipe the area with gauze, or fan the area with your hand. Place your remaining supplies within comfortable reach.
Principle. Using a circular motion helps carry foreign particles away from the puncture site. The site must be allowed to air-dry to allow the alcohol enough time to destroy microorganisms on the patient's skin. Residual alcohol entering the blood specimen can cause hemolysis, leading to inaccurate test results. In addition, residual alcohol causes the patient to experience a stinging sensation when the puncture is made. Touching or fanning the area causes contamination of the puncture site, and the cleansing process must be repeated. Items used during the procedure should be positioned so that you do not have to reach over the patient and possibly move the needle, resulting in patient pain, injury, or both.

13. **Procedural Step.** Reapply the tourniquet. Apply gloves. With the dominant hand, grasp the winged infusion set by pressing the butterfly tips together. Remove the protective sheath from the needle of the infusion set. The needle should be positioned with the bevel facing up.
Principle. Gloves provide a barrier against bloodborne pathogens. Positioning the needle with the bevel up allows easier entry into the skin and the vein, resulting in less pain for the patient.

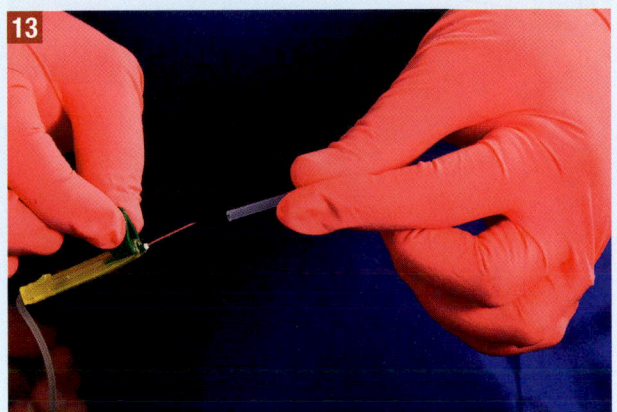
Remove the protective shield from the needle.

14. **Procedural Step.** Anchor the vein. Grasp the patient's arm with the nondominant hand. The thumb should be placed 1 to 2 inches below and to the side of the puncture site. Using the thumb, draw the skin taut over the vein in the direction of the patient's hand.
Principle. The thumb helps hold the skin taut for easier entry and helps stabilize the vein to be punctured. Placing the thumb to the side keeps it out of the way of the winged infusion setup so that you can maintain a 15-degree angle when entering the vein.

15. **Procedural Step.** Position the needle at a 15-degree angle to the arm. Rest the backs of the fingertips on the patient's skin. Make sure the needle points in the same direction as the vein to be entered. The needle should be positioned so that it enters the vein approximately $\frac{1}{8}$ inch below the place where the vein is to be entered.
Principle. An angle of less than 15 degrees may cause the needle to enter above the vein, preventing puncture. An angle of more than 15 degrees may cause the needle to go through the vein by puncturing the posterior wall. This could result in a hematoma.

Continued

16. Procedural Step. Tell the patient that he or she will "feel a small stick," and with one continuous steady motion, enter the skin and then the vein. You will feel a sensation of resistance followed by a "release" as the vein is entered. After penetrating the vein, decrease the angle of the needle to 5 degrees. If the needle is in the vein, a flash of blood appears at the top of the tubing.
Principle. Using one continuous motion reduces tissue damage.

Make the puncture.

17. Procedural Step. Seat the needle by threading it forward an additional ¼ inch inside the center of the vein so that it does not twist out of the vein, even if you let go of it. Open the butterfly wings and securely rest the wings flat against the skin. Ensure that the needle does not move.
Principle. Seating the needle anchors the needle in the center of the vein and allows the use of both hands for changing tubes. Moving the needle is painful for the patient.

Rest the butterfly wings flat against the patient's skin.

18. Procedural Step. Keep the tube and holder in a downward position so that the tube fills from the bottom up and not near the rubber stopper. Slowly push the tube forward to the end of the holder. This allows the needle to puncture the rubber stopper. Blood begins to flow into the tube. Allow the evacuated tube to fill to the exhaustion of the vacuum, as indicated by cessation of the blood flow into the tube. The suction of the evacuated tube automatically draws the blood into the tube.
Principle. The tube must fill from the bottom up to prevent venous reflux. If the evacuated tube is removed before the vacuum is exhausted, a rush of air enters the tube, damaging the red blood cells. Also, a tube containing an anticoagulant must be filled completely to ensure accurate test results.

Fill the tube in a downward position.

19. Procedural Step. Remove the tube from the plastic holder. If the tube contains a clot activator, gently invert the tube back and forth five times before laying it down. If the tube contains an anticoagulant, gently invert the tube 8 to 10 times.
Principle. The rubber sheath covers the point of the needle, stopping the flow of blood until the next tube is inserted. You must invert a tube containing an anticoagulant before laying it down, to prevent the blood from clotting. Careful mixing of the blood with a clot activator or an anticoagulant prevents hemolysis.

PROCEDURE 31-2   Venipuncture—Butterfly Method—cont'd

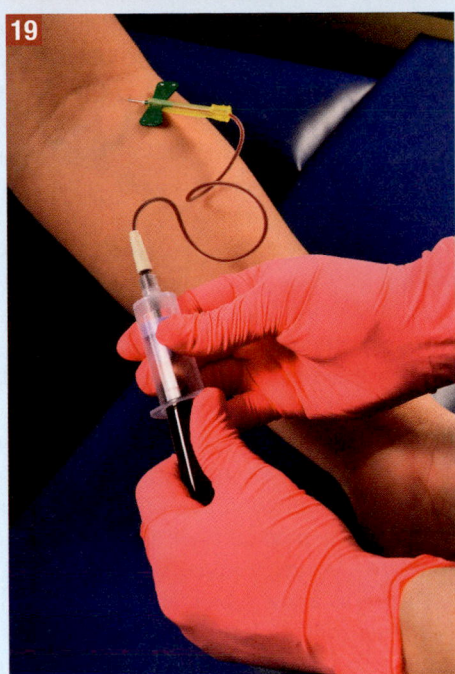

Remove the tube from the holder.

20. Procedural Step. Using the flange, carefully insert the next tube into the holder. Continue in this manner until the last tube has been filled.

21. Procedural Step. Remove the tension from the tourniquet by pulling upward on one of the flaps of the tourniquet. Ask the patient to unclench the fist.
Principle. The tourniquet tension must be removed before the needle. Otherwise, pressure on the vein from the tourniquet could cause internal and external bleeding around the puncture.

22. Procedural Step. Remove the last tube from the holder. Immediately invert the tube back and forth five times if it contains a clot activator and 8 to 10 times if it contains an anticoagulant.
Principle. Removing the last tube from the holder prevents blood from dripping out of the tip of the needle after it has been removed from the patient's arm.

23. Procedural Step. Place a sterile gauze pad slightly above the puncture site. Grasp the setup just below the wings, and slowly withdraw the needle at the same angle as for penetration. Immediately move the gauze over the puncture site, and apply firm pressure. (*Note:* Do not apply pressure to the puncture site until the needle has been completely removed.) Cooperative patients can be asked to assist by applying pressure with the gauze pad. Grasp the base of the needle's safety shield with the

thumb and index fingers of one hand, and with the other hand grasp either wing. Slide the wing back into the rear slot of the safety shield until you hear an audible click, which indicates the shield has locked into place (see Figure 31-18, *A, B*).
Principle. Placing the gauze pad above the puncture site helps prevent tissue movement as the needle is withdrawn and reduces patient discomfort. Careful withdrawal prevents further tissue damage.

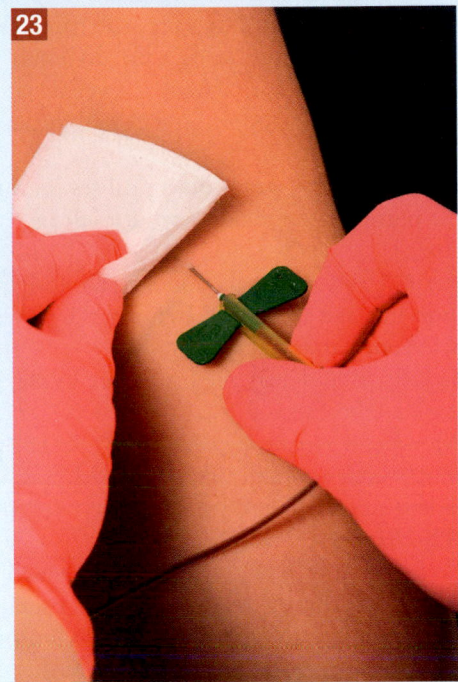

Release the tourniquet and remove the needle.

24. Procedural Step. Immediately discard the winged infusion set and attached plastic holder. Holding onto the plastic holder, first drop the needle into a biohazard sharps container, followed by the tubing and holder. Do not remove the plastic holder from the setup; the plastic holder must be discarded and not reused.
Principle. Proper disposal is required by the OSHA Standard to prevent a needlestick injury; even though the safety shield has been activated to encase the butterfly needle, a needlestick injury can still result from the posterior needle, which is covered with only a rubber sleeve. Plastic holders are often contaminated with blood and must not be reused.

25. Procedural Step. Continue to apply pressure with the gauze pad. The arm can be elevated to facilitate clot formation. Do not allow the patient to bend the arm at the elbow because this increases blood loss from the puncture site.

Continued

PROCEDURE 31-2   Venipuncture—Butterfly Method—cont'd

Principle. Applying pressure reduces the leakage of blood from the puncture site externally or internally. Internal leakage into the tissues could result in a hematoma.

26. Procedural Step. Stay with the patient until the bleeding has stopped. Remove pressure, and inspect the puncture site to ensure that the opening is sealed with a clot. Apply an adhesive bandage to the puncture site. As an alternative, the gauze pad can be folded into quarters and taped onto the puncture site to be used as a pressure bandage. Instruct the patient not to pick up anything heavy for about an hour. (*Note:* If swelling or discoloration occurs, apply an ice pack to the site after bandaging it.)

Principle. Lifting a heavy object causes pressure on the puncture site, which could result in bleeding.

27. Procedural Step. Place the tubes in an upright position in a test tube rack. Remove the gloves, and sanitize your hands.

28. Procedural Step. Chart the procedure in the patient's medical record.

   a. *Paper-based patient record:* Record the date and time, which arm and vein were used, unusual patient reactions, and your initials (refer to the PPR charting example).

   b. *Electronic medical record:* Document which arm and vein were used and any unusual patient reactions using the appropriate radio buttons, drop-down menus, and free text fields.

29. Procedural Step. If needed, process the specimen (e.g., centrifuging the specimen to separate serum from the cells). Test the specimen or prepare the specimen for transport to an outside laboratory for testing according to the medical office policy. If the specimen is to be transported to an outside laboratory, do the following:

   a. Place the specimen tube in a biohazard specimen bag.

   b. Place the laboratory request in the outside pocket of the specimen bag.

   c. Properly handle and store the specimen while awaiting pickup by a laboratory courier.

   d. Chart the date the specimen was transported to the laboratory in the patient's medical record.

Principle. The biohazard bag protects the laboratory courier from the possibility of an exposure incident. The outside laboratory must have the completed request form to know which laboratory tests have been ordered by the physician. The specimen must be handled and stored properly to maintain the in vivo characteristics of the specimen.

PPR CHARTING EXAMPLE

Date	
4/10/XX	10:30 a.m. Venous blood specimen collected from Ⓛ arm. Picked up by Medical Center Laboratory on 4/10/XX. ———
	———————— D. Glover, CMA (AAMA)

PROBLEMS ENCOUNTERED WITH VENIPUNCTURE

Sometimes the medical assistant encounters problems when attempting to draw blood from a patient. The appropriate response depends on the type of problem.

FAILURE TO OBTAIN BLOOD

Periodically, even individuals highly skilled at performing venipuncture have difficulty obtaining blood. Although large and prominent veins make it easier to collect the blood specimen, conditions often exist that make the procedure more difficult.

It is often difficult to draw blood from obese patients who have small, superficial veins and whose veins suitable for venipuncture are buried in adipose tissue. Elderly patients with arteriosclerosis may have veins that are thick and hard, making them difficult to puncture. Other patients have veins that are small or have a thin wall, making the veins likely to collapse. After two unsuccessful attempts at venipuncture, the medical assistant should seek assistance in obtaining the blood specimen.

Factors that result in failure to obtain blood after the needle has been inserted include not inserting the needle far enough, preventing it from entering the vein (Figure 31-21); insertion of the needle too far, causing it to go through the vein; and the bevel opening becoming lodged against the wall of the vein. In these instances, most authorities recommend removing the needle rather than trying to probe the vein. Probing is often uncomfortable for the patient and can affect the integrity of the blood specimen, leading to inaccurate test results. Occasionally, an evacuated tube loses its vacuum because of a manufacturing defect or through improper handling of the tube. If suspected, this problem can be corrected by removing the defective tube and inserting another vacuum tube.

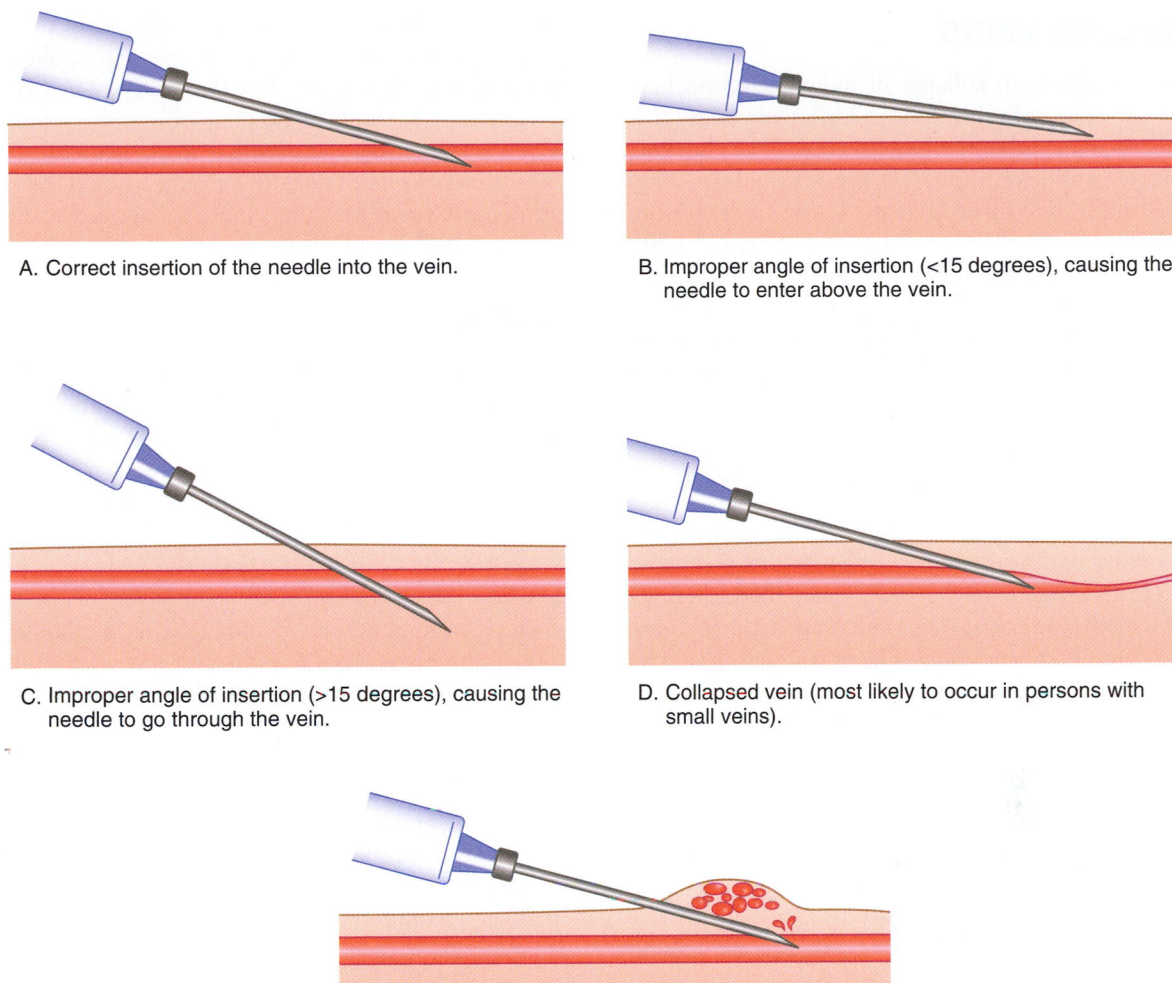

A. Correct insertion of the needle into the vein.

B. Improper angle of insertion (<15 degrees), causing the needle to enter above the vein.

C. Improper angle of insertion (>15 degrees), causing the needle to go through the vein.

D. Collapsed vein (most likely to occur in persons with small veins).

E. The beveled opening is partially within and partially outside of the vein, causing a hematoma.

Figure 31-21 Problems encountered with venipuncture.

INAPPROPRIATE PUNCTURE SITES

If a patient complains of pain or soreness in a potential venipuncture site, this area should be avoided. In addition, any skin areas that are scarred, bruised, burned, or adjacent to areas of infection should not be used. A venipuncture should not be performed on an arm with edema or an arm on the same side as a mastectomy. Swelling makes is more difficult to locate a vein and results in a longer time for healing of the puncture site to occur. Other sites to avoid include an arm that has a cast applied to it and an arm on the same side as a radical mastectomy.

SCARRED AND SCLEROSED VEINS

An individual who has had many venipunctures over a period of years often develops scar tissue in the wall of the vein. Elderly patients may have veins that have become thickened from arteriosclerosis. In both cases, the veins feel stiff and hard when palpated. A scarred or sclerosed vein is difficult to stick, and the blood return may be poor owing to a narrowed lumen; it is recommended that another vein be used for the venipuncture. If this is impossible, the needle should be inserted with careful pressure to avoid going completely through the vein.

ROLLING VEINS

The median cubital vein, located in the center of the antecubital space, is considered the best vein for a venipuncture. Sometimes it is impossible to use this vein, however, such as when it lies deep in the tissues and cannot be palpated or is scarred from repeated venipunctures. The veins on either side of the median cubital (cephalic or basilic) can be used, but they have a tendency to "roll," or move away from the needle, escaping puncture. To prevent rolling, firm pressure should be applied below and to the side of the vein to stabilize it as the needle is inserted.

COLLAPSING VEINS

Veins are most likely to collapse in individuals who have small veins or veins with thin walls. This is particularly true when the vacuum tube method is used. The "sucking action" exerted on the vein when the pressure in the vacuum is released causes the vein to collapse, blocking the flow of blood into the tube (see Figure 31-21). The typical result observed is that a small amount of blood enters the tube and then stops. Because better control and less pressure on the vein are possible, the butterfly method of venipuncture is recommended to obtain the specimen in patients with small veins.

PREMATURE NEEDLE WITHDRAWAL

Patient movement or improper venipuncture technique can cause the needle to come out of the vein prematurely. Because of the pressure exerted by the tourniquet, blood may be forced out of the puncture site, and immediate action is required to prevent a hematoma. The tourniquet should be removed at once, a gauze pad placed on the puncture site, and pressure applied until the bleeding has stopped.

HEMATOMA

A hematoma is caused by blood leaking from the puncture site of the vein and into the surrounding tissues, resulting in a bruise. A hematoma is caused by a needle that is inserted too far and goes through the vein, a bevel opening that is partially in the vein and partially out of the vein (see Figure 31-21), and insufficient pressure applied to the puncture site after removal of the needle. The first sign of a hematoma is a sudden swelling around the puncture site. If this occurs when the needle is in the patient's vein, first the tourniquet and then the needle should be removed immediately, and pressure should be applied to the puncture site until the bleeding stops.

HEMOLYSIS

The blood specimen should be handled carefully at all times. Blood cells are fragile, and rough handling may cause hemolysis, or breakdown of the blood cells. Hemolyzed blood specimens produce inaccurate test results. To prevent hemolysis, these guidelines should be followed:

1. Store the vacuum tubes at room temperature because chilled tubes can result in hemolysis.
2. Allow the alcohol to air-dry completely before performing the venipuncture. Alcohol entering a blood specimen can cause hemolysis.
3. Use an appropriate-gauge needle to collect the specimen. Using a small-gauge needle (e.g., 25 G) can cause the blood cells to rupture as they pass through the lumen of the needle.
4. Practice good technique in collecting the specimen; excessive trauma to the blood vessel can result in hemolysis.
5. Always handle the blood tube carefully; do not shake it or handle it roughly.

HIGHLIGHT on Vasovagal Syncope (Fainting)

Most people experience no change in their sense of well-being when they have blood taken. A very small percentage of individuals experience a type of fainting, however, known as *vasovagal syncope.*

Cause and Symptoms

Vasovagal syncope is caused by unpleasant physical or emotional stimuli, such as pain, fright, and the sight of blood. A sudden pooling of blood occurs, which results in a sudden decrease in blood pressure. This momentarily deprives the brain of blood, causing a temporary loss of consciousness, usually lasting only 1 to 2 minutes. Vasovagal syncope usually occurs when an individual is in an upright position, as in standing or sitting. Before fainting, the patient usually experiences some warning signals, such as sudden lightheadedness, nausea, weakness, yawning, paleness, blurred vision, a feeling of warmth, and sweating followed by drooping eyelids; a weak, rapid pulse; and finally unconsciousness.

Treatment

A person who is about to faint should be placed in a position that facilitates blood flow to the brain and told to breathe deeply. The preferred position is lying down (supine) with the legs elevated and the collar and clothing loosened. This position may not always be possible, such as when a patient is seated and the venipuncture needle has already been inserted. In this case, the tourniquet and then the needle should be removed, and the patient's head should be lowered between the legs. An individual who has fainted should be protected from injury from falling and should be placed in a position that facilitates blood flow to the brain, as just described.

Prevention

Fainting during or after venipuncture is more likely in the following individuals: patients having a venipuncture for the first time, young patients, thin patients, patients with a low diastolic or high systolic blood pressure, patients with a history of fainting, nervous and apprehensive patients, and patients who are very quiet or very talkative. Fainting often can be prevented by identifying and closely observing individuals who are more likely to faint (as described). Talking to the patient often helps relax the patient and divert attention from the venipuncture procedure. If a patient has a history of fainting, he or she should be in a semi-Fowler position for the venipuncture procedure because people rarely faint in this position. Other factors that contribute to fainting and that should be avoided include fatigue, lack of sleep, hunger, and environmental factors, such as a noisy, crowded, or overheated room. ■

FAINTING

Occasionally a patient experiences dizziness or fainting during or after a venipuncture. Should this occur, the most immediate concern is to protect the patient from injury—for example, by preventing the patient from falling. The patient should be placed in a position that promotes blood flow to the brain, and the physician should be notified for further treatment; see the box *Highlight on Vasovagal Syncope (Fainting).*

OBTAINING A SERUM SPECIMEN

SERUM

Serum is plasma from which the clotting factor fibrinogen has been removed.

Serum is normally clear in appearance and light yellow to yellow in color. Serum contains many dissolved substances, such as glucose, cholesterol, sodium, potassium, chloride, antibodies, hormones, and enzymes. As a result, many laboratory tests require a serum specimen to determine whether levels of these substances are within normal limits and to detect substances that should not normally be in the serum and that if present indicate a pathologic condition.

TUBE SELECTION

A tube without an anticoagulant (e.g., red-stoppered or SST) must be used to collect the blood specimen, to allow the specimen to separate into serum and clotted blood cells. Because the amount of serum recovered is only a portion of the specimen, a blood specimen must be drawn that is 2.5 times the amount required for the test. If 2 mL of serum is required, a 5-mL tube of blood must be collected; if 3 mL of serum is required, an 8-mL tube of blood is collected; and if 4 mL of serum is required, a 10-mL tube of blood is collected.

PREPARATION OF THE SPECIMEN

After the blood specimen has been collected, the red-stoppered tube or SST must be allowed to stand upright at room temperature for 30 to 45 minutes before being centrifuged. This allows clot formation of the blood cells, which yields more serum from the specimen. If the specimen is centrifuged too soon after collection of the blood specimen, the clotting factors do not have an opportunity to settle down into the cell layer to form a whole blood clot. The result of this is the formation of a *fibrin clot* in the serum layer. A fibrin clot is a spongy substance that occupies space, interfering with adequate serum collection (Figure 31-22). The blood specimen should not be allowed to stand for longer than 1 hour, however, because leaching of substances from the cell layer into the serum may occur. This leaching of substances changes the integrity of the serum, leading to inaccurate test results.

Serum

Fibrin clot

Figure 31-22 A fibrin clot may interfere with adequate collection of serum.

REMOVAL OF SERUM

After the specimen has been allowed to stand and the blood cells have clotted, the specimen is centrifuged for 10 minutes. If a red-stoppered tube has been used to collect the specimen, the serum is removed from the clot using a pipet and is placed in a separate transfer tube. It is important that proper technique be employed in removing the serum, to avoid disturbing the cell layer of the clot and drawing red blood cells into the serum layer. If cells do enter the serum, the entire specimen must be recentrifuged.

When the serum has been removed from the blood specimen, the medical assistant should hold the specimen in the transfer tube up to good light. The serum specimen should be inspected for the presence of intact red blood cells or hemolyzed blood; in both cases, the specimen has a reddish appearance. A specimen that has a reddish appearance must be recentrifuged. If the specimen contains intact red blood cells, they settle to the bottom of the tube, and the serum can be removed. If the blood is hemolyzed, recentrifugation would not make the red color disappear because the red blood cells have ruptured and released hemoglobin into the serum. Hemolyzed serum is unsuitable for laboratory tests because the results would be inaccurate; another blood specimen must be collected.

SERUM SEPARATOR TUBES

A serum separator tube (SST), also known as a *gel barrier tube,* is an evacuated tube specially designed to facilitate the collection of a serum specimen. The SST is identified by a red/gray stopper (or gold stopper for Hemogard tubes) and is used for collection and separation of blood. The SST

Figure 31-23 Serum separator tubes. **A,** An unused tube that contains the thixotropic gel in the bottom of the tube. **B,** A tube that has been used to collect a blood specimen. During centrifugation, the gel temporarily becomes fluid and moves to the dividing point between the serum and blood cells in a fibrin clot.

contains a thixotropic gel, which is in a solid state at the bottom of the unused tube (Figure 31-23, *A*).

The blood specimen is collected and processed following the appropriate venipuncture method. The specimen must be allowed to stand in an upright position for 30 to 45 minutes for proper clot formation of the blood cells and must be centrifuged as previously described. During centrifugation, the gel temporarily becomes fluid and moves to the dividing point between the serum and clotted cells, where it re-forms into a solid gel, serving as a physical and chemical barrier between the serum and the clot (Figure 31-23, *B*). It is important to centrifuge the specimen for the proper length of time (i.e., 10 minutes). Centrifuging the specimen for less than 10 minutes can result in an incomplete gel barrier between the serum and the clot.

The serum can be transported or stored in the separator tube; the medical assistant must inspect the tube carefully to ensure that the gel barrier is firmly attached to the glass wall. If a complete barrier has not formed, the serum specimen must be removed and placed in a properly labeled transfer tube to prevent leaching of substances from the cell layer into the serum, affecting the accuracy of the test results.

SKIN PUNCTURE

A skin puncture is used to obtain a capillary blood specimen and is also called a *capillary puncture.* Laboratory testing of a capillary blood specimen is usually performed at the

medical office. Examples of such tests are hemoglobin, hematocrit, blood glucose, mononucleosis, and prothrombin time.

A skin puncture is performed when a test requires only a small blood specimen. Skin puncture is the method preferred for obtaining blood from infants and young children. Collecting blood from patients in this age group by venipuncture is often difficult and may damage veins and surrounding tissues. In addition, infants and young children have such a small blood volume that removing large quantities of blood may cause anemia. A skin puncture also might be performed as a last resort on an adult when a blood specimen is needed and there are no acceptable veins. Before collecting a capillary blood specimen, the medical assistant must (1) select a puncture site, (2) select the skin puncture device, and (3) obtain the proper microcollection device to collect the specimen.

PUNCTURE SITES

The puncture site varies depending on the age of the patient. The fingertip of the third or fourth finger is the preferred site for a skin puncture in an adult. In the past, the earlobe also was recommended as a skin puncture site for an adult. This is no longer true. Blood obtained by puncturing the earlobe has been found to contain a higher concentration of hemoglobin than fingertip blood. In addition, the earlobe produces a slower flow of blood, making it more difficult to obtain a blood specimen.

In an infant (birth to 1 year old), the skin puncture should be performed on the plantar surface of the heel. A finger puncture should *never* be performed on infants. The amount of tissue between skin surface and bone is so small that an injury to the bone is likely. After a child has begun to walk, the skin puncture can be performed on the fingertip.

SKIN PUNCTURE DEVICES

According to OSHA, a skin puncture should be performed in the medical office using either a disposable or a reusable semiautomatic retractable lancet device. The device used to perform the skin puncture is a matter of personal preference, and the technique for performing the puncture depends on the device that is used. A description of skin puncture devices is presented next, and procedures for using them are presented at the end of this section.

Regardless of the skin puncture device, the puncture must not penetrate deeper than 3.1 mm in adults and 2.0 mm in infants (plantar surface of the heel) and children. If the puncture is deeper than this, the bone may be penetrated, which could result in the painful and serious conditions of osteochondritis or osteomyelitis. **Osteochondritis** is inflammation of bone and cartilage, and **osteomyelitis** is inflammation of the bone or bone marrow caused by bacterial infection. To avoid these complications, skin puncture devices with a spring-loaded blade (available in different lengths) are used to control the depth of puncture. The length of the blade used to perform a skin puncture is based on the sizes of the patient's fingers and the amount of blood specimen required. Adults with thin fingers and children require a shorter blade to avoid penetration of the bone. A longer blade must be used to obtain enough blood to fill a microcollection device, whereas a shorter blade can be used if only a drop of blood is needed.

OSHA does not recommend the use of lancets that are not retractable. A lancet that is not retractable increases the possibility that the medical assistant will stick himself or herself accidentally, resulting in an exposure incident. A disadvantage of a lancet that is spring-loaded and does not retract automatically is that some patients may become apprehensive and flinch when they see the point of the lancet. Children might pull their hands out of the medical assistant's grasp.

DISPOSABLE SEMIAUTOMATIC LANCET

A disposable semiautomatic retractable lancet consists of a spring-loaded plastic holder with a metal blade inside the holder. Disposable lancets are available in different lengths of blades to control the depth of the puncture. The plastic holder may be color-coded by the manufacturer for ease in identifying the blade length of the lancet device—for example, Surgilance Safety Lancet (Surgilance, Norcross, Ga) (Figure 31-24, *A*). The plastic holder conceals the blade so the patient cannot see it during the puncture, as with the CoaguChek Lancet (Roche Diagnostics, Branchburg, NJ) (Figure 31-24, *B*). Another example is the Quikheel Infant Lancet (Becton Dickinson), which is used for heel punctures in infants.

For the skin puncture, the lancet device is placed on the patient's skin, and the device is activated. Depending on the brand, this is accomplished by one of the following methods:

- Depressing an activation button located on the top of the lancet until an audible click is heard (e.g., CoaguChek Lancet)
- Pushing the lancet firmly onto the puncture site until an audible click is heard (e.g., Surgilance Safety Lancet)

When the device is activated, the spring forces the blade into the skin and retracts the blade into the holder. The concealed blade and automatic puncture tend to result in less patient apprehension. After the puncture, the entire lancet device is discarded in a biohazard sharps container. Procedure 31-3 describes the skin puncture procedure for use of a disposable semiautomatic lancet.

Figure 31-24 **A,** Surgilance color-coded lancet devices. **B,** CoaguChek Lancet device. **C,** Glucolet 2.

PROCEDURE 31-3

tissue surrounding the puncture firmly but gently to encourage blood flow.

Principle. Squeezing or massaging the site excessively causes dilution of the blood sample with tissue fluid, leading to inaccurate test results.

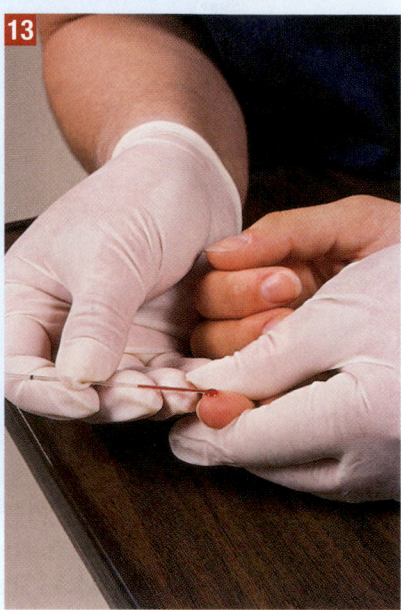

Collect the specimen.

14. **Procedural Step.** Collect the blood specimen on a test strip or in the appropriate microcollection device.
15. **Procedural Step.** Have the patient hold a gauze pad over the puncture and apply pressure until the bleeding stops. As a safety precaution, remain with the patient until the bleeding stops. If needed, apply an adhesive bandage.
16. **Procedural Step.** Test the blood specimen by following the manufacturer's instructions that accompany the blood analyzer or testing kit.
17. **Procedural Step.** Remove the gloves, and sanitize your hands.

MICROCOLLECTION DEVICES

After the skin has been punctured, a capillary blood specimen must be collected. The blood specimen can be collected directly onto a reagent strip, such as occurs with blood glucose monitors. It also can be collected in a small container known as a *microcollection device*. The device depends on the laboratory equipment running the test. Common microcollection devices are capillary tubes and microcollection tubes.

CAPILLARY TUBES

A capillary tube consists of a disposable glass or plastic tube (Figure 31-25, *A*). Depending on the size of the tube, it can hold 5 to 75 μL of blood. In the medical office, a capillary tube is used to collect a blood specimen for a hematocrit determination. This procedure is presented in Chapter 32.

MICROCOLLECTION TUBES

A microcollection tube consists of a small plastic tube with a removable blood collector tip. The tip is designed to collect capillary blood from a skin puncture, which results

in a relatively large blood specimen. After the specimen has been collected, the collector tip is removed, discarded, and replaced by a plastic plug. Microcollection tubes are available with or without anticoagulants. The plugs are color-coded and correspond to the color-coded evacuated tube system used in venipuncture. One such device is the Microtainer (Becton Dickinson) (Figure 31-25, *B*).

GUIDELINES FOR PERFORMING A FINGER PUNCTURE

1. If a laboratory test requires advance preparation, before you perform the finger puncture, verify that the patient has prepared properly. If this is not the case, do not collect the specimen unless directed otherwise by the physician. If the finger puncture is to be rescheduled, carefully review the preparation requirements with the patient.
2. The patient should be seated comfortably in a chair. The arm should be firmly supported and extended with the palmar surface of the hand facing up. Never perform a skin puncture with the patient sitting on a stool or standing. The patient may faint and injure himself or herself.

Capillary tubes   Microcollection tubes

Figure 31-25 Microcollection devices.

Middle finger

Figure 31-26 Recommended sites for a finger puncture.

3. Instruct the patient to remain still during the procedure. Explain to the patient that the procedure should be relatively quick and only slightly uncomfortable. Just before making the puncture, tell the patient that he or she will "feel a small stick." This prevents startling the patient, which could cause the patient to move.

4. Use the lateral part of the tip of the third or fourth finger (middle or ring finger) of the nondominant hand for the puncture site. The capillary beds in these fingers are large, and the skin is easy to penetrate. The puncture site should be free of lesions, scars, bruises, and edema. The index finger is not recommended as a puncture site. The index finger is more calloused, which makes it harder to penetrate than the other fingers. Also, the patient uses that finger more and would notice the pain longer. The little finger also should not be used as a puncture site. The amount of tissue between the skin surface and the bone is so small that using this finger as a puncture site could result in injury to the bone.

5. After selecting the puncture site, warm the site to increase the blood flow to the capillary bed. Warming the site can be accomplished by gently massaging the finger five or six times from base to tip, or by placing the hand in warm water for a few minutes (105° F [40° C]). Warming the site promotes bleeding after an effective puncture.

6. Cleanse the site with an antiseptic wipe, and allow it to dry thoroughly. The site must be dry to allow a round drop of blood to form on the finger. Otherwise, the drop would leach out onto the skin of the patient's finger and be difficult to collect. In addition, alcohol entering the capillary specimen contaminates it, leading to inaccurate test results. Alcohol also causes the patient to experience a stinging sensation when the puncture is made.

7. Firmly grasp the finger in front of the most distal knuckle joint. Apply enough pressure to cause the fin-

gertip to become hard and red so that adequate penetration and depth of puncture will occur.

8. Make the puncture in the fleshy portion of the fingertip, slightly to the side of center. To prevent injury to the bone, do not puncture the side or very tip of the finger. The blade of the lancet should be positioned so that the puncture is perpendicular to the lines of the fingerprint rather than parallel to the fingerprint (Figure 31-26). This facilitates the formation of a well-formed drop of blood that is easy to collect. A puncture that is not perpendicular causes the blood flow to follow the lines of the fingerprint and run down the finger, making it difficult to collect.

9. Firmly press the lancet device against the puncture site, and activate the spring-loaded puncturing device. If a good puncture has been made, the blood flows freely. When learning this procedure, many individuals do not apply enough pressure to obtain a puncture that is deep enough. If this occurs, a poor blood flow results and the patient has to be punctured again. A deep puncture hurts no more than a superficial one and provides a much better blood flow.

10. Wipe away the first drop of blood with a gauze pad. The first drop of blood is diluted with alcohol and tissue fluid and is not a suitable specimen for testing. Using the first drop of blood may lead to inaccurate test results.

11. Allow a large drop of blood to form by applying continual gentle pressure near the puncture site. Collect the blood specimen using a reagent strip or the appropriate microcollection device. If the required amount of blood is not obtained, you can gently massage the tissue surrounding the puncture site to promote blood flow. Do not squeeze or massage excessively because doing so causes dilution of the blood specimen with tissue fluids, which can affect the accuracy of the test results.

12. Check the puncture site to make sure the bleeding has stopped. Apply an adhesive bandage, if needed. A bandage is not recommended for children younger than 2 years. The bandage may irritate the skin of a young child, and the child might put the bandage in his or her mouth, aspirate it, and choke.

What Would You Do? What Would You *Not* Do? RESPONSES

Case Study 1
Page 824

What Did Dori Do?
❑ Told Angela that it was fine to have her friend there while she gets her blood drawn.
❑ Told Angela that she could not have the blood drawn out of her left arm because a good vein could not be located in that arm.
❑ Told Angela that using the hand veins is always the last choice when drawing blood. Explained to Angela that there will just be a small stick and that it will heal quickly, and there should be no reason it would affect her softball game this evening.
❑ Tried to relax and reassure Angela before the venipuncture. Carefully explained the procedure to her because it was her first one.
❑ Because Angela is nervous, took precautions to prevent her from fainting by placing her in a semi-Fowler position on the examining table.
❑ Had Angela's friend stand near the head of the table to help calm her down.

What Did Dori Not Do?
❑ Did not try to draw Angela's blood from her left arm or hand.
❑ Did not ignore the fact that Angela was nervous about the venipuncture.

Case Study 2
Page 828

What Did Dori Do?
❑ Told Buzz that when a butterfly setup is used, the air in the tubing alters the test results. Explained that the red tube is

used to get rid of the air, and because it is not needed for testing, it is thrown away.
❑ Stressed to Buzz how important it is to have his blood tested every week, which helps the physician determine if there is too much or too little Coumadin in his body. Explained to him again what might occur if his Coumadin were at the wrong level.
❑ Told Buzz that the office would help him locate a medical laboratory where he will be vacationing, so he can have his test done.
❑ Made sure that Buzz had a laboratory requisition so that he could have his test done while he was on vacation.

What Did Dori Not Do?
❑ Did not tell Buzz that it would be all right to skip his prothrombin test during his vacation.

Case Study 3
Page 837

What Did Dori Do?
❑ Told Mrs. Gabriel that the laboratory can accept only specimens drawn at the laboratory or at the medical office.
❑ Told Mrs. Gabriel that if it would make her feel more comfortable, the laboratory could drop off the blood-drawing supplies at the office, and her blood could be drawn tomorrow at the office.
❑ Informed the physician about Mrs. Gabriel's experience at the laboratory.

What Did Dori Not Do?
❑ Did not tell Mrs. Gabriel that probing a vein could cause the test results to be inaccurate.

↻ TERMINOLOGY REVIEW

Key Term	Word Parts	Definition
Antecubital space	*ante-:* before	The surface of the arm in front of the elbow.
Anticoagulant	*anti-:* against	A substance that inhibits blood clotting.
Buffy coat		A thin, light-colored layer of white blood cells and platelets that lies between a top layer of plasma and a bottom layer of red blood cells when an anticoagulant has been added to a blood specimen.
Evacuated tube		A closed glass or plastic tube that contains a premeasured vacuum.
Hematoma	*hemat/o:* blood *-oma:* tumor or swelling	A swelling or mass of coagulated blood caused by a break in a blood vessel.
Hemoconcentration	*hem/o:* blood	An increase in the concentration of the nonfilterable blood components in the blood vessels, such as red blood cells, enzymes, iron, and calcium, as a result of a decrease in the fluid content of the blood.
Hemolysis	*hem/o:* blood *-lysis:* breakdown	The breakdown of blood cells.

↻ TERMINOLOGY REVIEW—cont'd

Key Term	Word Parts	Definition
Osteochondritis	*oste/o:* bone *myel/o:* bone marrow *-itis:* inflammation	Inflammation of bone and cartilage.
Osteomyelitis	*oste/o:* bone *myel/o:* bone marrow *-itis:* inflammation	Inflammation of the bone or bone marrow as a result of bacterial infection.
Phlebotomist	*phleb/o:* vein *tomist:* specialist	A health care professional trained in the collection of blood specimens.
Phlebotomy	*phleb/o:* vein *-otomy:* incision	Incision of a vein for the removal of blood; the collection of blood.
Plasma		The liquid part of the blood consisting of a clear, straw-colored fluid that comprises approximately 55% of the blood volume.
Serum		Plasma from which the clotting factor fibrinogen has been removed.
Venipuncture	*ven/o:* vein	Puncturing of a vein.
Venous reflux	*ven/o:* vein *-ous:* pertaining to	The backflow of blood (from an evacuated tube) into the patient's vein.
Venous stasis	*ven/o:* vein *stasis:* control, stop	The temporary cessation or slowing of the venous blood flow.

ON THE WEB

For information on phlebotomy:

Clinical and Laboratory Standards Institute: www.clsi.org

Lab Explorer: www.labexplorer.com

American Society for Clinical Laboratory Science (ASCLS): www.ascls.org

American Society for Clinical Pathology (ASCP): www.ascp.org

American Society of Phlebotomy Technicians (ASPT): www.aspt.org

Becton Dickinson: www.bd.com

National Phlebotomy Association (NPA): www.nationalphlebotomy.org

The Safety Lady: www.safetylady.com

My Blood Draw: www.myblooddraw.com

Phlebotomy Pages: www.phlebotomypages.com

Center for Phlebotomy Education: www.phlebotomy.com

Outcome Perform a hematocrit determination

Equipment/Supplies

- Microhematocrit centrifuge
- Disposable gloves
- Lancet
- Antiseptic wipe
- Gauze pads

- Capillary tubes
- Sealing compound
- Adhesive bandage
- Biohazard sharps container

1. **Procedural Step.** Sanitize your hands. Greet the patient and introduce yourself. Identify the patient by full name and date of birth, and explain the procedure.

2. **Procedural Step.** Assemble equipment. Open the gauze packet. Cleanse the puncture site with an antiseptic wipe, and allow it to air-dry. Apply gloves and perform a finger puncture, then dispose of the lancet in a biohazard sharps container.
   Principle. Personal protective equipment and proper disposal of the lancet are required by the OSHA standard to prevent exposure to bloodborne pathogens.

3. **Procedural Step.** Wipe away the first drop of blood with a gauze pad. Fill the first capillary tube by holding one end of it horizontally, but slightly downward, next to the free-flowing puncture. Keep the tip of the capillary tube in the blood, but do not allow it to press against the patient's skin. Calibrated tubes are filled to the calibration line; uncalibrated tubes are filled approximately three quarters (within 10 to 20 mm of the end of the tube). The blood is drawn into the tube through capillary action. Fill a second tube using the method just described. Place a gauze pad over the puncture site and apply pressure.
   Principle. Not keeping the tip of the capillary tube in the blood can cause air bubbles in the stem of the tube, which leads to inaccurate test results. Allowing the capillary tube to press against the skin closes the opening of the capillary tubes and does not allow blood to enter. The type of tube (calibrated or uncalibrated) is based on the method used to read the test results. The hematocrit should be performed in duplicate to ensure accurate and reliable test results.

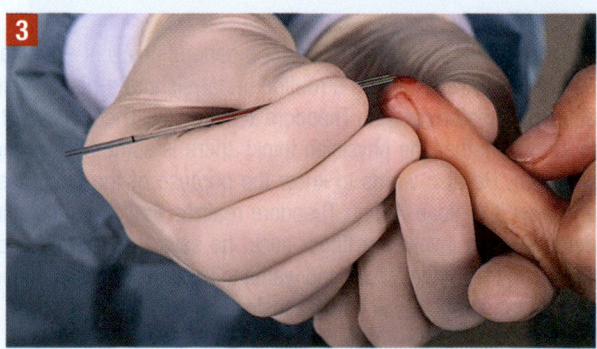
Fill the capillary tube.

4. **Procedural Step.** Push the dry end of the tube (end opposite the filling end that does not contain blood) down into the sealing compound. This seals the end of the capillary tube. The sealing compound can be used to hold the capillary tubes until they are ready to be placed in the microhematocrit centrifuge. To do this, place the sealing compound on a flat surface with the tubes in a vertical position. Before removing a capillary tube from the sealing compound, rotate the tube between the thumb and index finger to prevent the sealing compound from pulling out when the tube is lifted out of the sealing compound.
   Principle. Blood in the capillary tube at the end being sealed prevents a successful closure, which may cause leakage of the blood specimen, leading to inaccurate test results. Capillary tubes must be sealed properly to prevent leakage of the blood specimen during centrifugation.

Seal the end of the tube.

5. **Procedural Step.** Check the patient's puncture site for bleeding and apply an adhesive bandage, if needed.

6. **Procedural Step.** Place the capillary tubes in the microhematocrit centrifuge with the sealed end facing out. Balance one tube with the other capillary tube placed on the opposite side of the centrifuge.
   Principle. Placing the sealed end toward the outside prevents the blood specimen from spinning out of the capillary tube when the centrifuge is in operation.

PROCEDURE 32-1   Hematocrit—cont'd

Place the tube in the centrifuge.

Align the bottom of the red cell column with the 0 line.

Read the results.

7. Procedural Step. Place the cover on the centrifuge, and lock it securely. Centrifuge the blood specimen for 3 to 5 minutes at a speed of 10,000 rpm. *Principle.* Centrifuging the blood specimen causes the red blood cells to become packed and to settle on the bottom of the tube.

8. Procedural Step. Allow the centrifuge to come to a complete stop. Read the results, as follows:

Calibrated tube. If a capillary tube with a calibration line was used, read the results using the special graphic reading device that is part of the centrifuge. Adjust the capillary tube so that the bottom of the red blood cell column (just above the sealing compound) is placed on the 0 line. With a magnifying glass, read the results at the top of the packed red blood cell column, and you will see a percentage on the reading device.

Uncalibrated tube. If an uncalibrated tube was used, you must use a microhematocrit reader card to determine the results; place the top of the plasma column on the 100% mark and the bottom of the cell column on the 0 line. Read the results on the scale, which corresponds to the top of the packed cell column.

In both cases, the buffy coat should not be included in the reading. The answer represents the percentage of blood volume occupied by the red blood cells. (The hematocrit determination on this reading device is 38.)

Principle. Stopping the centrifuge with your hands can injure you and can damage the machine.

9. Procedural Step. Read the second tube in the manner just described; the results of the tubes should agree within 4 percentage points. If not, the hematocrit procedure must be repeated. If they are within 4 percentage points, the two values are averaged to derive the test results.

Continued

PROCEDURE 32-1   Hematocrit—cont'd

10. **Procedural Step.** Properly dispose of the capillary tubes in a biohazard sharps container. Remove gloves and sanitize your hands.

11. **Procedural Step.** Chart the results in the patient's medical record.

   a. *Paper-based patient record:* Record the date and time and the hematocrit results (refer to the PPR charting example).

   b. *Electronic medical record:* Document the hematocrit results using the appropriate radio buttons, drop-down menus, and free text fields.

12. **Procedural Step.** Return the equipment to its proper storage place. Store the sealing compound at room temperature. Exposing it to a temperature above 80° F adversely affects its consistency.

Reference Range for Hematocrit

Female: 37% to 47%
Male: 40% to 54%

PPR CHARTING EXAMPLE	
Date	
5/5/XX	11:15 a.m. Hct: 38%. —————— ——————— L. Sharpe, CMA (AAMA)

PATIENT TEACHING | **Iron-Deficiency Anemia**

Answer questions that patients have about iron-deficiency anemia.

What is anemia?

Anemia is a shortage of red blood cells or hemoglobin. Hemoglobin, the part of the blood that gives red blood cells their color, carries oxygen to all the cells in the body. There are many types of anemia, of which iron-deficiency anemia is the most common. Other types of anemia include pernicious anemia, sickle cell anemia, hemolytic anemia, and aplastic anemia.

What causes iron-deficiency anemia?

In general, iron-deficiency anemia is caused by conditions that deplete the iron stored in the body; it can result from an increased need for iron by the body or an increased loss of iron from the body. Iron-deficiency anemia may occur in children younger than 2 years if their diet does not include enough iron to meet the demands of rapid growth. This is especially true in children whose main source of nutrition during these years is breast milk or bottle milk, because milk contains very little iron. Adolescent girls are prone to iron-deficiency anemia because of growth spurts during puberty and blood loss through menstruation. In adults, the most common cause of anemia is chronic blood loss, such as from a bleeding ulcer or bleeding hemorrhoids and heavy menstrual bleeding. Pregnant women also are at increased risk because of the demands of the growing fetus.

What can be done for individuals at risk for iron-deficiency anemia?

Individuals prone to developing iron-deficiency anemia are encouraged to increase foods in their diet that contain iron, such as beef, liver, spinach, eggs, and iron-fortified breads and cereals. As a preventive measure, the physician usually prescribes vitamin supplements for individuals who are at increased risk for developing iron-deficiency anemia, such as pregnant women, infants, and young children. Infant formulas and cereals that have been supplemented with iron are also available.

What are the symptoms of anemia?

All types of anemia have the same general symptoms. Often these symptoms do not develop right away; when they do develop, feeling tired and run down may be the only sign of anemia. Other symptoms that may occur, particularly as the anemia becomes worse, are paleness of the skin, fingernail beds, and mucous membranes; shortness of breath, especially during physical activity; dizziness; headache; irritability; and inability to concentrate. These symptoms result from the diminished ability of the blood to carry oxygen to the cells of the body. Blood tests are necessary to diagnose anemia and to determine the specific type of anemia present.

How is iron-deficiency anemia treated?

The most important part of treating anemia is to determine its cause, such as not enough iron consumed in the diet or chronic blood loss, and to correct that condition. The physician usually prescribes an iron supplement to replace the iron that has been depleted from the body. It is typically prescribed in oral form, but it is given through an injection in special situations. An oral iron supplement causes the stool to turn a black, tarlike color. This is normal and should not be a cause for concern. Also, an effort should be made to consume foods high in iron content.

- For patients who have had a vitamin supplement prescribed to *prevent* iron-deficiency anemia, such as children younger than 2 years and pregnant women, emphasize to the patient (or parent) the importance of taking the vitamin supplement every day to prevent the development of iron-deficiency anemia.

- For patients who have had an iron supplement prescribed to *treat* iron-deficiency anemia, emphasize to the patient the importance of taking the iron supplement for the period of time prescribed by the physician, because replacement of iron takes time.

- Instruct patients to keep iron supplements out of the reach of children to prevent iron poisoning.

- Provide patients with written educational materials about anemia. ∎

Figure 32-4 Coulter blood cell counter. (Courtesy Holzer Health Systems, Athens, Ohio.)

WHITE BLOOD CELL COUNT

The white blood cell (WBC) count is used by the physician to assist in the diagnosis and prognosis of disease. The white blood cell count is an approximate measurement of the number of white blood cells in the circulating blood. The reference range for a white blood cell count is 4500 to 11,000 white blood cells per cubic millimeter of blood, which is expressed as 4.5 to 11 $(\times10^3/mm^3)$ on laboratory reports. An increase in the white blood cell count, or **leukocytosis,** is most commonly seen in acute infection such as appendicitis, chickenpox, diphtheria, infectious mononucleosis, meningitis, and rheumatic fever. Normal elevation of the white blood cell count can occur with pregnancy, strenuous exercise, stress, and treatment with corticosteroids. Conditions that result in **leukopenia,** or a decrease in the white blood cell count, include viral infections, chemotherapy, and radiation therapy.

If performed in the medical office, a CLIA-nonwaived automated blood cell counter must be used to obtain the WBC count, which is a moderately complex test. Blood cell counters also are able to perform a red blood cell count, platelet count, hemoglobin, hematocrit, and differential white blood cell count , as well as calculation of red blood cell indices. Examples of nonwaived blood cell counters include the QBC Autoread Plus (Becton, Dickinson), the Cell-Dyn (Abbott, Santa Clara, Calif.), and the Coulter (Beckman Coulter, Brea, Calif.) (Figure 32-4).

RED BLOOD CELL COUNT

The red blood cell (RBC) count is a measurement of the number of red blood cells in whole blood. The range for the red blood cell count in a healthy woman is 4 to 5.5 million red blood cells per cubic millimeter of blood, expressed on laboratory reports as 4 to 5.5 $(\times10^6/mm^3)$. The range for a healthy man is 4.5 to 6.2 million red blood cells per cubic millimeter of blood, expressed on a laboratory report as 4.5 to 6.2 $(\times10^6/mm^3)$. In the medical office, the red blood cell count is performed using a blood cell counter.

Conditions that cause a decrease in the RBC red blood cell count include anemia, Hodgkin disease, and leukemia; conditions that cause an increase in red blood cells include polycythemia, dehydration, and pulmonary fibrosis.

RED BLOOD CELL INDICES

The red blood cell (RBC) indices are measurements that are reported as part of the CBC (complete blood count) test. RBC indices provide the physician with information about the size and hemoglobin content of a patient's red blood cells. The RBC indices include the MCV (mean corpuscular volume), MCH (mean corpuscular hemoglobin), MCHC (mean cell hemoglobin concentration), and RDW (red cell distribution width). The RBC indices are obtained from calculations performed on certain test results included in a CBC—specifically, the RBC count, hemoglobin, and hematocrit. The calculation is automatically performed by the blood cell analyzer that performs the CBC.

A decrease in the number of red blood cells or in the amount of hemoglobin is known as *anemia*. More than 400 types of anemia have been identified, but many of them are rare conditions. Each of the various forms of anemia (e.g., iron-deficiency anemia, pernicious anemia) may alter one or more of the RBC indices in a particular way. This information is used by the physician to assist in the diagnosis of the type of anemia a patient has and in determination of its cause.

What Would You Do? What Would You *Not* Do?

Case Study 2

Baylee Frasure brings in her 6-month-old son, Travis, for a well-child visit. Mrs. Frasure has been breast feeding Travis since he was born, and he is not yet on solid food. She says that Travis has been doing just fine, but he did not like his liquid vitamins, so she stopped giving them to him. Mrs. Frasure says that she is eating a well-balanced diet and takes a multivitamin every day, so she did not think this would be a problem. Travis's hemoglobin is checked during the visit, and it is 8 g/dL. The physician prescribes ferrous sulfate drops for Travis. After the physician leaves the room, Mrs. Frasure becomes quite upset. She says she does not understand why Travis's hemoglobin is so low. She says that she thought that breast milk provided the best nutrition possible for infants. ■

Figure 32-5 Types of human blood cells. *1* to *7*, White blood cells (leukocytes) stained as they are in the laboratory to show the many types. They play the active role in immune response or in defense against disease. *1*, Neutrophil; *2*, neutrophilic band; *3*, eosinophil; *4*, basophil; *5*, lymphocyte; *6*, (large) lymphocyte; *7*, monocyte; *8*, platelets (thrombocytes), which are responsible for clotting; and *9*, red blood cells (erythrocytes), which carry oxygen. (From Custer RP: *An atlas of the blood and bone marrow*, ed 2, Philadelphia, 1974, Saunders.)

WHITE BLOOD CELL DIFFERENTIAL COUNT

There are five types of white blood cells, or leukocytes, each having a certain size, shape, appearance, and function (Figure 32-5). The purpose of the differential cell count is to identify and count the five types of white blood cells in a representative blood sample. An increase or decrease in one or more types may occur in pathologic conditions; this assists the physician in making a diagnosis.

The differential cell count can be performed automatically or manually. The automatic method is faster and more convenient; however, the manual method allows for closer inspection of abnormal white blood cells. If a differential cell count is performed on an automated analyzer at an outside laboratory and abnormalities are flagged by the analyzer, the laboratory will then perform a differential cell count by using the manual method.

AUTOMATIC METHOD

The automatic method involves the use of a blood cell counter, such as the Coulter cell counter (see Figure 32-4). The specimen requirement is an ethylenediaminetetraacetic acid (EDTA)–anticoagulated blood specimen, which is obtained through venipuncture using a lavender-stoppered tube. The blood cell counter automatically performs the differential cell count, and the results are printed on a laboratory report.

MANUAL METHOD

If a physician orders a manual differential cell count on a blood specimen, the medical assistant must prepare two blood smears at the medical office for transport to the outside laboratory. The preparation of a blood smear is outlined in Procedure 32-2. Fresh whole blood is preferred for blood smears; however, a satisfactory smear can be made from an EDTA-anticoagulated blood specimen, provided that the smear is made within 24 hours after collection. Other anticoagulants should not be used because they could alter the morphology and staining reaction of the white blood cells. After preparing the blood smear, the medical assistant places the slides in a protective slide container for transport to an outside laboratory.

The blood smear is evaluated at the laboratory by medical laboratory personnel. Because white blood cells are clear and colorless, they must be stained with an appropriate dye (usually Wright stain) before a differential count is performed. The nucleus, the cytoplasm, and any granules in the cytoplasm take on the characteristic color of their cell type; this aids in proper identification. A minimum of 100 white blood cells are identified on the blood smear using a microscope, and each cell is assigned to its appropriate category (neutrophil, eosinophil, basophil, lymphocyte, or monocyte). The number of each type of leukocyte is recorded as a percentage and reflects the overall distribution of white blood cells in the patient's bloodstream. During the manual evaluation of the blood smear, the laboratory technologist will also examine the slide for abnormalities in the morphology of the red blood cells, including their size, shape, and structure.

Reference Range

The healthy adult reference range for each type of white blood cell making up the total number of leukocytes is as follows:

Neutrophils: 40% to 75%
Eosinophils: 1% to 6%
Basophils: 0% to 2%
Lymphocytes: 20% to 40%
Monocytes: 3% to 10%

Memories *from* Practicum

Latisha Sharpe: During my practicum experience, I had a female patient who drank too much the night before and had been vomiting for 3 hours before coming to the physician's office. Although this incident was self-inflicted, I still found myself feeling deeply sorry for the patient. She was so weak she could not hold her head up, so I stayed with her and held her head up while she was vomiting. I stayed with her throughout this time, and my sympathy for her really made a difference. No matter what the situation is, I always let the patient know that I care. ∎

What Would You Do? | What Would You *Not* Do?

Case Study 3

Marjorie Merrick comes to the office for a follow-up visit to discuss her laboratory results with the physician. Marjorie is in perimenopause and has been having problems with heavy menstrual periods, hot flashes, insomnia, fatigue, and shortness of breath. Marjorie's laboratory tests indicate that she has iron-deficiency anemia. The physician orders an injection of iron dextran, Z-track technique, and instructs Marjorie to take an iron supplement every day and to return in 3 months for a recheck. Marjorie says she has heard that an iron injection can stain the skin and wants to know whether that is true. She says she has a friend who has anemia, and he has to go in every week for a vitamin B_{12} shot. Marjorie wants to know whether she will have to do that, too. Marjorie signed up to donate blood this week at her church's Red Cross blood drive. She wants to know whether it is all right for her to donate. ∎

PROCEDURE 32-2

PROCEDURE 32-2   Preparation of a Blood Smear for a Differential Cell Count

Outcome Prepare a blood smear for a differential white blood cell count

Equipment/Supplies

- Disposable gloves
- Supplies to perform a finger puncture or venipuncture
- Lavender-stoppered evacuated tube
- Slides with a frosted edge

- Slide container
- Biohazard specimen bag
- Laboratory request form
- Biohazard sharps container

1. **Procedural Step.** Sanitize your hands. Greet the patient and introduce yourself. Identify the patient by full name and date of birth, and explain the procedure.
2. **Procedural Step.** Assemble the equipment. Using a pencil, label two slides on the frosted edge with the patient's name and date of birth, and the date.
   Principle. Laboratories request the preparation of two blood smears as a means of quality control.

3. **Procedural Step.** Open the gauze packet. Cleanse the puncture site with an antiseptic wipe. Apply gloves, obtain a blood sample from the patient, and place a drop of fresh whole blood on each slide as follows:
   From a venipuncture. You can obtain the blood specimen from the fresh whole blood left in the needle immediately after performing a venipuncture for a CBC (using a

Continued

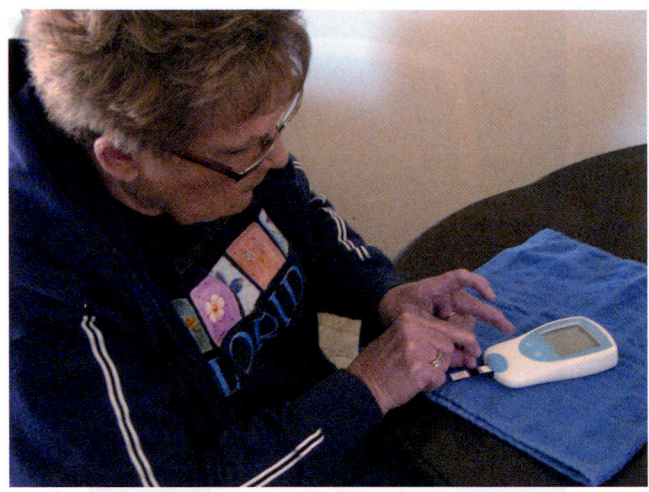

Figure 32-8 Patient performing a PT/INR test at home.

order from the physician. This provides a distinct advantage because patients are able to check their PT/INR immediately when conditions occur that might indicate a problem, such as nosebleeds, bleeding gums, or unexplained bruising. In these situations, treatment can be instituted immediately to prevent the problem from getting worse. Other factors that can affect the PT/INR results and cause them to be outside of the patient's ideal range include the following: a change in diet; use of prescription or over-the-counter medications that interact with warfarin; vitamins and herbal preparations; a change in the level of exercise; illness; smoking; and alcohol consumption. It is important that the patient keep his or her physician informed of any factors that may alter the body's response to warfarin.

What Would You Do? | What Would You *Not* Do? | RESPONSES

Case Study 1
Page 857

What Did Latisha Do?
❑ Told Theodore that the physician was running some routine screening tests on him to make sure he is in good health. Explained that all patients have these tests run as part of a physical examination.
❑ Told Theodore that it was not possible to get the specimen from the earlobe. Explained that the earlobe is not recommended as a good site from which to obtain blood.
❑ Reassured Theodore that the finger-stick would be made on the least sensitive part of his finger. Told him that it would hurt for just a second and then it would be all over and it would heal quickly.
❑ Told Theodore that the purpose of the blood test is early detection of anemia. Explained that if anemia is present, it can be caught early and treated before symptoms develop.

What Did Latisha Not Do?
❑ Did not collect the specimen from Theodore's earlobe.
❑ Did not tell Theodore that he is healthy and does not have anything wrong with him.

Case Study 2
Page 861

What Did Latisha Do?
❑ Commended Mrs. Frasure on eating nutritiously.
❑ Told Mrs. Frasure that breast milk does not contain very much iron. Explained that because of this, it is important to give Travis his liquid vitamins, which have iron in them.
❑ Reassured Mrs. Frasure that breast feeding does provide very good nutrition for Travis.

❑ Explained to Mrs. Frasure that the iron supplement may cause Travis's stool to be a dark, tarlike color, and she should not be alarmed because this is normal.

What Did Latisha Not Do?
❑ Did not criticize Mrs. Frasure for not giving Travis his vitamins or make her feel it was her fault that his hemoglobin was low.

Case Study 3
Page 863

What Did Latisha Do?
❑ Told Marjorie that the iron injection can stain the skin but that it would be given in a special way to prevent that from happening.
❑ Told Marjorie that vitamin B_{12} injections are given for pernicious anemia and that her type of anemia is iron-deficiency anemia.
❑ Gave Marjorie a patient education brochure on iron-deficiency anemia to take home with her.
❑ Told Marjorie that the Red Cross requires that a blood donor's hemoglobin level be within the normal range. Explained that she could not donate this time, but that when her hemoglobin is back to normal, she will be able to donate.
❑ Explained to Marjorie that the iron supplement may cause her stool to be a dark, tarlike color, and she should not be alarmed because this is normal.

What Did Latisha Not Do?
❑ Did not tell Marjorie that her friend has pernicious anemia because there is no way of knowing this.

↻ TERMINOLOGY REVIEW

Key Term	Word Parts	Definition
Anemia	*an-:* without or absence of *-emia:* blood condition	A condition in which there is a decrease in the erythrocytes or amount of hemoglobin in the blood.
Anticoagulant	*anti-:* against *-coagulant:* clotting	A substance that inhibits blood clotting.
Hematology	*hemat/o:* blood *-ology:* study of	The study of blood and blood-forming tissues.
Hemoglobin	*hem/o-:* blood *-globin:* protein	The protein- and iron-containing pigment of erythrocytes that transports oxygen in the body.
Leukocytosis	*leuk/o:* white *cyt/o:* cell *-osis:* abnormal condition (means "increased" when used with blood cell word parts)	An abnormal increase in the number of white blood cells (more than 11,000 per cubic millimeter of blood).
Leukopenia	*leuk/o:* white *-penia:* abnormal reduction in number	An abnormal decrease in the number of white blood cells (fewer than 4500 per cubic millimeter of blood).
Polycythemia	*poly-:* many *cyt/o:* cell *hem/o:* blood *-ia:* condition of diseased or abnormal state	A disorder in which there is an increase in the red blood cell mass.

ON THE WEB

For information on anemia:

National Anemia Action Council: www.anemia.org

Anemia Education: www.anemia.com

American Society of Hematology: www.hematology.org/patients/blood-disorders/anemia/5225.aspx

For information on leukemia:

Leukemia and Lymphoma Society: www.lls.org

Leukemia Research Foundation: www.leukemia-research.org

Leukemia: www.healthcommunities.com/health-topics/cancer.shtml

National Cancer Institute: Leukemia: www.cancer.gov/cancertopics/types/leukemia

American Cancer Society: Leukemia: www.cancer.org/cancer/leukemia-charoniclymphocyticcll/index

For information on clotting disorders:

American Society of Hematology Bleeding Disorders: www.hematology.org/patientsblood-disorders/5219.aspx

National Alliance for Thrombosis and Thrombophilia: www.stoptheclot.org

Clot Care Online Resource: www.clotcare.com

Blood Chemistry and Immunology

Ⓔ Check out the Evolve site at http://evolve.elsevier.com/Bonewit/today/ to access additional interactive activities and exercises to help you study and prepare for success.

LEARNING OBJECTIVES

Blood Chemistry

1. Explain the purpose of a blood chemistry test.
2. Explain the functions of glucose and insulin in the body.
3. State the patient preparation for a fasting blood glucose test.
4. Identify the reference range for a fasting blood glucose test.
5. State the purpose of each of the following tests: fasting blood glucose test, 2-hour postprandial glucose test, and oral glucose tolerance test.
6. Describe the procedure for a 2-hour postprandial blood glucose test.
7. Identify the patient preparation required for an oral glucose tolerance test.
8. State the restrictions that must be followed by the patient during an oral glucose tolerance test.
9. List three advantages of self-monitoring of blood glucose by diabetic patients.
10. Explain the purpose of the hemoglobin A_{1c} test.
11. State the hemoglobin A_{1c} level for an individual without diabetes.
12. State the recommended blood glucose level and hemoglobin A_{1c} percentage for an individual with diabetes.
13. Explain the storage requirements for blood glucose test strips.
14. Describe the functions of LDL cholesterol and HDL cholesterol in the body.
15. State the desirable ranges for each of the following tests: total cholesterol, LDL cholesterol, and HDL cholesterol.
16. State the patient preparation for a triglyceride test.

Immunology

17. Explain the purpose of each of the following immunologic tests: hepatitis test, HIV tests, syphilis tests, mononucleosis test, rheumatoid factor, antistreptolysin test, C-reactive protein, cold agglutinins, ABO and Rh blood typing, and Rh antibody titer.
18. List the symptoms of infectious mononucleosis.

PROCEDURES

Perform a fasting blood glucose test using a glucose monitor.
Instruct a patient on how to measure blood glucose using a glucose monitor.
Perform blood chemistry testing using an automated blood chemistry analyzer and operating manual.

Demonstrate the proper care and maintenance of a glucose monitor.
Perform a rapid mononucleosis test.

CHAPTER OUTLINE

INTRODUCTION TO BLOOD CHEMISTRY AND IMMUNOLOGY
BLOOD CHEMISTRY
COLLECTION OF A BLOOD CHEMISTRY SPECIMEN
AUTOMATED BLOOD CHEMISTRY ANALYZERS
Quality Control
Calibration
Controls
BLOOD GLUCOSE
Blood Glucose Testing
Fasting Blood Glucose Test

Two-Hour Postprandial Blood Glucose Test
Oral Glucose Tolerance Test
TESTS FOR MANAGEMENT OF DIABETES
Self-Monitoring of Blood Glucose
Frequency of Testing
Test Results
Advantages
Hemoglobin A_{1c} Test
Interpretation of Results

GLUCOSE METERS
Reagent Test Strips
Calibration Procedure
Control Procedure
Care and Maintenance
CHOLESTEROL
HDL and LDL Cholesterol
Cholesterol Testing
Interpretation of Results
Patient Preparation
CLIA-Waived Cholesterol Analyzers
TRIGLYCERIDES
BLOOD UREA NITROGEN

IMMUNOLOGY
IMMUNOLOGIC TESTS
Hepatitis Tests
HIV Tests
Syphilis Tests
Mononucleosis Test
Rheumatoid Factor
Antistreptolysin O Test
C-Reactive Protein
Cold Agglutinins
ABO and Rh Blood Typing
Rh Antibody Titer
RAPID MONONUCLEOSIS TESTING

KEY TERMS

agglutination (ah-gloo-ti-NAY-shun)
analyte (AN-uh-lyte)
antibody (AN-ti-bod-ee)
antigen (AN-ti-jen)
blood antigen

glycogen (GLIE-koe-jen)
glycosylation
HDL cholesterol
hemoglobin A_{1c}
hyperglycemia (hie-per-glie-SEE-me-ah)

hypoglycemia (hie-poe-glie-SEE-me-ah)
LDL cholesterol
lipoprotein (lie-poe-PROE-teen)

INTRODUCTION TO BLOOD CHEMISTRY AND IMMUNOLOGY

CLIA-waived blood chemistry and immunologic laboratory tests are often performed in the medical office. Advances in CLIA-waived automated blood analyzers and testing kits designed specifically for use in the medical office have made this possible. Automated blood analyzers perform laboratory tests in a short time with accurate test results.

This chapter is divided into two units. The first presents blood chemistry laboratory tests, and the second presents immunologic tests. The material in this chapter about blood testing is intended to serve only as a basic guide for the medical assistant and should be supplemented by much well-supervised practice in a classroom laboratory, the medical office, or both.

BLOOD CHEMISTRY

Blood chemistry testing involves the quantitative measurement of chemical substances in the blood. These chemicals are dissolved in the liquid portion (plasma) of the blood. Numerous types of blood chemistry tests are available; the type of test (or tests) the physician orders depends on the clinical diagnosis. Examples of common blood chemistry tests include alanine aminotransferase (ALT), alkaline phosphatase (ALP), aspartate aminotransferase (AST), blood urea nitrogen (BUN), calcium, chloride, cholesterol,

creatinine, globulin, glucose, lactate dehydrogenase (LD), phosphorus, potassium, sodium, total bilirubin, total protein, total thyroxine, triglycerides, and uric acid levels. The blood chemistry tests that are most frequently performed are described in greater detail in this chapter.

COLLECTION OF A BLOOD CHEMISTRY SPECIMEN

Most blood chemistry tests performed at an outside laboratory require a serum specimen for analysis (Figure 33-1). If the specimen is collected at the medical office, the medical assistant will need to perform a venipuncture using a serum separator tube (SST) or a red-stoppered tube. An example of a blood chemistry profile frequently ordered on patients in the medical office is a *comprehensive metabolic profile* (CMP). A CMP contains numerous blood chemistry tests and is used primarily in routine health screening of a patient. It is frequently used to detect any changes in the body's biologic processes that may be present, although the patient may not have had any symptoms to indicate that these changes have occurred. A comprehensive metabolic profile is also used when the patient's symptoms are so vague that the physician does not have enough concrete evidence to support a clinical diagnosis of a specific organ or disease state. Specimen collection and handling requirements for a comprehensive metabolic profile as presented in a laboratory directory are outlined in Figure 33-2.

Figure 33-1 Most blood chemistry tests are performed on a serum specimen collected in a serum separator tube (SST).

AUTOMATED BLOOD CHEMISTRY ANALYZERS

Automated blood chemistry analyzers are used to perform blood chemistry testing. A blood chemistry analyzer consists of a reflectance photometer that quantitatively measures the amount of chemical substances, or analytes, in the blood. An **analyte** is defined as a substance that is being identified or measured in a laboratory test. Specifically, a reflectance photometer measures light intensity to determine the exact amount of an analyte in a specimen.

Most physicians consider it too expensive in terms of equipment, supplies, and medical laboratory personnel to perform blood chemistry tests that are any more complex than waived tests in the medical office. These tests are usually performed at an outside laboratory. However, if moderately complex blood chemistry tests are performed in the medical office, a "benchtop" blood chemistry analyzer is typically used to run them; examples of these nonwaived benchtop analyzers include the ATAC lab system (Clinical Data, Newton, Mass) (Figure 33-3) and the Reflotron Chemistry Analyzer (Roche Diagnostics, Branchburg, NJ). Examples of CLIA-waived blood chemistry analyzers that are more commonly used to run blood chemistry tests in the medical office include the Accu-Chek Advantage blood glucose meter (Roche Diagnostics), A1cNow (Bayer, Morrisville, NJ), and the Cholestech LDX cholesterol system (Alere, Waltham, MA).

The manufacturer of each blood chemistry analyzer provides an operating manual (and sometimes an instructional video) with the instrument that includes information needed to collect and handle the specimen, perform quality control procedures, and test the specimen. The manufacturer also has personnel available for on-site training and service. Because most medical offices use CLIA-waived blood chemistry analyzers (rather than nonwaived analyzers), the remainder of this chapter focuses on CLIA-waived blood chemistry analyzers used in the medical office.

It is important that the medical assistant become completely familiar with all aspects of the CLIA-waived analyzer used to perform blood chemistry testing in his or her medical office. Medical offices running CLIA-waived tests are required to follow the manufacturer's instructions *exactly* for each testing procedure. Instructions include information on the quality control procedures that must be performed when running the test. Quality control procedures are of particular importance to ensure that the analyzer is functioning properly and that the test results are reliable and accurate. Additional information on quality control procedures is presented here (also refer to the quality control section in Chapter 29).

QUALITY CONTROL

The ultimate goal when performing blood chemistry testing is to ensure that the test accurately measures what it is supposed to measure; this involves practicing and maintaining a quality control program. Quality control consists of methods and means to ensure that test results are reliable and valid. Two important quality control measures must be performed routinely when a blood chemistry analyzer is used: calibration of the instrument and running controls.

Calibration

Calibration is a mechanism used to check the precision and accuracy of a blood chemistry analyzer to determine if the system is providing accurate results. A calibration check detects errors caused by laboratory equipment that is not working properly. Calibration is typically performed using a calibration device, often called a *standard*. The calibration device may come in the form of a calibration strip or cassette. The device is inserted into the analyzer (Figure 33-4, *A*) and the calibration results are displayed on the LCD screen of the analyzer. The calibration results are then compared with the expected results provided in the product insert or on the calibration device (Figure 33-4, *B*). If the calibration procedure does not perform as expected, patient testing should not be conducted until the problem has been identified and resolved. The frequency of performing a calibration check is indicated in the manufacturer's instructions. At a minimum, a calibration check should be performed when a new lot number of testing reagents is put into use.

Comprehensive Metabolic Profile

CPT Code: 80053

Tests included: albumin, albumin/globulin ratio (calculated), alkaline phosphatase, ALT, AST, BUN/creatinine ratio (calculated), calcium, carbon dioxide, chloride, creatinine, globulin, glucose, potassium, sodium, total bilirubin, total protein.

Type of specimen: Serum

Amount: 4 mL

Collection supplies: SST (send entire tube)

Collection techniques: Let SST stand for 30 minutes. Centrifuge SST within 45 minutes of collection to separate serum from cells with gel barrier.

Patient preparation: Patient should fast for 12 to 14 hours prior to collection.

Handling and storage: Refrigerate or store at room temperature. Stable at room temperature for 24 hours and stable in the refrigerator for 72 hours.

Causes for rejection: Nonfasting specimen, hemolysis, improper labeling of tube

Reference range: Values given with report.

Use:
The CMP is used as a screening test to assess the overall health of an individual. It is used to detect any changes in the body's biologic processes that may be present, although the patient may not have had any symptoms to indicate these changes have occurred. Also see uses of individual tests.

Limitations: See individual tests for limitations.

Methodology: See individual tests for methodologies.

Figure 33-2 Specimen collection and handling requirements for a comprehensive metabolic profile as presented in a laboratory directory.

Figure 33-3 Blood chemistry analyzer. (Courtesy of Holzer Health Systems, Athens, OH.)

Controls

A blood chemistry control consists of a solution that is used to monitor a blood chemistry analyzer to ensure the reliability and accuracy of the test results. Controls consist of commercially available solutions with known values. Controls usually come with a product insert, which lists the expected ranges for control results (Figure 33-5); however, expected ranges may sometimes be printed on the containers of the testing reagents. Controls are used to determine if the testing reagents are performing properly and to detect any errors in technique by the individual performing the test.

In general, two levels of controls must be performed on a blood chemistry analyzer. A *low-level control* (also known as a *Level 1 control*) produces results that fall below the reference range for the test; a *high-level control* (also known as a *Level 2 control*) produces results that fall above the reference

Calibration device

Calibration results

Expected results

Figure 33-4   A, Calibrating a blood chemistry analyzer using a calibration device. **B,** The calibration results are compared with the expected results on the calibration device.

Figure 33-5 Controls come with a product insert, which lists the expected ranges for control results.

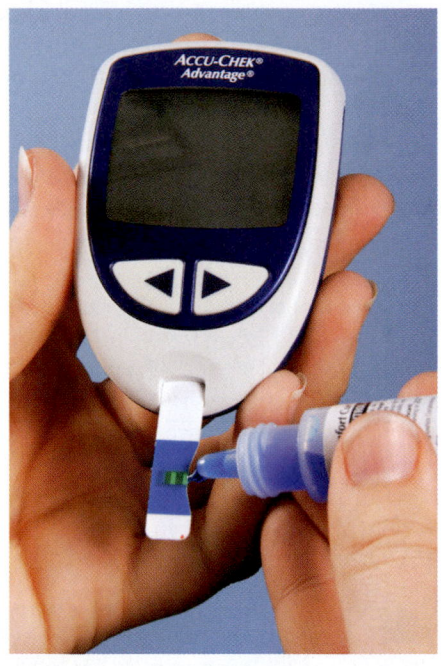

Figure 33-6 The control solution is added to a testing strip.

range for the test. The control procedure is performed in a similar manner to the procedure for performing the test on a specimen collected from a patient. Instead of the patient specimen being added to the testing device, however, the control is added to it (Figure 33-6). The control results are compared with expected results provided in the product insert (see Figure 33-5) or on the container of the testing reagents (Figure 33-7).

Failure of a control to produce expected results may be caused by the following: deterioration of testing components as a result of expiration or improper storage; improper environmental testing conditions; or errors in the technique used to perform the procedure. If the controls do not perform as expected, patient testing should not be conducted until the problem has been identified and resolved.

The frequency of performing controls is indicated in the manufacturer's instructions. At a minimum, they should be performed on each new lot number of testing reagents, and thereafter on a regular basis, such as monthly.

BLOOD GLUCOSE

Glucose is the end product of carbohydrate metabolism; it is the chief source of energy for the body. Energy is needed to perform normal functions and to maintain body

Figure 33-7 The control results are compared with the expected results.

temperature. The body maintains a constant blood glucose level to ensure a continuous source of energy for the body. Ingested glucose that is not needed for energy can be stored for later use in the form of **glycogen** in muscle and liver tissue. When no more tissue storage is possible, excess glycogen is converted to triglycerides (a form of fat) and is stored as adipose tissue.

Insulin is a hormone that is secreted by the beta cells of the pancreas and is required for normal use of glucose in the body. Insulin enables glucose to enter the body's cells and be converted to energy. Insulin also is needed for the proper storage of glycogen in liver and muscle cells.

BLOOD GLUCOSE TESTING

Measuring the amount of glucose in a blood specimen is one of the most commonly performed blood chemistry tests. It is used to detect abnormalities in carbohydrate metabolism such as those that occur in prediabetes, diabetes, gestational diabetes, **hypoglycemia,** and liver and adrenocortical dysfunction. Blood glucose is measured by several different testing methods, which include the fasting blood glucose, the 2-hour postprandial blood sugar test, and the oral glucose tolerance test. Each of these methods serves a specific role in diagnosing and evaluating abnormalities in carbohydrate metabolism, and each is described in greater detail here.

Fasting Blood Glucose Test

Blood glucose is usually measured when the patient is in a fasting state. This type of test, termed a *fasting blood glucose* (FBG) test, involves collecting a fasting blood sample and measuring the amount of glucose in it. The patient should not have anything to eat or drink except water for 12 hours preceding the test. Certain medications, such as oral contraceptives, salicylates, diuretics, and steroids, may affect the test results; the physician may place the patient on medication restrictions for a specific period before the test—usually 3 days. The patient should be scheduled for the test in the

morning to minimize the inconvenience of abstaining from food and fluid.

An FBG is often performed on patients diagnosed with diabetes to evaluate their progress and regulate treatment, and on other patients as a routine screening test to detect prediabetes and diabetes. *Prediabetes* is the term used to describe the condition in which glucose levels are higher than normal, but not high enough to be classified as diabetes. An individual with prediabetes has an increased risk of developing type 2 diabetes. The American Diabetes Association (ADA) recommends the following guidelines for interpretation of FBG test results:

70-99 mg/dL	Normal
100-125 mg/dL	Prediabetes (also termed *impaired fasting glucose*)
126 mg/dL or above	Diabetes (confirm by repeating the FBG test on another day)

Two-Hour Postprandial Blood Glucose Test

The 2-hour postprandial blood glucose (2-hour PPBG) test is used to screen for diabetes and to monitor the effects of insulin dosage in patients with diabetes. The patient is required to fast, beginning at midnight preceding the test and continuing until breakfast. For breakfast, the patient must consume a prescribed meal that contains 100 g of carbohydrate, which consists of orange juice, cereal with sugar, toast, and milk. An alternative to this is the consumption of a 100-g test-load glucose solution. A blood specimen is collected from the patient exactly 2 hours after consumption of the meal or glucose solution.

In a nondiabetic patient, the glucose level returns to the fasting level within $1\frac{1}{2}$ to 2 hours of glucose consumption, whereas the glucose level in a diabetic patient does not return to the fasting level. A postprandial glucose level of 140 g/dL or higher suggests diabetes and warrants further testing, such as the oral glucose tolerance test.

Putting It All Into Practice

My name is Michelle Villers, and I work for a physician in an internal medicine medical office. My primary job responsibility includes running the laboratory at the office. I mainly draw blood and perform blood chemistry tests. I also work up patients, run electrocardiograms, apply Holter monitors, and perform pulmonary function tests.

When performing a venipuncture, you need to make sure all the necessary equipment is on hand and ready. Sometimes you may have a tube that has no vacuum in it. In cases like these, it is always better to have a couple of spare tubes on hand. I recently had an experience in which one of my tubes had no vacuum. Luckily, I had a few extra tubes within arm's reach, so I did not have to interrupt the procedure to get a new one. I have learned that you can never be too prepared. ∎

Oral Glucose Tolerance Test

The oral glucose tolerance test (OGTT) provides more detailed information about the ability of the body to metabolize glucose by assessing the insulin response to a glucose load. The OGTT is used to assist in the diagnosis of prediabetes, diabetes, gestational diabetes, hypoglycemia, and liver and adrenocortical dysfunction. It provides a more thorough analysis of glucose use than is provided by the FBG or the 2-hour PPBG test.

Testing Requirements

The patient is usually required to consume a high-carbohydrate diet, consisting of 150 g of carbohydrate per day, for 3 days before the OGTT. The patient must be in a fasting state when the test begins. On the morning of the test, a blood specimen is drawn from the patient for an FBG. If the FBG indicates **hyperglycemia,** the physician should be notified because this situation is a contraindication to the administration of a large test load of glucose.

After the FBG has been performed, the patient is instructed to drink a solution containing 75 g of glucose within a 5-minute time frame. At regular intervals thereafter a blood specimen is taken to determine the patient's ability to handle the increased amount of glucose. Each blood specimen must be labeled carefully with the exact time of collection. The patient is permitted to eat and drink normally after completion of the test.

It is important that the patient adhere to certain restrictions during the test to ensure accurate results. Because food and fluid affect blood glucose levels, the patient must not eat or drink anything except water during the test. Smoking is not permitted during the test because tobacco is a stimulant that increases the blood glucose level. The patient should remain at the testing site so that he or she is present when needed for collection of blood specimens and to minimize activity. Activity affects the test results by using up glucose; the patient should remain relatively inactive during the test. Sitting and reading is an activity that would be recommended.

What Would You Do? What Would You *Not* Do?

Case Study 1

Crystal Louellen is at the medical office for an oral glucose tolerance test. She says that she tried not to eat anything, but she started shaking, so she stopped at McDonald's on the way over and got a sausage biscuit and orange juice. Crystal gets quite upset when she learns that she has to come back again to have her test run. She said that she hired a babysitter to watch her four preschool-age children. She demands to know why this test takes so long and why she can't have anything to eat before the test. Crystal wants to know if she can bring her children next time, so she doesn't have to hire a babysitter. Crystal says that she's a "nicotine" addict, and when she's not needed for testing, she could take the kids outside to play. She says that way the kids won't bother anyone and she can have a cigarette at the same time. ■

Side Effects

During the test, the patient may experience some normal side effects, including weakness, a feeling of faintness, and perspiration. These are considered normal reactions of the body to a decrease in the glucose level as insulin is secreted in response to the glucose load. The patient should be reassured that this is a temporary condition. Serious symptoms of severe hypoglycemia should be reported immediately to the physician; these may include headache; pale, cold, and clammy skin; irrational speech or behavior; profuse perspiration; and fainting.

Interpretation of Results

As glucose is absorbed into the bloodstream, the blood glucose level of a nondiabetic individual increases to a peak level of 160 to 180 mg/dL approximately 30 to 60 minutes after the glucose solution is consumed. The pancreas secretes insulin to compensate for this rise, and the blood glucose returns to the fasting level within 2 hours of ingestion of the glucose solution.

The individual with diabetes does not exhibit the normal use of glucose just described. This is because individuals with diabetes are unable to remove glucose from the bloodstream at the same rate as nondiabetic individuals. The blood glucose peaks at a much higher level. In addition, blood glucose levels are above normal throughout the test because of the lack of insulin.

Two hours after the glucose solution has been consumed, the test results are interpreted as follows, according to guidelines set forth by the American Diabetes Association (ADA):

139 and below	Normal
140-199 mg/dL	Prediabetes (also known as *impaired glucose tolerance*)
200 mg/dL or above	Diabetes (confirm by repeating the OGTT test on another day)

Hypoglycemia

Hypoglycemia is a condition in which the glucose in the blood is abnormally low (FBG below 70 mg/dL). During the OGTT, patients with this condition exhibit an abnormally low blood glucose level, beginning at the 2-hour interval and continuing for 4 or 5 hours. Hypoglycemia results from removal of glucose from the blood at an excessive rate, or from decreased secretion of glucose into the blood, which can be caused by an overdose of insulin, Addison disease, bacterial sepsis, carcinoma of the pancreas, hepatic necrosis, or hypothyroidism.

TESTS FOR MANAGEMENT OF DIABETES

It is important for individuals with diabetes to manage their condition effectively. This is best accomplished by keeping blood glucose levels as close to normal as possible. Diabetic patients who maintain good blood glucose control generally experience fewer symptoms and delay or prevent long-term complications of the disease; these results can lead to a longer life.

Two testing methods are used for the management of diabetes—self-monitoring of blood glucose (SMBG) and the hemoglobin A$_{1c}$ test. SMBG, which is performed by diabetic patients at home, measures day-to-day fluctuations in blood glucose levels. The hemoglobin A$_{1c}$ test must be ordered by the physician and provides an average or overall picture of the patient's blood glucose levels over time. These testing methods assist the patient and the physician in determining whether the diabetes management plan is working or whether it needs to be adjusted.

SELF-MONITORING OF BLOOD GLUCOSE

Individuals with diabetes cannot usually tell by the way they feel whether or not their blood glucose levels are within normal range. The only way for them to know for certain is by SMBG. SMBG not only provides diabetic patients with feedback for maintaining normal blood glucose levels, it also assists them in anticipating and treating day-to-day, or even hour-to-hour, fluctuations in glucose levels brought on by food, exercise, stress, and infection.

Diabetic patients who take insulin (insulin-dependent diabetes) must monitor their blood glucose levels each day. Based on the results of SMBG, decisions can be made regarding insulin and dietary adjustments that may be necessary to maintain normal glucose levels and to avoid the extremes of hypoglycemia and hyperglycemia (see Chapter 37). Satisfactory control of the blood glucose level on a day-to-day basis through SMBG reduces symptoms of the disease and helps delay or prevent long-term complications that can occur with diabetes.

Memories *from* **Practicum**

Michelle Villers: During my practicum experience, I was assigned to a four-physician pediatric practice. The office was constantly busy with screaming children. As if I were not nervous enough, I was asked to assist in the removal of sutures. When I walked into the room with the physician, beads of sweat began to form on my forehead. A child was lying on the examining table—a little boy no more than 7 years old. He was there to have sutures removed after a recent surgery. The sutures had been tied very well, and it was difficult for the physician to cut them. The little boy lay there with tears streaming down his cheeks. I reassured him and talked to him, and his tears began to subside. "A few more minutes and it will be all over," I told him. And within those next few minutes, the physician cut the last suture. The little boy eagerly hopped down off the examining table and gave me a big hug. I learned that day how a little reassurance can make everyone involved feel better. ■

PATIENT TEACHING | **Diabetes**

Answer questions that patients have about diabetes.

What is diabetes?

Diabetes is a lifelong condition that occurs when the body is not able to use glucose for energy because of a problem with insulin. Diabetes develops when the body produces little or no insulin, or when the body cannot use the insulin it does produce (known as *insulin resistance*). According to the American Diabetes Association, almost 26 million Americans have diabetes; of these, nearly 7 million are not yet diagnosed and are unaware that they have diabetes. An additional 79 million people have prediabetes. Prediabetes is a condition in which the glucose levels of an individual are higher than normal but not high enough to be classified as diabetes. An individual with prediabetes has an increased risk of developing type 2 diabetes.

The cause of diabetes is not completely understood, but it seems that the predisposition to develop diabetes is inherited. Diabetes increases the risk of developing serious complications, including heart disease, blindness (retinopathy), nerve damage (neuropathy), kidney damage (nephropathy), and poor circulation, which can result in amputation of a limb.

What is the function of insulin?

Insulin is a hormone produced and secreted by the beta cells of the pancreas. The pancreas is a gland located just behind the stomach and is about the size of a hand. Insulin is required for the normal use of glucose in the body. Through the process of digestion, carbohydrates are broken down into glucose. Shortly after a meal containing carbohydrates is consumed, glucose levels in the blood begin to increase. This sends a message to the pancreas to secrete insulin. Insulin "unlocks" the cells of the body and allows glucose to enter the cells. Inside the cells, glucose is converted into energy. Glucose is the main source of energy for the body and is needed to carry out normal body functions and to assist in maintaining body temperature.

What are the symptoms of diabetes?

Individuals with diabetes produce little or no insulin or cannot use the insulin they do produce. Without insulin, glucose cannot get into the cells of the body, and it builds up in the bloodstream, resulting in a high blood glucose level, known as *hyperglycemia*. Although blood glucose levels are increased, the body is unable to use the glucose for energy. This results in increased hunger,

Continued

weight loss, and fatigue. The body attempts to get rid of the excess glucose by expelling it in the urine. To be excreted, the glucose must be diluted in large amounts of water. This results in increased urination and increased thirst to replace the water being lost. A summary of the symptoms of diabetes follows:

- Increased urination
- Excessive thirst
- Weight loss
- Constant hunger
- Nausea and vomiting
- Abdominal pain
- Fatigue
- Blurred vision

What is the difference between type 1 diabetes and type 2 diabetes?

Two main categories of diabetes have been identified: type 1 diabetes and type 2 diabetes. Type 2 diabetes is the most common form of diabetes. Approximately 90% of individuals with diabetes have type 2 diabetes.

Type 1 Diabetes

Type 1 diabetes can occur at any age but is most apt to begin in childhood, adolescence, or early adulthood (before age 30). Type 1 diabetes is an autoimmune disease in which the body produces antibodies that attack and gradually destroy the insulin-producing beta cells of the pancreas. This results in an inability of the body to produce any insulin at all, or it may produce very little insulin. The symptoms are usually severe and occur rapidly—typically over weeks or months. Individuals with type 1 diabetes almost always require insulin therapy. The insulin is administered subcutaneously using an insulin syringe and needle or an insulin pen. An insulin pen is an insulin injection device that contains a needle and holds a vial of insulin. Insulin also can be administered through an insulin pump, which is a small, battery-operated device about the size of a cell phone that is clipped to a belt or carried in a pocket (see illustration). The pump is connected to plastic tubing that continuously delivers insulin into the subcutaneous tissue of the abdomen. An insulin pump also can be programmed to deliver varying doses of insulin as a patient's need for insulin changes during the day (e.g., before exercise or meals).

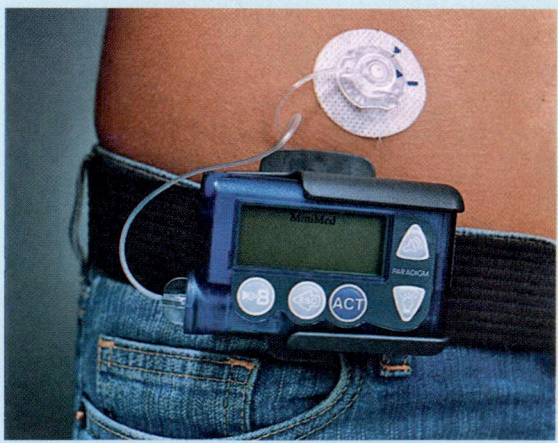

Insulin pump. (From Lewis S: *Medical-surgical nursing*, ed 9, St Louis, 2014, Mosby.)

Type 2 Diabetes

Type 2 diabetes can affect people at any age, but the chance of developing it increases with age, and it is more likely to occur in individuals who are 40 years of age or older. The biggest risk factor for developing type 2 diabetes is excess body weight. As a result of the recent increase in childhood obesity combined with a sedentary lifestyle, type 2 diabetes is starting to appear in younger age groups. Individuals with type 2 diabetes do not produce enough insulin or are not able to use the insulin they do produce (insulin resistance), resulting in high blood glucose levels. Type 2 diabetes almost always has a slow onset with mild symptoms that appear gradually over a long time (often years). Some individuals have no symptoms at all (except for high blood glucose levels). Because of this, they may be unaware that they have diabetes until a complication from prolonged hyperglycemia occurs, such as a vision problem or foot pain. Type 2 diabetes is first treated by dietary adjustments, weight reduction, and exercise. These changes sometimes can restore insulin sensitivity, even if the weight loss is modest. Approximately 20% of cases of type 2 diabetes can be managed by lifestyle changes alone. The next step, if necessary, is treatment with oral hypoglycemics, which are medications taken by mouth that stimulate the release of insulin from the pancreas, help the body use its own insulin better, or both. If this treatment is ineffective, insulin therapy becomes necessary to maintain normal or near-normal glucose levels.

What factors increase the risk of developing type 2 diabetes?

The cause of type 2 diabetes is unknown, although certain factors, known as *risk factors,* make a person more prone to developing type 2 diabetes. The more risk factors present, the more likely it is that an individual will develop type 2 diabetes. Some of these factors can be controlled, and others cannot.

Risk Factors That Can Be Controlled

1. *Weight.* The risk factor that contributes most to the development of type 2 diabetes is excess body weight. Approximately 80% of individuals with type 2 diabetes are overweight. Being overweight (body mass index of 25 or greater) makes it harder for the body to use insulin. A research study by the Diabetes Prevention Program showed that people who followed a low-fat, low-calorie diet; lost a moderate amount of weight; and engaged in regular physical activity (five times a week for 30 minutes) sharply reduced their chances of developing type 2 diabetes.
2. *Smoking.* Smoking makes it harder for the body to control the blood glucose level.
3. *Lack of physical activity.* Regular exercise helps the body to use insulin normally, whereas a sedentary lifestyle contributes to insulin resistance.
4. *High blood pressure, abnormal lipid profile, or both.* The following factors contribute to insulin resistance: blood pressure greater than 130/80 mm Hg, HDL cholesterol of 35 mg/dL or less, and triglyceride level of 250 mg/dL or greater. Decreasing blood pressure also can reduce the risk of cardiovascular complications.

PATIENT TEACHING | **Diabetes—cont'd**

Risk Factors That Cannot Be Controlled

1. *Family history.* The risk of developing type 2 diabetes is increased if a close relative (parent, brother, sister) has diabetes.
2. *Gestational diabetes or having given birth to a large infant.* Women who have diabetes during pregnancy or gave birth to an infant weighing more than 9 lb are at greater risk for developing type 2 diabetes.
3. *Age.* Type 2 diabetes is more common in people 40 years and older, but it is increasing among young people who are overweight and inactive.
4. *Ethnic group.* The following ethnic groups are more likely to develop type 2 diabetes: African Americans, Latinos,

Hispanics, Native Americans, Asian Americans, and Pacific Islanders.

Can diabetes be cured?

There is no cure for diabetes, but the outlook for individuals with this condition is improving. This is primarily because of better patient education, advances in blood glucose monitoring, and newer methods of insulin delivery that help simplify management of the disease. Today, most individuals with diabetes under good control have life expectancies comparable with those of individuals without diabetes. ■

What Would You Do? | What Would You *Not* Do?

Case Study 2

Dave Felden has recently been diagnosed with type 1 diabetes and is taking insulin. He has come to the office for a fasting blood glucose test. A finger-stick will be performed to collect the specimen, and a glucose meter will be used to test the specimen. Dave has been performing this test on himself at home now for 2 weeks and wants to know whether he can stick his own finger. Dave says that he's been having a few problems giving himself his insulin injections. He says that he has been getting some very large air bubbles in his syringe when he draws up the insulin. He says he's been having trouble getting them out and wants to know how important that is. Dave says he is on a limited income and wants to know whether he can use his needle and syringe for more than one injection. ■

Table 33-1 Recommended Blood Glucose Levels for Patients With Diabetes

Time of Day	Recommended Blood Glucose Level (mg/dL)
Before meals	80-120
1-2 hr after meals	100-180
At bedtime	100-140

physician in making decisions regarding the patient's diabetes management plan.

Advantages

Research shows that SMBG is the most effective way for a diabetic patient to maintain a normal blood glucose level and delay or prevent long-term complications associated with diabetes. High blood glucose levels (greater than 180 mg/dL) for a long time can cause progressive damage to the body organs, resulting in blindness, kidney disease, nerve damage, and circulation problems. Because of the necessity of performing a skin puncture and the fact that the patient must assume responsibility in self-management decisions, the medical assistant may need to reinforce the advantages of SMBG, as follows:

1. *Convenience of testing.* The patient is able to test his or her blood at any time of the day without a laboratory order from the physician. This provides a distinct advantage because patients are able to check their blood glucose level when a side effect common to diabetes, such as hypoglycemia, occurs. In these situations, treatment can be instituted immediately to prevent the problem from getting worse.
2. *Greater involvement in self-management decisions.* The patient is able to become more involved in self-management decisions regarding insulin dosage, meal planning, and physical activity. Initially some patients lack confidence in making insulin and dietary adjustments based on the blood glucose test results. The

Frequency of Testing

The frequency of blood glucose testing depends on numerous factors, including the severity of the diabetes, diet, activity level, and special conditions such as pregnancy. Ideally, the blood glucose level for an insulin-dependent diabetic patient should be measured four times a day: in the morning (after an 8-hour fast), before lunch, before dinner, and at bedtime. The FBG test result (obtained in the morning) is the best overall indicator of control, and the other determinations provide guidance for adjusting insulin dosage, diet, and exercise.

Test Results

Blood glucose levels are measured with a glucose meter, and the results are displayed in milligrams per deciliter (mg/dL). Table 33-1 lists recommended blood glucose levels for patients with diabetes based on when the testing is performed. Diabetic patients should be instructed to maintain a cumulative record of their daily SMBG test results for periodic review by the physician. This record assists the medical assistant should provide encouragement and stress the benefits to be derived in terms of improved regulation of the blood glucose level.

3. *Reliable decision making regarding insulin dosage.* More reliable decisions regarding insulin needs can be made during situations that affect the blood glucose level, such as illness, emotional stress, increased physical activity, or suspected hypoglycemia.

4. *Delay in or prevention of long-term complications.* The medical assistant should emphasize to patients how important it is to perform daily SMBG testing to increase their chances of staying healthy. As previously discussed, diabetic patients who maintain good blood glucose control generally experience fewer symptoms and a delay in or prevention of long-term complications of the disease.

HEMOGLOBIN A$_{1c}$ TEST

The hemoglobin A$_{1c}$ test (HbA$_{1c}$ test or A$_{1c}$ test) provides valuable information for determining whether a diabetic patient's blood glucose level is under control. The A$_{1c}$ test supplies the physician with an assessment of the average amount of glucose in the blood over a 3-month period.

When an individual consumes food containing glucose, the glucose is absorbed from the digestive tract and into the circulatory system. Glucose (sugar) has a "sticky" quality to it and thus has a tendency to stick to protein in the body. One of the proteins to which it attaches is the protein included in hemoglobin. Hemoglobin is found in red blood cells and functions in transporting oxygen in the body. The process of glucose attaching to hemoglobin is known as **glycosylation.**

When glucose attaches or glycosylates to the protein in hemoglobin, it forms a compound known as **hemoglobin A$_{1c}$.** Glycosylation occurs in all individuals—hemoglobin A$_{1c}$ is formed in diabetic patients and healthy individuals. The amount of glucose that attaches to hemoglobin is proportional to the amount of glucose in the blood; the more glucose in the blood, the more hemoglobin becomes glycated and the higher the A$_{1c}$ level. Individuals with undiagnosed or poorly controlled diabetes have a higher than normal blood glucose level, and more hemoglobin A$_{1c}$ forms in these individuals. The percentage of hemoglobin A$_{1c}$ in the blood can be measured by the A$_{1c}$ laboratory test. The attachment of the glucose to the hemoglobin is permanent for the life of the red blood cell (90 to 120 days); the A$_{1c}$ test result is able to provide an overall picture of the patient's blood glucose level for the past 3 months. CLIA-waived analyzers are available for performing a hemoglobin A$_{1c}$ test in the medical office; an example is the A1cNow test (Bayer Corporation).

Interpretation of Results

The normal A$_{1c}$ level for an individual without diabetes is 4% to 6%. Patients with diabetes usually have a higher A$_{1c}$ level than this. The American Diabetes Association (ADA)

Table 33-2 Comparison of Hemoglobin A$_{1c}$ Percentages With Average Blood Glucose Levels

Hemoglobin A$_{1c}$ (%)	Average Daily Blood Glucose Level (mg/dL)
4	65
5	100
6	135
7	170
8	205
9	240
10	275
11	310
12	345

strongly recommends that patients with diabetes maintain an A$_{1c}$ level of less than 7%. Table 33-2 shows the correlation between hemoglobin A$_{1c}$ percentages and average blood glucose levels. A change in a patient's diabetes management plan is almost always required if the A$_{1c}$ test result is greater than 8%.

Patients who keep their hemoglobin A$_{1c}$ levels close to 7% have a much better chance of delaying or preventing diabetic complications than do patients with A$_{1c}$ levels that are 8% or greater. Studies show that for every 1 percentage point drop in the A$_{1c}$ value, a 35% reduction in risk for diabetes-related complications occurs.

The physician orders an A$_{1c}$ test when a patient is first diagnosed with diabetes to determine how elevated the blood glucose level has been before the condition was diagnosed. The test is usually ordered several times after a diabetes management plan has been prescribed to verify that blood glucose control is being achieved. The A$_{1c}$ test is ordered periodically for patients already diagnosed with diabetes to evaluate the effectiveness of their diabetes management plan. For stable diabetic patients under good control, the test is typically ordered at least twice a year (every 6 months). The test is usually ordered on a more frequent basis for patients who have difficulty maintaining control of their blood glucose levels. The A$_{1c}$ test also is ordered when the physician makes an adjustment to a patient's diabetic management plan to assess the effectiveness of the change in treatment.

GLUCOSE METERS

In the medical office, a CLIA-waived glucose meter is often used to measure the blood glucose level quantitatively. The test most frequently performed using the glucose meter is the FBG, although some offices also perform the OGTT and the 2-hour postprandial test. By measuring the blood glucose concentration in the medical office, the physician can provide better patient care. On-site testing eliminates

Figure 33-8 Accu-Chek Advantage code key calibration procedure. **A,** The code key is inserted into the monitor. **B,** The code number must match the code number of the vial of test strips.

the time required for an outside laboratory to provide the results, allowing the physician to make decisions immediately regarding diagnosis, treatment, and follow-up care. Procedure 33-1 describes how to measure blood glucose using the Accu-Chek Advantage glucose meter.

REAGENT TEST STRIPS

A reagent test strip must be used with the glucose meter; it consists of a plastic strip with a reaction pad. The pad contains chemicals that react with the glucose in whole blood to determine the blood glucose level in milligrams per deciliter (mg/dL). Through an electronic signal, the glucose results are displayed as a digital readout. The manufacturer's instructions accompanying the glucose meter must be followed exactly to ensure accurate and reliable test results.

It is important to store the container of test strips properly to prevent their deterioration, which affects the test results. The chemical reagents on the strips are sensitive to heat, light, and moisture and must be stored in a cool, dry area at room temperature (below 90° F [32° C]) with the cap tightly closed. Strips that are discolored or that have darkened should be discarded to prevent inaccurate test results. The container of test strips includes a desiccant. Its purpose is to promote dryness by absorbing moisture.

CALIBRATION PROCEDURE

A calibration procedure may be required for a glucose meter. Because the Accu-Chek Advantage glucose meter is presented in Procedure 33-1, the calibration method discussed here relates specifically to this meter.

The calibration procedure is a coding procedure that is performed to ensure accurate and reliable test results; most glucose meters require this calibration procedure. The coding procedure must be performed each time a new container of test strips is opened. It is performed to compensate for variables that occur in the manufacturing process, which cause one batch of test strips to be a little different from another batch. The coding procedure programs the electronics of the glucose meter to match the reactivity of the container of strips that are in current use.

The coding procedure for the Accu-Chek Advantage is performed using a plastic code key that accompanies each container of Accu-Chek Advantage test strips (Figure 33-8). Accu-Chek requires lot-specific calibration, meaning that the calibration procedure needs to be performed only once per container of test strips. This is possible because the Accu-Chek glucose meter has a built-in memory system that enables it to retain a point of reference after it has been calibrated. This reference point is retained until the glucose meter is reprogrammed for a new container of test strips. The coding procedure delineated next should be followed when a new container of Accu-Chek test strips is opened:

1. Ensure that the meter is turned off.
2. Turn the meter over so that the back of the meter is facing you.
3. Remove the old code key, if one is installed, and discard it in a waste container.
4. Insert a new code key by sliding it into the code key slot until it snaps into place (see Figure 33-8, *A*).
5. Turn the meter on. A three-digit code number appears on the display screen. This number must match the code number of the vial of test strips (see Figure 33-8, *B*). If it does not, repeat steps 1 through 3.

Figure 33-9 Glucose controls.

CONTROL PROCEDURE

A control test should be run to ensure that test results are reliable and valid and that errors that might interfere with test results are detected and eliminated. A control check is performed on the Accu-Chek Advantage using commercially available glucose control solutions. Two levels of controls (high and low) (Figure 33-9) should be used.

The control solution is effective for 3 months from the date it is opened. When the control solution is opened, the medical assistant must write the date on the container label. The control solution can then be used for 3 months from that date (which should also be written on the container) or until the manufacturer's expiration date (stamped on the container) is reached, whichever comes first. The control solution is sensitive to heat, light, and moisture and must be stored with the cap tightly closed in a cool, dry area at room temperature between 36° F (2° C) and 86° F (30° C).

A control test should be performed under the following circumstances:
1. When the meter is new
2. Daily, before the meter is used for the first time
3. When a new container of test strips is opened
4. If the cap is left off the vial of test strips for any length of time

5. If the meter is dropped
6. If the test result does not agree with the way the patient feels
7. If a test has been repeated and the blood glucose result is still lower or higher than expected

If Level 1 or Level 2 control results are not within the acceptable range, the following should be performed:
1. Check the expiration date of the test strips and control solutions to make sure they are not outdated.
2. Determine whether the test strips and control solutions were stored at room temperature.
3. Make sure the container lids were tight on the test strips container and the control solution containers.
4. Check to make sure the code on the meter matches the code on the test strip vial.
5. Review the technique used to run the control to make sure it was followed correctly.

Any errors should be corrected, and the control should be run again. If the results are still not within acceptable range, the manufacturer of the glucose meter should be contacted.

CARE AND MAINTENANCE

The glucose meter must be handled carefully. It is a delicate instrument, and a severe physical jar could result in a malfunction. The glucose meter should not be placed in an area of high humidity, such as a bathroom. In addition, the meter should not be exposed to severe variations in environmental temperature, such as would occur if it were left in a closed vehicle on a hot or cold day.

Proper cleaning of the glucose meter is essential for its accurate and reliable operation. On a regular basis, the exterior of the glucose meter, including the display screen, should be cleaned with a soft, clean cloth slightly dampened with a mild cleaning agent, and it should be dried thoroughly. Acceptable cleaning agents include alcohol and mild dishwashing liquid mixed with water. Do not allow water or cleaning solution to run into the glucose meter; this could damage the internal components.

Because glucose meters are battery operated, periodic replacement of the battery is required. The glucose meter alerts the user to low battery voltage by displaying a special notation on the screen. The type of battery required is specified in the operating manual, along with directions for installation.

PATIENT TEACHING | **Obtaining a Capillary Blood Specimen**

The medical assistant may need to instruct the patient in the procedure for obtaining and testing a capillary blood specimen for blood glucose measurement. Properly educating the patient to perform the procedure is the most important factor in obtaining accurate test results.

1. *Obtaining the capillary blood specimen.* Inform the patient of the sites available for obtaining the blood specimen, including

the fingers and the side of the hand that has no calluses. Most patients prefer to use an automatic lancet to perform the skin puncture. Using such a device makes the puncture less painful, and the preset puncture depth generally ensures a successful stick. For a finger puncture, instruct the patient to obtain the blood specimen from the lateral side of the fingertip because this area contains fewer nerve endings, and less pain results. If the patient's hands are cold, tell him or her to rub them together or place them in warm water, which improves blood flow to the area. Instruct the patient in the proper procedure for obtaining enough blood to ensure accurate test results.

2. *Performing the blood glucose test.* The patient performs the test with a test strip using a glucose meter. Instruct the patient in the proper procedure for performing the test, making sure he or she understands that accurate test results assist in achieving greater glucose control. Patients also should be given detailed instructions on proper care and maintenance of the glucose meter.

3. *Recording results.* Instruct the patient to record each test result in a log book between office visits to provide a

permanent record. In addition, most glucose meters are equipped with a memory system that stores test results for later retrieval. Keeping track of these factors helps explain a shift in the blood glucose level and provides the basis for sound self-management decisions. The following information should be included with each recording:

- Date and time
- Number of hours since the patient last ate
- Time of the last insulin injection or oral hypoglycemic medication
- Any feeling of physical or emotional stress
- Amount of exercise the patient has had ■

PROCEDURE 33-1 Blood Glucose Measurement Using the Accu-Chek Advantage Glucose Meter

Outcome Perform a fasting blood glucose (FBG) test

Equipment/Supplies

- Disposable gloves
- Accu-Chek Advantage glucose meter
- Accu-Chek Advantage test strips
- Code key
- Control solutions

- Lancet
- Antiseptic wipe
- Gauze pad
- Biohazard sharps container

---

1. Procedural Step. Sanitize your hands. Assemble the equipment. Check the expiration date on the container of test strips. Check to make sure the environmental temperature falls between 57° F (14° C) and 104° F (40° C).

Principle. Outdated test strips can cause inaccurate test results. If the temperature is outside of the required range, the meter cannot perform the test, causing an error message to appear on the screen of the analyzer.

2. Procedural Step. If necessary, calibrate the glucose meter using the code key that accompanies the container of test strips.

a. Ensure that the meter is turned off.

b. Turn the meter over so that the back of the meter is facing you.

c. Insert the code key into the slot on the back of the meter.

Assemble the equipment.

Insert the code key.

Continued

d. Push on the code key until it snaps into place.

e. Turn on the meter.

f. A three-digit code number appears on the display screen. The number must match the code number on the container of test strips.

Check the code number.

Principle. Calibrating with the code key compensates for variables that occur in the manufacturing process of the test strips and must be performed before strips from a new container are used.

3. Procedural Step. Run a Level 1 (low) and Level 2 (high) control check on the glucose meter using Accu-Chek Advantage control solutions as follows:

a. Check the expiration date on the control solutions. (*Note:* The expiration date for the test strips was checked previously and therefore does not need to be checked again.)

b. Remove a test strip from the container and immediately recap the container.

c. Gently insert the end of the test strip with the silver-colored bars into the test strip guide with the yellow target area facing up. This automatically turns on the meter.

d. Check to make sure the code number matches the number displayed on the container of strips.

e. When the strip is inserted correctly, a blood drop symbol flashes on the display screen, indicating that it is ready to accept the control solution.

f. Roll the Level 1 low control solution between the palms of your hands to mix it.

g. Press and release the right arrow button once to select the Level 1 control.

h. Hold the control solution at an angle to the edge of the yellow target area of the test strip. Squeeze

the container, and touch and hold a drop of control solution to the edge (not the top) of the yellow target area. Promptly replace the cap for the control solution.

Apply the control solution.

i. After a short time, the control result is displayed on the screen of the glucose meter.

j. If the low control result is within the acceptable range, the result will alternate with the word *OK* on the display screen. The result will also fall within the expected range listed on the test strip container.

Control results should fall within the expected range.

PROCEDURE **33-1**   Blood Glucose Measurement Using the Accu-Chek Advantage Glucose Meter—cont'd

k. Repeat the control procedure outlined above using a Level 2 high control.

l. Record the control results in the quality control log.

Principle. Running a low and a high control check ensures that the test results are reliable and valid. Gloves do not need to be worn because the control consists of a glucose solution.

4. Procedural Step. Sanitize your hands. Greet and introduce yourself. Identify the patient by full name and date of birth. Explain the procedure.

5. Procedural Step. Ask the patient whether he or she has had anything to eat or drink (besides water) for the past 12 hours.

Principle. Consumption of food or fluid increases the blood glucose level, leading to inaccurate interpretation of FBG test results.

6. Procedural Step. Remove a test strip from the container. Promptly replace the lid of the container to prevent the strips from being exposed to moisture.

Principle. The reagent pads are moisture sensitive and could be affected by environmental moisture, leading to inaccurate test results.

7. Procedural Step. Gently insert the end of the test strip with the silver-colored bars into the test strip guide with the yellow target area facing up. Check that the code number displayed matches the code number on the vial of test strips that you are using. When the test strip symbol flashes on the display, the meter is ready to accept a blood specimen.

Principle. When the strip is correctly inserted, a blood drop symbol flashes on the display.

8. Procedural Step. Open the gauze packet. Cleanse the puncture site with an antiseptic wipe, and allow it to air-dry. Apply gloves, and perform a finger puncture. Dispose of the lancet in a biohazard sharps container.

Principle. The antiseptic must be allowed to dry to prevent it from reacting with the chemicals on the reagent pad, which would lead to inaccurate test results. Gloves provide a barrier against bloodborne pathogens.

9. Procedural Step. After the puncture has been made, wipe away the first drop of blood with a gauze pad. Place the hand in a dependent position (palm facing down), and gently massage the finger around the puncture site until a large drop of blood forms.

Principle. The first drop of blood contains a large amount of tissue fluid, which dilutes the specimen

and leads to inaccurate test results. A large drop of blood is needed to cover the target area of the test strip completely.

10. Procedural Step. Apply the drop of blood to the Comfort Curve test strip as follows:

a. Touch and hold a drop of blood to the edge (not the top) of the yellow target area.

b. Completely fill the yellow target area. You will hear a beeping sound when sufficient blood has been applied. If any yellow mesh is visible after you have applied the initial drop of blood, a second drop of blood may be applied to the target area within 15 seconds of the first drop. If more than 15 seconds has passed, the test result may be erroneous, and you should discard the test strip and repeat the test.

Principle. The entire yellow target area must be completely covered with blood to ensure accurate and reliable test results.

Apply a drop of blood.

11. Procedural Step. Have the patient hold a gauze pad over the puncture site and apply pressure until the bleeding stops.

12. Procedural Step. When the blood is correctly applied to the strip, an hourglass flashes on the screen while the meter analyzes the blood specimen. After a short time, the glucose value is displayed in milligrams per deciliter (mg/dL). If the glucose value is higher or lower than expected, or if the screen displays something other than the glucose value, see the Troubleshooting Guide section of the operator's manual to obtain instructions for correcting the problem. (The glucose result indicated on this glucose meter is 98 mg/dL.)

Continued

PROCEDURE 33-1

Read the glucose results.

13. Procedural Step. Remove the test strip from the meter, and discard it in a biohazard waste container. Turn the meter off.

14. Procedural Step. Check the puncture site and apply an adhesive bandage to the patient's finger if needed.

15. Procedural Step. Remove your gloves, and sanitize your hands.

16. Procedural Step. Chart the results in the patient's medical record.

 a. *Paper-based patient record:* Record the date and time, the type of glucose test (i.e., FBG), the glucose test results, and when the patient last ate. If the patient has diabetes, also record the time of his or her last insulin injection or last consumption of oral hypoglycemic medication (refer to the PPR charting example).

 b. *Electronic medical record:* Document the type of glucose test (i.e., FBG), the glucose test results, and when the patient last ate. If the patient has diabetes, also record the time of his or her last insulin injection or last consumption of oral hypoglycemic medication using the appropriate radio buttons, drop-down menus, and free text fields.

17. Procedural Step. Properly store the glucose meter according to the manufacturer's instructions.

PPR CHARTING EXAMPLE

Date	
5/18/XX	8:30 a.m. FBS: 98 mg/dL. Pt last ate on 5/17 @ 7:00 p.m. ——————
	—————— M. Villers, CMA (AAMA)

CHOLESTEROL

Cholesterol is a white, waxy, fatlike substance (lipid) that is essential for normal functioning of the body. It is an important component of all cell membranes in the body and is used in the production of essential hormones and bile. Most of the cholesterol circulating in the blood is manufactured by the liver; however, a portion of it comes from an individual's diet and is known as *dietary cholesterol.* Dietary cholesterol is found only in animal products, such as organ meats, egg yolk, and dairy products.

Having high blood cholesterol means an excessive amount of cholesterol is present in the blood. An individual's cholesterol level is determined by his or her genetic makeup and by the amounts of dietary cholesterol, saturated fat, and *trans* fat consumed. High blood cholesterol may cause fatty deposits, or plaque, to build up on the walls of the arteries, a condition known as *atherosclerosis.* As the atherosclerosis progresses, the arteries become more occluded, which eventually could lead to a heart attack or stroke. Because of this, high blood cholesterol is considered a risk factor for coronary artery disease (see *Highlight on Heart Disease With a Focus on Coronary Artery Disease*), and efforts should be made to reduce the cholesterol level (see *Highlight on Lowering Cholesterol*).

HDL AND LDL CHOLESTEROL

Cholesterol is transported in the blood as a complex molecule known as a **lipoprotein.** Two types of lipoproteins contain cholesterol: low-density lipoprotein (LDL) and high-density lipoprotein (HDL).

LDL picks up cholesterol from ingested fats and the liver and delivers it to blood vessels and muscles, where it is deposited in the cells. **LDL cholesterol** is often referred to as "bad" cholesterol because an excess amount of it in the blood can cause plaque to build up on the arterial walls, resulting in atherosclerosis. *HDL* removes excess cholesterol from the cells and carries it to the liver to be excreted. Because HDL removes excess cholesterol from the walls of the blood vessels, it is protective and beneficial to the body

HIGHLIGHT on Heart Disease With a Focus on Coronary Artery Disease

Heart disease is a general term used to refer to a variety of medical conditions that affect the heart. The primary forms of heart disease include coronary artery disease (CAD), high blood pressure, heart attacks, strokes, congestive heart failure, congenital heart disease, and rheumatic heart disease. These various forms of heart disease are interrelated and have elements in common—for example, atherosclerosis can lead to a stroke or heart attack.

Heart disease is the number one killer of adults in the United States today. Because of the national focus on heart disease and cholesterol reduction, since 1985 a decline in heart attacks by 25% has been reported, as well as a decline in strokes by nearly 40%; however, heart disease is likely to remain the number one cause of death until more Americans adopt a more heart-healthy lifestyle.

Coronary Artery Disease

The most common symptom of CAD is chest pain, which is known as *angina pectoris.* Angina pectoris is a symptom, or a set of symptoms, rather than a disease. Angina pectoris occurs when the muscle tissue of the heart does not receive enough oxygenated blood, resulting in discomfort or pain under the sternum.

Cause

For most patients, the cause of angina is atherosclerosis of the coronary arteries. *Atherosclerosis* of the coronary arteries is a condition in which fibrous plaques of fatty deposits and cholesterol build up on the inner walls of the coronary arteries. This causes narrowing and partial blockage of the lumen of these arteries, along with hardening of the arterial wall. CAD results in a reduction of oxygenated blood flow to the heart muscle. Despite the narrowing, enough oxygen may still reach the heart muscle for normal needs. More oxygen is needed, however, when situations occur that increase the workload of the heart, such as physical activity, emotional stress, a heavy meal, and exposure to cold weather. If the coronary arteries cannot deliver enough oxygen to the heart muscle during these times of increased need, angina pectoris may

result. Severe and prolonged anginal pain generally suggests a myocardial infarction (heart attack) caused by complete blockage of the coronary arteries and requires immediate medical attention.

Risk Factors

Not everyone is equal when it comes to CAD. Some individuals have a much higher risk of developing it than others. The following are risk factors for CAD:

- High total blood cholesterol (greater than 200 mg/dL confirmed by repeated measurement)
- High blood pressure
- Cigarette smoking (more than 10 cigarettes per day)
- Family history of premature CAD (definite heart attack or sudden death in a parent or sibling before age 55 years)
- Diabetes
- History of blood vessel disease
- Obesity and overweight
- Low HDL cholesterol (less than 40 mg/dL confirmed by repeated measurement)
- Elevated triglyceride level (greater than 150 mg/dL)
- Being a man older than 45 years
- Being a woman older than 55 years or postmenopausal

Some of these risk factors can be modified; others, such as age, gender, and a family history of CAD, cannot be modified or controlled. The three major risk factors for CAD are high total blood cholesterol, high blood pressure, and cigarette smoking, all of which are modifiable.

Each person's overall risk of CAD must be assessed individually by the physician, based on the type and number of risk factors present. A 47-year-old man with a cholesterol level of 220 mg/dL who smokes a pack of cigarettes a day and is overweight is at greater risk than a 28-year-old man who is within a normal weight range, does not smoke, and exercises regularly but has a cholesterol level of 250 mg/dL. ■

HIGHLIGHT on Lowering Cholesterol

Research has shown, beyond doubt, that high total blood cholesterol is a major risk factor for coronary artery disease, and the higher the cholesterol, the greater the risk. The National Institutes of Health (NIH) has established guidelines on safe levels of blood cholesterol. The NIH recommends that adults not exceed 200 mg/dL of blood cholesterol.

The National Cholesterol Educational Program (NCEP) was established in 1985 by the federal government to reduce the prevalence of elevated blood cholesterol levels in the United States by educating the public about the health risks associated with high blood cholesterol and to make recommendations for helping individuals reduce their cholesterol levels. It has been shown that for every 1% that an

individual lowers his or her total blood cholesterol, the risk of coronary artery disease is reduced by 2%. Taking the following measures can help individuals reduce their level of "bad" LDL cholesterol and increase their level of "good" HDL cholesterol.

Diet

Dietary therapy is the first line of treatment for high blood cholesterol. The NCEP recommends that all individuals older than 2 years of age reduce dietary cholesterol, *trans* fat, and saturated fats. Many foods high in fat tend to be high in cholesterol. Nutrition labels on packaged products provide information on the cholesterol and fat content of a food.

Continued

Dietary Cholesterol

The body manufactures all the cholesterol it needs for normal functioning, and dietary intake of cholesterol (in foods) serves only to increase the blood cholesterol. According to the NCEP, dietary cholesterol should be limited to less than 200 mg each day. Cholesterol is found only in animal foods and shellfish. Egg yolks, dairy products, and organ meats such as liver and kidneys are especially high in cholesterol.

Saturated and Unsaturated Fats

The intake of saturated fat is the most important dietary factor leading to high blood cholesterol, even more so than consuming dietary cholesterol. In general, the more saturated a fat is, the harder and more solid it is at room temperature. The main source of saturated fat is animal products, including meat fat, poultry skin, and the fat in dairy products (butter, cream, ice cream, cheese, whole milk). Unsaturated fats have little or no effect on the blood cholesterol level; they include olive oil, canola oil, peanut oil, and sunflower, safflower, and corn oils. The NCEP recommends that no more than 25% to 35% of the calories consumed each day come from total fat, with less than 7% of calories coming from saturated fat and with the remaining fat coming from unsaturated fat.

Soluble Fiber

Soluble fiber has been shown to lower the cholesterol level by keeping the cholesterol consumed from being absorbed by the body. Examples of foods high in soluble fiber include oatmeal, oat bran, barley, some fruits (e.g., apples and oranges), broccoli, and legumes. Weight Reduction

It is estimated that two out of every three Americans is overweight. It is recommended that these individuals follow a sensible eating plan along with an exercise program to reach and maintain desirable weight. Losing weight reduces total cholesterol and triglyceride levels. Overweight and obese people are at very high risk for heart disease because their hearts have to work harder to pump blood through the body.

Exercise

An aerobic exercise program is especially beneficial for weight control because it improves cardiovascular fitness and lowers blood cholesterol level. People who exercise regularly generally have higher HDL cholesterol levels and lower triglyceride levels in their blood. The American Heart Association recommends that healthy adults spend at least 150 minutes per week in moderate-intensity physical exercise (e.g., brisk walking).

Smoking Cessation

Smoking is one of the three main risk factors for coronary artery disease. By quitting smoking, an individual may be able to strengthen the heart and lower the cholesterol level. Also, non-smokers tend to have higher HDL levels in their blood. A variety of smoking cessation programs are usually available in the community. Some people have succeeded by using nicotine patches, which help them adjust gradually to lower levels of nicotine.

Summary

Generally, the cholesterol level begins to decrease 2 to 3 weeks after a cholesterol-lowering diet and other cholesterol-lowering measures are begun. Over time, it is possible to reduce the total cholesterol level by 30 to 55 mg/dL or even more through these lifestyle changes. If the blood cholesterol level cannot be lowered to an acceptable level, the physician may prescribe cholesterol-lowering medications along with continuation of the aforementioned measures. ■

and is often called "good" cholesterol. A high **HDL cholesterol** level has been shown to reduce the risk of coronary artery disease, whereas a low level of HDL cholesterol (less than 40 mg/dL) is a risk factor for coronary artery disease.

CHOLESTEROL TESTING

All adults older than 20 years should have a cholesterol test at least once every 5 years. Initial testing includes a *total cholesterol* determination, which is a combined measurement of LDL cholesterol and HDL cholesterol in the blood. To obtain a fuller picture of a patient's cholesterol status, physicians typically also order an HDL cholesterol determination, which measures only the HDL cholesterol in the blood. Cholesterol tests are considered screening tests, and elevated results usually require confirmation through repeat testing before a diagnosis of high blood cholesterol is made.

INTERPRETATION OF RESULTS

Cholesterol test results are interpreted as follows: Total cholesterol levels less than 200 mg/dL are desirable. Levels between 200 and 239 mg/dL are borderline high, and levels of 240 mg/dL and greater are high. Based on confirmed testing, individuals in the high category are clearly at increased risk for coronary artery disease, and individuals in the borderline high category are at increased risk if they have other risk factors, such as being overweight or smoking. According to the American Heart Association, an HDL cholesterol level less than 40 mg/dL for men and less than 50 mg/dL for women is considered a risk factor for coronary artery disease. An HDL cholesterol level between 40 and 50 mg/dL for men and between 50 and 60 mg/dL for women is desirable, whereas an HDL cholesterol level greater than 60 mg/dL is considered optimal and provides some protection against heart disease.

Although the primary use of cholesterol testing is to screen for the presence of high blood cholesterol related to coronary artery disease, this test also is used as a secondary aid in the study of thyroid and liver function.

PATIENT PREPARATION

Because total cholesterol and HDL cholesterol determinations are not affected significantly by food consumption, the patient usually is not required to fast before collection of the blood specimen. Some physicians prefer the patient to be in a fasting state, however.

If the total cholesterol level is 200 mg/dL or greater, the physician usually orders a *lipid profile,* which includes total cholesterol, HDL cholesterol, LDL cholesterol, and triglycerides. (The LDL cholesterol level is usually determined as a calculation from the triglyceride and HDL cholesterol levels.) Because triglyceride levels are affected by the consumption of food, the patient must be instructed to fast for at least 12 hours before the blood specimen is collected. An elevated triglyceride level (150 mg/dL or higher) is considered a risk factor for coronary artery disease, particularly when the LDL cholesterol is high and the HDL cholesterol is low.

Although the primary use of cholesterol testing is to screen for the presence of high blood cholesterol related to coronary artery disease, this test also is used as a secondary aid in the study of thyroid and liver function.

CLIA-WAIVED CHOLESTEROL ANALYZERS

CLIA-waived analyzers are available for performing cholesterol testing in the medical office; an example is the Cholestech LDX cholesterol system (Cholestech Corporation) (Figure 33-10).

The manufacturer of each cholesterol analyzer provides an operating manual (and sometimes an instructional video) with the instrument that includes information needed to collect and handle the specimen, perform quality control procedures, and test the specimen. The manufacturer may also have personnel available for on-site training.

Figure 33-10 Cholestech LDX cholesterol system.

It is important that the medical assistant become completely familiar with all aspects of the CLIA-waived analyzer used to perform cholesterol testing in his or her medical office. Medical offices running CLIA-waived tests are required to follow the manufacturer's instructions *exactly* for each testing procedure. These instructions include the quality control procedures that must be performed when the test is run. Quality control procedures are of particular importance to ensure that the analyzer is functioning properly and that the test results are reliable and accurate.

What Would You Do? What Would You *Not* Do?

Case Study 3

Karen Scrimshaw is at the office. She is 20 years old and is mildly obese. Karen had her cholesterol tested at a health fair, and it was 325. The physician orders a complete blood count, lipid profile, and thyroid profile on Karen and instructs her to return in 1 week for a follow-up visit to discuss the test results. Karen is very concerned about her cholesterol. She says that she had a candy bar and some potato chips before going to the health fair and wants to know whether that could have caused her cholesterol to be so high. She also wants to know the accuracy of machines that are used at health fairs. Karen says that if she has to go on cholesterol medication, it would be hard to decide between Lipitor and Zocor. She says she has seen them advertised on television, and they both seem pretty good to her. ∎

TRIGLYCERIDES

Triglycerides are the chemical form in which most fat exists in food, as well as in the body. Triglycerides are derived from two sources. The first is synthesis by the body. Ingested glucose that is not needed for energy can be stored in the form of **glycogen** in muscle and liver tissue for later use. When no more tissue storage is possible, most of the excess glycogen is synthesized by the body into triglycerides (a form of fat) and stored as adipose tissue. Excess protein not needed by the body is also converted to triglycerides and stored as adipose tissue. The second source of triglycerides is food. Excess triglycerides consumed by eating foods containing fat are also stored as adipose tissue.

Some of the triglycerides in the body are not stored as fat but remain in the bloodstream, specifically in the plasma. Most triglycerides in the bloodstream are carried by a lipoprotein known as very-low-density lipoprotein (VLDL). In normal amounts, triglycerides are essential to good health. Triglycerides carried by the blood serve as a major source of energy for the body. An excess of blood triglycerides, however, places an individual at increased risk for coronary artery disease, particularly when the LDL cholesterol is high and the HDL cholesterol is low. Triglyceride levels in the blood are usually measured as part of a lipid profile and are interpreted as follows:

Normal	Less than 150 mg/dL
Borderline high	150 to 199 mg/dL
High	200 to 499 mg/dL
Very high	500 mg/dL or higher

Conditions that result in elevated blood triglyceride levels include obesity, type 2 diabetes, physical inactivity, excessive alcohol consumption, smoking, hypothyroidism, kidney disease, and liver disease.

BLOOD UREA NITROGEN

The blood urea nitrogen (BUN) is a kidney function test. Urea is the end product of protein metabolism and is normally present in the blood. Certain kidney diseases may interfere with the ability of the body to excrete the urea properly, causing an increased level of urea in the blood.

IMMUNOLOGY

Immunology is the scientific study of antigen and antibody reactions. An **antigen** is a substance that is capable of stimulating the formation of antibodies in an individual. Antigens may consist of protein, glycoprotein, complex polysaccharides, or nucleic acid. Specific examples of antigens include bacteria and viruses, bacterial toxins, allergens, and **blood antigens.** An **antibody** is a substance that is capable of combining with an antigen, resulting in an antigen-antibody reaction.

Laboratory testing in immunology deals with studying antigen-antibody reactions to assess the presence of a substance (e.g., ABO blood typing) or to assist in the diagnosis of disease (e.g., mononucleosis testing). Immunologic tests are often used for the early diagnosis of disease and are used to follow the course of the disease.

IMMUNOLOGIC TESTS

Specific examples of immunologic tests are described next.

HEPATITIS TESTS

Hepatitis testing is performed to detect viral hepatitis. There are five types of viral hepatitis—A, B, C, D, and E—which are described in detail in Chapter 17. Hepatitis testing not only detects the presence of viral hepatitis, it also determines the type of hepatitis present.

HIV TESTS

The enzyme immunoassay (EIA) test and the enzyme-linked immunosorbent assay (ELISA) test are used as screening tests for the presence of HIV. Newer rapid screening HIV testing kits are also commercially available; brand names include Uni-Gold Recombigen HIV (Trinity Biotech, Bray County Wicklow, Ireland), Clearview Complete HIV (Inverness Medical Innovations, Waltham, Mass), and the OraQuick Advance Rapid HIV test (OraSure Technologies, Bethlehem, Pa). Because of the possibility of a false-positive result, a second screening test is always performed if a blood specimen tests positive. If the second test result also is positive, a more specific test, such as the Western blot test, is performed to confirm the test results. An individual who tests positive for HIV is seropositive.

A negative HIV test result is not conclusive for the absence of HIV infection. If an individual has recently been infected with HIV, the antibodies may not have had time to develop. It generally takes 2 to 12 weeks (but possibly as long as 6 months) for the HIV antibodies to appear in the blood.

SYPHILIS TESTS

Syphilis is a sexually transmitted disease (STD) caused by the microorganism *Treponema pallidum*. The most common tests used to detect the presence of syphilis are the Venereal Disease Research Laboratories (VDRL) test and the rapid plasma reagin (RPR) test. Test results are reported as nonreactive, weakly reactive, or reactive. Weakly reactive and reactive results are considered positive for the presence of syphilis antibodies. These tests are screening tests, and a positive result warrants more specific testing to arrive at a diagnosis of syphilis.

MONONUCLEOSIS TEST

The mononucleosis test ("mono test") is used to detect the presence of infectious mononucleosis. The theory and procedure for this test are discussed in detail later in this chapter.

RHEUMATOID FACTOR

Rheumatoid arthritis is a chronic inflammatory disease that affects the joints of the body. The blood of patients with rheumatoid arthritis contains a type of antibody called *rheumatoid factor* (RF). This test detects the presence of RF antibodies and assists in the diagnosis of rheumatoid arthritis.

ANTISTREPTOLYSIN O TEST

The antistreptolysin O (ASO) test is used to detect ASO antibodies in the serum. It is the most widely used immunologic test for the detection of conditions resulting from streptococcal infections and diseases that occur secondary to a streptococcal infection. This test is useful in assisting in the diagnosis of rheumatic fever, glomerulonephritis, bacterial endocarditis, and scarlet fever.

C-REACTIVE PROTEIN

During inflammation and tissue destruction, an abnormal protein called *C-reactive protein* (CRP) appears in the blood. Patients with inflammatory conditions or disorders accompanied by tissue destruction have positive results to this test. Because of this, the CRP test is used to assist in diagnosing or charting the progress of rheumatoid arthritis, acute rheumatic fever, widespread malignancy, and bacterial infections.

COLD AGGLUTININS

The cold agglutinins test is used to detect the presence of antibodies called *cold agglutinins*. This test is performed by incubating the patient's serum with erythrocytes at cold temperatures. If cold agglutinins are present, this causes **agglutination** of the erythrocytes. Cold agglutinins are found in patients with infectious mononucleosis, mycoplasmal pneumonia, chronic parasitic infections, and lymphoma.

ABO AND Rh BLOOD TYPING

Blood typing is performed to determine an individual's ABO and Rh blood type. Knowledge of blood type helps to prevent transfusion and transplant reactions and to identify problems such as hemolytic disease of the newborn.

Rh ANTIBODY TITER

The Rh antibody titer test detects the amount of circulating Rh antibodies in the blood. These antibodies can occur in a pregnant woman who is Rh negative and is carrying an Rh-positive fetus. This test is most frequently used to detect the presence of an Rh incompatibility problem with a mother and her unborn child.

RAPID MONONUCLEOSIS TESTING

Infectious mononucleosis is an acute infectious disease caused by the Epstein-Barr virus (EBV). Infectious mononucleosis most frequently affects children and young adults. It is transmitted through saliva by direct oral contact, and because of this it is often called the "kissing disease." Symptoms of infectious mononucleosis include mental and physical fatigue, fever, sore throat, severe weakness, headache, and swollen lymph nodes.

The (CLIA-waived) rapid mono test is often performed in the medical office and is used to assist in the diagnosis of infectious mononucleosis. Rapid mono tests are easy to perform and provide reliable results in a short time. Patients with infectious mononucleosis produce an antibody called *heterophile antibody,* usually by 6 to 10 days into the illness. Rapid mono tests detect this antibody. The presence of the heterophile antibody along with patient symptoms can provide the basis for the diagnosis of infectious mononucleosis.

Figure 33-11 illustrates the QuickVue+ mononucleosis test setup (Quidel Corporation, San Diego, Calif), and Figure 33-12 outlines the procedure for performing a rapid mono test using the QuickVue+ mononucleosis test. Figure 33-13 is an illustration of positive and negative test results for the QuickVue+ mononucleosis test.

Figure 33-11 QuickVue+ mononucleosis test setup. (From Garrels M, Oatis CS: *Laboratory and diagnostic care in ambulatory settings,* ed 3, St Louis, 2015, Saunders.)

Figure 33-12 Procedure for performing the QuickVue+ mononucleosis test. (Courtesy of and modified from Quidel Corporation, San Diego, Calif.)

Figure 33-13 QuickVue+ mononucleosis test results. The test results are interpreted as follows, starting at the top of the illustration: invalid, positive, and negative. (From Garrels M, Oatis CS: *Laboratory and diagnostic care in ambulatory settings,* ed 3, St Louis, 2015, Saunders.)

What Would You Do? What Would You *Not* Do? RESPONSES

Case Study 1
Page 876

What Did Michelle Do?
- ❏ Apologized to Crystal for the inconvenience. Explained to her that it takes 3 to 4 hours to run an oral glucose tolerance test because several specimens must be collected over time to see how her body handles sugar.
- ❏ Explained to Crystal that eating and smoking cause the test results to be inaccurate. Told her that she could eat and smoke as soon as the test was over.
- ❏ Told Crystal that she needs to sit quietly during the test, so it would not be possible for her to bring her children.
- ❏ Informed the physician of Crystal's situation to see whether he had any suggestions.

What Did Michelle* Not *Do?
- ❏ Did not become defensive or intimidated by Crystal's behavior.
- ❏ Did not tell Crystal that the staff would watch Crystal's children during the test.
- ❏ Did not tell Crystal that it was not a good idea for her to smoke around her children.

Case Study 2
Page 879

What Did Michelle Do?
- ❏ Told Dave that it would be fine for him to perform his own finger-stick.
- ❏ Made sure that his finger was cleansed with an antiseptic wipe and that he wipes away the first drop of blood.
- ❏ Explained to Dave that the air bubbles take up space that the insulin should occupy, and that if he does not get rid of them, he will not get his full dose of insulin.
- ❏ Demonstrated how to remove air bubbles, and have Dave practice it at the office.
- ❏ Told Dave he must not reuse his needle and syringe. Explained that a used needle could cause him to get an infection. Asked Dave whether he had checked to see if his insurance would cover the cost of the needles and syringes.

What Did Michelle* Not *Do?
- ❏ Did not tell Dave he didn't need to worry about the air bubbles in the syringe.

Continued

Case Study 3
Page 889

What Did Michelle Do?
❑ Tried to calm and reassure Karen.
❑ Explained to Karen that the cholesterol results are not affected by food, so eating before the health fair should not have affected her results.
❑ Told Karen that before a cholesterol analyzer is used, it is usually checked to ensure that it is working properly.
❑ Reassured Karen that the physician was checking her cholesterol again and is running some additional tests to determine whether she is having any problems.

❑ Told Karen that if she must take medication, the physician will determine what drug is best for her.

What Did Michelle Not *Do?*
❑ Did not tell Karen that her cholesterol is extremely high.
❑ Did not tell Karen that she should be more careful about what she eats because she is overweight.
❑ Did not tell Karen that there was no way to know whether the cholesterol analyzer used at the health fair was calibrated and had controls run on it.

TERMINOLOGY REVIEW

Key Term	Word Parts	Definition
Agglutination (as it pertains to blood)		Clumping of blood cells.
Analyte		A substance that is being identified or measured in a laboratory test.
Antibody	*anti-*: against	A substance that is capable of combining with an antigen, resulting in an antigen-antibody reaction.
Antigen	*anti-*: against *-gen*: substance or agent that produces or causes	A substance capable of stimulating the formation of antibodies.
Blood antigen	*anti-*: against *-gen*: substance or agent that produces or causes	A protein present on the surface of red blood cells that determines a person's blood type.
Glycogen	*glyc/o-*: sugar *-gen*: substance or agent that produces or causes	The form in which carbohydrate is stored in the body.
Glycosylation	*glyc/o-*: sugar	The process of glucose attaching to hemoglobin.
HDL cholesterol		A lipoprotein, consisting of protein and cholesterol, that removes excess cholesterol from the cells.
Hemoglobin A$_{1c}$	*hemo-*: blood	Compound formed when glucose attaches or glycosylates to the protein in hemoglobin.
Hyperglycemia	*hyper-*: above, excessive *glyc/o-*: sugar *-emia*: blood condition	An abnormally high level of glucose in the blood.
Hypoglycemia	*hypo-*: below, deficient *glyc/o-*: sugar *-emia*: blood condition	An abnormally low level of glucose in the blood.
LDL cholesterol		A lipoprotein, consisting of protein and cholesterol, that picks up cholesterol and delivers it to the cells.
Lipoprotein	*lip/o-*: fat	A complex molecule consisting of protein and a lipid fraction such as cholesterol. Lipoproteins function in transporting lipids in the blood.

ON THE WEB

For information on diabetes:

American Diabetes Association: www.diabetes.org

Joslin Diabetes Center: www.joslin.org

National Diabetes Education Initiative: www.ndei.org

The National Institute of Diabetes: www.2.niddk.nih.gov

Medical News Today: Diabetes: www.medicalnewstoday.com/info/diabetes

Diabetes: Medline Plus: http://www.nlm.nih.gov/medlineplus/diabetes.html

WebMD Diabetes: http://diabetes.webmd.com/

DLife: http://www.dlife.com/

34 Medical Microbiology

ℯ Check out the Evolve site at http://evolve.elsevier.com/Bonewit/today/ to access additional interactive activities and exercises to help you study and prepare for success.

LEARNING OBJECTIVES

Microorganisms and Disease

1. List and explain the stages of an infectious disease.
2. List and describe the three classifications of bacteria based on shape.
3. Give examples of infectious diseases caused by the following types of cocci:
   - Staphylococci
   - Streptococci
   - Diplococci
4. State examples of infectious diseases caused by bacilli, spirilla, and viruses.

Microscope

5. Explain the function of each of the following parts of a compound microscope: base, arm, stage, light source, substage condenser, iris diaphragm, body tube, coarse adjustment, and fine adjustment.
6. Identify the function of each of the following microscope lenses: low power, high power, and oil immersion.
7. List the guidelines for proper care of the microscope.

Microbiologic Specimen Collection

8. Explain the purpose of obtaining a specimen, and identify body areas from which a specimen can be taken for microbiologic examination.
9. List ways to prevent contamination of a specimen by extraneous microorganisms.
10. Explain the precautions a medical assistant should take to prevent infection from a pathogenic specimen.

Microbiologic Tests

11. Explain the importance of the early diagnosis of streptococcal pharyngitis.
12. Explain the purpose of and describe the procedure for a sensitivity test.
13. Explain the purpose of a microbiologic smear.
14. Explain the purpose of Gram staining.
15. Identify infectious diseases caused by gram-positive bacteria and gram-negative bacteria.
16. Give examples of methods to prevent and control infectious diseases in the community.

PROCEDURES

Use a microscope.
Properly handle and care for a microscope.

Collect a throat specimen.

Perform a streptococcus test using a rapid strep test.

CHAPTER OUTLINE

INTRODUCTION TO MICROBIOLOGY
NORMAL FLORA
INFECTION
Stages of an Infectious Disease
MICROORGANISMS AND DISEASE
Bacteria
Cocci
Bacilli
Spirilla

Viruses
MICROSCOPE
Support System
Frame
Stage
Light Source
Condenser
Diaphragm
Adjustment Knobs

Optical System
Eyepiece
Objective Lenses
Focus
Low and High Power
Oil Immersion
Care of the Microscope
MICROBIOLOGIC SPECIMEN COLLECTION
Handling and Transporting Microbiologic Specimens
Wound Specimens
Collection and Transport Systems

STREPTOCOCCUS TESTING
Rapid Streptococcus Tests
SENSITIVITY TESTING
MICROSCOPIC EXAMINATION OF MICROORGANISMS
Wet Mount Method
Smears
Gram Stain
**PREVENTION AND CONTROL OF INFECTIOUS
    DISEASES**

KEY TERMS

bacilli (bah-SILL-ie)
cocci (KOK-sie)
contagious (kon-TAE-jus)
culture
culture medium
false-negative result

incubate (IN-kyoo-bate)
incubation period
infectious disease
microbiology (mie-kroe-bie-OL-oe-jee)
mucous membrane (MYOO-kus
    MEM-brain)

normal flora
sequela (SEK-kwe-lah)
smear
specimen (SPESS-ih-men)
spirilla (spa-RILL-ah)

INTRODUCTION TO MICROBIOLOGY

Microbiology is the scientific study of microorganisms and their activities. As described in Chapter 17, microorganisms are tiny living plants and animals that cannot be seen by the naked eye, but must be viewed under a microscope. Anton van Leeuwenhoek (1632-1723) designed a magnifying glass strong enough for viewing microorganisms. He was the first individual to observe and describe protozoa and bacteria (Figure 34-1). Leeuwenhoek's magnifying glass was the precursor of modern microscopes used today to study microorganisms. A microscope allows the observer to see individual microbial cells and to differentiate and identify microorganisms.

For the most part, microbiology deals with unicellular, or one-celled, microscopic organisms. All of the life processes necessary to sustain the microbe are performed by one cell. Among them are the ingestion of food substances and their use for energy, growth, reproduction, and excretion.

Microorganisms are *ubiquitous;* they are found almost everywhere—in the air, in food and water, in the soil, and in association with plants, animals, and human life. Although vast numbers of microorganisms exist, only a relatively small number are pathogenic and able to cause disease.

When a pathogen infects a host, it often produces a set of symptoms peculiar to that disease. Scarlet fever is characterized by a sore throat, swelling of the lymph nodes in the neck, a red and swollen tongue, and a bright red rash

Figure 34-1 Bacteria drawn by van Leeuwenhoek in 1684. (From Fuerst R: *Frobisher and Fuert's microbiology in health and disease,* ed 15, Philadelphia, 1983, Saunders.)

covering the body. These symptoms aid the physician in diagnosing the disease. The medical assistant must be alert to all symptoms that the patient describes and must relay this information to the physician through careful and concise charting of these symptoms in the patient's medical record.

If the physician is not able to diagnose the disease from the patient's clinical signs and symptoms, laboratory tests may be used to help the physician identify the pathogen. Identification of the pathogen leads to proper treatment of the disease. Categories of laboratory tests used to identify a pathogen include the following:

- Microbial culture
- Biochemical tests
- Microscopy
- DNA testing (also known as polymerase chain reaction [PCR] testing)

Although most laboratory tests used to identify a pathogen are performed at an outside laboratory, the medical assistant is frequently responsible for collection of the specimen that will be transported to the outside laboratory.

This chapter provides an introduction to microbiology, including a description of proper microbiologic collection and handling techniques that must be followed to ensure a high-quality specimen. Identification of a pathogen using microbial culturing, biochemical testing, and microscopy is also discussed in this chapter. DNA testing to detect pathogens (e.g., those that cause chlamydia and gonorrhea) was previously described in Chapter 23. Before undertaking this study, the medical assistant should review Chapter 17, which discusses introductory concepts that are basic to this chapter.

NORMAL FLORA

Every individual has a **normal flora,** which consists of the harmless microorganisms that normally reside in many parts of the body but do not cause disease. The surface of the skin, the **mucous membrane** of the gastrointestinal tract, and parts of the respiratory and genitourinary tracts all have an abundant normal flora. Some microorganisms that make up the normal flora are beneficial to the body, such as those that inhabit the intestinal tract that feed on other potentially harmful microscopic organisms. Other examples are microorganisms found in the intestinal tract that synthesize vitamin K, an essential vitamin needed by the body for proper blood clotting. In rare instances, if the opportunity arises (e.g., lowered body resistance), certain microorganisms of the normal flora can become pathogenic and cause disease.

INFECTION

Invasion of the body by pathogenic microorganisms is known as *infection.* Under conditions favorable to the pathogens, they grow and multiply, resulting in an **infectious disease** (also known as a *communicable disease*) that produces harmful effects on the host. Not all pathogens that enter a host are able to cause disease, however. When a pathogen enters the body, it attempts to invade the tissues so that it can grow and multiply. The body tries to stop the invasion with its second line of natural defense mechanisms,* which includes inflammation, phagocytosis by white blood cells, and the production of antibodies. These defense mechanisms work to destroy the pathogen and remove it from the body. If the body is successful, the pathogens are destroyed, and the individual experiences no adverse effects. If the pathogen is able to overcome the body's natural defense mechanisms, an infectious disease results.

Many infectious diseases are **contagious,** meaning that the pathogen that causes the disease can be spread from one person to another directly or indirectly. Frequently, *droplet infection* is the mode of transmission of a contagious disease.

Droplet infection refers to an infection that is indirectly transmitted by tiny contaminated droplets of moisture expelled from the upper respiratory tract of an infected individual. When an individual exhales (as during breathing, talking, coughing, or sneezing), a fine spray of moisture droplets is emitted by that individual from the upper respiratory tract. If the individual has a contagious disease that is transmitted by droplet infection, the pathogens are carried into the air by these tiny moisture droplets. Another individual may inhale these contaminated droplets and become infected with the disease. To help prevent the spread of droplet infections, contagious individuals should cover their mouths and noses while coughing or sneezing. See Figure 17-1 for examples of other means of pathogen transmission.

STAGES OF AN INFECTIOUS DISEASE

When a pathogen becomes established in the host, a series of events usually ensues. The stages of an infectious disease are as follows:

1. The *infection* is the invasion and multiplication of pathogenic microorganisms in the body.
2. The *incubation period* is the interval of time between the invasion by a pathogenic microorganism and the appearance of the first symptoms of the disease. Depending on the type of disease, the **incubation period** may range from a few days to several months. During this time, the pathogen is growing and multiplying.
3. The *prodromal period* is a short period in which the first symptoms that indicate an approaching disease occur. Headache and a feeling of illness are common prodromal symptoms.
4. The *acute period* is when the disease is at its peak and symptoms are fully developed. Fever is a common symptom of many infectious diseases.
5. The *decline period* is when symptoms of the disease begin to subside.
6. The *convalescent period* is the stage in which the patient regains strength and returns to a state of good health.

---

*The first line of natural defense mechanisms, which work to prevent the entrance of pathogens into the body (e.g., coughing, sneezing), is described in Chapter 17.

MICROORGANISMS AND DISEASE

The groups of microorganisms known to contain species capable of causing human disease include bacteria, viruses, protozoa, fungi (including yeasts), and animal parasites. Bacteria and viruses are most frequently responsible for causing human diseases and are discussed next.

BACTERIA

Bacteria are microscopic single-celled organisms. Of the 1700 species known to dwell in humans, only approximately 100 produce human disease. The discovery of antibiotics has helped immensely in combating and controlling bacterial infections. Antibiotics are not effective against viral infections, however.

Bacteria can be classified according to their shape into three basic groups (Figure 34-2). Round bacteria are known as **cocci.** Cocci can be categorized further as diplococci, streptococci, or staphylococci, depending on their pattern of growth. Rod-shaped bacteria are **bacilli.** Spiral and curve-shaped bacteria are **spirilla,** and they include spirochetes and vibrios.

Cocci

Staphylococci are round bacteria that grow in grapelike clusters (Figure 34-3, *A*). The species *Staphylococcus epidermidis* is widely distributed and is normally present on the surface of the skin and the mucous membranes of the mouth, nose, throat, and intestines. *S. epidermidis* is usually nonpathogenic; however, a cut, abrasion, or other break in the skin can allow invasion of the tissues by the organism, resulting in a mild infection.

Staphylococcus aureus is commonly associated with pathologic conditions such as boils, carbuncles, pimples, impetigo, abscesses, *Staphylococcus* food poisoning, and wound infections. Infections caused by staphylococci usually cause much pus formation (suppuration) and are termed *pyogenic* infections.

Streptococci are round bacteria that grow in chains (Figure 34-3, *B*). Before the advent of antibiotics, streptococcal infections were a major cause of human death. Diseases caused by streptococci include streptococcal sore throat ("strep throat"), scarlet fever, rheumatic fever, pneumonia, puerperal sepsis, erysipelas, and skin conditions such as carbuncles and impetigo.

Diplococci are round bacteria that grow in pairs. Pneumonia, gonorrhea, and meningitis are infectious diseases caused by diplococci.

What Would You Do? | What Would You *Not* Do?

Case Study 1

Paula Hutchinson brings her 8-year-old daughter Caitlin to the medical office. Caitlin has had a fever and sore throat and has had difficulty eating for the past 2 days. The physician orders a rapid strep test. Caitlin refuses to open her mouth so that the specimen can be collected. She says that she doesn't want that "swab thing" in her mouth because she's afraid it will make her throw up. Paula wants to know why the strep test must be run. She says that Caitlin's throat is very red with white patches and wants to know why the physician doesn't just prescribe an antibiotic for her without running the test. ■

Bacilli

Bacilli are rod-shaped bacteria that are frequently found in the soil and air (Figure 34-3, *C*). Some bacilli are able to form spores, a characteristic that enables them to resist adverse conditions such as heat and disinfectants. Diseases caused by bacilli include botulism, tetanus, gas gangrene, gastroenteritis produced by *Salmonella* food poisoning, typhoid fever, pertussis (whooping cough), bacillary dysentery, diphtheria, tuberculosis, leprosy, and plague.

Escherichia coli is a species of bacillus that is found among the normal flora of the large intestine in enormous numbers (Figure 34-3, *D*). It is normally a harmless bacterium; however, if it enters the urinary tract as a result of lowered resistance, poor hygiene practices, or both, it may cause a urinary tract infection.

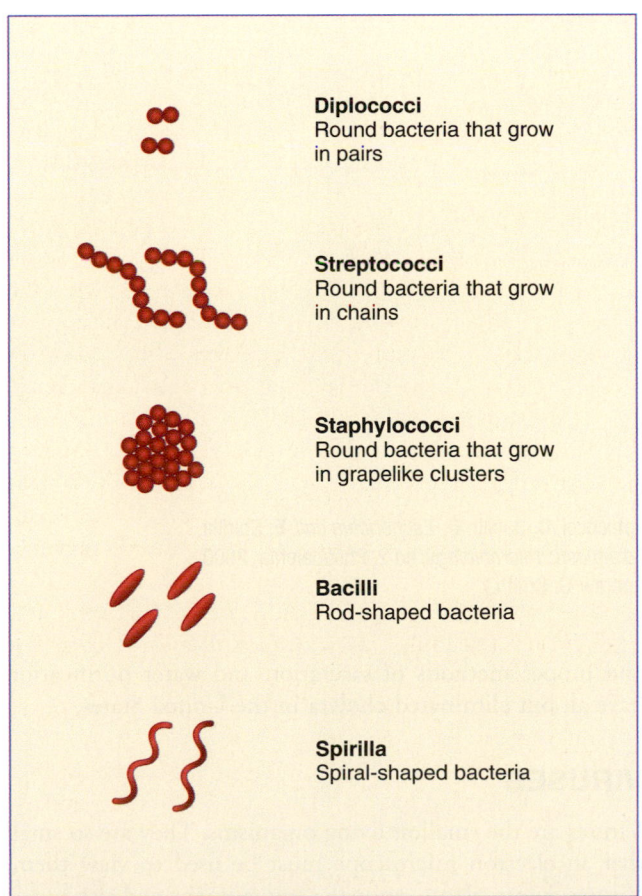

Diplococci
Round bacteria that grow in pairs

Streptococci
Round bacteria that grow in chains

Staphylococci
Round bacteria that grow in grapelike clusters

Bacilli
Rod-shaped bacteria

Spirilla
Spiral-shaped bacteria

Figure 34-2 Classification of bacteria based on shape.

Figure 34-3 Types of bacteria. **A,** Staphylococci. **B,** Streptococci. **C,** Bacilli. **D,** *Escherichia coli.* **E,** Spirilla. (**A, B,** and **D,** From Mahon CR, Manuselis G Jr: *Textbook of diagnostic microbiology,* ed 2, Philadelphia, 2000, Saunders; **C,** Courtesy Cathy Bissonette; **E,** Courtesy Dr. Andrew G. Smith.)

Spirilla

Spirilla are spiral or curve-shaped bacteria. *Treponema pallidum,* a spirochete, is the causative agent of syphilis (Figure 34-3, *E*). This microorganism cannot be grown in commonly available culture media; the diagnosis of syphilis is typically made using serologic tests. A serologic test is performed on the serum of the blood. Cholera is caused by another type of spirillum, *Vibrio cholerae.* Immunization

and proper methods of sanitation and water purification have all but eliminated cholera in the United States.

VIRUSES

Viruses are the smallest living organisms. They are so small that an electron microscope must be used to view them. Viruses infect plants, animals, and humans and use nutrients inside the host's cells for their metabolic and reproductive needs. Infectious diseases caused by viruses include influenza, chickenpox, rubeola (measles), rubella (German measles), mumps, poliomyelitis, smallpox, rabies, herpes simplex, herpes zoster, yellow fever, hepatitis, and most infectious diseases of the upper respiratory tract, including the common cold.

MICROSCOPE

Many kinds of microscopes are available, but the type used most often for office laboratory work is the *compound microscope.* The compound microscope consists of a two-lens system, and the magnification of one system is increased by the other. A source of bright light is required for proper illumination of the object to be viewed. This combination of lenses and light permits visualization of structures that cannot be seen with the unaided eye, such as microorganisms and cellular forms. The compound microscope consists of two main components—the support system and the optical system. The medical assistant should be able to identify the parts of a microscope (Figure 34-4) and should be able to use and care for it properly. Procedure 34-1 outlines the correct use and care of a microscope.

SUPPORT SYSTEM

Frame

The working parts of the microscope are supported by a sturdy frame consisting of a *base* for support and an *arm* for carrying it without damaging the delicate parts. The arm also is needed to support the magnifying and adjusting systems.

Stage

The *stage* of a microscope is the flat, horizontal platform on which the microscope slide is placed. It is located directly over the condenser and beneath the objective lenses. The stage has a small round opening in the center that permits light from below to pass through the object being viewed and up into the lenses above. The slide should be placed on the stage; the object to be viewed is positioned over this opening so that it is satisfactorily illuminated by the light source below. Standard microscope stages have metal clips attached to the stage to hold the glass slide securely in place. With this type of stage, the slide must be moved by hand for examination of various areas on it.

Other types of microscopes have a *mechanical stage* that allows movement of the slide in a vertical or horizontal position by use of adjustment knobs. The mechanical stage provides precise positioning of the slide, which is essential for performing certain procedures, such as differential white blood counts and inspection of Gram-stained smears.

Light Source

The light source is at the base of the microscope and consists of a built-in illuminator, along with a switch for turning it on and off. The light is directed to the condenser above it and then through the object to be viewed.

Condenser

Compound microscopes have a lens system between the light source and object, known as the *substage condenser.* A popular condenser is the *Abbe condenser,* which consists of two lenses used to illuminate objects with transmitted light. The condenser collects and concentrates the light rays and

Figure 34-4 Parts of the microscope.

PROCEDURE 34-2   Collecting a Throat Specimen

Outcome Collect a throat specimen for a rapid strep test

A throat specimen is obtained by using a sterile swab. It is commonly collected to aid in the diagnosis of infections such as streptococcal sore throat, pharyngitis, and tonsillitis. Less frequently, it is used to diagnose whooping cough and diphtheria. These latter diseases are not prevalent today because of the availability of immunizations against them. This procedure outlines the steps necessary to obtain a throat specimen to perform a rapid streptococcus test, which is discussed in this chapter.

Equipment/Supplies

- Disposable gloves
- Tongue depressor
- Sterile swab
- Waste container

1. **Procedural Step.** Sanitize your hands, and assemble the equipment.
2. **Procedural Step.** Greet the patient and introduce yourself. Identify the patient by full name and date of birth and explain the procedure.
3. **Procedural Step.** Position the patient, and adjust the light to provide clear visualization of the throat.
   Principle. The throat must be clearly visible so that the medical assistant is able to determine the proper area for obtaining the specimen.
4. **Procedural Step.** Apply gloves. Remove the sterile swab from its peel-apart package, being careful not to contaminate it.
   Principle. Contamination of the swab may lead to inaccurate test results.

Remove the swab.

5. **Procedural Step.** Depress the tongue with the tongue depressor.
   Principle. The tongue depressor holds the tongue down and facilitates access to the throat.
6. **Procedural Step.** Place the swab at the back of the throat (posterior pharynx), and firmly rub it over any lesions or white or inflamed areas of the mucous membrane of the tonsillar area and posterior pharyngeal wall. Rotate the swab constantly as you collect the specimen, making sure there is good contact with the tonsillar area. Do not allow the swab to touch any areas other than the throat, such as the inside of the mouth.

Principle. The swab should be rubbed over suspicious-looking areas where pathogens are likely to be found. A rotating motion is used to deposit the maximal amount of material possible on the swab. Touching it to any areas other than the throat contaminates the specimen with extraneous microorganisms.

Collect the specimen.

7. **Procedural Step.** Keeping the patient's tongue depressed, withdraw the swab, and remove the tongue depressor from the patient's mouth.
8. **Procedural Step.** Properly dispose of the tongue depressor in a regular waste container to prevent transmission of microorganisms.
9. **Procedural Step.** Process the swab according to the directions accompanying the rapid strep test.
10. **Procedural Step.** Remove gloves, and sanitize your hands. Chart the test results in the patient's medical record.

PPR CHARTING EXAMPLE

Date	
9/20/XX	10:30 a.m. Throat specimen collected.
	QuickVue Strep Test: Positive. ————
	———— N. Moorehead, CMA (AAMA)

STREPTOCOCCUS TESTING

The most common streptococcal condition is streptococcal sore throat, or *streptococcal pharyngitis,* which primarily affects children and young adults. The causative agent of streptococcal pharyngitis is a group A beta-hemolytic streptococcal species known as *Streptococcus pyogenes.*

Streptococcal pharyngitis is a potentially serious condition because some patients develop a poststreptococcal sequela. A **sequela** is a morbid secondary condition that occurs as a result of a less serious primary infection. A few patients with streptococcal pharyngitis (primary infection) develop rheumatic fever; the rheumatic fever is considered a poststreptococcal sequela. Owing to the risk of a sequela, early diagnosis of streptococcal pharyngitis and treatment with antibiotics are important. In the medical office, commercially available rapid streptococcus tests are often used for identification of group A beta-hemolytic streptococci. The specimen may also be sent to an outside laboratory for **culture** to determine the presence of group A streptococci. A culture is the growth and propagation of microorganisms in a **culture medium**. A culture medium is a mixture of nutrients on which microorganisms are grown in the laboratory.

RAPID STREPTOCOCCUS TESTS

Rapid streptococcus tests are biochemical tests that directly detect group A streptococci from a throat swab in a very short time. Most tests require only 4 to 10 minutes to process; diagnosis can often be made and antibiotics prescribed, if necessary, before the patient leaves the office.

The most frequently used rapid streptococcus test is the direct antigen identification test, which confirms the presence of group A streptococci through an antigen-antibody reaction. The test works by combining particles sensitized to the *Streptococcus* antibody with the throat specimen. If group A streptococcal antigen is in the specimen, it combines with the antibody-sensitized particles to produce a color change that can be observed with the unaided eye. Rapid streptococcus tests also include a control that determines whether the test results are accurate and reliable.

The advantage of the direct antigen identification test is that it provides the physician with immediate test results rather than requiring an overnight culture. Specific instructions are included with every commercially available antigen identification test; examples of these tests include Qtest Strep (Becton Dickinson), Clearview Strep A Exact (Wampole Laboratories, Princeton, NJ), and QuickVue In-Line Strep A Test (Quidel, San Diego, Calif) (Figure 34-6).

SENSITIVITY TESTING

The physician may request not only that the laboratory identify the infecting pathogen, but also that a sensitivity test be performed on it to determine the best antibiotic to treat the condition. A sensitivity test determines the susceptibility of pathogenic bacteria to various antibiotics.

The most common method for sensitivity testing is the *disc-diffusion method* (Figure 34-7). Commercially prepared discs impregnated with known concentrations of various antibiotics are dropped on the surface of a solid culture medium in a Petri plate containing the pathogen. The culture is incubated, allowing the antibiotics to diffuse into the culture medium. If the pathogen is susceptible or sensitive to an antibiotic, a clear zone without bacterial growth surrounds the disc. This indicates that the antibiotic was effective in destroying the pathogen. If the pathogen is unaffected by or resistant to the antibiotic, no clear zone is seen around the disc, indicating that the antibiotic was unable to kill the pathogen. Sensitivity testing enables the physician to decide which antibiotics would most likely be effective against the infectious disease in question.

MICROSCOPIC EXAMINATION OF MICROORGANISMS

Microorganisms can be examined under a microscope in the fixed state or in the living state. Examination in the fixed state involves the preparation of a smear through heat fixation, followed by a staining process such as Gram stain (see later). Most microorganisms are examined in the fixed state because it is easier to examine them when they are stained.

Some microorganisms require examination in the living state, however, owing to special circumstances, such as their inability to be readily stained or difficulty in culturing them. The living state also allows visualization of the movement of motile microorganisms. This is especially helpful in the identification of certain motile microorganisms, such as *Trichomonas vaginalis,* which is the causative agent of the vaginal infection trichomoniasis. To observe the motility of microorganisms, they first must be suspended in a liquid medium so that they are free to move about. The most common method of examining microorganisms in the living state is the wet mount method, which is described next.

WET MOUNT METHOD

In the wet mount method, the medical assistant places a drop of fluid containing the organism on a glass slide and covers it with a cover slip (Figure 34-8). The cover slip may be ringed with petroleum jelly to provide a seal between the slide and the cover slip. The purpose is to reduce the rate of evaporation through air currents that lead to drying and possible death of the specimen.

The slide is placed under the microscope for examination by the physician using the high-power objective. For satisfactory visualization, the intensity of the light must be diminished by partially closing the diaphragm of the

QuickVue® In-Line™ One-Step Strep A

Now "Fill to rim" instead of counting drops

Use this swab.

Insert completely.

Break.

Shake.

Quickly fill to rim.

Wait 5 minutes.

If liquid has not moved across the Result Window in 1 minute, completely remove the swab and reinsert.

Results

High Positive — QuickVue — C T — STREP A

Low Positive — QuickVue — C T — STREP A

Negative — QuickVue — C T — STREP A

Figure 34-6 Procedure for performing the QuickVue In-Line one-step strep A test. (Courtesy Quidel Corporation, San Diego, Calif.)

AZ:	Azithromycin
CE:	Cephalothin
CF:	Ciprofloxacin
CL:	Clarithromycin
CP:	Ciprozil
DX:	Doxycycline
E:	Erythromycin
NF:	Nitrofurantoin
NO:	Norfloxacin
P:	Penicillin
S:	Sulfisoxazole
T:	Tetracycline

Figure 34-7 Sensitivity testing. (From Mahon CR, Manuselis G Jr: *Textbook of diagnostic microbiology,* ed 2, Philadelphia, 2000, Saunders.)

Strep Throat

Answer questions that patients have about strep throat.

What is strep throat?

Strep throat is a contagious and acute infection that is medically known as *streptococcal pharyngitis*. It is caused by the bacterium group A *Streptococcus*. Strep throat is transmitted directly from one person to another through droplets of saliva or nasal secretions. It most frequently occurs in children 5 to 10 years old and during the months of October through April. Strep infections are different from most other infectious diseases because having one strep infection does not prevent the development of another at a future date.

What are the symptoms of strep throat?

The symptoms of strep throat are a sore throat with severe pain on swallowing, a bright red pharynx (called "beefy red pharynx"), fever, white patches on the tonsils, swollen glands in the neck, muscular aches and pains, and a feeling of tiredness.

How is strep throat diagnosed and treated?

Strep throat is diagnosed by taking a throat specimen and running a laboratory test on it to determine whether group A *Streptococcus*

is present. Strep throat usually is treated by antibiotics taken orally for 10 days. It is important to take all of the antibiotic prescribed by the physician to prevent complications that can occur from strep throat. A patient with strep throat should rest in bed and avoid contact with others to prevent spreading it.

What are the complications of strep throat?

Severe complications can result from strep throat if it is not adequately treated, including rheumatic fever and glomerulonephritis, which is a kidney disorder. These complications are rare because most patients seek early treatment for strep infections.

- Encourage the patient to complete the entire prescribed course of antibiotics.
- Instruct the patient to notify the physician if new symptoms develop.
- Provide the patient with educational materials about strep throat. ∎

What Would You Do? | What Would You *Not* Do?

Case Study 3

John Seimer calls the medical office. He says that he is not a patient at the office but would like some assistance. He says that for the past 3 days he has had a headache, fever, chills, and aching muscles. He says that a week ago he pulled a tick off his lower leg, and several days later he found a red rash around the tick bite. He says that he went on the Internet and looked up his symptoms, and he is sure that he has Lyme disease. The Internet site recommended taking doxycycline for 3 weeks to treat Lyme disease. John says that he does not like to go to the doctor and has not been to see a doctor for over 10 years. He wants to know whether the doctor could call in a prescription for doxycycline for him. He says that he has health insurance and the doctor could bill him for an appointment, just as long as he does not have to come in. ∎

A drop of fluid containing the organism is placed on a glass slide.

The specimen is covered with a coverslip ringed with petroleum jelly.

Figure 34-8 Wet mount method of slide preparation for examining microorganisms in the living state.

---

microscope. The slide and coverslip should be properly disposed of in a biohazard sharps container.

SMEARS

A **smear** consists of material spread on a slide for microscopic examination. It can be prepared directly from the specimen collected on the swab, or the specimen can be grown first on a culture medium and a smear then prepared. Most smears must be stained before they can be viewed under the microscope, using one of many staining techniques. Bacteria contained in a smear are colorless and usually are difficult to identify under the microscope unless some type of staining is used.

Smears are often helpful when time is a factor because a smear can be prepared immediately from the specimen. This procedure gives the physician a preliminary clue to the causative agent while other, more time-consuming tests are being performed.

GRAM STAIN

Gram stain is often used in combination with other tests to help in the diagnosis and treatment of infectious diseases. As already discussed, bacteria contained in a smear are colorless and usually are difficult to identify under the

CARBOHYDRATES
Classification of Carbohydrates
Dietary Fiber
FAT
Types of Dietary Fat
PROTEIN
Amino Acids
Classification of Protein
VITAMINS
Classification of Vitamins
Antioxidant Vitamins
MINERALS
Classification of Minerals
WATER
DIETARY SUPPLEMENTS
TOOLS FOR HEALTHY NUTRITION
NUTRITION GUIDES
MyPlate
2010 Dietary Guidelines for Americans
FOOD LABELS
Nutrition Facts Panel
Ingredient List

NUTRITION THERAPY
WEIGHT MANAGEMENT
Obesity
Treatment of Obesity
CARDIOVASCULAR DISEASE
Nutrition Therapy
HYPERTENSION
Nutrition Therapy
DIABETES
Type 1 Diabetes
Type 2 Diabetes
LACTOSE INTOLERANCE
Nutrition Therapy
GLUTEN INTOLERANCE
Celiac Disease
Non-Celiac Gluten Sensitivity
Symptoms of Gluten Intolerance
Nutrition Therapy
FOOD ALLERGIES
Nutrition Therapy
Medication and Supplements

KEY TERMS

antioxidant (an-tee-OCKS-i-dent)
atherosclerosis (ath-er-oh-skleh-ROH-sis)
bariatrics
cholesterol (ko-LES-ter-ol)
complete protein
disaccharide (die-SAK-a-ride)
empty calorie food
essential amino acid
gluten (GLOO-ten)

glycogen (GLIE-koe-jen)
incomplete protein
kilocalorie (KIL-o-cal-or-ee)
lactose (LAK-tos)
macronutrient (MAK-ro-noo-tree-ent)
micronutrient (MY-crow-noo-tree-ent)
mineral
monosaccharide (mah-no-SAK-a-ride)
nonessential amino acid
nutrient (NOO-tree-ent)

nutrition (noo-TRI-shun)
nutrition therapy
obesity (oh-BEE-si-tee)
percent daily value
saturated fat
triglycerides (tri-GLIS-eh-rides)
unsaturated fat
vitamin

INTRODUCTION TO NUTRITION

Nutrition is the study of nutrients in food including how the body uses them and their relationship to health. A **nutrient** is a chemical substance found in food that is needed by the body for survival and well-being. Good nutrition is an important component of the health and well-being of an individual. Inadequate nutrition can result in poor health and even disease. Some of the specific benefits derived from good nutrition include the following:

- Supports good physical and mental well-being
- Helps to maintain a healthy weight
- Boosts the functioning of the immune system
- Delays the effects of aging

- Lowers the risk of certain conditions and diseases (e.g., obesity, heart disease, cancer, diabetes)

The medical assistant should have a knowledge of basic nutrition principles and the recommended nutrition therapy for common conditions and diseases. The medical assistant uses this information when scheduling a patient for an appointment with a dietitian, relaying information to patients on dietary restrictions required for tests and procedures, providing patients with nutrition education handouts, and answering basic questions a patient may have regarding nutrition.

Medical assistants are not qualified to conduct nutritional assessments or recommend nutrition therapy. This is the responsibility of a registered dietitian. Medical assistants should make sure to adhere to these guidelines to stay within the scope of practice for a medical assistant.

DEFINITION OF TERMS

Terms that aid in understanding this chapter are listed and defined here.

Diet: A diet consists of the food and drink an individual consumes each day. To promote sound nutrition, an individual's diet should include the proper balance of nutrients.

Dietitian: A dietitian is a professional specially trained to assess the nutritional status of an individual and recommend appropriate nutrition therapy.

Digestion: The process by which food is broken down in the gastrointestinal tract into smaller components that can be absorbed by the bloodstream for use by the body.

Empty calorie food: A food that provides calories but few or no nutrients.

Enriched food: A food to which vitamins and minerals have been added to replace those lost during the processing of that food.

Fortified food: A food to which vitamins and minerals that were not there originally have been added to increase the nutritional quality of the food.

Malnutrition (or poor nutrition): A condition that can occur because of an excess or deficiency of one or more nutrients.

Nutrient density: Refers to the amount of nutrients in a food compared with the amount of calories. A food with a high nutrient density is low in calories and high in nutrients. A food with a low nutrient density (known as an *empty calorie food*) is high in calories and low in nutrients.

NUTRIENTS

Nutrients can be categorized into six classes according to their chemical structure and the role they play in nourishing the body. The six classes of nutrients include carbohydrates, fat, protein, vitamins, minerals, and water and are described in more detail in this section.

Each of the six classes of nutrients plays an important role in supporting good nutritional health. Nutrients provide three primary functions in the body as follows:
- Provide energy for the body
- Build, repair, and maintain body tissue
- Assist in the regulation of body processes

The National Academy of Sciences Food and Nutrition Board developed the Dietary Reference Intake (DRI) tables to assist individuals in determining their recommended daily intake of essential nutrients. Nutrient recommendations in the DRI tables are based on gender, age, and life stage and also allow for individual variation. The DRI tables can be accessed through the following website: www.nal.usda.gov/fnic/DRI/DRI_Energy/1319-1331.pdf.

Table 35-1 Energy Value of the Macronutrients

Macronutrient	Energy Value
Carbohydrate	4 kcal/gram
Fat	9 kcal/gram
Protein	4 kcal/gram

CLASSIFICATION OF NUTRIENTS

Nutrients can be further classified as macronutrients or micronutrients.

MACRONUTRIENTS

Macronutrients are nutrients needed in relatively large amounts by the body and include carbohydrates, fat, and protein. Macronutrients provide kilocalories to the body to yield energy in addition to performing other important body functions, which are discussed in this chapter. A **kilocalorie** (kcal), often referred to simply as a *calorie,* is a measurement unit of energy. A kilocalorie is defined as the amount of heat needed to raise the temperature of 1 kilogram of water 1° Celsius. The energy value provided by each of the macronutrients is outlined in Table 35-1.

The body uses carbohydrate as a short-term energy fuel and uses fat as a long-term fuel. Although protein provides 4 kcal of energy per gram and can be used as an energy source, the body would rather *not* use protein as an energy source. Instead the body prefers to use carbohydrate as an energy source to "spare" protein for its more important functions of building, maintaining, and repairing body tissues.

Macronutrient	Function	Food Sources
Carbohydrate	Chief source of energy for the body; Primary source of energy for the central nervous system	Pasta, rice, bread, cereal, potatoes, fruits, vegetables
Fat	Provides energy for the body; Transports fat-soluble vitamins in the body; Provides essential fatty acids for the body	Fatty meats, butter, cheese, cream, whole milk, egg yolk, vegetable oils, nuts, avocados
Protein	Builds, maintains, and repairs body tissue; Makes up enzymes, antibodies, and most hormones	Meat, fish, poultry, potatoes, eggs, milk, cheese, legumes, nuts

MICRONUTRIENTS

Micronutrients are nutrients required in very small amounts by the body and include vitamins and minerals. Vitamins and minerals are not broken down by the body and are used

Table 35-3 Water-Soluble Vitamins

Vitamin	Function	Food Sources	Deficiency Diseases and Conditions
Vitamin B_1 (thiamine)	Coenzyme in energy metabolism Normal functioning of the nervous system	Pork, beef, liver, eggs, fish, whole-grain and enriched breads, legumes	Beriberi Problems with the GI tract, nervous system, and cardiovascular system
Vitamin B_2 (Riboflavin)	Coenzyme in energy metabolism Normal vision and skin health	Milk, meats, green leafy green vegetables, whole-grain and enriched bread and cereals	Cheilosis Eye sensitivity Dermatitis Glossitis
Vitamin B_3 (niacin)	Coenzyme in energy metabolism Healthy skin Healthy nervous and digestive systems Skin health	Milk, eggs, meat, fish, poultry, whole-grain and enriched breads and cereals	Pellagra (dermatitis, neuritis, diarrhea)
Vitamin B_5 (pantothenic acid)	Coenzyme in energy metabolism Synthesis of fatty acids, cholesterol, steroid hormones	Eggs, liver, salmon, poultry, mushrooms, cauliflower, peanuts	Burning feet and other neurologic symptoms
Vitamin B_6 (pyridoxine)	Coenzyme in protein metabolism Assists in making red blood cells	Meat, fish, poultry, liver, milk, eggs, whole grains, legumes, soy products	Cheilosis Glossitis Dermatitis Confusion Depression Irritability
Vitamin B_7 (biotin)	Coenzyme in carbohydrate and protein metabolism	Milk, liver, egg yolk, legumes, yeast, soy flour, cereals, fruit	Dermatitis Nausea Anorexia Depression Hair loss
Vitamin B_9 (folic acid)	Synthesis of red blood cells Synthesis of DNA Development of fetal nervous system	Liver, leafy green vegetables, legumes, seeds, fruit, cereal and bread fortified with folate	Megaloblastic anemia Neural tube birth defects (anencephaly and spina bifida)
Vitamin B_{12} (cobalamin)	Synthesis of red blood cells Maintenance of myelin sheaths	Meat, poultry, fish seafood, liver, eggs, milk, cheese	Pernicious anemia Degeneration of myelin sheaths Sore mouth and tongue Neurologic disorders
Vitamin C (ascorbic acid)	Building and maintenance of strong tissues through collagen synthesis Wound healing Assists in absorption of iron Resistance to infection Antioxidant	Citrus fruits, broccoli, melons, strawberries, tomatoes, Brussels sprouts, potatoes, cabbage, green peppers	Scurvy Muscle cramps Bleeding and loose gums Tendency to bruise easily Poor wound healing Weakened bones

GI, Gastrointestinal.

include major minerals and trace minerals. Major minerals are required in the body in larger quantities, whereas trace minerals are required in very small amounts. Each of these mineral classifications is described in more detail in the following sections.

Major Minerals

Major minerals are required in the adult diet in amounts greater than 100 mg/day and are found in the body in levels of 5 grams or higher. They play important roles in bone and tooth health, blood pressure regulation, and water and acid-base balance. The major minerals include calcium (Figure 35-7), magnesium phosphorus, potassium, chloride, and sodium. Refer to Table 35-5 for the specific function, food sources, and deficiency diseases of major minerals.

Trace Minerals

Trace minerals are required in the adult diet in amounts less than 50 mg/day and are found in the body in levels of less than 5 grams. They are a diverse group of minerals that assist in proper metabolism and structure as well as immune and blood system functions. Trace minerals include iron, copper, zinc, manganese, fluoride, selenium, iodine, chromium, and molybdenum. Refer to Table 35-6 for the specific function, food sources, and deficiency diseases of trace minerals.

Table 35-4 Fat-Soluble Vitamins

Vitamin	Function	Food Sources	Deficiency Diseases and Conditions, and Toxicity Symptoms
Vitamin A (retinol)	Maintenance of vision in dim light Maintenance of mucous membranes and healthy skin Antioxidant	Liver, whole milk, butter, cream, fish liver oils, dark green leafy vegetables, deep orange fruits and vegetables	*Deficiency:* Night blindness Xerosis Xerophthalmia *Toxicity Symptoms:* Bone pain Dry skin Loss of hair Fatigue Anorexia
Vitamin D (calciferol)	Regulation of the absorption of calcium and phosphorus Calcification of bones and teeth	Fortified milk and margarine, liver, oily fish, fish liver oils Synthesized by the body using the ultraviolet rays of the sun	*Deficiency:* Rickets (in children) Osteomalacia Poorly developed bones and teeth Muscle spasms *Toxicity Symptoms:* Kidney stones Fragile bones Calcification of soft tissue
Vitamin E (tocopherol)	Protection of red blood cells Antioxidant	Vegetable oils, margarine, salad dressing, wheat germ, nuts, avocados	*Deficiency:* Hemolysis of red blood cells
Vitamin K (phylloquinone)	Formation of prothrombin for normal blood clotting Bone development	Green leafy vegetables, milk, meats, cabbage, broccoli, Brussels sprouts Synthesized by intestinal bacterial	*Deficiency:* Bleeding tendencies Poor bone growth *Toxicity Symptoms:* Prolonged blood clotting

Figure 35-6 Antioxidant Vitamins A and C food sources.

Figure 35-7 Calcium food sources.

WATER

Water is essential to the survival of an individual. This old adage still holds true: man can survive in the desert without food for more than 30 days but can make it only about 3 days without water. Water makes up approximately 60% to 65% of an adult's total body weight, and that percentage is even higher in young children.

Water serves many important functions in the body. Water is the universal solvent of the body; it allows nutrients such as glucose, vitamins, and minerals to dissolve in water and be transported by the circulatory system to the cells of the body. Water allows for transport of substances in and out of cells and is the basis of many chemical reactions in the body. In addition, water provides a solvent

HIGHLIGHT on Eating Disorders—cont'd

consuming only organic, raw, or plant-based foods. Ironically, such restrictive behavior often leads to an unbalanced and inadequate intake of nutrients. Patients with this disorder typically exhibit low self-esteem and a negative body image and often become increasingly socially isolated.

Compulsive Overeating
Compulsive overeating, also known as "food addiction," occurs when an individual engages in binging behaviors without purging. Compulsive overeaters report feeling "out of control" during eating binges. They spend large amounts of time thinking about food, planning their binge, and shopping for it. Uncontrolled eating behaviors typically occur in a frenzied manner and in private. Compulsive overeaters may continue to eat even after they become uncomfortably full. Like the bulimic, an overeater feels shame, embarrassment, and guilt after a binge episode. If left untreated, food addiction can lead to obesity and increase the risk of chronic diseases such as diabetes, high blood pressure, and heart disease. Depression and sleep apnea are also seen in these individuals.

Recovery and Prevention
What is the prognosis for eating disorders?
Recovery from an eating disorder is a gradual process with relapses often occurring. Approximately 50% of individuals with an eating disorder recover completely, and another 30% attain partial recovery. The remaining 20% continue to struggle with disordered eating throughout their lives. Suicide rates are more common in individuals with eating disorders than in the general population. If the medical assistant observes that a patient is exhibiting any of the physical or psychological symptoms of an eating disorder, he or she should inform the physician.

Are there methods for preventing eating disorders?
There are many strategies that help to decrease the risk of developing an eating disorder. These include the following:
- Strive for body acceptance. Focus on what your body can do, not how it looks.
- Avoid physical comparisons with others.
- Be mindful of your genetic influences on body type and embrace them.
- Avoid caloric restrictions that are below 1200 kcal daily.
- Be realistic with weight loss goals. The rate of healthy weight loss is 1 to 2 pounds weekly.
- Adopt a grazing type of eating style. Avoid going more than 4 hours without a meal or snack.
- Listen to your body. Eat when you are hungry and stop when you are full. ■

Table 35-7	Interpretation of Body Mass Index (BMI)
BMI	**Weight Status Category**
Less than 15	Very severely underweight
15-15.9	Severely underweight
16-8.49	Underweight
18.5-24.9	Healthy weight
25-29.9	Overweight
30-34.9	Obese Class I (Moderately obese)
35.0-39.9	Obese Class II (Severely obese)
40 or more	Obese Class III (Very severely obese)

Chapter 20 to review the methods for determining the BMI. The BMI of an adult is then interpreted using the weight status categories outlined in Table 35-7. It has been determined that as the BMI increases to greater than 25, there is an increased risk of developing certain diseases associated with overweight and obesity such as hypertension, coronary heart disease, stroke, type 2 diabetes, sleep apnea and respiratory problems, and osteoarthritis.

TREATMENT OF OBESITY

Obesity is considered a chronic condition that requires a multiple treatment approach consisting of the following three components: nutrition therapy, a physical exercise program, and a behavior modification plan. These three components are also key elements for the long-term maintenance of weight loss. Additional methods of treatment for obesity include prescription weight loss medications and bariatric surgery. Studies show that even a modest loss of weight results in improved health and the prevention of problems associated with obesity.

It should be emphasized that it is important for an individual to consult with his or her physician before beginning treatment for obesity. Primary care physicians often manage individuals with Class I obesity and Class II obesity, but patients with Class III obesity are usually referred to a bariatric specialist. **Bariatrics** is the branch of medicine that deals with the treatment and control of obesity and diseases associated with obesity.

Nutrition Therapy

Nutrition therapy for obesity involves the selection of an appropriate eating plan for weight loss. It is essential that the eating plan selected ensure an adequate intake of nutrients. The MyPlate nutrition guide and the 2010 Dietary Guidelines for Americans (previously discussed in this chapter) provide valuable recommendations for a healthy and balanced eating plan.

Before beginning a weight reduction program, it is important to first set reasonable and safe weight loss goals. Most weight loss authorities recommend a slow steady weight loss of no more than 1 to 2 pounds per week. This is accomplished by a moderate reduction in the total number of calories consumed to create what is known as a *caloric deficit.* A caloric deficit occurs when more calories are used for energy by the body (calories out) than are consumed (calories in), resulting in the burning of body fat, which leads to a loss of weight.

To completely understand the concept of a caloric deficit, it is important to have a knowledge of the relationship between calories and body fat. One pound of body fat is equal to 3500 kilocalories. Therefore a decrease of 500 kilocalories each day typically results in a loss of 1 pound each week (500 × 7 = 3500 kilocalories, or 1 pound). A decrease of 1000 kilocalories each day is needed to lose about 2 pounds each week (1000 × 7 = 7000 kilocalories, or 2 pounds). The total number of kilocalories consumed each day, however, should not fall below below 12000 kilocalories to ensure an individual is obtaining all the required nutrients. Most women lose weight safely on an eating plan consisting of 1200 to 1500 kcal/day, and most men lose weight safely by consuming 1500 to 1800 kcal/day.

Numerous weight loss programs are available to assist individuals in achieving their weight loss goals; examples include the DASH (Dietary Approaches to Stop Hypertension) eating plan, Weight Watchers, Jenny Craig, and the Mayo Clinic diet. When choosing a weight loss program, it is important for individuals to choose a program that is medically proven and is best suited to their particular needs and lifestyle. Fad diets should be avoided because they can be harmful to health and do not typically result in good long-term results; examples include the grapefruit diet, the cabbage soup diet, and the Scarsdale diet. Characteristics of fad diets typically include no exercise, a promise of quick and easy weight loss, a guarantee of a large amount of weight loss, and the elimination of one or more food groups.

Physical Exercise Program

Physical exercise plays a key role in the treatment of obesity. Exercise increases the number of calories the body burns for energy (calories out), contributing to a caloric deficit and loss of weight. Physical exercise offers additional benefits such as increased lean body mass, improved cardiorespiratory functioning, and an improved quality of life and general well-being. Studies show that individuals who exercise are also less likely to regain their weight after having lost it.

The AHA recommends that healthy adults spend at least 150 minutes per week in moderate-intensity physical exercise. The AHA further recommends that adults perform muscle-strengthening activities at least 2 days per week. Refer to the Patient Teaching box *Aerobic Exercise* in Chapter 19 for a more thorough discussion of physical exercise recommendations for adults.

Behavior Modification Plan

A behavior modification plan is an important component in the treatment of obesity. The purpose of such a plan is to assist individuals in changing behaviors that have contributed to their weight gain. An individual must first identify the behaviors that have contributed to his or her weight gain; examples include eating too fast, eating when not hungry, using food as a reward, eating while standing or watching television, and eating to relieve stress or boredom. Once an individual identifies these behaviors, he or she can then take steps to replace these unhealthy behaviors with behaviors that encourage weight loss such as chewing food more slowly, keeping tempting foods out of the house, using nonfood incentives as a reward, eating only while sitting at a table, and using techniques other than food to relieve stress and boredom.

CARDIOVASCULAR DISEASE

The leading cause of death in the United States is cardiovascular disease. The most common cause of cardiovascular disease is atherosclerosis of the coronary arteries. As previously described, atherosclerosis of the coronary arteries is a condition in which fibrous plaques of fatty deposits and cholesterol build up on the inner walls of the coronary arteries. This causes narrowing and partial blockage of the lumen of these arteries, along with hardening of the arterial wall, leading to coronary artery disease (CAD). As the atherosclerosis progresses, the coronary arteries become more occluded, which eventually could lead to a heart attack.

Research has shown, beyond doubt, that high total blood cholesterol is a major risk factor for CAD, and the higher the cholesterol, the greater the risk. The National Cholesterol Educational Program (NCEP) was established in 1985 by the federal government to reduce the prevalence of elevated blood cholesterol levels in the United States by educating the public about the health risks associated with high blood cholesterol and to make recommendations for helping individuals reduce their cholesterol levels. It has been shown that for every 1% that an individual lowers his or her total blood cholesterol, the risk of CAD is reduced by 2%. The NCEP recommendations are published as a set of guidelines known as the TLC (Therapeutic Lifestyle Changes) eating plan. The TLC plan provides numeric recommendations for a heart-healthy diet, which is presented in Table 35-8 and is described in more detail in the following section.

Table 35-8 Therapeutic Lifestyle Changes (TLC) Eating Plan	
Nutrient	**Daily Recommended Intake**
Total fat	25% to 35% of total calories
Saturated Fat	Less than 7% of total calories
Polyunsaturated fat	Up to 10% of total calories
Monounsaturated fat	Up to 20% of total calories
Carbohydrate	50% to 60% of total calories
Dietary fiber	20 to 30 grams/day (10 to 25 grams/day should consist of soluble fiber)
Protein	15 to 25% of total calories
Cholesterol	Less than 200 mg/day
Sodium	Less than 2,300 mg/day

NUTRITION THERAPY

TLC Eating Plan

Nutrition therapy is the first line of treatment for high blood cholesterol. The TLC eating plan recommends that all individuals older than 2 years reduce dietary cholesterol and saturated fats and increase their dietary fiber (refer to Table 35-8). Many foods high in fat tend to be high in cholesterol. Nutrition labels on packaged products provide information on the cholesterol, fat, and fiber content of a food. Following the nutrition therapy measures discussed later can help individuals reduce their level of "bad" LDL cholesterol and increase their level of "good" HDL cholesterol.

Dietary Cholesterol

The body manufactures all the cholesterol it needs for normal functioning, and dietary intake of cholesterol (in foods) serves only to increase the blood cholesterol. According to the TLC plan, dietary cholesterol should be limited to less than 200 mg each day. Cholesterol is found only in animal foods and shellfish. Egg yolks, dairy products, and organ meats such as liver and kidneys are especially high in cholesterol.

Saturated Fat

The intake of saturated fat is the most important dietary factor leading to high blood cholesterol, even more so than consuming dietary cholesterol. This is because a diet that is high in saturated fat raises the LDL cholesterol and lowers the HDL cholesterol. In general, the more saturated a fat is, the harder and more solid it is at room temperature. The main source of saturated fat is animal products, including meat fat, poultry skin, and the fat in dairy products (butter, cream, ice cream, cheese, whole milk). Plant sources that are high in saturated fat include palm oil and coconut oil.

The TLC eating plan recommends that no more than 25% to 35% of the calories consumed each day come from total fat, with less than 7% of calories coming from saturated fat and with the remaining fat coming from unsaturated (monounsaturated and polyunsaturated) fat. Refer to Table 35-8 for a summary of the TLC recommendations for daily fat consumption.

Soluble Fiber

Soluble fiber, in particular, has been shown to lower the cholesterol level by keeping the cholesterol consumed in food from being absorbed through the intestinal wall and into the body. Examples of foods high in soluble fiber include oatmeal, oat bran, barley, some fruits (e.g., apples and oranges), broccoli, and legumes. The TLC eating plan recommends that an individual consume 20 to 30 grams of dietary fiber each day, with 10 to 25 grams of that amount consisting of soluble fiber.

In general, the cholesterol level begins to decrease 2 to 3 weeks after a cholesterol-lowering diet and other cholesterol-lowering measures (such as exercise and weight loss) are begun. Over time, it is possible to reduce the total cholesterol level by 30 to 55 mg/dL or even more through these lifestyle changes. If the blood cholesterol level cannot be lowered to an acceptable level, the physician may prescribe cholesterol-lowering medications along with continuation of the aforementioned measures.

HYPERTENSION

Hypertension is the most common life-threatening disease among Americans. It is estimated that 68 million Americans age 18 and older (one in three adults) have high blood pressure. Another 70 million Americans have blood pressure in the prehypertension range. Without lifestyle modifications, individuals with prehypertension have an increased risk of developing hypertension. The incidence of hypertension in the United States has increased dramatically as a result of an aging population and an increased incidence of obesity.

If high blood pressure is not brought under control, it can cause severe damage to vital organs, such as the heart, brain, kidneys, and eyes. This damage can result in a heart attack or heart failure, stroke, kidney damage, or damaged vision. Early detection and treatment of hypertension can prevent these complications.

NUTRITION THERAPY

DASH Eating Plan

Hypertension can be prevented and controlled by following the DASH (Dietary Approaches to Stop Hypertension) eating plan (Table 35-9). Studies performed by the National Heart, Lung, and Blood Institute (NHLBI) show that individuals with normal blood pressure who follow the DASH eating plan can lower their systolic pressure by 6 mm and their diastolic pressure by 3 mm. Furthermore, prehypertensive and hypertensive patients following the DASH plan can actually lower their systolic pressure by 11 mm and their diastolic pressure by 6 mm.

Table 35-9 Dietary Approaches to Stop Hypertension (DASH) Eating Plan	
Food Group	**Frequency**
Whole grains	6 to 8 servings per day
Vegetables	4 to 5 servings per day
Fruits	4 to 5 servings per day
Low-fat or fat-free milk and milk products	2 to 3 servings per day
Lean meats, poultry, and fish	6 or fewer servings per day
Nuts, seeds and beans	4 to 5 servings per week
Fats and oils	2 to 3 servings per day
Sweets (preferably low-fat or fat-free)	5 or fewer per week
Sodium	Limit sodium intake to 1500-2300 mg daily

DASH Recommendations

The DASH eating plan is a lifelong approach to healthy eating that is recommended not only for individuals who have hypertension or prehypertension, but for all individuals. The DASH plan consists of a balanced diet that is low in saturated fat, total fat, cholesterol, and sodium. The DASH plan focuses on fruits, vegetables, whole grains, legumes, and low-fat dairy products. In addition to lowering blood pressure, the DASH eating plan can help prevent the development of certain conditions such as obesity, osteoporosis, diabetes, cancer, heart disease, and stroke. The comprehensive DASH diet plan is available at www.nhlbi.nih.gov/health/public/heart/hbp/dash/new_dash.pdf and is summarized in Table 35-9.

Sodium Intake

A small amount of sodium is needed in the diet; however, most Americans consume too much sodium. It is particularly important for individuals with hypertension to limit the amount of sodium in their diet, which assists in lowering blood pressure.

The relationship between sodium and water can be summarized as follows: "Where sodium goes, water follows." Because the plasma of the blood consists primarily of water, a decrease in sodium in the diet causes a decrease in the blood volume. When the blood volume is reduced, there is less resistance or force of the blood against artery walls. Less resistance translates into a lowered blood pressure. Refer to Box 35-2 for a list of foods that are high and low in sodium content.

DIABETES

Diabetes is a lifelong condition that occurs when the body is not able to use glucose for energy because of a problem with insulin. Diabetes develops when the body produces little or no insulin, or when the body cannot use the insulin it does produce effectively (known as *insulin resistance*). According to the American Diabetes Association, almost 26 million Americans have diabetes; of these, nearly 7 million are not yet diagnosed and are unaware that they have diabetes. An additional 79 million people have prediabetes. Prediabetes is a condition in which the glucose levels of an individual are higher than normal but not high enough to be classified as diabetes. An individual with prediabetes has an increased risk of developing type 2 diabetes.

TYPE 1 DIABETES

Type 1 diabetes is caused by an autoimmune defect that destroys the insulin-producing cells or beta cells of the pancreas. As a result, the body can no longer produce insulin and therefore it must be administered by injection. Refer to Chapter 33 of your textbook for a more in-depth discussion of type 1 diabetes.

BOX 35-2   Sodium Content of Food

High-Sodium Foods
- Many restaurant and fast food meals
- Cured meats such as ham, bologna, and hot dogs
- Canned foods such as soups, vegetables, vegetable juices, and meats
- Frozen meals
- Snack foods including pretzels, potato chips, salted crackers, and nuts
- Many condiments such as soy sauce, steak sauce, onion salt, garlic salt, salad dressings, marinades, and catsup
- Pickled foods such as pickles, relish, and sauerkraut

Low-Sodium Foods
- Fresh or frozen fruits and vegetables
- Dried beans, peas, and legumes
- Whole-grain products
- Fresh meat, fish, and poultry
- Dairy products including milk, yogurt, hard cheeses, and ice cream and frozen yogurt
- Most beverages including fruit juices and carbonated beverages
- Unsalted nuts and seeds
- Condiments such as herbs, spices, citrus, Tabasco, salsa, mustard, and chili sauce

---

Nutrition Therapy

The nutrition therapy for type 1 diabetes focuses on maintaining good control of the blood glucose level. This is accomplished by keeping track of the amount and type of carbohydrate consumed and when (time of day) the carbohydrate is consumed. Nutrition therapy for controlling a patient's blood glucose level includes the following methods: exchange lists, carbohydrate counting, and MyPlate. These methods are described here.

Exchange List System

The exchange list system categorizes foods into six groups according to their carbohydrate, protein, and fat content. The six food groups include starch, fruits, vegetables, meat, milk, and fat. Each food group lists examples of specifically portioned foods belonging to that group. An example of an exchange list for fruits is illustrated in Figure 35-13.

The term *exchange* is actually the same as a food serving. Each exchange or serving has a known or predictable blood glucose response. Any food within a given food group can be exchanged for another one in that group. For example, in the fruit group, a small orange is equivalent to or can be exchanged with one small banana (refer to Figure 35-13). Because of this, patients following the exchange system must become familiar with food serving sizes. The patient is provided with an individualized plan that specifies the number and type of exchanges that should be included for both meals and snacks. The exchange method provides a

Fruit	Serving Size
Each fruit exchange (one serving) contains about 15 grams of carbohydrate.	
Apple with skin (fresh)	1 small
Applesauce (unsweetened)	½ cup
Apricots (fresh)	4 apricots
Banana (fresh)	1 small
Blackberries (fresh)	¾ cup
Blueberries (fresh)	¾ cup
Cantaloupe (fresh)	1 cup
Cherries (fresh)	12 cherries
Grapefruit (fresh)	½ medium
Grapes	17 grapes
Orange (fresh)	1 small
Peaches (fresh)	1 medium
Peaches (canned)	½ cup
Pear (fresh)	½ large
Pears (canned)	½ cup
Pineapple (fresh)	¾ cup
Plums (fresh)	2 small
Raspberries (fresh)	1 cup
Strawberries (fresh)	1 ¼ cups
Tangerine	2 small
Watermelon (cubes)	1 ¼ cups

Figure 35-13 Diabetic exchange list for fruit.

balanced and portion-controlled nutrition plan that assists in nourishing the individual while controlling his or her blood glucose level.

Carbohydrate Counting Method

The carbohydrate counting method offers more flexibility in meal planning than the exchange method. With this method, the carbohydrate content of a food measured in grams is balanced against the amount of insulin administered. Typically 1 unit of insulin helps to process or metabolize 15 grams of carbohydrate. To balance the amount of insulin administered, women usually need to consume 45 to 60 grams of carbohydrate at each meal and men need 60 to 75 grams at each meal.

Individuals following the carbohydrate counting method must determine the carbohydrate content (in grams) of all of the foods they consume. This information can be obtained by referring to the data provided in the diabetic exchange lists or by referring to food labels and noting the total carbohydrate content of each food item consumed.

MyPlate Method

The MyPlate method (discussed earlier in this chapter) is the most basic dietary approach for controlling blood glucose (refer to Figure 35-9). It is ideal for the patient who has low literacy skills or may be mentally challenged. Patients are taught to visually divide their dinner plate in half. Fruits and vegetables should occupy 50% of the plate. The remaining 50% of the plate is then divided into two parts, one for the protein group, and the other for the starchy foods (grains). Starchy foods produce the highest blood glucose response and include grain-based foods such as pasta, rice, and bread. Starchy vegetables such as corn, peas, potatoes, winter squash, and lima beans are also included under this classification. By limiting the intake of starchy foods to one quarter of the plate, the individual can control the blood glucose level.

TYPE 2 DIABETES

Type 2 diabetes can affect people at any age, but the chance of developing it increases with age, and it is more likely to occur in individuals who are 40 years of age or older. The biggest risk factor for developing type 2 diabetes is excess body weight. As a result of the recent increase in childhood obesity combined with a sedentary lifestyle, type 2 diabetes is starting to appear in younger age groups. Individuals with type 2 diabetes may not produce enough insulin or they may have a condition known as *insulin resistance.*

Insulin resistance is a condition in which the body produces insulin but does not use it effectively. Normally, when the blood glucose level rises in the body, insulin is released by the pancreas. Insulin binds to the surface of the cells at a special receptor site, similar to a lock-and-key system. The cell recognizes the insulin and opens up so that the glucose in the blood can flow into the cell and be converted to energy. Obesity can interfere with this lock-and-key system, causing the cell to become insensitive or resistant to the presence of insulin. When this occurs, the pancreas produces more insulin in an attempt to lower the blood glucose level. Over time, the pancreas is unable to keep up with the increased demand for insulin. Without enough insulin, the blood glucose level rises above normal, resulting in hyperglycemia.

Nutrition Therapy

Weight management and carbohydrate control are the keys for the dietary management of type 2 diabetes. Individuals with type 2 diabetes should consume well-balanced meals and snacks that provide an even distribution of carbohydrates throughout the day. These individuals can also maintain good blood glucose labels by controlling portion size, limiting concentrated sweets, emphasizing low glycemic index foods, and increasing the amount of soluble fiber in the diet. Soluble fiber slows down the absorption of glucose, which helps in controlling blood glucose levels.

Another very important aspect of blood glucose management in individuals with type 2 diabetes is attaining a healthy body weight through caloric restriction and daily exercise. Lowering the calorie intake by 500 kcal each day usually results in a weight loss of about 1 pound each week. Caloric restriction should not fall lower than 1200 kcal/day, however, to ensure an adequate intake of nutrients.

LACTOSE INTOLERANCE

Lactose intolerance is not a food allergy but rather a condition in which the body is unable to fully digest lactose. **Lactose** (milk sugar) is a disaccharide that consists of two sugar units and is found in milk and milk products.

Lactose intolerance is caused by a deficiency of lactase, which is an enzyme produced by the lining of the small intestine. Lactase is needed to break down lactose into glucose and galactose, which are then absorbed into the bloodstream for use by the body. When the small intestine does not produce enough of the lactase enzyme, lactose is unable to be broken down and moves through the intestines in an undigested form. When this undigested lactose reaches the large intestine, it is broken down and used as a food source by bacteria normally found in the large intestine. The by-products that result from this breakdown include copious amounts of gas that cause the symptoms of lactose intolerance.

Lactose intolerance usually begins during late adolescence or adulthood. This is because the amount of lactase produced by the body gradually declines after childhood. Lactose intolerance can also be caused by intestinal disease or injury. Lactose intolerance is most common in individuals of Asian, African American, and Hispanic descent and much less common in individuals of European descent.

The symptoms of lactose intolerance vary based on the amount of lactose an individual can tolerate. Some individuals may be able to tolerate only very small amounts of lactose before they begin experiencing symptoms, whereas others may be able to consume larger amounts of lactose before experiencing symptoms. The symptoms of lactose intolerance can range from mild to severe and usually begin 30 minutes to 2 hours after consumption of foods containing lactose.

Common signs and symptoms of lactose intolerance include the following:
- Abdominal bloating and cramping
- Flatulence
- Diarrhea
- Borborygmi (gurgling or rumbling sounds in the abdomen)
- Nausea

NUTRITION THERAPY

Lactose intolerance is treated by limiting or avoiding foods containing lactose such as milk and milk products (Figure 35-14). Consuming a food containing lactose with a meal, instead of by itself, may help prevent or reduce symptoms. Other forms of treatment include consuming lactose-free dairy products (Figure 35-15) and substituting rice milk, soy milk, and soy cheese for milk and milk products. Cultured milk products such as yogurt contain bacteria that produce the enzyme for breaking down lactose. These products can usually be consumed by a lactose-intolerant individual without triggering symptoms. There are also over-the-counter lactase enzyme supplements available (e.g., Dairy Ease capsules, Lactaid Chewables) that assist in digesting lactose . These supplements must be taken before consuming foods that contain lactose. Although there is no cure for lactose intolerance, it is not a serious condition and can be treated effectively through careful dietary planning.

Figure 35-14 Foods containing lactose.

Figure 35-15 Lactose-free milk.

Consuming milk and milk products provides a convenient way to obtain enough calcium and vitamin D in the diet. Individuals who are lactose intolerant may need to ensure they are obtaining enough of these nutrients through careful menu planning. Nondairy foods that contain calcium include canned fish containing bones (e.g., salmon, sardines), broccoli, spinach, legumes, and calcium-fortified breads and cereals. Nondairy foods that contain vitamin D include fish liver oil, liver, and fortified cereals. The body also manufactures vitamin D when it is exposed to the ultraviolet rays of the sun.

GLUTEN INTOLERANCE

Gluten intolerance is a condition in which an individual cannot tolerate the ingestion of a substance known as gluten. **Gluten** consists of a protein found in certain grains such as wheat, rye, barley, and triticale (a cross between wheat and rye). Gluten intolerance most commonly occurs with celiac disease and non-celiac gluten sensitivity (NCGS), which are discussed in more detail in the following sections.

CELIAC DISEASE

Celiac disease is an autoimmune disorder of the digestive tract in which the immune system launches an attack against gluten. The ingestion of gluten irritates the small intestine, which causes damage to the villi. Villi are finger-like extensions that line the small intestine and increase its surface area, providing for increased absorption of nutrients into the bloodstream. Damage to the villi results in a decreased surface area for absorption, which leads to malabsorption of nutrients.

NON-CELIAC GLUTEN SENSITIVITY

NCGS is also a disorder in which the body cannot tolerate gluten. Unlike celiac disease, however, NCGS does not cause damage to the villi of the small intestine. Before a diagnosis of NCGS is made, the patient is first tested for celiac disease to rule out that condition. Research estimates that approximately 18 million individuals in the United States have NCGS, which is six times the number of individuals with celiac disease.

SYMPTOMS OF GLUTEN INTOLERANCE

Celiac disease and NCGS share many of the same symptoms; however, the symptoms of NCGS are usually less severe. Symptoms of gluten intolerance tend to vary widely among patients and can include the following:
- Abdominal bloating
- Abdominal pain
- Weight loss
- Flatulence
- Diarrhea
- Constipation
- Foul-smelling stools
- Headache
- Fatigue
- Joint pain
- Brain fog
- Depression

NUTRITION THERAPY

The treatment for gluten intolerance is to follow a gluten-free diet, which excludes the consumption of all foods containing wheat, barley, rye, and triticale. Foods that frequently contain gluten include bread, cereal, crackers, pasta, salad dressing, baked goods, soups, sauces, and beer (Figure

Figure 35-16 **A,** Foods containing gluten. **B,** Gluten-free foods.

Figure 35-17 Common food allergens.

35-16, *A*). Foods that are gluten free include beans, seeds, nuts, eggs, meat, poultry, fish, seafood, fruits, vegetables, and dairy products (Figure 35-16, *B*). Grains that are gluten free include buckwheat, cornmeal, flax, quinoa, rice, soy, and gluten-free oats. There are also many gluten-free food products available that can be used as alternatives to foods that contain gluten.

FOOD ALLERGIES

In the United States, food allergies affect approximately 6% to 8% of young children and about 4% of adults. Common food allergens include milk, eggs, wheat, fish and shellfish, peanuts, soybeans, and tree nuts (Figure 35-17). Examples of tree nuts include cashews, pecans, walnuts, Brazil nuts, hazelnuts, almonds, and coconut. Food allergies may also be triggered by certain fruits and vegetables such as strawberries, tomatoes, and peppers.

It is important to recognize the signs and symptoms of food allergies so that proper treatment can be obtained. The symptoms of a food allergy commonly occur within 2 hours after ingestion of the food. The skin and the respiratory and GI systems are often affected. Common symptoms include skin rash, hives, and swelling. In addition, swelling and itching of the face, tongue, ears, eyelids, and lips may occur. Respiratory symptoms include wheezing, shortness of

breath, or difficulty breathing. GI symptoms may occur, such as abdominal cramping and pain, nausea, vomiting, or diarrhea.

NUTRITION THERAPY

Food allergies are most commonly treated with special diets. The response of the body to a food allergen can range from mild to moderate to severe. The specific treatment recommended depends, in large part, on the severity of the allergy.

Common methods of treatment for food allergies are as follows.

Elimination Diet

An elimination diet involves removing the offending food from the diet and is typically recommended when an individual is allergic to only one or two foods. Removing the offending food(s) from the diet is an easy way to prevent an allergic reaction. An elimination diet is also necessary when an individual has a very severe allergy to a food (e.g., peanuts) that might result in an anaphylactic reaction if the food were consumed. Food allergies are typically more severe earlier in life and tend to diminish in intensity as aging occurs. Reintroduction of that food allergen should be conducted only under a physician's guidance.

Rotation Diet

The allergic response to a food is often increased when a food is repeatedly consumed. A rotation diet (use of a rotation schedule) limits the number of times a food is ingested. This typically leads to a gradual desensitization to the food allergen, which lowers the allergic response to that food. A rotation diet is usually recommended for mild or moderate food allergies.

The most commonly used food rotation interval is 4 to 5 days. This means that the problem food (as well as foods belonging to the same food family) are consumed only every 4 to 5 days. A rotational schedule not only allows for the consumption of a known food allergen on a rotational basis, but may also minimize the development of a new food allergy.

Denaturation

Exposing a food to heat will denature or alter the chemical structure of the food allergen protein, so that the body no longer recognizes it as an invader. A child who is allergic to milk may be able to tolerate milk if it is heated in hot chocolate because of this denaturing process. An individual's tolerance to cooked or canned fruits and vegetables is typically much better than to fresh fruits and vegetables. Exposing the food allergen to acid has the same result. For example, adding tomato or lemon juice to food allergens may significantly reduce the allergic response.

MEDICATION AND SUPPLEMENTS

Medications that suppress the allergic response may be prescribed to treat the food allergy. Because such medications treat only the symptoms and not the cause of the allergy, the food allergy may actually become worse over time.

The oral intake of supplemental digestive enzymes can assist in treating food allergies. Digestive enzymes help break down the food into smaller, less allergenic molecules. This, in turn, decreases the allergenic response of the body. With continued intake, however, the individual may actually become allergic to the enzymes themselves.

Antacids that contain bicarbonate are used to treat food reactions. The pH of the blood becomes more acidic during an allergic reaction. Bicarbonate antacids cause the blood to become more alkaline, which works to neutralize the acid pH and helps to relieve the allergic symptoms.

There are several vitamins that assist in controlling food allergies; they include vitamin C and vitamin B_5 (pantothenic acid). Vitamin C exerts a stabilizing effect on mast cells, resulting in a reduction in the amount of histamine released by the body. Vitamin B_5 (pantothenic acid) functions in steroidal hormone production, which can lower the allergic response. Both of these vitamins are water soluble and therefore can be administered as a supplement without danger of toxicity or overdose.

↻ TERMINOLOGY REVIEW

Key Term	Word Parts	Definition
Antioxidant	*anti-:* against *ox/i:* oxygen	A molecule that inhibits the oxidation of other molecules.
Atherosclerosis	*ather/o:* yellowish, fatty plaque *-sclerosis:* hardening	Buildup of fibrous plaques of fatty deposits and cholesterol on the inner walls of an artery that causes narrowing, obstruction, and hardening of the artery.
Bariatrics	*bar/o:* weight *-iatrics:* a branch of medicine	The branch of medicine that deals with the treatment and control of obesity and diseases associated with obesity.
Cholesterol		A white, waxy, fatlike substance that is essential for normal functioning of the body.
Complete protein		A protein that contains all the essential amino acids needed by the body.
Disaccharide	*di-:* two *-saccharide:* containing sugar	A simple carbohydrate consisting of two sugar units.
Empty calorie food		A food that provides calories but few or no nutrients. Also known as a low–nutrient density food.
Essential amino acid		An amino acid that is required by the body but cannot be manufactured by the body and must be obtained from food.
Gluten		A type of protein found in certain grains such as wheat, rye, and barley.
Glycogen	*glyc/o-:* sugar *-gen:* substance or agent that produces or causes	The form in which carbohydrate is stored in the body.
Incomplete protein		A protein that lacks one or more of the essential amino acids needed by the body.
Kilocalorie	*kilo-:* thousand	The amount of heat needed to raise the temperature of 1 kilogram of water 1 degree Celsius. (Often referred to as a *calorie*.)
Lactose	*lact/o:* milk *-ose:* full of (sugar)	A disaccharide that consists of two sugar units and is found in milk and milk products.
Macronutrient	*macro-:* large *nutriti/o:* nourishing	A nutrient required in relatively large amounts by the body. Includes carbohydrates, fat, and protein.

TERMINOLOGY REVIEW—cont'd

Key Term	Word Parts	Definition
Micronutrient	*micro-:* small *nutriti/o:* nourishing	A nutrient required in very small amounts by the body. Includes vitamins and minerals.
Mineral		A naturally occurring inorganic substance that is essential to the proper functioning of the body.
Monosaccharide	*mono-:* one	A simple carbohydrate consisting of one sugar unit.
Nonessential amino acid	*non-:* not	An amino acid required by the body that can be synthesized by the body in sufficient quantities to meet its needs.
Nutrient	*nutriti/o:* nourishing	A chemical substance found in food that is needed by the body for survival and well-being.
Nutrition	*nutriti/o:* nourishing *-ion:* condition of	Nutrition is the study of nutrients in food including how the body uses them and their relationship to health.
Nutrition therapy	*nutriti/o:* nourishing *-ion:* condition of	The application of the science of nutrition to promote optimal heath and treat illness.
Obesity		A medical condition in which there is an excessive accumulation of body fat to the extent to which it may have an adverse effect on the health and well-being of an individual.
Percent daily value		The percentage of a nutrient provided by a single serving of a food item compared with how much is required for the entire day.
Saturated fat	*satur-:* full, well-fed	A type of fat that is solid at room temperature and comes primarily from animal sources.
Triglycerides	*tri-:* three	The chemical form in which most fat exists in food, as well as in the body.
Unsaturated fat	*un-:* not *satur-:* full, well-fed	A type of fat that is liquid at room temperature and comes primarily from plant sources.
Vitamin	*vit/a:* life	An organic compound that is required in small amounts by the body for normal growth and development.

ON THE WEB

For information on nutrition:

Nutrition.gov: www.nutrition.gov

ChooseMyPlate: www.choosemyplate.gov

Academy of Nutrition and Dietetics: www.eatright.org

Nutrition Facts: www.nutritionfacts.org

American Diabetic Association: www.diabetes.org

American Society for Nutrition: www.nutrition.org

CDC Nutrition: www.cdc.gov/nutrition

The Nutrition Source: www.hsph.harvard.edu/nutrit

Super Kids Nutrition: www.superkidsnutrition.com

Food and Nutrition Information Center: fnic.nal.usda.gov

Obesity Society: www.obesity.org

American Society for Metabolic and Bariatric Surgery: asmbs.org

American Diabetic Association: www.diabetes.org

Vegegarian Nutrition: vegetariannutrition.net

The Eating Disorder Foundation: www.eatingdisorderfoundation.org

36 Emergency Preparedness and Protective Practices

e Check out the Evolve site at http://evolve.elsevier.com/Bonewit/today/ to access additional interactive activities and exercises to help you study and prepare for success.

LEARNING OBJECTIVES   PROCEDURES

Disasters
1. State the effects a disaster or serious emergency can have on a health care facility.
2. Explain the difference between a natural disaster and a man-made disaster and list examples of each.

Psychological Effects of Emergencies
3. List the characteristics of a disaster that tend to cause the most serious psychological effects.
4. List and describe the three phases of the generalized adaptation syndrome.
5. List and describe the stages of anxiety and the intervention that should be employed for each.

Emergency Preparedness
6. State the purpose of an emergency action plan.
7. List and describe the six elements that must be included in an emergency action plan.
8. List and describe the three components of an emergency evacuation plan.
9. Identify the information that should be included on an evacuation floor plan.
10. State the duties that may be performed by evacuation wardens in the medical office.

Develop an emergency action plan for a natural or man-made disaster.

Fire Safety and Prevention
11. List and describe the elements of a fire.
12. State the five elements that must be included in a fire prevention plan.
13. Identify methods of fire prevention for the medical office.
14. List and describe safety measures used for fire protection in the medical office.
15. List and describe the five classes of fire.
16. Identify the steps included in the RACE response.

Demonstrate methods of fire prevention in the health care setting.
Demonstrate proper use of a fire extinguisher.

Employee Training
17. Identify the education and training that must be provided to medical assistants related to medical office emergency situations.
18. State the purpose of emergency practice drills.
19. Describe the role of the medical assistant in disasters and serious emergencies.

Participate in a mock exposure event, and document the steps taken.

CHAPTER OUTLINE

INTRODUCTION TO DISASTER AND EMERGENCY PLANNING
CATEGORIES OF DISASTERS
Natural Disasters
Man-made Disasters
PSYCHOLOGICAL EFFECTS OF SERIOUS EMERGENCIES
The Stress Response
Alarm Phase
Resistance Phase
Recovery or Exhaustion Phase

Managing Anxiety
EMERGENCY PREPAREDNESS IN THE MEDICAL OFFICE
Emergency Action Plan
Components of an Emergency Action Plan
FIRE SAFETY IN THE MEDICAL OFFICE
ELEMENTS OF A FIRE
Fuel Source
Ignition Source (Heat)
Oxygen
FIRE PREVENTION PLAN

Components of a Fire Prevention Plan
Fire Protection in the Medical Office
Sprinkler Systems
Fire Doors
Fire-Resistant Cabinets
Fire Alarms
Smoke Detectors

Fire Extinguisher
Emergency Response to a Fire
EMPLOYEE TRAINING AND EDUCATION
EMERGENCY PRACTICE DRILLS
Fire Drill
Disaster Drills
MEDICAL ASSISTANT'S ROLE

KEY TERMS

anxiety
disaster
emergency action plan
emergency preparedness
evacuation

evacuation procedures
exit route
fire extinguisher
fire prevention plan
fire protection

HAZMAT
man-made disaster
natural disaster
stress

INTRODUCTION TO DISASTER AND EMERGENCY PLANNING

Every health care facility faces the possibility that a disaster or serious emergency may occur, resulting in injuries, loss of life, property damage, and the inability to provide usual services. Medical offices must plan ahead to minimize the damage from any disaster or serious emergency and facilitate recovery so that services can be restored as efficiently as possible.

This chapter presents an overview of the various types of disasters and serious emergencies that may affect the medical office along with the psychological effects that emergency situations can have on an individual. Also presented in this chapter is a discussion of emergency preparedness and protective practice guidelines including the OSHA requirements for developing an emergency action plan and a fire prevention plan.

CATEGORIES OF DISASTERS

A **disaster** is defined as a sudden adverse event that can cause damage or loss of life. Disasters can be categorized as natural or man-made.

NATURAL DISASTERS

A **natural disaster** is a catastrophic event that is caused by nature or the natural processes of the earth (Figure 36-1). Examples of natural disasters include floods, tornados, hurricanes, earthquakes, tsunamis, blizzards, volcanic

eruptions, and epidemics. Natural disasters may cause injuries and loss of life as well as significant damage to the environment. Natural disasters may occur with or with or without warning. For example, a hurricane develops over a period of days, which allows for some preparation. On the other hand, an earthquake usually occurs without warning. The impact of a natural disaster may be random. For example, the exact strength and path of a hurricane are difficult to predict. This often requires numerous communities to prepare for this type of disaster in the event the hurricane hits their community.

MAN-MADE DISASTERS

A **man-made disaster** is an event that causes serious damage through intentional or negligent human actions or the failure of a man-made system (Figure 36-2). Examples of man-made disasters include fire, power outages, bomb explosions, terrorism, structural collapse, radiation accidents, chemical spills, and bioterrorism.

The amount of threat or damage from man-made disasters can vary considerably. For example, a fire in a wastebasket is usually quickly contained. On the other hand, a hazardous chemical spill may involve an entire city or area. The type of emergency personnel who respond to a man-made disaster depends on the nature of the disaster. Municipal fire departments and police departments provide rapid assistance for fires, injury, structural collapse, and criminal activity. The National Response Center of the Environmental Protection Agency (EPA) responds to the release, or potential release, of oil, radioactive materials, or hazardous chemicals into the air, land, or water (Figure 36-3).

Figure 36-1 A tornado is an example of a natural disaster. (Copyright © 2015 PhanXuanHuong, iStock, Thinkstock.com. All rights reserved.)

Figure 36-2 A fire is an example of a man-made disaster. (Copyright © 2015 Steinbergpix, iStock, Thinkstock.com. All rights reserved.)

PSYCHOLOGICAL EFFECTS OF EMERGENCIES

Whenever an emergency situation occurs that causes serious damage or interruption of the normal daily routine, individuals react positively and negatively to the loss of property or disruption of service. Positive reactions involve the triggering of resources, both internal and external, to meet the challenges. For example, when a serious flood threatens an area, individuals usually mobilize quickly to fill and place sandbags to minimize the anticipated damage. When physical and emotional resources are depleted, however, individuals react negatively. Disasters that tend to cause the most serious psychological effects include those with the following characteristics:

- Occur without warning
- Pose a serious threat to personal safety or have unknown health effects
- Have an uncertain duration (such as serious floods of major rivers)
- Result from malicious intent or human error
- Have symbolic significance (such as the 9/11 attacks)

THE STRESS RESPONSE

Stress is the body's response to threat or change. When a disaster or serious emergency occurs, individuals who are affected by it frequently experience stress. Hans Selye was an Austrian physician who practiced medicine in the middle of the twentieth century. Selye described the body's reaction to stress as a three-part general adaptation syndrome (GAS), which is illustrated in Figure 36-4. The three stages of the GAS include the alarm phase, the resistance phase, and the recovery or exhaustion phase.

Alarm Phase

This phase is often called the *fight-or-flight response.* In this phase, the body senses a stressor and begins to react to combat it. Epinephrine is released from the adrenal medulla, which stimulates the sympathetic nervous system, triggering the following changes in the body: dilation of the pupils, increase in heart rate, increase in respirations and perspiration, and increase in the blood pressure. These changes prepare the body to fight or to run away. In addition, the

Figure 36-3 Teams responding to disasters involving a hazardous material (HAZMAT) must wear protective clothing and initiate decontamination of casualties.

muscles tense in preparation for action, and the attention becomes narrowly focused on the perceived threat or significant task. This phase does not last very long; in some instances it may only last a matter of seconds. Some people experience the alarm phase as energizing, whereas others quickly become extremely anxious.

Example: If a serious fire erupts in a medical office, employees typically experience the alarm phase. The fight-or-flight response helps employees to remain focused and allows them to quickly and effectively evacuate themselves and others from the burning building and perform other types of rescue duties.

Resistance Phase

The resistance phase begins almost immediately after the alarm phase. In this phase, the stress remains but the body adapts in an effort to cope with the stressor. The resistance phase may last hours, days, or even months depending on the circumstances. During this phase, the adrenal cortex secretes cortisol. Cortisol increases the blood glucose level to sustain energy because more energy is required to maintain the stage of resistance than the normal state. The body constantly remains "on guard" and is not in a state of balance (homeostasis) but is able to carry on its normal functions. Individuals may experience a number of stress-related symptoms during this phase such as fatigue, irritability, lethargy, and lapses in concentration.

Example: If a medical office employee temporarily becomes trapped by the fire (described in the earlier example), he or she may be unable to cope with the stress of that experience. In this case, the employee enters the resistance phase and constantly feels on guard but is still able to function normally. If the resistance phase lasts for a period of time, the employee may begin experiencing stress-related symptoms.

Recovery or Exhaustion Phase

If the stress is removed, the body enters the recovery phase. However, if the stress continues, the body's ability to resist stress is lost and the individual enters the exhaustion phase.

General Adaptation Syndrome

Figure 36-4 The general adaptation syndrome (GAS) developed by Hans Selye.

Figure 36-5 In the exhaustion phase, the body's resources to combat stress become depleted.

a. *Recovery phase*: In the recovery phase, the stress has been removed and the parasympathetic nervous system begins to regain control. Eventually the body returns to its normal level of function (homeostasis).

b. *Exhaustion phase*: If stress is chronic and excessive, the body's resources to combat it become depleted. Eventually the immune system is compromised, and the individual becomes more susceptible to a variety of illnesses ranging all the way from colds and flu to cancer.

Example: If the employee learns to cope with the stress of being trapped in the fire, the body enters the recovery phase and returns to a normal level of functioning. If the employee is unable to cope, the stress becomes chronic and he or she will enter the exhaustion phase and begin to experience stress-related illnesses (Figure 36-5).

MANAGING ANXIETY

Anxiety is defined as a feeling of worry or uneasiness, often triggered by an event that is perceived as having an uncertain outcome. There are four levels of anxiety that range in degree from fleeting worried thoughts to a full-blown panic attack. The four levels of anxiety are outlined Figure 36-6.

An individual's level of anxiety has a direct influence on his or her ability to function effectively in an emergency situation. For example, a medical assistant with moderate anxiety is not able to notice details and think as clearly in an emergency situation. However, emergency procedures that have been thoroughly learned through practice drills help the medical assistant decide what to do without having to think through all the possibilities. In addition, practice drills tend to keep the anxiety level from rising because he or she feels more confident when there is a structured plan to respond to in an emergency situation.

LEVELS OF RISING ANXIETY

Panic

Severe state of psycholgic stess. Person unable to focus or cope. May focus on small details which are totally blown out of proportion.

Manifestations: incoherent speech, ineffective communication, sweating, rapid pulse and breathing, muscle tremors, increased muscle tension, elevated blood pressure.

Interventions: The panic state usually subsides fairly quickly because the body cannot sustain it. Interventions are the same for severe anxiety. It may be necessary to make transportation arrangements for the patient.

Severe anxiety

Painful level of anxiety produces loss of abstract thinking and consumes almost all of a person's energy. The person cannot notice what is going on even if it is pointed out.

Manifestations: crying, confused speech, dry mouth, sweating, rapid pulse and breathing, muscle tremors, increased muscle tension, elevated blood pressure.

Interventions: Provide a quiet area for the person to regain control. A calm manner is reassuring. Encourage the patient to take slow deep breaths. Seek guidance from the physician if the patient is breathing faster than 22-24 breaths per minute.

Moderate anxiety

Attention is restricted to a particular task or problem rather than entire situation (called selective inattention). Still able to think fairly clearly but focuses on only one thing at a time.

Manifestations: sweating, rapid pulse and breathing, muscle tension and possible stomach pain, frequent urination and/or diarrhea

Interventions: A calm manner is reassuring. Acknowledge that the patient appears anxious. Focus on one thing at a time. Encourage the patient to take slow deep breaths.

Mild anxiety

Manifestations: The body functions well in this state. The person may feel a little nervous.

Figure 36-6 Levels of anxiety.

Severe anxiety can be problematic in an emergency situation because it tends to immobilize an individual and stimulate anxiety in others. Symptoms of severe anxiety include the following: hyperventilation, rapid pulse rate, excessive perspiration, and confused speech. In an emergency situation, a patient with severe anxiety may lose control of his or her emotions and cry or scream. This behavior can be minimized by the medical assistant giving the patient directions in a calm and reassuring voice. It may first be necessary to touch the patient to gain his or her attention, and then directions should be given in short sentences, speaking a little more slowly than usual. Helping the patient to breathe deeply helps to reduce anxiety, but it is also important to direct the person exactly where to go if a dangerous area must be evacuated.

If an emergency occurs in the workplace, the medical assistant should immediately focus on responding to the immediate situation, implementing established procedures, and helping others. Deep breaths will help to control anxiety, which should be seen as a normal response. Even in disasters that have caused enormous amounts of damage, lives have been saved and injury has been minimized when people have been able to stay reasonably calm and follow established emergency procedures.

Putting It All Into Practice

My name is Beth Ann Wilson, and I am a Certified Medical Assistant. I have been assisting the office manager in updating the equipment in our office that might be used in case of fire or natural disaster. We recently purchased an additional fire extinguisher for the staff break room, where we have a microwave and coffee maker. In addition, we have purchased an office disaster kit which has emergency supplies for 10 people for a few days including food, water, a flashlight, a radio, batteries, a first aid kit, and other supplies that might be useful in a building collapse. Of course we hope that we will never have to use these things. I was also one of the staff members from our office who participated recently as a "victim" in a mock disaster drill that was held for emergency personnel in our town. I pretended to be a victim with fractures of my arm and leg. I had never been in a situation where there were many people injured or been transported in an ambulance. The experience increased my understanding of the problems that emergency personnel face, and now I have a more personal understanding of how important it is to be prepared with training and equipment. ■

What Would You Do? What Would You *Not* Do?

Case Study 1

Julie Manning, who is sitting in the waiting room, receives a telephone call, speaks on the telephone for a few minutes, and rushes to the front desk window. She tells Beth Ann that she has to leave immediately because she has just learned that there is a fire at her son's school. Mrs. Manning speaks very quickly, but her story seems disconnected. It is also clear that she is breathing very rapidly and is perspiring excessively. ■

EMERGENCY PREPAREDNESS IN THE MEDICAL OFFICE

Large clinics and small medical offices alike may experience emergencies such as fires, floods, earthquakes, power outages, workplace violence, and a variety of other emergency situations. **Emergency preparedness** is the process of making plans to prevent, respond, and recover from an emergency situation. To protect employees from fire and other emergencies and to prevent property loss, medical offices should develop emergency preparedness plans. Emergency preparedness plans, as stipulated by OSHA, must include an emergency action plan (EAP) and a fire prevention plan. These plans are discussed in more detail on the following pages.

EMERGENCY ACTION PLAN

An **emergency action plan** (EAP) is a written document that describes the actions that employees should take to ensure their safety if a fire or other emergency situation occurs. The purpose of an EAP is to prevent fatalities, injuries, and property damage during an emergency situation. Almost all medical offices are required by OSHA to develop an EAP. The EAP must be in writing, be kept in in the workplace, and be available for employee review.

Before development of the EAP, an assessment must be performed by the medical office to determine the potential emergencies that could affect the office. Some emergencies may occur within the medical office; examples include a fire, workplace violence, or a medical emergency (e.g., patient having a heart attack). Other emergencies may arise from situations occurring outside of the facility; examples include a flood, tornado, and earthquake. The EAP should outline the actions that should be taken for each of the potential emergency situations identified by the office.

Components of an Emergency Action Plan

There are six elements (as required by OSHA) that must be included in an EAP; these are listed and described in the following paragraphs. Other EAP elements that are recommended by OSHA (but not required) include a description of the alarm system to notify employees to evacuate, the site of an alternative communication center to be used in the event of a fire or explosion, and a secure location to store originals or duplicate copies of essential records.

The six elements required in an EAP are as follows.

1. *The preferred means of reporting fires and other emergencies*
   In the event of an emergency situation, it is important to report the situation and alert employees immediately. Emergency situations, such as fires, can reach dangerous levels very quickly, and a delay in summoning emergency responders and alerting employees may result in the loss of life and property. One or more of the following methods are typically used to report the emergency and/

or alert employees to the presence of an emergency situation:

a. *Dialing 911:* This is a common and preferred method for reporting emergencies.

b. *Dialing an internal emergency phone numbers:* If internal ("in-house") numbers are used for reporting emergencies, they should be posted on or near each phone. Internal emergency numbers are sometimes connected to an intercom system so that coded announcements may be made throughout the facility. For example, a facility may indicate a patient is having a heart attack by an announcement of "Code Blue" or that there is a fire in the facility by an announcement of "Code Red."

c. *Activation of a manual alarm system:* OSHA requires that employers provide an early warning system so that employees can safely escape the workplace. The most common means to alert employees (and other building occupants) are audible and visual alarms. In offices with 10 or fewer employees, it is acceptable to use direct voice communication for alerting employees, provided that all employees can hear the voice alarm. OSHA requires that the alarm be distinctive and recognized by all employees as a signal to evacuate the workplace or to begin implementing emergency actions.

2. *Emergency evacuation plan*

An **evacuation** is a planned systematic retreat of people to safety in an emergency situation. According to OSHA, the emergency evacuation plan for the medical office must include the following three components:

a. *Emergency evacuation procedures:* **Evacuation procedures** consist of clear step-by-step procedures for the rapid, efficient, and safe removal of individuals from a building during an emergency. It is recommended that an *emergency evacuation coordinator* be assigned to take charge of and manage the evacuation procedures during an emergency. In high-rise buildings, the office evacuation procedures should coordinate with the building evacuation procedures. Evacuation procedures should include the following:

- The conditions that would require evacuation of the area
- The chain of command showing who can authorize an evacuation
- The actions employees should take during the evacuation (e.g., shutting windows, turning off equipment, closing doors)
- Procedures for evacuating individuals with disabilities or who do not speak English

b. *Type of evacuation:* The type of evacuation ordered during an emergency depends on the type of emergency situation. For example, the immediate and complete evacuation of a building to a safe area is typically required in the event of a large fire On the other hand, a small fire in a wastebasket may require only a partial evacuation of employees from the immediate area. In some instances, the evacuation of occupants from the building may not be the best response. In the event of a tornado, for example, employees are typically required to evacuate to a safe part of the building such as a designated shelter area (known as a *shelter-in-place* evacuation). The EAP should specify the type of evacuation recommended for each type of emergency identified in the plan.

c. *Exit routes:* An **exit route** is a continuous and unobstructed path of travel from any point within a workplace to a place of safety. OSHA requires that specific guidelines be followed with respect to exit routes. Some of these guidelines (that most affect the medical office) are as follows:

- Exits should be clearly marked and well lit.
- Exit routes must be at least 28 inches wide at all points.
- Exit routes should be unobstructed and free of clutter at all times.
- Exit signs should be posted indicating the nearest emergency exit.
- Exit doors must be free of decorations or signs that obscure visibility of the exit
- route door.
- Doors that cannot be used to leave the facility should be clearly labeled "Not an Exit" or identified by a sign indicating the door's actual use (e.g., "Storeroom").
- An exit door must be unlocked from the inside.
- An exit door must open outward.

Evacuation floor plan: Exit routes should be clearly identified and marked on an evacuation floor plan (Figure 36-7). It is recommended (if possible) that both a primary and a secondary exit route be identified on the floor plan. A *primary exit route* is the quickest and easiest way to exit a building during an evacuation and is usually represented on the floor plan by a continuous solid red line with a directional arrow. A *secondary exit route* provides a secondary means of escape in the event the primary route becomes blocked by smoke or fire. It is often represented by a continuous dashed blue line with a directional arrow on the evacuation floor plan.

The floor plan of a multiple-story building should show the locations of stairways and elevators and must indicate that the stairs (not the elevators) should be used as a means of exit in an emergency. Evacuation floor plans should be posted in multiple locations throughout the medical office including each examining room, the waiting room, rest rooms, the break room, and offices.

An evacuation floor plan should include the location of the following:

- Employee's current location
- Primary and secondary exit routes
- Manual fire alarm boxes
- Portable fire extinguishers
- Emergency exit doors
- Wheelchair accessible exits

Figure 36-7 Evacuation floor plan.

- Shelter-in-place areas
- Assembly areas

3. *Procedures for employees who remain behind to perform critical operations before evacuation*

   If necessary, some employees may be designated to stay behind briefly to operate fire extinguishers or shut down electrical equipment or special equipment that could be damaged if left operating or create additional hazards to emergency responders. The EAP should identify each of these employees and describe in detail the procedure that he or she is to perform. Any employee remaining behind must be capable of recognizing when to abandon the operation or task and evacuate to a safe area.

4. *Procedures to account for all employees after an evacuation*

   The EAP should identify an assembly area for employees to meet after an evacuation. The assembly area should be a safe distance from the building and have enough space to accommodate all of the employees. Assembly areas typically include parking lots and other open areas away from busy streets.

   The EAP should include a mechanism for accounting for all employees after an evacuation. The purpose of accounting for building occupants following an evacuation is to help determine if someone is still in the building in need of rescue. This can be accomplished by taking a head count or through the use of an employee roster checklist. A mechanism also needs to be established for accounting for non-employees such as patients and visitors (e.g., pharmaceutical company representatives). Most offices designate the patient log-in sheet as a means of accounting for patients in the event of an evacuation. The name and last known location of any individual not accounted for need to be relayed to an emergency official. It is important that the building occupants be instructed not to leave the assembly area until everyone has been accounted for and dismissed.

5. *Procedures for employees performing rescue or medical duties*
   During an emergency situation, various rescue or medical duties may need to be performed by employees. These employees are often referred to as *evacuation wardens.* The type of duties vary depend on the emergency situation. The EAP should specify these duties including the type of duty to be performed and the name of the employee who is to perform it. Each employee evacuation warden must be thoroughly trained in the duty he or she is to perform. Duties that may need to be performed by evacuation wardens during a fire are discussed later in this chapter and are outlined in Table 36-2.

6. *The names or job titles of individuals who can be contacted for further information or explanation of duties under the plan*
   At times, an employee may need additional information or further clarification of the duties to perform under the plan. The EAP should list the names or job titles of the individuals, both within and outside of the facility, who can be contacted to provide this information.

FIRE SAFETY IN THE MEDICAL OFFICE

Fire is the most common type of emergency situation that occurs in the workplace. Each year there are approximately 70,000 to 80,000 serious workplace fires in the United States that result in the deaths of more than 200 workers and injures 5000 more workers. It has been shown that approximately 85% of workplace fires are the result of human behavior, whereas only 15% are caused by catastrophic failure of equipment. Overall, fire is third leading cause of accidental death in the United States. In addition to the human cost, a fire can also cause structural damage to the medical facility as well as the loss of valuable documents and information.

There are numerous ways for fires to start in the medical office. Examples include overloaded electrical outlets; heat-producing equipment that is too close to combustible materials; improper use of appliances (e.g., coffee makers, microwave ovens, stoves); improper handling and storage of chemicals, cleaning supplies, and other combustible materials; and arson. If the medical office processes its own laundry, poorly maintained washers and dryers can also cause fires, especially if the dryer is vented improperly or if the lint trap is not kept clean.

ELEMENTS OF A FIRE

A fire is a chemical reaction that involves the rapid burning of a fuel. A fire needs three elements to occur: a fuel source, an ignition source (heat), and oxygen. Once a fire has started, it will grow hotter and it will not stop until at least one of these three elements has been removed.

FUEL SOURCE

A fuel source consists of any flammable or combustible material. A *flammable* material catches on fire easily (e.g., propane, gasoline), whereas a *combustible* material is any material that will burn (e.g., paper, wood). All flammable materials are combustible, but not all combustible materials are flammable. A tiny spark may cause a flammable material to ignite but would not cause a combustible material to ignite. Many items can provide fuel for a fire, such as paper, cardboard, wood, plastic, fabric, and flammable liquids. Common examples of fuel sources found in the medical office include the following:

- Patient charts
- Furniture
- Drapes and rugs
- Office equipment
- Chemicals used for sterilization and disinfection
- Laboratory testing chemicals
- Trash

IGNITION SOURCE (HEAT)

An ignition source provides the energy necessary to increase the temperature of the fuel source to a point at which it ignites. Once the fuel source has ignited, it produces heat. As long as enough fuel and oxygen are present, the heat generated by the fuel source will continue the combustion process. Examples of common ignition sources include the following:

- Open flames (e.g., burning candle)
- Faulty electrical equipment
- Hot surfaces (e.g., examination light)
- Sparks (e.g., burning cigarette)

OXYGEN

The air around us has about a 21% oxygen content, and most fires only require an atmosphere of 16% to burn. Many medical offices store oxygen in their facilities to administer to patients if necessary. This stored oxygen is a safe gas as long as it is stored and used properly. Oxygen stored in the medical office is not flammable, nor will it explode; however, it greatly increases the combustion rate of a fire. If something catches fire, oxygen will make the flame hotter and cause it to burn faster and more vigorously. The result is that a fire involving oxygen can appear explosive-like.

FIRE PREVENTION PLAN

A **fire prevention plan** is a written document that identifies flammable and combustible materials stored in the workplace and ways to control workplace fire hazards. A fire prevention plan reduces the probability that a workplace fire will ignite or spread, which helps prevent injury or death, keeps the workplace safe, and helps to prevent financial losses to the medical office. Almost all medical offices are required by OSHA to develop a fire prevention plan. The fire prevention plan must be in writing, be kept in in the workplace, and be available for employee review.

COMPONENTS OF A FIRE PREVENTION PLAN

Five elements (as required by OSHA) must be included in a fire prevention plan; these are as follows:
1. A list of all major fire hazards including:
   a. Proper handling and storage of fire hazards
   b. Potential ignition sources and controls
   c. Type of fire protection equipment necessary to control each fire hazard

2. Procedures to control accumulation of flammable and combustible waste materials
3. Procedures for regular maintenance of safeguards installed on heat-producing equipment to prevent accidental ignition of combustible materials
4. Name or job title of employees responsible for maintaining equipment to prevent or control ignition sources or fires
5. Name or job title of employees responsible for the control of fuel source hazards

Methods of fire prevention for the medical office (which incorporate many of the elements listed above) are presented in Box 36-1.

FIRE PROTECTION IN THE MEDICAL OFFICE

Fire protection involves the implementation of safety measures to reduce the unwanted effects of fire. The purpose of fire protection is to prevent the spread of fire from one area of a building to another, allow for the safe exit of building occupants, and prevent or reduce the amount of property damage. Fire protection for an office building is specified by fire code requirements and is the responsibility of the

---

BOX 36-1   Methods of Fire Prevention in the Medical Office

Flammable and Combustible Materials
1. Keep the medical office free of clutter.
2. Keep flammable and combustible materials away from ignition sources.
3. Read the label and safety data sheet (SDS) accompanying medical office supplies (e.g., laboratory testing kits, hazardous chemicals, printer toner cartridges) to determine how to properly handle, store, and use these items.
4. Do not allow trash to accumulate.
5. Store trash awaiting removal in a safe location away from heat-producing equipment.
6. Safely dispose of flammable and combustible waste.
7. Clean up any spill of flammable liquids immediately.
8. Do not allow the use of open flames (e.g., burning candles) in the medical office.
9. Ensure that smoking bans are enforced in the workplace.
10. Designate an area outside the building for smoking with fire-resistant containers.

Electrical Equipment and Appliances
1. Make sure equipment and appliances are properly plugged into wall outlets.
2. Use only grounded appliances plugged into grounded outlets (three-prong plug).
3. Do not overload electrical outlets.
4. Promptly disconnect and replace cracked, frayed, or broken electrical cords.

5. Keep heat-producing equipment (e.g., coffee makers, copy machines) away from flammable or combustible materials.
6. Turn off all heat-producing equipment (e.g., examination lights, autoclave) and appliances (e.g., coffee makers) at the end of each work day.
7. Shut down electrical equipment that malfunctions or gives off a strange odor.
8. Avoid the use of extension cords.
9. Avoid the use of space heaters.

Inspection and Maintenance
1. Store oxygen in a clean, dry, well ventilated room.
2. Keep compressed oxygen cylinders and liquid oxygen tanks upright at all times.
3. Ensure that fire alarms and fire extinguishers are clearly visible and not blocked by equipment, decorations, coats, or other objects.
4. Ensure that fire extinguishers are properly stored in their designated locations.
5. Ensure that authorized personnel perform yearly inspections and maintenance of medical equipment (e.g., autoclave, electrocardiograph).
6. Test smoke detectors every month and replace batteries every 6 months.
7. Have authorized personnel perform regular inspections, maintenance, and testing of fire alarms, sprinkler systems, and fire extinguishers.
8. Report fire hazards you cannot correct yourself.

owner of the building; however, fire protection for the contents of the office is the responsibility of office staff. Some of the important safety measures employed in fire protection are listed and described in the following paragraphs.

Sprinkler Systems

Sprinkler systems are one of the best measures available to extinguish a fire in its early stages. Sprinkler systems are usually located at ceiling level and use water to put out or slow the progress of a fire. Sprinklers are activated by the build-up of heat in the fire area, which causes a glass component in the sprinkler head to melt or break, releasing water from the sprinkler. Only those sprinklers closest to the fire area are activated, which reduces water damage to the contents of the building. For example, just one or two activated sprinklers may be able to quickly extinguish a fire that has just started in an office laboratory. Most sprinkler systems include an alarm system that alerts both building occupants and emergency responders when sprinkler activation occurs.

Many states require sprinkler systems in commercial and office buildings. Some states that require sprinklers for larger office buildings do not require them for smaller offices (e.g., physician's office that has been converted from a house).

Fire Doors

A fire door is a fire-resistant door that is designed to prevent the spread of fire from one area of a building to another (Figure 36-8). Fire doors assist in the safe escape of occupants from a building during a fire and help to reduce property damage. In a large office or freestanding clinic, fire doors are typically located at certain points in the corridors. Fire doors should never be propped open; instead they should be allowed to shut to their naturally closed position.

Fire-Resistant Cabinets

Whenever possible, records should be stored in fire-resistant file cabinets. If the office uses a physical system to back up computer files (instead of a network or an Internet system), the backup drives should be stored in a fire-resistant file cabinet or fire-resistant box-type safe. It is always preferable to store a backup copy on the Internet or at another location.

Fire Alarms

A fire alarm is a device that warns building occupants of the presence of a fire (Figure 36-9). Once a fire alarm has been activated, a loud noise and flashing lights are broadcasted to alert building occupants of the fire and to provide them with enough time to safely evacuate the building. The alarm also notifies the fire department so that firefighters can quickly respond to the fire. Fire alarm pull stations are frequently located in the corridors of buildings. It is important for employees to be trained in the proper activation of a fire alarm and what conditions necessitate activating the alarm.

Smoke Detectors

A smoke detector is a device that detects and automatically provides a warning of the presence of smoke. Smoke detector laws vary by state in terms of how many must be in an office and where they must be located. In many buildings,

Figure 36-8 A fire door prevents the spread of fire from one area of a building to another.

Figure 36-9 Fire alarm pull stations are commonly found in the corridors of an office building.

smoke detectors are wired into the building's security and fire alarm system. If the office has battery-operated smoke detectors, these should be tested monthly by pressing the test button. Batteries should be changed every 6 months, and the date should be noted on the detector.

Fire Extinguisher

A **fire extinguisher** is a portable device that discharges an agent designed to extinguish a fire (Figure 36-10, *A*). Common examples of extinguishing agents include dry chemicals, foam, carbon dioxide, and water. Portable fire extinguishers are considered a first line of defense in the early stages of a fire and have two primary functions: to control or extinguish a small fire that has just started and to protect an evacuation route that a fire may block with smoke or burning materials. A fire extinguisher should

never be used to fight a large fire that is out of control; instead, the building occupants should evacuate the premises immediately and call the fire department.

Fires are classified into five categories according to the type of fuel that is burning. For example, a class A fire involves the burning of ordinary combustible materials. Fire extinguishers are marked with a label indicating the type of fire classification they are designed to handle. Newer types of fire extinguishers are labeled with a pictogram illustrating the type of fuel that can be extinguished by that particular extinguisher. Older types of extinguishers are labeled with colored geometric shapes with letter designations. Table 36-1 lists and describes the five fire classifications along with the type of extinguisher (by label) that can be used to extinguish each class of fire. Most fire extinguishers are designed to handle more than one fire classification. For example, a

Figure 36-10 **A,** Fire extinguisher with parts labeled. **B,** A multipurpose fire extinguisher is labeled with three pictograms indicating the A, B, and C fire classifications it is designed to extinguish.

Table 36-1 Extinguishers Used to Extinguish Various Classifications of Fire

Extinguisher Label: Pictogram	Extinguisher Label: Geometric Symbol	Works on: Fire Classification
	A	**Class A: Ordinary Combustibles** Paper, wood, cloth, rubber, and many plastics
	B	**Class B: Flammable Liquids** Gasoline, oil, grease, tar, oil-based paints, solvents, lacquers, alcohols, flammable gases
	C	**Class C: Electrical Equipment** Equipment and appliances that are plugged into an outlet, wiring, circuit breakers, and electrical outlets
	D	**Class D: Combustible Metals** Magnesium, titanium, zirconium, sodium, lithium and potassium
	K	**Class K: Cooking Media** Vegetable oil, animal oil, fats in cooking appliances involving these substances

Figure 36-11 A fire extinguisher installed in a wall cabinet.

multipurpose fire extinguisher is labeled with three pictograms (Figure 36-10, *B*) and is designed to extinguish class A, B, and C fires. Most medical offices have multipurpose fire extinguishers in their facilities because this type of extinguisher can put out most types of fire.

Fire extinguishers must be properly identified (Figure 36-11) and readily accessible in an emergency situation. Fire code requirements specify the size, number, location, and type of fire extinguishers within a facility. These requirements are based on the protection level that is appropriate for the hazard class of the building and the types (classes) of fire most likely to occur in that facility. Fire extinguishers are mounted on brackets or installed in wall cabinets (Figure 36-11) and are usually located along normal paths of travel and near building exits. If a fire extinguisher is mounted in a room, it is placed near the door so that the fire does not get between an individual and an exit. There should always be a fire extinguisher within a 50-foot travel distance of flammable liquids that are stored in containers. Fire extinguishers must be stored in their designated place at all times except during operation.

Fire extinguishers must be properly maintained to ensure that they are safe to use and will operate properly when needed. Most medical offices use maintenance personnel and a certified fire extinguisher agency to inspect, maintain, and test their fire extinguishers on a regular basis (monthly and yearly). A durable tag is attached to each fire extinguisher to document each service check, including the date

of the service and the signature of the individual performing the service.

Small fires can often be put out quickly by an employee using a portable fire extinguisher, ending the threat of a major fire. To do this safely, however, the employee must know how to properly operate a fire extinguisher. OSHA requires that any employee responsible for operating a portable fire extinguisher be thoroughly trained in the use of the fire extinguisher as well as the hazards associated with fighting a fire. The acronym *PASS* is used to help remember the steps involved in operating a fire extinguisher:

P: Pull out the pin.
A: Aim the nozzle at the base of the fire.
S: Squeeze the handle.
S: Sweep the nozzle from side to side at the base of the fire.

Procedure 36-1 outlines in more detail the procedure for operating a fire extinguisher

EMERGENCY RESPONSE TO A FIRE

It is important to respond immediately to a fire. Most fires start out small but can quickly increase in size and intensity and become life-threatening in just a matter of minutes. The heat, smoke, and toxic gases from a fire that is spreading are often more dangerous than the flames.

The acronym *RACE* can be used to identify the basic steps to follow in responding to a fire (RACE against fire). These steps are as follows:

R: Rescue anyone in immediate danger of the fire.
A: Activate the alarm.
C: Confine the fire by closing doors and windows.
E: Extinguish the fire or evacuate the area. If the fire is small, use a fire extinguisher to put the fire out. If the fire cannot be extinguished, evacuate the area.

Procedure 36-2 presents a more detailed emergency plan for responding to a fire, incorporating the RACE response outlined here.

What Would You Do? What Would You *Not* Do?

Case Study 2

Brie Matthews is at the medical office for an evaluation of her diabetes. Mary Beth enters the examining room to measure Brie's vital signs. As Mary Beth enters the room, she notices that Brie is studying the fire extinguisher mounted on brackets near the door and turning the service tag over to read the information on it. Brie indicates that she needs to get a fire extinguisher for her home and wants to know the meaning of the three pictures on the extinguisher and why the extinguisher has a tag attached to it. Brie wants to know who is allowed to operate the fire extinguisher and how long the extinguisher lasts before it gets "used up." Brie also wants to know why there are fire extinguishers in the office, because she noticed that the office has sprinklers in the ceiling. ■

PROCEDURE 36-1   Demonstrating Proper Use of a Fire Extinguisher

Outcome Demonstrate proper use of a fire extinguisher in a role-playing situation

Equipment/Supplies

- Portable office-size multipurpose (ABC) fire extinguisher that has been discharged

1. Procedural Step. Identify a safe evacuation route before approaching the fire.
Principle. A clear evacuation route allows for immediate escape if the fire gets worse.

2. Procedural Step. Remove the multipurpose fire extinguisher from its mounting device and hold it upright with the nozzle pointing away from you. Stand 6 to 8 feet from the fire, keeping your back to the exit at all times.
Principle. Standing at 6 to 8 feet prevents being burned or being hit by splattering material or sparks. Keeping the back to the exit allows for constant monitoring of the situation and immediate awareness if the fire begins to flare up or spread.

3. Procedural Step. Perform a quick assessment of the fire to determine if it is small enough to extinguish with a fire extinguisher (while continuing to stand at a distance of 6 to 8 feet). *Do not* attempt to extinguish the fire if it is too large or if there is excessive smoke or heat. In these instances, close the door to contain the fire then evacuate immediately.
Principle. A fire extinguisher is designed to handle only small fires in the beginning stages.

4. Procedural Step. Operate the fire extinguisher using the PASS technique:

a. *Pull* the safety pin straight out from the handle located at the top of the extinguisher. This will also break the tamper-proof seal. Make sure the fire extinguisher is held in an upright position at all times.
Principle. The tamper-proof seal holds the safety pin in place. The safety pin provides a locking mechanism that prevents the fire extinguisher from accidentally discharging.

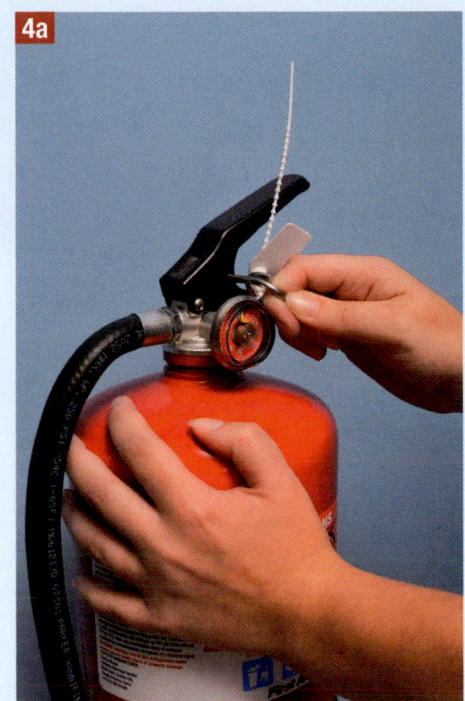

4a

Pull the safety pin straight out from the handle.

b. *Aim* the nozzle at the base of the fire (not the flames) with your dominant hand.
Principle. Aiming the nozzle at the base of the fire allows the extinguishing agent to deprive the fire of fuel. Aiming the nozzle at the flames causes the extinguishing agent to pass through the flames without stopping the fire.

c. *Squeeze* the handle slowly and continuously to release the extinguishing agent. Letting go of the pressure on the handle causes the discharge of the extinguishing to cease.
Principle. Squeezing the handle opens a valve that releases the pressurized extinguishing agent from the fire extinguisher.

Continued

PROCEDURE 36-1

PROCEDURE 36-1 Demonstrating Proper Use of a Fire Extinguisher—cont'd

Squeeze the handle slowly and continuously.

d. *Sweep* the nozzle of the extinguisher evenly from side to side at the base of the fire. Gradually move closer to the fire as it begins to smolder. Continue to discharge the extinguishing agent until the fire is completely out. Evacuate immediately if the fire grows larger or if the extinguisher is empty and the fire is not out. Fire extinguishers use up their extinguishing agent within 10 to 30 seconds, depending on the size of the extinguisher.
Principle. A sweeping motion helps to extinguish the fire. Even distribution of the agent helps to put out the fire at a faster rate.

6 to 8 feet

Sweep the nozzle of the extinguisher at the base of the fire.

5. **Procedural Step.** Back away from the extinguished fire in case it flares up again. Continue to watch the area to be sure that flames do not recur after having been extinguished.
Principle. Material that has been burning can remain hot enough that flames will reignite.

PROCEDURE 36-2 Participating in a Mock Exposure Event

Outcome Participate in a mock environmental exposure event and document the steps taken

Scenario

A fire has erupted in an examining room at your medical office. The fire, caused by faulty electrical wiring, has ignited several boxes of disposable drapes. (Place a poster, flashing light, or other indicator at the location of the "fire"). A disabled patient in a wheelchair is located in the room where the fire erupts. The emergency evacuation coordinator determines that an evacuation of the facility is necessary.

Equipment/Supplies

- Scenario
- Emergency evacuation floor plan
- Employee roster
- Patient log-in sheet
- Pen and paper

Predrill Activities

1. **Procedural Step.** Make a list of the names and phone numbers of the following resources that may be needed in the event of a fire:
   a. Emergency responders (911)
   b. Fire department
   c. Police department
   d. Local hospital
   e. Insurance carrier

2. **Procedural Step.** Review the location and purpose of fire protection safety measures.
   a. Locate and review the purpose of the following in your facility using the evacuation floor plan as a reference:
   - The path of the primary exit route
   - The path of the secondary exit route
   - Manual fire alarm pull stations
   - Portable fire extinguishers
   - Emergency exit doors
   - Wheelchair accessible exits
   - Assembly area
   - Shelter-in-place areas

Locate the path of the primary and secondary exit routes.

   b. Locate and review the purpose of the following through visual inspection of the facility:
   - Sprinklers
   - Smoke detectors
   - Fire doors
   - Exit signs
   Principle. The medical assistant should know the location and purpose of the fire protection safety measures in his or her facility.

3. **Procedural Step.** Evaluate primary and secondary exit routes for the following:
   a. Exits are clearly marked and well lit.
   b. Exit routes are unobstructed and free of clutter.
   c. Exit doors are free of decorations or signs that obscure the visibility of the exit.
   d. Exit doors are unlocked from the inside.
   e. Exit doors open outward.
   f. Fire extinguishers are in place and clearly identified.
   g. Evacuation floor plans are posted in multiple locations throughout the facility.

4. **Procedural Step.** Assign an emergency evacuation coordinator to assume overall charge and responsibility for the evacuation process including the following:
   a. Calling emergency responders (911)
   b. Identifying safe evacuation routes
   c. Ensuring that evacuation wardens are performing their duties
   d. Coordinating with the emergency responders
   Principle. The emergency evacuation coordinator is responsible for taking charge of the evacuation process.

5. **Procedural Step.** Compile an employee roster and assign evacuation wardens to perform one or more of the duties outlined in Table 36-2. Make sure each evacuation warden understands his or her roles and responsibilities and is well trained in his or her assigned duties.

Continued

PROCEDURE 36-2

Principle. Evacuation wardens are responsible for performing rescue duties during an evacuation.

6. **Procedural Step.** Assign individuals to play the role of patients and compile a patient log-in sheet. Patients with special needs should be included, such as:
   a. Mother with a young child with an illness
   b. Patient with emphysema on oxygen
   c. Pregnant patient in the last trimester of her pregnancy
   d. Patient with crutches wearing a leg cast
   e. Elderly patient with a heart condition
   f. Patient with dementia
   g. Disabled patient in a wheelchair
   h. Patient with severe anxiety
   i. Hearing-impaired patient
   j. Patient with a visual impairment

Conduct the Fire Drill

(The emergency evacuation coordinator and evacuation wardens should perform their assigned duties during the fire drill).

1. **Procedural Step.** Rescue anyone in immediate danger of the fire. If an individual's clothes catch on fire, the following can be performed to extinguish the flames:
   a. Instruct the person to stop, drop, and roll.
   b. Cover the person with a blanket or clothing to help extinguish the flames.

Cover the person with a blanket or clothes to extinguish flames.

2. **Procedural Step.** Activate the alarm. The employee who first discovers the fire should activate the nearest fire alarm pull station by pulling down on the lever. *Principle.* Activating the alarm warns building occupants of the presence of a fire to provide them with enough time to safely evacuate the building.

Activate the alarm.

3. **Procedural Step.** Immediately notify emergency responders by dialing 911. Speak clearly and calmly to the emergency medical dispatcher. Identify the problem as accurately and concisely as possible so that proper equipment and personnel can be sent. Do not hang up until the dispatcher gives you permission to do so. Information that should be relayed (if known) to the emergency dispatcher includes the following:
   a. Type of fire (e.g., electrical, combustibles, flammable liquids)
   b. Exact location of the fire
   c. Extent of the fire
   d. Whether an evacuation is in process
   e. Other information requested by the dispatcher
   Principle. Calling 911 allows the fire department to be on its way while other activities are being performed. Any delay may allow the fire to grow and further endanger the building occupants and property.

4. **Procedural Step.** Confine the fire by closing doors and windows in the immediate area of the fire. *Principle.* Closing doors and windows helps prevent the spread of smoke and fire throughout the building.

5. **Procedural Step.** Extinguish the fire with a portable fire extinguisher if it is small and confined, following the steps outlined in Procedure 36-1. *Do not* attempt to extinguish the fire if it is too large or if there is excessive smoke or heat. In these instances, close the door to contain the fire then evacuate immediately.

6. **Procedural Step.** Evacuate the area immediately. The evacuation wardens should perform their evacuation duties as assigned in Table 36-2. Important evacuation guidelines include the following:
   a. Shut down all electrical equipment and appliances in the immediate area

PROCEDURE 36-2 Participating in a Mock Exposure Event—cont'd

b. Before exiting a room, feel the door with the back of your hand. If the door is warm:
- Do not open the door.
- Call 911 to report your location or place a signal in the window.
- Place clothing or towels along the bottom of the door to keep out smoke.
- Stay calm and wait to be rescued.
- Do not break the window. Smoke entering from the outside may hamper rescue.

Feel the door with the back of your hand before exiting the room.

Place clothing along the bottom of the door.

c. Use the primary exit route if possible. If the primary exit route is blocked by fire or smoke, use the secondary exit route.

d. Exit by stairways only. Do not use elevators.

Do not use elevators.

e. Close doors after a room is evacuated and place an X on the door with chalk or a marker to indicate the room has been evacuated

Principle: The size of a fire can double every 30 seconds; therefore it is important to evacuate immediately. The primary exit route is the quickest and easiest way to exit a building during an evacuation. Elevators may fail during a fire trapping occupants.

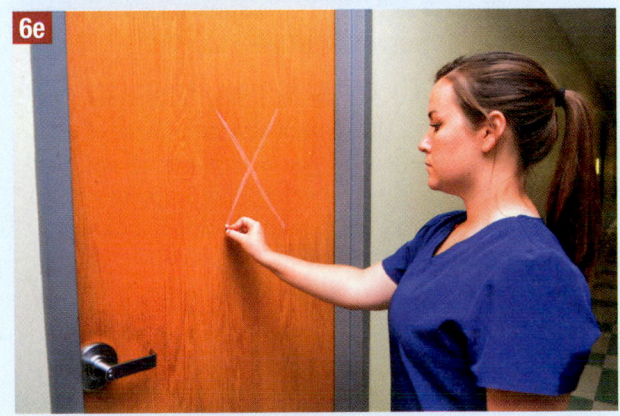

Place an X on the door.

Continued

PROCEDURE **36-2** Participating in a Mock Exposure Event—cont'd

7. Procedural Step. Escort patients to the designated assembly area. Check to make sure everyone is accounted for by completing the following:

a. Account for all employees using the employee roster checklist.

b. Account for all patients using the patient log-in sheet.
   Principle. Accounting for building occupants helps to determine if someone is still in the building and in need of rescue.

Account for all employees.

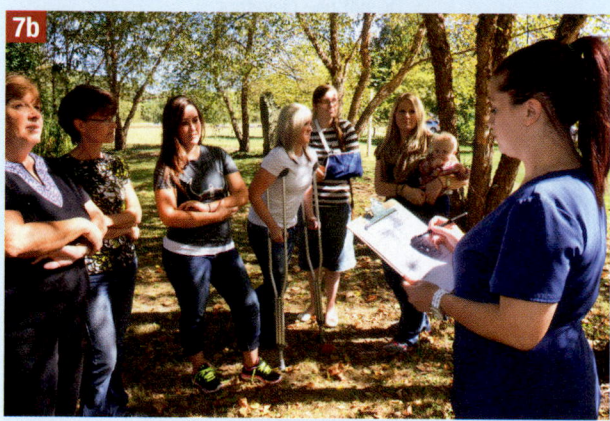

Account for all patients.

8. Procedural Step. Keep the building occupants together in the assembly area at a safe distance from the building. Make sure that occupants do not block access to the building by emergency responders. Do not allow anyone to reenter the building unless directed to do so by emergency officials. Instruct occupants not to leave until everyone has been accounted for and dismissed.

9. Procedural Step. Provide emergency responders with the following information:

a. The name and last known location of any individual not accounted for during the head count.

b. Special hazards in the building that may endanger emergency responders such as oxygen tanks and hazardous chemicals.

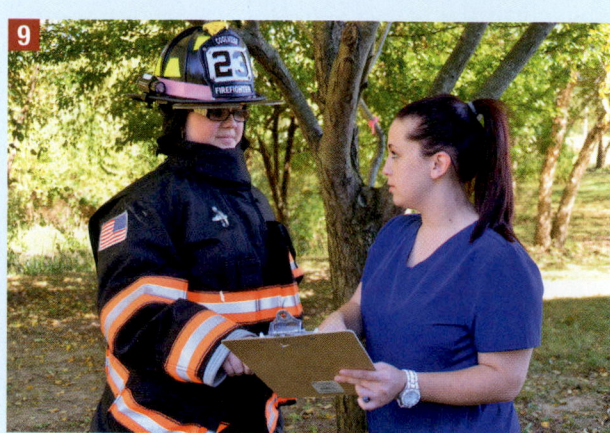

Provide emergency responders with information.

Postdrill Activities

1. Procedural Step. Critique the effectiveness of the fire drill (in terms of strengths, concerns, and means of improvement) by evaluating the following:

a. The evacuation was completed in an orderly, efficient, and timely manner.

b. Building occupants and emergency responders were immediately alerted of the situation.

c. Evacuation wardens effectively completed their duties.

d. Patients and visitors were escorted to the nearest exit and assembly area.

e. Each building occupant was accounted for after the evacuation.

f. Emergency responders were provided with appropriate information.

2. Procedural Step. Document the results of the fire drill including your role and the effectiveness of the group as a whole in carrying out the evacuation.
Principle. Evaluation of the fire drill identifies strengths, concerns, and means of improvement.

Table 36-2 Evacuation Warden Duties During a Fire

Evacuation Warden Duties	Guidelines and Key Points
Activate the nearest fire alarm pull station	The employee who first discovers the fire should activate the nearest fire alarm pull station.
Operate a fire extinguisher	A fire extinguisher can be used to extinguish a small fire in the beginning stages. *Do not* attempt to extinguish a fire if it is too large or if there is excessive smoke or heat.
Alert patients to the presence of a fire	Alert patients using a calm and firm manner so as not to cause panic. Use a clear and distinct voice to instruct patients during the evacuation.
Evacuate patients and visitors from each room and close windows and doors in each room	Closing windows and doors reduces the amount of oxygen that is able to get to the fire and helps to limit the spread of smoke and fire throughout the building.
Escort patients and visitors to the nearest exit and assembly area according to the evacuation floor plan	Use the primary exit route if available. If the primary exit route is blocked, use the secondary exit route. If smoke is present, stay low and close to the floor while evacuating because the air is fresher nearer to the ground. Proceed (walk, do not run) through the escape route in a quiet, orderly manner.
Assist patients with disabilities	If it is not possible to evacuate a disabled patient, take the patient to a shelter-in-place area and notify emergency personnel of the patient's location.
Direct patients to stairways that are free of smoke	Instruct individuals to not push, rush, or jostle other individuals when exiting by way of a stairway.
Keep people out of elevators	Elevators should not be used during a fire because: a. Elevator may fail during a fire, trapping the occupants. b. Elevator shafts may fill with smoke. c. Elevators need to be available to emergency responders.
Perform a final check of each room (examining rooms, rest rooms, offices, break room, storage rooms) to make sure everyone has been evacuated	A final check ensures that all occupants have been evacuated from the building.
Make sure fire doors are closed when exiting	Fire doors prevent spread of fire from one area to another.
Instruct building occupants not to leave the assembly area or to go back into the building	Building occupants need to remain in the assembly area so that they can be accounted for by the emergency evacuation coordinator. Occupants should not go back into the building until given permission to do so by emergency officials.
Direct emergency responders to the location of the fire	Use a clear and distinct voice to direct emergency responders to the location of the fire.
Notify emergency responders of hazardous materials (e.g., oxygen tanks, hazardous chemicals) in the building	Providing information on hazardous materials is essential to the safety of emergency responders.

EMPLOYEE EDUCATION AND TRAINING

Medical assisting employees must know what types of emergencies may occur in their medical office and what course of action they should take. OSHA requires that employees be provided with education and training on the EAP. The training should include the following:

- Individual roles and responsibilities
- Threats, hazards, and protective actions
- Location and operation of manually activated pull stations and communication equipment
- Emergency response procedures
- Evacuation, shelter, and accountability procedures
- Location and use of common emergency equipment
- Emergency shutdown procedures

The EAP must be reviewed with each employee at the following times:

- When the initial plan is developed
- When new employees are hired
- When the employee's responsibilities or designated actions under the plan change
- Whenever the plan is changed

EMERGENCY PRACTICE DRILLS

Once employees have reviewed and been trained in the EAP, it is important to hold emergency practice drills. The purpose of a practice drill is to provide employees with the opportunity to practice their assigned duties in a simulated emergency situation. This increases the probability that employees will perform their duties safely and effectively in the event of an actual disaster or serious emergency. Emergency practice drills also provide the opportunity to evaluate the effectiveness of the EAP and determine any necessary changes or adjustments needed for improving performance. There are two types of emergency practice drills—fire drills and disaster drills—which are discussed in more detail in the following sections.

FIRE DRILLS

Fire drills may be required at specific intervals depending on the municipal or state laws for the type of building and insurance requirements. Fire drills may be announced or unannounced. They assist employees of a medical facility to review emergency escape routes and procedures to respond to a fire. Fire drills provide employees with the opportunity to become familiar with exit routes under nonthreatening conditions. This increases the probability of an organized and smooth evacuation during an actual emergency.

DISASTER DRILLS

Disaster drills are usually more comprehensive than fire drills. Disaster drills often involve several community agencies depending on the severity of the disaster scenario that will be simulated. Disaster drills are time-consuming, but they allow all participants to practice skills that would be needed in the event of a disaster. In addition, they allow organizations and communities to evaluate the effectiveness of their systems and identify potential weaknesses in the ability to respond to an actual disaster.

MEDICAL ASSISTANT'S ROLE

The medical assistant is an important team member in developing and implementing the EAP for a health care setting and can also contribute to emergency preparedness in the community. He or she may make recommendations to supplement emergency equipment or facilities in the office, serve on a committee to review or revise the emergency plan, participate actively in all fire drills and disaster drills, and participate in the review of the effectiveness of any drill. In addition, the medical assistant must be prepared to provide emergency first aid or cardiopulmonary resuscitation (CPR), both in the workplace and in the community (see Chapter 37). In an actual disaster, medical assistants might assist by providing emergency first aid, conducting patient interviews, helping to calm victims, documenting services provided, and performing phlebotomy or other procedures as directed.

The medical assistant should be aware of community resources for emergency preparedness The medical office may keep a list of local organizations with telephone numbers or other contact information in the following areas:

- Emergency Medical Services (911)
- Poison Control Center
- Telephone numbers of local hospitals
- Telephone numbers of local and state health departments
- Telephone number for the state HAZMAT response team (**HAZMAT** is an acronym constructed from "*haz*ardous *mat*erials." It refers to materials that pose a danger to health or the environment and for which protective clothing is required for cleanup.)

The medical assistant should also be aware of community disaster plans and community organizations that might assist in a disaster. The website of the state emergency medical agency often includes helpful articles related to the disasters that occur most frequently in that state. It is helpful to develop a list of useful resources for the medical office and update it regularly.

What Would You Do? | What Would You *Not* Do?

Case Study 3

Jordan Mendels, 32 years of age, is at the medical office complaining of headaches, fatigue, and insomnia. Jordan tearfully relays that her brother's house burned down 2 weeks ago. Jordan is now concerned about a fire in her own home. She wants to know the best way to prevent that from happening and also wants to know if her family should hold fire drills. Jordan says that she knows she should get a fire extinguisher but she doesn't know how to use one. ■

Memories *from* Practicum

Beth Ann Wilson: The office where I did my practicum was a clinic in a large city hospital. While I was there, I was allowed to attend a hands-on fire training session for hospital employees. We met at a training facility at the fire department where we saw two training videos. One of them showed how to test a door for warmth and emphasized that a warm door or a door with smoke leaking around the edge should never be opened. In the film, a fireman did open the door, and we saw how the flames and smoke gushed out when the fire received the new supply of oxygen. Someone asked what you should do if you knew there was a patient in the room behind a warm door. The fireman answered that if possible, you should wait for a firefighter, who would be prepared to handle the flame and smoke. After the videos, we were dressed in protective equipment and allowed to discharge fire extinguishers to put out small fires. Even though the fires were small, it was still a scary experience. I hope I never have to deal with a fire, even a small one, but I know that this experience helped to prepare me if it ever happens. ■

Case Study 1
Page 949

What Did Beth Ann Do?
❑ Told Mrs. Manning to stop and breathe, and encouraged her to take several deep breaths.
❑ Recognized that Mrs. Manning was showing signs of severe anxiety, which would make it difficult for her to focus on driving safely.
❑ Told Mrs. Manning that she seemed very upset by the news, reassured her that the fire department would respond promptly, and encouraged her to sit down and relax for a minute until she collects herself.
❑ Asked Mrs. Manning if there was a family member or friend she could call to pick her up and drive her to her son's school.
❑ Listened attentively to Mrs. Manning's concerns.

What Did Beth Ann **Not** *Do?*
❑ Did not allow Mrs. Manning to leave and drive an automobile while in a state of severe anxiety.
❑ Did not tell Mrs. Manning to calm down because she was overreacting.
❑ Did not give Mrs. Manning a detailed explanation of the effects of anxiety.

Case Study 2
Page 956

What Did Beth Ann Do?
❑ Told Brie that the pictures indicate the type of fires the extinguisher can handle and that this extinguisher is a multipurpose extinguisher and can put out fires caused by ordinary combustibles such as paper or wood, flammable liquids, and electrical equipment.
❑ Explained to Brie that each fire extinguisher must be inspected and maintained on a regular basis and the tag documents the date of each service check.
❑ Informed Brie that only employees with the proper training and knowledge are permitted to operate the fire extinguishers in the office in the event of a fire.
❑ Told Brie that fire extinguishers use up their extinguishing agent within 10 to 30 seconds depending on the size of the extinguisher.

❑ Relayed to Brie that fire code requirements, which often include a variety of safety measures, specify the type of fire protection safety measures that must be present in a building.

What Did Beth Ann **Not** *Do?*
❑ Did not let Brie remove the fire extinguisher from its mounting brackets.
❑ Did not scold Brie for not already having a fire extinguisher in her home.

Case Study 3
Page 964

What Did Beth Ann Do?
❑ Listened empathetically to Jordan and allow her to express her fears and concerns.
❑ Reassured Jordan that practicing fire prevention methods in the home is the best way to reduce the possibility of a fire.
❑ Provided Jordan with the names of websites (FEMA, American Red Cross, National Fire Protection Association, ready.gov) that she could use to access information on fire prevention and protective measures in the home.
❑ Told Jordan that it is a very good idea to hold fire drills in the home to make sure everyone knows what to do in the event of a fire and how to evacuate quickly and safely.
❑ Explained to Jordan that fire extinguishers are not difficult to operate and that each fire extinguisher comes with step-by-step instructions.
❑ Informed the physician of the situation so that he could provide the best treatment for Jordan.
❑ Reminded Jordan that fires in the home do happen, but they are not regular occurrences.

What Did Beth Ann **Not** *Do?*
❑ Did not say or imply that Jordan was overreacting or worrying for no reason.
❑ Did not push Jordan to accept her suggestions, but rather just offered information.
❑ Did not alarm Jordan about the possibility of a home fire.

TERMINOLOGY REVIEW

Key Term	Definition
Anxiety	A feeling of worry or uneasiness, often triggered by an event that is perceived as having an uncertain outcome.
Disaster	A sudden event that causes damage or loss of life.
Emergency action plan	A written document that describes the actions that employees should take to ensure their safety if a fire or other emergency situation occurs.
Emergency preparedness	The process of making plans to prevent, respond to, and recover from an emergency situation.
Evacuation	A planned systematic retreat of people to safety in an emergency situation.
Evacuation procedures	Clear step-by-step procedures for the rapid, efficient, and safe removal of individuals from a building during an emergency.
Exit route	A continuous and unobstructed path of travel from any point within a workplace to a place of safety.
Fire extinguisher	A portable device that discharges an agent designed to extinguish a fire.
Fire prevention plan	A written document that identifies flammable and combustible materials stored in the workplace and ways to control workplace fire hazards.
Fire protection	The implementation of safety measures to reduce the unwanted effects of fire.
HAZMAT	An acronym constructed from the beginnings of the two words "*haz*ardous *mat*erials." It refers to materials that pose a danger to health or the environment and must be handled with protective equipment.
Man-made disaster	An event that causes serious damage through intentional or negligent human actions or the failure of a man-made system.
Natural disaster	A catastrophic event that is caused by nature or the natural process of the earth.
Stress	The body's response to threat or change.

ON THE WEB

For information on fire safety:

OSHA Fire Safety: www.osha.gov/SLTC/firesafety

U.S. Fire Administration: www.usfa.fema.gov

National Fire Protection Association: www.nfpa.org

For information on evacuation plans:

OSHA Evacuation Plans and Procedures: www.osha.gov/SLTC/etools/evacuation

For information on emergency and disaster planning:

American Red Cross: www.americanredcross.org

CDC Emergency Preparedness: www.bt.cdc.gov/preparedness

Citizen Corps: www.ready.gov/citizen-corps

FEMA (Federal Emergency Management Agency): www.fema.gov/

Disaster help and resources: www.disasterassistance.gov

State agencies: www.fema.gov/state-offices-and-agencies-emergency-management

To find local emergency preparedness programs:

National Office of Citizen Corps: http://www.ready.gov/citizen-corps

Emergency Medical Procedures and First Aid

37

Check out the Evolve site at http://evolve.elsevier.com/Bonewit/today/ to access additional interactive activities and exercises to help you study and prepare for success.

LEARNING OBJECTIVES

First Aid

1. State the purpose of first aid.
2. Explain the purpose of the emergency medical services (EMS) system.
3. List the OSHA standards for administering first aid.
4. List the guidelines that should be followed when providing emergency care.

Common Emergency Situations

5. List and describe conditions that cause respiratory distress.
6. List the symptoms of a heart attack and a stroke.
7. Explain the causes of each of the following types of shock: cardiogenic, neurogenic, anaphylactic, and psychogenic.
8. Identify and describe the three classifications of external bleeding.
9. Explain the difference between an open wound and a closed wound.
10. Describe the characteristics of each of the following fractures: impacted, greenstick, transverse, oblique, comminuted, and spiral.
11. Identify the characteristics of each of the following burns: superficial, partial thickness, and full thickness.
12. Explain the difference between a partial seizure and a generalized seizure.
13. List examples of each of the following types of poisoning: ingested, inhaled, absorbed, and injected.
14. Identify factors that place an individual at higher risk for developing heat-related and cold-related injuries.
15. Describe the differences between type 1 and type 2 diabetes mellitus.
16. Explain the causes of insulin shock and diabetic coma.
17. Identify the symptoms and describe emergency care for each of the following conditions: respiratory distress, heart attack, stroke, shock, bleeding, wounds, musculoskeletal injuries, burns, seizures, poisoning, heat and cold exposure, and diabetic emergencies.

PROCEDURES

Respond to common emergency situations.

CHAPTER OUTLINE

INTRODUCTION TO EMERGENCY MEDICAL
 PROCEDURES
OFFICE CRASH CART
EMERGENCY MEDICAL SERVICES SYSTEM
FIRST AID KIT
OSHA SAFETY PRECAUTIONS
GUIDELINES FOR PROVIDING EMERGENCY CARE
Respiratory Distress
Asthma
Emphysema
Hyperventilation

Heart Attack
Stroke
Shock
Hypovolemic Shock
Cardiogenic Shock
Neurogenic Shock
Anaphylactic Shock
Psychogenic Shock
Bleeding
External Bleeding
Internal Bleeding

hyperventilation. More recent studies no longer recommend this practice because it could be harmful if an underlying medical condition exists or if the patient is not actually hyperventilating. If the medical assistant suspects that hyperventilation has been caused by an organic problem, EMS should be activated immediately.

HEART ATTACK

A heart attack, also known as a *myocardial infarction* (MI), is caused by partial or complete obstruction of one or both of the coronary arteries or their branches. In most cases, the severity of the attack depends on the size of the obstructed artery and the amount of myocardial tissue nourished by that artery. If a small branch of a coronary artery is obstructed, myocardial damage and symptoms may be mild, whereas the damage is usually extensive and the symptoms intense if a coronary artery is completely blocked.

The principal symptom of a heart attack is chest pain or discomfort. Patients describe the chest pain as squeezing or crushing pressure, severe indigestion or burning, heaviness, or aching. Chest discomfort can range in severity from only mildly uncomfortable to intense and accompanied by a feeling of suffocation and doom. The pain is usually felt behind the sternum and may radiate to the neck, throat, or jaw or to both shoulders and both arms. The pain associated with a heart attack is prolonged and usually is not relieved by resting or taking nitroglycerin. Other signs and symptoms of a heart attack include shortness of breath, profuse perspiration, nausea, and fainting.

If the medical assistant suspects that the patient is having a heart attack, EMS should be activated immediately. Meanwhile, loosen tight clothing and have the patient rest in a comfortable position that facilitates breathing. If cardiac arrest occurs, the medical assistant should begin cardiopulmonary resuscitation (CPR) immediately.

STROKE

A stroke, also called a *cerebrovascular accident* (CVA), results when an artery to the brain is blocked or ruptures, causing an interruption of blood flow to the brain. The signs and symptoms of a stroke include sudden weakness or numbness of the face, arm, or leg on one side of the body; difficulty in speaking; dimmed vision or loss of vision in one eye; double vision; dizziness; confusion; severe headache; and loss of consciousness.

If the medical assistant suspects that the patient is having a stroke, EMS should be activated immediately. Meanwhile, loosen tight clothing and have the patient rest in a comfortable position. If respiratory arrest, cardiac arrest, or both occur, begin rescue breathing and CPR as required.

SHOCK

For the body to function properly, adequate blood flow must be maintained to all of the vital organs. This is accomplished by the three important cardiovascular functions, as follows:

- Adequate pumping action of the heart
- Sufficient blood circulating in the blood vessels
- Blood vessels being able to respond to blood flow

When an individual experiences a severe injury or illness, one or more of these cardiovascular functions may be affected, which can lead to shock.

Shock is defined as the failure of the cardiovascular system to deliver enough blood to all of the body's vital organs. Shock accompanies different types of emergency situations, such as hemorrhaging, MI, and severe allergic reaction. The five major types of shock are categorized according to cause: hypovolemic, cardiogenic, neurogenic, anaphylactic, and psychogenic. Each type of shock is described in this section. If not treated, most types of shock become life-threatening. This is because shock is progressive—when it reaches a certain point, it becomes irreversible, and the patient's life cannot be saved.

The signs and symptoms of shock are caused by the failure of the vital organs to receive enough oxygen and nutrients. The organs most affected are the heart, brain, and lungs, which can be irreparably damaged in 4 to 6 minutes. The general signs and symptoms of shock are weakness, restlessness, anxiety, disorientation, pallor, cold and clammy skin, rapid breathing, and rapid pulse.

If not treated, these symptoms can progress rapidly to a significant drop in blood pressure, cyanosis, loss of consciousness, and death. The signs and symptoms of shock may be subtle or pronounced. In addition, no single sign or symptom determines accurately the presence or severity of the shock. Because of this, it is crucial to consider the nature of the illness or injury in determining whether the patient is a possible victim of shock. If a patient has a traumatic injury to the abdomen, shock should be considered a possibility, even if the patient's signs and symptoms do not suggest shock.

Shock (with the exception of psychogenic shock) requires immediate medical care. The medical assistant should activate EMS without delay so that proper medical care can be obtained as soon as possible.

Hypovolemic Shock

Hypovolemic shock is caused by loss of blood or other body fluids. Conditions that result in this type of shock include external and internal hemorrhaging; plasma loss from severe burns; and severe dehydration from vomiting, diarrhea, or profuse perspiration. The first priority in hypovolemic shock is to control bleeding. A patient in hypovolemic shock must have the volume of fluid that was lost replaced and must be transported to an emergency care facility immediately.

Cardiogenic Shock

Cardiogenic shock is caused by the failure of the heart to pump blood adequately to all of the body's vital organs. This type of shock occurs when the heart has been injured or damaged. Cardiogenic shock is most frequently seen with

MI. Other causes include dysrhythmias, severe congestive heart failure, acute valvular damage, and pulmonary embolism. When a patient develops cardiogenic shock, it is difficult to reverse and has a high fatality rate (80% to 90%).

Neurogenic Shock

Neurogenic shock occurs when the nervous system is unable to control the diameter of the blood vessels. In normal situations, the nervous system instructs the blood vessels to constrict or dilate, which controls blood pressure. In neurogenic shock, that control is lost, and the blood vessels dilate, causing the blood to pool in peripheral areas of the body away from vital organs.

This type of shock is most often seen with brain and spinal injuries. The blood vessels become dilated, and not enough blood is present in the circulatory system to fill the dilated vessels, which causes the blood pressure to drop significantly.

Anaphylactic Shock

Anaphylactic shock is a life-threatening reaction of the body to a substance to which an individual is highly allergic. Allergens that are most apt to result in anaphylaxis are drugs (e.g., penicillin), insect venoms, foods, and allergen extracts used in hyposensitization injections.

An anaphylactic reaction causes the release of large amounts of histamine, resulting in dilation of the blood vessels throughout the entire body and a decrease in blood pressure. The symptoms of anaphylactic shock begin with sneezing, hives, itching, angioedema, erythema, and disorientation and progress to difficulty in breathing, dizziness, fainting, and loss of consciousness. Medical care should be obtained immediately because most fatalities occur within the first 2 hours.

The emergency care for anaphylactic shock is the administration of epinephrine. Because time is a factor, individuals known to have a severe allergy carry an anaphylactic emergency treatment kit that contains injectable epinephrine (Figure 37-2) and oral antihistamines. With the kit, treatment for a severe allergic reaction can be started immediately.

Psychogenic Shock

Psychogenic shock is the least serious type of shock. It is caused by unpleasant physical or emotional stimuli, such as pain, fright, and the sight of blood. With psychogenic shock, sudden dilation of the blood vessels causes blood to pool in the abdomen and extremities. This temporarily deprives the brain of blood, causing a temporary loss of consciousness (fainting), usually lasting 1 to 2 minutes. In general, fainting occurs when an individual is in an upright position. Before fainting, the patient usually experiences some warning signals such as sudden lightheadedness, pallor, nausea, weakness, yawning, blurred vision, a feeling of warmth, and sweating.

An individual who is about to faint should be placed in a position that facilitates blood flow to the brain and told

Figure 37-2 Anaphylactic emergency epinephrine injector.

Figure 37-3 Prevention and treatment of fainting.

to breathe deeply. The preferred position is to move the patient into a supine position with the legs elevated approximately 12 inches and the collar and clothing loosened (Figure 37-3). This position is not always possible, such as when a patient is seated; in this case, the patient's head should be lowered between the legs (Figure 37-4). A patient who has fainted should be placed in the supine position with the legs elevated. It is recommended that a patient who has fainted should contact her or his physician for further evaluation.

BLEEDING

Bleeding, or hemorrhaging, is the escape of blood from a severed blood vessel. Bleeding can range from very minor to very serious, leading to shock and death. The amount of blood that can be lost before bleeding becomes life-threatening varies according to each individual. In general, loss of 25% to 40% of an individual's total blood volume can be fatal. This equates to approximately 2 to 4 pints of blood for the average adult.

External Bleeding

External bleeding is bleeding that can be seen coming from a wound. Common examples of external bleeding include bleeding from open fractures, lacerations, and the nose. Individuals with serious external bleeding exhibit the following symptoms: obvious bleeding, restlessness, cold and clammy skin, thirst, increased and thready pulse, rapid and

PROCEDURE 38-2

patient's signature by signing your name in the appropriate space on the form.

Principle. For information to be released, the form must be signed by the patient or patient's representative authorizing the disclosure of medical information. The signature validates the required patient consent under the Health Insurance Portability and Accountability Act (HIPAA).

5. **Procedural Step.** Provide the patient with a copy of the medical records release form for his or her files.

6. **Procedural Step.** Copy the information requested on the form or print the information from the electronic medical record (EMR). Release only the information requested. Include a copy of the completed release form with the medical information.

7. **Procedural Step.** Document what information is being released and the date of its release on the medical records release form or in a progress note in the medical record. Sign the release of information form with your name and credentials verifying you were the individual releasing the information.

8. **Procedural Step.** File the original document and the release of medical information form in the paper medical record or scan into the EMR.

Principle. Maintaining the release form provides legal documentation that the patient gave permission for the release of his or her medical information.

9. **Procedural Step.** Send the medical information to the appropriate site according to your medical office policy.

Mailed or Faxed Requests for Release of Medical Information

These steps should be followed when a completed medical records release form has been mailed or faxed to the medical office:

1. **Procedural Step.** Check the expiration date on the medical records release form. If the authorization is outdated, a new release form needs to be completed.

2. **Procedural Step.** Verify the authenticity of the signature on the form. This can be accomplished by comparing the patient's signature on the form with the patient's signature in his or her medical record. If you have any doubt as to the authenticity of the signature, do not release the records.

3. **Procedural Step.** Copy or print the information requested on the form. Release only the information requested. Include a copy of the completed release form with the medical information.

4. **Procedural Step.** Document what information is being released and the date of its release on the release of information form.

5. **Procedural Step.** File the release of medical information form or scan it and save it in the patient's medical record.

6. **Procedural Step.** Send the medical information according to your medical office policy.

CLINICAL SECTION OF THE MEDICAL RECORD

The clinical section of the medical record includes a variety of records and reports that assist the physician in the care and treatment of the patient. Common clinical records are listed and described next. Paper forms filled out by the patient or received in the mail are always filed in a patient's paper-based medical record. If there is an EMR, paper records are usually scanned into it, and the original is either shredded or retained in a patient file with other paper records.

DATABASE

Health History

A **health history** is a collection of subjective data about the patient. Most of this information is obtained by having the patient complete a preprinted form that is then reviewed for completeness by the medical assistant. Some of the

information included in the health history is obtained by the physician or medical assistant by interviewing the patient. Although not yet in widespread use, computer-guided questionnaires are available so that patients can enter their own health histories. The medical office must provide a private area for the patient to complete the questionnaire, and the medical assistant must be available to answer questions.

Along with the physical examination and laboratory and diagnostic tests, the health history is used for the following reasons: to determine the patient's general state of health, to arrive at a diagnosis and to prescribe treatment, and to document any change in a patient's illness after treatment has been instituted. The term **diagnosis** refers to the scientific method of determining and identifying a patient's condition. Before there is enough information to make a definitive diagnosis, the provider uses terms such as *medical impression, provisional diagnosis, preliminary diagnosis,* or *tentative diagnosis.*

A thorough history of personal health is obtained for each new patient, and subsequent office visits provide additional information regarding changes in the patient's condition or treatment. A complete discussion of the health history is presented later in this chapter.

Physical Examination

A **physical examination** is an assessment of each part of the patient's body. The purpose of the physical examination is to obtain objective data about the patient, which assists the physician in determining the patient's state of health. (The physical examination is described in detail in Chapter 20.)

The physician's findings from the head-to-toe assessment of each part of the patient's body are included in the paper medical record as a history and physical examination report. In the EMR, there may be a separate section to document the results of the physical examination, or it may be documented as a progress note. Each type of EMR is set up individually, and there are many methods to enter information.

Allergies

The patient usually includes all known allergies on the patient history form. For paper-based patient records, serious allergies are often noted on the chart folder using red or orange stickers. The EMR usually has an easily accessible record of patient allergies including medication, food, and environmental allergies. This is found in the database section of the record. For each allergen it is noted if the allergy is active, the reaction type, and the severity of reactions. This should be updated at every visit as needed. There may be a check-box in the EMR to indicate that the medical assistant has reviewed allergies with the patient.

One of the advantages of the EMR related to allergies is its ability to cross-check allergies with new medications that might be ordered, including immunizations. For example, if a patient has a recorded allergy to eggs, an alert will be issued if the physician orders an immunization that contains (or may contain) egg proteins. An alert is also triggered for new prescriptions if they contain medications or food products to which the patient is allergic.

Medication Record

A medication record consists of detailed information related to a patient's medications. The record usually includes one or more of the following categories: prescription medications, over-the-counter (OTC) medications, herbal and natural remedy products, immunizations, and other medications administered at the medical office. In the paper-based medical record most medical offices use separate forms to record current prescription and OTC medications and immunizations and an additional form to keep a record of medications administered to the patient at the medical office. In the EMR there will be separate screens for each of these areas depending on the type of EMR that is used. If a new medication is added, the program often has drop-down menus that facilitate this (Figure 38-6). The record of immunizations includes the name of the vaccine, type,

dose, date, provider, route and site, manufacturer and lot number, and expiration date and any reaction.

EMR software includes a prescription program, which greatly reduces the amount of time needed to prescribe and refill medication. The prescription program can print a prescription for the physician to sign, or it can transmit the prescription electronically (by e-fax or e-mail) to the patient's pharmacy. Both of these features eliminate the need of the pharmacist to decipher the physician's handwriting. If the medical office uses a paper medical record, physicians may still have the ability to send prescriptions directly to the patient's pharmacy by using a handheld device, such as a smartphone.

The EMR automatically checks any new medication against any drug allergies the patient may have. It also checks for potential interactions with other medications being taken by the patient. Once the physician has entered the prescription into the computer, the medication is recorded in the patient's medication list. The EMR usually provides access to extensive and current product information on all medications approved by the U.S. Food and Drug Administration (FDA. It may also have the capability of comparing the prescription with the formulary or list of drugs covered by the patient's insurance plan. If the prescription is not in the patient's formulary, the physician is advised of alternative drugs that are covered by the patient's insurance plan.

PROBLEM LIST

The problem list is updated at every visit so that active problems can be identified. In the EMR, it is usually possible to add the diagnosis code directly on the problem list to assist with billing. There is usually a separate screen for active and inactive problems. The problem list helps the provider organize and plan appropriate care for the patient.

PROGRESS NOTES

Progress notes update the medical record with new information each time the patient visits or telephones the medical office. With an EMR the physician or medical assistant enters this information directly into the computer using free text entry, drop-down lists, and check-boxes. Most EMR programs require a person entering data to finalize each entry. This may be done automatically when information is saved, or an additional step may be required such as checking a box or entering a digital signature (such as a password). Once the entry is finalized, it is automatically linked to a specific date and time, and it cannot be changed. (See Chapter 40 for a more complete discussion of computer features and passwords). It is important that the date and time be included with each progress note in the paper-based medical record, along with the signature and credentials of the individual making the entry. A thorough discussion of documenting progress notes is presented later in this chapter.

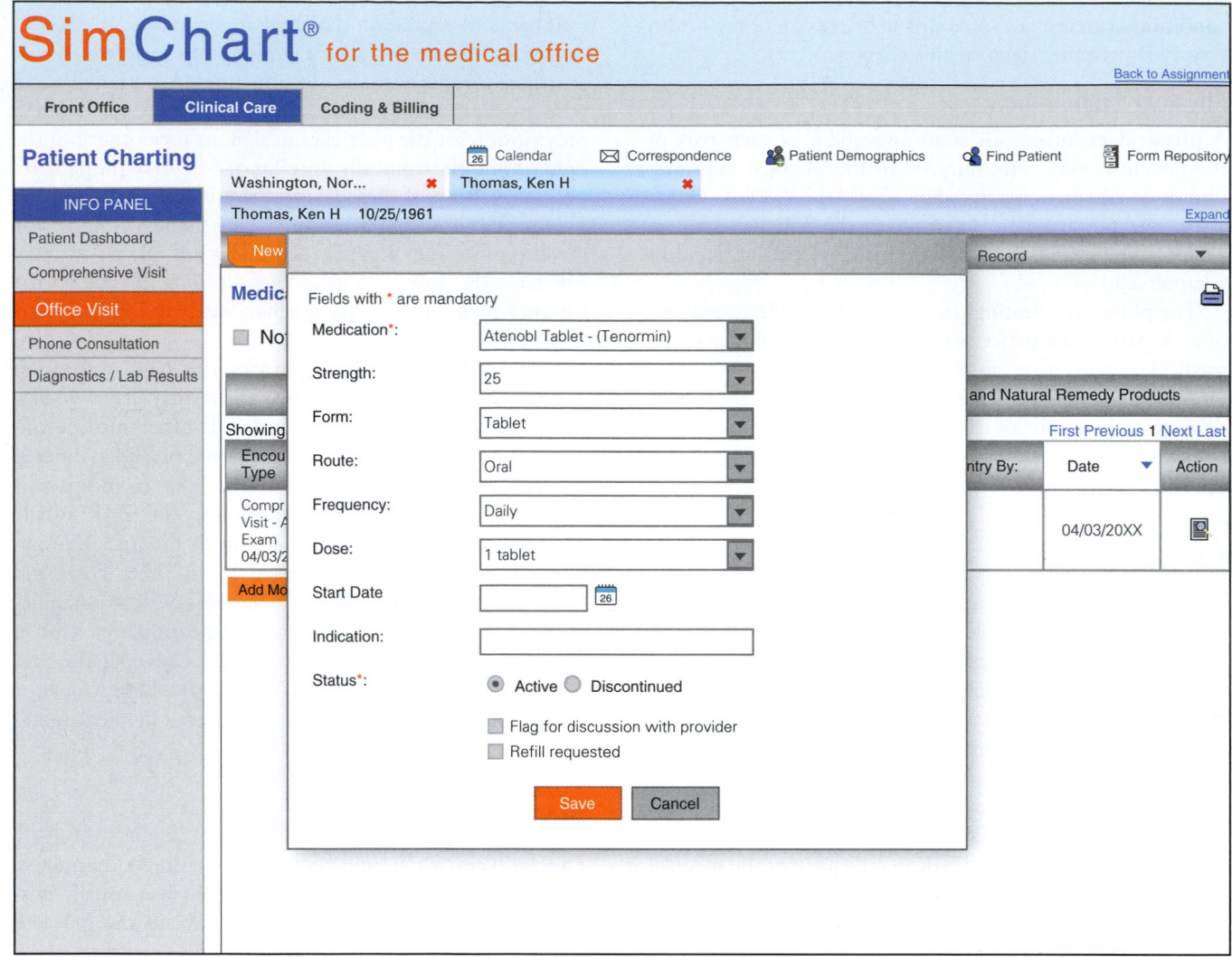

Figure 38-6 Adding a medication in SimChart® for the Medical Office.

LABORATORY DATA

In the POR, laboratory data obtained at the initial visit and the physical examination findings are considered part of the database, whereas laboratory reports related to specific problems are to be filed with other reports related to the problem. Laboratory reports are usually filed together in a paper-based medical record and accessed from one tab in an EMR. Many medical offices already communicate with outside laboratories electronically using a computer system that interfaces with the computer of the outside laboratory. This provides distinct advantages for the medical office using an EMR. Laboratory requisition forms can be completed on a request form displayed on the computer screen using fill-in boxes, drop-down lists, and check-boxes. The form can then be transmitted electronically to the medical laboratory. Once the patient's tests have been completed, the laboratory test results can be sent electronically to

patient's medical record in the medical office. At the same time, a notification that there are new laboratory data is placed in the physician's "electronic review bin" for his or her review and electronic signature. Abnormal values are highlighted on the report; for example, a high value may be highlighted in red and a low value in green. If a critical result appears on the laboratory report, an urgent message is e-mailed to the physician.

An advantage of the EMR is the ability to quickly view laboratory results in a chronological order. In addition, the results of laboratory tests performed on a routine basis (e.g., blood glucose) can usually be accessed by the computer and graphed. This permits an abnormal trend to be identified early so that appropriate action can be taken.

If the medical office is not networked through computers with an outside laboratory, the laboratory reports received by the office must either be scanned into the computer or filed in the patient's paper-based medical record.

DIAGNOSTIC PROCEDURES

A **diagnostic procedure** is a type of procedure performed to assist in the diagnosis, management, or treatment of a patient's condition. The procedure may be performed by a physician, the medical assistant, or a technician specially trained in the procedure. A physician is responsible for interpreting the results of the diagnostic procedure and completing the written report. In the paper-based medical record, a report is filed in the record with a paper copy of test results that can be printed on paper (such as electrocardiogram [ECG], spirometry results). The image of a diagnostic procedure (e.g., x-ray study, computed tomography [CT] scan, magnetic resonance imaging [MRI] scan, ECG) can be stored in the EMR as a digital image. A **digital image** is a picture that is stored electronically to allow viewing on a computer. EMR software can then display the digital image. The machine used for a procedure performed in the medical office (e.g., ECG, spirometry) must be interfaced with the office's computer system for the image to be directly transmitted to the EMR.

A diagnostic procedure report consists of a narrative description and interpretation of a diagnostic procedure. Diagnostic procedure reports completed by an outside facility may be sent electronically to the medical office.

Electrocardiogram Report

An ECG report is a narrative description of a cardiologist's interpretation of an ECG, including the implications for the patient. The graphic tracing is usually included with the report either in paper form or as a digital image.

Holter Monitor Report

A Holter monitor report is a narrative description of the interpretation of a 24- to 48-hour ambulatory ECG, including the evaluator's impressions. Portions of the graphic tracing are usually included with the report.

Spirometry Report

A spirometry report is a narrative and graphic description of the interpretation of a patient's breathing capacity as measured with a spirometer.

Radiology Report

A radiology report is a narrative description of a diagnostic or therapeutic radiologic procedure. If the procedure is done outside the medical office, a radiologist examines the radiograph and provides a written report, which includes a detailed interpretation of the radiograph and his or her impressions. If the office EMR has an interface to the facility where the study was done, the digital image will also be available in the patient's record.

Diagnostic Imaging Report

A diagnostic imaging report is a narrative description of a diagnostic imaging procedure. The report includes a detailed interpretation of the diagnostic image, along with the practitioner's impressions. Examples of common diagnostic imaging procedures include ultrasonography, CT scan, and MRI.

CONTINUITY OF CARE

Continuity of care measures are an important part of the Stage 2 Meaningful Use Measures for the EMR. Core objectives for Stage 2 include a requirement for a summary care record when patients are referred to another setting of care or provider of care. A percentage of these records must be electronically transmitted to the recipient following specified guidelines. Other data must also be transferred electronically, including immunization data to immunization registries and clinical data related to public health (e.g., reporting cancer cases to a public health central cancer registry).

Reports of services received from other providers, hospitals, home health agencies, or other health care providers may be included in a paper-based medical record or an EMR in the office of the primary care provider. This also facilitates continuity of care for the patient.

Consultation Report

A **consultation report** is a narrative report of a clinical opinion about a patient's condition by a practitioner other than the primary physician, known as a *consultant*. The consultant is usually a specialist in a certain field of medicine (e.g., cardiology, endocrinology, urology). The consultant's opinion of the patient's condition is based on a review of the patient's record and an examination of the patient. The consultation report must include the following:

- Documentation that the consultant reviewed the patient's health history
- Documentation that the consultant examined the patient
- A report of the consultant's impressions
- Any care or treatment provided by the consultant
- A report of the consultant's recommendations

Home Health Care Report

Home health care is the provision of medical and nonmedical care in a patient's home or place of residence. The purpose of home health care is to minimize the effect of disease or disability by promoting, maintaining, and restoring the patient's health. There is a growing preference for home health care over equivalent health care options. Research shows that familiar surroundings contribute positively to a patient's emotional and physical well-being.

Home health care must be ordered by the patient's physician and is provided by skilled professionals. Home health care professionals include nurses, home health aides, dietitians, physical therapists, occupational therapists, speech therapists, and social workers. Examples of specialized services available through home health care include cardiac home care, intravenous (IV) therapy, respiratory therapy, pain management, diabetes management, rehabilitation, and maternal-child care. Home health care providers must periodically provide a summary report to the patient's physician that includes the following:

- Observations and evaluations
- Type of care or service provided
- Instructions given to the patient on medications
- Safety measures recommended for the home
- Diet
- Activities permitted

Therapeutic Service Documents

A therapeutic service report documents the assessments and treatments designed to restore a patient's ability to function. Examples of therapeutic services are physical therapy, occupational therapy, and speech therapy.

Physical therapy involves the use of therapeutic exercise, thermal modalities, cold, hydrotherapy, electrical stimulation, massage, and other physical agents to restore function and promote healing after an illness or injury. A physical therapist might help a football player with a knee injury to regain normal functioning of the knee or assist a patient recovering from a stroke to use his or her legs to walk again.

Occupational therapy helps a patient learn new skills to adapt to a physically, developmentally, emotionally, or mentally disabling condition. This enables the patient to perform activities of daily living and to achieve as much independence as possible. An occupational therapist might help an individual with a physical disability learn how to get dressed and how to prepare meals.

Speech therapy refers to treatment for the correction of a speech impairment resulting from birth, disease, injury, or previous medical treatment.

Hospital Documents

Hospital documents are prepared by the physician responsible for the care of a patient while at the hospital; this physician is known as the **attending physician.** The attending physician may be the patient's regular physician or a different physician. An example of the latter is a physician attending a patient at an urgent care center or in the emergency department of a hospital.

Hospital documents are prepared by the attending physician at the hospital. The original document is filed in the patient's hospital medical record, and a copy is sent to the patient's primary care provider. Hospital documents assist the patient's physician in reviewing the patient's hospital visit and in providing follow-up care. They include a history and the physical examination findings from the inpatient stay, a discharge summary, and any operative reports. If a patient is seen at an emergency department, a copy of the emergency department report will also be sent to the patient's primary care provider.

The term **inpatient** refers to a patient who has been admitted to the hospital for at least one overnight stay. A health history must be obtained and a physical examination performed on all inpatients. There is one exception to this: If a patient history was obtained and a physical examination performed at the medical office within 1 week before

admission, a copy of these documents may be used. In the event that a reliable health history cannot be obtained from the patient, it must be obtained from the person best able to relay the facts.

An operative report must be completed for all patients who have undergone a surgical procedure. This report describes the surgical procedure and must be completed and signed by the surgeon who performed the operation. If tissue was removed for microscopic examination, a pathology report will also be generated.

The **discharge summary report** is a brief (usually one-page) summary of the significant events of a patient's hospitalization. The report must be completed and signed by the attending physician. The discharge summary report includes a concise account of the patient's illness, course of treatment, and response to treatment, as well as the condition of the patient at the time of discharge from the hospital. The purpose of this report is to document information needed by the patient's physician to provide for the continuity of future care. It also is used to respond to authorized requests for information regarding the patient's hospitalization.

The emergency department report is a record of the significant information obtained during an emergency department visit. The report is prepared and signed by the emergency department physician, and a copy is sent to the primary care provider for the purpose of providing follow-up care.

Memories *from* Practicum

Dawn Bennett: During my practicum as a medical assisting student, I was placed in a family practice clinic. I was very nervous my first day, wondering how in the world I would be able to remember everything I had learned in school. My first patients were an elderly couple. The wife was there for some test results for cancer. I looked at the results, and they were positive. After the physician relayed the results, the husband broke down. He had just lost his granddaughter after a car accident and his son-in-law to a stroke. You could tell that he just could not bear losing his wife too.

One week later, the elderly man's wife was placed in a nursing home. He came into our office for an appointment. As I was working him up, he was telling me stories about himself and his wife when they were first married. He looked so sad. I sat with him for a few minutes after completing his workup and gave his stories my full attention. As I was leaving the room, a smile came across his face, and he thanked me for listening to him. I realized that working in a physician's office is more than just knowing what I learned in school. Compassion and showing patients you really do care about them are just as important. I felt good about myself that day. ■

TAKING A HEALTH HISTORY

The health history is a collection of subjective health data obtained by interviewing. A thorough history is taken for each new patient as a baseline. Progress notes recorded at subsequent office visits provide information regarding changes in the patient's illness or treatment, but the health history is usually reviewed and updated annually. A quiet, comfortable room that allows for privacy encourages the patient to communicate honestly and openly. Showing genuine interest in and concern for the patient reduces apprehension and facilitates the collection of data.

COMPONENTS OF THE HEALTH HISTORY

The health history is taken before the physical examination is performed, providing the physician the opportunity to compare findings. The health history consists of several parts or sections.

Identification Data

The identification data section is included at the beginning of a paper health history form to obtain basic demographic data regarding the patient. The patient completes the identification data section. If the office uses an EMR, selecting the correct patient automatically links history information to the patient demographic data.

Chief Complaint

The **chief complaint** (CC) identifies the patient's reason for seeking care—that is, the symptom that is causing the patient the most trouble. The CC is used as a foundation for the more detailed information obtained for the present illness and review of systems sections of the health history. The medical assistant is usually responsible for obtaining the CC from the patient and recording it in the patient's chart. This information may be recorded on a paper form or entered directly into an EMR (Figure 38-7). Certain guidelines must be followed in obtaining and recording the CC, as follows:

- An open-ended question should be used to elicit the CC from the patient: What seems to be the problem? How can we help you today? What brings you to the doctor today?
- The CC should be limited to one or two symptoms and should refer to a specific rather than a vague symptom.
- The CC should be recorded concisely and briefly, using the patient's own words as much as possible.
- The duration of the symptom (onset) should be included in the CC.
- The medical assistant should avoid using names of diseases or diagnostic terms to record the CC.

Recording Chief Complaints

Following are correct and incorrect examples of recording chief complaints.

Correct Examples
- Burning during urination that has lasted for 2 days
- Pain in the shoulder that started 2 weeks ago
- Shortness of breath for the past month

Incorrect Examples
- Has not felt well for the past 2 weeks (This statement refers to a vague rather than a specific complaint.)
- Ear pain and fever (The duration of the symptoms is not listed.)
- Pain on urination indicative of a urinary tract infection (Names of diseases should not be used to record the chief complaint; the duration of the symptom is not listed.)

Present Illness

The present illness (PI) is an expansion of the chief complaint and includes a full description of the patient's current

Chief Complaint *:

| Dizziness when standing up X 2 weeks |

History of Present Illness

Location:	Generalized	Timing:	"It happens when I stand up"
Quality:	"I feel dizzy and weak"	Context:	"If I have been sitting or lying down"
Severity:	Moderate dizziness for a few seconds	Modifying Factors:	"It is worse if I stand up fast"
Duration:	2 weeks	Associated Signs and Symptoms:	None

Figure 38-7 Recording the chief complaint in SimChart® for the Medical Office.

illness from the time of its onset. The medical assistant is often responsible for completing this section of the health history, which is recorded on the same form as the chief complaint in the EMR (see Figure 38-7). To complete this section of the health history, the medical assistant asks the patient questions to obtain a detailed description of the symptom causing the greatest problem. The medical assistant is encouraged to use the patient's own words if possible. Much skill and practice in asking the proper questions are required to elicit detailed information.

Allergies, Current Medications, and Immunizations

The lists of allergies, current medications, and immunizations, as discussed earlier, are usually on separate screens in the EMR. The information is often collected from patients on a paper patient history form.

Past History

The past medical history is a review of the patient's past medical status (Figure 38-8, *B*). Obtaining information on past medical care assists the physician in providing optimal care for the current problem. Most medical offices ask the patient to complete this section of the health history through a checklist type of form. The medical assistant should assist the patient with this section as necessary by offering to answer any questions regarding the information required. The information may be transferred to an EMR either at the beginning of the visit or during the patient visit. The past history includes the following areas:
- Major illnesses and/or previous health problems
- Hospitalizations and operations
- Previous surgeries

Family History

The family history is a review of the health status of the patient's blood relatives (see Figure 38-8, *C*). This section of the health history focuses on diseases that tend to be familial. A **familial** disease is one that occurs in or affects blood relatives more frequently than would be expected by chance. Examples of familial diseases include hypertension, heart disease, allergies, and diabetes mellitus. The patient usually completes this section of the health history and is asked to provide the following information about each blood relative:
- State of health
- Presence of any significant disease
- If deceased, cause of death

Paternal relatives include a patient's father and his parents and/or siblings. Maternal relatives include a patient's mother and her parents and/or siblings. The patient's own siblings should also be entered. Aunts and uncles are usually entered only if they have familial or hereditary diseases.

Social History

The social history section of the health history includes information on the patient's lifestyle, such as health habits and living environment (see Figure 38-8, *D*). The social history is important because the patient's lifestyle may have an impact on his or her condition and may influence the course of treatment chosen by the physician. The social history also provides the physician with information regarding the effect that the illness may have on the patient's daily living pattern. If it is necessary for the individual to make a major lifestyle adjustment (e.g., stop smoking, reduce working hours), the physician may recommend support services to assist in this transition. This section of the history is usually completed by the patient and includes the following areas:
- Education
- Occupation (past and present)
- Living environment (including whether the patient feels safe at home)
- Diet
- Personal history
- Use of tobacco, caffeine, drugs
- Exercise

Review of Systems

A review of systems (ROS) is a systematic review of each body system to detect any symptoms that have not yet been revealed. The importance of the ROS is that it assists in identifying symptoms that might otherwise remain undetected. The physician usually completes the ROS by asking a series of detailed and direct questions related to each body system; the results of this section of the health history assist the physician in a preliminary assessment of the type and extent of physical examination required. If an EMR is being used, the information is usually entered into the computer as the questions are asked (Figure 38-9).

What Would You Do? What Would You *Not* Do?

Case Study 3

Brett Oberlin is 21 years old and lives at home. He commutes to a local college and is a junior majoring in art education. His mother and father have come to the medical office and ask to see his medical record. The physician is attending a medical conference and will not return for another 4 days. Mr. and Mrs. Oberlin found some medications in Brett's room and looked them up on the Internet. They found out that they are used to treat human immunodeficiency virus (HIV) infection. Brett would not talk to them about the medications and told them he is an adult and it is none of their business. Mr. and Mrs. Oberlin are very concerned about Brett's health and well-being. They say that because they are supporting him, they should be allowed to see his record. ∎

PATIENT HEALTH HISTORY

A

IDENTIFICATION DATA   Please print the following information.

Today's date _____

Name _____

_____ Male _____ Female

Address _____

_____ Married _____ Separated _____ Divorced _____ Widowed _____ Single

_____

Date of Birth _____

Telephone _____   _____
　　　　　　　Home number　　　　　Work number

B

PAST HISTORY

Have you ever had the following: (Circle "no" or "yes", leave blank if uncertain)

Measles _____ no yes	Heart Disease _____ no yes	Diabetes _____ no yes	Hemorrhoids _____ no yes
Mumps _____ no yes	Arthritis _____ no yes	Cancer _____ no yes	Asthma _____ no yes
Chickenpox _____ no yes	Sexually Transmitted Disease _____ no yes	Polio _____ no yes	Allergies _____ no yes
Whooping Cough _____ no yes	Anemia _____ no yes	Glaucoma _____ no yes	Eczema _____ no yes
Scarlet Fever _____ no yes	Bladder Infections _____ no yes	Hernia _____ no yes	AIDS or HIV+ _____ no yes
Diphtheria _____ no yes	Epilepsy _____ no yes	Blood or Plasma Transfusions _____ no yes	Infectious Mono _____ no yes
Pneumonia _____ no yes	Migraine Headaches _____ no yes	Back Trouble _____ no yes	Bronchitis _____ no yes
Rheumatic Fever _____ no yes	Tuberculosis _____ no yes	High Blood Pressure _____ no yes	Mitral Valve Prolapse no yes
Stroke _____ no yes	Ulcer _____ no yes	Thyroid Disease _____ no yes	Any other disease _____ no yes
Hepatitis _____ no yes	Kidney Disease _____ no yes	Bleeding Tendency _____ no yes	Please list: _____

MAJOR HOSPITALIZATIONS: If you have ever been hospitalized for any major medical illness or operation, write in your most recent hospitalizations below.

Hospitalizations	Year	Operation or illness	Name of hospital	City and state
1st Hospitalization				
2nd Hospitalization				
3rd Hospitalization				
4th Hospitalization				

TESTS AND IMMUNIZATIONS: Mark an X next to those that you have had.

Tests:

☐ TB Test
☐ Rectal/Hemoccult
☐ Sigmoidoscopy
☐ Colonoscopy

☐ Electrocardiogram
☐ Chest x-ray
☐ Mammogram
☐ Pap Test

Immunizations:

☐ Influenza
☐ Hepatitis B
☐ Tetanus
☐ MMR
☐ Polio

ALLERGIES: List all allergies (foods, drugs, environment). ☐ None

_____
_____
_____
_____

CURRENT MEDICATIONS: List the following that you are currently taking: Prescription medications, over-the-counter (OTC) medications, vitamin supplements, and herbal supplements. ☐ None

Medication	Frequency

ACCIDENTS/ INJURIES: Describe all serious accidents, severe injuries, head injury, or fractures. Include the date each occurred. ☐ None

Accident/Injury: _____   Date: _____

Figure 38-8 Health history form.

Continued

C   FAMILY HISTORY

For each member of your family, follow the purple or blue line across the page and check boxes for:
1. His or her present state of health
2. Any illnesses he or she has had

If deceased, write in age and cause of death.

	Good Health	Poor Health	Deceased	Allergies or Asthma	Diabetes	Heart Disease	Stroke	Cancer	High Blood Pressure	Glaucoma	Arthritis	Ulcer	Kidney Disease	Mental Health Problems	Alcohol/Drug Abuse	Obesity	High Cholesterol	Thyroid Disease
Father:																		
Mother:																		
Brothers/Sisters:																		

D   SOCIAL HISTORY

EDUCATION _____ High school   _____ College   _____ Postgraduate

Occupation _____ Years _____

Previous occupations _____ Years _____

_____ Years _____

Have you ever been exposed to any of the following in your environment?

☐ Excess dust (coal, lime, rock)   ☐ Cleaning fluids/solvents   ☐ Radiation   ☐ Other toxic materials

☐ Sand   ☐ Hair spray   ☐ Insecticides

☐ Chemicals   ☐ Smoke or auto exhaust fumes   ☐ Paints

Please answer the follwing questions by placing an X in the box in front of the word Yes or No, except where you are asked for specific information. This information is obviously highly confidential and will be released to other healthcare professionals or insurance carriers ONLY with your consent.

DIET:

Do you eat a good breakfast?   ☐ Yes ☐ No

Do you snack between meals (soft drinks, chips, candy bars)?   ☐ Yes ☐ No

Do you eat fresh fruits and vegetables each day?   ☐ Yes ☐ No

Do you eat whole grain breads and cereals?   ☐ Yes ☐ No

Is your diet high in fat content?   ☐ Yes ☐ No

Is your diet high in cholesterol content?   ☐ Yes ☐ No

Is your diet high in salt content?   ☐ Yes ☐ No

Are you allergic to any foods?   ☐ Yes ☐ No

How many glasses of water do you drink each day? _____

How would you describe your overall eating habits?   ☐ Excellent
☐ Good
☐ Fair
☐ Poor

PERSONAL HISTORY:

Do you find it hard to make decisions?   ☐ Yes ☐ No

Do you find it hard to concentrate or remember?   ☐ Yes ☐ No

Do you feel depressed?   ☐ Yes ☐ No

Do you have difficulty relaxing?   ☐ Yes ☐ No

Do you have a tendency to worry a lot?   ☐ Yes ☐ No

Have you gained or lost much weight recently?   ☐ Yes ☐ No

Do you lose your temper often?   ☐ Yes ☐ No

Are you disturbed by any work or family problems?   ☐ Yes ☐ No

Are you having sexual difficulties?   ☐ Yes ☐ No

Have you ever considered committing suicide?   ☐ Yes ☐ No

Have you ever desired or sought psychiatric help?   ☐ Yes ☐ No

EXERCISE:

Do you exercise on a regular basis?   ☐ Yes ☐ No

Does your job require strenuous, sustained physical work?   ☐ Yes ☐ No

SLEEP PATTERNS:

Do you seem to feel exhausted or fatigued most of the time?   ☐ Yes ☐ No

Do you have difficulty either falling asleep or staying asleep?   ☐ Yes ☐ No

USE OF TOBACCO/ALCOHOL/CAFFEINE/DRUGS: Amt:

How much do you smoke per day?   ☐ Cigarettes __

☐ Don't smoke   ☐ Cigars/pipes __

Do you take two or more alcoholic drinks per day?   ☐ Yes ☐ No

Do you drink six or more cups of coffee or tea per day?   ☐ Yes ☐ No

Are you a regular user of sleeping pills, marijuana, tranquilizers, pain killers, etc?   ☐ Yes ☐ No

Have you ever used heroin, cocaine, LSD, PCP, etc?   ☐ Yes ☐ No

List any country outside the USA you have visited in the past six months. _____

When did you have your last physical examination? _____

Figure 38-8, cont'd

Figure 38-9 Review of systems in SimChart® for the Medical Office.

DOCUMENTATION IN THE MEDICAL RECORD

Documenting is the process of making written entries about a patient in the medical record and is performed by medical office personnel who are directly involved with the health care of the patient. The medical record is considered a legal document; the information must be documented as completely and accurately as possible. Developing good documentation skills requires a thorough knowledge of the guidelines combined with much repeated practice. To provide guidance in attaining this important skill, general guidelines for documenting in both the EMR and the paper-based medical record are presented in this section, followed by specific guidelines with examples of entries documented properly.

GENERAL GUIDELINES FOR DOCUMENTATION

To ensure accurate and concise documentation, specific guidelines must be followed. These are listed and described as follows:

1. *Check the name and date of birth on the EMR or paper chart before making an entry to ensure you have the correct*

record. If the medical assistant records in the wrong patient's record by mistake, information such as a procedure that was performed on a patient may be excluded from the correct patient's record. As previously stated, from a legal standpoint, a procedure not documented was not performed.

2. *Document information accurately in a logical order, using clear and concise phrases.*
   - The medical assistant should be brief but thorough and should avoid vagueness and duplication of information.
   - It is not necessary to include the patient's name in the entry because the entire medical record centers on one patient; it is assumed the information refers to that patient.
   - Each phrase should begin with a capital letter and end with a period.
   - Standard abbreviations, medical terms, and symbols can be used to help save time and space. It is *crucial* that the medical assistant first check the office policy to determine the abbreviations, medical terms, and symbols that are commonly used in that office. Using abbreviations that can be substantiated in a medical dictionary avoids confusing others who read the record. A list of abbreviations and symbols commonly used in medical offices is presented in Table 38-1.

Table 38-1 Abbreviations and Symbols Commonly Used in the Medical Office*

Abbreviations Used to Document Symptoms and Procedures			
$\overline{aa}$	of each	H$_2$O	water
Ab	abortion	HR	heart rate
ac	before meals	HRT	hormone replacement therapy
ad lib	as desired	ht	height
AM or a.m.	before noon	ID	intradermal
amt	amount	IM	intramuscular
AP	apical pulse	IPV	inactivated polio vaccine
approx	approximately	IV	intravenous
appt	appointment	lab	laboratory
ASAP	as soon as possible	lac	laceration
BA	backache	lat	lateral
BC	birth control	lax	laxative
bid	twice a day	liq	liquid
BM	bowel movement	LMP	last menstrual period
BP	blood pressure	med, meds	medication, medications
BPM	beats per minute	min	minute
BSE	breast self-examination	MMR	measles, mumps, and rubella
$\overline{c}$	with	mod	moderate
caps	capsules	N/A	not applicable
cath	catheter, catheterize	neg	negative
CC	chief complaint	NICU	newborn intensive care unit
chemo	chemotherapy	NKA	no known allergies
CMA (AAMA)	certified medical assistant (American Association of Medical Assistants)	NKDA	no known drug allergies
c/o	complains of	noct	nocturnal
CS	cesarean section	NS	normal saline
Cx	cervix	N&V	nausea and vomiting
d	day	NVA	near visual acuity
/d	per day	OB	obstetrics
d/c	discontinue	occ	occasionally
disch	discharge	oint	ointment
DNKA	did not keep appointment	OR	operating room
DOB	date of birth	OT	occupational therapy
DRE	digital rectal examination	OTC	over-the-counter (nonprescription medication)
DTaP	diphtheria and tetanus toxoids and acellular pertussis vaccine	OV	office visit
DVA	distance visual acuity	P	pulse
ED	emergency department	Pap	Papanicolaou (Pap) test
EDD	expected date of delivery	path	pathology
Fe	iron	pc	after meals
F/U	follow-up	peds	pediatrics
Fx	fracture	per	by or through
GYN	gynecology	pharm	pharmacy
h or hr	hour	PM or p.m.	afternoon
H/A	headache	PMS	premenstrual syndrome
HBP	high blood pressure	po or PO	by mouth
Hep B	hepatitis B vaccine	pos	positive
Hg	mercury	postop	postoperative (after surgery)
		preop	preoperative (before surgery)
		prep	preparation

Table 38-1 Abbreviations and Symbols Commonly Used in the Medical Office—cont'd

prn	as needed		RLQ	right lower quadrant
PT	physical therapy, prothrombin time		RUQ	right upper quadrant
Pt or pt	patient		**Abbreviations Used to Document Measurement**	
qh	every hour		C	Celsius
q(2,3,4)h	every (2, 3, 4) hours		cm	centimeter
qid	four times a day		dL	deciliter
R	respiration		F	Fahrenheit
reg	regular		g	gram
rehab	rehabilitation		kg	kilogram
RMA	registered medical assistant		L	liter
Rx	prescription		lb	pound
$\overline{s}$	without		m	meter
S/E	side effects		mcg	microgram
SOB	shortness of breath		mg	milligram
sol	solution		mL or ml	milliliter
spec	specimen		mm	millimeter
STAT	immediately		oz	ounce
surg	surgery		pt	pint
T	temperature		qt	quart
tab, tabs	tablet, tablets		ss	one half
temp	temperature		T	tablespoon
tid	three times a day		tsp	teaspoon
TLC	total lung capacity, tender loving care		**Miscellaneous Abbreviations**	
TPR	temperature, pulse, and respiration		*Patient Examination*	
tr	trace		Dx	diagnosis
TSE	testicular self-examination		H/O	history of
VO	verbal order		H&P	history and physical
VS	vital signs		Hx	history
WNL	within normal limits		PE or Px	physical examination
WO	written order		Sx	symptoms
w/o	without		Tx	treatment
wt	weight			
Abbreviations Used to Document Body Parts and Locations			*Conditions*	
abd	abdomen		BPH	benign prostatic hyperplasia
EENT	eye, ear, nose, and throat		CA	cancer
GI	gastrointestinal		CAD	coronary artery disease
GU	genitourinary		CHF	congestive heart failure
(L) or lt	left		COPD	chronic obstructive pulmonary disease
(LA)	left arm		CRC	colorectal cancer
(LL)	left leg		CVA	cerebrovascular accident
LLQ	lower left quadrant		DM	diabetes mellitus
LRQ	lower right quadrant		DVT	deep vein thrombosis
LUQ	left upper quadrant		GC	gonorrhea
(R) or rt	right		GDM	gestational diabetes mellitus
(RA)	right arm		HTN	hypertension
(RL)	right leg		IBS	irritable bowel syndrome
			MI	myocardial infarction

Continued

Table 38-1 Abbreviations and Symbols Commonly Used in the Medical Office—cont'd

MS	multiple sclerosis		FBG	fasting blood glucose
OA	osteoarthritis		FBS	fasting blood sugar
OM	otitis media		GCT	glucose challenge test
PID	pelvic inflammatory disease		GTT	glucose tolerance test
RA	rheumatoid arthritis		Hct	hematocrit
RF	rheumatic fever		Hgb	hemoglobin
STD (STI)	sexually transmitted disease (sexually transmitted infection)		PSA	prostate-specific antigen
			PT, PT/INR	prothrombin time
TB	tuberculosis		RBC	red blood cell
URI	upper respiratory infection		RBS	random blood sugar
UTI	urinary tract infection		SG	specific gravity
			UA	urinalysis
Diagnostic Procedures			WBC	white blood cell
CT, CAT	computed axial tomography			
CXR	chest x-ray		***Symbols***	
ECG	electrocardiogram		Ø	none, no
Echo	echocardiogram		✓	check
EEG	electroencephalogram		↑	increase
FOBT	fecal occult blood test		↓	decrease
IVP	intravenous pyelogram		♀	female
LP	lumbar puncture		♂	male
MRI	magnetic resonance imaging		°	degree
NST	nonstress test		×	times
PET	positron emission tomography		p̄	after
PFT	pulmonary function test		#	number
US	ultrasound		1°	primary
			2°	secondary
Laboratory Tests			+	positive
ABG	arterial blood gas		−	negative
BG	blood glucose		Ⓡ	rectal temperature
Bx	biopsy		Ⓐ	axillary temperature
CBC	complete blood count		"	inches
C&S	culture and sensitivity		'	feet
diff	differential			
ESR	erythrocyte sedimentation rate			

*Note: This table follows The Joint Commission's list of "Do Not Use" abbreviations and symbols. The Joint Commission requirements do not currently apply to pre-programmed health information technology systems such as electronic medical records.

3. *Spell correctly.* Correct spelling is essential for accuracy in documentation. A dictionary should be consulted as needed.

4. *Document immediately after performing a procedure.* When a procedure has been performed, it should be documented without delay. The name of the provider who ordered the procedure or who is going to be cosigning the note must be included. If a time lapse occurs between performing the procedure and documenting it, the medical assistant may not remember certain aspects of the procedure, such as the results of the treatment or the patient's reaction.

5. *Procedures should never be documented in advance.* The individual performing the procedure should be the one to document it after the procedure has been completed.

DOCUMENTING IN THE PAPER-BASED MEDICAL RECORD

1. *Use black ink to make entries in the paper medical record.* Black ink must be used to provide a permanent record. In addition, entries made in black ink are easier to reproduce when a record must be duplicated for insurance company purposes and patient referral.

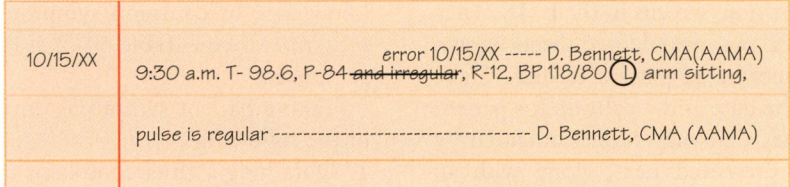

10/15/XX	error 10/15/XX ----- D. Bennett, CMA(AAMA) 9:30 a.m. T- 98.6, P-84 ~~and irregular~~, R-12, BP 118/80 Ⓛ arm sitting, pulse is regular ----------------------------------- D. Bennett, CMA (AAMA)

Figure 38-10 Correction of handwritten documentation error.

2. *Write in legible handwriting or print.* For the medical record to be meaningful to others, the medical assistant must document information legibly. If the medical assistant's cursive script is not legible, the information should be printed.

3. *Begin each new entry on a separate line but do not leave blank lines.* Each new entry should begin on a separate line and be dated with the month, day, year, and time (either AM/PM or military time). If the entire line is not needed, draw a single line through unneeded space so that nothing can be added at a later date.

4. *Each entry should be signed by the person making it.* The signature should include the medical assistant's first initial, full last name, and title (e.g., D. Bennett, CMA [AAMA]). The following title abbreviations are often used for medical assistants:
   a. *CMA (AAMA):* certified medical assistant
   b. *RMA:* registered medical assistant
   c. *MA:* medical assistant
   d. *SMA:* student medical assistant

5. *Never erase or obliterate an entry.* If an error is made in a paper record, the medical assistant must never erase or obliterate it. Should the physician or medical staff be involved in litigation, erased or obliterated entries tend to reduce credibility. If incorrect information is documented, the medical assistant should draw a single line through the incorrect information, permitting it to remain legible. The word *error* or *correction* is then written above the incorrect data, including the date and the medical assistant's first initial, last name, and credentials. If the correct information can be entered on the same line, it can be added next to the deleted entry. Otherwise it should be entered on the next blank line (not above or below the line). It is impossible to know when a correction that is not on the main line of writing was actually made (Figure 38-10).

UPDATING ALLERGIES AND MEDICATIONS

At the beginning of every office visit, the medical assistant should review a patient's allergies and current medications with a patient and record any changes. A list of current medications is often printed from the EMR, and the patient is asked to review and update the list. The medical assistant may update the list of current medications either on the paper printout or in the EMR, but in many offices the

Figure 38-11 Medical assistant documenting patient vital signs in the electronic medical record.

physician must review and approve any updates. It is important for the physician to be aware of any changes in the medications that the patient is actually taking.

DOCUMENTING ON FLOW SHEETS

Much of the documentation done by medical assistants in the EMR is done on **flow sheets,** records or computer screens that allow similar data to be recorded and viewed chronologically. These data include vital signs, growth charts, and immunization records. Complete information should be entered on these screens (Figure 38-11). For example, a drop-down box must be selected when entering a temperature to identify the method used to measure the temperature.

DOCUMENTATION IN PROGRESS NOTES

After completion of the initial health history, a system is needed to update the medical record with new information each time the patient visits the medical office. Most offices use progress notes to fulfill this function. Progress notes document the patient's health status and the care and treatment being received by the patient in chronological order. Progress notes provide effective communication among medical office personnel and serve as a legal document.

The medical assistant is frequently responsible for creating progress notes in the medical record. They are entered in SOAP format on progress note screens in the EMR. They are usually entered on special preprinted lined sheets known as *progress note sheets* in paper-based patient records. These sheets have a column for the date and a column for patient information. Types of notes that may be documented by the medical assistant are presented next, along with an example of each.

DOCUMENTING PATIENT SYMPTOMS

The medical assistant records patient symptoms during office visits and telephone conversations. Information conveyed during a telephone conversation helps the medical assistant determine whether the patient needs to be seen and the immediacy of the situation.

A **symptom** is any change in the body or its functioning that indicates the presence of disease. Symptoms can be classified as subjective or objective. A **subjective symptom** is one that is felt by the patient and cannot be observed by another person. Pain, pruritus, vertigo, and nausea are examples of subjective symptoms. An **objective symptom** is one that can be observed by another person and by the patient. Rash, coughing, and cyanosis are objective symptoms. The medical assistant should have a thorough knowledge of common symptoms and should be able to recognize them. Table 38-2 lists and describes common symptoms.

Taking patient symptoms during an office visit consists of the following:
1. Obtaining a chief complaint (see earlier discussion)
2. Obtaining additional information about the chief complaint

If the patient complains of pain in the abdomen that has lasted for 2 days (chief complaint), additional information is needed to describe the pain, including its location, quality, severity, duration, timing, and context; modifying factors; and associated signs and symptoms. The procedure for taking and recording the patient's chief complaint during an office visit is outlined in Procedure 38-3. Additional skills and practice in taking patient symptoms are included in Chapter 38 of the *Study Guide*.

OTHER ACTIVITIES THAT NEED TO BE DOCUMENTED

Procedures

The medical assistant frequently documents procedures performed on the patient, including vital signs, weight and

Table 38-2 Common Symptoms	
Symptom	**Definition**
Integumentary System	
Diaphoresis	Excessive perspiration.
Flushing	A red appearance to the skin, which typically affects the face and neck. A flushed appearance is commonly present with a fever.
Jaundice	A yellow appearance to the skin, first evident in the whites of the eyes.
Rash	An eruption on the skin.
Circulatory System	
Bradycardia	An abnormally slow pulse rate.
Dehydration	A decrease in the amount of water in the body. The patient has a flushed appearance, dry skin, and decreased output of urine.
Edema	The retention of fluid in the tissues, resulting in swelling. Skin over the area is tight. Edema is most easily observed in the extremities.
Tachycardia	An abnormally fast pulse rate.
Gastrointestinal System	
Anorexia	A loss of appetite and a lack of interest in food.
Constipation	A condition in which the stool becomes hard and dry, resulting in difficult passage from the rectum. The consistency of the stool, rather than the frequency of defecation, is used as a guide in determining the presence of constipation. (Frequency of bowel movements varies with the individual; some people have a bowel movement only every 2 to 3 days but are not constipated.) Other symptoms of constipation include headache, nausea, and general malaise.
Diarrhea	The passage of an increased number of loose, watery stools. The fecal material moves rapidly through the intestinal tract, resulting in decreased absorption by the body of water, electrolytes, and nutrients. Other symptoms usually associated with diarrhea are intestinal cramping and general weakness.
Flatulence	The presence of excessive gas in the stomach or intestines.
Nausea and vomiting	Nausea is a sensation of discomfort in the stomach with a feeling that vomiting may occur. Vomiting is the ejection of the stomach contents through the mouth, also known as *emesis*. The ejected content is known as *vomitus*.

Table 38-2   Common Symptoms—cont'd

Symptom	Definition
Respiratory System	
Cough	An involuntary and forceful exhalation of air followed by a deep inhalation. A cough may be productive (meaning a discharge is produced) or nonproductive (no discharge is present).
Cyanosis	A bluish discoloration of the skin caused by lack of oxygen.
Dyspnea	Labored or difficult breathing.
Epistaxis	Hemorrhaging from the nose (nosebleed).
Nervous System	
Chills	A feeling of coldness accompanied by shivering. In general, chills are present with a fever.
Convulsions	Involuntary contractions of the muscles.
Fever or pyrexia	A body temperature that is higher than normal.
Headache	A feeling of pain or aching in the head. It is a common symptom that accompanies many illnesses. Tension, fatigue, and eyestrain can result in a headache.
Malaise	A vague sense of body discomfort, weakness, and fatigue, often marking the onset of a disease and continuing through the course of the illness.
Pain	Irritation of pain receptors, resulting in a feeling of distress or suffering. Pain is an important indication that a part of the body is not working properly.
Pruritus	Severe itching.
Vertigo	A feeling of dizziness or lightheadedness.

PROCEDURE 38-3

PROCEDURE 38-3   Obtaining Patient History and Formulating Chief Complaint

Outcomes

1. Obtain a patient history using reflection, restatement, and clarification techniques
2. Formulate and document the patient's chief complaint and/or patient symptoms

Equipment/Supplies

- Medical record of the patient to be interviewed
- Patient history form
- Black ink pen
- Computer or laptop with access to electronic medical record (EMR)

1. **Procedural Step.** Assemble the equipment. Ensure that you have the correct patient's record in the form of either an electronic record or a paper record. If using a paper record, be sure you have a black ink pen for entering patient information. *Principle.* Black ink must be used to provide a permanent record.

2. **Procedural Step.** Escort the patient to a quiet examination room or other room. *Principle.* Information related to patient health should be taken in a room that encourages communication and maintains privacy.

3. **Procedural Step.** In a calm and friendly manner, greet the patient and introduce yourself. Identify the patient by his or her full name and date of birth. *Principle.* A warm introduction sets a positive tone for the remainder of the interview.

4. **Procedural Step.** Ask the patient to be seated. You should seat yourself so that you face the patient at a distance of 3 to 4 feet. *Principle.* This type of seating arrangement facilitates open communication and respects a patient's personal boundaries.

5. **Procedural Step.** Use effective communication skills to interact with the patient. These include the following:
   a. Use the patient's name of choice.
   b. Show genuine interest and concern for the patient.
   c. Maintain appropriate eye contact.
   d. Adjust terminology based on the patient's age, education, and English competency.
   e. Listen carefully and attentively to the patient.
   f. Pay attention to the patient's nonverbal messages.

Continued

g. Avoid judgmental comments.

h. Avoid rushing the patient.

i. Use reflection, restatement, and clarification techniques as necessary.

6. **Procedural Step.** If it is a new patient or a physical examination, record or review the following information on the patient history form (paper-based medical record) or in the EMR: past history, family history, social history, and pregnancy history (for a female patient). Be sure to include information about the use of tobacco products and smoking status. If using SimChart® for the Medical Office, fill in or review each field and save your work on each screen before progressing to the next part of the history.

    Principle: A complete medical history is obtained from a new patient and updated during the physical examination of an established patient. Smoking status is required to demonstrate meaningful use of the EMR.

7. **Procedural Step.** Ask the patient if he or she has any allergies to medications or other substances; record the patient's allergies for a new patient, or review them for an established patient and add any new allergies. If using a paper-based medical record, allergies may be recorded in red, and a sticker is usually applied to the front of the medical record that contains the name of the allergen. If using SimChart® for the Medical Office, click the *Add Allergy* button on the *Allergy* screen to add each allergy and follow directions, saving every screen as indicated.

8. **Procedural Step.** Review the patient's current medications and repeat that all prescription medications, over-the-counter medications, and vitamins or supplements should be included. If using SimChart® for the Medical Office, click the *Add Medication* button on the *Medication* screen to add each medication, saving entries as indicated.

9. **Procedural Step.** Locate the screen for chief complaint in the EMR or the progress note sheet in the paper medical record. If documenting in a paper record, write the date and time and the abbreviation for chief complaint (CC).

10. **Procedural Step.** Use an open-ended question to elicit the chief complaint, such as "What seems to be the problem?"

    Principle. An open-ended question allows the patient to verbalize freely.

11. **Procedural Step.** Document the chief complaint while following the documentation guidelines that are outlined beginning on the next page. In addition, these guidelines should be followed:

a. Limit the chief complaint to one or two symptoms, and refer to a specific rather than a vague symptom.

b. Document the chief complaint concisely and briefly, using the patient's own words as much as possible.

c. Fill in boxes.

d. Avoid using names of diseases or diagnostic terms to record the chief complaint.

Principle. Medical assistants should use correct terminology but may not use diagnostic terms in documentation.

12. **Procedural Step.** Obtain additional information regarding the chief complaint using *what, when,* and *where* questions. Fill in boxes in the EMR for location, quality, severity, duration, timing, context, modifying factors, associated signs and symptoms in the EMR or summarize this information in a paper medical record.

What Questions

- What does it feel like when the symptom occurs?
- Does the symptom occur suddenly or gradually?
- Does anything make it worse?
- What else do you experience when the symptom occurs?

Where Question

- Where is the symptom located?

When Questions

- When did the symptom first occur?
- How long does it last?
- How frequently does it occur?

Principle. This information provides a complete description of the chief complaint.

13. **Procedural Step.** Clarify as needed using reflection, restatement, or summarizing what the patient has said. Repeat in simpler language if the patient does not seem to understand you.

    Principle. Effective communication requires continuous feedback to be sure that there is mutual understanding of what is being communicated.

14. **Procedural Step.** Thank the patient and proceed to the next step in the patient workup. (This may include measuring vital signs and height and weight and preparing the patient as needed for the physical examination [see Chapters 19 and 20].)

15. **Procedural Step.** Inform the patient approximately how long he or she will have to wait for the physician.

    Principle. Patients have a right to a realistic estimate of projected waiting time.

height, visual acuity, and ear irrigations. Procedures should be documented immediately after they are performed; from a legal standpoint, a procedure that is not documented was not performed. In the EMR, procedures are usually documented as orders instead of notes. In general, the following information should be included: the type of procedure, the ordering physician, the outcome, and the patient reaction. In a paper record, the date and time should also be recorded. The specific information to be documented is included with each procedure presented in this text.

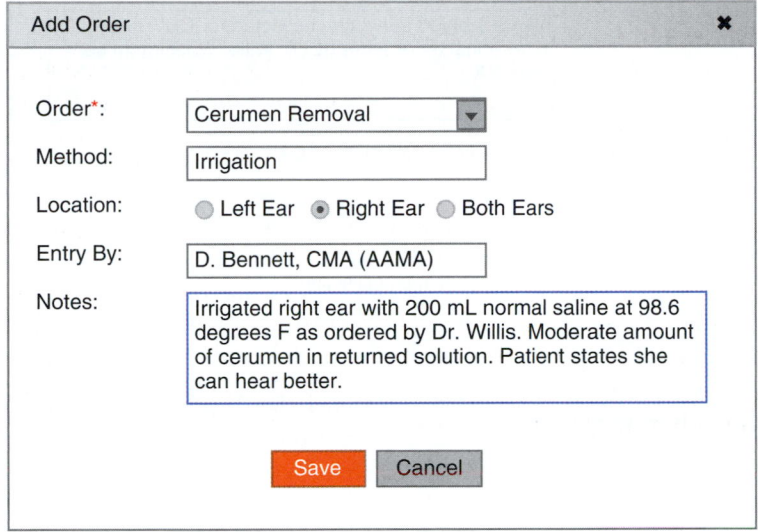

Procedure.

Administration of Medication

Documenting medications and immunizations administered to the patient is an important responsibility in the medical office. The recording should include the name of the medication, the ordering physician, the lot number (if required), the dosage given, the route of administration, the injection site used (for parenteral medication), and any significant observations or patient reactions. In a paper record, the date and time should be recorded. In an EMR, the information may be entered on a flow sheet or in a progress note depending on the type of EMR used by the medical office.

Specimen Collection

Each time a specimen is collected from a patient, the medical assistant should document the date and time of the collection, the type of specimen, and the area of the body from which the specimen was obtained. If the specimen is to be sent to an outside laboratory for testing, this information also should be recorded, including the tests requested, the ordering physician, the date the specimen was sent, and where it was sent. Thus the physician would know that the specimen was collected and sent to the laboratory when test results are not back yet.

Administration of immunization.

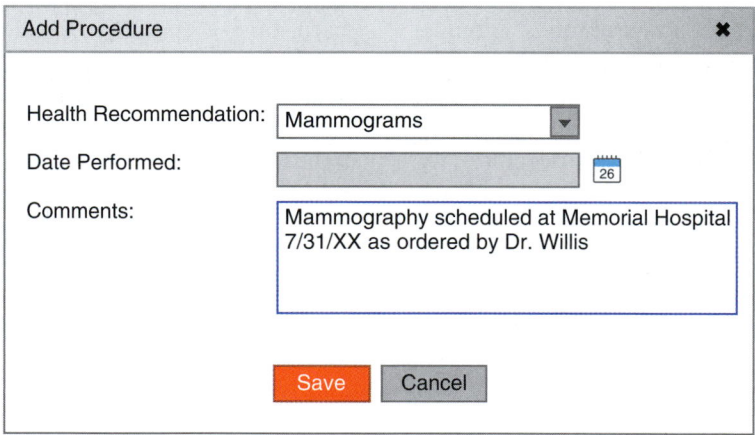

Specimen collection.

Diagnostic Procedures and Laboratory Tests

Diagnostic procedures and laboratory tests ordered for a patient should always be documented in the medical record. If the patient does not undergo the test, documented proof exists that the test was ordered. Recording that diagnostic procedures and laboratory tests were ordered protects the physician legally and refreshes the physician's memory of the procedures and tests being run on the patient when results are not yet back from the testing facility. Information to include in the entry consists of the date and time, the type of procedure or test ordered, the ordering physician, the scheduling date, and where the procedure is being performed.

Diagnostic or laboratory tests.

Results of Laboratory Tests

It is usually unnecessary to document results from laboratory reports returned from outside laboratories because the report itself is filed in the patient's record. In case of a STAT request or critical findings, the test results may be telephoned to the medical office, requiring the medical assistant to record the results on a report form. Careful recording is essential to avoid errors, which could affect the patient's diagnosis. Results of laboratory tests performed by the medical assistant in the office should be documented in the medical record. There are usually specific screens to enter test results in the EMR. The EMR identifies all entries by date, time, and person entering the information.

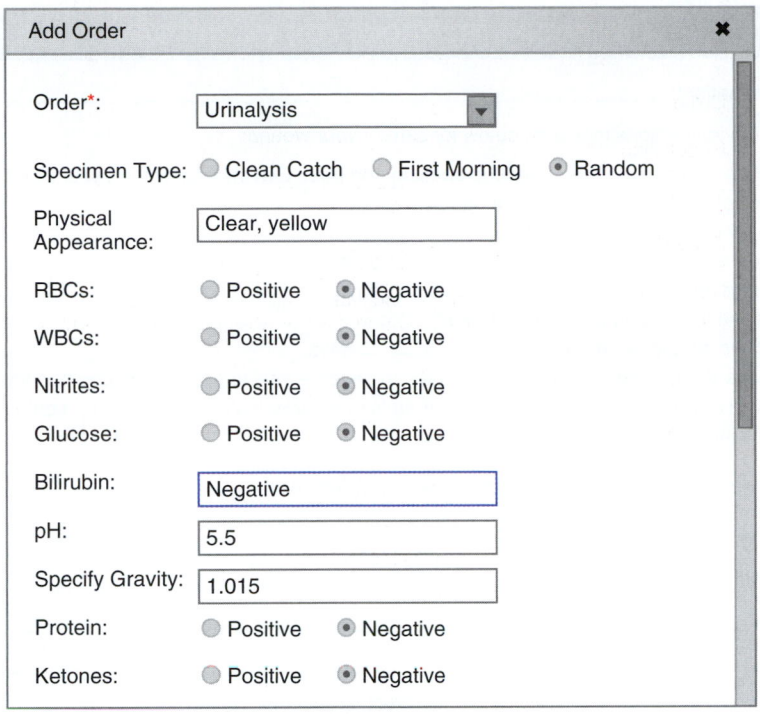

Laboratory test results.

Patient Instructions

It often is necessary to relay instructions to a patient regarding medical care (e.g., wound care, cast care, care of sutures). The medical assistant should document this information, taking care to include the date and time and the type of instructions relayed to the patient. Many medical offices have printed instruction sheets that are given to the patient. The patient may be asked to sign a form, which is filed in or scanned into the patient's record, indicating that he or she has read and understands the instructions (Figure 38-12). The form also should be signed by the medical assistant, who functions as a signature witness. This protects the physician legally in the event that the patient fails to follow the instructions and causes further harm or damage to a body part.

Other items that the medical assistant is responsible for documenting in the medical record include missed or canceled appointments, telephone calls from patients, medication refills, and changes in medication or dosage ordered by the physician. Information related to routine teaching can usually be entered on a patient instruction screen in the EMR. Information related to telephone calls from patients or medication refills can usually be entered into a message screen.

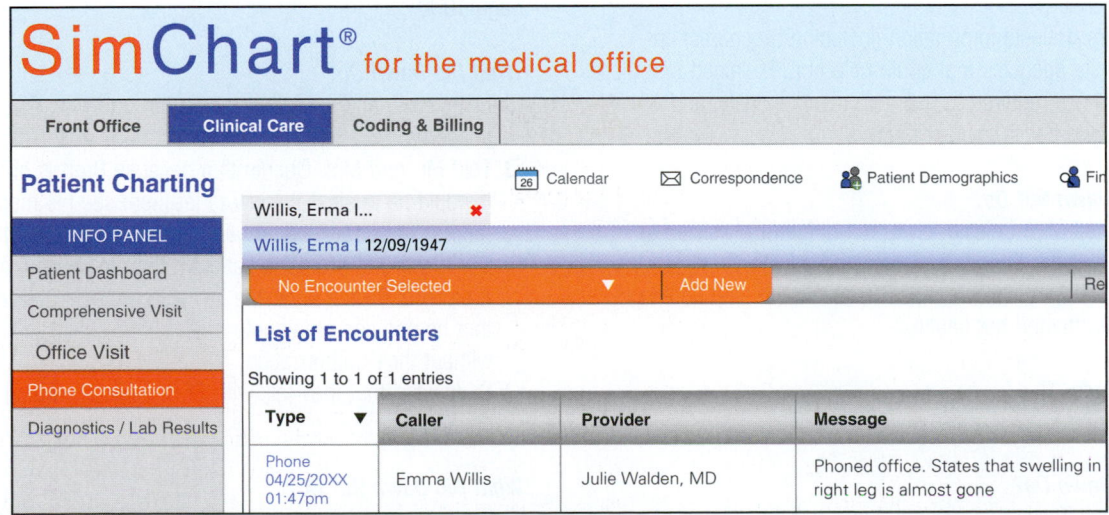

Telephone call.

PATIENT INSTRUCTIONS FOR WOUND CARE

Name of patient: _____

Follow the instructions indicated below for care of your wound:

1. Use ice bag and elevate to reduce swelling and pain. Elevate higher than your heart.
2. You may take aspirin/Tylenol for pain.
3. Keep the dressing clean and dry.
4. Replace the dressing within _____ days.
5. Discard the dressing within _____ days.
6. Cleanse the wound daily as instructed.
7. Stitches should be removed in _____ days.
8. Despite the greatest of care, any wound can become infected. If your wound becomes red or swollen, shows pus or red streaks, or feels more sore instead of less sore, contact the physician **immediately.**

I have received and understand the above instructions:

Patient (or representative): _____

Relationship to patient: _____

Witness: _____   Time and date: _____

Figure 38-12 Instruction sheet for patients.

What Would You Do? What Would You *Not* Do? RESPONSES

Case Study 1
Page 996

What Did Dawn Do?
- ❏ Listened carefully to Mrs. Celeste and relayed concern through both verbal and nonverbal behavior.
- ❏ Reassured Mrs. Celeste that her information would be kept completely confidential. Explained to Mrs. Celeste that health care professionals are required by law to keep all patient information confidential.
- ❏ Told Mrs. Celeste how important it is to record information that relates to her health. Explained that the physician must have accurate data to diagnose and treat her. Stressed that certain medications can be harmful to a patient if consumed with alcohol.
- ❏ Gave Mrs. Celeste information (including brochures) on community agencies that could help her. Explained that these agencies are required to maintain confidentiality, and encouraged her to contact them.

What Did Dawn Not *Do?*
- ❏ Did not tell Mrs. Celeste to go to a different physician to ensure that her information remained private.
- ❏ Did not tell Mrs. Celeste that she needed to stop drinking before it affected her health.

Case Study 2
Page 999

What Did Dawn Do?
- ❏ Reassured Tessa that she and her family have been good patients, and apologized for the inconvenience.

- ❏ Told Tessa that it is against the law to transfer medical records without the patient's written authorization. Explained that the reason for the law is to safeguard a patient's privacy.
- ❏ Asked Tessa if she had a fax machine because the forms could be faxed to her for signing and then faxed back to the office. If not, explained that Tessa and her husband would need to come to the office to sign release forms.

What Did Dawn Not *Do?*
- ❏ Did not get defensive about Tessa being so annoyed.
- ❏ Did not send their medical records to the new physician without the signed release forms.

Case Study 3
Page 1008

What Did Dawn Do?
- ❏ Listened to and empathized with Mr. and Mrs. Oberlin's concerns.
- ❏ Told Mr. and Mrs. Oberlin that because Brett is of adult age, it would be against the law to let them see his medical record without his written authorization. Explained that the law is there to protect a patient's right to privacy, and just as it protects Brett's right, the law also protects their right, so that no one can obtain information from their medical records without their authorization.
- ❏ Suggested that they talk with Brett again regarding the situation.

What Did Dawn Not *Do?*
- ❏ Did not give them any information from Brett's medical record.

TERMINOLOGY REVIEW

Key Term	Word Parts	Definition
Attending physician		The physician responsible for the care of a hospitalized patient.
Chief complaint		A statement of the most important symptom or symptoms for which a patient is seeking care.
Consultation report		A narrative report of an opinion about a patient's condition by a practitioner other than the attending physician.
Diagnosis	*dia-:* through, complete *-gnosis:* knowledge	The scientific method of determining and identifying a patient's condition.
Diagnostic procedure	*dia-:* through, complete *gnos/o:* knowledge *-ic:* pertaining to	A procedure performed to assist in the diagnosis, management, or treatment of a patient's condition.
Digital image		A picture that is stored electronically to allow viewing on a computer.
Discharge summary report		A brief summary of the significant events of a patient's hospitalization.
Documenting		The process of making written or electronic entries about a patient in the medical record.
Electronic medical record (EMR)		A patient health record that is stored on a computer. It may also be called an electronic health record (EHR).
Familial	*famil:* family *-al:* pertaining to	Occurring in or affecting members of a family more frequently than would be expected by chance.
Flow sheet		A paper document or electronic screen that allows similar data to be recorded and viewed chronologically.
Health history		A collection of subjective data about a patient.
Home health care		The provision of medical and nonmedical care in a patient's home or place of residence.
Inpatient		A patient who has been admitted to a hospital for at least one overnight stay.
Medical record		A written record of important information regarding a patient, including the care of that individual and the progress of the patient's condition.
Medical record format		The way a medical record is organized. The two main types of medical record formats are the source-oriented record and the problem-oriented record.
Objective symptom		A symptom that can be observed by an examiner.
Paper-based patient record		A medical record in paper form.
Physical examination		An assessment of each part of the patient's body to obtain objective data about the patient that assists the physician in determining the patient's state of health.
Problem		Any condition that requires further observation, diagnosis, management, or patient education.
Reverse chronological order		Arranging documents with the most recent document on top or in the front, which means that the oldest document is on the bottom or at the back of a section or file.
SOAP		A method of organization for recording progress notes. The SOAP note includes the following categories: subjective data, objective data, assessment, and plan.
Subjective symptom		A symptom that is felt by the patient but is not observable by an examiner.
Symptom		Any change in the body or its functioning that indicates the presence of disease.

ON THE WEB

For information on the medical record:

American Health Information Management Association: www.ahima.org

Privacy Rights Clearinghouse: www.privacyrights.org

Electronic medical Records: www.healthit.gov

For information on Medicare and Medicaid Financial Incentives and Meaningful Use:

Centers for Medicare and Medicaid Services: http://www.cms.gov/Regulations-and-Guidance/Legislation/EHRIncentive
    Programs/index.html

Patient Reception

ⓔ Check out the Evolve site at http://evolve.elsevier.com/Bonewit/today/ to access additional interactive activities and exercises to help you study and prepare for success.

LEARNING OBJECTIVES

1. Describe how to open the medical office and prepare for the day's activities.
2. Compare and contrast the tasks necessary to open and close the medical office.
3. Discuss measures to protect the confidentiality of patients in the reception areas.
4. List information that must be obtained from new patients.
5. Describe the proper procedure to check in a new or established patient.
6. Discuss procedures that are necessary to validate that a patient's insurance will pay the bill.
7. List information that must be given to a new patient about the practice.
8. Describe different types of informational materials for new and prospective patients.

PROCEDURES

Open the office.
Close the office.

Obtain new patient information.

Explain general office policies and procedures.

CHAPTER OUTLINE

INTRODUCTION TO PATIENT RECEPTION
PREPARING FOR PATIENTS
Opening the Medical Office
Checking for Messages and/or Faxes
Preparing for the Day's Activities
Making Sure Patient Charts Are Prepared
Checking the Office and Waiting Room
Checking Equipment and Supplies
Closing the Medical Office
PATIENT CHECK-IN
Maintaining Confidentiality
New Patients

Acknowledgement of Receipt of Notice of Privacy Practices
Patient History Form
Verifying Insurance and Obtaining Authorizations
Verifying a Managed Care Referral
Established Patients
Accepting Copayments
Indicating That the Patient Is in the Waiting Room
ORIENTING PATIENTS TO THE MEDICAL OFFICE
Information for New or Prospective Patients
Selecting a Physician for a New Patient
Considerations to Facilitate Patient Understanding
Patient Informational Materials

KEY TERMS

assignment (ah-SIGN-ment) of benefits
call-in times

copayment
Medicaid (MEH-dih-kayed)

tickler file

INTRODUCTION TO PATIENT RECEPTION

The medical assistant may be responsible for opening the office, preparing for patients, and processing patients as they arrive for appointments. It is important to be sure that all parts of the office are prepared for patients because there is little time to pick up or arrange facilities once patient appointments begin. There are several forms that new patients must fill out, and the patient signature must be kept on file as permission to provide treatment, bill insurance, and verify that the patient has been given an opportunity to read the office's Notice of Privacy Practices. At the end of the day, the medical assistant must prepare for the next day and close the medical office.

PREPARING FOR PATIENTS

OPENING THE MEDICAL OFFICE

Office staff need to arrive at the medical office early enough to make sure the office is prepared for the patients. The medical assistant is often responsible for opening the office (Procedure 39-1). Several activities must be performed immediately:

- Disarming the alarm system (if the office has one)
- Turning on the lights
- Unlocking the door through which patients enter
- Unlocking file cabinets, medication cabinets, and medical record files (if paper records are used)
- Turning on all of the office equipment that will be used during the day, such as computers and copy machines

Depending on the way the medical office is organized, there may be several other tasks that should be completed before the first patient arrives.

Checking for Messages and/or Faxes

Someone must review messages and prepare the telephone system for the day's activities. The telephone message must be switched from the night and weekend message to the telephone system used during the day. Usually the night and weekend message states that the office is closed, gives an emergency telephone number, and directs the caller to leave a message if the matter is not urgent. During the day, the medical assistant may answer the telephone directly or the caller may have to select an option from a menu before being connected to a member of the office staff.

If the medical office uses an answering service, the medical assistant should call the service to indicate that the office is open. The medical assistant must also obtain any messages that have come in within the past hour or nonurgent messages left during the night. For calls relating to illness, the answering service would have contacted the physician on call overnight.

After checking the message mailbox or answering machine, the medical assistant usually checks for faxes that have arrived overnight and routes the messages and faxes to the appropriate person.

A separate mailbox or answering machine may be used for prescription refill requests. If this is the case, the medical assistant should retrieve the messages from this mailbox before the physician arrives.

Preparing for the Day's Activities

It is helpful to take a minute at the beginning of the day to organize the day's tasks. This includes reviewing the appointment schedule and noting deviations from the routine schedule, such as physicians who are out of the office for all or part of the day. Reminders about the day's activities may be stored using an electronic task system and/or a physical **tickler file.** A tickler file is a set of 43 file folders, one for each month (for a total of 12 folders) and an additional set of 31 folders for the days of the current month. Written notes, bills to be paid, receipts, or other items are filed in these folders to "tickle" the memory at the time when they must be handled. (Tickler files are also discussed in Chapter 43.)

The medical assistant usually counts the cash in the cash drawer, a fixed amount of money used to make change when patients pay in cash. The cash drawer (change fund) is usually kept locked except when the medical assistant is actually sitting at the reception desk.

Making Sure Patient Charts Are Prepared

Paper-based patient records are usually pulled the evening before the next appointment day or are prepared in the morning before the patients arrive. Even if the office uses an electronic medical record (EMR), some providers will want to be able to consult a patient's old paper medical record. Paper charts must be arranged for each physician in order of the arrival of the patient. A separate appointment schedule is usually prepared for each physician. A charge slip may be created for each person before the visit, or the entire billing and charging system may be electronic. Some offices also print other sheets, for example, a list of medications for the patient to review and update.

Copies of the appointment schedule(s) are usually printed and placed at designated locations, although most medical office staff are more likely to refer to the schedule in the computer. The medical assistant usually places a schedule in each physician's office, at the reception desk, and at the medical assistant's desk. The schedule may be printed the evening before in case of a power outage or server problem, but it is usually updated with new appointments in the early morning, so a new schedule should be printed just before patients start arriving.

Paper medical records or other forms for the day are usually kept at the front desk. Some physicians prefer to have all paper medical records for their scheduled patients on their private desk when they start to see patients.

Checking the Office and Waiting Room

The waiting room, reception area, and examination and treatment rooms all need to be checked for the following: cleanliness, neatness, correct temperature, and appropriate reading material. The medical assistant should make sure that the cleaning service has cleaned all parts of the office and emptied the trash. The medical assistant may need to turn on a television, radio, and/or DVD player in the patient waiting room. Magazines should be stored neatly and replaced with current issues as needed. If there are toys in the waiting room, they should be cleaned regularly and stored neatly. Holders in the waiting room that contain information brochures for patients should be restocked and arranged neatly (Figure 39-1).

Checking Equipment and Supplies

The medical assistant should perform a visual safety check of the medical office daily. This includes removing any hazards that might block hallways or exits and making sure that all equipment is performing correctly. It is helpful to

Figure 39-1 The waiting area should be kept tidy for patients.

fill the paper trays of the copier, printer, and fax machine every morning.

The reception area and examination rooms should be tidied and restocked daily, either in the morning or at closing and sometimes again at a specified time during the day. Biohazard waste containers should be checked, and waste discarded properly if necessary. The medical assistant may need to turn on or set up equipment used for clinical procedures, run controls in the laboratory, and/or remove items from a battery charger. It may also be necessary to unload the autoclave and put away items that were sterilized the evening before.

CLOSING THE MEDICAL OFFICE

At the end of the day, the activities of the morning are reversed. Many medical offices run the autoclave in the afternoon so that items can dry thoroughly overnight. If paper-based medical records are used, they are usually prepared for new patients and removed from the files for established patients in the late afternoon because it leaves more time in the morning. Before leaving the office, the medical assistant must perform the following tasks (Procedure 39-2):

- Prepare the bank deposit and balance the cash drawer. At the end of the day, the money in the cash drawer must be balanced against cash receipts. Any amount above the usual change fund is added to the bank deposit (see Chapter 46).
- Make a backup copy of the main computer hard drive if the office does not subscribe to an online computer backup service.
- Check the fax machine for faxes that have come in during the day.
- Turn off computers, printers, copiers, and other equipment (with the exception of the fax machine).
- Change the telephone to the night message or call the answering service to tell them the office is closing.
- Lock the door through which patients enter.
- Lock file cabinets, medical record files, and medication cabinets.
- Make sure the coffee machine or other kitchen equipment is turned off.
- Unplug equipment, such as a toaster, that might be a fire hazard.
- Turn off the lights.
- The last person to leave the medical office makes sure the door is locked and sets the alarm system.

PROCEDURE 39-1   Opening the Medical Office

Outcome Open the medical office

Equipment/Supplies

- Medical office

1. **Procedural Step.** Enter the office and disarm any alarm system immediately.
2. **Procedural Step.** Turn on the lights.
3. **Procedural Step.** Adjust heat or air conditioning to a comfortable setting.
4. **Procedural Step.** Unlock the door through which patients and visitors will enter the office.
   Principle. Medical office staff usually enter the office through a different door than patients and visitors.
5. **Procedural Step.** Turn on machines that will be used all day, including computers, printers, and copier.

6. **Procedural Step.** Set the telephone system to the day setting and get messages from the electronic mailbox, telephone answering machine, or answering service.
   Principle. Callers to a business expect calls to be picked up as soon as the business opens. An important telephone message may need attention.
7. **Procedural Step.** Listen to any messages in order, writing down the pertinent information for each message on a message pad. (See Chapter 41, Procedure 41-2: Taking a Telephone Message.) Fill in the information, including the name of the caller,

Continued

PROCEDURE 39-2

PROCEDURE 39-1 Opening the Medical Office—cont'd

business affiliation (if any), date, time of the call, telephone number including area code, and information the caller wishes to leave about the reason for the call. Place your initials on the message in case there are questions. Messages may also be taken using the computer.

Principle. Complete information is necessary for the appropriate person to return the call.

8. **Procedural Step.** Arrange the messages in order of importance. Deal with any urgent calls at once, then work through other calls. Pull medical records (if paper records are used) for calls from patients and place the messages in the appropriate locations for various office staff to review.

9. **Procedural Step.** Review the day's activities and note any special tasks that must be completed that day.

10. **Procedural Step.** Count the money in the cash drawer and record the amount.

11. **Procedural Step.** Check the office for safety hazards including frayed wires, items blocking corridors or walkways, and other hazards.

12. **Procedural Step.** Straighten up the waiting room, including reading material; clean children's toys as needed; turn on radio, television, and/or DVD player; and restock patient information brochures.

13. **Procedural Step.** Print appointment lists and make sure all paper patient medical records have been pulled and arranged in order as needed. Print or stamp today's date on the progress notes and place the medical records in the designated location. If an electronic medical record system is used, be sure any necessary paperwork has been printed.

14. **Procedural Step.** If it is office policy, prepare charge slips and clip to each patient's medical record or paperwork.

15. **Procedural Step.** Check biohazard waste containers and discard properly.

16. **Procedural Step.** Check examination rooms to be sure they are clean and contain all needed supplies and equipment.

17. **Procedural Step.** Run the autoclave as needed, or empty the autoclave if it was run the evening before.

PROCEDURE 39-2 Closing the Medical Office

Outcome Close the medical office

Equipment/Supplies

• Medical office

1. **Procedural Step.** Make sure examination rooms are clean and contain all necessary supplies.

2. **Procedural Step.** Run the autoclave if needed.
   Principle. If the autoclave is run at the end of the day, supplies can dry overnight.

3. **Procedural Step.** Print a patient schedule for the next day, and pull paper medical records if needed. Print charge slips and clip to each patient's medical record if it is office policy.

4. **Procedural Step.** Make sure all cabinets or rooms containing medical records are locked.

5. **Procedural Step.** Balance the cash drawer and prepare the bank deposit. Lock the cash drawer or place the change fund in the office safe. If possible, make the bank deposit at the end of the day.
   Principle. It is best to leave as little money in the office as possible. The change fund should be kept under lock and key.

6. **Procedural Step.** Make sure the night system for the telephones is activated. Switch the message on the electronic telephone system or answering machine, and call the answering service as needed.

7. **Procedural Step.** Turn off all machines throughout the medical office that are used only during the day. Exceptions include the fax machine and telephone system. Unplug machines such as a coffee maker or toaster oven that might pose a fire hazard.
   Principle. Machines that generate heat such as coffee makers can pose a fire hazard. Unplugging these machines is also an extra reminder to make sure they do not remain on overnight.

8. **Procedural Step.** Lock the door through which patients and visitors enter the medical office.

9. **Procedural Step.** Turn the heat or air conditioning to the night setting.

10. **Procedural Step.** Turn off the lights.

11. **Procedural Step.** Arm the security system and make sure the door is securely locked as you leave the medical office.

Putting It All Into Practice

My name is Keisha White, and I work in a small office with two internists. We are the primary care providers for most of our patients. I am responsible for opening the office every day, and I usually arrive at about 8:00 AM. I leave before the office closes every day except Friday. Gerri, another medical assistant, is responsible for closing the office. We had an alarm system put in about 5 years ago, so as soon as I enter the office, I go to the keypad and enter the code so that the alarm won't go off. Then I have a look around as I turn on the lights. Sometimes the air seems a little stale, so I either open a window or turn up the air conditioning, depending on how hot it is outside. After I turn on the copier and the computers, I call the answering service to tell them that I have arrived. I take down any messages and handle them. Then I make sure the telephones are set so that patients can call. Next I turn on the lights in the patient waiting area, make sure everything is tidy, and unlock the door for patients. We like to have music in the waiting room, so I make sure there are six CDs in the player and turn it on. I usually change the selection every day because we get tired of hearing the same music all the time. We have shifted over to an electronic medical record. In the morning we print a medication list from the medical record of each scheduled patient. Once the computers are warmed up, I check the electronic calendar to see if there is anything special to do that day, and I print appointment schedules. We keep one schedule at the front desk, and I put one on each physician's desk. When patients arrive, we give them their medication list to review. Then we call the patient when the physician is ready to escort him or her to the examination room. The first appointment is scheduled for 8:30, so I really have to keep moving to be ready for the day. ∎

Figure 39-2 If an open desk is used for reception, the waiting room should be large enough to prevent other patients from overhearing the conversation at the desk.

PATIENT CHECK-IN

It is important to acknowledge each person who enters the office as soon as possible to prevent that person from feeling awkward. The medical assistant or a receptionist usually sits at the reception desk. This person should greet everyone who enters the office. If a sign-in sheet is used, it is recommended that this sign-in sheet have adhesive peel-off strips for each line so that the medical assistant can remove the patient's name immediately after check-in.

MAINTAINING CONFIDENTIALITY

Many offices have a sliding glass window. This prevents people in the waiting room from hearing telephone conversations or other discussions in the reception area. In some facilities, the medical assistant sits behind a reception desk that is recessed but open (Figure 39-2). Because patients standing near the desk can hear any conversation behind the desk, these offices usually have a separate room for scheduling appointments. When a patient is at the desk, the medical assistant should not carry on a telephone conversation with another patient. Only one patient should be at the desk or window at a time. The medical assistant can instruct other patients and/or family members to have a seat in the waiting room.

If it is necessary to discuss sensitive or personal information, the patient should be taken to a private area.

NEW PATIENTS

The office must obtain several types of information about new patients. Personal and insurance information is obtained either when the appointment is made or at the first visit. It may be obtained on a paper form, the patient may be asked to call a specific telephone number to register, or the information may be taken by a staff member at a computer. It is important to maintain patient confidentiality when discussing personal information. The information is entered into the office practice management system. It is important to remember that many office computer systems combine a practice management system (for patient demographic data, appointments, and billing) with an EMR for medical information either in one program or using two programs that interact.

The patient is usually asked to sign a statement that allows the office to release information to the insurance company for billing purposes. This consent may be part of the patient information form or may be a separate sheet. For the office to receive payments directly from the insurance company (called **assignment of benefits**), the patient must also sign a form authorizing this. The assignment of benefits statement is usually included with the consent to release information to insurance companies. The patient signature authorizes the physician or medical practice to release information to the insurance company and authorizes the insurance company to pay the medical practice directly. In addition, the patient usually agrees to be responsible for charges not covered by insurance.

If a paper form is used to obtain information it includes the following:

- Patient information (personal and demographic)
- Guarantor information (personal and employment information for the individual who will be financially responsible)
- Provider information (primary care provider and/or referring physician)
- Insurance information (insurance company, policy holder, ID number and group number for primary and any other insurance)
- Assignment of benefits consent
- Authorization to release information to insurance
- Agreement to pay costs that insurance does not cover

In addition to the new patient information form (Figure 39-3), the medical office may also use an additional form to obtain other information as needed. For example, to meet criteria for meaningful use of the EMR, an office must collect demographic data about patients related to ethnicity, race, and preferred language that may not be requested on traditional patient information forms. Until new forms are ordered, the office may collect these and other data on an additional form (Figure 39-4). Paper forms may be scanned into the office computer system to preserve the patient's signature (Figure 39-5).

> The Forms Repository in SimChart® for the Medical Office contains a Patient Information Form and Notice of Privacy Practices that can be printed for patients.

Acknowledgement of Receipt of Notice of Privacy Practices

The Health Insurance Portability and Accountability Act (HIPAA) requires that patients sign a form acknowledging that they were given the opportunity to read or were given a copy of the office Notice of Privacy Practices (Figure 39-6). The Notice of Privacy Practices itself is usually very detailed. It may be given to patients or be posted in an accessible location.

Patient History Form

Most offices also have a history form for the patient to fill out before being seen by the physician (see Chapter 38. It may be mailed to the new patient before the first appointment, or the patient may fill it out in the waiting room. The medical assistant goes over this form with the patient in the examination room to be sure that all of the relevant information has been included. Medical information should not be discussed at the front desk.

Verifying Insurance and Obtaining Authorizations

After a new patient has filled out the patient information sheet, the medical assistant should ask for his or her insurance card. After making a photocopy of both sides or scanning the card, the medical assistant stores the copy with the patient's medical record. The card verifies the information given by the patient and sometimes gives additional information needed for billing. An insurance card scanner at the front desk may be used to read both sides of the insurance card and scan it into the computer. Information from the card can be transferred to the practice management software, and an image of the card can be saved to the patient's EMR.

It may also be office policy to verify a patient's identity at every visit by asking for photo ID or two other forms of identification and retaining photocopies. Medical identity theft has become a more common problem in the past decade. It can result in incorrect information in the medical record as well as fraudulent charges to insurance companies.

Some types of insurance require authorization every time the patient visits the primary care physician. Patients with Medicaid must usually have their coverage verified and/or must receive prior authorization for each visit. **Medicaid** is an insurance program established by the federal government that pays for low-income patients' medical needs. Each state administers Medicaid independently, and the program has a different name in each state. The cost is split between the state and the federal governments. In some states, some patients on Medicaid receive new identification cards each month; in other states, patients' insurance coverage can be verified by telephone, fax, or an electronic card reader. An electronic card reader is a small machine in the physician's office that is connected via telephone to the insurance company's database and can verify insurance benefits while the patient is in the office. Many offices use a card reader that can read not only the patient's insurance card, but also several types of credit cards (Figure 39-7).

For other types of insurance, it may be necessary to call the patient's insurance company to obtain authorization for treatment (especially if the patient needs minor surgery or

REGISTRATION
(PLEASE PRINT)

Home Phone: _____   Today's Date: _____

PATIENT INFORMATION

Name _____ Soc. Sec.# _____
    Last Name   First Name   Initial

Address _____

City _____ State _____ Zip _____

Single ___ Married ___ Widowed ___ Separated ___ Divorced ___ Sex M___ F___ Age ___ Birthdate _____

Patient Employed by _____ Occupation _____

Business Address _____ Business Phone _____

By whom were you referred? _____

In case of emergency who should be notified? _____ Phone _____
    Last Name   Relationship to Patient

PRIMARY INSURANCE

Person Responsible for Account _____
    Last Name   First Name   Initial

Relation to Patient _____ Birthdate _____ Soc. Sec.# _____

Address (if different from patient's) _____ Phone _____

City _____ State _____ Zip _____

Person Responsible Employed by _____ Occupation _____

Business Address _____ Business Phone _____

Insurance Company _____

Contract # _____ Group # _____ Subscriber # _____

Name of other dependents covered under this plan _____

ADDITIONAL INSURANCE

Is patient covered by additional insurance? ___ Yes ___ No

Subscriber Name _____ Relationship to Patient _____ Birthdate _____

Address (if different from patient's) _____ Phone _____

City _____ State _____ Zip _____

Subscriber Employed by _____ Business Phone _____

Insurance Company _____

Contract # _____ Group # _____ Subscriber # _____

Name of other dependents covered under this plan _____

ASSIGNMENT AND RELEASE

I, the undersigned, certify that I (or my dependent) have insurance coverage with _____
    Name of Insurance Company(ies)
and assign directly to Dr. _____ insurance benefits, if any, otherwise payable to me for services rendered. I understand that I am financially responsible for all charges whether or not paid by insurance. I hereby authorize the doctor to release all information necessary to secure the payment of benefits. I authorize the use of this signature on all insurance submissions.

_____ _____ _____
Responsible Party Signature   Relationship   Date

ORDER# 58-8426 • © 1996 BIBBERO SYSTEMS, INC. • PETALUMA, CALIFORNIA • TO REORDER CALL TOLL FREE: (800) 242-9330

Figure 39-3 New patient information form. (Courtesy Bibbero Systems, Petaluma, Calif.)

11. Procedural Step. Transfer the information from the new patient information form to the patient's computer account, or validate that information obtained by telephone is correct.
Principle. Demographic information must be entered into the computer system for billing and appointment scheduling, in addition to the recording of health information. An electronic medical record (EMR) often includes a practice management system (patient demographic information, billing, scheduling) as well as patients' clinical information.

12. Procedural Step. Scan the new patient information form, insurance card, and other consent forms if it is office policy (usually if the office uses an EMR).
Principle. If the office stores a patient's health information electronically in addition to billing records, all new paper forms must be scanned into the computer.

INDICATING THAT THE PATIENT IS IN THE WAITING ROOM

After the patient has been checked in at the front desk, any paperwork such as a form for patients to update current medications and/or medical history may be located or printed. If paper charge slips are used, these are also printed, and they may be clipped to the patient's paper-based medical record, if that is still used. Any paperwork is placed in the designated space for patients who are ready to be seen. Most offices also automatically print patient labels for use on laboratory requisitions and specimens.

ORIENTING PATIENTS TO THE MEDICAL OFFICE

INFORMATION FOR NEW OR PROSPECTIVE PATIENTS

The medical assistant may be responsible for informing new patients and prospective patients about the medical office and its policies and procedures (Procedure 39-4). The medical assistant should be familiar with all of the following information:
- A brief description of the physicians, how long each has been in practice, each physician's credentials, and whether each physician is accepting new patients.
- Specialties of the physicians in the practice, types of patients seen, and basic philosophy of the physician(s).
- Information about languages spoken by staff, whether the physician practices alternative therapies (e.g., acupuncture), or whether the physician insists that patients stop smoking.
- Location of the main office and satellite offices, directions to each office, and a description of available parking and access to public transportation, if applicable.
- The types of insurance that the practice accepts, whether the patient's insurance will be accepted, and whether payment is required at each visit.
- How to make appointments and the policy regarding canceling appointments. Patients are normally asked to give 24 hours' notice if possible for a cancellation.
- The telephone procedure and whether the physician has **call-in times** (when the physician takes telephone calls).
- What hospital(s) each physician is affiliated with; some patients might also want to know whether the physician makes nursing home visits.
- How medication refills are handled.
- How to sign up to use an online medical record and/or appointment request system

SELECTING A PHYSICIAN FOR A NEW PATIENT

New patients are assigned to practice physicians who are accepting new patients. If there is more than one, a new patient will appreciate a brief description of each. A physician might not be accepting new patients for a few reasons:
- A physician may have so many patients that he or she cannot in all fairness accept new patients. If the patient load decreases, the physician may begin to accept new patients again.
- The physician may be returning from a maternity, family, or personal disability leave and be working a reduced schedule.
- The physician may be easing back before retiring.

The medical assistant should also be able to tell prospective patients how much time to allow for a first (new patient) visit. Most physicians see new patients only on certain days and at certain times. Medical assistants should be sure to remind new patients to bring a complete list of their medications to the initial appointment, as well as a written list of concerns.

CONSIDERATIONS TO FACILITATE PATIENT UNDERSTANDING

When coaching new or prospective patients about the medical office, the medical assistant must take into account the patient's cultural or ethnic background, the patient's developmental stage, and any communication barriers that may exist. Depending on the patient's cultural background and preferred language, it may be desirable to have a medical interpreter or translator follow up with the patient to be

What Would You Do? What Would You *Not* Do?

Case Study 3

Donna Pohl calls the office to ask about the medical practice. An acquaintance has recommended Dr. Sylvia Lawrence. She says that she prefers a female physician. She asks for information about her and her specialty. Dr. Lawrence specializes in general internal medicine. At the current time the doctor is pregnant, and her due date is 2 months away. Although Dr. Lawrence is still seeing established patients, she has instructed Keisha not to make any appointments for her with new patients for the next 4 months. The other physician in the practice, Dr. William Rudner, also specializes in general internal medicine. ∎

sure there are no unanswered questions. It may also be necessary to simplify explanations or increase the amount of information provided if the patient appears to be unfamiliar with a typical medical office. If the patient is hard of hearing, the medical assistant should speak clearly, use short sentences, and repeat as needed. At the first office visit, the medical assistant should always speak using language appropriate for the patient's developmental stage and should implement additional safety measures as needed for very young or elderly patients.

PATIENT INFORMATIONAL MATERIALS

An increasing number of practices today have a website that contains the previously mentioned information. There are also often photographs of the office and office staff. Pages on the website usually include information about the practice as well as directions to the main facility and any satellite facilities. There may be a section related to health and wellness with information about specific medical conditions, especially those related to the specialty of the practice. Maintaining the website is usually not the responsibility of the medical assistant, but he or she can remind the office administrator if certain information needs to be updated. Photographs of patients should be used only if the patient has signed a release form. The Web address of the practice website can be added to the business cards of the practice physicians.

In addition to a practice website, there is usually information about each physician available on the website of the hospital(s) where the physician has privileges as well as the website of any large group with which the medical practice is affiliated. Most of these websites have a "find a doctor" feature for all their physicians, and these usually link to an information page about each physician. These links may need updating if the physician obtains new credentials or if the physician starts or stops accepting new patients.

Patient informational booklets are another very successful marketing and public relations tool, but they must be kept up to date. A patient information booklet should include all the information for new patients that was discussed previously. Patients appreciate having something in writing to which they can refer. A patient information booklet should be given to a new patient at the first visit and should be on display for established patients to request if they want one.

PROCEDURE 39-4 Explaining Office Policies and Procedures

Outcome Coach a patient regarding office policies and procedures

Equipment/Supplies

- Patient information booklet (if available)
- Map
- List of points to cover

1. **Procedural Step.** Offer to give or send the patient a patient information booklet if one is available.
   Principle. A patient information booklet provides a handy resource to answer questions about a medical practice.
2. **Procedural Step.** Take a patient's cultural background, developmental life stage, and potential barriers to communication into consideration when coaching the patient about office policies.
3. **Procedural Step.** Identify the name, credentials, and specialties of physicians who are accepting patients in the medical office.
   Principle. Some physicians may not currently be accepting patients.

4. **Procedural Step.** Offer information as required about languages spoken by staff in the medical office and additional services or specialized complementary practices.
5. **Procedural Step.** Identify the location of the office and/or satellite offices and give directions as needed. Identify where the patient can park if necessary.
6. **Procedural Step.** Tell the patient whether the office accepts his or her medical insurance plan and discuss expectations for payment of the patient's bill.
   Principle. The patient has a right to know what his or her financial obligation will be before receiving service.

Continued

PROCEDURE **39-4** Explaining Office Policies and Procedures—cont'd

7. Procedural Step. Describe how far in advance to make appointments and the office policy on canceling appointments.
Principle. Most offices reserve the right to charge the patient if the appointment is not cancelled at least 24 hours in advance.

8. Procedural Step. Tell the patient when and how to contact the office, and notify the patient if the physician has specific call-in times (times when he or she takes telephone calls.)

9. Procedural Step. Explain how prescriptions and prescription refills are handled as needed.

10. Procedural Step. Explain and/or provide written information about how to sign up for and use any patient access to an online health record or appointment request system.

11. Procedural Step. Identify the hospital(s) with which each physician is affiliated. Answer any questions about other services (e.g., nursing home visits) that each physician may provide.

What Would You Do? | What Would You *Not* Do? | RESPONSES

Case Study 1
Page 1030

What Did Keisha Do?
❏ Checked to see if there were other patients in the waiting room. Because there were, she took Ms. Harris to a private area.
❏ Asked Ms. Harris for each piece of information on the new patient information form and filled it in for her.
❏ Read each statement at the bottom of the form out loud and showed Ms. Harris where to sign the form.
❏ Explained that Ms. Harris could read the Notice of Privacy Practices at a later time when she had her glasses, but asked her to sign the form acknowledging receipt of the Notice of Privacy Practices.

What Did Keisha Not Do?
❏ Did not tell the patient that she should have realized she might need her reading glasses.
❏ Did not tell the patient to sign any of the consents without reading them to her.
❏ Did not ask for protected health information where another patient could hear the conversation.

Case Study 2
Page 1034

What Did Keisha Do?
❏ Looked up the policy number for Mr. Ritano in the computer and handed it to him in writing so that he could write it on the form.
❏ Attempted to call the insurance company to verify his coverage.
❏ Explained that she needed to make a photocopy of his insurance card and asked him to bring it in as soon as possible.

❏ Accepted his check for $20.00 for his copayment.
❏ Explained that if it turned out that his insurance did not cover this visit or if he needed an authorization or referral, he would be responsible for paying the charges for the visit.
❏ Gave him an estimate of the cost of the visit.
❏ Allowed him to reschedule if he wanted to wait until he had his insurance card.

What Did Keisha Not Do?
❏ Did not refuse to let Mr. Ritano see the physician until he brought his insurance card.
❏ Did not make negative comments about forgetting the insurance card or imply that she does not believe he has insurance.
❏ Did not discuss his protected health information in front of other patients.
❏ Did not talk to other staff members about the forgotten insurance card unless he stated he would bring the card when she did not expect to be in the office.

Case Study 3
Page 1037

What Did Keisha Do?
❏ Explained that Dr. Sylvia Lawrence would be out on leave and could not accept appointments for 4 months.
❏ Offered to make an appointment with Dr. Lawrence after the 4-month period.
❏ Offered to make an appointment with Dr. Rudner as soon as he had one available.
❏ Listened sympathetically if Ms. Pohl was displeased about not being able to be seen more promptly by a female physician.
❏ Responded calmly and in a normal speaking voice if the patient became irritated or upset.

What Would You Do? | What Would You *Not* Do? RESPONSES—cont'd

❏ Made a recommendation about another female physician only if specifically instructed to do so by Dr. Lawrence.

What Did Keisha* Not *Do?
❏ Did not agree to make an appointment with Dr. Lawrence before the end of the 4-month period just this once.

❏ Did not become defensive or imply that Ms. Pohl's preference for a female physician is silly.
❏ Did not become irritated or upset with Ms. Pohl.
❏ Did not talk about the telephone conversation later with other office staff.

⟳ TERMINOLOGY REVIEW

Key Term	Definition
Assignment of benefits	Authorization given by the patient to allow the insurance company to make payments directly to the health care provider instead of to the patient.
Call-in times	Blocks of time when a physician accepts telephone calls from patients.
Copayment	A fixed amount of money that the patient is responsible to pay at each visit.
Medicaid	A federal and state insurance program for low-income patients. The Medicaid program has a different name in each state.
Tickler file	A chronological file containing reminders of things to be done.

ON THE WEB

For information on HIPAA:

U.S. Department of Health and Human Services, Office for Civil Rights—HIPAA: www.hhs.gov/ocr/hipaa

Sample Notice of Privacy Practices at Medicare.gov: www.medicare.gov/privacypractices.asp

40 Medical Office Computerization

Check out the Evolve site at http://evolve.elsevier.com/Bonewit/today/ to access additional interactive activities and exercises to help you study and prepare for success.

LEARNING OBJECTIVES   PROCEDURES

Computer Concepts

1. Explain the difference between data and a program.
2. Explain the purpose of each of the following parts of the data processing cycle: input, processing, and output.
3. List examples of input and output devices.
4. Explain the difference between software and hardware.
5. Explain the function of an operating system.
6. State the function of application software.
7. List common types of application software and describe how each works.
8. Describe the care and maintenance of the main computer unit.
9. Describe the function, care, maintenance, and ergonomics of the computer monitor.
10. List and describe the function of the special keys on a computer keyboard.
11. Describe the care, maintenance, and ergonomics of a computer keyboard.
12. Identify the guidelines to follow in the care and maintenance of a printer.
13. List and describe the storage devices used with microcomputer systems.

Medical Office Computerization

14. Explain why it is important to have a foundation in computer concepts before engaging in hands-on computer operations.
15. List and explain the advantages and disadvantages of medical office computerization.
16. List and describe measures that can be taken to promote the efficient running of a computerized medical office.
17. Describe the processes for obtaining information from the Internet and sharing information electronically.

Computer Maintenance and Security

18. Describe the methods used to maintain security of the medical office computer system.
19. List and describe methods used to back up computer data in the medical office.
20. State the various types of system maintenance that should be performed on a computer system.
21. List the various types of service agreements available for a computer system.

CHAPTER OUTLINE

INTRODUCTION TO MEDICAL OFFICE COMPUTERIZATION
COMPUTER CONCEPTS
DATA PROCESSING CYCLE
Input
Processing
Output
COMPONENTS OF THE COMPUTER SYSTEM
Software
System Software
Application Software

Entering Data
File Format
Documentation
Hardware
MAIN COMPUTER UNIT
Microprocessor
Main Computer Memory
Storage Capacity
Care and Maintenance of the Main Computer Unit
COMPUTER MONITOR

Types of Monitors
Monitor Ergonomics
Monitor Care and Maintenance
INPUT DEVICES
Computer Keyboard
Special Keys
Mouse
Touchscreen
Keyboard Ergonomics
Keyboard Care and Maintenance
PRINTER
Inkjet Printer
Laser Printer
Wireless Printing
Printer Care and Maintenance
STORAGE DEVICES
Hard Disk Drives
Solid State Drives
Optical Discs
USB Flash Drive
MEDICAL OFFICE COMPUTERIZATION
Prerequisite Computer Concepts
Impact of Medical Office Computerization
Advantages of Computerization
Speed and Productivity
Efficiency
Accessibility
Audit Trail
Reduced Costs
Disadvantages of Computerization
Initial Cost and Maintenance
Time Investment
Start-up Tasks

Computer System Malfunctions
Measures to Promote Efficient Computer Operation
Selection of Hardware and Software
Qualified Personnel
Proper Care and Maintenance of the Computer System
ELECTRONIC INFORMATION TRANSFER
Internet
E-Mail
Secure Messaging Within the Electronic
    Medical Record
Patient Portals
Electronic Transmission of Billing and Insurance
    Information
E-Prescribing
MEDICAL ASSISTANT'S USE OF THE ELECTRONIC
    MEDICAL RECORD
Functions Performed by the Medical Assistant
PHYSICIAN'S USE OF THE ELECTRONIC
    MEDICAL RECORD
COMPUTER NETWORK SECURITY
Authentication
Levels of Authorization
Automatic Logoff
Audit Controls
Antivirus Software
Firewall
BACKUPS
SYSTEM MAINTENANCE
Disk Cleanup
Disk Defragmentation
System Administration
SERVICE AGREEMENTS

KEY TERMS

app
application software
backup
bit
broadband
byte
cloud computing
computer
computer system
data
data processing
digital subscriber line (DSL)
documentation
e-mail
encryption
firewall
gigabyte (GB)
hard copy
hard disk drive

hardware
input
input device
Internet
kilobyte (KB)
main computer memory
medical practice management program
megabyte (MB)
microcomputer
microprocessor
network
operating system
optical disc
optical disc drive
output
output device
patient portal
printing speed
processing

program
random-access memory (RAM)
router
server
software
solid state drive
special keys
storage capacity
storage device
system software
terabyte (TB)
touchscreen
URL
USB port
user
Web browser
World Wide Web

INTRODUCTION TO MEDICAL OFFICE COMPUTERIZATION

The computer is the most frequently used piece of equipment in today's medical office. It may be used to schedule appointments, process patient statements and insurance claims, order supplies, maintain computerized medical records, prescribe medications, receive e-mail, and/or create reports, to mention only a few common functions. The medical assistant must be very familiar with the computer system used in his or her office and the programs (e.g., medical practice management program, electronic medical record [EMR] program) being run on that computer system.

This chapter presents an overview of the parts of the medical office computer system, as well as important information about maintenance and data storage.

COMPUTER CONCEPTS

A **computer** is a device consisting of electronic components that has the ability to process data according to a program to produce a desired result. The primary advantage of using a computer to perform administrative procedures in the medical office is that these tasks are performed with greater speed and accuracy than with other types of devices (e.g., typewriter, pegboard system, calculator). In addition, computers are versatile: Rather than performing only one function (e.g., typing, posting a payment, math calculations), a computer can perform many different types of tasks.

Computers are useful tools because they can perform the same tasks repeatedly while maintaining the same level of efficiency. It should always be remembered, however, that the computer does not have a mind of its own. You are always in charge, and the computer will never do anything without your direction.

Most medical offices use **microcomputers** (also known as *personal computers* or *desktop computers*) linked together to form a **network,** a collection of computers that can share data and resources (Box 40-1). The number of computers in a network varies based on the size of the medical practice and the type and number of tasks performed on the computer. For example, a two-physician medical office using a practice management program typically has four to eight networked computers. A small network is called a *local area network* (LAN). In a larger system, the computers in a medical office may be linked to a hospital and possibly other offices. LANs may be linked to form larger networks. A *wide area network* (WAN), such as the Internet, is a collection of connected LANs. Networks for large systems usually contain one or more **servers,** large computers that store data and manage tasks for the computers on the network.

Increasingly, computer networks use **cloud computing,** a model in which the Internet is used to store and access data and programs, and servers are not physically located at

---

BOX 40-1   Types of Computers

Desktop Computer
A desktop computer, so named because it can fit on and under a desk, usually consists of a plastic case containing the CPU (central processing unit), storage devices (e.g., hard disk, DVD/CD-ROM discs), other personal computer (PC) components (e.g., video card, sound card), a monitor, a keyboard, and a mouse.

Workstation
A workstation designates a desktop computer that is more powerful than a typical desktop computer and is normally devoted to one task. The term may also be used to indicate an area for a single worker in an office or laboratory setting.

Laptop Computer
A laptop computer (also called a *notebook*) usually weighs less than 5 lb and contains the processor, screen, other PC components, storage devices, and a means to input data, all contained in one portable unit.

Tablet Computer or Tablet
A tablet computer is a complete computer with a touchscreen contained in one portable unit. This may be a modified laptop that folds so that the screen faces out.

Handheld Devices
Smartphones, personal digital assistants (PDAs), and palmtop or handheld PCs are small devices with less powerful computing capabilities but greater portability than other types of computers.

---

the same site as the computer. The term *cloud* is reflected in the cloudlike symbol that is used in network diagrams around entry and exit points when the network architecture is not specifically delineated. The information being accessed is found "in the clouds," and the user can access it from many different locations.

DATA PROCESSING CYCLE

As previously described, computers function by processing data. **Data processing** is the term applied to changing raw facts or data into an organized, recognizable form. To fully comprehend data processing, it is important to have a thorough understanding of the terms *data* and *program*. **Data** is a general term used to describe the raw, unorganized facts presented to the computer for processing. Patients' names, addresses, and telephone numbers are examples of data frequently entered into the computer in the medical office.

A **program** is defined as a set of instructions organized in a logical step-by-step sequence that tells the computer how to perform a specific function. As in cooking, when a recipe is required to explain how to mix ingredients, a computer requires a program to tell it how to process data.

Computers process data in a logical three-part sequence known as the *data processing cycle* (Figure 40-1). The data processing cycle includes the following phases: input, processing, and output. Each phase of the data processing cycle involves a specific activity, which is described as follows.

The terms *input* and *output* have slightly different meanings depending on how they are used. When referring to the data processing cycle, they are used from the "computer's point of view" as verbs to describe the transfer of information. Input and output are also used as nouns to describe the data that have been entered into the computer (input) and the information that has been generated by the computer (output). As these terms appear throughout this chapter, you will become familiar with their different meanings.

INPUT

The **input** of data is the transfer of data to the computer for processing. Input includes both the entering of data into the computer and the conversion of it into an electronic form that can be understood by the computer. Because computers cannot understand the written word in the form used in communication among humans, the data must first be translated into an electronic code that can then be processed by the computer. Once the computer is finished working on the "electronic" data, the result must be converted back into a form that can be understood by the user. A **user** is defined as the individual operating the computer.

Data must be entered into the computer through an **input device** (see Figure 40-1). The most common examples of input devices are the computer keyboard and the mouse, which are usually used together. They convert data into the electronic code that can be understood and processed very quickly by the computer. Other examples of input devices include a scanner, a digital camera, and a microphone.

PROCESSING

The **processing** of data is the computer's handling and arranging of the electronic data according to a program; in other words, the data undergo some type of manipulation or change to produce useful information. Depending on the result, the processing phase may include one or more of the

following: classifying, sorting, calculating, summarizing, or listing of the data (see Figure 40-1).

OUTPUT

The final phase of the data processing sequence is the output of the processed data. **Output** is the transfer of usable information back to the user. Because the computer works with an electronic code, an output device must be used to communicate with the user. The **output device** converts the electronic code into a form that can be understood by the user. The most common output devices are the monitor and the printer (see Figure 40-1).

COMPONENTS OF THE COMPUTER SYSTEM

All of the components making up the computer are collectively known as the **computer system** (Figure 40-2). Computer systems include two major divisions: software and hardware.

SOFTWARE

Software is a general term for the programs or instructions that tell a computer what to do. Software tells the computer how to perform specific tasks in a series of step-by-step instructions organized in a logical sequence. Two categories of software exist: system software and application software. System software assists the computer in carrying out its tasks, whereas application software assists the user in carrying out his or her computer tasks. Each software category is described in more detail next.

System Software

System software is made up of a group of special programs that control or maintain the operations of a computer. The

Figure 40-1 Data processing cycle.

Figure 40-2 Computer system.

most important type of system software is the **operating system.** The operating system is installed on the hard disk of the computer and is automatically loaded into the computer's main memory (random-access memory [RAM]) when the computer is turned on. An example of an operating system frequently used in the medical office is Windows (Microsoft Corporation). The operating system performs "housekeeping" chores required by the computer system to operate itself. The most important function performed by an operating system is to serve as an intermediary to tell the hardware how to run an application program. Hence, application programs are useless without an operating system.

HIGHLIGHT on Operating Systems

Almost all of today's medical office computers run on a Windows operating system. The Windows operating system was introduced in the 1980s as a more intuitive system than the command-based interface (DOS) that had been used before. An operating system allows interactions between the computer and the user, between the computer and peripheral equipment, and between computer and computer. The interaction may occur through a direct connection, a wireless network, a telephone line, or the Internet. Each time a new operating system is developed, it allows for more complex computer system interactions.

Windows and the Mac OS are based on the concept of the graphical user interface (GUI, pronounced "gooey"). The theory behind this type of operating system is that it operates the way people think—it is intuitive. When the computer is turned on, a start screen (Windows 8) or desktop (Windows 7) appears. These are the starting place for the user to open and view programs and files, to perform operations, and to create and store files.

An individual item, such as a patient record, a daily appointment list, or a medical record, is called a *file.* A file is a set of computer data that has been saved to disk. Files are collected in folders, indicated by an icon of a file folder. Folders can be displayed individually either within a window or on the desktop. When a folder is opened, it appears as a window, and all the files that reside in the folder are in the window. Files can be moved from one folder to another, just as they might be at a desk with papers, folders, and files.

Arranged on the desktop screen in Windows 7 are icons. Icons are small graphics that provide a link to files, folders, or applications. The start screen in Windows 8 has tiles that link to programs or apps by a touch or mouse click, depending on the type of computer. An **app** is a specialized program, often small enough to run on a mobile device. Windows 8.1 Update has a tile that links to a desktop, which is often preferred when a mouse is used. ■

Application Software

Software designed to allow a user to accomplish a specific task is **application software,** also known as an *application program* or *software program.* Application software

constitutes the greatest proportion of the software available for use with a computer.

Office suites are collections of programs used to facilitate general tasks in all kinds of offices. They often contain at least four types of application programs: word processing, spreadsheets, telecommunications, and database management. More detail about these application programs is found below.

A **medical practice management program** provides instruction to the computer for performing medical practice management procedures including appointment scheduling and managing practice finances. It facilitates the day-to-day administrative operations of a medical office. It uses database capabilities to store demographic information about patients, physicians, insurance providers, and procedure and diagnosis codes. It uses spreadsheet and database capabilities to manage financial records, generate patient statements, and perform insurance billing. It also maintains the appointment schedule, which interfaces with patient information. EMRs may be linked to a medical practice management program, or practice management and word processing functions may be embedded in the EMR.

Word Processing

Word processing software allows the user to enter, edit, format, and file (store) text. Microsoft Word is an example of a commercially available word processing application program. A medical practice management program can produce letters, statements, receipts, and insurance forms using data from its database.

Spreadsheet

A spreadsheet is an electronic ledger designed to perform mathematic calculations quickly. Spreadsheet programs are used to produce financial reports and to analyze and process statistics. An example of a commercially available spreadsheet application program is Microsoft Excel. A medical practice management program or EMR can generate financial reports for the office and revise the data quickly in the same way as a spreadsheet application program.

Telecommunications

A telecommunications application provides the means for one computer to "talk" with another computer. Electronic communication between computers greatly reduces the time it takes to send information. A medical practice management program and/or EMR incorporates a telecommunications application for the electronic submission of insurance claims.

In addition, telecommunications software is used to send letters and messages as electronic mail (e-mail). A common telecommunications program is Microsoft Outlook.

Many EMRs have an internal messaging system that allows patient records to be linked with the messages. If the messages stay within the EMR, they are as secure as the EMR itself.

Database Management

Database management is the storing and retrieving of data in and from a database. Database management allows the user to store large amounts of data on a storage device (e.g., hard disk). The data can then be easily retrieved and manipulated. An example of a commercially available database management software program is Microsoft Access. The data in the database of the medical office computers can be accessed by both the medical practice management program and the EMR. Database management increases efficiency in recordkeeping and eliminates numerous time-consuming repetitive tasks. The database for a medical practice consists of patient records, patient transactions, diagnosis codes, procedure codes, insurance carriers, and so on. This information is stored on the hard disk of the computer or server for later retrieval and use as needed. A database also provides the ability to add new information, modify existing information, and delete unneeded information. The most significant aspect of a database is that the computer can cross-reference all the information stored in its database. The medical practice database can be thought of as a large pool of information that the computer can access in a multitude of ways according to the task being performed.

Entering Data

There are a variety of methods to enter data into practice management programs and/or EMRs. The user may fill in information in text boxes. Screens may be set up to select one option using a check-box or radio button. When new data, such as a new patient, new appointment, or new medication, are entered, a popup window may appear to allow entry of the information with a save button at the bottom of the window. A drop-down menu allows the user to choose one value from a list, which is usually activated by clicking on a down arrow to the right of the list. Progress notes are usually entered using free text boxes, although it is possible to set up templates with some information already filled in (Figure 40-3). As stated earlier, it is possible to dictate information for free text boxes using voice recognition software.

Voice Recognition

Voice recognition software or speech recognition software is built into Windows 7 (or higher) and many mobile devices, or a separate program may be purchased. By speaking into the microphone, the user can say commands that instruct the computer or other device what to do. It is also possible to dictate information that the computer transforms into text. The user must usually work with this feature to learn the commands and to give the computer an opportunity to learn to recognize the user's speech patterns. Many physicians now use this method to dictate progress notes and reports instead of traditional transcription.

File Format

When files are saved, the extension attached to the file name indicates the way that the information is encoded for storage. For example, if a letter is be saved as Letter1.docx,

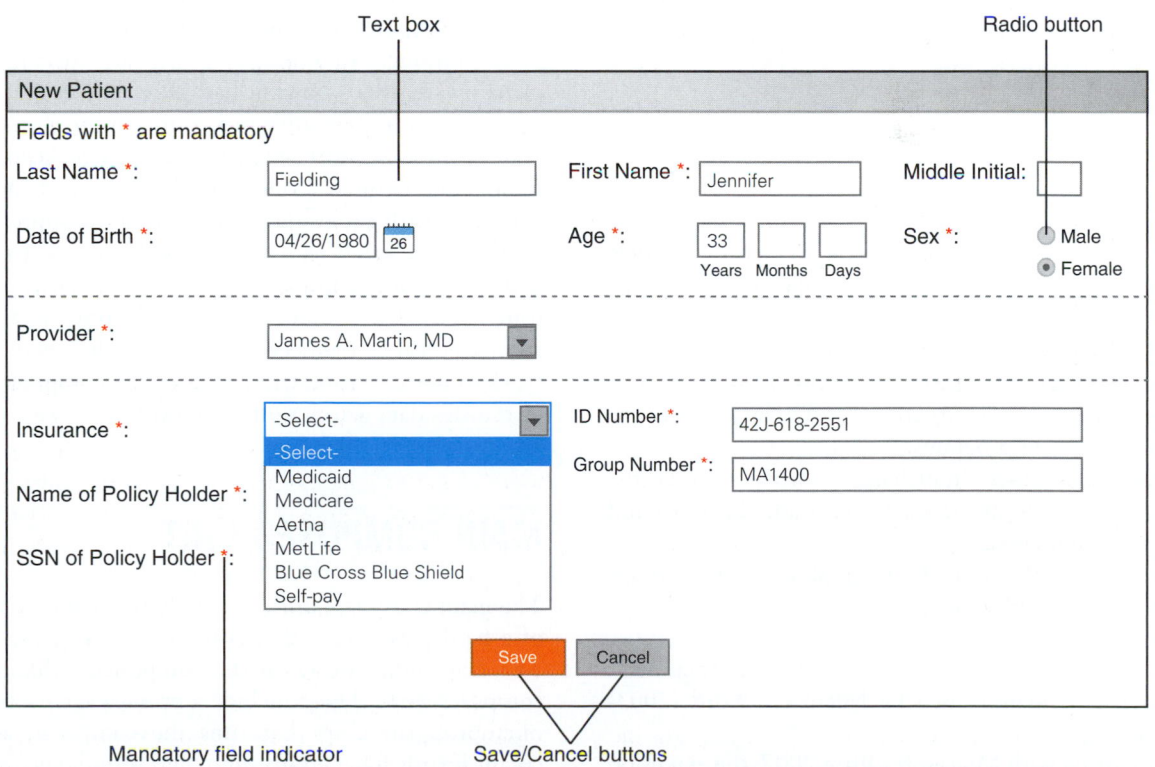

Figure 40-3 Pop-up window in SimChart® for the Medical Office.

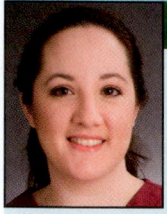

Putting It All Into Practice

My name is Emma Hayes, and I am a Certified Medical Assistant. Since I graduated, I have been working at the main office of an internal medicine practice. Our office manager is very interested in computers, and we have been using integrated practice management and EMR software for the past 2 years. When a new patient calls for an appointment, we obtain all his or her personal and insurance information and enter it into the computer during that first conversation. When patients first come to the office, we have them sit at a computer terminal in a private room next to the waiting room and enter their medical history. If the patient is not comfortable with the computer, we have the patient complete a paper form, and then I enter the data from the form into the computer. We have a scanner at the front desk to scan the patients' insurance cards and all the forms they sign at the first visit. We keep a folder for our patients with forms that they have signed, but everything is also available in electronic form.

One of the things our patients really like is that our physicians send all prescriptions to the pharmacy electronically. At the first visit, we ask patients for the name, address, and telephone number of the pharmacy they want to use. Some patients like to get their prescriptions by mail order, and we can also indicate that. I also ask the patient what medications he or she is taking and enter them into the computer. After that, the physician can go to the patient's EMR, enter the information about the medication he wants to prescribe, and automatically send the prescription directly to the patient's pharmacy. The EMR program checks for drug interactions with all the medications that the patient is taking. Our physicians believe that this saves time and is actually more accurate, because the pharmacist doesn't have to read the handwritten prescriptions. ■

docx is file extension. It is then possible to identify the type of file from the file extension. The following are a few common graphic file formats:

- bmp: BMP (Windows bitmaps) handles graphics files within the Microsoft operating system. They tend to be large files, but their structure is simple and can be handled by many programs.
- gif: GIF (Graphics Interchange Format) limits the number of colors and is used for simple diagrams and cartoon style images.
- jpg: JPG or JPEG (Joint Photographic Experts Group) is often used for photographs.
  The following are file formats:
- doc: The file extension .doc signifies a document, although it is mainly used by Microsoft Word (2003-2007 versions).
- docx: Starting with Microsoft Office 2007, the extension .docx became the file format for Microsoft Word when

Microsoft adopted file formats based on XML (Extensible Markup Language).
- rtf: The file extension .rtf (rich text format) signifies a document that can be used by many word processing programs.
- txt: The extension .txt signifies plain text that can be used by all word processing programs.
  The following are spreadsheet file formats.
- xls and xlsx: The file extension for Microsoft Excel spreadsheets was .xls until 2007 when it was changed to .xlsx.

Documentation

In the context of computer systems, **documentation** is a written set of instructions designed to assist the user in understanding how to operate an application program. Clear, concise, and easy-to-understand documentation makes it much easier to learn and use the program. Documentation includes the following: (1) the program user manual, which can usually be downloaded and printed or stored on the computer's hard drive; (2) online help screens displayed on the computer monitor; and (3) reference cards containing frequently needed details for quick reference. It is important to learn to seek out and rely on the documentation that comes with any program you are using. This results in more efficient operation of the computer system and less frustration in solving computer problems when they arise.

HARDWARE

Hardware is the term for the physical equipment making up the computer system—that is, the tangible computer parts. Although a computer system may include a variety of hardware, the following hardware devices are necessary to perform administrative procedures in the medical office: main computer unit, monitor, computer keyboard and mouse, and printer. External devices are connected to the computer with cables that attach to the computer at a specialized port (such as a printer port), a jack (usually for audio components), a USB (Universal Serial Bus) port or using a wireless connection, A **USB port** is a standard computer cable connection interface that allows several types to devices to be connected to the computer in order to transfer data across short distances.

MAIN COMPUTER UNIT

The main computer unit, or simply the main unit, consists of a hard plastic case that is usually rectangular in shape. The main unit houses all the components that make the computer work. These include a primary circuit board; the microprocessor chip that runs the computer; additional circuit boards for memory, graphics, sound, and so on; and storage devices.

MICROPROCESSOR

The **microprocessor** or central processing unit (CPU) is the functional core or "brain" of the computer and is the most complex computer component. The microprocessor is a chip that resides on the mainboard housed in the main unit of the computer. More so than any other computer component, it determines how fast a computer can process information. The speed of the microprocessor is expressed in gigahertz (abbreviated GHz); the higher the value, the faster the computer. For example, a computer with a 3-GHz microprocessor chip can process information approximately twice as fast as a computer with a 1.5-GHz chip. The power of the microprocessor is determined by the number of bits it contains. A **bit** is the smallest amount of computer storage. Modern computers usually have 32-bit or 64-bit microprocessors. Examples of manufacturers of these microprocessor chips are Intel and Advanced Micro Devices (AMD).

MAIN COMPUTER MEMORY

Main computer memory (or simply *main memory*) consists of computer chips mounted on a small board that connects to the mainboard. Main memory is responsible for temporarily storing information.

In a microcomputer, main computer memory has a special name: **random-access memory (RAM).**

It is called *random access* because the computer can get to any part of the information stored in its memory directly, rather than having to look through all the rest of the stored information.

One very important aspect of RAM is that it provides only *temporary* storage, not permanent storage. When the computer is turned off, all of the items stored in RAM are "dumped out"; in other words, RAM will be empty when the computer is turned back on and therefore ready to accept more storage items. Because of this, you *must be sure* to permanently store information that you do not want to lose before turning off the computer. In the medical office, this information is stored either on the hard disk of the computer or on the server by way of the network. Other common storage devices include Universal Serial Bus (USB) flash drives and optical disc drives, which are described later in this chapter.

Storage Capacity

Storage capacity (the amount of information that can be stored) is measured in units of storage known as **bytes.** One byte, usually 8 bits, is approximately equal to one character, such as a letter or number. Stating the capacity of RAM in bytes, however, results in astronomically high numbers. Therefore it is more convenient to use larger units, such as kilobytes, megabytes, gigabytes, and terabytes. A **kilobyte (KB)** is equal to 1024 bytes, which is usually rounded off to 1000 bytes. A **megabyte (MB)** is equal to a little more than 1 million bytes; in terms of kilobytes, 1 MB is equal to 1000 KB. An even larger measure than a megabyte is a **gigabyte (GB);** 1 GB is equal to 1 billion bytes or 1000 MB. The largest measure in current use is a **terabyte (TB)**; 1 TB is equal to 1 trillion bytes or 1000 GB. There are names for even larger units (petabyte—1000^5 bytes; exabyte—1000^6 bytes; zettabyte—1000^7 bytes), and as storage capacity increases, these units will come into more common usage.

As you would imagine, the larger the capacity of RAM, the more information it can hold at one time. For example, a computer with 2 GB of RAM has the ability to hold more than 2 billion bytes. Most microcomputers now come with a main memory of 2 GB or more.

The capacity of a computer's memory (RAM) correlates directly with the level of complexity of the programs it can run. A program takes up a certain amount of space in RAM. A small and simple application program that performs a limited number of tasks occupies much less space in RAM than a large, complex, and powerful program that performs numerous complicated tasks, such as a medical practice management program. The capacity of RAM is an important criterion to consider when working with or purchasing a computer or an application program. A computer with less than the required memory for a particular program would not have enough storage space to hold that program. Hence, that program could not be run on that particular computer. The packaging of the application program is labeled with information on *computer system requirements*. System requirements tell you what your computer system must have (e.g., type of operating system, microprocessor speed, amount of memory, hard disk space) to run the program. Storage devices are discussed later in the chapter.

CARE AND MAINTENANCE OF THE MAIN COMPUTER UNIT

The main computer unit should be placed on a flat, stable surface, such as a computer desk. This prevents excessive vibration during operation, which could loosen the electronic circuit boards. If the main unit is found in a tower, it is designed to be placed in a vertical position. Information on proper positioning is always indicated in the instruction manual accompanying the computer. Laptops should also be placed on a flat, stable surface if possible, and they should be lifted by the base, not the screen.

Computers operate best in a moderately cool temperature environment. Extreme heat and inadequate ventilation increase the chance of malfunction. As a precautionary measure, the main unit should not be placed near a window or other areas that receive direct sunlight. In addition, to prevent overheating, the ventilation slots on the main unit should not be obstructed.

A common cause of improper functioning of the computer is exposure to environmental contaminants, such as dust, dirt, and smoke. For this reason, rooms with computers should be kept clean with no smoking permitted. The casing of the main unit should be periodically wiped

45-70 cm (18-28 in.)

Shoulders relaxed

Forearms and hands in a straight line

Forearms level or tilted up slightly

Lower back supported

Thighs horizontal

Top of the screen at or slightly below eye level (You may need to adjust the height of your computer by placing something under it or by raising your work surface.)

Screen positioned to avoid reflected glare

Clearance under work surface

Feet flat on the floor

Figure 40-5 Keyboard ergonomics.

to attain the proper typing height for each individual working with the computer (Figure 40-5).

For entering data, a light touch should be used and the hands and fingers should be kept as relaxed as possible. If using a mouse, position it at the same height as the keyboard. Be sure to allow adequate workspace to use both the keyboard and mouse comfortably. These measures help to prevent strain on the wrists and hands.

An adequate working space should be available to position the material being entered into the computer. The material should be placed so that it can be viewed easily, either by positioning it lying flat on the work surface or vertically in a copy holder.

KEYBOARD CARE AND MAINTENANCE

With extended use, a residue may build up on the surface of the keyboard. This residue, often referred to as *grime,* should be cleaned with an antiseptic wipe or a slightly damp, lint-free cloth. Aerosol sprays should never be used to clean the keyboard because liquid may drip down into the keyboard, damaging its electrical components. The keyboard interior can be "dusted" by using a compressed inert gas that comes in a pressurized can and is available from computer supply stores. Alternatively, a vacuum cleaner with a small brush attachment may be used to clean the keyboard interior.

The following steps should be followed when cleaning the computer keyboard:

1. Shut down the computer.
2. Disconnect the keyboard cable.
3. Hold the keyboard upside down and shake it to remove any dust, dirt, or crumbs that may be stuck in the keyboard.
4. Clean the keyboard using a can of compressed air following the manufacturer's instructions. Use the can in an upright position. Do not tilt or shake the can.

5. Clean the top and side of the keys with an antiseptic wipe or a damp, lint-free cloth to remove grime. A cotton swab moistened with alcohol can be used to clean between the keys.
6. Allow the keyboard to dry completely (about 30 minutes) before reconnecting it to the computer.

Because of their electronic components, computer keyboards can be damaged if liquids spill into them, particularly liquids that are sweet or sticky, such as soft drinks. Therefore it is best not to place beverages close to the keyboard. If a liquid is accidentally spilled into the keyboard, the computer should immediately be turned off. If the liquid spilled is thin and clear, such as water, unplug the keyboard, turn it upside down and shake it gently to get as much liquid out as possible. Keep the keyboard inverted to allow additional liquid to drain out, and use a paper towel or cloth to wipe off the top of the keyboard. Let the keyboard dry in an inverted position for 24 hours at room temperature. If after these steps have been taken the keyboard does not work, it should be replaced. A greasy, sweet, or sticky liquid such as a soft drink spilled into the keyboard usually causes permanent damage and the keyboard must be replaced.

PRINTER

A printer is an output device capable of printing text and graphics on paper. Printers convert processed data from a combination of electronic impulses into a printed form called **hard copy.** In the medical office, a hard copy of the computer input is frequently required; examples include patient reminders, patient receipts, prescriptions, patient statements, and office reports.

Some printers can also double as fax machines and photocopiers, but this is practical only when there is a small volume of work. A printer can be dedicated to one computer or can be networked to a number of computers.

The printers most commonly used in the medical office are inkjet and laser printers.

INKJET PRINTER

An inkjet printer uses droplets of ink to form text characters and graphics. This type of printer contains nozzles that spray tiny drops of ink onto the paper to create an image. Inkjet printers are lightweight and inexpensive and can produce text and graphics in both black and white and color on a variety of paper types.

Printing speed refers to the number of pages per minute (ppm) generated by the printer. Printing speed for an inkjet printer ranges from 8 to 36 ppm. Pages that contain text print at a faster rate than pages that are in color or contain graphics.

Although the initial cost of an inkjet printer is low, operating costs are higher than those of a laser printer. The ink used by an inkjet printer is contained in cartridges, which are expensive and must be replaced frequently. Most inkjet printers have at least two ink cartridges—one containing black ink, and one or more containing colored ink.

LASER PRINTER

The most significant feature of a laser printer (Figure 40-6) is that it has a "computer of its own" to direct its functioning. Laser printers use a micro-thin beam of light (laser beam), electric charges, and a toner powder to produce each page of text. Under direction of the printer's computer, the laser beam is bounced off a series of mirrors onto a positively charged rotating drum. The pulses of the beam correspond to the characters making up the document being printed. The areas where the laser beam hits the drum become neutral, which enables the toner powder to stick to them and form characters. Finally, the characters are transferred from the rotating drum to paper with the use of pressure and heat to solidify the toner powder on the paper. This process is similar to that of a photocopy machine.

The toner powder used with a laser printer is housed in a plastic cartridge and must be replaced when it runs out. Although the initial cost of a laser printer is more than that of an inkjet printer, the operating cost is less than an inkjet's. This is because the cost per page of using toner powder (laser printer) is less than the cost per page of using ink cartridges (inkjet printer).

The print quality of laser printers is superb, nearly attaining the quality of typesetting seen in textbooks. Laser printers are available in both black-and-white and color models. Other advantages of laser printers include their fast printing speed and quiet mode of operation. The printing speed of laser printers is faster than that of inkjet printers. Depending on the model of laser printer, the printing speed ranges

Figure 40-6 Laser printer.

from 12 to 35 or more ppm. Text prints at a faster rate and color and graphics print at a slower rate. Laser printers do not have as many mechanical moving parts as other types of printers, which usually reduces their frequency of repair.

WIRELESS PRINTING

Many modern printers contain WiFi transceivers and are able to print without a cable connection from any computer connected to the network. The printer must be installed on the wireless network. Smartphones and tablets can also be connected to the network using the requested login credentials so that documents can be printed. It may be necessary to download printing apps such as AirPrint for Apple devices.

PRINTER CARE AND MAINTENANCE

Proper maintenance keeps the printer operating at its best and prolongs its life. Some general guidelines that should be followed to properly care for and maintain an inkjet and a laser printer are as follows:

1. Place the printer on a flat, stable surface.
2. Avoid placing the printer in a location that would expose it to direct sunlight, excessive heat, moisture, or dust.
3. Sufficient room should be left around the printer to allow for easy access for such tasks as adding paper and replacing ink or toner cartridges.

4. Add paper when needed, following the manufacturer's instructions. Inkjet and laser printers use individual sheets of paper stored in a tray in the printer's casing.

5. Replace ink cartridges in inkjet printers and toner cartridges in laser printers as required, following the manufacturer's instructions.

6. After turning off the printer, wait at least 5 seconds before turning it back on. Rapid switching of the power off and on can damage the printer.

7. The printer should be cleaned regularly to remove accumulated dust and dirt. The outside case should be cleaned with a soft clean cloth dampened with a mild detergent solution. Never use strong detergents or solvents on the casing because they could damage the finish. Clean the platen glass, inside of the document cover, and document feeder with a lint-free cloth moistened with water to prevent streaks. The inside of the printer should be cleaned according to the instructions in the printer's user manual.

STORAGE DEVICES

A **storage device** consists of a storage medium that permanently stores information for later retrieval by the computer. A storage device retains its information after the power has been removed and is used to store both programs and data. Examples of storage devices available for microcomputer systems include hard disks, CDs, DVDs, and USB flash drives, which are discussed on the following pages.

Storage capacity varies widely based on the type of storage device and usually is related to the cost of the device. For example, a flash drive can hold from 4 to over 100 GB, whereas the hard disk drive of a new computer often has a storage capacity of 500 GB to 1 TB.

HARD DISK DRIVES

A **hard disk drive** is a storage device consisting of one or more rigid, nonflexible platters coated with a magnetically sensitive material and encased in a permanently sealed, airtight container (Figure 40-7). The composition of a hard

Read/write head

Hard disk platters

Figure 40-7 Hard disk drive.

disk is designed to maximize its important functions: the storage and retrieval of information. To accommodate the storage of information, hard disks are coated with a magnetically sensitive material. Data are stored on the disk as magnetic particles.

The hard disk drive rotates a hard disk at a high rate of speed. A read/write head mounted on an arm floats on a layer of air above the spinning disk and has instant access to all the tracks and sectors on the disk. Desktop computers have an internal hard disk drive, meaning it is located inside the main computer unit. Portable hard disk drives can be attached to the computer using a USB port for additional data storage or backups. Because a hard disk is very sensitive to dirt, dust, and smoke, the entire disk unit is encased in a permanently sealed, airtight container to protect it from these contaminants. The entire disk unit (consisting of the hard disks and read/write heads) makes up the hard disk drive.

SOLID STATE DRIVES

Solid state drives use integrated circuit assemblies to store data permanently, and they have no actual "disks" or motors. They usually use nonvolatile semiconductor-based integrated circuits (flash memory) on a memory chip to store information. Although solid state drives are more expensive than hard disks, they are faster and more durable. They are commonly found in laptop computers and tablets as well as other portable devices.

OPTICAL DISCS

Optical discs are storage devices that store data using laser technology. They have replaced floppy disks, which were once commonly used storage devices for microcomputers. Optical discs are used to store system software, application software, data, photographs, music, and movies. An optical disc consists of a flat, round portable disc made of metal, plastic, and lacquer. It is usually $4\frac{3}{4}$ inches in diameter and less than $\frac{1}{20}$ inch thick.

An optical disc may be *read only*, which means that data can only be read (retrieved) from the disc; data cannot be written (saved) on the disc. An example of a read-only disc is a CD-ROM. The data on a CD-ROM are stored as microscopic pits along a spiral groove that runs along the surface of the disc. Data are read from a CD-ROM with a beam of laser light known as a *laser diode*.

Application software may come on a CD-ROM, and it is installed onto a computer's hard drive to operate. CD-ROMs hold about 650 MB of information. Sometimes the CD must be in the CD-ROM optical disc drive for the program to be successfully run.

Optical discs may also be *read/write*, which means that data can be read from the disc and written onto the disc. Writing on an optical disc is often termed *burning* a disc. An example of a read/write disc is a CD-RW (compact disc rewritable).

A DVD (digital versatile disc or digital video disc) uses another type of optical disc technology. This type of disc can hold about six times as much information as a CD-ROM, and therefore it has become popular as a means of storing music and movies, both of which require large amounts of storage space.

An **optical disc drive** uses a laser to read an optical disc or write onto an optical disc. Today's computers usually include one or more optical disc drives that can read and write both CD-ROM discs and DVD discs. The optical disc drives are installed in drive bays on the main computer unit. For an optical disc drive to be used, a button is pushed to slide out a tray; the optical disc is then inserted into the tray (label-side up), and the same button is pushed to close the tray.

USB FLASH DRIVE

A USB flash drive is a portable storage device that consists of a small circuit board in a plastic case. Other terms for a flash drive include a *jump drive* and a *thumb drive* (Figure 40-8). It is called a flash drive because it uses flash memory. For a flash drive to be used, it must be inserted into a USB port on the main unit. A USB flash drive has a storage capacity that usually ranges from 4 GB to 100 GB, although some flash drives have considerably more memory.

MEDICAL OFFICE COMPUTERIZATION

Medical office computerization is the use of the computer to perform medical office administrative procedures. With the advent of the microcomputer, medical offices now use computers to perform administrative procedures that were previously performed manually. This, in turn, has increased the demand for qualified individuals trained in medical office computerization, not only to perform the administrative tasks on the computer, but also to instruct other staff members in computer operations.

PREREQUISITE COMPUTER CONCEPTS

Before beginning to work with medical practice management software and/or an EMR, it is important to first acquire a thorough knowledge of computer concepts. Just as medical terminology is a necessary prerequisite to clinical procedure courses, knowledge of computer concepts is necessary to effectively operate a computer system in the front office.

The benefits of understanding computer concepts include increased confidence and ease when working on the computer and the ability to understand the computer terminology presented in the program user manual. Furthermore, a computer concepts base facilitates communication with computer software specialists, such as the technical support staff for the medical practice management program. Working with technical support is often necessary when first learning a new program or when a problem occurs. To build this foundation, the beginning of this chapter provides a presentation of computer concepts.

IMPACT OF MEDICAL OFFICE COMPUTERIZATION

Almost all medical offices use computers to perform at least some functions. Although there are distinct advantages to using a computer, it should be realized that there are also some disadvantages that can lead to difficulties. It is important to be aware of these problem areas so that steps can be taken to either prevent them altogether or be better prepared for them if they occur. Adequate preparation will result in the least amount of disruption to the efficient running of a computerized front office. The following discussion outlines both advantages and disadvantages of medical management computerization.

Figure 40-8 Flash drive.

What Would You Do? | What Would You *Not* Do?

Case Study 1

Olivia Young has moved to the community and has come to the medical office for a new patient appointment for her chronic asthma. Olivia is leaving the office and is quite upset. She says that she doesn't like having computers in the examining rooms—that it's not natural. She feels like the physician and medical assistant are ignoring her and interacting more with the computer than with her. Olivia says it's like there's a barrier between her and the doctor. She says that the medical office she used to go to didn't have computers in the examination rooms and the doctor really paid attention to her and listened to what she had to say. She says she's thinking of looking for another doctor so that she doesn't have to play second fiddle to a computer. ■

ADVANTAGES OF COMPUTERIZATION

The advantages of computerizing the front office include the following.

Speed and Productivity

One of the principal advantages of a computer is that it can process a large amount of data quickly. For example, if a physician requests a list of all patients with a diagnosis of hypertension, accomplishing this task by hand would require considerable time and effort. However, with a computer an inquiry search can be performed in which the computer searches all the patient files and automatically generates a list of patients with hypertension. Billing and health insurance requirements have placed a tremendous burden on the medical office of today. In addition, the completion of insurance claims becomes ever more complicated. Therefore a large portion of front office responsibility is often devoted to preparing and submitting patient statements and insurance claims. Because they can prepare and process items in a short period of time, computers provide much assistance in this area. In addition, faster computer processing of data related to overdue accounts often leads to better collections for the medical office.

Efficiency

Computers are particularly good at performing repetitive tasks in which information is used over and over again but in a different format. For example, once a patient's name and address have been entered into the computer's database, they can be used on a number of different forms without the need to reenter them. The computer automatically transfers this information where needed, based on the task being performed. The patient's name and address can be automatically transferred by the computer to a patient statement, insurance form, and mailing label depending on the task being performed. Medical practice management programs also keep track of the status of functions that have been executed in the office, such as the submission of insurance claims.

Accessibility

Information that has been entered into the computer system is easy to retrieve when needed. For example, after a patient registration record has been entered, it is quite simple to request information about that patient and have it instantly displayed on the screen of the monitor. This avoids having to perform the much more time-consuming task of manually hunting through a file storage system to locate the patient's chart.

Audit Trail

The computer can keep track of data entry. When new information is entered or existing information is changed, a log is created to record the time and date of the entry, as well as the name of the computer operator. This log is stored and can be retrieved by the practice manager to detect irregularities. If an error was made, the program lists the name of the operator and the date the information was entered.

Reduced Costs

After the initial cost of purchasing the hardware and software, computerization of the front office helps to decrease operating costs by reducing the amount of time required to perform front office procedures.

DISADVANTAGES OF COMPUTERIZATION

The disadvantages presented by computers in the medical office include the following.

Initial Cost and Maintenance

The combined expense of initially purchasing hardware and software can easily amount to thousands of dollars. In addition, an office must periodically upgrade its computer system and software or even purchase an entirely new system altogether, leading to further expenses.

Time Investment

Because medical management programs perform highly sophisticated tasks, it takes considerable time to learn a program and use it with ease. Most software vendors provide on-site training of staff for a newly purchased program, as well as technical support when problems are encountered with the program. Even with all of this assistance, however, learning a medical management program, an electronic record program, or even an updated version of either can easily take a month or more. During this time, the medical assistant may experience much frustration when difficulty is encountered in executing a task. However, once the initial training period has been completed, most individuals agree that the time and patience expended are worth the outcome.

Start-up Tasks

Certain tasks must be performed before a medical practice management program or EMR becomes operational—in other words, before a new program can be used in its intended manner. Examples of start-up tasks include (1) entering background information that the program will use, such as diagnosis and procedure codes or customized menus, and (2) entering patient information such as demographic information and/or health history. In implementing an EMR, a decision must be made about how much of the old medical record to enter into the new electronic record. The start-up data need to be entered only once. Later, additional information can be added as needed, and the length of input time is greatly diminished.

COMPUTER SYSTEM MALFUNCTIONS

Even the best hardware and software systems can and will occasionally fail, and one or more of the front office procedures will come to an abrupt halt. Some problems have no explanations, whereas others are directly related to a specific event, such as operator error, a software bug, or a hardware malfunction. To minimize computer downtime, most medical offices are connected to some kind of network or server that stores information and provides backup systems.

MEASURES TO PROMOTE EFFICIENT COMPUTER OPERATION

The challenges presented by computerizing the front office can for the most part be overcome by implementing the following preventative measures. These measures work to reduce computer frustration and promote the efficient running of a computerized medical office.

Selection of Hardware and Software

Hardware and software should be selected from experienced and established vendors. Some medical offices use a consultant to assist with this process.

Qualified Personnel

Individuals working on the computer should be well trained in computer concepts and hands-on computer operation. This can be accomplished by employing office staff who have graduated from a formal educational program or by having the front office staff attend computer workshops and seminars. Untrained staff can adversely affect the efficient operation of a computer system.

Proper Care and Maintenance of the Computer System

Proper care and maintenance of the computer system are undoubtedly directly related to reliable operation of the system. The beginning of this chapter presents the proper care and maintenance for each component in the computer system. Make sure you thoroughly review this information before working with a computer system. In addition to providing many years of reliable service, a well-cared-for system is much less likely to malfunction.

Memories *from* Practicum

Emma Hayes: When I did my practicum, it was the first time I really realized how much a modern medical office relies on its computer system. At that time, the office where I was placed was using a computer program to schedule appointments and manage the patient billing, but they were using a traditional paper medical record. There were four computers in the office, and they were networked together with two laser printers. The night before, we printed a list of patients scheduled for the next day, and we used that list to pull the medical records. In the evening, we also backed up all the computer files from that day. We were using a magnetic tape drive at that time to make a copy of all the files from the financial management software and appointment program. Individuals who did word processing or used a spreadsheet program had to back up their own files. I think that there wouldn't be enough storage space for most offices to do backups this way today. One day, the office computer system was not working, and we couldn't look anything up. It was very frustrating because we didn't know how much the patient's copayment was and we couldn't enter information about the visit. We did have the paper charge slips that the physicians had filled out, and by the next day everything was working again. I think it would be even more difficult now because we are using an electronic medical record as well. ∎

ELECTRONIC INFORMATION TRANSFER

One of the major developments of the past 25 years has been the significant increase in the use of the Internet to transfer data over great distances. The first network of computers sharing information by telephone lines was set up in 1969, but the Internet as we know it first became available to commercial users and the general public in the 1990s. In the medical office, electronic data sharing is primarily used for e-mail, transfer of billing and insurance information, banking, and e-prescribing, in addition to local network capabilities that allow for communication of data within the office itself or between different facilities of the same organization.

INTERNET

The **Internet** is a global system of interconnected computer networks that use the Internet protocol (TCP/IP)

What Would You Do? What Would You *Not* Do? RESPONSES—cont'd

❑ Did not promise to call the pharmacy to make sure they have received the prescription.

Case Study 3
Page 1059

What Did Emma Do?

❑ Reassured John that it is a legitimate concern to want to make sure his medical information is kept confidential.
❑ Explained to John that something called a "firewall" protects the office computers from unauthorized access by computer hackers.
❑ Told John that each staff member has to enter a password to log onto the computer and that a patient would not have a password and would not be able to log onto the computer.

❑ Explained to John that the office places a lot of emphasis on maintaining security of the computer system and preventing loss of data. Told John that the office has antivirus software running all the time to protect the computer from viruses and that the office also has a backup system so that even if data were lost, there would be a backup of the data.

What Did Emma Not Do?

❑ Did not minimize John's concerns.
❑ Did not criticize John for not having an antivirus program on his home computer.

↻ TERMINOLOGY REVIEW

Key Term	Word Parts	Definition
App		A specialized program, often small enough to run on a mobile device.
Application software		Software designed to accomplish a specific task (e.g., word processing); also called *application program* and *software program.*
Backup		A duplicate copy of a program or data kept for reference in case the original is damaged, lost, or destroyed.
Bit		The smallest unit of computer storage capacity.
Broadband		A method of transmitting electronic data that handles a wide range of frequencies.
Byte		A unit of computer storage capacity, usually eight bits. One byte is approximately equal to one character.
Cloud computing		A model in which the Internet is used to store and access data and programs, and servers are not physically located at the same site as the computer.
Computer		An electronic machine that has the ability to process data according to a program to produce a desired result.
Computer system		All of the hardware and software components making up the computer.
Data		Raw, unorganized facts about subject matter presented to the computer for processing.
Data processing		The changing of raw facts or data into usable information by following a three-part sequence: input, processing, output.
Digital subscriber line (DSL)		Technology that allows digital signals to be transmitted over telephone lines at high speed even if the telephone line is also being used for voice transmission.
Documentation		A written set of instructions accompanying an application program, designed to assist the user in understanding how to operate the program. Examples include the user manual, help screens, and reference cards.
E-mail		A method of composing, sending, receiving, and storing messages that are sent over the Internet.
Encryption	*crypt-:* secret	A process by which electronic information is changed into an unreadable form that requires the original encryption software to reverse the process.
Firewall		A system that protects a computer network from unauthorized access by users on its own network or another network, such as the Internet.
Gigabyte (GB)	*giga-:* one billion	A unit of computer storage capacity. One gigabyte is equal to a little more than 1 billion bytes or 1000 megabytes.
Hard copy		Printed output from a computer.

↻ TERMINOLOGY REVIEW—cont'd

Key Term	Word Parts	Definition
Hard disk drive		A storage device consisting of one or more rigid, nonflexible platters coated with a magnetically sensitive material and encased in a permanently sealed, airtight container.
Hardware		The physical devices making up a computer system (e.g., main computer unit, keyboard, monitor, printer).
Input		1. (noun) Data that have been entered into the computer. 2. (verb) The transfer of data to the computer for processing.
Input device		A device for entering data into the computer (e.g., keyboard, mouse, scanner).
Internet		A global system of interconnected computer networks that use the Internet protocol (TCP/IP) to transmit and exchange data.
Kilobyte (KB)	*kilo-*: one thousand	A unit of computer storage capacity. One kilobyte is equal to 1024 bytes (characters).
Main computer memory		The part of the CPU that is responsible for temporarily storing information until it is needed for processing by the computer. Main memory in a microcomputer is known as *RAM.*
Medical practice management program		A program that provides instructions to the computer for performing medical practice management procedures.
Megabyte (MB)	*mega-*: one million	A unit of computer storage capacity. One megabyte is equal to a little more than 1 million bytes or 1000 kilobytes.
Microcomputer	*micro-*: small	A small general-purpose computer that relies on a tiny microprocessor chip to perform its processing functions.
Microprocessor	*micro-*: small	The "brain" of the computer housed in the main unit that interprets and executes the instructions that operate the computer. The microprocessor is a chip that resides on the mainboard in the main unit of the computer.
Network		A group of computers that share data and resources.
Operating system		A type of system software that performs tasks required by the computer to operate itself.
Optical disc		A storage device consisting of a flat, round portable disk that stores data using laser technology.
Optical disc drive		A device installed in a drive bay on the main computer unit that uses a laser to read an optical disc or write onto (burn) an optical disc.
Output		1. (noun) Information that has been generated by the computer. 2. (verb) The transfer of processed data back to the user.
Output device		A device that transfers processed data to the user (e.g., computer monitor, printer).
Patient portal		An online application that allows patients to interact with and communicate with their health care providers
Printing speed		The number of pages per minute (ppm) generated by a printer.
Processing		The manipulation and reorganization of data according to the instructions in a program.
Program		A set of instructions organized in a logical step-by-step sequence, which tells the computer how to perform a specific function.
Random-access memory (RAM)		The main computer memory of a microcomputer, which is used to temporarily store items until needed by the computer for processing. Also known as *main computer memory.*
Router		A wired or wireless device used to form or connect networks.
Server		A large computer that stores data and manages tasks for other computers on a network.
Software		A general term for the programs or instructions that tell a computer what to do.
Solid state drive		Drive that uses integrated circuits (flash memory) to store data permanently.
Special keys		Keys that issue commands to the computer to perform specific functions on the information displayed on the screen.

Continued

↻ TERMINOLOGY REVIEW—cont'd

Key Term	Word Parts	Definition
Storage capacity		The maximum amount of information that a device can hold, measured in bytes.
Storage device		A device that permanently stores information for later retrieval by the computer.
System software		A group of programs that control or maintain the operations of a computer.
Terabyte (TB)	*tera-*: one trillion	A unit of computer storage. One terabyte is equivalent to a little more than a trillion bytes or 1000 gigabytes.
Touchscreen		A visual display unit that the user can touch to input data using the fingers or a stylus
URL		The characters and/or words used to access a specific website or file on the World Wide Web.
USB port		A standard computer cable connection interface that allows several types to devices to be connected to the computer in order to transfer data across short distances.
User		The individual operating a computer.
Web browser		A software program used to access the World Wide Web.
World Wide Web		A series of interlinked websites or files accessed via the Internet.

ON THE WEB

For information on medical office computerization:

American Health Information Management Association (AHIMA): www.ahima.org

Department of Health and Human Services HIPAA website: www.hhs.gov/ocr/hipaa

Microsoft Windows: www.microsoft.com/windows

Microsoft Office: www.microsoft.com/office

Telephone Techniques

ⓔ Check out the Evolve site at http://evolve.elsevier.com/Bonewit/today/ to access additional interactive activities and exercises to help you study and prepare for success.

LEARNING OBJECTIVES

PROCEDURES

1. Describe the importance of effective telephone courtesy and a pleasing telephone personality for the medical assistant.
2. Explain the use of multiline telephones, cell phones, smartphones, and pagers in the medical office.
3. Differentiate between incoming telephone calls the medical assistant can handle and other incoming calls.
4. Describe the correct procedure for screening incoming calls.

Perform telephone screening.

5. Describe the correct procedure for taking messages and transcribing messages recorded on an answering machine or voicemail.

Take a telephone message.
Take requests for medication or prescription refills.

6. Identify the correct steps to respond to a telephone call regarding an emergency or urgent medical problem.
7. Describe how to deal with problem calls.
8. Explain how the medical assistant should make outgoing telephone calls.

Call a patient for follow-up.

CHAPTER OUTLINE

INTRODUCTION TO TELEPHONE TECHNIQUES
USING THE TELEPHONE EFFECTIVELY
Telephone Courtesy
Telephone Personality
Maintaining Patient Privacy
Effective Telephone Communication
TELEPHONE TECHNOLOGY
Multiline Phones
Special Features
Answering Machines and Voicemail
Cell Phones and Smartphones
Pagers
INCOMING CALLS
Centralized or Electronic Routing
Managing Incoming Calls
Performing Telephone Screening

Calls the Medical Assistant Usually Handles
Taking Messages on a Paper Message Form
Taking Messages on the Computer
Calls from Other Physicians
Calls from Salespeople
Urgent or Emergency Calls
Dealing With Problem Calls
The Caller Who Refuses to Give Information
Complaints
Patients with Special Problems
OUTGOING CALLS
Local Calls
Appointment Reminders
Long-Distance Calls
Conference Calls

KEY TERMS

enunciation (ee-nun-see-AY-shun)
pager

smartphone

voicemail

INTRODUCTION TO TELEPHONE TECHNIQUES

Contact with a patient takes many forms. In addition to face-to-face contact, medical assistants often speak to patients and other callers over the telephone. The telephone is often the first contact between the medical office and a patient. In addition, the telephone is used throughout the day to make and receive referrals, request laboratory results, call in prescriptions for patients, and respond to patient questions.

Managing the phone is one of the most important jobs in the office. It is the first chance the medical assistant has to project a positive attitude and image to a patient. One never has a second chance to make a first impression.

USING THE TELEPHONE EFFECTIVELY

TELEPHONE COURTESY

The telephone in a medical office should always be answered promptly. Some offices have a policy that every phone call should be answered within three rings. The medical assistant identifies the office, gives his or her name, then finds out who is calling. If the call will be transferred, the staff member needs to know who will be on the other end of the call.

The medical assistant should always speak before putting someone on hold. It is not courteous to immediately place a call on hold before speaking to the caller. The caller cannot even be sure that he or she has reached the correct telephone number. It is far more polite to obtain the caller's name and purpose for calling before putting the caller on hold. It is helpful to keep a written record of each caller's name, with the number of the line on which he or she is holding. A physician should not be placed on hold if it can be avoided. The medical assistant should check back about every 30 seconds or so with a person who is on hold. This reassures the caller that the medical assistant is aware of the call. The medical assistant should also try to give an idea of how long it will take before the call will be answered.

When handling a call, the medical assistant should not chew gum or eat. Paying close attention during the telephone call is also important. A caller can tell if the medical assistant is distracted.

TELEPHONE PERSONALITY

In addition to words, many nonverbal cues are given in the quality of a medical assistant's voice on the telephone. The "telephone personality" is important. It is important to stay focused on the call and smile. The medical assistant should use the same volume as when speaking in person and should speak naturally. An artificial telephone voice may be perceived as cold and "fake."

All words should be spoken clearly so that they are easy to understand. **Enunciation** is the act of speaking so that the message can be easily understood. It may be necessary to speak a little more slowly on the telephone, and it is very important to avoid mumbling. It may be helpful for a medical assistant to record a telephone greeting and analyze the quality of his or her voice and the personality that is projected.

Qualities such as interest, friendliness, concern, and understanding are clearly communicated over the telephone. So too are boredom, anxiety, and indifference.

MAINTAINING PATIENT PRIVACY

When speaking on the telephone, the medical assistant must take measures to maintain patient privacy and confidentiality as required by the Health Insurance Portability and Accountability Act (HIPAA). When the telephone located at the front desk is used, the privacy window should be closed, if there is one. Otherwise, waiting patients should stand away from the intake area, and the medical assistant's voice should be low enough to avoid being overheard. The telephone used for responding to patient calls and scheduling urgent appointments is often located in a separate area so that patients cannot overhear conversations. The medical assistant should remember to maintain a professional tone in all telephone conversations.

EFFECTIVE TELEPHONE COMMUNICATION

When speaking on the telephone, the medical assistant should try to complete the call without interruption. If it is necessary to put someone on hold, the medical assistant should give a reason and apologize to the caller when the call is resumed. Information and materials should be readily available to handle calls and take messages. These include message slips or a computer messaging system, a pen, the office computer appointment program, and a resource for frequently used telephone numbers. A desk clock, computer clock, or wristwatch should be visible to note the time when taking messages.

The medical assistant begins the conversation by identifying the practice—for example, "Primary Care Associates, Channa speaking." If the caller asks a question or asks for a staff member without identifying himself or herself, the medical assistant asks politely for the caller's name: "With whom am I speaking?" or "May I ask who is calling?" Using complete sentences is important because the medical assistant does not want to sound abrupt or rude.

The medical assistant should sit with the back supported and the head in a neutral position (not forward or to one side). The feet should be flat on the floor or supported on a foot stool. Figure 41-1 shows proper body position for answering the telephone. If the receiver is tucked between the head and shoulder, it places strain on the shoulder muscles and may change the voice quality, so this should be

Figure 41-1 Good posture when answering the telephone improves voice quality and prevents muscle strain.

Figure 41-3 A multiline telephone is commonly used in a medical office.

Figure 41-2 A telephone headset leaves the hands free and facilitates good body posture.

avoided. A headset, which consists of an earpiece that fits over the ear and a mouthpiece in front of the mouth, allows for good body posture and leaves the hands free. This is recommended if the medical assistant spends a lot of time on the telephone. Figure 41-2 shows such a headset.

The medical assistant should be clear with callers who leave messages about when they can expect their calls to be returned. Many physicians have specific times when they return nonurgent telephone calls, such as late morning, lunch time, or the end of the day.

One should avoid cutting into a person's replies, even if he or she rambles on and repeats information. When the medical assistant gets the chance to speak, he or she should try to give a focused answer that lets the caller know what can be done and what the medical assistant is going to do.

TELEPHONE TECHNOLOGY

Advances in telephone technology have given medical offices many options to maintain contact with patients, physicians, pharmacies, laboratories, and hospitals.

MULTILINE PHONES

Most offices have a multiline telephone, with several extensions. It is important for the medical assistant to learn how to determine which line is ringing, how to place calls on hold, and how to transfer calls to all parts of the medical office. Figure 41-3 illustrates a multiline telephone.

A flashing light usually identifies a line that is ringing; it flashes at a different rate on a line where a person is on hold. The medical assistant answers a call by pressing the button on the telephone that corresponds to the line that is ringing. If a second call comes in while the medical assistant is speaking to a caller, the medical assistant should tell the first caller that he or she needs to place the caller on hold, then he or she presses the hold button. The medical assistant answers the second call, identifies the caller, and usually places that caller on hold before returning to the first caller and apologizing for the interruption. The calls are then handled in order.

If the caller asks to be connected to another extension or person, the medical assistant should first obtain the caller's name. To transfer a call, the medical assistant may need to press another button and/or dial an extension number, depending on the type of telephone system. Knowing the caller's name allows the medical assistant to announce the caller when the call is connected, and it is also helpful if the call is disconnected for some reason.

While a caller is on hold, the light on that line will flash. If the light continues to flash, the medical assistant should pick up that line about every 30 seconds and ask if the person would like to continue holding or leave a message. Sometimes transfers do not go through or the call is not picked up.

Special Features

Multiline telephone systems come with many other features, including speed dialing, call forwarding, call park, and caller ID.

Speed dialing allows storage of frequently called telephone numbers in the telephone system's memory. These numbers can be called by pressing a button or a one- or two-digit code.

Call forwarding allows forwarding of incoming calls to another telephone number. This service is turned on and off by dialing a sequence of numbers and activity keys.

Call park allows a call to be placed on hold and retrieved from another telephone.

Caller ID identifies the caller's telephone number before the telephone is answered. This feature may be available on some, but not all, telephones within a telephone system.

The medical assistant must learn how to use these and other features of the telephone system efficiently.

ANSWERING MACHINES AND VOICEMAIL

Physicians have always needed to be available at all times. Most physicians' offices still use an answering service for getting messages to physicians during hours when the office is normally closed. This is an independent company that answers telephones for a number of clients. Some offices also have an answering machine or voicemail system, which has a message with a number to call outside of office hours and gives people the option to leave a nonurgent message. **Voicemail** is a method for message delivery, storage, and retrieval that is built into the telephone system. It is usually attached to each individual extension. Answering services and answering machines are activated whenever the office is closed, including during lunch break if no one is assigned to take phone calls during that time. The answering service should be notified if the office is closed, although the service will usually pick up phones after a predetermined number of rings.

Increasingly, physicians' offices use voicemail systems instead of or in addition to answering machines. Voicemail is a system provided by the office's telephone carrier that allows for messages to be left in a number of "mailboxes" for different people. Each physician might have his or her own voicemail box, as well as each medical assistant, the business manager, and so on. If a call is not answered, many telephone systems will give a caller the option of leaving a message in a voicemail box. Each box has a two- to four-number extension. Many voicemail systems have a directory by which people can find voicemail box numbers by using their touch-tone phone to type in some or all of the letters of the last name of the person with whom they would like to speak.

Even if an office has a voicemail system, most medical offices will still need to have a contract with an answering

service. The answering service provides a medical office with coverage outside of normal business hours. The service either answers all of the office's telephone calls or takes calls that are forwarded to it by individuals who listen to the voicemail system message and press the appropriate message code for an urgent message. The answering service must be informed how to deal with urgent calls.

Putting It All Into Practice

My name is Channa Eng, and I am a Certified Medical Assistant. I work for an internal medical practice with two physicians and two nurse practitioners in an urban area. We have many Asian and Hispanic patients. I don't speak much Spanish, but I do speak Cambodian and some Vietnamese. Another medical assistant speaks Spanish, and we both help with translating telephone calls from patients who have difficulty in English. When patients call our office, they get three choices right away. They can hear the message in English, Spanish, or Cambodian. Most patients like this because they can hear the instructions in a language they are comfortable with. On Tuesdays and Thursdays, I spend most of the day on the telephone making appointments and responding to patients who call with medical problems. I don't usually sit at the front desk. Instead, we have a telephone room with three telephones. When it is very busy, there are usually two of us. When a patient calls for an appointment, I ask for his or her name and date of birth. Then I locate the patient in the electronic medical record. Our system coordinates the clinical record with the appointment system. In addition, I can take messages through the EMR, which are attached to the patient's record and routed to the patient's physician or another staff member. My goal is to handle each call as quickly and efficiently as possible while still making the patients feel that their needs were met. In our office we think that telephone conversations are very important. We try very hard to answer all telephone calls promptly and to avoid putting patients on hold. ∎

CELL PHONES AND SMARTPHONES

Cell phones allow two individuals to speak to each other as they would using regular telephones, but the cell phone uses radio signals instead of telephone wires. A **smartphone** is a device that adds computer capabilities to the cell phone, with a drug reference, address book, and other tools; an Internet connection; the ability to send and receive e-mails; and sometimes even access to the electronic medical record (EMR) system used by the health care facility. Many physicians use cell phones or smartphones to remain in contact with the medical office when they are in other locations. The physicians' cell phone numbers should never be given to patients, but they should be available to office staff so that physicians can be contacted as needed.

Health care organizations recognize that excellent service is an important part of providing high-quality health care. Because the first contact with a patient is often a telephone contact, it is vital for a medical assistant to be aware of the importance of good customer service.

Internal customers include other departments within the health care facility as well as physician employers and fellow employees. External customers include patients, referring or consulting physicians, visitors, third-party payors, and suppliers. Both types of customers must be treated with respect on the telephone as well as in person. Medical assistants should follow guidelines to be sure that telephone calls are answered promptly, that accurate and complete information is given and received, and that any complaints or concerns are met with an understanding and appropriate response.

There are several service expectations when using the telephone.

- Use a four-part greeting: Answer the telephone using a greeting, introduce yourself, identify your department, and ask how you can help.
- Address the patient by *Miss, Mrs., Ms.,* or *Mr.*
- Ask for permission before putting the caller on hold.
- Ask the caller for permission to transfer the call.
- Repeat information such as an appointment date and time before ending the call.
- Ask the caller if there is anything else you can do before ending the call.
- Listen attentively.
- Smile and use a friendly tone of voice.

An acronym that is often recommended to provide excellent customer service to patients is *AIDET*. It stands for Acknowledge, Introduce, Duration, Explanation, Thank You. This is not only important for telephone calls, but also in all interactions with patients.

- *Acknowledge:* Acknowledge patients or other customers promptly and greet them as the first step in building a connection.
- *Introduce:* Identify yourself and then identify the customer, especially if it is a patient.
- *Duration:* Reduce anxiety by setting time expectations. On the telephone, ask permission before placing a caller on hold, and return to the call at regular intervals. Offer timely appointments.
- *Explanation:* Explain procedures or other information in terms that the patient can understand. Good explanations are a cornerstone of good health care.
- *Thank You:* Thank the caller before ending the call.

If a customer has a complaint, it is important to listen carefully and address the problem. If necessary, staff should have tools available to amend the situation for a patient who is present in person, such as food or parking vouchers. For patients on the telephone, a caring attitude and careful listening are the main tools available to the medical assistant. A four-part service recovery model called *LEAD* is sometimes recommended.

- *Listen:* Allow the patient and/or family to feel heard.
- *Empathize:* Notice and acknowledge feelings.
- *Apologize:* Acknowledge the situation without blame and apologize on behalf of the health care organization.
- *Do the Right Thing:* Determine the best solution and be timely with corrective action.

It may be necessary to report a situation to the manager if it cannot be resolved on the spot. Inform a telephone caller of the action that will be taken, and be sure to follow through. ■

PAGERS

Pagers are used in areas with unreliable cell phone service and sometimes in large institutions such as hospitals. A **pager** (also called a *beeper*) is like a radio that is always tuned in to a single station. When it "hears" its unique access code signal, it lights up, beeps, or vibrates to indicate that a message is being received. Some pagers are also linked to voicemail. Pagers used by physicians or other health professionals are either numeric or alphanumeric. A numeric pager's message is a telephone number (e.g., the answering service, the office, the emergency department, home, a colleague). The physician then returns the call to the number on the display. An alphanumeric pager displays an entire message, so the physician can return a phone call or act on the information that is relayed to the pager. Some pagers also include e-mail so that a return message can be sent. If the physicians use pagers, the office staff should have the pager numbers for each physician in the practice.

A simple type of pager may also be used for patients in ambulatory care areas of hospitals or clinics. It is similar to pagers used in restaurants and lights up and/or vibrates to notify patients when it is their turn. Patients can leave the waiting area and be notified when to return. This type of pager provides patient confidentiality because it eliminates the need to call the patient by name.

INCOMING CALLS

An incoming telephone call sounds like a routine event. But breaking down the process, it becomes clear that a number of different elements go into answering a routine call.

CENTRALIZED OR ELECTRONIC ROUTING

Many offices use an electronic routing system to direct calls. At each extension, the telephone may be answered or the call will go to voicemail, and the caller can leave a message for office staff members who are not available. By offering the caller several options (e.g., scheduling an appointment, speaking with the medical assistant, discussing a billing question), the electronic routing system directs the call to the appropriate part of the office, saving the expense of a staff person who would otherwise be answering the call. It also keeps patients from being put on hold, which some people appreciate.

However, other patients find electronic routing of messages confusing and frustrating, especially if the person they need to speak with is not available and does not return calls promptly.

If electronic routing is used, the message should be kept up to date and should be as clear and concise as possible.

In other offices, incoming calls are answered directly by the medical assistant. Although the personal touch is appreciated by many patients, when several calls come in at the same time, some callers end up on hold. If the office has several staff members, many of the calls end up being transferred anyway.

MANAGING INCOMING CALLS

Performing Telephone Screening

The first step in handling telephone calls is to find out how urgent the call is and what is necessary to handle the call.

Most calls are routine and can be taken in the order in which they come. In most cases a new call is placed on hold while the previous call is handled. However, there are some exceptions:

- Calls from other physicians are put through at once.
- Emergency calls are treated as urgent and receive top priority. They will be discussed in detail later in this chapter.
- If the caller is a relative of the physician, the medical assistant either puts the caller through or speaks to the physician via intercom to determine how to handle the call.

When answering calls, it is polite to obtain the caller's name and ask permission to place the caller on hold. This gives the caller the opportunity to identify the call as urgent.

After the caller's name has been obtained, the caller usually states the reason for the call or asks for a staff member or department. When the caller asks for a staff member by name, the medical assistant usually transfers the call. If that staff member is with a patient, the medical assistant may offer to take a message or transfer the call to voicemail. Often the caller asks for the physician. Most physicians do not take calls while they are seeing patients. Additional questions may show that the medical assistant can handle the call, or it may be necessary to take a message for the physician (Procedure 41-1).

Calls the Medical Assistant Usually Handles

The medical assistant usually handles four kinds of calls.

1. *Requests to schedule appointments.* The medical assistant will usually schedule appointments and tests, either in the office or at an outside laboratory or the hospital. This topic is discussed in Chapter 42.

2. *Billing inquiries.* The medical assistant may handle inquiries about a patient bill or insurance. For this type of call, the medical assistant refers to the patient account in the computer and gives the caller the information requested. If the caller's question is complicated, the call may be referred to a billing specialist or the office manager.

3. *Receiving diagnostic test and laboratory results.* The medical assistant can also take calls regarding diagnostic test and laboratory results. Most laboratory results today are sent to physicians' offices by fax or directly through the computer system. But if a laboratory calls in test results, the medical assistant needs to have a blank laboratory slip so that the results can be filled in, along with the patient's name and the date the tests were taken. After taking the results, the medical assistant places them for the physician to review. If a paper medical record system is used, the report is clipped to the patient's medical record. Taking all results accurately is very important.

4. *Requests for information.* Finally, the medical assistant can handle calls requesting information, such as directions to get to the office, office hours, and the office's medical specialty.

What Would You Do? What Would You *Not* Do?

Case Study 1

Channa has answered a telephone call from Jane Weston, who has called to make a routine appointment. Although the patient has been offered several different appointment days and times, none of the choices has been satisfactory. A low buzz indicates a call on another telephone line. Channa is the only person available to take the call. She tells Mrs. Weston that she will need to put her on hold for a minute. Mrs. Weston says, "Please don't put me on hold. I'll take that last appointment. What time was it for?" ■

Taking Messages on a Paper Message Form

The medical assistant may take messages on a paper message form. Some forms are pressure sensitive so that a copy is created with the original message. The originals stay in the message book and form a telephone log. If the message form does not create a copy, it is helpful to keep a separate telephone log for future reference. In some offices a form is used that has a space for the physician to write orders or desired follow-up on the bottom of the form. The medical assistant should not write in this space when taking the message. If telephone messages are filed in the patient's medical record after the physician or other recipient has responded to the message, a form with a peel-off backing is preferable.

Taking Messages on the Computer

The medical assistant may work in a facility where telephone messages are taken using the computer, either using a stand-alone computer messaging program or using the clinical messaging feature within the EMR. Built-in message templates facilitate taking the message during the telephone call and forwarding the message to one or more recipients. When this feature is part of the EMR, the patient's medical record can be attached to the message, and the transmission is secure. This can be very useful for questions about laboratory results and requests to renew prescriptions.

When taking a message about a patient, include the following information in the message:

- Date and time.
- Name of the physician or staff member.
- Patient's full name and date of birth.
- Name of the caller (if not the patient).
- Message or question that indicates clearly what the patient wants (e.g., prescription, laboratory results, medical advice).
- Additional information to clarify the message, such as symptoms, medication and pharmacy information, and actions that have already been taken.
- If the patient is ill or requests medication, any medication allergies should be noted.
- Telephone number.
- Initials of the person taking the message.

When a medical assistant transcribes messages from an answering machine or from voicemail, the same paper or electronic message form should be used as for ordinary telephone calls. The time the call was recorded should be used. The medical assistant may need to play the message more than once to record all information (Procedure 41-2).

Patients Requesting Test Results

When a patient calls requesting test results, the medical assistant should find out when and where the test was done and take a message for the physician. Some offices choose to send patients letters about laboratory results, which cuts down on the number of telephone calls requesting information, especially for routine tests. After reviewing the laboratory or diagnostic test results, the physician may instruct the medical assistant to call the patient back to give the results, to schedule follow-up testing, and/or to ask the patient to schedule an appointment to discuss the results.

Patients Reporting Satisfactory or Unsatisfactory Progress

Physicians often tell a patient to call and check at a specified interval after a visit, to report on how a condition is resolving after treatment. If the patient reports satisfactory progress, the medical assistant should take a brief message and leave it for the physician. An unsatisfactory report should generate a more complete message. When a patient gives a progress report on the telephone, either the original message should be filed in the patient record or the medical assistant should document the telephone conversation in the record. Messages taken through the EMR are usually automatically recorded with other information related to an individual patient.

Requests for Medication or Prescription Refills

Often patients or pharmacies call with requests to have prescriptions refilled or renewed. When the pharmacy calls, it is important to get the patient's name and date of birth, name of the medication, dosage, and amount of medication prescribed. When the patient calls, it is important to get the name of the medication, dosage, and how often the patient takes it. In addition, it is important to determine how the patient wants to receive the medication (from the pharmacy or by mail). It is helpful to verify the information in the patient's medical record when an EMR is used. Otherwise the message should include the name, telephone number, and location of the pharmacy or mail-order company. It is more common for a physician to prescribe using a computer program, but if this is not the case, a written prescription should be sent to the patient if mail-order is specified. If the medication is an antibiotic or a controlled substance used for pain relief, the medical assistant should ask about symptoms that would require a refill. The medical assistant should tell patients to check with the pharmacy the next day unless they hear from the physician or office. A message to request medication is also attached to the patient's medical record. Physicians often follow up directly with the pharmacy, especially if they are using an electronic prescription routing service, but in some offices the physician writes the prescribing information on the bottom of a paper message for the medical assistant to fax or call in to the pharmacy. If a medical assistants telephones a prescriptions, it should always be noted in the progress notes and/or medication record (Procedure 41-3).

Calls for Referrals or Requesting Laboratory or Diagnostic Tests

A patient may call to say he or she needs a referral (because of a particular insurance company's policy) to see a specialist outside the medical group or to have a laboratory test or diagnostic procedure done.

The medical assistant takes the necessary information (what type of referral, for what, to whom) as a message for the physician. If a referral is appropriate—or necessary because of an insurance company or health maintenance organization policy—the medical assistant may complete a paper or electronic form. If the patient is asking for a laboratory test, such as a throat culture, the medical assistant should fill out the laboratory form for the patient to pick up or should enter the information into the computer, after verifying with the physician that the requested test is appropriate. The physician may ask the medical assistant to call the patient and schedule an appointment before authorizing the referral.

Patients with Medical Questions

For patients with medical questions, the medical assistant takes a message for a physician or refers the call to another staff member designated by the office to handle such calls. The office should have written guidelines to follow if a medical assistant screens medical questions. The medical assistant should follow the written guidelines closely and take a message for the physician about any concern or question that falls outside the preset guidelines.

What Would You Do? What Would You *Not* Do?

Case Study 2

Mary Woodward, a 62-year-old woman with hypertension, has called because she has run out of her blood pressure medication. Mrs. Woodward tells Channa that the medication is atenolol and she is pretty sure that the dose is 50 mg every morning. When Channa asks for the pharmacy name, Mrs. Woodward says, "It's the Best Buy Pharmacy in Whittier, but that doesn't matter because I will come in and pick up the prescription." Channa checks the electronic medical record (EMR) in the computer and finds that the office has a different preferred pharmacy recorded for this patient. ■

Calls from Other Physicians

Calls from other physicians are usually put through right away, even if the physician is examining a patient. If the medical assistant has to find the physician, this may be given as a reason to place the caller on hold briefly, but the medical assistant should locate the physician as quickly as possible and explain which physician is calling. The physician may ask the medical assistant to transfer the call to another extension to avoid talking in front of a patient.

Calls from Salespeople

Often a sales representative from a pharmaceutical company or equipment company calls before visiting the physician's office. Salespeople are usually seen by the office manager, who gives the information to the physician. Drug company representatives sometimes drop by, but if they hope to talk to the physician they usually must call and ask for an appointment. Physicians usually schedule sales representatives during lunch. The physician has to agree to see the representative before a medical assistant makes an appointment.

URGENT OR EMERGENCY CALLS

If a patient calls with a medical problem, the medical assistant asks questions to determine how urgent the problem is. After obtaining the caller's name and telephone number and identifying who has the problem (the patient's name, age or date of birth, and relationship to the caller), the medical assistant should obtain the patient's symptoms and current condition. In most offices there is a guide to telephone screening in the office procedure manual. This helps the medical assistant identify which questions to ask to determine how urgent the problem is. In the next chapter, there is a more complete discussion of the kind of appointment to offer a patient based on the symptoms the patient reports.

If the medical assistant determines that the call represents an urgent problem or emergency, he or she should follow office policy. The call should be referred to a physician if one is in the office; in a group practice, one physician may be assigned at all times to take urgent calls. If there is no physician in the office, a nurse practitioner, physician's assistant, or registered nurse may be assigned to take urgent calls. If no licensed professional is present in the office, the medical assistant must advise the caller or contact the on-call physician. The following are the guidelines for dealing with such a call:

1. If the emergency is serious or life-threatening, the caller should be instructed to call an ambulance by dialing 911. This activates the emergency medical services (EMS) system. If the caller is a child or seems upset or confused, the medical assistant can offer to call an ambulance for the caller.
2. If the emergency is a case of poisoning, the caller should be instructed to call the Poison Help number. The telephone number of the Poison Help number (1-800-222-1222) should be placed next to every telephone in the medical office. Even if it is a case of poisoning, if the patient is unconscious or not breathing, the caller should be instructed to call an ambulance.
3. If the patient has a problem that requires treatment in an emergency department but is conscious and able to walk (e.g., a bleeding wound), the caller should be instructed to take the patient to the nearest emergency department or call an ambulance. If the patient is alone, an ambulance should be called.
4. If the patient's problem is usually treated in the office, the patient should be given an appointment for that day.
5. If the condition of the patient is not life-threatening and/or the medical assistant is unsure how urgent the problem is, the physician should be contacted for instructions either by cell phone or pager. If there is any doubt about how serious the patient's condition is, it is safer to instruct the patient to call an ambulance and/or go to the hospital emergency department.

Whenever an urgent call is handled, the medical assistant should fill out a message form to be sure that the information has been written down. Either the message form or the instructions given to the patient should later be documented in the medical record. If a patient has been instructed to go to the emergency department, the physician should be notified promptly.

DEALING WITH PROBLEM CALLS

The Caller Who Refuses to Give Information

When callers ask for a physician and refuse to identify themselves, it is probably because they want to speak to the physician but suspect that if they give a name, they will be asked to leave a message. The medical assistant should explain politely that the physician is not available and offer to take a message. If the caller still refuses to give information, the medical assistant can instruct the caller to write a letter to the physician and mark it "personal."

Complaints

The medical assistant should listen carefully to callers with complaints, avoid getting defensive or angry, and ask for specific information. It is important to remain calm so that a professional demeanor is maintained. The medical assistant should state clearly what he or she can and will do. It may be necessary to refer the matter to the office manager or the physician, but the medical assistant should get as much information as possible at the initial contact.

It is important to avoid hanging up on an angry caller. It is usually possible to calm a caller down as long as the medical assistant does not raise his or her voice and does not become defensive. The caller should be told a specific time when he or she can expect to hear back from someone in the office.

Patients with Special Problems

If a patient calls who is confused or has difficulty with English, the medical assistant should listen carefully and try as hard as possible to understand. The medical assistant may speak more slowly than usual but should not speak more loudly. If it is impossible to communicate, even using simple language, the medical assistant should try to at least obtain the caller's name and telephone number. Then it may be possible to find out from the medical record if the patient speaks a different language or if there is an emergency contact number. If the person seems confused, the medical assistant should ask if there is another person with whom he or she can speak because this may be a medical emergency. The medical assistant may need to ask for guidance from the physician or office manager.

PROCEDURE 41-1 Performing Telephone Screening

Outcome Screen incoming telephone calls

Equipment/Supplies

- Telephone
- Message pad
- Pen or pencil
- Computer terminal or manual appointment book
- Clock or watch

1. **Procedural Step.** Answer every telephone call within the first three rings.
   Principle. Good customer service requires prompt acknowledgment of an internal or external customer.
2. **Procedural Step.** Identify the medical office and give your name. Each practice will have a preferred way for all employees to answer the telephone. Example: "Hello, this is Channa at Primary Care Associates. How can I help you?" Do not rush through the greeting. The caller needs to hear this greeting clearly.
   Principle. Callers need to know what business they have reached and with whom they are speaking. Good customer service involves an offer to be of assistance.
3. **Procedural Step.** Listen carefully to what the caller says, and decide as soon as possible whether this is a call you can handle, whether you need to take a message, or whether the call should be transferred to someone else in the office.
   Principle. The caller does not want to have to repeat all the details if the call must be transferred. If you need to take a message, begin recording it.
4. **Procedural Step.** Ask for the caller's name. "May I ask who is calling?"
   Principle. You will need the caller's name to address the caller by name, to take a message, or to identify the caller before transferring the call.

5. **Procedural Step.** Clarify whether the caller is a patient or calling about a patient. Obtain the patient's name (if not the caller) and date of birth.
6. **Procedural Step.** If you can handle the call, such as a call for an appointment, do so promptly.
7. **Procedural Step.** If you need to take a message, see Procedure 41-2: Taking a Telephone Message.
8. **Procedural Step.** If you need to transfer the call to someone else in the office, place the caller on hold, noting the caller's name and the extension. Tell the person to whom you are transferring the call who is calling and what extension the call is on.
   Principle. It is a courtesy to tell the person to whom you transfer a call who is calling; the call recipient must be able to locate the call if more than one line has a call on hold.
9. **Procedural Step.** If the caller describes symptoms that require immediate care, ask questions to assess the problem, following guidelines in the office procedure manual. If there is a physician or other licensed professional in the office, transfer the call immediately. Otherwise, assess the urgency of the problem and follow up according to office guidelines. If the patient's health is at risk, instruct the caller to call 911.
   Principle. Patients expect correct medical advice from a health care facility when they have urgent medical problems.

Continued

PROCEDURE 41-1   Performing Telephone Screening—cont'd

10. Procedural Step. If your telephone has more than two lines, it is helpful to keep a list of the names of callers and extensions. When a call is on hold, the light for that telephone line blinks. If you have transferred a call but the caller remains on hold, within 30 to 45 seconds you should determine if the caller is still holding; if so, you should try to transfer the call again or take a message.
Principle. Sometimes a transfer does not go through or the call is not picked up. The caller has no way to get back in contact with you to leave a message or to ask to speak to someone else.

11. Procedural Step. If the telephone rings for another call, ask if you may put the caller to whom you are speaking on hold and wait for the caller to agree. After pressing the hold button, answer the other call and explain that you are speaking to a caller on another line. Give the second caller the option to

hold and wait for you or take his or her number and offer to call back as soon as you are finished.
Principle. In general, calls are handled in the order they are received. By asking for permission to put the caller on hold, you give the caller a chance to tell you if it is an emergency. Some callers prefer to hold; others prefer to be called back. Time passes slowly when a caller is on hold, and the caller may become tired of waiting and wish to leave a message.

12. Procedural Step. At the end of the call, repeat any information you have discussed (such as the date and time of an appointment). End the call politely by thanking the caller and saying goodbye.
Principle. Confirmation helps avoid misunderstandings. Thanking the caller and closing the conversation demonstrates good customer service.

PROCEDURE 41-2   Taking a Telephone Message

Outcome Take a telephone message

Equipment/Supplies

- Telephone
- Computer
- Message pad

- Pen or pencil
- Clock or watch

1. Procedural Step. If you determine that the person to whom a telephone caller wants to speak is not available, offer to take a message.
Principle. A message is a way of communicating to a person who is not available to speak on the telephone.

2. Procedural Step. Give the caller a reason why the person cannot take the call. Acceptable reasons are as follows: busy with a patient, not at his or her desk, not in the office, on another line. In general, physicians do not take calls except possibly during specified hours. Patients who ask for the physician are told that the physician is not in the office or that the physician is busy with patients.
Principle. Most callers are willing to leave a message if they understand why their call is not being answered.

3. Procedural Step. Fill in the information in the computer messaging program or on a paper message

form, including the name of the caller, business affiliation (if any), patient name (if not the caller) and patient date of birth, date of the call, time of the call, telephone number including area code, and information the caller wishes to leave about the reason for the call. Place your initials on the message in case there are questions. If there is a section at the bottom of a paper message form for a response to the message, leave that area blank.
Principle. Complete information is necessary for a call to be returned.

4. Procedural Step. Verify the information. If possible, give a time when the call might be returned. If the message recipient does not have a scheduled time to return messages, say, "I will give him (or her) the message."
Principle. Callers like to know when to expect a return call.

PROCEDURE 41-2   Taking a Telephone Message—cont'd

4

MESSAGE FROM								
For Dr. *Lawler*	Name of Caller *Anne Richards*	Ref. to pt. *mother*	Patient *Janice*	Pt. Age. *4*	Pt. Temp. *101°*	Message Date *10/13/XX*	Message Time *9:00* AM PM	Urgent ☐ Yes ☐ No

Message: *Child has been on antibiotic for two days — still has fever. Should she come in again?*   Allergies *∅*   DOB *4/2/XX*

| Respond to Phone # *814-322-6510* | Best Time to Call *any* AM PM | Pharmacy Name / # *WestSide* *814-754-9817* | Patient's Chart Attached ☒ Yes ☐ No | Patient's chart # | Initials *KJ* |

DOCTOR - STAFF RESPONSE

Doctor's / Staff Orders / Follow-up Action

| Call Back ☐ Yes ☐ No | Chart. Mes. ☐ Yes ☐ No | Follow-up Date / / | Follow-up Completed-Date/Time / / | AM PM | Response By: |

Product # 78-9156-Pkg, #78-9157-Pads, Bibbero Systems, Inc., Petaluma, CA. To order, call toll free 800-BIBBERO (800 242-2376) OR FAX 800-242-9330.

Fill in the information on the message form.

5. Procedural Step. End the call politely.

6. Procedural Step. If the call is from a patient or concerns a patient, attach the message to the patient medical record in a clinical messaging computer program or attach a paper medical record if a paper record system is used. Be sure to select the correct EHR or paper medical record.
Principle. This ensures that information about the patient is available and the action taken on the call can be documented if necessary.

7. Procedural Step. Place the message (with the patient record, if needed) where the person for whom it is intended expects to find messages. This may be on a desk or in a mailbox. If a computer messaging program was used, send the message to the intended recipient(s) using secure messaging.

8. Procedural Step. Perform follow-up according to office procedure.
Principle. This ensures that important issues do not fall through the cracks.

PROCEDURE 41-3   Taking Requests for Medication or Prescription Refills

Outcome Take a message requesting medication or a prescription refill

Equipment/Supplies

- Telephone
- Computer
- Message pad
- Pen or pencil
- Medical record
- Clock or watch

1. Procedural Step. Identify the caller and telephone number.

2. Procedural Step. Identify whether the caller is a patient or a pharmacy employee.

3. Procedural Step. If the caller is a patient, identify the patient and date of birth. Take the information about the medication requested, dose, and number of times a day the patient takes the medication. Write down or enter into the computer the name and telephone number of the patient's preferred pharmacy or mail order supplier.

4. Procedural Step. If the caller is a pharmacy employee, usually the medical assistant takes a message, including the name and address of the patient, the medication requested, and the dosage and amount of medication to be prescribed. Inform the pharmacy when the physician is likely to approve the refill so that the pharmacy can tell the patient.
Principle. Usually physicians have specific times when they review tend respond to messages.

5. Procedural Step. End the call politely.

Continued

PROCEDURE 41-3   Taking Requests for Medication or Prescription Refills—cont'd

6. **Procedural Step.** Follow usual procedures to attach the patient's medical record to the message (either manually or electronically) and place the message where the physician can review it, or send the message electronically.
   Principle. The physician will need to review information about the patient before agreeing to refill or prescribe medication.

7. **Procedural Step.** Usually the physician fills the prescription directly by computer, indicates on the message slip whether the prescription may be refilled, or writes a new prescription on the message slip for the medical assistant to call or fax the pharmacy with the information. Read the prescription from the message slip exactly as the physician has written it.
   Principle. The medical assistant functions as an agent of the physician in this case. He or she must give the exact information the physician has indicated.

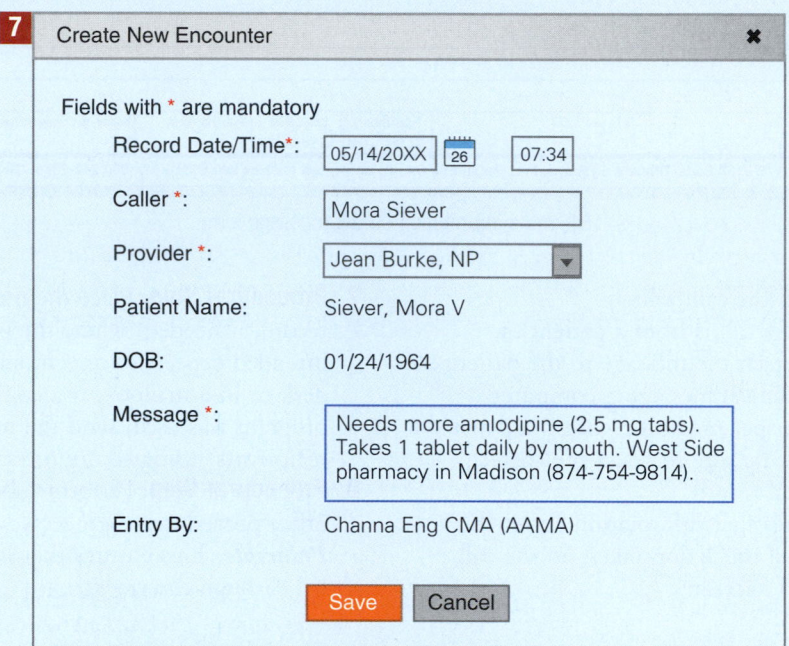

7   Create New Encounter   ✖

Fields with * are mandatory

Record Date/Time*:	05/14/20XX 📅 26 07:34
Caller *:	Mora Siever
Provider *:	Jean Burke, NP ▼
Patient Name:	Siever, Mora V
DOB:	01/24/1964
Message *:	Needs more amlodipine (2.5 mg tabs). Takes 1 tablet daily by mouth. West Side pharmacy in Madison (874-754-9814).
Entry By:	Channa Eng CMA (AAMA)

Save   Cancel

The physician may write prescription information on the message form in SimChart® for the Medical Office.

8. **Procedural Step.** Verify that the refill or prescription has been documented in the patient's medical record. In some offices the message itself is filed in the medical record. See Chapter 38 to review common abbreviations used when documenting medications.

   Principle. Any treatment of the patient must be documented in the medical record as part of the continuous record of care given.

OUTGOING CALLS

More calls come into the office than go out. But there are certainly enough outgoing calls. Medical assistants make many of them. Outgoing calls a medical assistant may make include calls to patients, suppliers, insurance companies, other medical offices, laboratories, pharmacies, and hospitals. In some systems it is necessary to dial the number 9 before the telephone number to get an outside line. Telephone numbers of businesses can be looked up using the Internet, but it is helpful to keep an office directory of frequently called numbers.

LOCAL CALLS

Calls to patients, whether the matter is medical or financial, should be made from the front desk only if the privacy window is closed. The medical assistant must prepare information and supplies before making the call. If the medical assistant is calling a patient, the patient's medical record should be at hand with any notes from the physician. If the call is picked up by an answering machine, it is permissible to leave your name, practice name, and telephone number for the patient to call back. Because the patient's family members may have access to the answering machine or voicemail, no medical information should be included in the message (Procedure 41-4).

It may be necessary to call a patient about an overdue account. The medical assistant should not call the patient at work for this type of call or discuss billing information with anyone other than the person responsible for the bill.

For calls to laboratories, hospitals, or suppliers, the medical assistant should be sure to have organized the information necessary to complete the call before dialing the telephone number.

If the medical assistant places a call for one of the office's physicians, the physician must be ready to talk before the call is placed. As soon as the physician being called is located, the medical assistant connects the physician placing the call.

Medical assistants and other office staff should not make or receive personal calls using the office telephone system except for emergencies, both to avoid tying up the telephone and because telephone calls take time away from work. The medical assistant can check messages and make outgoing calls during breaks or at lunchtime using a pay phone or personal cell phone. Although permission may be given to make an urgent call using the office telephone, a personal long-distance call is never appropriate. In most offices medical assistants are not allowed to carry cell phones while they are working even if the phones are set to vibrate instead of ringing. Cell phones can interfere with medical equipment, such as electrocardiographs. They can also be a distraction, even if they do not make a noise.

What Would You Do? What Would You *Not* Do?

Case Study 3
The physician asks Channa to schedule an appointment for Andrew Page, a 35-year-old man whose recent lipid profile shows an elevated cholesterol and triglyceride level. This is a change from previous laboratory work. The physician says to tell the patient that he wants to discuss the recent blood work in person. When Channa calls the patient, his wife answers the telephone. Channa identifies herself and the medical office and asks to leave a message for Mr. Page to return her call. Mrs. Page says, "He's away on a business trip until Thursday. What is this about? Is it really important?" ∎

APPOINTMENT REMINDERS

Medical assistants may be asked to place reminder telephone calls to patients 24 to 48 hours before their scheduled appointments. The HIPAA Privacy Rule allows health care providers to call patients and leave messages regarding their care as long as the patient has not requested confidential communication. It is recommended to limit the information left in a message to the minimum required to confirm the appointment.

Medical offices have begun to use computer programs that interface with scheduling programs and call patients automatically 24 to 48 hours before a scheduled appointment. They provide a recorded message about the appointment and will leave a message if no one answers the telephone. It may be possible for the person who answers the call to confirm or cancel the appointment after listening to the recorded message. The patient is instructed to call the office with any questions or to change the appointment.

LONG-DISTANCE CALLS

Long-distance calls are almost always dialed directly. The telephone number for a long-distance call can be obtained from directory assistance (411). When calling distant locations, it is important to be aware of the different time zones. To make international calls, the medical assistant should dial 1, then the country code, then the telephone number. To prevent unauthorized long-distance calls, most offices have a code that must be used to access the long-distance system, especially for international calls. Long-distance services may also be limited to one or two extensions.

CONFERENCE CALLS

Some phone systems allow conference calls among three or more parties, such as a physician and other individuals who are being called at different telephone numbers. If the telephone system allows this, the medical assistant should learn how to set up such calls for the physicians. Conference calls among several parties are sometimes scheduled using a special service.

Memories *from* Practicum

Channa Eng: I was terrified of the telephone when I first started my practicum. It was a busy clinic, and I started out in adult medicine. In the morning, I sat at the front desk to check patients in, take copayments, and answer the telephone. I was always afraid that I wouldn't know what to say. We got the callers who wanted to speak to someone in person, so you never knew what to expect. My supervisor told me to answer each call by saying "hello" followed by my name and the name of the clinic, and then ask how I could help the caller. If I didn't know how to handle the call, I was supposed to put the caller on hold and ask Mary Lynn, the other medical assistant, for guidance. One call that I remember particularly was from an older woman who seemed lonely and confused. She asked for her physician, but she was willing to leave a message when I told her that the physician didn't take calls while he was seeing patients. She said that she couldn't remember if she was supposed to take her blood pressure medication once a day or twice a day and she wasn't sure if it was one pill or two pills. She told me that her daughter set up her pills in a pill container every week but she had forgotten if she should take them both in the morning or one in the morning and one at night. I told her to get the bottle of medication and read the label to me. From the label we determined that she was supposed to take two pills every morning. She thanked me, and I indicated on the message form that we had clarified the problem. After the call, Mary Lynn complimented me for being so helpful and for handling the call by myself. After that I began to feel more confident about taking telephone calls. ∎

PROCEDURE 41-4 Telephoning a Patient for Follow-Up

Outcome Place an outgoing telephone call to a patient for follow-up

Equipment/Supplies

- Telephone
- Scratch paper
- Pen or pencil

- Material necessary to place the call, including the telephone number, instructions from physician, and/or patient medical record

1. **Procedural Step.** Organize all materials that may be necessary during the telephone call. Schedule calls during business hours.
   Principle. Preparation allows calls to be made more efficiently.

2. **Procedural Step.** Write the telephone number on a piece of paper. Include the area code and a country code, if necessary.
   Principle. It may be difficult to remember the number, especially if you do not reach the number on the first attempt.

3. **Procedural Step.** Place the call. When it is answered, ask for your party. Identify yourself with your practice's name and your name ("This is Channa from Primary Care Associates").

4. **Procedural Step.** If you reach an answering machine, identify yourself with your practice name and your name and ask the intended recipient to call you back. Leave your telephone number with area code.

Principle. Unless it is an appointment reminder, the subject of the telephone call should not be left on an answering machine to protect patient confidentiality.

5. **Procedural Step.** If you are speaking to the patient, give the information requested by the physician. This may be an instruction to make an appointment or may include laboratory results. Do not give more information than the physician has authorized.
   Principle. As an agent of the physician, you have limited authorization to provide information.

6. **Procedural Step.** If the patient has additional questions, offer to take a message for the physician.

7. **Procedural Step.** Close the call politely. Repeat instructions if any were given.

8. **Procedural Step.** Document the telephone call including the name of the physician who instructed you to make the call (if any). Include any specific instructions given to the patient in the documentation.

What Would You Do? | What Would You *Not* Do? | RESPONSES

Case Study 1
Page 1068

What Did Channa Do?
- ❑ Spoke politely, and told Mrs. Weston that she needed to pick up the other call.
- ❑ Gave Mrs. Weston the choice of being placed on hold or being called back.
- ❑ Assured Mrs. Weston that she would get back to the telephone call with her as soon as possible.
- ❑ Kept her voice calm and friendly.

What Did Channa Not Do?
- ❑ Did not let the second telephone call ring more than three times.
- ❑ Did not promise Mrs. Weston that she would put the other call on hold immediately.
- ❑ Did not try to rush through the call with Mrs. Weston without making sure that she is clear about the appointment date and time.

Case Study 2
Page 1070

What Did Channa Do?
- ❑ Told Mrs. Woodward to get the bottle of pills, which has a record of the dose and exact name of the pharmacy.
- ❑ Told Mrs. Woodward she would place her on hold; instructed Mrs. Woodward to stay on the line after finding the medication bottle.
- ❑ Gave Mrs. Woodward the option of calling back when she had found the bottle of pills.
- ❑ Told Mrs. Woodward that the physician would be glad to send the prescription directly to the pharmacy, and instructed her to check with the pharmacy the next day.
- ❑ Remained calm and friendly.
- ❑ Made sure to follow up and complete the message.
- ❑ Updated the pharmacy information in the EMR if it has changed.

What Did Channa Not Do?
- ❑ Did not become impatient or tell Mrs. Woodward that she should know she needed her bottle of medication ready when she called to ask for a refill.
- ❑ Did not pass on the message without confirming that Mrs. Woodward had asked for the correct dose of medication.
- ❑ Did not pass on the message without confirming the name and location of the pharmacy.

What Would You Do? | What Would You *Not* Do? | RESPONSES—cont'd

Case Study 3
Page 1075

What Did Channa Do?
- ❑ Reassured Mrs. Page that it was not an urgent matter, but said she hoped Mr. Page would return her call after his trip.
- ❑ Told Mrs. Page politely that she could not discuss the matter with anyone but Mr. Page.

What Did Channa Not Do?
- ❑ Did not tell Mrs. Page exactly why she was calling her husband.
- ❑ Did not tell Mrs. Page that the matter was not important.
- ❑ Did not ask Mrs. Page to contact her husband before he returned from his business trip.
- ❑ Did not tell Mrs. Page that the physician could give her more information about the matter.

↻ TERMINOLOGY REVIEW

Key Term	Definition
Enunciation	The act of speaking clearly and concisely.
Pager	An electronic device that notifies the recipient to receive a message or return a telephone call.
Smartphone	A cell phone with computer capabilities.
Voicemail	A method for delivery, storage, and retrieval of telephone messages that is built into the telephone system.

ON THE WEB

For information on HIPAA (Health Insurance Portability and Accountability Act) and appointment reminders:

U. S. Department of Health and Human Services: www.hhs.gov/ocr/privacy/hipaa/faq/smaller_providers_and_businesses/286.html

For information on poison control centers:

American Association of Poison Control Centers: www.aapcc.org

National Capital Poison Center: www.poison.org

For information on time zones:

The Official U.S. Time: www.time.gov

42 Scheduling Appointments

(e) Check out the Evolve site at http://evolve.elsevier.com/Bonewit/today/ to access additional interactive activities and exercises to help you study and prepare for success.

LEARNING OBJECTIVES   PROCEDURES

Methods of Scheduling
1. Describe how scheduling appointments efficiently meets the needs of both physicians and patients.
2. Describe the correct use of computer scheduling to make appointments.
3. Explain why the medical office must retain an official record of patients seen each day (daily appointment schedule).

Types of Scheduling
4. Describe several types of scheduling, including stream scheduling, wave scheduling, modified wave scheduling, double booking, open booking, and patient self-scheduling.
5. Identify types of patient appointments that may be clustered in the appointment schedule.

Setting up the Appointment Schedule
6. Identify factors to be considered when setting up the appointment schedule.   Set up the appointment schedule.
7. Explain how to set up the appointment schedule.

Making an Appointment
8. Differentiate between the information needed to make an appointment for a new patient   Make an appointment.
   and for an established patient.
9. Differentiate among medical conditions that require emergency care, urgent care, and routine care.
10. Describe how to schedule appointments for individuals who are not patients.

Managing the Appointment Schedule
11. Describe the method for changing or canceling appointments.   Manage the appointment schedule.
12. Describe how to document changes to the appointment schedule and cancellations or no-shows in the medical record.
13. Identify three methods to remind patients to make or keep appointments.
14. Discuss the storage of appointment schedules and/or daily schedules.

Scheduling Diagnostic Tests, Procedures, and Admissions
15. Identify how to schedule inpatient and outpatient diagnostic tests and procedures.   Schedule inpatient and outpatient diagnostic tests or procedures.
16. Identify how to schedule hospital admissions and surgery.   Schedule inpatient or outpatient admissions.

CHAPTER OUTLINE

INTRODUCTION TO APPOINTMENT SCHEDULING
GUIDELINES FOR APPOINTMENT SCHEDULING
SCHEDULING APPOINTMENTS
DAILY APPOINTMENT SCHEDULE
TYPES OF SCHEDULING

Time-Specified (Stream) Scheduling
Wave Scheduling
Modified Wave Scheduling
Double Booking
Open Booking

Patient Appointment Requests and Self-Scheduling
Clustering or Categorization
Multiple Offices
SETTING UP THE APPOINTMENT SCHEDULE
Appointment Intervals
Physician's Preferences and Needs
Facility and Equipment Requirements
GUIDELINES FOR SCHEDULING
Established Patients
Special Situations
New Patients
Same-Day Appointments
Urgent Care and Emergencies
Walk-in Patients
Individuals Who Are Not Patients

MANAGING THE APPOINTMENT SCHEDULE
Changing Appointments
Late Patients
Appointment Reminders
Storing Appointment Books and Daily Schedules
SCHEDULING REFERRAL APPOINTMENTS, DIAGNOSTIC
    TESTS, PROCEDURES, AND ADMISSIONS
Referrals
Scheduling Diagnostic Procedures and Hospital
    Admissions
Scheduling a Diagnostic Procedure
Scheduling an Inpatient Admission
Scheduling Surgery
Giving a Patient Instructions Before Surgery
Documenting an Appointment for Surgery

KEY TERMS

appointment matrix (MAY-trix)
blocked
clustering
double booking
established patient
fixed appointment scheduling
hospice (HOSS-piss)

modified wave scheduling
new patient
no-show
patient self-scheduling
preadmission testing (PAT)
preauthorization
    (pree-awe-thur-eye-ZAY-shun)

referral
single booking
stream scheduling
time-specified scheduling
triage (TREE-ahzh)
wave scheduling

INTRODUCTION TO APPOINTMENT SCHEDULING

Scheduling appointments is one of the most important administrative responsibilities performed in the medical office. Until the 1970s, people went to a medical office expecting to wait as long as an hour or more. Most physicians liked to see a full waiting room; it reassured them that their practice was healthy.

In the twenty-first century, people have little tolerance for waiting in a medical office. Lifestyles have changed and people have busy lives. Many have to take personal time away from work to go to the medical office, and they feel that their time is as valuable as the physician's time. In the patient-centered medical home (PCMH) one of the key goals is to reduce patient wait time and provide same-day appointments if needed. PCMH is discussed in more detail in Chapter 1.

Scheduling appointments correctly and efficiently is crucial to the smooth operation of the medical office. Many factors must be taken into consideration when scheduling appointments. The patient who has made an appointment weeks or even months in advance wants to be seen within 15 minutes after arriving at the medical office. The physician wants a smooth flow of patients during the time

scheduled for seeing patients. Patients who are ill or have accidents want to be able to see their physician on the day of the illness or injury. They prefer to be given a specific time, even if it is later in the day, rather than come into the office and wait for an open moment.

GUIDELINES FOR APPOINTMENT SCHEDULING

When scheduling appointments, it is important for the medical assistant to use good interpersonal skills and to minimize the amount of time a patient has to wait to see the physician. To accomplish this, the medical assistant should follow seven guidelines:
1. Maintain the confidentiality of the patient. For example, do not discuss protected health information within hearing distance of other patients.
2. Speak clearly and do not appear rushed. Make sure the tone of your voice is friendly and courteous.
3. Concentrate only on the person to whom you are speaking.
4. Obtain all the necessary information from the patient. Make sure the information is both correct and complete.

5. Repeat the information relayed to you by the patient. This avoids errors.
6. Schedule the proper amount of time for the type of appointment you are scheduling. For example, a new patient requires more time than an established patient.
7. Document all of the necessary information correctly in the appointment schedule.

SCHEDULING APPOINTMENTS

Appointments are almost always scheduled using a computerized appointment scheduling program. Using a computer to schedule appointments offers advantages. The computer allows the medical assistant to designate appointment intervals. The appointment interval can be adjusted to 10, 15, or 20 minutes depending on the needs of the practice. The computer makes it easy to add, delete, or change appointments; set up repeating appointments; and set up a recall system. A recall system identifies patients that need to be contacted when it is time for them to schedule another appointment.

The medical assistant enters the patient's appointment into a data entry screen (Figure 42-1). This screen requires the entry of the same information as a paper appointment book, although all information linked to an appointment may not be visible on the main screen. The computer also allows the medical assistant to print out a daily appointment schedule of patients to be seen that day.

Appointment Book Scheduling

Appointment books are usually spiral-bound, so they will lie flat when opened. Occasionally a paper appointment book is used in the medical office as a back-up to the computer schedule. Appointment books are available in the following formats: pages for a single day, pages that display a week when open (over two pages), or pages with two or three physicians' schedules for a single day. The pages are further divided into time intervals. The pages are typically divided into 10- or 15-minute intervals.

Figure 42-1 Medical assistant making an appointment.

DAILY APPOINTMENT SCHEDULE

In a computer appointment scheduling program, the daily appointment schedule can be viewed on the computer, and an updated hard copy can be printed as needed. It may be used as a guide for pulling patients' paper medical records or appointment reminder calls. A printed appointment schedule usually contains the patients' names and telephone numbers and the reasons for their visits (e.g., new patient, physical examination, recheck) (Figure 42-2). According to Health Insurance Portability and Accountability Act (HIPAA) requirements, the daily appointment schedule should never be posted in an office area accessible to patients. The office must keep an updated record either on paper or electronically to verify tax returns and insurance claims.

TYPES OF SCHEDULING

Several methods are available to schedule appointments in the medical office. They include time-specified scheduling, wave scheduling, modified wave scheduling, double booking, and open booking. Many offices allow established patients to request appointments or schedule appointments using the Internet. In addition, appointments may be clustered or categorized depending on the type of patient or type of examination or treatment. The method an office uses to schedule appointments is based on the needs of the practice and physician preference.

TIME-SPECIFIED (STREAM) SCHEDULING

Time-specified scheduling, also known as **stream scheduling,** involves scheduling appointments at a specific time. Most offices use this method for scheduling appointments. The goal of time-specified appointments is to minimize the waiting time for the patient and at the same time to keep a steady flow of patients moving through the office (like a stream of water). The amount of time allotted for a time-specified appointment depends on the reason for the visit. In general, the following times are allotted:

- New patient: 30 to 45 minutes
- Complete physical examination: 30 to 45 minutes
- Established patient: 10 to 20 minutes

When using the time-specified method, the medical assistant needs to make sure to allow time in the schedule to accommodate urgent visits, such as from ill or injured patients. There are two other terms that may be used for this type of scheduling: **fixed appointment scheduling** and **single booking.**

WAVE SCHEDULING

With **wave scheduling,** three or four patients are scheduled every hour and are seen in the order in which they arrive

Western Medical Center

Richard Warner, MD
Schedule for May 30, 20XX

Time	Name	Reason	Home Phone	Work Phone
9:00 AM	ROBERT RICIGLIANO	Physical exam	(490) 459-2811	(490) 459-6217
9:10 AM	*			
9:20 AM	*			
9:30 AM	JUNE ST. JAMES	BP & ECG	(490) 459-5807	(490) 459-9222
9:40 AM	*			
9:50 AM	DARLA SISSLE	Influenza vaccine	(490) 220-1156	
10:00 AM	Catch-up			
10:10 AM	*			
10:20 AM	LLOYD RIDLON	Recheck	(490) 459-4242	(490) 459-0419
10:30 AM	ESTELLE JORDAN	New patient	(490) 459-8249	(490) 459-1062
10:40 AM	*			
10:50 AM	*			
11:00 AM	MARIA SANTOS	Physical exam	(490) 459-0022	
11:10 AM	*			
11:20 AM	THOMAS MAXWELL	Recheck	(490) 459-4123	(490) 459-9201
11:30 AM	*			
11:40 AM	ROBIN SOTO	Well baby	(490) 459-1349	
11:50 AM	*			
12:00 PM	LUNCH			
12:10 PM	*			
12:20 PM	*			
12:30 PM	*			
12:40 PM	*			
12:50 PM	*			
1:00 PM	LUCILLE MORENA	Chem screen	(490) 459-6677	(490) 459-1566
1:10 PM	*			
1:20 PM	*			
1:30 PM	*			

Figure 42-2 Daily appointment schedule.

at the office. The goal is for patients to arrive in "waves" so that there is always a patient waiting to be seen. Sometimes, ill patients are seen before those with routine appointments.

This scheduling system assumes that some patients will need to be worked into the schedule. Sometimes patients become uncomfortable when they realize that another patient was given the same appointment time, but a simple explanation can usually reassure the patient. The medical assistant might say, "We schedule all our patients on the hour, and then they are seen in the order they arrive. There is always a patient to be seen, and we find that patient don't really arrive all at once."

MODIFIED WAVE SCHEDULING

The wave system can be changed in several ways. This is called **modified wave scheduling.** The office may schedule patients at specific times during the first half of each hour,

and keep the second half-hour open for special circumstances. This may include working in patients, seeing patients who arrived late, or finishing up with patients from the first half-hour.

Another modification to the wave system is to schedule one appointment that is expected to take longer (e.g., physical examination) on the hour and to schedule three or four follow-up appointments on the half-hour (Figure 42-3).

DOUBLE BOOKING

When two patients are given the same appointment time, the practice is called **double booking.** Double booking means that two patients are scheduled into a single time slot. Double booking may be used when a patient can be fitted in around a patient undergoing a diagnostic procedure such as an electrocardiogram (ECG). It is also used for siblings in a pediatric practice or when a patient with an injury or acute illness must be added to an already-full schedule.

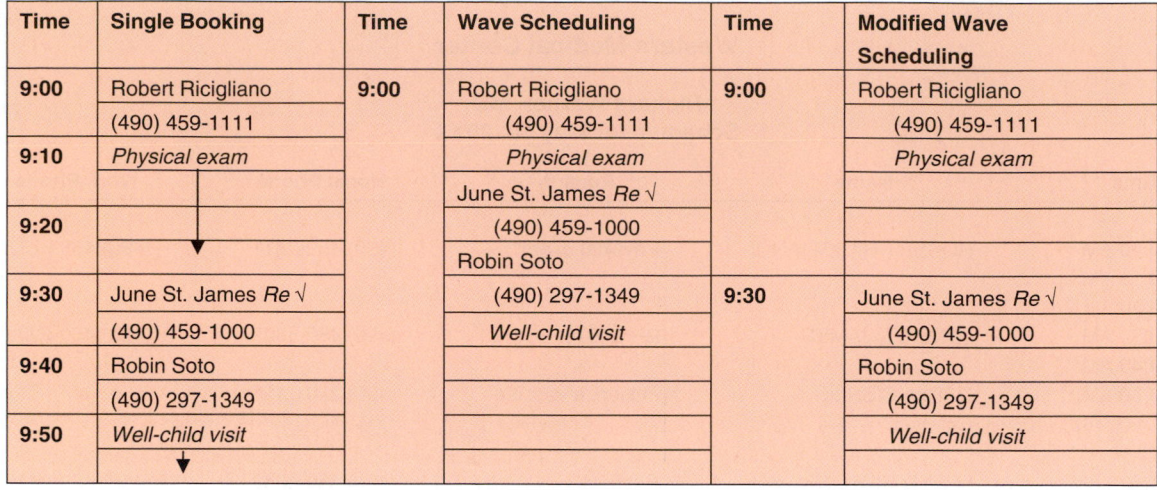

Time	Single Booking	Time	Wave Scheduling	Time	Modified Wave Scheduling
9:00	Robert Ricigliano	9:00	Robert Ricigliano	9:00	Robert Ricigliano
	(490) 459-1111		(490) 459-1111		(490) 459-1111
9:10	*Physical exam*		*Physical exam*		*Physical exam*
			June St. James *Re* √		
9:20			(490) 459-1000		
			Robin Soto		
9:30	June St. James *Re* √		(490) 297-1349	9:30	June St. James *Re* √
	(490) 459-1000		*Well-child visit*		(490) 459-1000
9:40	Robin Soto				Robin Soto
	(490) 297-1349				(490) 297-1349
9:50	*Well-child visit*				*Well-child visit*

Figure 42-3 Comparison of single booking, wave scheduling, and modified wave scheduling.

OPEN BOOKING

Sometimes patients are not given a specific appointment time but are told to come in during a time range, such as between 9:00 AM and 11:00 AM. The patients are then seen in the order in which they arrive. In an open-booking system, patients with an injury or an acute illness may be seen ahead of patients with less significant complaints.

Sometimes medical offices and clinics have walk-in hours designated for urgent care before regular office hours. In this situation, patients are seen in the order of arrival.

Open booking works best when there is a constant stream of patients or when a practice is not busy. Because patient flow is unpredictable, patients often have to wait a long time.

PATIENT APPOINTMENT REQUESTS AND SELF-SCHEDULING

Many medical practices allow patients to request routine appointments from the practice website. Office staff usually schedules the appointment, making every effort to accommodate the patient's request. After the appointment has been made, staff notifies the patient either electronically or by a letter. Some practices even give patients limited access to their appointment scheduling software so that patients can schedule their own appointments if a desired time is available. This is called **patient self-scheduling.**

CLUSTERING OR CATEGORIZATION

Clustering involves scheduling patients with similar problems or conditions into groups. Each group is seen on a certain day or within a certain time block during the day. This scheduling method is also called *categorization.*

Examples of conditions that can easily be clustered into a day or portion of a day are as follows:
- Physical examinations
- Prenatal patient visits in an obstetrics and gynecology (OB/GYN) practice
- Diagnostic procedures

MULTIPLE OFFICES

Some physicians see patients in more than one office. Appointments may be scheduled in each office or through a central system. In this case, it is important to clarify which office the patient wants to visit. When there are multiple offices, it is an advantage to have an electronic medical record (EMR). If a paper record system is used, patients are encouraged to choose one location where their record will be stored.

SETTING UP THE APPOINTMENT SCHEDULE

Appointments are usually scheduled up to 6 months in advance. Before scheduling can begin, the appointment book or computer software must be set up to indicate the times when the physician will see patients. Times when the physician is not available to see patients must be **blocked** out. The appointment schedule showing only available times for appointments is sometimes called the **appointment matrix** because it is the basic pattern of available patient appointment times (Procedure 42-1).

How the times are blocked out depends on the scheduling method used by the office. If the office uses an appointment book, the times are blocked out by drawing lines through the blocked times. If a computer is used to schedule appointments, the times are blocked out by setting aside blocks of time. Various types of color-coding are used in a computer scheduling program, but blocked times are different colors than open appointment times (Figure 42-4).

The appointment schedule must take three variables into consideration: the scheduling system, the physician's preferences and needs, and the facility and equipment requirements. Each of these is discussed later.

APPOINTMENT INTERVALS

Appointments are usually scheduled at intervals of 10 minutes, 15 minutes, or 20 minutes. An appointment may be scheduled for more than one block, depending on the type of appointment. For example, if a 10-minute interval is used, an established patient coming to have his blood pressure checked might be scheduled for one 10-minute interval and a new patient might be scheduled for three

10-minute intervals. In this case, a 10-minute interval uses one line and a new patient uses three lines in the schedule. If a 15-minute interval is used, all appointments are scheduled in multiples of 15 minutes. In general, more time must be allotted for new patients, physical examinations, and special procedures than for routine follow-up visits.

PHYSICIAN'S PREFERENCES AND NEEDS

The second variable influencing the appointment schedule is the physician's preferences and needs. Physicians may prefer to do physical examinations and/or procedures at specific times as well as a certain number of either during a day. The appointment slots for those times would need to indicate the type of visit (such as a physical). If there are multiple physicians, their preferences may vary and certain rooms may need to be shared.

Figure 42-4 Appointment Schedule from SimChart® for the Medical Office.

At times during the day the physician is not able to see patients, and therefore these times must be blocked out on the schedule. Time must be blocked out when the physician has another obligation, such as hospital rounds and nursing-home visits. Time may also need to be blocked out for lunch, pharmaceutical representative visits, and catch-up. Days are also blocked out of the schedule for vacation, days off, attendance at conferences, lectures to be given, and other professional activities. Protocols for each physician should be kept available for those setting up the appointment schedule.

FACILITY AND EQUIPMENT REQUIREMENTS

The third variable affecting the appointment schedule is the availability of facilities and equipment. The appointment schedule must be set up so that examination rooms and rooms with equipment required for certain procedures are available to all physicians who are seeing patients. For optimal use of resources, one or more physicians should be available to see patients whenever the office is open. Physicians like to have at least two examination rooms available for seeing patients, preferably side by side. This improves efficiency and time management for examining patients. In many scheduling programs, the examination room can be scheduled with the visit. In other types of programs, the examination room number is added to the appointment after the patient arrives and has been escorted to the room.

PROCEDURE 42-1 Setting up the Appointment Schedule

Outcome

1. Set up an appointment schedule
2. Implement time management principles to maintain effective office functions

Equipment/Supplies

- Computer appointment schedule or appointment book
- Pen
- Physician schedule
- Office calendar

1. **Procedural Step.** Block times when the office is not open to see patients. This includes times before office hours begin, lunch and/or breaks for all office staff, afternoons or days when the office is closed, and holidays when the office will be closed. Some offices set up the appointment schedule 6 months in advance, whereas others do it for a year in advance. In a computer schedule, either set up the schedule so that only times when the office is open appear on the schedule, or block times when the office is closed. In an appointment book, draw an X through times when the office is closed.
   Principle. In an effective appointment schedule, only available appointment times are blank.

2. **Procedural Step.** Block times when each individual physician is not available to see patients, including lunch (if the office does not close for lunch) and hospital rounds. In addition, block days when each

physician will be away from the office for vacations, conferences, or other anticipated absences. If the physician has regular meetings or other regular commitments (such as nursing home visits), mark these also. In a computer schedule, schedule the meeting, vacation, or other anticipated absence like an appointment, using color-coding to show that the times are unavailable. In an appointment book, draw an X through the times when the physician is not available.

3. **Procedural Step.** For each physician, mark times when the physician does certain types of examinations, procedures (e.g., physical examinations, obstetric visits), or surgery. In a computer schedule these times may be set up as if for a separate physician (e.g., "Dr. Gomez and Dr. Gomez—OB visits"), or a color-coding system can be used. In an appointment book these are often highlighted with a marker or given a written title at the beginning of the time block.

PROCEDURE 42-1   Setting up the Appointment Schedule—cont'd

4. Procedural Step. Depending on office policy, block out as much time as is anticipated for same-day appointments, catch-up time, and unexpected needs. Depending on the practice, catch-up time may be 15 minutes in the morning and afternoon for each doctor, and time for same-day appointments may be an hour or longer for all physicians or one particular physician on a rotating basis. These times can be marked in various ways as long as it is generally understood that they must be saved until the scheduled day.

Example. On this day, the office will be open from 9 to 5, but Dr. Martin will be available to see patients only from 9 to 12 because he plans to attend a conference in the afternoon. The appointment interval is 15 minutes. Dr. Warner likes to have 15 minutes set aside for catch-up time at 10:30 in the morning.

4 | **James A. Martin, MD**
- 8am — Office closed: All Staff
- 9am
- 10am
- Catch-up: James A. Martin, MD
- 11am
- 12pm — Out-of-office: James A. Martin, MD

In SimChart® for the Medical Office, block times when the physician is not available using a colored background. (*Note:* "Catch-up" may also be called "buffer time.")

PROCEDURE 42-1

GUIDELINES FOR SCHEDULING

When scheduling an appointment, the medical assistant needs to obtain the proper information from the patient, document it accurately, and confirm it with the patient. The procedure for scheduling appointments varies depending on whether the patient is an established patient or a new patient.

ESTABLISHED PATIENTS

For insurance billing, an **established patient** is defined as a patient who has received services from the physician or another physician of the same specialty in the same group practice within the past 3 years. If the patient has been seen by a physician in the group who specializes in primary care (internal medicine, family practice, or pediatrics), this does not make the patient an established patient for other specialties. For example, a patient has been treated for several years by a family practice physician who refers the patient to an orthopedic surgeon within the group. The patient is a new patient for the orthopedic surgeon. If the patient is seen by a different family practice physician for an urgent care appointment, the patient is an established patient for that physician. Patients who have not been seen within the past 3 years are typically treated as new patients, although their old medical records should be found if possible.

If an established patient is scheduling a return appointment after a visit, the physician usually specifies a time interval for the return visit (e.g., 1 week, 2 weeks, 1 month, 6 months). The appointment should be scheduled as close

as possible to the interval specified by the physician. The appointment must also be scheduled for the length of time preferred by the physician, which is usually 10 to 15 minutes. Before locating available appointment times to offer the patient, the medical assistant should ask what day of the week and what time of day are convenient for the patient. For an established patient, it is necessary to obtain the patient's name, date of birth, and physician. When the correct patient is selected, other demographic information (e.g., telephone number, address) is automatically linked to the appointment.

If the patient is at the office, the medical assistant should complete an appointment reminder card and give it to the patient. The medical assistant enters the patient's name, the name of the physician, and the date and time of the new appointment on the card.

If the patient has submitted an appointment request electronically, the medical assistant should attempt to accommodate the patient's wishes when scheduling the appointment or should make the appointment as close to the time requested as possible. The patient should receive an email or letter verifying the date and time of the appointment.

Special Situations

Some situations require special attention when scheduling an appointment for an established patient. The most common situation is when a patient visits the medical office and the physician orders laboratory tests to be performed at a medical laboratory. The physician will want to review the results of these tests before the patient comes in for a return visit. When scheduling the patient's return visit, the medical assistant must be sure to allow enough time for the patient to have these tests performed and the results to be entered into the computer system or returned to the office.

Patients who must undergo a laboratory test at the medical office that requires fasting (e.g., fasting blood sugar) should be scheduled early in the morning and provided with written instructions. This provides the least amount of inconvenience for the patient, who must abstain from food and fluids until the specimen has been collected.

Sometimes the patient needs to be scheduled for an appointment for a date later than can be accommodated by the appointment schedule. In this situation, the medical assistant can either tell the patient the date when he or she can request the appointment or the patient's name can be put on a recall list. When the patient's name comes up, the medical assistant either schedules the appointment and notifies the patient or sends a letter reminding the patient to schedule the appointment.

NEW PATIENTS

Specific information needs to be obtained when scheduling an appointment for a **new patient.** This includes the patient's full name and daytime telephone number and the reason for the visit or type of visit (e.g., sick visit, physical examination, diagnostic procedure). The medical assistant should ask the patient if he or she has been referred by another physician and determine the patient's insurance and if that insurance requires preauthorization (precertification). The process for verifying that insurance requirements have been met is discussed later in the chapter.

Most offices schedule new patients for 30 to 45 minutes. The medical assistant should set aside the correct amount of time for the appointment depending on the physician's preference.

The medical assistant may need to relay directions to the office location to the patient. Some offices mail the health history form to new patients and instruct them to bring the completed form to the first appointment. An office brochure containing information about the practice may also be mailed to the patient or given to the patient at the first appointment.

When the patient has been referred by another physician, the patient should be given an appointment as soon as possible, especially if the patient has urgent symptoms or if the patient's primary physician's office is calling to make the appointment (Procedure 42-2).

SAME-DAY APPOINTMENTS

The following problems are usually treated in the medical office and are usually scheduled the same day as the patient calls. The medical assistant should be familiar with office policy because each office varies in the degree of complexity of care it offers.
- Wounds without fracture or dislocation
- Sprains and strains

- Nausea, vomiting, or diarrhea that has persisted for more than 2 or 3 days
- Fever (defined by office guidelines)
- Sudden illness or severe pain without bleeding, fainting, or loss of consciousness
- Sore throat, especially with fever
- Burning, frequency, or urgency associated with urination, especially if accompanied by fever or blood in the urine
- Vaginal bleeding in a pregnant woman (who may also be sent to the emergency department)

If a patient's primary physician's schedule is booked, patients with these types of conditions may need to be scheduled with a practitioner who has a more flexible schedule. When there are several practitioners in an office, a period of time may be blocked off in one physician's schedule to accommodate same-day appointments.

Putting It All Into Practice

My name is Elaine Wyatt, and I am a Certified Medical Assistant. My primary responsibility is to schedule routine and urgent care appointments, although sometimes I sit at the front desk and check patients in. I work in an office with five internists and two nurse practitioners. Calls from patients who select "make an appointment" from our telephone menu will end up with me or another medical assistant, or the receptionist may transfer a call to me. I also check patients out after they have been seen and make follow-up appointments using our computer system. Sometimes the telephone is ringing off the hook, and I really have to concentrate to keep track of each call. Our office has a procedure manual with guidelines for handling urgent calls, and we try very hard to give patients appointments the same day if they are sick. We leave several open appointments for this, but even if we have to double book, we will fit them in because our physicians want to be sure that everyone receives the care they need. All of our physicians and nurse practitioners are accepting new patients, and we always ask new patients to arrive at the office about 15 minutes early to fill out a patient history form. Usually our appointment system works pretty well and patients do not have to wait more than 10 or 15 minutes—at least, that is our goal. There are days, of course, when the physicians get behind, but through trial and error, we have developed a system that works pretty well for us. ■

URGENT CARE AND EMERGENCIES

The majority of appointments are made well in advance of the date a patient will see the physician, but there are times when urgent or emergency situations occur. A patient calling the office with an emergency presents a challenging situation for the medical assistant. It is important to give a caller a chance to tell you that it is an urgent situation before putting the call on hold. A life-threatening or serious medical problem should be immediately referred to the physician. The physician will make the decision about the appropriate course of action to take. If the physician is not present, the caller should be referred to the emergency medical services system, usually activated by calling 911 (Box 42-1). The office procedure manual should be used when responding to emergencies.

WALK-IN PATIENTS

Sometimes patients come to the office without an appointment and ask to be seen. If the patient is experiencing an

emergency or urgent problem, the physician may ask the medical assistant to work the patient into the schedule. In routine situations, however, the patient is asked to return at a later date and is offered an appointment. In these situations the medical assistant should tactfully inform the patient of the medical office policy with respect to scheduling appointments.

INDIVIDUALS WHO ARE NOT PATIENTS

During office hours the physician may see various individuals who are not patients. Time should be blocked from the schedule to accommodate these appointments. Many offices have a specific time slot, often during the lunch hour, to schedule representatives of pharmaceutical companies or representatives of companies with medical equipment or computer equipment that the office may be thinking of purchasing. There is usually a maximum of one or two appointments set aside for each physician for this type of appointment each week.

BOX 42-1   Medical Conditions Referred to Emergency Medical Services (911)

1. Conditions that may result in damage to body structures. This is especially important for problems that can cause a significant decrease in oxygen to the body because of breathing or circulation disorders:
   - Breathing problems or respiratory arrest
   - Severe chest pain or cardiac arrest
   - Bleeding that cannot be controlled
   - Large open wounds
   - Any condition that raises the suspicion of internal bleeding
   - Potential poisoning or overdose
   - Bleeding in, or injury to, a pregnant woman

2. Conditions that result in very low blood pressure:
   - Shock
   - Serious burns
   - Severe bleeding
3. Conditions that result in a change in the level of consciousness (loss of consciousness, disorientation, confusion, loss of alertness)
4. Fractures or large wounds that require the equipment found in an emergency department

---

HIGHLIGHT on Triage

Triage is the process of sorting patients according to their need for care. When a disaster occurs, health care workers choose which patients to treat first, depending both on the severity of their injuries and the likelihood the person will survive.

Victims are sorted into three groups—hence the word *triage*, from a French word meaning "sort." Some victims' injuries are minor and can wait for treatment; some victims have injuries so severe that they will probably not survive no matter what effort is put into their treatment; and some have severe injuries but will probably survive if prompt treatment is given.

This system has been adapted to office and appointment scheduling to decide if a patient can wait for the next available appointment, if the patient should be seen immediately, or if the patient should be sent to the emergency department. Triage in the

medical office setting is rarely a case of life or death, and the term *triage* is usually reserved for screening performed by licensed health care personnel with the education needed to assess the medical needs of ill patients.

The medical assistant does screen calls and make decisions on the basis of guidelines established by the physicians where he or she works. The medical assistant must remember that if there is any question about a patient needing immediate care, either the telephone call should be referred to a qualified person in the office or the patient should be directed to an emergency department or other facility where care can be obtained. The medical assistant should be familiar with the policies of his or her employer and work within them, both to avoid injuring the patient and to protect against liability in a potential lawsuit. ∎

What Would You Do? | What Would You *Not* Do?

Case Study 2

On a winter afternoon, there is only one physician in the office. He must leave promptly at 3:45 because he is scheduled to give a lecture to medical students at a nearby hospital shortly after 4:00. The physician has been running behind because two extra patients have been worked into the schedule. At 2:30, in addition to three patients in the waiting room, he still has four established patients scheduled, as well as one new patient scheduled for 3:15, the last appointment of the day. ∎

PROCEDURE **42-2** Making an Appointment

Outcome Make an appointment for a patient

Equipment/Supplies

- Computer appointment schedule or appointment book
- Pencil

1. **Procedural Step.** Identify the patient using the full name and date of birth. Obtain information from the patient: the provider, the purpose of the appointment, and any scheduling preference. Referrals are usually offered the first available appointment. If you do not find the patient in the computer database, ask if he or she has been seen before. New patients may be encouraged to choose a physician who has joined the practice recently if no physician preference is mentioned. Established patients are usually booked with their primary physician, but if it is an urgent problem the patient may accept an appointment with another provider in the practice.

2. **Procedural Step.** Offer the patient a date and time for the appointment. Keep locating appointments until an acceptable date and time have been found. The more urgent the appointment, the more the patient must adapt to the office schedule.

3. **Procedural Step.** For a new patient, obtain the patient's demographic data (e.g., address, telephone number, date of birth), the name of the patient's insurance company, the name of the insured, the patient's insurance group number and ID number, a prior authorization (precertification) number, or other information related to insurance. Be sure to discuss the cost of the visit or procedure if the patient does not have insurance. Inform the patient if a referral form from the primary physician is necessary. Enter this information directly into the computer as you obtain it from the patient.

   Principle. Before making an appointment for a new patient, it is important to be sure that the patient can pay the bill. Information about insurance and referral provides a basis to inform the patient what his or her personal financial liability is likely to be.

4. **Procedural Step.** For an established patient, obtain the information to make the appointment. After identifying the patient, this includes the reason for the visit, the provider, and the desired date and time.

5. **Procedural Step.** Repeat the information to the patient to confirm the appointment. Offer to tell a new patient where the office is located.

6. **Procedural Step.** Enter the patient's name, the correct amount of time for the appointment, and the reason for the visit. If using an appointment book, enter the information in pencil and block out the correct amount of time.

   Example. The appointment schedule shows a 30-minute appointment for Norma Washington, who complains of back pain; a 30-minute appointment to evaluate shortness of breath for Carl Bowden; and a 45-minute appointment for a new patient, Estelle Jordan.

6	**James A. Martin, MD**
8am	**Office closed:** All Staff
9am	**Washington, Norma B:** James A. Martin, MD: Back pain
	Bowden, Carl C: James A. Martin, MD: Shortness of Breat...
10am	**Jordan, Estelle:** James A. Martin, MD: Physical Examinati...

In SimChart® for the Medical Office, schedule appointment times for the correct amount of time.

MANAGING THE APPOINTMENT SCHEDULE

CHANGING APPOINTMENTS

The most frequent modification required in the appointment schedule is to change an appointment from one time slot to another. In the computer appointment schedule, the original appointment can usually be changed by altering the date and time within the appointment pop-up window. In some systems, the appointment should be copied and pasted to the new time.

Occasionally an entire block of patients has to be rescheduled. This occurs when the physician is unexpectedly absent or delayed during office hours. The absence or delay may be the result of an emergency, a delay at the hospital, or personal illness. Every effort must be made to accommodate scheduled patients by giving them a new appointment as quickly as possible. If there are patients in the office when a physician is severely delayed or must leave, it is important to tell patients how long they can expect to wait. The patients should be given the option of waiting or rescheduling their appointments.

If the physician is running seriously behind schedule, patients often become impatient. Some may wish to reschedule, and this should be done willingly. Usually the physician is willing to stay late to finish the day's appointments, but if the physician must leave at a particular time, appointments set for late in the day may need to be rescheduled.

No-shows are patients who simply do not show up for their appointment. No-shows and cancellations on the day of the appointment should be noted on the official appointment schedule. The information should also be documented in the patient's medical record. This provides a permanent record in case the patient's condition becomes worse and the patient claims that the physician would not see him or her (Procedure 42-3).

Most offices have a policy of reviewing records of patients after three consecutively missed appointments. If the patient is not motivated to adhere to the treatment plan, the physician may wish to terminate the relationship with the patient.

LATE PATIENTS

The office should have a policy regarding late patients. Traffic problems or other incidents can delay even the most punctual person, and usually the office attempts to work the patient into the schedule. If a patient telephones to say that he will be unexpectedly delayed, either the schedule can be adjusted or the patient can be offered a new appointment. Patients who habitually arrive late can cause delays in the appointment schedule. They may be given the last appointment of the day when the physician is most likely to be running late. In some practices habitual latecomers are given an appointment time that is 15 to 30 minutes earlier than the appointment is actually scheduled.

APPOINTMENT REMINDERS

It is easy to print an appointment reminder for a patient who makes an appointment before leaving the office, or a card may be filled out manually. Appointment reminders help patients remember the exact date and time of their next appointment.

Most offices also send reminder letters, emails, and text messages and/or call patients 1 or 2 days before the appointment. The patient's preference should be noted, and permission obtained if email or text messages are used. The medical assistant may place a personal call to each patient scheduled for an appointment (see Chapter 41), or the office may use a computer-generated appointment reminder system. The computer may also be used to generate letters or emails reminding patients to make appointments for periodic routine examinations such as a physical examination or a mammogram.

Text messages to patients may be used for appointment and laboratory reminders, but text message systems are usually not secure and should not contain protected health information. If a medical office uses text messaging, it should inform patients at the time that cell phone numbers are collected how they will be used and allow patients to opt out of receiving text messages.

STORING APPOINTMENT BOOKS AND DAILY SCHEDULES

When computer appointment schedules are used as official schedules, backups should be made according to the guidelines in Chapter 40). If a paper schedule or appointment book (maintained in ink) is used as the official schedule, it should be stored in a secure area.

Memories *from* Practicum

Elaine Wyatt: The office where I did my practicum was always very busy. I remember one afternoon when one of the physicians had to leave suddenly. She was expected to be gone about 2 hours. I was told to call the list of afternoon patients and tell them that the physician had been called away from the office and would be delayed about 2 hours. If the patient wanted to reschedule, I had to put him or her on hold and transfer the call to the appointment scheduler. If the patient wanted to be seen that day, I had to give him or her a time from the revised list. I was surprised that about half of the patients were completely willing to reschedule, so there did end up being enough appointment times for the patients who still wanted to be seen. The major problems occurred when we could not reach the patients by telephone. There were about five of them, and they all came. Two of them were during the 2-hour delay, and both of them decided to reschedule. The other three had appointments after the physician returned. We managed to fit them in close to their original appointment times, and they never even knew that the physician had been out of the office unexpectedly. ∎

PROCEDURE 42-3 Managing the Appointment Schedule

Outcomes

1. Review the daily appointment schedule
2. Cancel a patient appointment
3. Change a patient appointment
4. Indicate a missed appointment
5. Document cancellations and missed appointments on the day of the appointment

Equipment/Supplies

- Computer appointment schedule or appointment book
- Pen

1. **Procedural Step.** Review the daily appointment schedule and be sure that all paperwork and/or paper medical records have been prepared.
2. **Procedural Step.** Check patients in as they arrive. Depending on office procedure, you may check them in using the electronic appointment schedule or a paper appointment schedule.
3. **Procedural Step.** If a patient calls to cancel an appointment, locate the appointment on the appointment schedule, in the appointment book, and/or in the computer appointment program. Ask whether the patient wants to reschedule the appointment.
   Principle. The patient may have a schedule conflict with the original appointment.
4. **Procedural Step.** To cancel an appointment without rescheduling, delete the appointment. If using a paper schedule, if the appointment is canceled on the day of the appointment, draw a line through the patient's name on the schedule.
   Principle. If a paper schedule is used as the official schedule, it is a legal document so changes must be made in ink.
5. **Procedural Step.** If the patient cancels an appointment and declines or postpones making a new appointment, document the cancellation in the patient's medical record. This can be done as a telephone message filed in the medical record or as a progress note.

Principle. Documentation of cancelled or missed appointments makes it readily apparent if this behavior is a common pattern for the patient.

6. **Procedural Step.** If the patient wants to change or reschedule an appointment, find an acceptable time to reschedule.
7. **Procedural Step.** Change the appointment in the computer program by finding the appointment at the originally scheduled date and time and changing to the new date and time. Enter the new appointment in a manual appointment book, then erase the original appointment after checking to make sure all information was copied correctly.
   Principle. Changing the appointment in the computer (instead of deleting) makes it unnecessary to reenter the appointment information.
8. **Procedural Step.** Repeat the information to the patient if speaking on the telephone, or fill out an appointment reminder if the patient is present in the office.
9. **Procedural Step.** If the patient misses an appointment without canceling, draw a line in ink through the appointment on the daily appointment sheet and label the appointment "No Show." If the official schedule is maintained in the computer, indicate that the appointment was not kept by marking the appointment as a missed appointment or no-show or adding a comment that the patient did not keep the

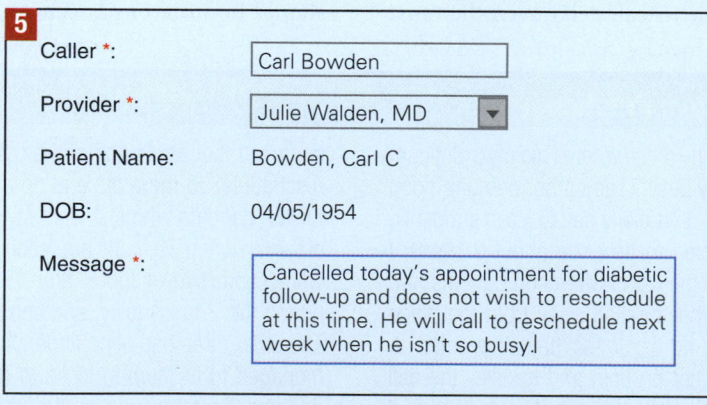

5		
Caller *:	Carl Bowden	
Provider *:	Julie Walden, MD	▾
Patient Name:	Bowden, Carl C	
DOB:	04/05/1954	
Message *:	Cancelled today's appointment for diabetic follow-up and does not wish to reschedule at this time. He will call to reschedule next week when he isn't so busy.	

appointment, depending on the computer program.

Principle. Computer scheduling programs often give the opportunity to track no-show or missed appointments. If it becomes a pattern for an individual patient, it is easy to identify the problem.

10. **Procedural Step.** It may be office policy to telephone the patient to determine why the appointment was missed and offer another appointment.

11. **Procedural Step.** Document the no-show appointment in the medical record, and indicate whether any follow-up was done.

SCHEDULING REFERRAL APPOINTMENTS, DIAGNOSTIC TESTS, PROCEDURES, AND ADMISSIONS

REFERRALS

A **referral** is an authorization for a visit to another physician, usually a specialist. A referral is made by the patient's primary care physician. It may be necessary to obtain **preauthorization** (official permission from the patient's insurance company) before the patient can see the specialist. The physician determines the type and amount of service needed, but the medical assistant usually obtains the necessary insurance authorization (see Chapter 48).

After obtaining all necessary information and insurance authorization, the medical assistant either instructs the patient to make the appointment or calls to make the appointment for the patient. Some managed care plans require the referring provider's office to make the appointment. If the medical assistant calls from the office, the patient may be able to obtain an earlier appointment, but it is important to verify the date and time with the patient. Figure 42-5 is an example of an approved electronic request for referral to a medical specialist.

For a referral to a community resource, the medical assistant must know the patient's name, address, and telephone number, as well as the particular resource needed, the diagnosis, and the reason for the service. Community services include home health care and **hospice** care (a range of services provided to an individual with a terminal illness). Most community agencies do an intake evaluation of the patient, but others depend on the primary care or other physician and staff to tell them what resources the patient needs.

SCHEDULING DIAGNOSTIC PROCEDURES AND HOSPITAL ADMISSIONS

It is often easier for a physician's office to schedule a diagnostic procedure or laboratory test for a patient than to have the patient schedule it. Hospital admissions are always scheduled by the physician's office. Scheduling procedures and admissions can be performed while the patient is at the office or when the patient is at home. If the patient is at home, the details of the appointment and any special patient instructions must be mailed to the patient and confirmed with a follow-up telephone call.

Scheduling a Diagnostic Procedure

Before scheduling a diagnostic procedure for a patient with an outside facility, the medical assistant should compile all of the information that needs to be relayed to the facility. This includes the patient's name and telephone number, the type of procedure being performed, the reason for the procedure, the time frame within which the procedure must be performed, the physician's National Provider Identifier (NPI) number and contact information, and insurance information including any preauthorization number.

After an appointment has been made, the medical assistant must contact the patient to relay when and where the procedure will be performed. The medical assistant may also need to provide directions to the facility. Patients are often required to prepare for a diagnostic procedure. For example, a patient undergoing a colonoscopy needs to perform procedures at home to cleanse the colon of gas and fecal material. These instructions must be relayed to the patient by the medical assistant. If written instructions are available, they should be given or sent to the patient. The medical assistant should document in the patient chart the type of verbal and written instructions provided to the patient. After the procedure, the medical assistant should document when and how the patient was notified of the results of the diagnostic procedure. Precise documentation in patient charts is necessary to avoid later claims of malpractice or abandonment (Procedure 42-4).

Scheduling an Inpatient Admission

The medical assistant has several tasks that must be performed when a patient is admitted to the hospital. The medical assistant must contact the patient's insurance company to obtain preauthorization. The next step is to call the hospital's admitting department to schedule the admission.

The medical assistant must provide the admitting department with the patient's name, address, date of birth, admitting diagnosis, and insurance information and

SH9999999 Detail Approved			Mary Patient SH123456789		
			Request Information		
Patient	MARY PATIENT	Requesting provider	RICHARD WARNER (1234567890 NPI)	Contact info	(490) 555-6464
Diagnosis	I145.10 RT BUNDLE BRANCH BLOCK	Servicing provider	THOMAS HIGHT (2345678901 NPI)	Contact info	(490) 222-3232
Requested service	Specialist consult			Units	1 visit approved
Procedure code				Procedure date	
Start date	4/5/XX	End date	9/5/XX	Delay reason	
Level of service		Related causes		Release of information	Signed statement/ claims
Remarks	Transaction approved				
Procedures and Services					

Status	Reason	Follow-up	Description
Approved (Transaction approved)			Consult

Additional Information		
Additional information requested	Identification code	Description
No paper work at this time		

Edit   Cancel

Figure 42-5 Approved electronic request for referral to a specialist.

preauthorization number. A patient must be seen by his or her physician within the first 24 hours after admission. Because of this, the hospital may ask when the physician is coming to see the patient. In addition, admitting orders must be sent (electronically or by mail) or faxed before the patient is admitted to the hospital.

The procedure for admitting a patient to the hospital is modified somewhat if the patient is first seen in the emergency department and then admitted to the hospital. In this situation, the hospital obtains the information from the patient and then contacts the physician to obtain admitting orders (Procedure 42-5).

SCHEDULING SURGERY

Scheduling a surgery is similar to scheduling a diagnostic procedure; however, more information is necessary to schedule a patient for surgery. In addition to the patient's name, date of birth, and telephone number, the medical assistant must also know the type of surgery to be performed, the time frame within which the surgery is to be performed, who the surgeon and any assistant surgeons will be, who the anesthesiologist will be, and the name of the hospital or outpatient center at which the surgery will be performed.

Before scheduling the surgery, the medical assistant must call the patient's insurance company and obtain preauthorization (prior approval by the insurance company). The preauthorization number must be relayed when scheduling surgery. This number facilitates payment by the insurance company for the procedure. The patient's insurance may require the patient to undergo the surgery at specific hospitals or outpatient facilities.

Before a patient undergoes a surgical procedure, **preadmission testing (PAT)** is performed. PAT includes blood tests, an ECG, and a chest x-ray examination. A physical examination must also be performed within 6 months of the surgery and may be done by the physician or as part of PAT. The purposes of PAT are to obtain data about the patient's health before surgery, to be sure that the patient can tolerate the proposed surgical procedure and anesthesia, and to obtain baseline data for comparison during and after the surgical procedure. The medical assistant helps the patient to schedule this testing.

PAT may be performed in the hospital or medical office, depending on the requirements of the facility where the surgery will be done. If performed in the medical office, the PAT is done either at the surgeon's office or at the office of the patient's primary care physician.

A patient may also need to be scheduled to donate one or more units of his or her own blood. This blood would then be available if a patient needs a transfusion during or after surgery.

Giving a Patient Instructions Before Surgery

The medical assistant is often responsible for providing the patient with specific instructions before the surgery. The office usually gives the patient a set of written instructions so that the patient will remember everything. If the patient is receiving a general anesthetic, he or she must fast for a period of time before the surgery. Fasting requires that the patient have nothing to eat or drink for approximately 12 hours before the surgery. If the patient takes medication for hypertension or heart problems, the surgeon may allow the patient to take his or her morning medication with a sip of water. Other examples of preparation that may be required before a surgical operation include washing with an antibiotic soap and removing body piercings. Patients should be instructed not to bring valuables with them on the day of surgery. If they are having outpatient surgery, they need to have someone available to drive them home after the surgery.

Documenting an Appointment for Surgery

It is important for the medical assistant to carefully document all information relayed to the patient regarding the surgery. Other information that should be documented includes the interactions with the surgical team members, patient, and facilities.

PROCEDURE 42-4 Scheduling Inpatient or Outpatient Diagnostic Tests or Procedures

Outcome Schedule an inpatient or outpatient diagnostic test or procedure

Equipment/Supplies

- The patient's computer or paper medical record and insurance information
- Name of the test or procedure to be scheduled
- Telephone

- Telephone number of the facility and name of the appropriate department with which to schedule the test or procedure
- Pen

---

1. **Procedural Step.** Assemble necessary information about the patient, including the patient's demographic and insurance information.
2. **Procedural Step.** From the patient's medical record and/or a diagnostic test or procedure requisition filled out by the physician, determine the facility and department to call for scheduling. If the office uses a computerized system, be sure the test, procedure, or hospital admission has been ordered in the computer. *Principle.* Any admission, diagnostic test, or diagnostic procedure must have a valid physician order. For insurance reimbursement, a facility that participates in the patient's insurance plan must be used.
3. **Procedural Step.** Determine the time frame for scheduling and, if possible, discuss with the patient preferred days and times.

4. **Procedural Step.** Obtain preauthorization from the patient's insurance, if necessary. *Principle.* The patient's medical condition must justify the service requested. Failure to obtain preauthorization required by the insurance company will result in denial of the patient's insurance claim.
5. **Procedural Step.** Call the department of the facility where the procedure will be performed.
6. **Procedural Step.** Provide the patient's name and demographic and insurance information as needed and a preauthorization number if needed. Identify the test or procedure to be scheduled, and set up a specific day and time.

Continued

PROCEDURE 42-4

PROCEDURE 42-5

PROCEDURE 42-4 Scheduling Inpatient or Outpatient Diagnostic Tests or Procedures—cont'd

7. Procedural Step. Inform the patient of the date and time for the test or procedure and provide verbal and written instructions, including preparation for the test, special instructions, and/or dietary restrictions. *Principle.* The patient must know how to prepare for the test or procedure. Written instructions reinforce verbal explanations.

8. Procedural Step. Send a computer or paper requisition to the facility, or give a paper requisition to the patient to take to the test.

9. Procedural Step. Document the scheduled diagnostic test or procedure and instructions given to the patient in the patient's medical record.

Go over any instructions with the patient before the test.

9 Objective:	Barium enema scheduled at Memorial Hospital at 9:15 AM as ordered by Dr. Martin. Pt. given Instruction sheet for bowel preparation and directions to Memorial Hospital x-ray department.
Assessment:	Patient demonstrated understanding of each step of the bowel preparation by reading the instructions out loud and restating in her own words.

PROCEDURE 42-5 Scheduling Inpatient or Outpatient Admissions

Outcome Schedule an inpatient or outpatient admission for a patient

Equipment/Supplies

- The patient's computer or paper medical record and insurance information
- Name of the procedure to be scheduled or reason for the hospital admission
- Telephone
- Telephone number of the facility and the admitting department
- Pen

1. Procedural Step. Assemble necessary information about the patient, including the patient's demographic and insurance information.

2. Procedural Step. From the patient's medical record and/or directions from the physician, determine the reason for the inpatient or outpatient admission. *Principle.* Any admission must have a valid physician order. For insurance reimbursement, a facility that participates in the patient's insurance plan must be used.

3. Procedural Step. Determine the time frame for the admission. If it is for an elective procedure or surgery, discuss with the patient preferred days and times.

4. Procedural Step. Obtain preauthorization from the patient's insurance company.

Principle. The patient's medical condition must justify the service requested. Failure to obtain preauthorization required by the insurance company will result in denial of the patient's insurance claim.

5. Procedural Step. Call the admissions department to schedule the admission. *Principle.* The patient must be entered into the facility's computer system with all demographic and insurance information for an inpatient or outpatient hospital admission.

6. Procedural Step. Provide all necessary information including demographic and insurance information about the patient, preauthorization number (if any), diagnosis or reason for the admission, and date of the admission.

PROCEDURE 42-5   Scheduling Inpatient or Outpatient Admissions—cont'd

7. Procedural Step. For an inpatient admission, provide admitting orders as needed or fill out admitting orders according to the patient's medical record and fax to the department or nursing floor.

8. Procedural Step. If the patient is to be admitted to the hospital directly from the physician's office, help the patient notify a family member, prepare a patient transfer form, obtain consent forms to release information, and make arrangements for the patient to be transported to the hospital.

9. Procedural Step. If the patient is to be admitted for a procedure or surgery in the future, inform the patient of the date and time of the test or procedure and provide verbal and written instructions, including preparation, special instructions, and dietary restrictions.

Principle. The patient must know how to prepare for the procedure or surgery. Written instructions reinforce verbal explanations.

10. Procedural Step. Document in the patient's medical record the admission, other pertinent information, and instructions given to the patient. For a hospital admission, identify any documents sent with the patient.

10

Plan: Apply oxygen at 2 L/min per order Dr. Martin. To be transferred to Memorial Hospital by ambulance. Admitting orders and copies of medical records will be sent with the patient. Patient's son notified and states he will meet his mother at the hospital.

Evaluation:

Entry By: Elaine Wyatt, RMA

What Would You Do? What Would You *Not* Do? RESPONSES

Case Study 1
Page 1086

What Did Elaine Do?
- Listened to Sandra's concerns without interrupting.
- Apologized for the delay and agreed that it is difficult to wait when you have other obligations.
- Informed Sandra that the physician was running behind schedule and that there were two patients ahead of her. Gave her a realistic estimate of when she would be taken to an examination room.
- Offered to reschedule the appointment if Sandra said that she really could not wait to see the physician that day.

What Did Elaine Not Do?
- Did not tell Sandra that she would be taken to an examination room in just a minute.
- Did not give a long explanation about why the physician was delayed.
- Did not give exaggerated or made-up excuses to imply that this was a one-time crisis.
- Did not become defensive or interrupt Sandra.

Case Study 2
Page 1088

What Did Elaine Do?
- Asked the physician if it would be a good idea to reschedule the new patient or some of the other patients for another appointment in the next few days.
- If instructed to do so, called patients, explained that the physician was going to have to leave the office early, and asked if they would be willing to reschedule.
- If instructed to do so, explained to the patients in the waiting room that the physician was delayed, and asked if they would like to reschedule.
- Evaluated all patients carefully to be sure that everything was prepared to make their examinations go smoothly.

What Did Elaine Not Do?
- Did not reschedule patients without discussing it with the physician.
- Did not tell the patients specific information about the physician's commitments.

Continued

What Would You Do? What Would You *Not* Do? RESPONSES—cont'd

Case Study 3
Page 1092

What Did Elaine Do?
❑ Made a general statement that the physician thought the test was important, and it would help the physician to provide the best care for Anna.
❑ Asked Mrs. Greene and Anna to wait to see if the physician could give them more information about the reason and need for the test.
❑ Offered to call the insurance company to determine whether Mrs. Greene's insurance would cover the cost of the test.
❑ Explained that the office preferred to schedule this type of test to be sure that the testing facility had all necessary information from the physician.
❑ Documented the interaction with the patient in detail.

What Did Elaine Not *Do?*
❑ Did not give a reason for the test unless authorized by the physician.
❑ Did not imply that the mother cared more about the money than her daughter.
❑ Did not say that the physician knows what he is doing.
❑ Did not insist on scheduling the test even if Mrs. Greene did not agree to it.

↻ TERMINOLOGY REVIEW

Key Term	Definition
Appointment matrix	Basic pattern of available appointment times.
Blocked	Times in the appointment schedule when physicians are not available to see patients.
Clustering	Scheduling similar types of patients or examinations on the same day or part of the day.
Double booking	Scheduling two patients for the same appointment time.
Established patient	A patient who has been seen by one of the physicians in the practice of the same specialty within the past 3 years.
Fixed appointment scheduling	An appointment scheduling method in which each patient is given a different, specific appointment time. Also called *stream scheduling, time-specified scheduling,* or *single booking.*
Hospice	Palliative service provided for patients whose life expectancy is less than 6 months. Services may be provided in the patient's home, a nursing home, or a special hospice facility.
Modified wave scheduling	An appointment system that has some fixed appointments and some appointment times during which patients are seen in order of arrival.
New patient	For billing purposes, a patient who has not received services during the previous 3 years from any physician of the same specialty in a medical practice.
No-show	A patient who does not keep a scheduled appointment.
Patient self-scheduling	The practice of allowing patients to have access to the computer scheduling program so that they can schedule their own appointments.
Preadmission testing (PAT)	A series of diagnostic tests done before surgery to establish the patient's health status and identify any potential problems that may occur during surgery.
Preauthorization	Permission from a patient's insurance company for a test, procedure, or surgery.
Referral	The directing of a patient to a medical specialist by a primary care physician.
Single booking	An appointment scheduling method in which each patient is given a different, specific appointment time. Also called *stream scheduling* or *fixed appointment scheduling.*
Stream scheduling	An appointment scheduling method in which each patient is given a different, specific appointment time. Also called *fixed appointment scheduling, time-specified scheduling,* or *single booking.*
Time-specified scheduling	An appointment scheduling method in which each patient is given a different, specific appointment time. Also called *stream scheduling, fixed appointment scheduling,* or *single booking.*
Triage	The process of separating patients by the urgency of their need for care.
Wave scheduling	A method of scheduling appointments in which several patients are given the same appointment time and are seen in the order in which they arrive.

ON THE WEB

For information on Health Insurance Portability and Accountability Act (HIPAA) regulations:

U.S. Department of Health and Human Services, Office for Civil Rights—HIPAA: www.hhs.gov/ocr/hipaa

Center for Medicare and Medicaid Services HIPAA website: www.cms.hhs.gov/HIPAAGenInfo

For information on open access (same-day) appointment scheduling:

U.S. Department of Health and Human Services Agency for Healthcare Research and Quality: https://cahps.ahrq.gov/quality-improvement/improvement-guide/browse-interventions/Access/Open-Access.html

43 Medical Record Management

e Check out the Evolve site at http://evolve.elsevier.com/Bonewit/today/ to access additional interactive activities and exercises to help you study and prepare for success.

LEARNING OBJECTIVES

1. Identify supplies and equipment needed to create and store paper-based medical records.
2. Describe how to create a new paper-based medical record.

3. Describe different types of filing systems.
4. List principles of alphabetic and numeric filing.

5. Describe the process of filing reports and paper-based medical records.

6. Compare and contrast advantages and disadvantages of alphabetic and numeric filing systems for paper-based medical records.
7. Describe the implications of the paper-based medical record and the electronic medical record for medical record management.
8. Differentiate between storage of active and inactive records.
9. Identify methods for retention and disposition of paper-based medical records.

PROCEDURES

Prepare a medical record.

File patient records: alphabetic.
File patient records: numeric.

File reports.

CHAPTER OUTLINE

INTRODUCTION TO MEDICAL RECORDS
PAPER-BASED MEDICAL RECORDS
EQUIPMENT AND SUPPLIES FOR PAPER-BASED MEDICAL
   RECORDS
Storage Equipment
File Cabinets
Shelf Filing Units
Filing Supplies
File Folders
Folder Labels
Chart Dividers
Mounting Sheets
Other Supplies
PREPARING A PAPER-BASED MEDICAL RECORD FOR A NEW
   PATIENT
FILING SYSTEMS
Alphabetic Filing
Rule 1: Individual Names
Rule 2: Prefixes
Rule 3: Abbreviations and Nicknames
Rule 4: Hyphenation
Rule 5: Titles and Seniority Terms

Rule 6: Names of Married Women
Rule 7: Companies and Businesses
Rule 8: Identical Names
Numeric Filing
Terminal Digit Filing Systems
Consecutive Filing Systems
Subject Filing
Chronologic Filing
Choosing a Filing System
RETRIEVING OR FILING A PAPER-BASED MEDICAL RECORD
Retrieving Patient Records
Filing Records
Filing Reports and Correspondence
Measures to Ensure Accuracy or Locate Misplaced
   Records
ELECTRONIC MEDICAL RECORD
STORING MEDICAL RECORDS
Active Records
Inactive Records
Retention of Records
Storing Computerized Records

KEY TERMS

acronym (AK-row-nim)
active record
cross-index
electronic signature
filing system

inactive record
indexing units
medical record management
outguide
sorter

surname (SIR-name)
tab
terminal digit filing

INTRODUCTION TO MEDICAL RECORDS

A medical record (also known as a *patient chart*) contains the important information related to an individual patient in written or electronic form. It includes the care given to that patient and the progress of the patient's condition. **Medical record management** is the process of controlling and handling medical records from the time a record is created until it is placed in permanent storage or destroyed. In addition to recording the care given to patients, both paper-based records and electronic medical records (EMRs) may be used to review quality of care and for recording statistical information.

It is impossible for a physician or other professional to remember every detail of care, such as the results of a physical examination or doses of particular medications. Many people in the primary care physician's office have contact with a patient, as well as consulting professionals, laboratories, and hospitals. It is important that each interaction be recorded in the patient's medical record. This provides an ongoing record of both the patient's state of health and the service provided by the medical office.

Medical records are also legal documents, available if there are questions about the care given. If a patient sues a physician, the court will require documentary evidence, such as a medical record, to be presented in court. The court will take the position that whatever is documented in the record is the care that was given. If something is not documented, officially it never happened. To protect the legal interests of the physician's office, it is therefore important to keep complete medical records. The EMR is discussed in Chapter 38. This chapter focuses on principles of record management and the paper-based medical record.

PAPER-BASED MEDICAL RECORDS

Many medical offices still rely on paper-based medical records to document care. A manila file folder is created for each patient, containing all documents related to the care of that patient. These records are maintained in files to be available each time the patient is seen at the office. After

the transition to an EMR, the old paper record may be destroyed if the entire record has been scanned. In some offices, most of the paper record is scanned into the new electronic record system, and the old record is placed in storage. In most offices, however, only baseline data and very recent information are entered into the new electronic record, because large charts are time-consuming to scan, and too much information tends to overwhelm the system. For at least 2 to 3 years after the transition to an EMR, the old paper chart is made available to the physician for each patient visit.

EQUIPMENT AND SUPPLIES FOR PAPER-BASED MEDICAL RECORDS

STORAGE EQUIPMENT

Paper-based medical records may be kept in various types of file cabinets or on open shelves. The choice of equipment depends on the following: the number of people who need to access the medical records, the office layout, and the amount of floor space available. Usually the records are stored with the files side to side. The files may take up part or all of a room. In a rotary system, the medical assistant can move sections of shelving to access other shelves behind. Large offices may even use an automated system, which stores more records and brings the record to the medical assistant.

File Cabinets

Cabinets or shelves used to store medical records should always be of heavy construction, with proper weighting on the bottom so that they will not tip over, especially if the drawers or shelves pull out. File cabinets should have a locking system. Lateral drawer file cabinets are more common than vertical file cabinets for medical records, although vertical file cabinets may be used for storing other types of information. Lateral drawer file cabinets have drawers that open from the long side, resembling a chest of drawers.

Shelf Filing Units

Shelf filing units consist of shelves arranged horizontally similar to bookshelves. Shelf units are often used to store

Putting It All Into Practice

My name is Ellen McDonald, and I am a Certified Medical Assistant. I have been working for a cardiologist for about a year. Although our office uses a computer-based billing and appointment system, our patient medical records are still in paper-based format. We file our records alphabetically. The physician plans to change to an electronic system this year, but we will be using the paper system during the transition. There is always a big stack of reports, correspondence, and other paperwork to be filed. We are not allowed to file any report unless the physician has seen it. In addition, our physician still dictates the progress notes, which are sent electronically to a transcription service. Every day we print the dictation that the transcription service has returned to us electronically, and we stamp them for the physician to initial after he reads them and makes any corrections. I am responsible for making sure the files of medical records are kept in good order.

In addition to pulling records and putting them away, I sometimes have to look for a misplaced record. If I can't find a patient's medical record, I begin to look for it. First I check the stacks of records for patients who will be seen that day or the next day. Sometimes a medical record gets caught on another record, so it is important to check through the stacks thoroughly. Next I check the computer to find out when the patient was last seen. I check on and behind the desks of the physician the patient last saw, as well as the billing desk. I also check through the files looking for a record that has been misfiled. We use color-coded labels, so it is usually easy to see when a record is out of place. These measures are usually enough to find the record, although sometimes it may take as long as a week before the record turns up. One time we looked for a record for 3 weeks before we found it. Whenever I am filing, I am very careful, because I remember how much work it is to find a record that has been misfiled. ∎

medical records because the records can be accessed without having to open and close drawers. Adjustable metal shelf dividers that interlock at the back of the shelves come with the units. Their function is to keep the records in an upright position, thus preventing the records from slumping or sliding under one another.

File folders with side tabs (described later in this chapter) must be used with shelf units to permit the patient's name to be visible on the shelf. A record is placed on the shelf with the bottom edges of the folder down and the side tabs facing outward. This means that the record is accessed from the side, rather than the top, as with drawer filing cabinets.

Shelf files are preferred because they allow easier access to records, and a number of people can have access to the shelves at the same time. For example, a medical assistant may need to retrieve the medical records of patients to be seen that day, while at the same time another medical assistant may need to look up information for an insurance company or to document a patient telephone call.

Shelf units are available in two styles: open-shelf units or pull-down front units. As the name suggests, open-shelf units are open to the environment and cannot be closed. They must be in a room that can be locked separately from other parts of the office. The pull-down front units have lids that can be pulled over the front of the shelves and locked. This protects the records from environmental factors and allows each part of the file to be locked. It must always be possible to lock either the entire medical record room or individual shelving units.

FILING SUPPLIES

File Folders

A file folder is a protective cover used to hold paper-based medical record documents in an organized format. Usually file folders are made of manila card stock. Flexible metal fasteners at the top of the inside of the folder hold documents in place. Although the folders expand as the number of documents increases, it is recommended that the folder be broken down into two folders after attaining a width of ¾ inch.

Folders are available with tabs. A **tab** is a projection of a folder that extends beyond the top or side edge of the folder. Folders for a file cabinet with drawers have tabs on the top, whereas folders for shelf units have tabs at the side of the file folder. In the medical office with shelf filing cabinets, a folder with a full-cut side tab is used. Indentations at intervals along the tab indicate the placement of adhesive labels. This ensures that all the labels on all the medical records are affixed at the same place on the file folders (Figure 43-1).

Folder Labels

Labels are used to identify the paper-based medical record and are commercially available in rolls or continuous folded strips. Most offices use pressure-sensitive self-adhesive labels. The labels for an alphabetic system assign colors to letters in either the first third or first half of the alphabet, and the remaining letters are assigned the same colors along with some type of distinguishing mark, such as one or two white stripes. If the office uses a numeric filing system, each digit from zero to nine is assigned a specific color. Color-coded year labels are often used to identify the last year a patient was seen at the office. The current year label is placed on a new record and updated the first time a patient has an office visit each year. This allows the records of patients who have not been seen for some time to be removed from the active files and placed in inactive storage.

Chart Dividers

Chart dividers are used to identify each section of the paper-based medical record by subject. Chart dividers are made

Figure 43-1 File folders for shelf units have a full-cut side tab. Color labels are affixed in the same position on each folder.

of a heavy material such as manila card stock. Each divider has a tab for identification. Common categories include Progress Notes, History/Physical, Lab Reports, Diagnostic Testing, Hospital Reports, Immunizations/Medications, and Correspondence, but this varies according to medical office requirements.

Mounting Sheets

Laboratory reports, copies of prescriptions, and telephone messages are often filed on mounting sheets with adhesive strips. Usually several items can be filed on the same sheet. The medical assistant files the first item at the bottom, with each succeeding item shingled up the mounting sheet. With this system the most recent item is always on top. Figure 43-2 shows this type of mounting sheet.

Other Supplies

Outguides, shown in Figure 43-3, are placed in the file to mark the place where a folder has been removed. Each guide has a pocket for a card indicating who removed the record and/or items that accumulate while the record is out of its storage area. Another type of outguide is made of heavy cardboard and has lines to write the name of the individual removing the record.

A **sorter** is a device that facilitates placing documents in alphabetic or numeric order. It has pockets or dividers for each letter or number.

Figure 43-2 Laboratory reports are often mounted one above another so that the most recent is visible on top. (Courtesy Bibbero Systems, Petaluma, Calif., 1-800-242-2376; fax 1-800-242-9330; www.bibbero.com.)

What Would You Do? | What would You *Not* Do?

Case Study 1

A patient has come to the office to request that a copy of her medical record be sent to another physician. She says that her name is Anna Soubrette and her birth date is April 25, 1952. She says that she has not been seen for 4 years, but her current physician had asked about various medications she had taken for a heart problem in the past. Ellen looks the patient up on the computer under Soubrette, but she does not find the patient listed. ■

Figure 43-3 Outguides. (Courtesy Bibbero Systems, Petaluma, Calif., 1-800-242-2376; fax 1-800-242-9330; www.bibbero.com.)

PREPARING A PAPER-BASED MEDICAL RECORD FOR A NEW PATIENT

When a patient comes to the medical office for his or her first visit, a medical record must be prepared for that patient (Procedure 43-1). The method used to prepare the record depends on the following criteria: the format used to organize the record, the filing system, and the type of storage equipment. Most medical offices use the source-oriented format to organize their medical records, the alphabetic filing system to arrange the records, and shelf filing units to store the medical records. Many offices keep partially prepared medical records at the front desk and add the patient's name and labels on the day before or day of a new patient's first appointment.

PROCEDURE 43-1 Preparing a Medical Record

Outcome

1. Prepare a medical record
2. Organize a patient's medical record

The following procedure outlines the method for preparing a paper-based medical record for a new patient using the following organization: a source-oriented format stored in shelf files using a color-coded alphabetic filing system.

Equipment/Supplies

- New Patient Information Form
- Notice of Privacy Practices (NPP)
- NPP acknowledgment form
- File folder with a full-cut side tab
- Metal fasteners
- Name labels

- Color-coded alphabetic bar labels
- Miscellaneous chart labels
- Set of chart dividers
- Blank preprinted forms
- Two-hole punch

---

1. **Procedural Step.** Greet the patient when he or she arrives at the medical office. Introduce yourself and identify the patient. Verify that the patient is a new patient.

2. **Procedural Step.** Ask the patient to do the following:
   a. Complete a patient registration form.
   b. Read a Notice of Privacy Practices (NPP).
   c. Sign an NPP acknowledgment form.

3. **Procedural Step.** When the patient returns the completed forms, check the new patient information form for accuracy, and make sure that you can read the patient's handwriting. If you have any questions regarding the information on the form, ask the

patient for clarification. Ask the patient for his or her insurance card and make a copy of it.
   Principle. A copy of the patient's insurance card is used for third-party billing.

4. **Procedural Step.** Enter into the computer the data on the completed new patient information form.

5. **Procedural Step.** Assemble supplies needed to prepare the medical record. Enter the patient's full name into the computer for printing on a name label, following these guidelines:
   a. Enter the patient's name in transposed order as follows: last name, first name, middle name (or initial).

PROCEDURE 43-1   Preparing a Medical Record—cont'd

b. Enter the patient's name two or three spaces from the left edge of the label and one line down from the top of the label.

c. Ensure that the patient's name is spelled correctly. **Principle.** Following these guidelines facilitates the accurate and efficient filing of the patient's medical record.

6. **Procedural Step.** Determine the first two letters of the patient's last name and select the appropriate alphabetic color-coded labels. Attach the color-coded labels to the (full-cut) side tab. The labels should be affixed to the folder using the label placement indentations on the tab.
Principle. Using the label placement indentations ensures that all labels on medical records are affixed at the same place.

7. **Procedural Step.** Affix the name label immediately above the first color-coded alphabetic label.

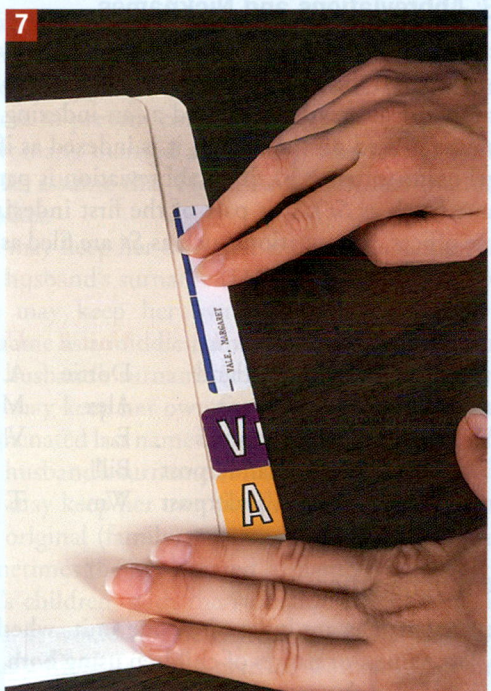

Affix the name label.

8. **Procedural Step.** Attach any additional chart labels, such as a year label and miscellaneous chart labels (e.g., allergy, insurance), to the folder according to the office policy.

9. **Procedural Step.** Insert the chart dividers onto the metal fasteners of the file folder.

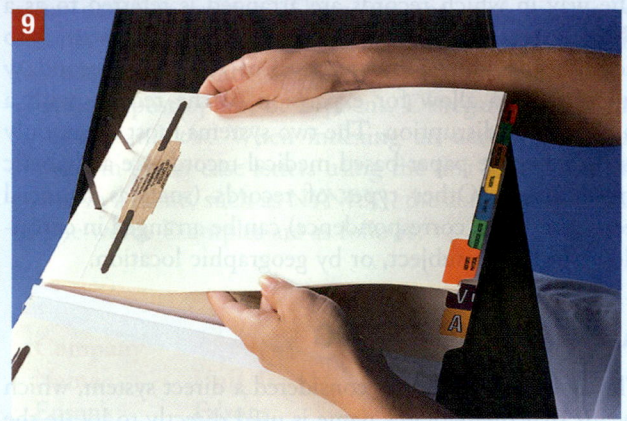

Insert the chart dividers into the metal fasteners.

10. **Procedural Step.** Place the original patient registration form in the front of the medical record. Place the signed NPP acknowledgment form and the copy of the patient's insurance card in the appropriate section of the record.

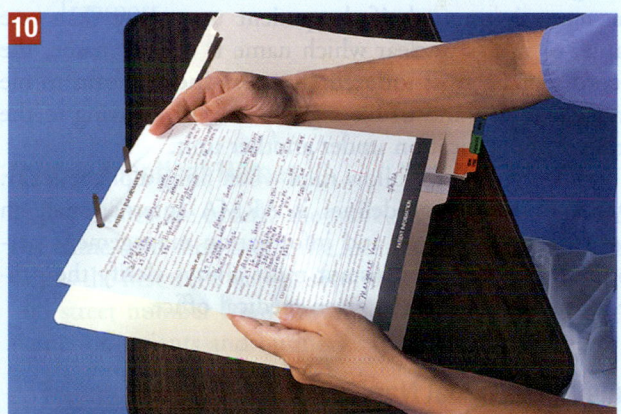

Place the patient registration form in the front of the medical record.

11. **Procedural Step.** Label preprinted forms to be placed in the record with required information such as the patient's name and date. These forms typically include the medical history form, the physical examination form, progress note sheets, and a medication record form. If the forms are not prepunched, the medical assistant must use a two-hole punch to insert two holes into the top or side of the form.

12. **Procedural Step.** Insert each form under its proper chart divider.

13. **Procedural Step.** Check the medical record to ensure that it has been prepared properly.

PROCEDURE 43-3

PROCEDURE 43-3   Filing Patient Records: Numeric

Outcome

1. File patient records correctly using a terminal digit filing system
2. Maintain organization by filing

Equipment/Supplies

- Patient records with terminal digit labels
- File cabinet or shelves
- Numeric sorter

- Outguides
- Index cards

1. **Procedural Step.** Gather the records that are ready to be filed and remove any elastic bands or paper clips. *Principle.* Paper clips, elastic bands, and so on prevent the record from sliding easily into and out of the file.
2. **Procedural Step.** Check the records to be sure that no loose sheets of paper are present. If loose sheets are found, insert them in the record.
3. **Procedural Step.** Sort the records according to the terminal digit indexing units, using the sorter if available.
4. **Procedural Step.** Find the correct location in the file for the first record, based on the final group of numbers. Refine your search based on the middle group of numbers and then the first group of numbers. At the correct location for the record, pull

the outguide halfway out, slide the record in front of the outguide, and finish removing the outguide. If your office does not use outguides, use your hand to make a space between the record before and the record after the one you are filing.

5. **Procedural Step.** If there is an index card in the outguide showing who had the record from the outguide, remove it. Place the outguide with other unused outguides. Some offices keep index cards for the physicians in separate boxes so that new cards do not need to be written; some offices cross out the name and reuse the index cards; some offices use slips of paper that are discarded after each use.
6. **Procedural Step.** File each record in the same way until all records have been filed.

RETRIEVING OR FILING A PAPER-BASED MEDICAL RECORD

RETRIEVING PATIENT RECORDS

A paper-based patient record has to be removed from its proper location in the file whenever someone in the office wants to look at it (e.g., for an appointment, when a patient leaves a message).

The record is located using the filing guidelines of the particular office. Paper-based medical records needed for patients with appointments on a particular day are usually pulled the afternoon before the appointments, using the printed appointment list. Each time a record is taken from storage, an outguide is placed exactly where the record was removed, as illustrated in Figure 43-4.

The person removing the record fills in a card with the name or number on the record and the name of the person who will have the record. Although it seems cumbersome to fill in a card for every record removed, in the long run it is much less frustrating than searching the entire office for a record when the patient is in the waiting room.

FILING RECORDS

Each day, several records need to be returned to the file when a paper-based record system is used. In most offices, records ready for filing are placed in one location.

Figure 43-4 Placing an outguide.

Before filing records or documents, the medical assistant should be sure that the records are ready to file. To condition a record, the medical assistant takes several steps:

- All clips, pins, or other extraneous material should be removed.
- Any tears or broken punch holes should be repaired with tape.
- Any sticky notes or other loose papers should be either removed or filed in the record in the correct location.

A sorter is used to arrange the records so that they can be filed efficiently according to name or medical record number. It is important to locate the correct position to replace the record and remove the outguide. Any items to be filed in the pocket of the outguide should be filed in the record at this time.

FILING REPORTS AND CORRESPONDENCE

All reports, letters, and other materials that come into the office should be reviewed by the physician, initialed, and then filed in the patient record. A date stamp is often used to identify exactly when a report or letter was received. If the physician dictates progress notes, these must also be reviewed and initialed before filing. With the paper medical record, there is no end to the number of papers that the physician must review. Even if an EMR is used, the medical office receives many paper reports and letters that must be reviewed and scanned. Sometimes physicians even come into the office on the weekend to catch up on all their paperwork. Because of this, there is often a stack of material to be filed on Monday. The physician may indicate an action for the medical assistant to take on a message form or sticky note. These actions can range from arranging laboratory or diagnostic follow-up to notifying a patient of results of laboratory or diagnostic tests to calling a pharmacy with a prescription. The medical assistant must complete any follow-up before filing the report (or record) (Procedure 43-4).

Several steps facilitate filing reports or other items in the paper medical record:

- Each report or note to be filed should be initialed by the physician, and any required action should be completed.
- Reports should be sorted before filing according to name or medical record number.
- Once the correct record has been located, the report is filed at the front of the appropriate section. It may be necessary to remove a section of the record to insert the new item.

- The record should be reassembled before being replaced in the file.
- Reports for items that are not in their correct locations should be set aside. After all other reports have been filed, if time permits, the medical assistant can search for the missing records.

MEASURES TO ENSURE ACCURACY OR LOCATE MISPLACED RECORDS

Seven steps can ensure accuracy in filing or locating a misplaced record. A missing paper record creates multiple problems. Working carefully can help avoid lost records.

1. The medical assistant should work slowly and carefully when filing records.
2. It is recommended to use outguides to keep track of the record.
3. Medical records should be returned to storage after use and not just handed to others in the medical office. If it is necessary to give a record to the physician, the outguide should be updated.
4. Physicians and other personnel should be discouraged from hoarding records. The medical assistant should encourage the physician(s) to finish all dictation each day, review laboratory reports, and sign off on them.
5. Records should be kept in orderly stacks when they are out of the files. This makes it easier to scan for one particular record.
6. If the medical assistant notices a misfiled record in the files, it should be removed and filed correctly without delay.
7. Hunting for "missing" records and being alert to find them in unexpected places are important. After all possible measures fail to locate a missing record, it may be necessary to create a second record for a patient until the record can be found.

What Would You Do? | **What Would You *Not* Do?**

Case Study 3

When Ellen is pulling paper-based medical records for the next day's appointments, she does not find the medical record for Alan DuBois under "Dubois." The file also has no outguide. Ellen remembers that the patient was seen within the past week or two. She also checks under "Bois," but the record is not filed there, either. ∎

PROCEDURE 43-4 Filing Reports

Outcome

1. File reports, correspondence, and other material in a patient record
2. Organize a patient's medical record

Equipment/Supplies

- Medical records
- Assorted reports
- Letters or other material to be filed
- Hole punch
- Tape
- Stapler
- Sorter

1. **Procedural Step.** Assemble materials to be filed and necessary supplies to assist in the filing process.
2. **Procedural Step.** Remove extraneous materials, such as paper clips or pins; mend any tears with tape; and staple related pages together. Punch holes if necessary. **Principle.** Preparation before filing allows all materials in the record to be maintained in good condition.
3. **Procedural Step.** Verify that each report is ready to be filed. In most offices the physician initials reports after he or she has seen them. If the initials are missing, the report should go back to him or her. **Principle.** The physician must see each report that comes to the medical office. A procedure verifying that the physician has seen the report before filing prevents reports from being accidentally overlooked.
4. **Procedural Step.** Sort the reports using the sorter alphabetically or numerically, depending on the filing system. Sort by letters, numbers, or number groups first, then sort within each letter or number group. **Principle.** Even in a small office, large numbers of reports need to be filed in patient records if a paper-based record system is used. It is more efficient to file in order, especially when patients have more than one report to be filed.
5. **Procedural Step.** Gather all reports for a particular patient, find the correct record, and insert the report(s) into the record in the correct location. In any section, reports are filed chronologically with the most recent reports at the front of the section. When several reports are shingled on a page, the oldest report goes at the bottom with newer reports

progressing up the page and in front of the older reports. You may need to place a divider in the record if you are filing the first report in a given section. **Principle.** The record usually contains several sections in a specific order. Reports need to be in the correct section to be easily located.

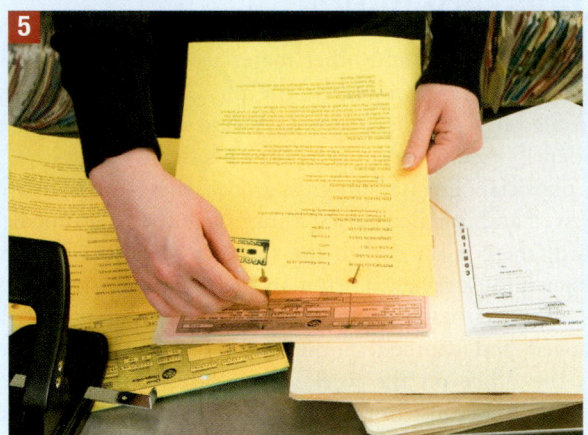

Insert the report(s) into the medical record.

6. **Procedural Step.** Put the record back together if necessary, and file with other medical records. **Principle.** It is easier to file reports in the wrong record when several records are out.
7. **Procedural Step.** If the record is not in the file, place the report back in the sorter or in the pocket of the outguide. **Principle.** It is more efficient to file reports in records you can find easily than to hunt for records just to file reports.

ELECTRONIC MEDICAL RECORD

The EMR is usually updated immediately by medical assistants, physicians, or other staff members who interact with patients. The physician may use voice recognition software to generate reports, or a transcription service may be used that links the transcribed reports directly into the patient's record. Use of the EMR greatly reduces the need for filing, although paper reports, correspondence, and consent forms are usually scanned into the record as soon as possible. The originals may be shredded or stored in a paper record depending on the office.

EMRs are password protected, and patient data are compartmentalized so that access can be limited to the information that any given staff member needs to view. A system administrator should authorize users and remove them from the system as appropriate. Data should be encrypted between the server and the user, and the infrastructure for access should be secure. The medical assistant should never allow other personnel to access patient information with his or her password.

STORING MEDICAL RECORDS

The storage area for paper medical records should be well lit and climate controlled. It is important to maintain the relative humidity at 48% to 52% to prevent deterioration of the records. Basement storage is not recommended unless the humidity is well controlled. The records should also be protected from dust, insects, rodents, fires, and floods. As discussed earlier, records should be secure when the office is closed so that unauthorized personnel do not have access to them. The Occupational Health and Safety Administration (OSHA) requires that main aisles leading out of a room or to a fire exit be a minimum of 5 feet wide, and secondary aisles, such as between shelving units, be a minimum of 3 feet wide.

The shelf files should be full enough to allow the folders to stand upright but loose enough to allow folders to be easily stored and retrieved.

HIGHLIGHT on Electronic Signatures

When talking about electronic signatures, it is important to distinguish between actual signatures that are captured electronically and an electronic entry specific to one individual that authenticates identity and can be linked to a specific date and time.

When a medical office uses an electronic medical record (EMR), the staff can use two ways to handle actual patient signatures. With the first method, the patient signs a paper consent form and the paper consent form is then scanned into the electronic record. With the second method, the patient reads the consent form, either in a paper version or on a computer screen, and then the patient signs an electronic signature pad that captures an image of the actual signature and inserts it into an electronic version of the form being signed.

Physicians and other staff in the medical office usually use an **electronic signature,** an electronic sound, symbol, or process added to an electronic record that indicates intent to sign. These processes are built into the software with safeguards to validate the time of the entry and the identity of the individual making the entry. Electronic signatures are also used for transmitting insurance claims and for validating entries to the EMR. Electronic signatures are valid in all states and are accepted by the Health Insurance Portability and Accountability Act (HIPAA), provided that the software being used validates identity, validates that the document was not altered later, and provides that the user cannot later repudiate the electronic signature.

The term *digital signature* is used for a form of encryption that binds electronic records to an "electronic fingerprint." Digital signatures require validation by private companies called *certification authorities.* The entire document is encrypted and decrypted using public and private keys (mathematic formulas). Digital signatures are used for transferring money and signing legal documents electronically. This level of security is currently not required for EMRs. ■

Memories *from* Practicum

Ellen McDonald: I did my practicum in a clinic affiliated with a large hospital that had made the transition from paper medical records to an electronic medical record (EMR). When a patient checked in, we entered the data from the patient information sheet into the computer immediately, and we used a signature pad at the front desk to obtain electronic signatures from the patient for consent to treatment, authorization to disclose information for billing, and acknowledgement of receipt of HIPAA confidentiality information.

Each medical assistant had to log into the system to enter information in the medical record. Even as a student, I was given a password so that I could check patients in, enter vital signs, and enter other information. For example, the machine for electrocardiograms (ECGs) looked like a laptop computer attached to the ECG cables. It was also connected to the EMR. We entered patient information using a computer keyboard. I learned how to print the ECG as a hard copy, but the physician could also view the tracing on the computer.

When the clinic made the transition to the EMR, the records of active patients were scanned into the system, but they kept the paper records for inactive patients. I remember one time when a patient who had not been seen for about 6 years made an appointment. He was experiencing medical problems that he thought might be connected to earlier radiation therapy. I was instructed to create a new electronic record for him, and then I was sent to find the old paper record. Several rooms were full of paper medical records, arranged in order by clinic number. I found it confusing because I was not very familiar with the terminal digit method of filing, but one of the staff members helped me to find the record. After the appointment, I had to return the record to storage. ■

ON THE WEB

For information on record management:

American Health Information Management Association (AHIMA): www.ahima.org

ARMA International: www.arma.org

U.S. Department of Health and Human Services—Office of the National Coordinator for Health Information Technology (OCN): healthit.gov

For information on record retention and destruction:

American Health Information Management Association (AHIMA)—Retention and Destruction of Health Information: http://library.ahima.org/xpedio/groups/public/documents/ahima/bok1_049252.hcsp?dDocName=bok1_049252

American Medical Association—Retention of Medical Records: www.ama-assn.org/ama/pub/physician-resources/medical-ethics/code-medical-ethics/opinion705.page

For information on legal processes and electronic medical records:

American Health Information Management Association (AHIMA)—The Legal Process and Electronic Health Records: http://library.ahima.org/xpedio/groups/public/documents/ahima/bok1_028134.hcsp?dDocName=bok1_028134

Written Communications

ⓔ Check out the Evolve site at http://evolve.elsevier.com/Bonewit/today/ to access additional interactive activities and exercises to help you study and prepare for success.

LEARNING OBJECTIVES

PROCEDURES

Business Letters

1. Define the parts of a business letter.
2. Identify different formats for preparing business letters.
3. Explain how to format and compose a business letter.

Compose a business letter.

Responding to Written Communication

4. Identify how to respond to written communication from businesses and patients.
5. Discuss the importance of using correct grammar and spelling in written communication.

Memoranda and Other Documents

6. Describe the process of creating memoranda.
7. Explain how to prepare and proofread documents.

E-mail or Other Electronic Transmission

8. Compare the use and style of business letters and electronic communication, such as e-mail or secure messaging within the EMR.
9. Explain how to use e-mail and attachments for business communication.
10. Explain how to transmit information using a fax machine.

Send a fax.

Photocopying Documents

11. Describe how to make copies of multiple-page documents.

CHAPTER OUTLINE

INTRODUCTION TO WRITTEN COMMUNICATION
BUSINESS LETTERS
Equipment and Supplies
Parts of a Business Letter
Heading
Inside Address
Salutation or Greeting
Body of the Letter
Complimentary Closing
Signature, Printed Signature, and Title
End Notations
Format of Business Letters
Setting up a Letter
Letter Styles
Composing a Business Letter
Responding to Written Communication
PREPARING MEMORANDA

GRAMMAR AND PUNCTUATION
Parts of Speech
Sentence Structure
Sentence Errors
Comma Rules
SPELLING AND PROOFREADING
Spelling
Proofreading
ELECTRONIC DATA TRANSMISSION
E-mail
Secure messaging Within the Electronic Medical Record
E-mail Attachments
Fax Transmissions
Fax Machine
Sending a Fax
PHOTOCOPYING

KEY TERMS

collate (cull-LATE)	grammar	right justified
complimentary closing	left justified	salutation
duplex	letterhead	semiblock style
e-mail	memo (memorandum)	simplified letter style
fax	modified block style	template
full block style	proofread	

INTRODUCTION TO WRITTEN COMMUNICATION

Until 20 years ago, almost all written communication between the medical office and other parties was managed by letters or forms and mailed through the U.S. Postal Service. Today, it is also common to transmit data electronically or by fax, and these data can be viewed and/or printed in paper form. Regardless of how the written material is transmitted, however, written communication must still adhere to professional standards. The medical assistant is often responsible for preparing letters, e-mails, memoranda, reports, and other types of written communication. To do this professionally requires thorough knowledge of grammar, spelling, format, and the technology that supports modern methods of producing written documents. In addition, the medical assistant must be familiar with the implications of Health Insurance Portability and Accountability Act (HIPAA) regulations regulating access to patient health information. These regulations are covered in detail in Chapter 3. The procedure for obtaining consent to release information from the medical record is discussed in Chapter 38.

BUSINESS LETTERS

Letters leaving the medical office—whether sent to a referring physician, a patient, an attorney, another business, or an insurance company—require proper formatting. Some letters may be dictated by the physician and prepared by the medical assistant. The medical assistant may also compose and send letters independently. The medical office may also use form letters and/or templates for routine matters. A **template** is a standard form to which additional data can be added as needed.

EQUIPMENT AND SUPPLIES

Business letters are usually created using a computer and printer. A word processing program is used to create the letter so that formatting can easily be adjusted and any necessary corrections can be made.

The medical office orders stationery and envelopes preprinted with the practice name, address, telephone number, and business logo. Individual physician names are also often included. A sheet of this type of stationery is called **letterhead**. Blank sheets of the paper of exactly the same type and weight must be purchased for letters that are longer than one page. Photocopies of letters printed on letterhead are often retained for office records in addition to the computer file used to create the letter.

PARTS OF A BUSINESS LETTER

Heading

The heading includes the return address and the date line. The return address is composed of the name and address of the business sending the letter. If office letterhead is used, no return address needs to be added. The date line is the date the letter is mailed in month, day, year order. The month is written out in full on the date line. It is usually entered on the second or third line below the return address. On letterhead stationery, it is placed to fall a few spaces below the bottom of the letterhead.

Inside Address

The inside address includes the name and address of the party to whom the letter is being sent. Beginning with the inside address, information is single spaced with one or two blank lines between the separate parts of the letter. The inside address should be located in a position such that the body of the letter is centered top to bottom on the page. If the body of the letter is small, there should be more blank lines between the date line and the beginning of the inside address. If the letter is long enough to require two pages, the inside address begins on the second or third line below the date line.

Salutation or Greeting

The **salutation** (the greeting that begins a letter) is found below the inside address separated by one or two blank lines. A business letter is formal, so the recipient's last name and title (e.g., Mr., Ms., Miss, Dr.) should be used. The salutation is punctuated with a colon. Correct examples include the following:

Dear Ms. Wilson:
Dear Dr. Taylor:
Dear Mrs. Porto:

Titles or initials indicating credentials (such as MD or RN) are not used after names. The following are *incorrect*:

Dear Amy,
Dear William Taylor, MD:

If the recipient's name is not known, it is permissible to use "Dear Sir," "Dear Madam," "Dear Sir or Madam," or "To Whom It May Concern." At least one line is left blank after the salutation.

Body of the Letter

The body of the letter contains the content, which should be presented clearly and concisely. A subject line may be used to begin this section. Within a paragraph the letter is single spaced, but one or two blank lines should separate each new paragraph.

Complimentary Closing

The **complimentary closing** (or *complimentary close*) is a term for the words used as a polite ending to a letter just before the writer's signature. It is a sign of respect and can be adjusted depending on how well the letter's author and the party being addressed know each other. "Sincerely" is the standard closing. A more formal closing is "Yours truly" or "Very truly yours." It is followed by a comma and separated from the body of the letter by one or two blank lines.

Signature, Printed Signature, and Title

The signature is the actual written signature of the individual sending the letter. It is added after the letter has been printed. The signature line contains the printed signature of the individual sending the letter, with credentials (e.g., MD). It is entered four to five lines below the complimentary closing to leave room for the written signature. A business title (e.g., Office Manager) is capitalized if used and is entered on the line below the printed signature.

The medical assistant uses his or her own name and signature for a letter to a supplier or a letter to a patient responding to a billing question. Any letter dictated or composed by a physician will be signed by the physician.

End Notations

Various pieces of information may be given in notations at the bottom of the letter, usually beginning one or two lines below the typed signature. The order of the end notations may vary according to the preference of the office. A reference notation notes the initials of the person who composed the letter (in uppercase) followed by the initials of the person who typed or keyed the letter (in lowercase). The two sets of initials are separated by a colon or a slash. If the letter contains enclosures, such as a log of visits and/or billing records, this is noted in the enclosure notation, on the second line below the title. *Enclosure* or *Enc.* may be used for one enclosure. *Enclosures* followed by the number in parentheses is used for more than one enclosure. This

alerts the recipient to make sure that everything the sender intended to include actually accompanies the letter. A copy notation (distribution notation) identifies the recipient(s). The letters "cc" are used, followed by a colon and the name(s) of those who are receiving copies. If a copy is sent to an individual without the knowledge of the recipient or the original letter it is called a *blind copy* (bcc). For a printed letter, the blind copy notation must be added after the original is printed. In an e-mail, the notation *Bcc* can be chosen, and a copy will be sent to the identified recipient or recipients, but there will be no notation of these copies on the original e-mail. Figure 44-1 shows a business letter with the parts of the letter identified.

FORMAT OF BUSINESS LETTERS

Setting up a Letter

When preparing letters using a word processing program, the first step is to set the margins. The top margin of the letter should be large enough to accommodate the letterhead (usually 2 to $2\frac{1}{2}$ inches). The side margins may be 1 to 2 inches. Wider margins are used for a short letter. The body of the letter is single spaced.

In writing a business letter, a standard font should be used, such as Times New Roman 12 point. The entire letter should be created in the same font. The word processing program may include a letter wizard, which formats the letter automatically. It is also possible to use or create a letter template so that all letters from the office have the same format.

If the letter has two pages, a header should be placed at the left top margin of the second page with the name of the recipient, the page number, and the date.

Letter Styles

- **Full block style:** The letterhead may be centered, but all other lines are **left justified,** which means that they start at the left margin on the page. This allows rapid entry of information and easy formatting. One or two blank lines should be left between paragraphs (Figure 44-2).
- **Modified block style:** All lines in the inside address, salutation, and body of the letter and reference lines are left justified, and there are one or two blank lines between paragraphs. However, the date line, complimentary closing, and signature lines begin in the center of the letter or are sometimes **right justified** (aligned with the right margin) (Figure 44-3).
- **Semiblock style** (also called *modified block with indented paragraphs*): All lines in the inside address, salutation, and body of the letter and reference lines are left justified. Paragraphs are indented five to eight spaces, and there are double spaces between paragraphs. The date line, complimentary closing, and signature lines begin in the center of the letter or are sometimes right justified. Semiblock style is the same as modified block style, except that the first sentence of each new paragraph is indented (Figure 44-4).

WALDEN-MARTIN
FAMILY MEDICAL CLINIC
1234 ANYSTREET ANYTOWN, ANYSTATE 1234
PHONE 123-123-1234   FAX 123-123-5678

Letterhead →

⇓

Date Line → April 10, 20XX   (Enter spaces after the date line to center the body
⇓   of the letter in the middle of the page)
⇓
⇓

Inside Address → Ms. Danielle Kessens
878 Lippert Avenue
Anytown, AL 12345
⇓

Salutation → Dear Ms. Kessens:
⇓

Body
Paragraph 1 → I have received the results of your thyroid function tests that were done on March 30, and I am
pleased to say that the results were within normal limits.
⇓

Paragraph 2 → These results indicate that your hypothyroidism is now well under control and your current
dosage of thyroid medication is appropriate and should be continued. Feel free to call me at my
office if you have any questions or if I may be of any further assistance.
⇓

Complimentary close → Sincerely,
⇓

Handwritten signature → ⇓ *James Martin*
⇓

Signature Line → James Martin, MD
⇓

Reference Notation → JM/cw

Figure 44-1 Sample business letter with the parts of the letter identified.

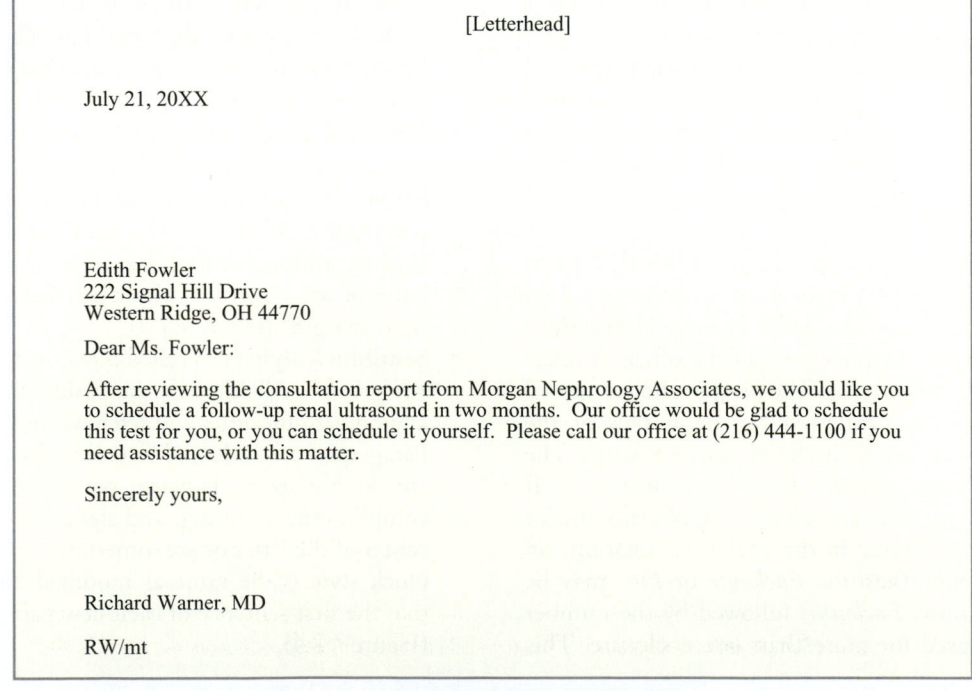

[Letterhead]

July 21, 20XX

Edith Fowler
222 Signal Hill Drive
Western Ridge, OH 44770

Dear Ms. Fowler:

After reviewing the consultation report from Morgan Nephrology Associates, we would like you
to schedule a follow-up renal ultrasound in two months. Our office would be glad to schedule
this test for you, or you can schedule it yourself. Please call our office at (216) 444-1100 if you
need assistance with this matter.

Sincerely yours,

Richard Warner, MD

RW/mt

Figure 44-2 Sample letter—full block style.

[Letterhead]

July 21, 20XX

Edith Fowler
222 Signal Hill Drive
Western Ridge, OH 44770

Dear Ms. Fowler:

After reviewing the consultation report from Morgan Nephrology Associates, we would like you to schedule a follow-up renal ultrasound in two months. Our office would be glad to schedule this test for you, or you can schedule it yourself. Please call our office at (216) 444-1100 if you need assistance with this matter.

Sincerely yours,

Richard Warner, MD

RW/mt

Figure 44-3 Sample letter—modified block style.

[Letterhead]

July 21, 20XX

Edith Fowler
222 Signal Hill Drive
Western Ridge, OH 44770

Dear Ms. Fowler:

After reviewing the consultation report from Morgan Nephrology Associates, we would like you to schedule a follow-up renal ultrasound in two months. Our office would be glad to schedule this test for you, or you can schedule it yourself. Please call our office at (216) 444-1100 if you need assistance with this matter.

Sincerely yours,

Richard Warner, MD

RW/mt

Figure 44-4 Sample letter—semiblock style (also called *modified block with indented paragraphs*).

SENTENCE STRUCTURE

Sentences are composed of various combinations of independent and dependent clauses. A clause contains a subject (noun or pronoun) and a verb. If it can stand alone, it is called an *independent clause.* If it requires an additional clause in order to be meaningful, it is called a *dependent* or *subordinate clause.* Sentence classifications are as follows:

1. *Simple sentence:* A sentence composed of one independent clause. Example: *The dog was very hungry.*
2. *Compound sentence:* A sentence composed of two independent clauses connected by a conjunction. A comma separates the two clauses. Example: *The dog returned from its walk, and it drank all the water in its bowl.*
3. *Complex sentence:* A sentence composed of one independent clause and one or more dependent clauses. If the dependent clause begins the sentence, it is followed by a comma. Example: *When it returned from its walk, the dog drank all the water in its bowl.* If the dependent clause comes after the independent clause, the dependent clause is not separated by a comma. Example: *The dog drank all the water in its bowl when it returned from its walk.*

Sentence Errors

1. *Sentence fragment:* A sentence fragment is a dependent clause used to stand alone as a sentence. In this case, an additional independent clause is necessary for meaning.
   Sentence fragment: When I arrive for my appointment.
   Correct sentence: When I arrive for my appointment, I will bring my insurance card.
2. *Run-on sentence:* A run-on sentence is a sentence in which two or more independent clauses are joined without a conjunction.
   Run-on sentence: My appointment is on Thursday I will bring my insurance card.
   Correct sentence: My appointment is on Thursday, and I will bring my insurance card.
3. *Comma splice:* A comma splice is the incorrect use of a comma to separate two sentences. The sentences should be separated by using a period and beginning a new sentence or by using a semicolon. It is also permitted to separate the sentences with a comma and a conjunction.

COMMA RULES

1. Use a comma to separate the elements in a series of three or more things. The comma before the conjunction "and" is optional.
   Example: The patient complained of abdominal pain, difficulty breathing, and headache.
   Example: This 40-year-old, well-nourished, Caucasian woman was seen on 12/22/15.
2. Use a comma before a conjunction, such as *and, but,* or *or,* when the conjunction connects two independent clauses. An independent clause could be used as a complete sentence.

   Example: The patient called an ambulance, and the ambulance brought her to Memorial Hospital.
   Example: We gave the patient furosemide intravenously, but after an hour her urine output was still poor.
3. Use a comma to set off introductory elements such as prepositional phrases or dependent clauses.
   Example: After the upper GI, the patient continued to experience epigastric pain.
   Example: Because we were planning surgery for next week, I did not want to prescribe any new medications.
4. Use a comma to set off information that could be omitted or placed in parentheses without changing the meaning of the sentence.
   Example: The patient, who was referred by Dr. Jenkins, is a 40-year-old woman in good health.
   Example: We will follow this patient closely in the clinic, which is open on Tuesdays and Thursdays.
5. Use a comma before quotation marks except at the end of the sentence where a period precedes the close quotation marks. Do not use a comma to introduce quoted elements introduced by the word *that.*
   Example: The patient said, "My incision burns like fire."
   Example: "My incision burns like fire," said the patient.
   Example: The patient states that her incision burns like fire.
6. Use a comma to avoid confusion.
   Example: For most the year is already finished.
   Example: For most, the year is already finished.
7. Use a comma between the city and the state, the date and the year, a name and a title, and in long numbers. No comma is necessary when only the month and year are used.
   Example: The patient was admitted to Memorial Hospital, Westford, Massachusetts in late July 20XX.
   Example: On July 5, 20XX, the patient was burned severely in a fire in Las Vegas, Nevada.
8. Use commas with terms like *not, however,* and *but* to express contrast.
   Example: The wound was large, but healing well.
   Example: The patient, however, had obtained antibiotics from another physician.
9. Use a comma to separate appositives, nouns of direct address, titles that follow a person's name, and introductory words from the rest of the sentence.
   Example: We will make an appointment with Dr. Cannon, a gynecologist, sometime next week.
   Example: Doctor, there is something else I wanted to ask you.
10. Separate parenthetical expressions from the rest of the sentence using commas. These expressions include the following: *I believe, I am sure, on the contrary, indeed, of course, nevertheless, in my opinion,* and *in fact.*
    Example: The report, I hope, will give you more information about multiple sclerosis.

BOX 44-1 Confusing Pairs of Words

Nouns and Adjectives

affect (mood) and *effect* (result)

councilor (member of a council) and *counselor* (someone who gives guidance)

ileum (last part of the small intestine) and *ilium* (a bone in the pelvis)

principal (head of a school; most important) and *principle* (basis of a system of belief)

stationary (fixed in place) and *stationery* (paper and other writing materials)

Verbs, Adjectives, and Adverbs

accept (agree or believe in) and *except* (verb: exclude; preposition or conjunction: other than)

adverse (unfavorable or bad) and *averse* (strongly disliking)

affect (to make a difference to) and *effect* (to bring about a difference)

complement (to contribute extra features) and *compliment* (to praise)

continual (happening frequently) and *continuous* (without interruption)

eminent (distinguished) and *imminent* (about to occur)

fewer (not as many) and *less* (not as much)

imply (to suggest) and *infer* (to deduce)

loose (to set free; not tight) and *lose* (to be unable to find)

precede (to go before) and *proceed* (to continue)

Pronouns

whose (shows possession) and *who's* (contraction of "who is")

your (shows possession) and *you're* (contraction of "you are")

its (shows possession) and *it's* (contraction of "it is")

their (shows possession) and *there* (shows location)

Example: An inadequate supply of oxygen to the myocardium, for example, is caused by narrowing of the coronary arteries.

SPELLING AND PROOFREADING

SPELLING

Although word processing programs usually provide a spell-check feature, the medical assistant must still proofread all documents for spelling. The spell-check function verifies the spelling of a given word but cannot confirm that it is the intended word or that it is used correctly in context. See Box 44-1 for a list of pairs of words that are commonly confused.

A tool to improve spelling is a personal list of words that cause difficulty. It is important to make an effort to learn these words, and remember to spell-check these words every time they are used. The medical office may purchase a medical dictionary program that can be installed on office computers for reference.

PROOFREADING

After preparing any letter or document, the medical assistant should spell-check or look up any unfamiliar words to spell them correctly. Abbreviations for medical conditions should be avoided, but abbreviations for medication times, measurements, and vital signs are usually acceptable.

It is helpful to use medical spell-check software, which is available from several companies. An ordinary spell-check program can also be personalized over time by adding medical words and abbreviations that the program does not recognize; however, additions should always be checked for correctness. After the document or letter has been keyed,

What Would You Do? What Would You *Not* Do?

Case Study 2

Christine is proofreading a letter created by voice recognition software related to the examination of a patient with hematuria (blood in the urine). She has no difficulty proofreading the patient's history and presenting symptoms, but in the section related to diagnostic testing, there is an abbreviation that is clearly incorrect. She also does not understand the sentence in which the unknown abbreviation occurs. She proofreads the rest of the report and then returns to the section that caused difficulty. She is still unable to make any sense of the abbreviation and the rest of the sentence. ■

the medical assistant should print a copy, **proofread** it (read it carefully and make corrections), and then correct it and print out a final copy. If there is an unintelligible word, a space can be left and marked in pencil for the physician to fill in before the final copy is printed.

ELECTRONIC DATA TRANSMISSION

E-MAIL

E-mail (electronic mail) has become an accepted means of communication throughout the business world. **E-mail is the exchange of information from one computer to another.** As described in Chapter 40, a computer with an Internet connection is used to send e-mail. Medical assistants may use e-mail to communicate with business contacts as well as patients. It is usually faster and more efficient to send an e-mail for a short message.

An e-mail message should contain an informative subject line. Successive e-mails relating to the same subject are usually created as a reply so that the recipient can read the previous correspondence related to the subject. It is polite to acknowledge receipt of an e-mail, even if there is no reply, so the sender knows that the e-mail has been received.

The tone of an e-mail is somewhat less formal than that of a letter, but correct grammar and spelling should be used without any of the abbreviated forms or emoticons that are sometimes used in personal e-mails. Many e-mail programs have spelling tools that should be used. Humor should be avoided because the recipient does not have the nonverbal cues to know when a message is meant to be humorous. The medical assistant should also avoid sending an e-mail containing criticism or other negative content because it is easier to be more negative than intended in writing than when speaking directly to an individual.

E-mails usually use plain text. At the foot of the message, the medical assistant should include the business name, contact information, and e-mail address and telephone number. Most e-mail programs allow the medical assistant to create an e-mail signature with the contact information to be included at the bottom of every e-mail.

It is important to remember that e-mails are not private. Even after messages have been deleted, they can often be recovered from the computer or network used to create them. E-mail should be used only for business communications that are straightforward and not confidential. It is also always important to be sure that the e-mail is being sent to the correct recipient. It is a good policy to review the recipient name(s) before hitting the "send" button. The account should be set up so that sent messages are saved, but the medical assistant may also want to create printed copies of e-mails related to orders or billing problems.

SECURE MESSAGING WITHIN THE ELECTRONIC MEDICAL RECORD

Secure messaging is a common feature within an electronic medical record (EMR) system. It is also called *clinical messaging* or *clinical e-mail*. Messages sent within the EMR are considered as secure as the EMR itself. The record of an individual patient can be attached to the message. The format and tone are the same as in an ordinary e-mail. Messages can be sent only to users of the EMR system, however.

E-MAIL ATTACHMENTS

Programs for sending e-mail allow documents, images, and other types of files to be attached and transmitted with the e-mail. Unfortunately, many computer viruses are spread through e-mail attachments, so attachments should not be opened unless they are from a trusted source and/or are expected. If an attachment does contain a virus, opening the attachment launches the virus. Any e-mail with an attachment from an unknown recipient should be deleted immediately. If a medical assistant sends a file as an attachment, the recipient may also be hesitant to open the file for the same reason.

The format of an attachment may also pose a problem. The recipient may be unable to open the attachment without the software that was used to create the file in the attachment. Document files can always be saved in text format if there is any question about compatible software. Most files can also be saved as webpages, which the recipient can view with his or her Web browser.

FAX TRANSMISSIONS

Fax Machine

Paper copies of documents can be sent quickly from one location to another using a fax machine. The word **fax** is a short form of *facsimile* and is a method of sending images over telephone lines. The original document is fed into the fax machine, which encodes the images on the paper into signals to be sent over the phone. At the other end, a second fax machine prints black dots on a piece of paper that correspond to the information received. There should be a dedicated telephone line and telephone number for the fax machine, which is shown in Figure 44-7. The phone number for the fax machine should be listed next to each telephone so that any caller can be told how to fax information to the office.

Sending a Fax

The fax is useful for doing business (e.g., ordering supplies) and for sending out meeting agendas or receiving résumés when hiring. To protect confidentiality, fax transmissions of patient health information should be made only when patient consent has been obtained or in an emergency situation when prompt information transfer is required. A cover sheet should be used for privacy, and the recipient should be notified by telephone when the fax is being sent so that he or she can remove it from the receiving fax machine promptly (Procedure 44-2). The cover sheet should contain a confidentiality statement similar to the one in Figure 44-8.

Figure 44-7 A fax machine allows transmission of images from one location to another using a telephone line.

CONFIDENTIALITY STATEMENT:

The documents accompanying this transmission may contain confidential information that is protected under the Privacy Act of 1974. It is being faxed to you after appropriate patient authorization or under circumstances that do not require patient authorization. This information is intended only for the use of the intended recipient(s). The authorized recipient(s) of this information is/are prohibited from disclosing this information to any other party unless permitted to do so by law or regulation.

If the reader of this message is not the intended recipient(s) or the employee or agent responsible for delivering the attached information to the intended recipient(s), please note that any dissemination, distribution, or copying of this information is strictly prohibited. **Anyone who receives this information in error should notify the sender immediately and arrange for the return or destruction of the transmitted information.**

Figure 44-8 A medical office should include a confidentiality statement on the cover sheet for fax transmissions.

PROCEDURE 44-2   Sending a Fax

Outcome

1. Send a fax
2. Apply Health Insurance Portability and Accountability Act (HIPAA) rules regarding privacy and release of information

Equipment/Supplies

- Fax machine
- Cover sheet with a confidentiality statement
- Document to be faxed

1. **Procedural Step.** Prepare the cover sheet including the name, address, and fax number of the recipient; fax number of the sender; and number of pages (including the cover sheet). If there is a message to the sender, include it on the bottom of the cover sheet.

Continued

PROCEDURE 44-2   Sending a Fax—cont'd

2. **Procedural Step.** Organize all pages to be faxed with the cover sheet first.
   Principle. Pages should be in order and all facing the same direction. The cover sheet with a confidentiality statement protects information in the fax transmission from being visible as the upper page to protect confidentiality.

3. **Procedural Step.** Place pages in the fax machine, face up or face down as is correct for the machine being used.

4. **Procedural Step.** Enter the fax number. Include any extra digits as required, such as a 9 to obtain an outside line, a 1 for long-distance, and an area code if required.
   Principle. Some areas of the country have introduced so-called *overlay area codes* requiring all telephone numbers to be dialed with an area code.

5. **Procedural Step.** Verify the fax number as it appears in the window or on the computer screen to be sure the number is correct.
   Principle. To maintain confidentiality, always be sure the fax number has been entered correctly.

6. **Procedural Step.** Press the correct button to send the fax.

7. **Procedural Step.** If the fax contains patient health information, place a telephone call to the recipient so that the fax can be removed from the recipient's fax machine as soon as it is received.

8. **Procedural Step.** Check back to be sure the fax has been sent. Some machines print a confirmation for every fax, and some print a written report only if the fax does not go through.

9. **Procedural Step.** File the original document appropriately.

PHOTOCOPYING

It may be necessary to use a copy machine to copy documents of one or several pages (e.g., an article or paper written by a physician) or to make several copies of a document (e.g., a report to be discussed at a staff meeting). To copy efficiently, the medical assistant should become familiar with special features of the available copy machine. Before copying, staples should be removed from the document to be copied, the pages should be arranged in order, and the copy machine should be checked to ensure it has enough paper.

When several copies of a multiple-page document are needed, the machine should be preset to **collate** (arrange each copy in sequence) or sort the pages if the machine has this feature. Some machines will also staple documents.

For a machine that copies only single pages, the desired number of copies of each page must be copied, arranged in order, and stapled manually. The medical assistant should avoid distractions when copying and should be careful to copy each page correctly and place pages in the correct order.

Another feature of many photocopiers is the ability to **duplex,** or store images from both sides of a page in memory to produce two-sided copies.

When copying a patient's medical record, the medical assistant must preserve the confidentiality of the information. Before beginning to make a copy, verify that the patient has signed an authorization for the release of information. After copying, it is important to double-check that no originals or copies were left at the machine. The medical assistant is responsible for shredding any spoiled copies.

What Would You Do? What Would You *Not* Do? RESPONSES

Case Study 1
Page 1123

What Did Christine Do?
❑ Looked up the two companies mentioned by the physician using the Internet to obtain the exact business names and addresses and model numbers of machines in which the physician might be interested.
❑ Also looked for other companies that might manufacture similar machines.

❑ Prepared letters to each company requesting information using the usual format for office letters.
❑ Used the salutation "Dear Sir or Madam."
❑ Proofread and signed the letters before mailing.
❑ Made a note to follow up after a week.

What Did Christine Not *Do*?
❑ Did not ask the physician how to find the addresses.
❑ Did not initiate a contact that would result in a call by a salesperson.

What Would You Do? What Would You *Not* Do? RESPONSES—cont'd

❑ Did not send the letters out with an incomplete address or with errors.

Case Study 2
Page 1125

What Did Christine Do?
❑ Asked another medical assistant in the office if she knew what the abbreviation should be.
❑ Tried to look it up in a dictionary of abbreviations to make sense of the sentence.
❑ If still unable to identify an appropriate abbreviation, left a blank line in the letter and indicated on a sticky note that the physician should fill in the blank.
❑ After the letter was reviewed by the physician, corrected the letter and printed a new copy for the physician to sign.

What Did Christine Not *Do?*
❑ Did not leave the abbreviation if it did not make sense, hoping that the physician would not notice.
❑ Did not mail the letter without correcting and reprinting it.
❑ Did not interrupt the physician to ask about the confusing abbreviation and sentence.
❑ Did not complain to other office staff about the voice recognition software program.

Case Study 3
Page 1126

What Did Christine Do?
❑ Used either office e-mail or the contact button on the website to send an e-mail about the missing box of test strips.
❑ Used the same professional tone in the e-mail that she would have used in a letter or telephone call.
❑ In the e-mail, included the order number, billing name and address, number of boxes of test strips ordered, and number of boxes of test strips received.
❑ In the e-mail, stated clearly that the company should send an additional box of test strips.
❑ Because the bill indicated that the office was being charged for only the one package of paper that was shipped, decided to order the other four packages of paper for the Clinitek machine from a more reliable company.

What Did Christine Not *Do?*
❑ Did not cross out the charge for 10 boxes and test strips and change it to nine boxes when approving the bill for payment without contacting the company.
❑ Did not ignore the missing box of strips when approving the bill for payment, assuming that the company would send another box automatically.
❑ Did not use casual, critical, or hostile language in the e-mail.

TERMINOLOGY REVIEW

Key Term	Definition
Collate	To assemble the pages of a document in numeric order.
Complimentary closing	Words used as a polite ending to a letter just before the writer's signature.
Duplex	To produce double-sided copies by storing images from both sides of the original in the memory of a photocopier.
E-mail	The exchange of information from one computer to another using telecommunication.
Fax	Transmission of scanned, printed material by telephone. A short form of the word *facsimile*.
Full block style	A letter format in which all parts of the letter are left justified.
Grammar	The study of accepted rules used to create meaning in a language.
Left justified	Lines of type that begin at the left margin of a document.
Letterhead	A sheet of stationery preprinted with information about a business, including name, address, telephone number, and other information as needed.
Memo (memorandum)	A form of communication within a company that is usually short and limited to one subject.
Modified block style	A format for business letters in which the date line, complimentary closing, and printed signature line are on a tab at the center or right justified and all other parts of the letter are left justified.
Proofread	To identify and correct errors in a document.
Right justified	Type that is aligned with the right margin of a document.
Salutation	The greeting that begins a letter.
Semiblock style	A letter format in which the date line, complimentary closing, and printed signature line are on a tab at the center or right justified, all paragraphs are indented five to eight spaces, and the other parts of the letter are left justified.
Simplified letter style	A letter format in which all elements are left justified. The greeting is replaced by a subject line in all capital letters. The complimentary closing and typed signature are replaced by a typed signature in all capital letters.
Template	A standard form to which additional information can be added as needed.

ON THE WEB

For information on improving written communication:

Grammar and Spelling—The Purdue Online Writing Lab (OWL): http://owl.english.purdue.edu/owl/section/1/5/

For information on patient confidentiality in written communication:

Centers for Medicare and Medicaid Services—HIPAA Privacy Rule: www.hhs.gov/ocr/hipaa

Mail 45

 Check out the Evolve site at http://evolve.elsevier.com/Bonewit/today/ to access additional interactive activities and exercises to help you study and prepare for success.

LEARNING OBJECTIVES	PROCEDURES

U.S. Mail
1. Identify the function of the U.S. Postal Service (USPS).
2. State the purpose of the ZIP and ZIP+4 systems.
3. Describe the use of the following USPS mail classifications: Priority Mail Express, Priority Mail, First-Class Mail, Standard Post, and Media Mail.
4. Correlate available insurance and delivery confirmation services with their appropriate use in the medical office.

Other Package Delivery Services
5. Compare and contrast the use of private package delivery services with the use of the USPS.

Processing Incoming Mail
6. List and describe the steps for processing incoming mail.

Process incoming mail.

Preparing Envelopes for Mailing
7. List and describe the USPS recommended addressing standards that should be followed to prepare mail.
8. Describe how to prepare labels and envelopes for mailing.
9. Compare and contrast postage meters and online postage services.

Look up a ZIP code for automated processing.
Prepare envelopes for mailing.

CHAPTER OUTLINE

INTRODUCTION TO MAIL AND SHIPPING
U.S. POSTAL SYSTEM
ZIP Code and Bar Code Systems
Classifications of Domestic Mail
Priority Mail Express
First-Class Mail
Priority Mail
Standard Post
Media Mail
Insurance and Delivery Confirmation Services
Certified Mail
Return Receipt
Signature Confirmation
Certificate of Mailing
Restricted Delivery
Registered Mail
Insured Mail
Special Handling
Collect on Delivery
Postal Money Orders

OTHER PACKAGE DELIVERY SERVICES
PROCESSING INCOMING MAIL
Opening Mail
AUTOMATED MAIL PROCESSING
POSTAL ADDRESSING STANDARDS
Letters and Large Envelopes
Complete Address
Address Format
Return Address
OUTGOING MAIL
Preparing Envelopes or Mailing Labels
Folding and Inserting Letters Into Envelopes
No. 10 Envelope
No. 6¾ Envelope
Window Envelope
Adding Postage
Postage Meters
Online Postage Services

INTRODUCTION TO MAIL AND SHIPPING

Mail communication is an important aspect of the efficient operation of the medical office. Every day the medical assistant processes incoming mail to facilitate delivery to physicians and other employees in the medical office. Preparing outgoing mail is also important. Most of this chapter is devoted to the services and postal addressing standards of the U.S. Postal Service (USPS), which is used to send the bulk of outgoing mail.

U.S. POSTAL SYSTEM

The USPS is an independent agency with an official monopoly on the delivery of mail within the United States. It is financed primarily through the sale of postage and postage stamps. The postal service processes an average of 554 million pieces of mail daily and is one of the largest employers in the United States. The USPS provides a variety of ways for mail to be transported from sender to receiver. The cost of these various services depends on the urgency with which mail must be received, as well as any special handling services provided.

ZIP CODE AND BAR CODE SYSTEMS

In 1963 the USPS introduced the Zone Improvement Plan (ZIP) code system. This system enables the postal service to process mail more accurately, quickly, and economically with automated equipment. A **ZIP code** consists of a five-digit code that identifies the post office to which a piece of mail is to be delivered. In 1967 it became mandatory to use the ZIP code for second- and third-class bulk mailing.

The **ZIP+4 code,** which was introduced in 1983, consists of the original five-digit code followed by a hyphen and four additional digits. These digits identify a specific geographic segment within the five-digit delivery area, such as a city block, an office building, or a group of post office boxes. The plus-four code is required for certain presorted mailings. The USPS maintains a ZIP code lookup service that makes it easy to use the Internet to look up the ZIP+4 code for any address in the United States.

For bulk mailing, the ZIP code is translated into a postal bar code that is printed on the piece of mail by the sender. A computer program is used to add the bar code to pieces of mail, mailing labels, and mailing lists. For ordinary letters, the postal service may add the postal bar code because it makes the mail easier to sort. Unlike supermarket bar codes, which consist of wide and narrow bars, the **postal bar code** consists of long and short bars. Each individual digit in the ZIP code is represented by five bars, and a check digit is used after the ZIP code or ZIP+4 code. The postal bar code may be printed in the address block above or below the mailing address. When not included in the address block, the postal bar code is placed in the **bar code clear zone,** a blank rectangular area at the lower right of the card or envelope (Figure 45-1).

CLASSIFICATIONS OF DOMESTIC MAIL

Domestic mail includes mail that is collected and distributed within, among, and between the United States, its territories and possession, the military service, and the United Nations. Classifications are based on speed of delivery, weight of individual pieces of mail, and number of pieces of mail in the mailing.

Priority Mail Express

Priority Mail Express provides overnight delivery including on Saturday to most U.S. locations. Sunday delivery can be provided for an extra charge. Priory Mail Express can be used for letters and packages weighing up to 70 pounds. Envelopes and packing materials are available from the post office. Medical offices may use Priority Mail Express to send laboratory specimens to an outside laboratory for testing. The postage rates for this service are considerably higher than other services, but they do include insurance against loss or damage.

First-Class Mail

First-Class Mail is used for letters or other lightweight items up to 13 ounces. The postage is based on weight, with a base rate for 1 ounce and additional postage for each additional ounce. The medical office uses this mail classification to send letters, postcards, patient statements, and sometimes insurance claim forms (if the office has permission to submit paper claims).

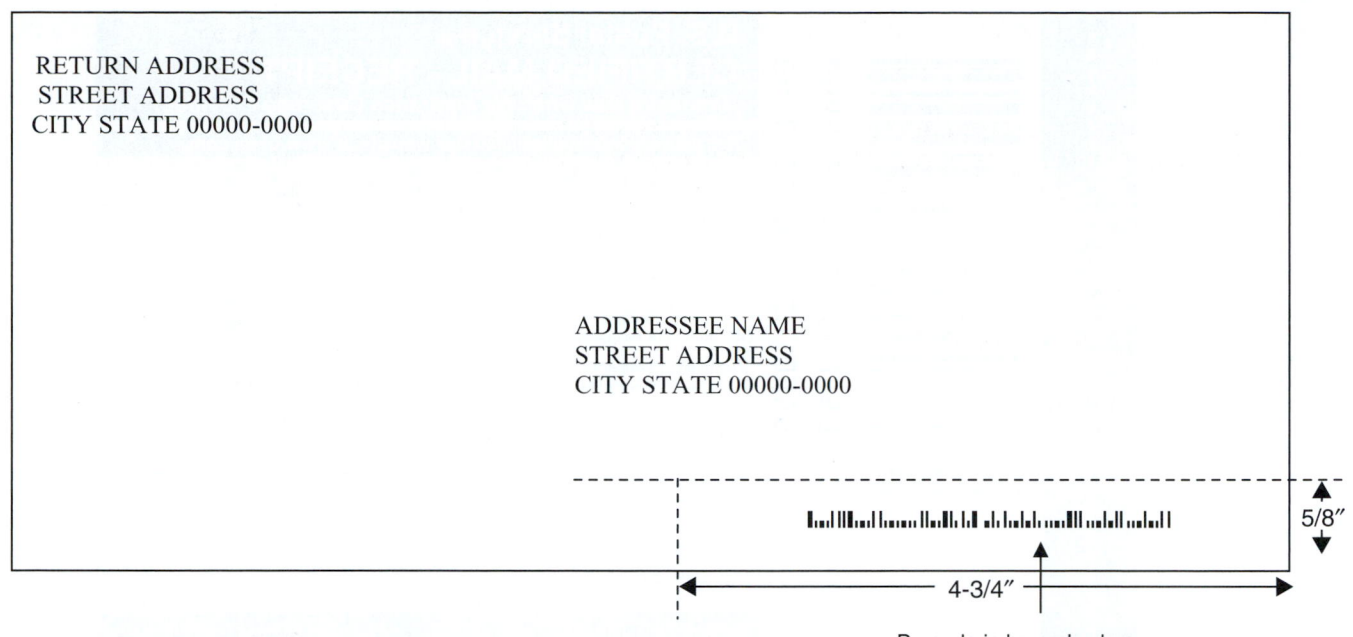

RETURN ADDRESS
STREET ADDRESS
CITY STATE 00000-0000

ADDRESSEE NAME
STREET ADDRESS
CITY STATE 00000-0000

5/8″

4-3/4″

Barcode in barcode clear zone

Figure 45-1 The postal bar code is a series of long and short lines that is either printed by the sender above or below the address or added by the post office in the bar code clear zone at the lower right of the envelope.

Sending an item First Class usually results in overnight service to local cities and second-day service nationwide. Delivery by the third day can be anticipated for some outlying areas. All First-Class Mail should be sealed, and it may not be opened for postal inspection without a federal search warrant.

Additional extra mailing services can be purchased for First-Class Mail, such as Certificates of Mailing, Certified Mail, Registered Mail, Collect on Delivery (COD), and Restricted Delivery. If the item that is being sent First Class is letter size, no additional designation is required on the letter. However, if the item is not letter size, it must be clearly marked "First Class."

Priority Mail

Priority Mail is used for mail weighing more than 13 ounces and up to 70 pounds that will be delivered in the same time frame as First-Class Mail. It will be delivered anywhere in the United States within 2 to 3 days. The USPS has a set rate for items up to 1 pound, and flat rate envelopes and boxes are available. For an item over 1 pound in ordinary packaging, the rate depends on both the weight of the item and the distance it must be transported. For an additional charge Priority Mail can be combined with Insured Mail, Registered Mail, Certified Mail, COD, or other services. An example of an item that might be sent from the medical office by Priority Mail is a copy of medical records.

Standard Post

The Standard Post classification is used for less than urgent delivery and for oversized packages. Expected time for delivery is 2 to 8 days. The medical office rarely sends items using this service, but it may receive shipments of medical or office supplies sent by Standard Post.

Media Mail

Media Mail is a special classification for packages containing printed or digital educational material. It may not contain advertising, computer games, or digital drives of any kind.

INSURANCE AND DELIVERY CONFIRMATION SERVICES

The USPS offers a number of extra mailing services. These services must be purchased in addition to the regular postage required to send an item. The medical assistant must understand these extra services, particularly those that are used most frequently in the medical office, such as Certified Mail and Return Receipt.

Certified Mail

Certified Mail is available for First-Class Mail and Priority Mail. It serves as legal evidence that an item was mailed by providing the sender with a mailing receipt. In addition, a record of delivery of the certified item is maintained for 2 years. A green certified mail sticker affixed to the envelope identifies the envelope as Certified Mail. The recipient must sign on delivery of a piece of Certified Mail. This service can also be combined with a Return Receipt for an additional fee (Figure 45-2).

Return Receipt

A Return Receipt provides the sender with proof of delivery of a piece of mail and the signature of the person receiving

Figure 45-2 A Certified Mail Receipt form must be filled out by the sender and signed by the recipient.

Putting It All Into Practice

My name is Diane Waters, and I am a Certified Medical Assistant. I have been working for a group practice with three general surgeons for the past 6 years. A few years ago the hospital where our surgeons operate went to an electronic medical record. The operative reports and discharge summaries are now entered into the electronic medical record automatically, and the physicians review them online. That means that we get significantly less mail because not only those reports but also most laboratory reports, pathology reports, and other types of reports no longer come to the office. As a result, we don't have as much filing, either. Our office still gets piles of journals, magazines, and other printed matter, however. Every day when I am sorting the mail, I have to separate the professional journals that our physicians want to read from magazines, catalogs, circulars, and other items that they would look at only if we found some item of special interest to them. One physician likes to look through this material if it comes with his name on it, but the others don't even want it to show up on their desks. ■

the mail. This may be done through a postcard signed by the recipient and returned to the sender or by an e-mail with an attachment containing the recipient's signature. The sender then has a copy of the signature of the person who signed for the piece of mail. This service can be combined with other services. It is often used with Certified Mail to establish proof of mailing, as well as proof of receipt (Figure 45-3).

Signature Confirmation

Signature Confirmation provides a record of the date and time an item was delivered, as well as the name of the person who signed for the item. A delivery record, including the signature of the recipient, is available by fax or mail on request. The medical office usually uses Return Receipt instead of Signature Confirmation for evidence of delivery because the return postcard or e-mail will be sent automatically.

Certificate of Mailing

A Certificate of Mailing provides evidence of the date and time an item was mailed, but there is no legal proof that the item was actually delivered to the recipient. A certificate of mailing might be used when proof of timely mailing is required, such as a tax return. No record is maintained at the post office, so the sender is responsible for keeping the form.

Restricted Delivery

If an item is strictly confidential, Restricted Delivery limits delivery to the addressee, the individual authorized in writing to sign for the addressee, or a parent or guardian. In general, it is not necessary to use this service for letters from the medical office, but if a legal case is pending, it might be advisable.

Registered Mail

Registered Mail is available for First-Class and Priority Mail, to insure the contents up to $25,000.00. Registered Mail is used when the contents of the item mailed are valuable. The items are tracked, and the date and time of delivery or

UNITED STATES POSTAL SERVICE

||||

First-Class Mail
Postage & Fees Paid
USPS
Permit No. G-10

• Sender: Please print your name, address, and ZIP+4 in this box •

SENDER: *COMPLETE THIS SECTION*

■ Complete items 1, 2, and 3. Also complete item 4 if Restricted Delivery is desired.
■ Print your name and address on the reverse so that we can return the card to you.
■ Attach this card to the back of the mailpiece, or on the front if space permits.

1. Article Addressed to:

COMPLETE THIS SECTION ON DELIVERY

A. Signature

X

☐ Agent
☐ Addressee

B. Received by (*Printed Name*)   C. Date of Delivery

D. Is delivery address different from item 1?   ☐ Yes
   If YES, enter delivery address below: ☐ No

3. Service Type
   ☐ Certified Mail   ☐ Express Mail
   ☐ Registered   ☐ Return Receipt for Merchandise
   ☐ Insured Mail   ☐ C.O.D.

4. Restricted Delivery? *(Extra Fee)*   ☐ Yes

2. Article Number
   (Transfer from service label)

PS Form 3811, February 2004   Domestic Return Receipt   102595-02-M-1540

Figure 45-3 The sender must fill out a Return Receipt form.

delivery attempts can be verified online. The cost depends on the value of the item being sent. The sender receives a receipt that is kept until the recipient receives the item. The recipient must sign a form acknowledging receipt. For an additional fee, the sender can receive a Return Receipt.

Insured Mail

Insurance can be purchased on the contents of mail up to $5000.00. The cost depends on the declared value of the contents. If the mail is lost or damaged, the sender presents the receipt to make a claim for reimbursement of the declared value.

Special Handling

Special Handling is used for unusual items that require special treatment, such as a shipment of live bees. Ordinary packages with breakable items can be marked "FRAGILE" and do not require Special Handling provided they are packed with adequate packing material to protect the contents. This service is not usually used by the medical office.

Collect on Delivery

COD is a special mailing service that allows a sender to collect for merchandise and postage on delivery. The amount due is collected by the postal carrier and returned to the sender by a postal money order. This service is rarely used by the medical office.

Postal Money Orders

Postal money orders are a safe way to send money through the mail within the United States. They may be purchased in an amount up to $1000.00. The sender is given a customer receipt. If the money order is lost or stolen, the sender presents the receipt to the post office for replacement. Some patients may pay bills with postal money orders.

OTHER PACKAGE DELIVERY SERVICES

Private carriers compete with the USPS to provide delivery of letters and packages. Many companies use United Parcel Service (UPS), FedEx, or DHL for next-day and 2-day delivery service. Larger packages that are not time sensitive can be shipped via UPS or FedEx Ground service. A shipping service company will pick items up from an office and offer continuous item tracking over the company's website. Each company also provides mailing envelopes and small boxes at no cost to the customer. Once an account has been established, shipping can be arranged and paid for using the Internet.

Private carriers often deliver packages to the medical office. Examples include business supplies and laboratory reagents requiring refrigeration. The medical office may use a private delivery service to send some laboratory specimens to a laboratory for testing if the specimen must go to a special laboratory or cannot wait for the regular laboratory pickup service.

What Would You Do? What Would You *Not* Do?

Case Study 1
Jerome Stone, a 68-year-old man who has had two laparoscopic surgeries in the past, calls the office and asks to have a copy of his medical record sent to his new surgeon in another state because he needs to have another surgery for the same condition. He tells Diane that the surgery is scheduled for the following week and asks if she can send the copy of the record immediately. He states that he can come into the office the following day to sign the form giving permission to release the record. He gives her the name, address, and telephone number of the new physician. ■

PROCESSING INCOMING MAIL

Mail is delivered to the medical office in various ways. The postal carrier may deliver the mail directly to the office, or it may be placed in an outside mailbox. Some medical offices use a post office box. In this case the medical assistant must go to the post office to collect the mail each day. In a large clinic the mail may be delivered to a central mailroom, where it is sorted and distributed to each department or individual mailbox.

Once the mail is received by the medical office, it must be processed according to the preferences of individual physicians. One physician may want to see all the incoming mail, whereas another physician may want the medical assistant to screen the mail and remove circulars, patient and insurance payments, and magazines for the waiting room (Procedure 45-1).

Incoming mail should be sorted in the following way. If the mail is addressed to a particular physician, it goes into that physician's mailbox or pile. Mail from another physician's office that is not addressed to a particular physician should go into the box or pile of the managing partner, medical director, or office manager.

The medical assistant handles patient and insurance payments, mail from insurance companies, and catalogs from business and medical supply companies. Table 45-1 provides a guide for sorting incoming mail.

Table 45-1 Sorting Incoming Mail

Mail Category	Recipient
First-Class Mail	
Correspondence addressed to the physician marked "Confidential" or "Personal"	Physician
Correspondence from an attorney	Physician
Laboratory reports	Physician (attach laboratory report to patient's paper-based medical record)
Patient records	Physician
Patient payments	Medical assistant
Insurance payments	Medical assistant
Bills for office supplies and equipment	Medical assistant
Bank statements	Medical assistant
Letters from insurance companies	Medical assistant
Résumés for employment	Medical assistant
Periodicals, Circulars, Catalogs	
Professional journals	Physician
Medical convention and seminar information	Physician
Pharmaceutical advertising	Physician
Advertisements for equipment and supplies	Physician or medical assistant
Magazines for the waiting room	Medical assistant
Catalogs for equipment and supplies	Medical assistant
Drug Samples and Packages	
Overnight packages	Screen appropriately
Administrative and clinical office supplies	Medical assistant
Drug samples	Medical assistant (place in drug sample storage area)

OPENING MAIL

Once the mail has been sorted, it must be opened. The medical assistant must know which mail he or she is to open and which is to go to the individual who must deal with it unopened. Some physicians like to open their own mail, whereas others like to have the mail opened, organized, and ready for them to read and respond to. Clearly, any mail marked "personal" or "confidential" should not be opened.

If the physician or physicians prefer mail to be opened, the medical assistant should use a letter opener to open each piece carefully at the top edge. An automated letter opener facilitates this process in a larger office or clinic where there is a lot of mail. Each letter or report is stamped with the receipt date and then alphabetized by the patient's last name. The pages of each report should be stapled together, if they are not already that way. A letter or report containing patient information should be attached to the patient's medical record with a paper clip. Some offices use a cover sheet on the top of each report, on which the physician can check off the action he or she wishes to occur with regard to the report (e.g., file, respond, call the patient).

Non–patient-related items are stacked together to be dealt with by the medical assistant or another member of the staff. Medical journals addressed to a particular physician can be put in his or her mail pile; those addressed to the practice can be put into the medical library or staff lounge. If the office is large, each staff member may have a cubicle in a central location, as shown in Figure 45-4.

Some physicians may instruct the medical assistant to annotate letters. To **annotate** means to underline or highlight important words or phrases in the correspondence. This saves the physician time when reading and responding to the mail. The medical assistant may also be instructed to underline or highlight abnormal values on laboratory reports or diagnostic tests.

When a physician is on vacation, someone on the office staff is delegated to review his or her mail and refer any urgent mail to the physician by telephone or e-mail at the vacation location or to a covering physician. Arrange non-urgent mail by date received for the physician to review when he or she returns to the office.

What Would You Do? **What Would You *Not* Do?**

Case Study 2

Diane is preparing an envelope to mail a letter that the physician has dictated to a colleague named Dr. Leonie. She uses the U.S. Postal Service (USPS) website to look up the ZIP code. Although a five-digit ZIP code is displayed, it is accompanied by a message that says, "This address may be nondeliverable." ■

PROCEDURE 45-1 Processing Incoming Mail

Outcome

1. Process incoming mail
2. Implement time management principles to maintain effective office function

Equipment/Supplies

- Letter opener
- Date stamp
- Paper clips
- Stapler
- Pen or highlighter
- Transparent tape

1. **Procedural Step.** Assemble supplies in a work area large enough to make several piles of mail.
2. **Procedural Step.** Stack all the envelopes so that they face in the same direction. Place any envelopes marked "personal" or confidential to the side.
   Principle. Letters marked "personal" or "confidential" should be opened only by the person to whom they are addressed.
3. **Procedural Step.** Tap the lower edge of the first envelope on the desk so that the contents fall to the bottom.

Principle. Tapping the envelope prevents cutting the contents when opening the envelope.

4. **Procedural Step.** Using a letter opener, open the envelope along its top edge.
   Principle. Using a letter opener makes it easier to open the envelope neatly and preserves the return address should it be needed.
5. **Procedural Step.** Remove the contents of the envelope. Check to be sure the envelope is empty.

Continued

PROCEDURE 45-1

6. **Procedural Step.** Unfold and flatten letters. Date stamp each letter, preferably in the upper right-hand corner of the letter.
Principle. A date stamp provides a record of when the letter was received.

Date stamp each letter.

7. **Procedural Step.** Check to make sure that the letter contains an inside address. If not, staple the envelope to the letter. Discard the envelope if it is not needed, unless office policy states otherwise.

8. **Procedural Step.** Fasten enclosures to the letter with a paper clip. If a letter indicates an enclosure, but it is missing, write "No" next to the enclosure notation and circle or highlight it.

9. **Procedural Step.** Mend any torn paper with transparent tape to prevent further damage.

10. **Procedural Step.** If directed by the physician, annotate the correspondence by underlining or highlighting important words and phrases in the correspondence. Attach a sticky note indicating any action that should be taken in response to the correspondence.
Principle. Annotating saves the physician time in reading and responding to incoming mail.

11. **Procedural Step.** Follow the same steps to open each piece of mail as described earlier, and separate the pieces of mail into categories: urgent or very important, other letters, letters or reports containing patient information or results, medical journals, and circulars or advertising.

12. **Procedural Step.** Arrange letters and reports containing patient information in alphabetic order. If the office uses paper-based medical records, find the appropriate medical record and attach each letter or report to the medical record with a paper clip.

13. **Procedural Step.** Arrange the mail for each physician with the most important mail on top and the least important on the bottom.

14. **Procedural Step.** Distribute each stack of mail to the appropriate individual.

15. **Procedural Step.** Explain why efficient mail sorting helps maintain office effectiveness.

Figure 45-4 In a large office, each staff member may have a mailbox at a central location.

AUTOMATED MAIL PROCESSING

Since the early 1980s the methods used to process the mail have evolved from manual and mechanized processing to automated processing. Automated equipment can read and sort mail more than six times faster than manual mail sorting. Machine-addressed letters are processed using optical character recognition (OCR), the mechanical or electronic recognition and interpretation of text.

Mail that is prepared for automated processing facilitates the sorting process. As an incentive, the USPS offers lower rates to high-volume mailers who prepare their mail for automation by adding postal bar codes and presorting mail. Most medical offices do not qualify for the lower rates because they are not high-volume mailers. To qualify for a lower rate on First-Class Mail, the mailer must send out 500 letters in one mailing.

HIGHLIGHT on Automated Postal Equipment

Automated postal equipment can handle most letters and process them without human intervention. At a Processing and Distribution Center, packages and large pieces of mail are diverted from the stream of mail. All other mail enters the Advanced Facer Canceler System (AFCS), which rotates the mail so that it faces in the proper direction to postmark and cancel the postage stamp. If a piece of mail has a printed address, it goes to the Multiline Optical Character Reader (MLOCR), which reads the delivery address, translates this information into a bar code, and prints the bar code in the lower right-hand corner of the envelope. If the MLOCR cannot read the address, it sprays an identifying code on the back of the envelope. An operator at a distant site reads the address on a video screen, transmits a ZIP code back to the envelope, and a bar code is sprayed onto the envelope without it leaving the automated stream. Once a bar code has been added to the piece of mail, it goes to a Delivery Bar Code Sorter (DBCS), which reads and interprets the bar code and sorts it accordingly. Items for local delivery are retained, but other mail is shipped either by air or by truck to a destination station, where it is passed through another DBCS. At the local destination station the mail is sorted right down to arranging the mail in the order of a carrier's delivery route. Automated equipment is continuously updated and improved by the U.S. Postal Service. ■

POSTAL ADDRESSING STANDARDS

Specific standards must be met to prepare a piece of mail so that it can be processed by automated equipment. The medical assistant should be familiar with these standards and put them into practice to ensure the most efficient and timely delivery of outgoing mail.

LETTERS AND LARGE ENVELOPES

To be mailed as a letter, an envelope must be $3\frac{1}{2}$ to $6\frac{1}{8}$ to inches in height and 5 to $11\frac{1}{2}$ inches in length. The two most common sizes for business envelopes are the No. 10 envelope ($4\frac{1}{8} \times 9\frac{1}{2}$ inches) and the smaller No. $6\frac{3}{4}$ envelope ($3\frac{5}{8} \times 6\frac{1}{2}$ inches), but other sizes may be used. Square letters and letters that are too thick to pass through automated equipment require additional postage. The address may be printed directly on an envelope or on a label that will be attached to the envelope.

A large envelope requires more postage. It may be $6\frac{1}{8}$ to 12 inches in height and $11\frac{1}{2}$ to 15 inches in length. Large manila or white envelopes may be used to send patient medical records or other documents that have too many pages to fold.

COMPLETE ADDRESS

The USPS defines a complete address as one that includes all elements necessary for delivery. To be complete, the address block should include the following elements in the following order:

Recipient line (and/or)
Organization name
Street address or postal box number
Apartment or suite number (if needed; separate line if needed)
City, state, and ZIP code

The post office recommends that the address be printed legibly without punctuation except for the hyphen after the first five digits in the ZIP+4 (Procedure 45-2). Recommended abbreviations for elements of the address are found in Box 45-1. Abbreviations for individual states are found in Table 45-2.

ADDRESS FORMAT

Address format refers to how the various address elements appear on an envelope. The following standards are recommended:

1. The address should be machine printed or hand-printed using plain block letters. A typeface without serifs (cross strokes at the end of the main strokes of the letter), such as Helvetica or Arial, is preferred. Script and italic styles should be avoided.
2. All lines of the address should be formatted with a uniform left margin.
3. All lines of the address should be parallel to the bottom of the envelope.
4. No punctuation should be used in the address except the hyphen in the ZIP+4 code.
5. If a window envelope is used, the entire address must be visible through the window. At least $\frac{1}{8}$-inch clearance ($\frac{1}{4}$ inch is preferred) must be maintained between the address and the edges of the window to distinguish the address from the edge of the window. No other print should show through the window.
6. Delivery instructions (e.g., "personal," "confidential") should be placed immediately below the return address. Special services (e.g., Registered Mail, Certified Mail, Insured Mail) should be indicated above the address and to the right of the return address below or to the left of the area where stamps or postage will be affixed.
7. Address labels should be applied using methods and materials that prevent them from becoming damaged or removed during high-speed automated processing.
8. The address should be placed within an area that extends from $\frac{5}{8}$ inch to $2\frac{3}{4}$ inches from the bottom edge of the envelope with a $\frac{1}{2}$-inch margin on each side. This is called the *OCR read area* (Figure 45-5).

BOX 45-1 Specific Delivery Address Standards

1. Use common Postal Service standard abbreviations as much as possible.

AVE	Avenue
BLVD	Boulevard
CIR	Circle
CTR	Center
DR	Drive
EXT	Extension
HWY	Highway
IS	Island
JCT	Junction
LN	Lane
MTN	Mountain
PARK	Park
PKWY	Parkway
RD	Road
RIV	River
SQ	Square
ST	Street
TER	Terrace
VLG	Village
VLY	Valley

2. Use secondary address directional abbreviations (e.g., N, S, NE, SW).
3. Include secondary address locators, such as apartment numbers, suite numbers, and room numbers, at the end of the delivery address line or on the line below the street address.

APT	Apartment
BLDG	Building
STE	Suite
UNIT	Unit

Table 45-2 Two-Letter State and Territory Abbreviations

AL	Alabama	MT	Montana
AK	Alaska	NE	Nebraska
AZ	Arizona	NV	Nevada
AR	Arkansas	NH	New Hampshire
CA	California	NM	New Mexico
CO	Colorado	NY	New York
CT	Connecticut	NC	North Carolina
DE	Delaware	ND	North Dakota
DC	District of Columbia	OH	Ohio
FL	Florida	OK	Oklahoma
GA	Georgia	OR	Oregon
GU	Guam	PA	Pennsylvania
HI	Hawaii	PR	Puerto Rico
ID	Idaho	RI	Rhode Island
IL	Illinois	SC	South Carolina
IN	Indiana	SD	South Dakota
IA	Iowa	TN	Tennessee
KS	Kansas	TX	Texas
KY	Kentucky	UT	Utah
LA	Louisiana	VT	Vermont
ME	Maine	VI	Virgin Islands
MD	Maryland	VA	Virginia
MA	Massachusetts	WA	Washington
MI	Michigan	WV	West Virginia
MN	Minnesota	WI	Wisconsin
MS	Mississippi	WY	Wyoming
MO	Missouri		

9. The bar code clear zone is the area on an envelope where a bar code is printed by the automated equipment. It represents an area that is $\frac{5}{8}$ inch high × $\frac{3}{4}$ inches long. It must remain free of all printing, markings, or colored borders.

RETURN ADDRESS

The return address identifies the location to which a piece of mail should be returned if it cannot be delivered. It must be located in the upper left corner of the envelope and must not extend into the OCR read area. The return address should include the following elements:

Sender's name (optional)
Sender's delivery address
Sender's city, state, and ZIP code

Letterhead envelopes or envelopes preprinted with the return address are usually used.

PROCEDURE 45-2 Looking up a ZIP Code

Outcome Use the Internet to find the correct ZIP+4 code for a given address

Equipment/Supplies

- Computer with Internet access
- Pen and pencil

- Address with incorrect and/or incomplete ZIP code

1. **Procedural Step.** Open the computer's Web browser and enter the Web address for the USPS.
2. **Procedural Step.** From the USPS home page, click on the link labeled "Look up a ZIP code."
3. **Procedural Step.** In the address popup window, enter the delivery address, city, and state abbreviation of the address for which a ZIP code is sought. (It is also possible to search for a ZIP code if only the city and state are known.)
4. **Procedural Step.** Copy the ZIP+4 code on a piece of paper to use in preparing a label or envelope or use the computer "copy" function to copy and paste into a computer file.

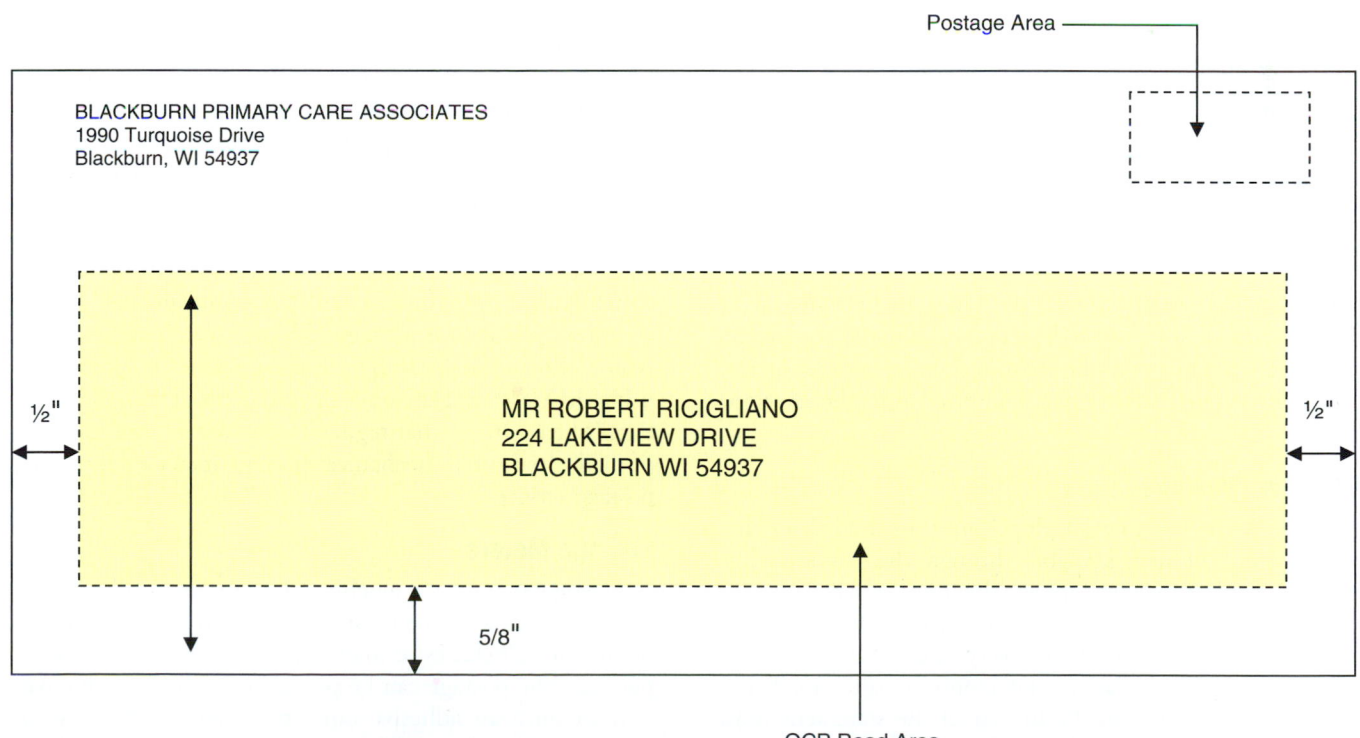

Figure 45-5 Envelope showing address in the optical character recognition (*OCR*) read area.

OUTGOING MAIL

The process of preparing items for mailing may include addressing envelopes, preparing mailing labels, folding letters or statements to place into envelopes, calculating and adding postage, and mailing items either in mailboxes or at the post office.

PREPARING ENVELOPES OR MAILING LABELS

Most word processing programs have a feature that creates and prints an address (and return address if desired) on various sizes of envelope. The medical assistant selects the envelope function and enters the delivery address (and return address if not preprinted on the envelope). A single envelope can then be placed in the manual feed tray for printing. Some printers have an optional envelope feed tray for processing several envelopes. When several addresses must be printed, it is more common to use labels. These come in pages and can be printed from lists using the mail merge feature.

FOLDING AND INSERTING LETTERS INTO ENVELOPES

The medical assistant should fold letters so that they can be inserted into envelopes easily. It is also important to use standard methods of folding so that letters are not damaged during opening.

No. 10 Envelope

To fold a letter in thirds, bring the bottom third of the letter up and form a crease. Then fold the top third down and make a crease. The second crease of the letter is inserted into the envelope first.

No. 6¾ Envelope

For a smaller envelope, fold the letter in half and make a crease. Then fold the right third in and make a crease. Fold the left third over the right and make another crease. The final crease of the letter is inserted into the envelope first.

Window Envelope

A letter for a window envelope must be folded so that the delivery address is visible through the window. The bottom third of the envelope is folded up to make a crease. The top third of the envelope is then folded back from the previous crease so that the delivery address shows on the outside of the letter. Patient statements are often mailed in window envelopes, and the format of the statement must be adjusted to the specific envelopes that the office uses (Figure 45-6).

Figure 45-6 Correct methods of folding letters for envelopes.

ADDING POSTAGE

The medical assistant may add postage using stamps or postage meters or by printing postage from the computer (Procedure 45-3).

Postage stamps can be purchased at the post office or by telephone or mail from the USPS. Stamps can also be printed from the computer using software and stamp labels. The postage for a stamp printer is purchased online. Patient statements, which are usually sent First Class, require one First-Class stamp. Letters that weigh more than 1 ounce and envelopes that are larger than $6\frac{1}{8} \times 11\frac{1}{2}$ inches require additional postage. For these letters, an office would require either stamps of various values or a stamp printer, as well as a postage scale, for postage to be calculated accurately. It is not difficult to look up the correct amount of postage using the USPS website once the weight of an item has been established. Offices that regularly send out a steady volume of mail often use a mechanical postage meter or an online postage service.

Postage Meters

A **postage meter** is a machine that automatically stamps outgoing mail with the proper postage. Postage meters may be used for all classes of mail and for any denomination of postage. The postage can be printed directly onto an envelope or onto an adhesive tape strip that is affixed to an envelope or package. Mail that has been stamped by a postage meter is known as **metered mail**.

Memories *from* Practicum

Diane Waters: My practicum was at a large clinic with many departments. I spent the majority of the time in the internal medicine department, but to get experience with all the aspects of medical assisting, I spent time in other departments, including the mailroom. In the morning the mail was sorted. There was usually one or two bags of mail, and we sorted it into small storage crates using one crate for two departments. If the department was indicated on the piece of mail, it was easy to place in the correct crate, but if there was only a name, I had to use a list to identify which department the person worked in. After the mail was sorted, we placed the crates on a mail cart and delivered the mail to the separate departments. In the administration area, we also placed the mail into mailboxes for the staff in that department, but in the clinical areas, we just gave all the mail for the department to the secretary at the front window. In the afternoon, we prepared the outgoing mail. We collected the crates of outgoing mail from all the departments. In the mailroom, we separated letters in standard envelopes from any large envelopes and packages. I was taught to use the postage meter to print the postage directly on envelopes. The postage meter had a built-in scale, so we could run any letter in a standard envelope through the meter. The large envelopes were weighed and correct postage was printed using strips from the postage meter. John, who was in charge of the mailroom, took the mail to the post office every afternoon because there were always items that needed special services. He said that the other mail would go out faster if it was sent directly from the post office. ∎

Postage meters cannot be purchased. Instead, they must be leased from one of the postal service's approved vendors. The amount of postage that can be stamped with the meter is predetermined and prepaid either on a regular basis, such as monthly, or when the amount remaining is getting low. Postage can be purchased online, by telephone, or from the post office. To use a postage meter for bulk mailings, the medical office must apply for a bulk mailing permit and pay an annual fee.

Many different types of postage meters are available, ranging from simple to complex models. The simplest model has only the ability to stamp the mail. More complex models, on the other hand, have security features and may automatically weigh the mail, fold and insert letters into envelopes, seal the envelopes, and catch envelopes in a stacker tray. Complex models typically consist of two separate components: the meter that adds the postage and a base that performs the other functions. A base that is compatible with the chosen model of postage meter can be purchased outright by the medical office.

Safety Precautions

Certain safety precautions should be followed when using a postage meter:

1. Read the operating guide carefully before operating the postage meter.
2. Do not touch any moving parts of the postage meter when it is in operation.
3. Make sure to keep loose clothing, jewelry, and long hair away from all moving parts of the postage meter.
4. Do not cover the ventilation slots on the machine, to prevent overheating.
5. If a paper jam occurs, unplug the machine and make sure all machine mechanisms have come to a stop before clearing the jam.
6. Never attempt to disassemble the machine for repair. If service is required, contact the manufacturer's service representative.

Online Postage Services

The medical office may also subscribe to a service that allows the medical assistant to purchase, calculate, and print postage directly from the computer. These services usually allow the client to print stamps, print shipping labels, print postage directly on envelopes, and add special services (e.g., insurance, delivery confirmation, Return Receipt requested). The computer program can also check the accuracy of the address. Postal scales can be integrated with the computer software to calculate postage automatically. Online postage services offer increased versatility with respect to printing and personalizing labels, but if an office has a large volume of First-Class envelopes, a postage meter with envelope handling features may provide more efficient mail handling.

What Would You Do?   What Would You *Not* Do?

Case Study 3

The medical office where Diane works has been using the same postage meter to prepare the mail for several years, and most of the staff is familiar with it. It usually works well when operated by someone who is familiar with it, but new staff members complain that it is "difficult." Diane is familiar with this postage meter and has used another model of postage meter, but she does not know anything specific about online postage services. At a staff meeting, the office manager suggests that it may be time to update the postage meter to a newer model. One of the physicians says that he has heard that the office could save money and handle the mail more efficiently using an online postage service. He asks Diane for her opinion. ∎

PROCEDURE 45-3

PROCEDURE 45-3   Preparing Envelopes for Mailing   ⓔ

Outcome Address an envelope, and process envelopes to be mailed

Equipment/Supplies

- Envelope
- Other items to be mailed
- Pen
- Typewriter

- Computer and printer
- Postal scale
- Postage meter (optional)
- Stamps

1. **Procedural Step.** Determine the exact address to be used to address the envelope. Addresses may be kept in a computer file or manually in an index card box or circular card file (e.g., Rolodex).

2. **Procedural Step.** Select an envelope of the appropriate size. For business letters a No. 10 envelope is most commonly used. A large manila envelope may be used for documents containing several pages.

3. **Procedural Step.** Decide on a means to address the envelope (e.g., typewriter, computer, label printer). The address may be printed directly on the envelope or on a label. Avoid addressing ordinary correspondence by hand.
   Principle. Standard business correspondence appears more professional if addressed using a typewriter or computer.

4. **Procedural Step.** Key the address near the center of the envelope in the OCR read area with the name of the recipient on the first line, the street address and apartment or suite on the second (or second and third) line, and the city, state, and nine-number ZIP code on the bottom line. Punctuation is not required except for a hyphen after the first five numbers of the ZIP+4 code. If using an envelope without letterhead, key the return address in the upper left corner using the same guidelines.
   Principle. These are guidelines recommended by the U.S. Postal Service (USPS).

5. **Procedural Step.** Add any special notations, such as "Personal" or "Confidential," below the return address and above the address at the left side of the envelope.
   Principle. Nothing must be placed below the address, so the post office equipment can read the envelope correctly.

6. **Procedural Step.** Add any mailing instructions or special services (e.g., "Certified") on the right side of

the envelope above the address, leaving room for a postage label above.

7. **Procedural Step.** Place the item to be mailed in the envelope, folding it as needed, and seal the envelope (unless a postage meter with a sealer will be used).

8. **Procedural Step.** Weigh the piece of mail if it contains more than two sheets of paper or if an envelope larger than $6\frac{1}{8} \times 11\frac{1}{2}$ is used.
   Principle. Large envelopes, rigid envelopes, and envelopes that are not rectangular require more postage than First-Class letters weighing less than 1 oz.

9. **Procedural Step.** Calculate and apply the correct amount of postage. One First-Class stamp or equivalent is required for First-Class letters weighing less than 1 oz. Postage for other items may be calculated from the USPS website, using a postage meter, or using an online postage service. If a postage meter is used, all envelopes to be mailed in one day may be processed together.

10. **Procedural Step.** Assemble all letters and other items to be mailed.

11. **Procedural Step.** Sort envelopes according to size.

12. **Procedural Step.** Separate any items with special mailing instructions that must be taken to the post office. If necessary, add instructions to the envelopes. If the office does not have a postal scale, include any letters that may need extra postage.

13. **Procedural Step.** Place items with postage in a mailbox, or request a pickup from the postal service.

14. **Procedural Step.** Take special items to the post office. This may include items that are to be sent Return Receipt, Certified Mail, Registered Mail, or Insured Mail and stamped items weighing more than 13 oz.
    Principle. Stamped mail and Priority Mail weighing more than 13 oz will not be accepted from a mailbox even if proper postage is attached.

What Would You Do? What Would You *Not* Do? RESPONSES

Case Study 1
Page 1136

What Did Diane Do?
- Asked Mr. Stone if he wanted her to send the form to sign for release of the medical record as an e-mail attachment.
- Informed Mr. Stone of the standard charge for copying a medical record and also whether he would be required to pay for postage.
- After receiving the consent form, took precautions to maintain privacy of Mr. Stone's record while photocopying it.
- Determined the best way to send the record so that it would arrive in time. Obtained authorization to send the record Priority Mail Express or Priority Mail if it was not office policy to charge the patient for postage.

What Did Diane *Not* Do?
- Did not tell Mr. Stone that his request could not be granted because there wasn't enough time.
- Did not send the record before receiving the signed consent form to release the record.
- Did not criticize Mr. Stone for making an unreasonable request.
- Did not fail to follow up on this request.

Case Study 2
Page 1137

What Did Diane Do?
- Searched for the correct (or complete) address of Dr. Leonie using other methods, such as looking up the address in the office's address file, looking at previous correspondence,

looking up the address using the Internet, or calling Dr. Leonie's office.
- After locating the correct (or complete) address, looked up the ZIP code again until a complete ZIP+4 code was found.
- Finished preparing the envelope using the correct address and ZIP+4 code.

What Did Diane *Not* Do?
- Did not ask the physician to find Dr. Leonie's address for her.
- Did not send the letter using the five-digit ZIP she found on the first search.

Case Study 3
Page 1143

What Did Diane Do?
- Stated that she was familiar with postage meters but that she did not know about online postage services.
- Gave her honest opinion about the ease of using the current postage meter.
- Offered to research the benefits and costs of an online postage service versus updating the postage meter.
- Offered to try to find out how much time it would take to orient staff to a new method of preparing the mail.

What Did Diane *Not* Do?
- Did not give a negative opinion of online postage services just because she did not want to cope with a system change.
- Did not automatically agree with the physician that changing to an online postage system would be a good idea.
- Did not say that the current postage meter worked very well if a person just took the time to try to understand it.

TERMINOLOGY REVIEW

Key Term	Definition
Annotate	To underline or highlight important words and phrases in correspondence.
Bar code clear zone	The area on the lower right-hand corner of a card or envelope that is left clear for the postal bar code to be printed.
Metered mail	Mail for which the postage has been applied using a postage meter.
Postage meter	A machine that automatically stamps a piece of mail with the correct postage.
Postal bar code	A series of vertical bars of two lengths, which represent the delivery address of a piece of mail. The bar code facilitates automated sorting of mail.
ZIP code	A five-digit code that identifies the post office to which a given piece of mail is to be delivered.
ZIP+4 code	A more detailed mailing code consisting of the original five-digit ZIP code followed by a hyphen and four additional digits. These digits identify a specific geographic segment within the delivery area.

ON THE WEB

For information on the U.S. Postal Service:

Calculate postage and look up ZIP codes: www.usps.com

Domestic mail manual: pe.usps.gov

Postage options: www.usps.com/business/postage-options.htm

46 Managing Practice Finances

ⓔ Check out the Evolve site at http://evolve.elsevier.com/Bonewit/today/ to access additional interactive activities and exercises to help you study and prepare for success.

LEARNING OBJECTIVES

1. Describe manual and computerized methods of maintaining patient accounts.
2. Differentiate between a simple charge slip and a charge slip with diagnosis and procedure codes (superbill).
3. Describe how charges are entered on a charge slip or a superbill.
4. Identify the information contained on a fee schedule, and describe how it is used.
5. Describe the information contained in a patient account ledger.
6. List the steps to post charges, payments, and/or adjustments to the patient account.
7. Describe the process to print patient ledgers, day sheets, or other reports using a practice management computer system.
8. Differentiate between accounts receivable and accounts payable.
9. Identify various types of bank accounts.
10. Discuss the information printed on a check.
11. Describe various methods to write checks.
12. Describe precautions to take when accepting checks, credit cards, or debit cards.
13. Discuss methods to transfer funds electronically.
14. Describe how to balance a cash drawer.
15. Describe how a bank deposit is prepared and made.
16. Describe how entries are made in the cash disbursement journal.
17. Describe how to maintain a petty cash fund.

PROCEDURES

Complete a patient charge slip.

Post charges to the patient ledger.
Post payments and/or adjustments.

Write a check.

Prepare a bank deposit.

CHAPTER OUTLINE

INTRODUCTION TO DAILY FINANCIAL ACTIVITIES
MAINTAINING PATIENT ACCOUNTS
COMPONENTS OF A PATIENT ACCOUNT
Charge Slip
Computerized Charge Entry
Fee Schedule
Patient Account Ledger
Posting Payments to the Patient Account
Posting Adjustments to the Patient Account
Day Sheet
Printing Day Sheets and Other Reports
OTHER FINANCIAL ACCOUNTS
BANKING ACTIVITIES
Types of Accounts
Checking Account
Savings Account
Money Market Account

Checks
Types of Checks
Preparing a Check
Precautions for Accepting Checks, Credit Cards, and/or Debit Cards
Electronic Transfer of Funds
Bank Deposits
Balancing the Cash Drawer
Preparing a Bank Deposit
Endorsing Checks
Making a Deposit
Reconciling a Bank Statement
ACCOUNTS PAYABLE OR RECORD OF CASH DISBURSEMENTS
PETTY CASH

KEY TERMS

ABA routing number
accounting
accounts payable
accounts receivable
accrual (ah-KREW-ul) basis of
   accounting
adjustment
assets
bookkeeping

cash basis of accounting
cashier's check
certified check
charge slip
credit
day sheet
debit
disbursements
fee schedule

invoice
ledger
liabilities
MICR line
payee (pay-EE)
petty cash
reconciling
superbill

INTRODUCTION TO DAILY FINANCIAL ACTIVITIES

A medical office is a business. The business of a medical office is providing medical services—one of the most important services in the entire economy. Because the medical office is a business, daily management of the practice's finances is key to the physicians' ability to provide the best services possible for patients. If the practice's bills are not paid and fees are not collected, the practice will cease to be a viable business and the patients will suffer.

Accounting is the term for systematic recording and reporting of financial transactions. The **cash basis of accounting,** which is usually used by medical offices, enters income when payment is received for services. This contrasts with the **accrual basis of accounting,** in which income is entered at the time of sale, even if payment has not yet been received. Companies that sell merchandise usually use the accrual basis of accounting. In both systems, expenses are entered when they are incurred, even if they have not yet been paid.

Bookkeeping refers to the process of keeping detailed records of financial transactions. Managing the daily finances is a task that often falls to a medical assistant. Professional accountants are usually responsible for general aspects of financial management, such as preparing detailed financial reports, financial planning, and preparing tax returns.

This chapter focuses on the parts of the daily financial activities involved in charging patients for the services provided each day, maintaining patient accounts and other **accounts receivable** (money owed to the practice), and managing the **accounts payable** (money the practice owes).

MAINTAINING PATIENT ACCOUNTS

Patient accounts make up the bulk of the medical practice's income. Some income might come from rental of space—

for instance, to a particular laboratory for a specimen collection station or to a social worker, psychologist, or other specialist who consults for the practice. Other income may come from royalties—from a particular medical instrument that one or more of the physicians developed, for instance, or from a book written by the professionals in the practice. But the bulk of the practice's income will be earned on a daily basis from the charges for services to patients.

Patient accounts may be recorded manually or using a computer. Most medical offices use a computerized medical billing system, although they may maintain some manual records, such as a day sheet. If there is an electronic medical record (EMR), the billing system is usually linked to or part of it. A manual bookkeeping system uses the following:

- A daily journal, commonly called a *day sheet,* to record all transactions that occurred on that day.
- An accounts receivable ledger for each patient, to keep a record of transactions related to that patient.
- A cumulative record of financial activity, both for the practice as a whole and for each individual physician; this information is recorded on the day sheet, and cumulative totals are carried forward throughout the month.

In a computerized billing system, the same types of records are maintained. When procedures are performed, charges for individual patients are entered into the medical computer billing program and automatically posted to the patient's account and the daily record of charges. In a modern practice management program that coordinates with the EMR, the physician can enter the services provided at the end of the patient visit, specify the diagnosis (and diagnosis code) that applies, and link them to the billing system. In a similar way, payments made by the patient (or an insurance company) are posted to both the patient account and the daily record of charges. The computer program can access data to generate patient bills, insurance claims, and a variety of reports, including monthly statements, activity of individual physicians, and the number of specific procedures billed.

HIGHLIGHT on Bookkeeping Systems

The two most common systems for keeping records of accounts are single-entry and double-entry systems. Historically, financial transactions were recorded in a book called a *ledger* with separate pages for individual accounts. In medical offices, separate cards began to be used for individual accounts (instead of pages of a book). These cards came to be called *ledger cards,* and in medical computer billing programs, a screen showing cumulative charges and payments for a single patient is called a *patient ledger.*

The Accounting Principle

A common formulation of the accounting principle is as follows:

$$Assets=Liabilities+Owner's\ equity$$

where assets are property owned by the business, liabilities are debts, and owner's equity is the amount by which the owner's assets exceed liabilities.

Single-Entry Bookkeeping System

The single-entry bookkeeping system is the simplest system and is usually used in individual medical offices. It requires at least three records:

1. A chronologic journal that keeps track of all charges and patient payments, such as a daily journal.
2. A journal that keeps track of payments made by the medical office, traditionally a checkbook but now usually an electronic check register.
3. A method to keep track of individual patient accounts. These used to be recorded on pages of a book, index cards, or

ledger cards, but today they are usually accounts in a computerized billing program.

Although the single-entry system is simple, its methods for cross-checking to prevent and/or detect errors are incomplete.

Double-Entry Bookkeeping System

The double-entry system is the most complete type of book-keeping system. It is used by manufacturing or retail businesses, hospitals, and other large health care institutions. However, it usually requires a trained bookkeeper or accountant to be used effectively.

Every transaction is posted into two different records, as a credit in one and a debit in the other. A credit is a posting that is subtracted from the balance, and a debit is a posting that is added. Records of **assets**—money and property owned by the business and money owed to the business—are balanced against records of **liabilities**—money owed to others by the business.

A charge for service to a patient, for example, is a credit (added to the balance) in the records of assets because it increases the total assets, but it is a debit (subtracted from the balance) in the records of liabilities because it decreases the amount owed by the business.

If a double-entry bookkeeping system is used by a medical practice—for example, if the practice is owned by a hospital or other large health care institution—the medical assistant is usually responsible only for keeping the daily journal and entering charges, payments, and adjustments in the computer. The actual records of assets and liabilities are kept by an accountant. ■

Putting It All Into Practice

My name is Maria Hernandez, and I am a Registered Medical Assistant. I work at the office of three physicians who specialize in internal medicine. One of my duties is to manage patient accounts. The physicians enter the service provided into the electronic medical record (EMR) at the time of the visit, and we verify the charges and enter payments and copayments. I also enter almost all of the payments we receive in the mail including checks from patients, as well as posting insurance payments that are received by electronic transfer to individual patient accounts. I am also responsible for paying the bills for the practice. Our patient billing is linked to our EMR, but we have another computer program to manage our accounts payable and pay bills. We also use online banking, and we have set up automatic bill payment for those bills that occur every month including our mortgage, condominium fee, electricity, telephone, and answering service bills. We usually pay our other bills by check. The computer accounting program tracks all payments and prints checks. All of the physicians are authorized to sign checks under $500.00. If we purchase an item that costs more than $500.00, the check must be signed by any two physicians. When I was in school, I didn't appreciate what a big job it is to manage financial accounts. I really enjoy this part of my job now, and I have come to understand that it always saves time to work carefully and avoid mistakes. ■

COMPONENTS OF A PATIENT ACCOUNT

Four components are used to maintain a patient account, whether a manual or computer accounting system is used:
- Charge slip or computerized charge entry
- Fee schedule
- Patient account ledger
- Daily journal (day sheet)

CHARGE SLIP

A **charge slip** is a means of keeping track of charges for services and payments made at the time of the patient visit. A paper charge slip, if used, is usually prepared before the patient visit and completed after the patient has been seen. In its simplest form, the charge slip contains the patient's name, the date of the service rendered, any procedures performed (including the visit itself), the total charges, and the amount the patient paid.

In traditional medical office manual accounting systems, a "one-write" or "write-it-once" system (also called a *pegboard system*) is used. All necessary forms are held in place on a metal or plastic board by a row of pegs across the left side. In this type of system, information from the top form is transferred to the forms below. Entering information once generates a charge slip and receipt, an entry on the patient's ledger card, and an entry on the daily journal (day sheet) (Figure 46-1).

Pegboard charge slips, paper ledger cards, and paper day sheets are rarely used today because most offices use a medical computer billing program (practice management program) to keep track of individual patient accounts. The format of computer billing programs is based on the old pegboard system, however. A pegboard system may also be used to write checks and keep a check register if not done electronically.

When insurance companies began requiring numeric codes for procedures and diagnoses, a new type of charge slip was developed so that these codes could be identified at the time of service. A **superbill** (sometimes called a *billing encounter form*) is a form containing both diagnosis and procedure codes in addition to charges and payments.

Most medical offices use a customized superbill as a charge slip, if a paper charge slip is still used. The top section of the form is filled out with patient information by using a printed label, filling it out manually, printing the information on the form from the computer, or entering the information into the computer. Figure 46-2 shows an example of a completed paper superbill.

Figure 46-1 Medical assistant using a pegboard system.

When the patient is seen, the physician or other provider who sees the patient checks off the boxes next to the correct code for the type of visit (problem focused, straightforward, detailed, low complexity, comprehensive, moderately complex, and so forth), as well as any other procedures performed, and also fills in the patient's diagnosis.

Using the fee schedule, the medical assistant adds charges and enters any payments made by the patient. The completed superbill is used to enter billing information into the computer. For this reason, it is extremely important to be sure that the superbill is filled out accurately.

COMPUTERIZED CHARGE ENTRY

When the computerized billing system is linked to the EMR, the physician specifies the services provided and links each service to a diagnosis at the time of the visit. The front desk staff then formalizes the charge entry by creating an electronic superbill or using a transaction entry function. Each service must be linked in the computer to a procedure code and a diagnosis code for insurance billing purposes. Coding is discussed in Chapter 47. Computerized billing programs usually contain the most commonly used codes so that they do not need to be entered for each patient.

FEE SCHEDULE

A **fee schedule** is a list of charges for the various procedures a physician performs. In a hospital system, it is commonly called a chargemaster. Years ago, a physician had one set of fees that he or she charged patients for office visits, procedures, and/or treatments. Today, however, a medical practice may have to accept different amounts as payment for each service it performs, depending on which insurance provider is paying for the service. The reimbursement varies from a fixed percentage of the physician's charges to a set amount for a given service. Insurance is discussed in detail in Chapter 48.

The medical office usually has a basic fee schedule that lists the usual charges for office visits and procedures. The fee schedule is used to fill out charges on the charge slip or electronic superbill. Some computer billing programs can link a patient's fees to the fee schedules of his or her specific insurance provider, such as Medicare or Medicaid (Procedure 46-1).

What Would You Do? What Would You *Not* Do?

Case Study 1

In the afternoon, Maria is entering charges and payments into the patient computer accounts. She is using itemized paper charge slips (superbills) to do this. In Maria's office the superbills are numbered consecutively, and Maria notices that there are two gaps in the numbers of the superbills. The office records all transactions using a manual day sheet, and Maria verifies that one of the physicians saw two patients for whom she does not have charge slips. ∎

Western Medical Center
109 River Street
Western, OH 44770-0421
(490) 555-6464

Richard Warner, MD   NPI # 23456781XX
Maria Gomez, MD   NPI # 34567891XX
                          Tax ID 52-XX63777

Patient Name and Address	Birthdate	Subscriber Name	MD Name	Today's Date
DARLA SISSLE 10 MAPLE STREET WESTERN, OH 44770	2/17/52	DARLA SISSLE	WARNER	6/26/XX
	Account #	Insurance Company	Insurance Phone #	Time
	1015	SHHMO	(490) 565-2000	10:00 AM
Telephone No.		Insurance ID #	Group/Plan #	Sex
(490) 220-1156		21-58624	8300099	Male ☐ Female ☒

√	DESCRIPTION	CPT	FEE	√	DESCRIPTION	CPT	FEE	√	DESCRIPTION	CPT	FEE
	OFFICE VISIT				**IMMUNIZATIONS**				**PROCEDURES**		
	NEW PATIENT				Imm. admin, one	90471		√	ECG w/interpretation	93000	65--
	Problem Focused	99201			Imm. admin, each add'l	90472			Spirometry	94010	
	Exp. Prob. Focused	99202			Influenza < 3	90657			Inhalation treatment	94640	
	Detailed	99203			Influenza 3 and >	90658			Remove skin tag <15	11200	
	Comp/Mod MDM	99204			Medicare code	G0008			Cerumen removal	69210	
	Comp./High MDM	99205			Varicella	90716			Wart destruction < 14	17110	
	ESTABLISHED PATIENT				DTaP	90700			I & D abscess	10060	
	Minimal/Nurse Visit	99211			Td adult	90718					
	Problem Focused	99212			Rubella	90706					
√	Exp. Problem Focused	99213	65--		MMR	90707			**OTHER**		
	Detailed	99214			Hep B Child	90744					
	Comprehensive	99215			Hep B Adult	90746					
	Post-op Exam	99024	0.00		IPV	90713					
	WELL VISIT				**WELL VISIT**				**LABORATORY**		
	NEW PATIENT				ESTABLISHED PATIENT				Blood collection Vein	36415	
	Infant–1 year	99381			Infant–1 year	99391			Venipuncture, Medicare	G0001	
	1 yr–4 yr	99382			1 yr–4 yr	99392			Finger stick, glucose	82948	
	5 yr – 11 yr	99383			5 yr –11 yr	99393			Hemoccult, guaiac	82270	
	12 yr–17 yr	99384			12 yr–17 yr	99394			Strep, rapid	87880	
	18 yr –39 yr	99385			18 yr –39 yr	99395			UA, dipstick (manual)	81000	
	40 yr –64 yr	99386			40 yr –64 yr	99396			UA, automated	81003	
	65 yr and over	99387			65 yr and over	99397			Urine pregnancy	81025	

DIAGNOSTIC CODES (ICD-10-CM)

☐ R10.9 Abdominal Pain	☐ E11.9 Diabetes II–Non Ins	☐ H66.9_ Otitis Media	☐ Z23 Immunization Encounter
☐ E63.4 AllergicReaction	☐ K57.92 Diverticulitis	☐ J02.9 Pharyngitis	☐ Z00.12_ Well Child Check
☐ D64.9 Anemia	☐ K57.90 Diverticulosis	☐ M06.9 Rheumatoid Arthritis	☐ Z00.0_ Well Adult
☐ D51.0 Anemia, Pernicious	☐ R60.9 Edema	☐ R06.02 Short of Breath	☐ _____
■ I12.9 Angina Pectoris	☐ R51 Headache	☐ J32.9 Sinusitis	☐ _____
☐ I49.9 Arrhythmia, Cardiac	☐ R31.9 Hematuria	☐ L19.8 Skin Tag(s)	☐ _____
☐ I70.0 Atherosclerosis, Aorta	☐ B00.9 Herpes Zoster	☐ J02.0 Streptococcal Sore Throat	☐ _____
☐ J45.909 Asthma	☐ I10 Hypertension	☐ N39.0 Urinary Tract Infection	☐ _____
☐ M54.9 Back Pain	☐ E03.9 Hypothyroidism		
☐ J20._ Bronchitis, Acute	☐ H61.2_ Impacted Cerumen	**RETURN APPOINTMENT**	**BALANCE DUE**
☐ J42 Bronchitis, Chronic	☐ J10.1 Influenza	_____ Days	Total Charge $ 130.00
☐ R07.9 Chest Pain	☐ K58.9 Irritable Bowel Syndrome	_____ Weeks	Amount Paid $ 20.00
☐ J44.9 COPD	☐ M19.0 Osteoarthritis	_____ Months	Previous Bal $ 35.00
☐ E10.0 Diabetes I–Ins. Dep	☐ M19.0 Osteoarthritis	_____ PRN	Adjustment $ 0.00
			Balance Due $ 145.00

Figure 46-2 Completed charge slip (superbill) containing procedure and diagnosis codes (ICD-10).

PATIENT ACCOUNT LEDGER

Each patient has his or her own account. It is important to verify that all information about the account is current when the patient arrives at the office, because address information and insurance information can change between visits. A cumulative record of charges and payments is kept, usually using a computer program. It is also possible to keep account records manually. This record of charges and payments is called the patient account **ledger.** In a practice management program, the patient account ledger is linked to the patient demographic and insurance information so that periodic bills and insurance claims can be generated. Information about services provided to an individual patient and payments received for that patient show up in chronologic order on the patient ledger (Figure 46-3). Traditionally patient ledger cards recorded a running balance, but computerized ledgers may record the balance for each line (entry) with the total patient balance at the end of the ledger.

After the charge slip has been completed, the charges are posted to the patient ledger (Procedure 46-2).

Posting Payments to the Patient Account

Payment for services performed can be received in four ways:
1. The patient pays at the time of service, in full or in part (e.g., a copayment for managed care insurance). The office will accept cash and checks, and most offices also accept credit and debit cards.
2. The patient may make a payment through the mail in response to a bill.
3. The patient may make an online payment using a credit or debit card through the medical practice website or the online patient portal.
4. An insurance company may make a payment either by mail or, usually, by electronic transfer.

All payments must be posted to the account of the patient for whom they are made. Some computer programs have different codes for each method of payment. Cash and checks must match daily bank deposits. Payments using credit cards, online banking, or electronic transfer must later be matched to bank statements or online banking records. If checks are deposited remotely by scanning them, they must also be matched to bank statements or online banking records.

Posting Adjustments to the Patient Account

A change to the patient account that is neither a charge for services nor a payment is called an **adjustment. Credit** (negative) adjustments are subtracted from the patient balance. These are the most common type of adjustments. Examples of credit adjustments include discounts for payment at the time of service, professional courtesy discounts, and discounts given to insurance companies (also called *insurance write-offs*). Credit adjustments are usually discounts that are given in specific circumstances. (See Box 46-1 for common terminology used in accounting.)

Debit (positive) adjustments are added to the patient balance. Debit adjustments are discussed in more detail in Chapter 49. In most computer billing programs, the medical assistant selects a code for each charge, payment, or adjustment. The correct mathematical operation is linked to the transaction code so that the computer automatically adds charges and debit adjustments (such as a returned check) to the patient balance and subtracts payments and credit adjustments (such as an insurance write-off) (Procedure 46-3).

DAY SHEET

The **day sheet** (daily journal) keeps a running tally of the practice's income for that day and is a record of daily transactions. Manual day sheets are rarely used, but the principle of keeping transactions from each individual day is maintained in a practice management program, and the daily journal is still called a day sheet.

WALDEN-MARTIN
FAMILY MEDICAL CLINIC
1234 ANYSTREET ANYTOWN, ANYSTATE 1234
PHONE 123-123-1234   FAX 123-123-5678

Ledger for Guarantor: Mora Siever

Home phone: 123-914-3584

Address: 1 Trinity Lane
            Anytown
            AL 12345

Account #:   72534

DOB: 01/24/1964

Date	Patient	Service	Charges	Payment	ADJUSTMENT	Balance
12/02/20XX	Mora Siever	99396	$ 105.00	$ 20.00	$ 0.00	$ 85.00
12/02/20XX	Mora Siever	99300	$ 89.00	$ 0.00	$ 0.00	$ 89.00
10/22/20XX	Mora Siever	Ins payment	$ 0.00	$ 35.00	$ 15.00	$ −50.00
10/07/20XX	Mora Siever	99203	$ 70.00	$ 20.00	$ 0.00	$ 50.00
					Total:	$ 174.00

Figure 46-3 Patient ledger from SimChart® for the Medical Office.

PROCEDURE 46-1

BOX 46-1   Common Terminology Used in Accounting

Account balance: The amount remaining in the account after all entries have been totaled.

Accounts receivable control: A summary of all unpaid accounts.

Adjustment: An entry to change an account balance that is not a charge for services or a payment, often a discount.

Credit: An entry that reduces an account balance, usually a payment.

Credit balance: The balance on an account when payments exceed charges.

Day sheet: The record of daily financial transactions (daily journal in a pegboard accounting system).

Debit: An entry that increases an account balance, usually a charge.

Disbursements: Money paid out.

Invoice: A bill or written statement describing a purchase or service and the amount due.

Journal: The original record of financial transactions that identifies the accounts to which they belong.

Ledger: A card, book, or computer database in which financial transactions are recorded.

Payables: Amounts owed to others.

Posting: Recording financial transactions or transferring information from one record to another.

Proof: Validation of calculations.

Receivables: Amounts of money owed by others.

ROA (received on account): Designation used for payments that reduce the amount owed but are not payment in full.

Trial balance: A method of checking the accuracy of calculations of accounts.

For each individual patient seen, the manual day sheet records charges, payments, previous balance, adjustments, and the new balance.

Each transaction is recorded on the manual day sheet in the order in which was recorded or entered into the computer. This includes not only patient visits but also all checks received in the mail that day. Even though the checks pay all or part of a patient balance from a previous day, they are posted to the patient account on the day they are received and deposited. At the end of the day, the day is closed (i.e., no further transactions are allowed for that day).

The use of practice management computer programs has eliminated the need for manual checking of calculations and entries that used to be done on the *proof of posting* section of a manual day sheet. Practice management programs can make all necessary calculations and use them to generate a variety of reports.

PRINTING DAY SHEETS AND OTHER REPORTS

When a computer billing program is used, the day sheet can usually be printed at the end of the day. Most computer billing programs allow the day to be closed (so that additional entries cannot be entered using that date). Usually only one day sheet can be printed for a given date. This prevents later alterations to the financial records. If an account must be corrected at a later time, any adjustments are entered on a new screen dated the day the correction is made. The original entry should never be altered after the day has been closed. Many other types of reports can be produced using billing software, including patient ledgers and various activity reports. The computer billing program contains a report menu with standard formats, and the practice can create custom reports depending on its needs.

What Would You Do? **What Would You *Not* Do?**

Case Study 2

When posting charges and payments for a new patient named Linda Harris, Maria notices that the physician has written in an amount on the paper charge slip for the patient's office visit that is $15.00 less than the usual charge for the service. The physician has also written an amount for a flu shot that was given that is $10.00 less than the usual charge. Maria notices that the patient has paid $75.00 on the account, which is about half the amount of the bill. In Maria's office the usual charge for every procedure is entered for every patient. On the rare occasions when charges are reduced, any reduction is posted as a write-off. ■

PROCEDURE 46-1   Completing a Patient Charge Slip

Outcome Complete an itemized charge slip or superbill for a patient by using a fee schedule

Equipment/Supplies

- Blank charge slip
- Computer with SimChart® for the Medical Office
- Patient information form or computer data

- Daily patient schedule
- Calculator
- Fee schedule

PROCEDURE 46-1   Completing a Patient Charge Slip—cont'd

1. Procedural Step. Before the patient is seen by the physician, complete the top part of an itemized charge slip with the information requested including the patient's name, date of birth, insurance, insurance group, and subscriber numbers and the name of the subscriber (insured person). This may be done manually from information on a ledger card or computer account, by attaching a label printed by the computer, or by printing charge slips using the computer billing program. *Principle.* Complete information about the patient and his or her insurance facilitates the billing process. *Example:*

Western Medical Center
109 River Street
Western, OH 44770-0421
(490) 555-6464

Richard Warner, MD   NPI # 23456781XX
Maria Gomez, MD   NPI # 34567891XX
    Tax ID 52-XX63777

Patient Name and Address	Birthdate	Subscriber Name	MD Name	Today's Date
DARLA SISSLE 10 MAPLE STREET WESTERN, OH 44770	2/17/52	DARLA SISSLE	WARNER	6/26/XX
	Account #	Insurance Company	Insurance Phone #	Time
	1015	SHHMO	(490) 565-2000	10:00 AM
Telephone No.		Insurance ID #	Group/Plan #	Sex
(490) 220-1156		21-58624	8300099	Male ☐ Female ☒

Top part of the charge slip.

2. Procedural Step. Before the patient is seen by the physician, enter the patient's previous balance on the bottom of the paper charge slip. *Principle.* The patient's account balance includes the previous balance plus new charges minus any payment made at the time of the visit. *Example:*

		RETURN APPOINTMENT	BALANCE DUE	
☐ M54.9 Back Pain	☐ E03.9 Hypothyroidism		Total Charge	$
☐ J20._ Bronchitis, Acute	☐ H61.2_ Impacted Cerumen	_____ Days	Amount Paid	$
☐ J42 Bronchitis, Chronic	☐ J10.1 Influenza	_____ Weeks	Previous Bal	$ 35.00
☐ R07.9 Chest Pain	☐ K58.9 Irritable Bowel Syndrome	_____ Months	Adjustment	$
☐ J44.9 COPD	☐ M19.0 Osteoarthritis	_____ PRN	Balance Due	$
☐ E10.0 Diabetes I–Ins. Dep	☐ M19.0 Osteoarthritis			

Enter previous balance on the charge slip.

3. Procedural Step. Using the fee schedule, fill in the charges on the charge slip by writing the fee for each service provided beside the line containing the correct code and procedure name (if the physician has not already done so). *Example:*

√	DESCRIPTION	CPT	FEE	√	DESCRIPTION	CPT	FEE	√	DESCRIPTION	CPT	FEE
	OFFICE VISIT				**IMMUNIZATIONS**				**PROCEDURES**		
	NEW PATIENT				Imm. admin, one	90471		√	ECG w// interpretation	93000	65--
	Problem Focused	99201			Imm. admin, each add'l	90472			Spirometry	94010	
	Exp. Prob. Focused	99202			Influenza < 3	90657			Inhalation treatment	94640	
	Detailed	99203			Influenza 3 and >	90658			Remove skin tag < 15	11200	
	Comp/ Mod MDM	99204			Medicare code	G0008			Cerumen removal	69210	
	Comp./ High MDM	99205			Varicella	90716			Wart destruction < 14	17110	
	ESTABLISHED PATIENT				DTaP	90700			I & D abscess	10060	
	Minimal / Nurse Visit	99211			Td adult	90718					
	Problem Focused	99212			Rubella	90706					
√	Exp. Problem Focused	99213	65--		MMR	90707			**OTHER**		
	Detailed	99214			Hep B Child	90744					
	Comprehensive	99215			Hep B Adult	90746					
	Post-op Exam	99024	0.00		IPV	90713					

Enter charges on charge slip.

Continued

PROCEDURE 46-1   Completing a Patient Charge Slip—cont'd

4. Procedural Step. Complete the remainder of the charge slip by entering the total charges and payment made, and then calculate the new balance. The new balance is the sum of the total charges and previous balance minus any payment.

5. Procedural Step. Complete other information requested on the charge slip, such as the place of service and check number and/or method of payment.

Principle. The information on the charge slip must be complete and accurate because it will be used to post the charges and payment to the patient's account.

Example:

5		RETURN APPOINTMENT	BALANCE DUE	
☐ M54.9 Back Pain	☐ E03.9 Hypothyroidism	_____ Days	Total Charge $	130.00
☐ J20._ Bronchitis, Acute	☐ H61.2_ Impacted Cerumen	_____ Weeks	Amount Paid $	20.00
☐ J42 Bronchitis, Chronic	☐ J10.1 Influenza	_____ Months	Previous Bal $	35.00
☐ R07.9 Chest Pain	☐ K58.9 Irritable Bowel Syndrome	_____ PRN	Adjustment $	0.00
☐ J44.9 COPD	☐ M19.0 Osteoarthritis		Balance Due $	145.00
☐ E10.0 Diabetes I–Ins. Dep	☐ M19.0 Osteoarthritis			

Enter totals on charge slip.

Superbill in SimChart® for the Medical Office

These steps should be followed to create a superbill in SimChart® for the Medical Office.

1. Procedural Step. If completing the superbill in SimChart® for the Medical Office, click on the *Coding & Billing* tab. Search for and select the correct patient. If an encounter has been created, selecting the encounter will populate the top of the superbill with the patient information.

Example:

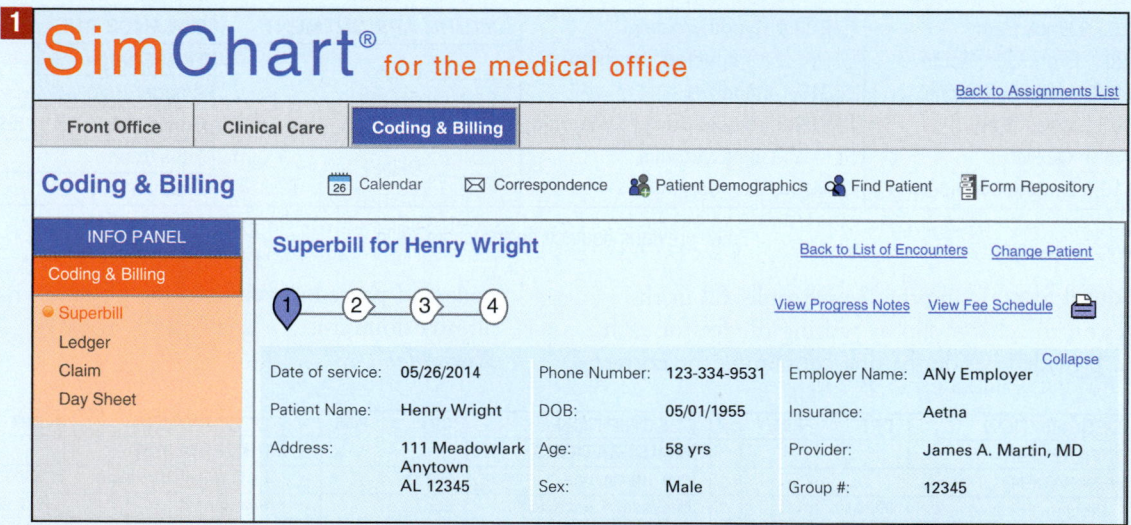

Top part of superbill from SimChart® for the Medical Office.

2. Procedural Step. Document the copayment amount in the *Copay* field.

3. Procedural Step. Document the amount the patient paid in the *Today's Payment* field.

4. Procedural Step. Click on the *Fee Schedule* link in the top right corner and calculate the total charges for the visit. Enter the charges in the *Today's Charges* field.

5. Procedural Step. Calculate and enter the amount the patient owes in the *Balance Due* field Complete the first page of the superbill as needed, click the *Save* button, and click *Next* to proceed to the second page of the superbill.

6. Procedural Step. Look up and enter the correct code for the main diagnosis in the Rank 1 row of the *Diagnoses* box. Click the correct radio button to

---

PROCEDURE 46-1 Completing a Patient Charge Slip—cont'd

indicate if you are using ICD-9 or ICD-10 codes. Enter other diagnoses as indicated in the Rank 2 to 6 rows.

7. **Procedural Step.** Select the first service and document *1* in the Rank column (assuming that the main diagnosis is the reason for the service). Find the correct CPT code and fee for the service. If the service is a *Well Visit* or an *Office Visit,* enter the correct fee and CPT code in the *New* box for a new patient or in the *Est* box for an established patient. Enter the fee and CPT code for each service provided in the correct box, and click the *Save* button before progressing to a new page.

8. **Procedural Step.** When all services have been entered, click the *Next* button until you reach the fourth and final page of the superbill. Select the *I am ready to submit the superbill* check-box.

9. **Procedural Step.** Scroll down and select the *Yes* radio button to indicate that there is a *Signature on File.* Enter today's date for a new patient, or the date of the first visit for an established patient, in the *Date* field.

10. **Procedural Step.** Select *Save,* click *OK,* then click the *Submit Superbill* button.

PROCEDURE 46-2 Posting Charges

Outcome Using the information from the completed charge slip, post patient charges to a patient account

Equipment/Supplies

- Patient charge slip
- Patient ledger or computer with SimChart® for the Medical Office
- Patient day sheet (optional)
- Fee schedule
- Pen or computer

1. **Procedural Step.** If using a manual system, post the charges from a completed patient charge slip on the patient ledger and paper day sheet or SimChart® day sheet (optional) using one line for one day's services. Place the total charges for the services in the column labeled *Charges.* If using SimChart® for the Medical Office, post the first service on the first line. Enter the date, patient name, CPT code, charges (from the fee schedule), payment, and adjustment. The computer will calculate the balance.

2. **Procedural Step.** If using SimChart® for the Medical Office, click the *Add Row* button to post each additional charge on a new line.

3. **Procedural Step.** If using a manual system, enter the total charge in the balance column. If using SimChart® for the Medical Office, click the *Save* button after all charges have been posted. *Example:*

	DATE*	PATIENT*	SERVICE*	CHARGES*	PAYMENT*	ADJMT*	BALANCE
☐	05/26/201📅	Henry Wright	99203	$ 70.00	$ 0.00	$ 0.00	$ 70.00

Add Row   Delete   TOTAL: $ 70.00

Outcome Post payments and/or adjustments to a patient account

Equipment/Supplies

- Patient ledger card or computer with SimChart® for the Medical Office
- Check or cash from the patient or payment from the insurance carrier

- Calculator
- Stamp with restrictive endorsement
- Stamp pad

1. **Procedural Step.** When a payment has been made, locate the patient ledger in the computer or select the patient ledger card.
   Principle. Both payments received at the patient visit and checks received in the mail must be entered to the correct patient account.

2. **Procedural Step.** Compare the amount of the payment against the total amount owed.

   Principle. The total amount owed will be the balance due and charges for new services.

3. **Procedural Step.** If using a manual system, post the payment from a completed patient charge slip on the patient ledger on the same line as the day's charges. If it is a check, record the number of the check. If using a computer program, post the patient payment on the same line as the charges from the day's visit.

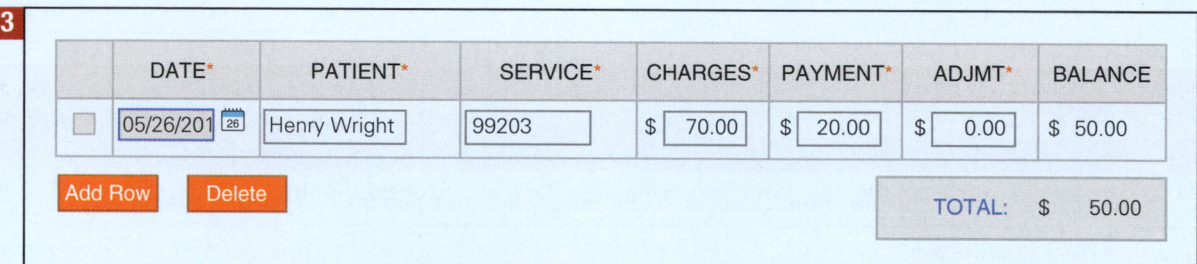

	DATE*	PATIENT*	SERVICE*	CHARGES*	PAYMENT*	ADJMT*	BALANCE
☐	05/26/201 📅	Henry Wright	99203	$ 70.00	$ 20.00	$ 0.00	$ 50.00

Add Row   Delete   TOTAL: $ 50.00

Charges and payments entered into the computer.

4. **Procedural Step.** If posting an insurance payment, use a new line on a ledger card and a new line on a patient ledger in SimChart® for the Medical Office.
   Principle. All payments are posted using the date of posting. In the case of insurance payments, this is not the same as the date of service.

5. **Procedural Step.** If using a computer program to post an insurance payment, identify it in the service column (or use a code if the computer program requires it).

6. **Procedural Step.** Determine if the amount excluded by the insurance company can be billed to the patient. If it cannot, enter the amount excluded by

the insurance company as a credit adjustment in the credit column. On a ledger card, enter in the adjustment column.
   Principle. Insurance adjustments are amounts that the insurance does not allow. The insurance company provides a code to indicate them. They are credit adjustments because they are subtracted from the balance owed by the patient.
   Example. The statement from the insurance company shows that the insurance company paid $57.00 on the claim for Michael Lee. It excluded $23.00, which must be entered as a credit adjustment or write-off. The patient's copayment is $20.00.

6

UNITED WESTERN BENEFIT
1220 SIXTH STREET
WESTERN RIDGE, OH 45770

FOR SERVICES PROVIDED BY: WESTERN MEDICAL CENTER

Name of Insured: Michael Lee

Patient/ Service	Service Date(s)	Total Charge	Excluded Amounts	Patient Copayment	Plan Paid Amount
Office Visit	11/24/20XX	$ 65.00	$ 15.00 EAC	$ 20.00	$ 30.00
Cerumen Removal	11/24/20XX	$ 35.00	$ 8.00 EAC		$ 27.00
Total		**$ 100.00**	**$ 23.00**	**$ 20.00**	**$ 57.00**

EAC: This amount exceeds the allowable charge for the service. The provider is prohibited by law from billing the patient for this amount.

Insurance explanation of benefits.

PROCEDURE 46-3   Posting Payments and/or Adjustments—cont'd

7. Procedural Step. Calculate the balance.
Example. The insurance payment of $57.00 has been entered as an insurance payment in the payment column, and the excluded amount has been entered in the adjustment column. The total amount subtracted from the patient's balance is $80.00.

	DATE	PATIENT	SERVICE	CHARGES	PAYMENT	ADJMT	BALANCE
7	12/01/20XX	Michael Lee	Ins. pay & adjust	$ 0.00	$ 57.00	$ −23.00	$ −80.00

Insurance payment and insurance adjustment entered into the computer.

8. Procedural Step. Endorse a check using a stamp containing the practice name, the statement "For deposit only," and the number of the checking account.
Principle. This type of endorsement only allows the bank to deposit the check and prevents anyone from cashing the check or using it in any other way.

9. Procedural Step. Place cash or a processed check in the designated drawer or money box for later deposit.

OTHER FINANCIAL ACCOUNTS

In addition to taking money in, a practice pays money out. Some of this is done on a regular basis—for example, taking care of weekly or biweekly salaries, mortgage or rent, equipment leases, and utilities. Other payments are made in relation to specific invoices for materials or equipment.

Unless a bill is paid immediately when presented, it becomes part of the accounts payable (money owed by the business). A complete bookkeeping system notes each month any outstanding accounts payable, as well as the **disbursements** (payments) made during the month.

In addition, many offices keep a **petty cash** account, a small amount of cash available for everyday expenses. Again, petty cash must be recorded.

BANKING ACTIVITIES

If the medical practice is to pay its bills, including salaries for medical assistants and other employees, it must have money in the bank. Part of the responsibility of the individual who handles the office's financial management is maintaining the practice's bank accounts.

TYPES OF ACCOUNTS

Businesses such as medical practices will typically have one or more of the following types of bank accounts—checking, savings, or money market accounts.

Checking Account

A checking account is an account in which the money held can be withdrawn by simply writing a check against the funds available. Many banks allow businesses to earn interest on their checking accounts as long as a certain amount of money remains in the account (the minimum balance).

The minimum balance can range from as little as $500 to as much as $2500. Interest is the payment the bank makes to the owner of the money on deposit for the privilege of being able to use the depositor's money to make loans to other bank customers.

If the checking account balance falls below the minimum, the account does not earn interest and there is usually a monthly service charge and a charge for each check written against the account for the entire monthly reporting period in which the balance was below the minimum. Sometimes a bank will waive the minimum balance in the practice's checking account if the practice agrees to keep a higher minimum balance in either a savings account or a money market account.

Savings Account

A practice may want to keep cash that is not necessary to pay expenses in a savings account, which usually earns interest at a slightly higher rate than an interest-bearing checking account. A savings account does not have any check-writing privileges, but money can be withdrawn or transferred to the checking account if necessary.

Money Market Account

A money market account offers features of both savings and checking accounts. Money market accounts usually require a fairly high minimum balance (often $2500). However, they may earn interest at the money market rate—the rate at which major corporations lend to or borrow from one another for 10- to 30-day periods.

Money market accounts let the owner draw a specified number of checks per month without a processing fee. They often require checks to be for at least $500.

A medical practice might want to maintain a money market account to hold money for regular but infrequent expenses, such as quarterly, semiannual, or annual payments for malpractice insurance; licenses for physicians and other licensed professionals on the staff; or dues to the state, county, or local medical association or chamber of commerce.

CHECKS

Types of Checks

Checks are slips of paper used by a checking account owner to authorize payments to a third party (**payee**) for the amount of money written on the check. Paying by checks allows the medical practice to maintain a permanent record of the payments it makes for goods and services.

In addition to the checks from the practice's checkbook or money market account, the practice may have occasion to ask its bank to prepare a cashier's check to assure the payee (person or company being paid) that funds are available. A **cashier's check** is a check drawn on the bank itself rather than on an individual account. Because the bank assumes liability for payment of the check, a cashier's check is considered more reliable than the check of an individual or business. This might be the case if the office were purchasing a large piece of equipment for which the seller is unwilling to accept a simple business check. The bank may also guarantee a personal or business check by withdrawing the funds from the checking account at the time the check is issued. This is called a **certified check.**

Check Format

At the top of each check toward the right, under the check number, is a fractional number that identifies the bank on which the check is drawn. This ABA number, which is assigned by the American Bankers Association, designates the federal reserve bank zone, the state or territory, and the unique identification number for the bank on which the check is drawn. Across the bottom of checks is a set of numbers called the **MICR line,** written in magnetic ink. When checks are processed and "cleared" for payment from the issuing bank to the account of the individual making the deposit, this set of numbers is read by a magnetic ink character recognition (MICR) system. The MICR line contains the **ABA routing number** (the unique number of the bank), the account number, and the check number. Other information that is usually printed on a check includes the name and address of the account holder and the name of the bank.

Business Checkbook with Stubs

One type of business checkbook that is commonly used has three checks to a page, with check stubs on the left on which to record the same information that is recorded on the check when it is written (Figure 46-4). The checks and matching stubs are preprinted in order. In addition, the stubs have room in which to write in the amount of deposits made; the stubs therefore act as a running checkbook ledger.

Computer-Generated Checks

A number of business accounting computer programs will generate checks and immediately post the payment to the accounts payable ledger. To use these systems, the practice will need to buy compatible blank checks for computer printing. The software can also generate the fractional bank number and MICR numbers, or they may be preprinted on the check forms.

Online Payment

Most medical offices pay bills online either as a single payment or every month. This is also popular with suppliers, who create online accounts and accept payments directly using a pay-by-computer system.

Because some businesses still do not accept online payment, a medical practice will still need to write or print some checks. If an office handles its own payroll, it may encourage employees to use direct deposit instead of paper checks. Some practices may do all of their bill paying to regular suppliers, medical associations, liability insurance carriers, and other creditors online and have their payroll checks written by an outside service provider, so checks are written only occasionally.

Preparing a Check

Checks are produced on watermarked paper to make it difficult for people to erase and then overwrite part of the check. The bank has the right to refuse to honor a check with erasures, overwrites, or other alterations. Minor corrections may be accepted if initialed by the person who signs the check. This protects the account holder from having people to whom checks are written cross out the amount and write in a larger amount. However, this also makes it important that checks be written carefully.

Most checks have at least one memo line—a line on which to write the purpose of the check. If the check is for payment of a bill or **invoice** (itemized bill), the invoice number or the account number for that particular vendor would go on the memo line.

If a mistake is made on a check, the medical assistant should write *void* on the check and check stub. The voided check should not be destroyed. It should be filed with bank statements and other account records so that it is available for the practice's auditors. When writing a check, the medical assistant should begin the amount in numbers immediately after the printed dollar sign and write the amount in words at the left side of the check. Legally, the amount in words is accepted as the amount for which the check is written if there is a discrepancy. After all the checks for a particular period (week or month) have been written, they are attached to the supporting invoices and placed in a folder or envelope on the desk of the physician who is to sign the checks that week. In many practices, two physicians have check-signing privileges so that one can sign if the other is on vacation. Also, in some practices, checks exceeding a certain amount (e.g., $500, $1000) must be signed by two people; this is often a provision of that part of the practice's general liability insurance policy that covers employee theft (Procedure 46-4).

HIGHLIGHT on Check Security Features

Because of the prevalence of color copiers, many security features are built into the paper used to print checks. The paper usually has a watermark that cannot be photocopied and/or invisible florescent fibers that can be viewed under black light. The paper should have erasure protection so that the background color fades if writing or printing is altered. The paper of the check may also have a chemical stain that reacts if chemicals are used to alter information. A word such as *nonnegotiable* or *void* may appear if the check is passed through a photocopier or treated with chemicals. Various parts of the check usually have also been treated in a special way so that they will not be reproduced if the check is photocopied. The border and endorsement line usually include microprinting that will not be reproduced if the check is photocopied. ■

Figure 46-4 A business checkbook is often arranged with three checks per page and check stubs to record transactions.

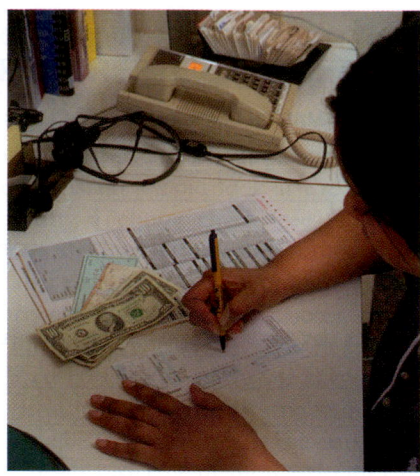

Figure 46-6 Medical assistant preparing a bank deposit.

bank statement equal each other after adjusting for checks that were written but have not yet cleared through the bank and deposits recorded after the statement period ended.

Each month the bank will send the practice a statement of account activity, or the practice may access this statement online. The account balance at the end of the statement period will almost always be different from the account balance in the office's checking account ledger.

There are several reasons for this discrepancy. First, it usually takes about a week from the time the statement period ends until the office receives the statement, during which time more checks have been written. Second, checks written near the end of the statement period usually will not have cleared the account when the period ends. Third, some vendors and others do not promptly deposit or cash checks; thus some checks will not clear the account for a month or more. Fourth, bank charges are added to the statement for such things as checks returned for insufficient funds, per-check fees, and lockbox fees. Finally, interest may accrue on the balance during the month.

For these reasons, it is important to reconcile the bank statement with the office's checkbook to verify the arithmetic used by those who have written checks. Before reconciling, enter and subtract any bank fees in the office's checking account ledger and add any interest. The amount of all outstanding checks (checks that have not cleared the bank) should be totaled and subtracted from the "new balance" shown on the bank statement. The amount of any deposits made during the month that do not appear on the statement should be added to obtain a true balance. The figures may be taken from a paper statement or an online statement using a form such as the one shown in Figure 46-7. This true balance should match the balance in the office's checking account ledger).

Memories *from* Practicum

Maria Hernandez: There was only one doctor in the office where I did my practicum, and in that office they used both a manual system to record patient accounts and a computer system. The office manager had been in charge for many years, and she said that she didn't trust the computer. Every morning we set up the pegboard by placing a day sheet on the bottom and receipts above. The receipts had carbon strips so that anything written would be duplicated on the layer below. As each patient checked out, we placed his or her ledger card between the receipt and the day sheet so that the next open line was directly above the next open line on the day sheet. The ledger cards we used were made of a special kind of carbonless paper called *NCR paper*. NCR stands for "no carbon required." When we filled in the date and charges on the receipt, it automatically was copied on the ledger card and then on the day sheet. The challenges were to be sure all three forms were lined up correctly and also to be sure to apply enough pressure with the pen. The other big challenge was to add up the entries on the day sheet at the end of the day and make sure that everything balanced. The office manager said that sometimes it would take a long time to find and fix every mistake. I don't think there are very many offices left that record patient accounts this way, but I am glad I saw how it was done. It makes me appreciate how useful the computer is in managing office finances. ∎

THIS WORKSHEET IS PROVIDED TO HELP YOU BALANCE YOUR ACCOUNT

1. Go through your register and mark each check, withdrawal, Express ATM transaction, payment, deposit or other credit listed on this statement. Be sure that your register shows any interest paid into your account, and any service charges, automatic payments, or Express Transfers withdrawn from your account during this statement period.

2. Using the chart below, list any outstanding checks, Express ATM withdrawals, payments or any other withdrawals (including any from previous months) that are listed in your register but are not shown on this statement.

3. Balance your account by filling in the spaces below.

ITEMS OUTSTANDING		
NUMBER	**AMOUNT**	
TOTAL	$	

ENTER

The NEW BALANCE shown on
this statement_____$

ADD

Any deposits listed in your register $
or transfers into your account $
which are not shown on this $
statement.   + $ _____

                                     TOTAL

CALCULATE THE SUBTOTAL_____$

SUBTRACT

The total outstanding checks and
withdrawals from the chart at left_____ - $

CALCULATE THE ENDING BALANCE

This amount should be the same
as the current balance shown in
your check register_____$

PROCEDURE 46-4

Figure 46-7 Bank statement reconciliation form.

PROCEDURE 46-4 Writing a Check

Outcome Write checks to pay bills for a medical office, and record them in the checkbook or check register

Equipment/Supplies

- Checks with check register or check stubs
- Monthly bills to be paid
- Pen

1. **Procedural Step.** Organize bills to be paid by opening envelopes and/or arranging invoices. Use a pen to prepare a check for each bill or invoice.

Principle. This prevents alterations after the check has been written.

Continued

PROCEDURE 46-4 Writing a Check—cont'd

2. **Procedural Step.** Write the date on the line that says *Date*.
   Principle. The date identifies when the check was written. Banks have specific policies that specify for how long the check is valid.
3. **Procedural Step.** Write the name of the payee on the line of the check that says *Pay to the order of*.
4. **Procedural Step.** Write the amount of the check in numbers in the box next to the dollar sign. When writing the numbers, use a decimal between the number of dollars and the number of cents.
   Example. $1568.42
5. **Procedural Step.** Write the amount of the check in words on the line below the name of the payee. Begin writing at the beginning of the line. When writing the words, remember that *and* is used only before the number of cents. Numbers such as 25 contain a hyphen when written in words (e.g., *twenty-five*). Write the number of cents as a fraction over 100. Draw a line from the end of the fraction to the word *dollars*.
   Example:
   One thousand five hundred sixty-eight and 42/100————————DOLLARS
   Principle. Writing the amount in numbers, as well as words, helps prevent alteration of the amount of the check.
6. **Procedural Step.** Write the invoice number, account number, and/or purpose of the check on the line marked *for* or *memo*.
   Principle. If the check is separated from the payment slip, this helps the payee identify what the check is for. It may also assist in record keeping after the check is returned by the bank.
7. **Procedural Step.** Record the date, check number (if not preprinted), payee, amount of the check, and reason the check was written on the check stub in the checkbook or in the check register.
   Principle. A record is kept of every check that is written.
8. **Procedural Step.** Subtract the amount of each check from the balance on the check stub or in the check register. If completing a check stub, enter and add any deposits since the previous check and add them to the previous balance. Then subtract the amount of the check and enter the new balance. Write the new balance on the stub of the check below in the box labeled *Balance carried forward*.

Principle. Keeping a running balance makes it possible to determine easily how much money is present in the checking account.
Example. Completed check stub for a check to D&D Medical Supply.

8	1837	
DATE	3/12/XX	
TO	D & D Med. Supply	
FOR	Invoice #JTS006	
BALANCE BROUGHT FORWARD	4,482	21
DEPOSITS		
BALANCE	4,482	21
AMT. THIS CHECK	1,000	00
BALANCE CARRIED FORWARD	3,482	21

Filling out a check stub.

9. **Procedural Step.** If you make a mistake, draw a single line through the mistake, correct the error, and initial the correction.
10. **Procedural Step.** If the check cannot be used, write the word *Void* across the check and enter the word *Void* in the check register. Place the voided check in the folder where accounts payable records are kept.
    Principle. Keeping voided checks instead of destroying them facilitates accurate record keeping and provides proof that the check was voided.
11. **Procedural Step.** Prepare an envelope to mail the payment, or use a window envelope supplied by the vendor.
12. **Procedural Step.** Clip the prepared check to the envelope with the payment slip, and place it in the designated place for review and signature by the physician authorized to sign office checks.

PROCEDURE 46-5   Preparing a Bank Deposit

Outcome Prepare a bank deposit

Equipment/Supplies

- Account deposit slip
- Deposit slip itemization record from the day sheet (optional)
- Cash and checks received as payments
- Calculator or adding machine
- Bank deposit envelope or bag

1. **Procedural Step.** Obtain an account deposit slip and place today's date on it. If the deposit slip from a day sheet is used, write the name of the medical practice and the bank account number at the top.
   Principle. The date, practice name, and account number must appear on the deposit slip so that the bank can credit the deposit correctly.

2. **Procedural Step.** Write the amount of currency and the amount in coins on the correct lines.

3. **Procedural Step.** Stamp each check with the restrictive endorsement, and write the amount of each check on the bank deposit detail with either the numerator of the fractional ABA number or the check number. If a deposit slip has been created as part of the day sheet, it can be used as itemization and clipped to the bank's deposit slip.
   Principle. A reference number for each check allows the bank to verify individual items if questions arise.

4. **Procedural Step.** Total all the checks and place that total on a deposit slip in the box for checks.

5. **Procedural Step.** Total the cash and total amount of checks for the total amount of the bank deposit. The total amount of this deposit should be equal to the

amount in the payments column on the day sheet or accounts receivable record for the given day.

6. **Procedural Step.** Make a copy of the deposit slip if a duplicate deposit record was not made when creating the day sheet.
   Principle. The office should keep a copy of information regarding the checks and cash included in a deposit in case there are questions at a later date.

7. **Procedural Step.** Place the cash, checks, and deposit slip in a bank envelope or bank deposit bag and take or send it to the bank.

8. **Procedural Step.** Record the amount of the deposit on the accounts payable record and in the check register or on the check stub nearest to the date of deposit.
   Principle. This provides information on the amount of money in the checking account against which checks can be written.

9. **Procedural Step.** File the bank deposit receipt and copy of the bank deposit detail in a labeled file folder.
   Principle. All bank records must be saved for a period of time for tax and accounting purposes.

ACCOUNTS PAYABLE OR RECORD OF CASH DISBURSEMENTS

The record of cash disbursements is called the *cash disbursement journal.* The simplest form of this type of journal is a check register. In a one-write or pegboard system, cash disbursements are automatically recorded at the time each check is written out. In a computerized bookkeeping system, the cash disbursement journal is also automatically updated, or posted, when a check is drawn. In a single- or double-entry system, the cash disbursement journal must be separately maintained.

Each line of the cash disbursement journal has columns to record information about payments. Usually there are also columns to track expenses by categories. These features are also found in computer accounting programs.

PETTY CASH

Petty cash is the cash kept on hand to pay for small, miscellaneous items, such as tips for a delivery, postage due, reimbursement to a staff member for parking at a meeting, or even a box of Girl Scout cookies for the office break room.

A check for a predetermined amount—usually $100 to $200—is drawn to cash to establish the petty cash account. It is important to keep each office account separate. Thus, cash should never be taken from any patient payment and put into petty cash. The petty cash account should always be funded via a check drawn on the practice's checking account.

A petty cash journal should be located near the cash box so that each disbursement can be recorded. Also, a

Table 47-1 Selected CPT Modifiers Used in the Medical Office
(See the Current Procedural Terminology manual, Appendix A, for a complete list of modifiers.)

Modifier	Description
–22	Increased Procedural Services (not used for E/M services)
–23	Unusual anesthesia
–26	Professional Component
–32	Mandated Services
–33	Preventative Services
–47	Anesthesia by Surgeon (not including local anesthesia)
–50	Bilateral Procedure—This code is added to the second (bilateral) procedure performed at the same operation
–57	Decision for Surgery (added to an E/M [Evaluation and Management] code when the physician makes the decision for surgery during an E/M visit)
–59	Distinct Procedural Service
–80	Assistant Surgeon
–81	Minimum Assistant Surgeon
–82	Assistant Surgeon (when qualified resident surgeon not available)
–90	Reference (Outside) Laboratory
–91	Repeat Clinical Diagnostic Laboratory Test
–92	Alternative Laboratory Platform Testing
–99	Multiple Modifiers

Figure 47-2 Examples of terms in the index of the CPT manual when looking up the diagnosis *Incision and drainage of a bursa of the foot.*

main term. Each level of modifying term is indented further than the level above it. For example, the main term is the main word in the procedure. The first modifying term would identify a subterm, an anatomic location, or a procedure (such as *Lesion, Nerve,* or *Repair*). When a procedure is listed in the index (as the main term or any level of modifying term), it is followed by a code or range of codes (e.g., *Excision, Nerve, Foot* ...... 28055). Both main terms or anatomic terms and modifying terms may point to a cross-reference using the word *See.* (See Figure 47-2.)

Several pieces of information may be significant when choosing the correct code for a procedure:

- Location
- Size of lesion or repair
- Method of performing the procedure, test, or surgery
- Number of minutes allotted for a treatment (e.g., acupuncture)
- Complexity of the procedure or service

SELECTING A SPECIFIC CPT CODE

After identifying a code or code range from the index, the medical assistant should read all relevant codes carefully in the main text. It may also be necessary to review the guidelines at the beginning of the appropriate section of the CPT manual to obtain additional information that can be helpful

in choosing a code. The medical assistant should select the code that is the best match for the medical documentation and determine if it is necessary to use a modifier or an add-on code.

There are two types of CPT codes: stand-alone codes and indented codes. The stand-alone code contains a semicolon (e.g., 93000 Electrocardiogram, routine ECG with at least 12 leads; with interpretation and report). The indented code, which follows a stand-alone code or another indented code, provides only text to replace the words after the semicolon in the stand-alone code (e.g., 93005 [indent] tracing only, without interpretation and report). In the example given, the code 93000 would be used if the electrocardiogram (ECG) tracing is made and the physician interprets the tracing in the same medical office. The code 93005 would be used if the ECG tracing is made in one office, but insurance should not be billed for the interpretation because it will be done by another physician and billed from another office (Procedure 47-1).

Evaluation and Management

The E/M section contains codes for office visits provided by primary care practitioners and specialists. E/M codes cover the service-oriented, rather than the procedure-oriented, parts of medical care. It is important to determine where the service was provided when selecting the correct E/M code.

Although procedures are fairly easy to define—for instance, incision and drainage of a cyst—the amount of service provided by a physician during an office visit is more difficult to describe. One physician may consider 20 minutes an appropriate amount of time for a visit, whereas another may consider 30 minutes the minimum amount of time to spend with a patient. One physician may focus strictly on the patient's presenting problem, whereas another may want to examine the patient more completely, especially if he or she has not been seen for several months.

The codes in the E/M section attempt to link reimbursement to the completeness of the examination and the amount of skill required to manage the patient's problems. Unfortunately, this may push the physician to limit the time spent with patients. If the patient does not have well defined, complex medical problems, the visit is reimbursed as uncomplicated, no matter how much time the visit took. For example, if a patient is in the office for a recheck of an ear infection, the visit would not usually take a significant amount of time. If the patient has several questions about methods other than antibiotics that could be used to treat ear infections, it will take more time for the physician to complete the examination, even though there is no additional medical problem or complication.

When determining the proper code for E/M services, the medical assistant must consider a number of factors.

1. For coding purposes, the patient is either an **established patient** (one who has been seen in the previous 3 years) or a **new patient** (one who has not had services performed by any provider in the medical office in the previous 3 years). There are separate groups of codes for each type of patient. New patients are expected to take longer to examine and are reimbursed at a higher rate. The patient is also either an **outpatient** (one who has not been admitted to a health care facility) or an **inpatient** (a patient who has been formally admitted to a health care facility). Although most services for patients who are inpatients are billed by the health care facility itself, physicians who are not employees of that facility bill for visits to the patient during a hospital admission, for inpatient consultations, for providing reports for some diagnostic tests performed at the hospital (such as cardiac stress tests), for critical care and intensive care services, and for care for visits to patients in nursing homes.

2. There are separate groups of codes, depending on where the service is provided and whether the physician is the patient's primary care provider or a consultant. A medical service could have been provided in the office, in a nursing home, in a hospital to a patient who has been admitted, or in a hospital emergency department. The E/M section of the CPT manual is divided into several subsections, and it is important to select a code from the correct subsection, depending on the service that the physician provided and the location where the service was provided.

3. The level of service depends primarily on three key factors:
   - The extent of the medical history (number of body systems discussed)
   - The extent of the physical examination (number of body systems examined)
   - The complexity of medical decision making

Medical History

History taking consists of four levels: (1) problem focused, (2) expanded problem focused, (3) detailed, and (4) comprehensive.

- A problem-focused history is one that addresses the chief complaint, with a brief history of the illness or problem. It would be used for a straightforward problem, such as a sore throat.
- An expanded problem-focused history addresses the chief complaint, a brief history of the present illness or problem, and a review of systems that have to do with the chief complaint. It might be used for a somewhat more complicated problem, or a single diagnosis that involves more than one body system or location, such as a patient with an established diagnosis of psoriasis with lesions on the elbows, an itchy scalp, and thickening and discolorations of the fingernails.
- A detailed history addresses the chief complaint, an extended history of the present illness, and a review of body systems, including other systems beyond those related to the chief complaint. Family history is also reviewed as it relates to the present problem. If a patient has more complicated medical problems and/or multiple problems, it may be necessary to obtain a detailed history.
- A comprehensive history includes a chief complaint; an extended history of the present illness; a review of all body systems, especially those directly related to the present problem; and a complete family history. This type of history is taken when a patient has a severe, acute medical condition or serious changes in a long-term condition.

Physical Examination

- A problem-focused examination is limited to the affected body system or organ.
- An expanded problem-focused examination is related to the affected body system, as well as other organs or systems that might be symptomatic. For example, the patient may be followed for angina (recurrent chest pain) and have a new complaint of calf pain when walking.
- A detailed examination includes the affected body systems or organs and other related systems or organs.
- A comprehensive examination is a multisystem examination, or a complete examination of one system.

Medical Decision Making

Medical decision making can be straightforward or have a low, moderate, or high level of complexity. If a patient has one problem, medical decision making is usually straightforward. When a patient has multiple problems, especially if they are causing severe or life-threatening symptoms, the decision-making process is more complex. For example, if a new patient has poorly controlled diabetes mellitus type 1, fever, and an increased white blood count, the decision-making process for the physician would be highly complex.

Looking up Diagnosis Codes in the Alphabetic Index

When coding in the outpatient setting, the medical assistant should try to find the most specific code that matches each diagnosis given by the provider. The first-listed diagnosis describes the primary reason that the patient has sought care. This may be a disease or condition, if diagnostic testing has confirmed the diagnosis. It may be one or more symptoms, if a confirmed diagnosis is pending. It may also be a reason for seeking health care when the patient is not ill (such as a routine physical examination). In addition, the provider may list other diagnoses if the patient has complications or coexisting conditions, especially if they are the reason for procedures or diagnostic tests.

The first step is to locate the first-listed diagnosis in the alphabetic index. As an example, assume that the physician lists the patient's first diagnosis as *Salmonella* gastroenteritis. If the medical assistant looks under *Salmonella,* he or she is referred to *Infection, Salmonella* and the code listed is A02.9. If the medical assistant looks under *Gastroenteritis,* a subheading is found for *Salmonella* with the identical code. After locating the code in the index, the medical assistant should always follow up by reviewing the code in the tabular list to be sure that he or she has located the most specific code and has chosen a code with the required number of characters. It is not always possible to know from the index how many characters a specific code will require.

Codes for Individuals Who Do Not Have a Disease or Injury (Z01 to Z99)

Codes from Chapter 21 (Factors Influencing Health Status and Contact with Health Services) are used when the patient does not have a disease or injury and are referred to as *Z codes.* This code may be used as the first-listed diagnosis if the patient has sought health care to receive an immunization or for a physical examination. If the physician lists a diagnosis of family history of diabetes, the medical assistant would look up *History, family (of), diabetes mellitus* to find the code, Z83.3. Checking the tabular list would confirm that this is an acceptable first-listed or secondary diagnosis. The medical history alone justifies periodic examinations. It is important to note that even a code such as Z00.00 (Encounter for general adult medical examination without abnormal findings) is a diagnosis code, and it must be accompanied by a valid procedure code (CPT code) when billing the insurance company.

A Z code may also be used as a secondary code when a patient seeks care for a specific disease or condition. For example, a patient may seek care for an infection, but the care given may be influenced by the fact that the patient has a penicillin allergy that influences the care for the current condition. To code for the allergy, the medical assistant would look in the index under *History, personal allergy to, penicillin.*

External Cause Codes (V01 to Y99)

External cause codes cover external causes of injury or poisoning, such as injury resulting from collision of a motor vehicle with another motor vehicle. They facilitate the collection of statistics about causes and severity of injuries. These codes are used only in combination with other diagnosis codes to give more information about the cause of a medical problem. They are never the first-listed diagnosis. The External Cause Index is located before the Table of Drugs and Chemicals.

USING THE ALPHABETIC INDEX

When looking up diagnosis codes, the medical assistant must always keep in mind that insurance companies will be using the diagnosis code to pay for services. If the diagnosis codes are incorrect or incomplete, the insurance carrier may refuse to pay for the services provided.

To find the diagnosis in the index, the medical assistant may look under the main word of the patient's diagnosis. It is also possible to start from the anatomic location of the medical problem, which will be cross-referenced to the main term. The index is arranged with headings and subheadings. Each level of subheadings is also arranged alphabetically. In the examples that follow, a comma indicates that the next term is a subheading of the previous term.

Memories *from* **Practicum**

John Grant: My practicum was performed in a large clinic where I spent some time in several departments. I was placed in the medical records department for 4 days, and I didn't understand why I needed to be there for such a long time. I was surprised to learn that not only was this department responsible for filing and taking care of the medical records, but they also did a considerable amount of coding. They asked me to look up diagnosis codes one day, and I spent all morning and part of the afternoon doing this. They gave me a stack of referral forms and told me to look up and write the diagnosis code on each form. If I couldn't find it or if I wasn't sure, I should put the form to one side so that someone could help me later. I was told to find the diagnosis in the index, and then look up the best code in the tabular list. I had had some practice in school, so this wasn't completely new to me. I have to admit that my pile of codes I was sure of was smaller than the pile I had questions about. I never realized that coding could be so complicated. There were some I couldn't find at all and others where I just couldn't decide what the best code was. For example, when the diagnosis was "unequal arm length due to old fracture" I found out that I should look up "Deformity, limb, unequal length, short site is …" in the index. I also found out that I would have to look at the medical record to identify the specific bone that had been previously fractured to select a specific code. This experience showed me that coding requires real attention to detail. ∎

Diagnosis:	Right shoulder pain, R/O bursitis

Index:	**Pain** (*main term*)
	      joint (*subterm*) M25.50
	         shoulder (*subterm*) M25.51-

Index:	**Shoulder** – *see* condition (*cross-reference*)
Tabular:	**M25 Other joint disorder not elsewhere specified** (*category code*) **M25.5 Pain in joint** (*subcategory code*) **M25.51 Pain in joint** (*subclassification code*) **M25.511 Pain in right shoulder** (*specific code*)
Code:	M25.511 Pain in right shoulder

Figure 47-4 To code a diagnosis, look up the condition or location in the index, then find the most specific code in the tabular list.

During the period when the physician is still trying to determine exactly what the patient's diagnosis is, symptoms may be listed on the charge sheet. These should be coded exactly as written. If the physician writes *rule out (R/O)* with a diagnosis or condition, that condition may *not* be used for coding. Only the patient symptoms should be coded. If a patient has received ambulatory surgery, the medical assistant should look up the condition for which the surgery was done or the postoperative diagnosis, if it is different from the preoperative diagnosis.

Examples

1. If the progress note describes the patient's problem as "recurrent right shoulder pain, rule out bursitis," the code can be located in the index under: *Pain(s), joint, shoulder* (M25.51-). The dash at the end of the code in the index indicates that at least one additional character is required (in this case to indicate if it is the right shoulder, left shoulder, or unspecified shoulder). If the medical assistant looks up *Shoulder* in the index, the following instruction is given: *see condition* (Figure 47-4). The medical assistant should start again, and look up the patient's condition, which is pain in the shoulder.

2. If the patient's diagnosis is given on the charge slip as "diabetic neuropathy," the medical assistant should look in the index under *Neuropathy, diabetic*. The code range is listed as E09-E13 with .40. This means that types of diabetic neuropathy are listed under E09.40, E10.40, E11.40, and so on. It turns out that it is necessary to correlate the underlying type of diabetes (drug induced, type 1, type 2, or other) to the neuropathy. The medical assistant would find this information either in the medical record or by asking the physician. It is also possible to locate the code by looking in the index under *Diabetes, diabetic, with, neuropathy*, although the code given here refers specifically to type 2 diabetes mellitus.

USING THE TABULAR LIST

Once a code or range of codes has been identified, the medical assistant should find the correct section and determine the best code to match the information on the patient's charge slip or in the medical record. It is important to look at the additional information given relating to the diagnosis.

In the tabular list, the medical assistant should always look for the most specific code possible, remembering that the code must be supported by the information in the medical record. Parentheses are used in the index and tabular list to identify words that may be found in the diagnosis but are not required. When symbols indicate that codes require additional characters or cannot be used as a first-listed diagnosis, it is necessary to continue to look for a correct code. Codes may be identified as NOS or NEC as used in the ICD-9. A code that is identified by a symbol indicating that it is used for a complication or a comorbidity (additional disease or condition) should always follow another code related to the reason the patient has sought treatment (see Figure 47-4).

Instructional Notes

The word *Includes* may be used under a category and will identify additional names for conditions in the category or a description of conditions. For example, under the category code for *Mumps* (B26), the tabular list states, "Includes epidemic parotitis and infectious parotitis." The word *Excludes* identifies specific conditions that are not included in a category and usually points to an alternative code. *Excludes 1* means that the condition is not coded here, and the patient cannot have both the excluded condition and the condition listed above it. *Excludes 2* means that the condition is not included in this code, but the patient may have two conditions, the one included in the current code, as well as the condition using the correct code for the excluded condition. For example, in the category *Allergic contact dermatitis* (L23), the patient cannot have a diagnosis of contact dermatitis that does not specify allergy (Excludes 1), and conditions such as dermatitis caused by substances taken internally are not included (Excludes 2). (See Figure 47-5.)

More than one code may be required for a single disease or condition when a condition affects multiple body systems or is caused by or results from an underlying condition in

GOVERNMENT PLANS

Medicare

Medicare is a federally funded plan administered by the Centers for Medicare and Medicaid Services (CMS). It pays for health care services for the following individuals:

- Individuals older than 65 who are eligible for Social Security
- Retired railroad employees and some retired federal employees
- Individuals who have been permanently disabled for 2 years
- Blind individuals
- Individuals with chronic renal disease who require dialysis or kidney transplant
- Kidney donors

The Medicare plan has several parts. Medicare Part A provides coverage for hospitalization services. Medicare Part B covers physician and other provider services. Together these two parts make up what is called the *Original Medicare Plan.* The patient's Medicare card identifies what type of coverage the patient has (Figure 48-1). Medicare was expanded to provide more choice in the types of available plans in 1997 (also known as *Part C*). Several Medicare Advantage Plans, including managed care plans and fee-for-service plans, replace the Original Medicare Plan if recipients choose them. Medicare Part D was passed in 2003 and went into effect in 2006. It adds a prescription drug benefit to the Original Medicare Plan and Medicare Advantage Plans that did not include this benefit. If the patient is enrolled in a Medicare Advantage plan, the physician must be a member physician of that plan for services to be covered.

Individuals aged 65 and older on Social Security, those younger than 65 but who collect Social Security disability benefits, and those who receive railroad retirement benefits are automatically enrolled in Medicare Part A. Most people do not pay a premium for participation in Medicare Part A. There is a Part A deductible, and the amount the patient is required to pay is adjusted annually. Medicare Part A is funded through a tax paid by working individuals on all of their earned income.

Anyone eligible for Medicare Part A may also obtain Part B coverage. However, they must apply and pay a premium to obtain Medicare Part B or to enroll in one of the Medicare Advantage Plans. Former federal employees, who receive federal employee pensions rather than Social Security and who are not covered by Medicare Part A, can purchase Medicare Part B coverage.

Each Medicare claim is submitted by the medical office or other health care facility to a **Medicare Administrative Contractor (MAC),** a multistate, regional business that administers both Part A and Part B claims under a contract with CMS. The amount of payment for any service is standardized nationally.

Payment for hospitals for claims under Part A is based on **diagnosis-related groups (DRGs),** a system that classifies patients according to the diagnosis, treatment, and length of hospital stay. The patient is assigned a DRG based on the primary diagnosis, and the payment made by Medicare to a hospital is determined by the DRG rather than the length of time the patient remains in the hospital.

Since 1992, payments for services under Part B have been based on a **resource-based relative value scale (RBRVS)** developed by researchers at Harvard University. This system establishes relative value units for each procedure based on the amount of work involved, overhead expenses, and cost of malpractice insurance. The amount Medicare pays for each relative value unit is then adjusted annually; it is also adjusted for different geographic areas (because overhead and malpractice cost may vary). An annual fee schedule is available online for identifying the amount Medicare pays for specific procedures. A similar system is used by most commercial insurance carriers today.

A participating provider in the Medicare program must bill for the patient, accept assignment of benefits, and accept Medicare's determination of the allowable charge for the service. Under Part B, after paying an annual deductible, the patient is responsible for 20% of the allowable charge. The amount of the deductible is adjusted yearly. If the physician, medical office, or other health care facility has any reason to believe that Medicare payment may be denied for a covered service under original Medicare Part B, the patient must be given an **Advanced Beneficiary Notice of Noncoverage (ABN)**. This form, which can be downloaded from the CMS website, informs the patient in writing that he or she will be required to pay for a covered service if the claim is denied by Medicare as medically unnecessary. The form is not required for services that Medicare never covers (e.g., cosmetic surgery).

If a physician does not participate in the Medicare program (nonPAR), usually he or she does not accept assignment of benefits but collects the bill from the patient up to a limiting charge (percent limit on fees above the fee-schedule amount) set by legislation.

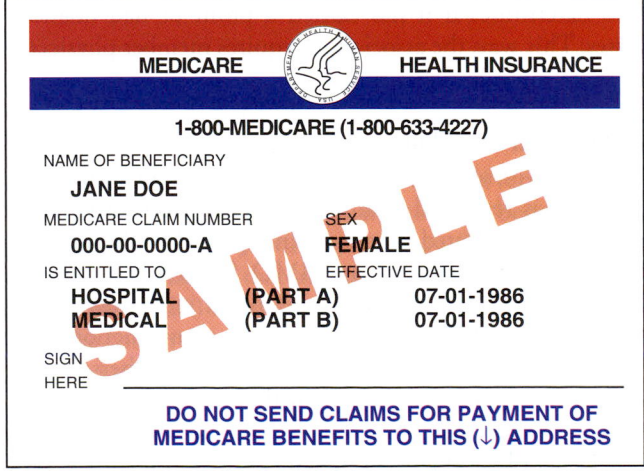

Figure 48-1 Identification card for Medicare.

Many patients purchase additional insurance (known as *Medicare supplemental* or *Medigap insurance*) that covers the annual deductible and 20% coinsurance for Part B, as well as the deductible for Part A. Patients in most Medicare Advantage plans do not need supplemental insurance. Some patients may also be covered by employment plans after retirement. In this case, Medicare is the primary insurance and the Medigap or employment retiree plan is secondary. If a person continues to work after 65 and obtains insurance through employment, that insurance is the primary insurance for that individual and Medicare is the secondary insurance.

Medicaid

Medicaid, formally Title XIX (Title 19) of the 1965 amendments to the Social Security laws, provides for the federal government to give each state a grant to be used toward care of low-income residents. Along with the federal government's basic funding comes an obligation for the states to provide basic health care. States may add coverage for other care to their Medicaid laws but must pay for most of those costs, with the federal government paying a portion. The name of the Medicaid program, as well as procedures for gaining access to it, vary from state to state.

A patient's Medicaid eligibility must be checked at every office visit. In many states patients have a Medicaid card similar to a credit card with a magnetic stripe. The medical assistant uses a machine similar to a credit card reader to verify the patient's eligibility, as discussed in Chapter 39.

Physicians may agree or decline to provide services to Medicaid patients. If they agree to treat Medicaid patients, they must accept all patients with Medicaid insurance. In addition, physicians must agree to accept the state's payment for services, without billing patients for any difference between the state's payment and the actual charge.

Adults and children receiving basic welfare grants from a state are automatically eligible for Medicaid. Also, the children in many working households are eligible for Medicaid benefits if the parents' pay is low enough to put the family below the poverty line or if employee-provided medical insurance covers only the employed parent.

In addition to paying for medical services, Medicaid also covers the cost of long-term nursing home care for low-income elderly and disabled individuals. Because nursing home care is so expensive, 20% of Medicaid beneficiaries—elderly residents of nursing homes—account for 70% to 80% of the cost of the Medicaid program.

Children's Health Insurance Program

The Children's Health Insurance Program (CHIP), established in 1997, is overseen by the CMS as part of Medicaid, but it is managed by the individual states. The program was reauthorized and expanded in 2009 and extended again until 2019 as part of the Affordable Care Act of 2010. The CHIP program is administered and partially funded on a statewide basis. Depending on the state, eligible children are enrolled in the state's Medicaid plan or a separate CHIP

program, or a combination of the two approaches is used. The medical assistant should familiarize himself or herself with the state requirements for this plan.

Insurance Plans for Dependents of Members of the Armed Services and Veterans

TRICARE is the federal insurance program that provides health benefits for the dependent spouses and children of active military personnel when receiving care from civilian physicians and health facilities. The name was changed to TRICARE with the addition of managed care services because there are three plans available to members of the armed services: TRICARE Standard (formerly CHAMPUS), TRICARE Prime, and TRICARE Extra.

TRICARE Standard benefits are available to dependent spouses and children of active-duty military personnel, dependent spouses and children of military personnel who died while on active duty, and military retirees (and their dependents) who are not old enough to be eligible for Medicare. It is a standard fee-for-service plan.

TRICARE Prime is an HMO-type plan with optional participation. In addition to the services covered by TRICARE Standard, it includes preventive and primary care services.

TRICARE Extra allows an individual to seek care from a network provider on a visit-by-visit basis, with a discount on medical services provided and a lower copayment than when using TRICARE Standard.

In 1973 the federal government created CHAMPVA to provide both inpatient and outpatient medical benefits for the dependent spouses and children of veterans who have sustained total, permanent, service-connected disabilities and for surviving spouses and children of veterans who have died as a result of those service-connected disabilities. The nearest VA Medical Center determines eligibility and issues an identification card, but the CHAMPVA-covered patients are allowed to choose their own physicians and other medical service providers.

Workers' Compensation

Workers' compensation insurance covers lost wages and the cost of medical treatment for workers injured on the job or who fall ill as a result of workplace hazards or disease. Each state has its own workers' compensation program. The cost of workers' compensation insurance is paid by employers. The premium for a given employer depends on how many previous employees have made claims under workers' compensation.

Workers are required to make a prompt claim for workers' compensation coverage after an accident or the onset of an illness. In many states the employer and the insurance company issuing the policy have the right to choose the physician who treats the patient.

If a patient visits his or her regular primary care physician and says the illness or injury is workplace related, the medical assistant should check promptly with the employer to verify that the employee has made a report and that the care will be covered by the company's workers' compensation plan.

If a patient of the medical practice is seen for a workers' compensation case, separate medical and financial records should be established for that patient. Laws require that requests for medical records for compensation cases must contain only information associated with the work-related injury. If a workers' appeal board needs work-related injury records, it is important that no other medical information about the patient be released.

For a workers' compensation case, the physician must file a Physician's First Report of Injury. In most states this must be done electronically within 72 hours of the patient's initial visit for a workplace injury. Four copies are prepared: one for the employer's compensation insurance carrier, one for the employer, one for the state compensation board, and one for the patient's medical record. A sample form can be printed or completed online using SimChart® for the Medical Office and saved to a simulated patient's medical record.

In addition to the report, the physician submits a statement of services to the insurance carrier. As is the case for most government programs, the physician must accept the payment provided as payment in full. The physician submits a report and a statement monthly until care is completed.

INSURANCE AND MANAGED CARE POLICIES AND PROCEDURES

MEETING REQUIREMENTS FOR INSURANCE AND MANAGED CARE PLANS

To obtain the maximum third-party reimbursement for services provided to patients, it is very important to be familiar with the requirements of each insurance carrier and HMO that provides insurance for the practice's patients. In addition, the same carrier may support more than one insurance plan. Each insurance plan works in its own way, and each one has a handbook for providers. This is available in hard copy and can also usually be accessed via the Internet and downloaded to the office network. The medical assistant should familiarize himself or herself with the various requirements of each particular insurance plan, including such things as whether a referral to a specialist must be in writing (hard copy or electronic) or can be given over the telephone. Each precertification and most referrals must be authorized by the HMO, and the authorization number should be noted on all of the certification or referral paperwork or electronic forms.

The medical assistant must also know which laboratory can do laboratory work for each plan and where patients can be referred for diagnostic follow-up. Most HMOs, for example, have contracts with a limited number of laboratories and/or medical facilities and will pay only for services provided by an approved facility.

Because many patients have prescription drug benefits, the medical assistant should also learn the pharmacies that should be used for each plan and be sure that pharmacy information has been entered along with insurance plan information for each patient. The patient may have a separate pharmacy insurance card with specific information. This card should be copied for the patient file or scanned into the office computer system.

VERIFYING ELIGIBILITY AND OBTAINING PREAUTHORIZATION (PRECERTIFICATION)

Most insurance companies have a process for reviewing services such as surgery, treatment by a specialist, physical therapy, certain diagnostic tests, and so on. The services and specific requirements vary greatly and tend to be stricter for managed care plans. The medical assistant must be able to obtain and interpret information on the patient's insurance card (Procedure 48-1). The patient's insurance card identifies telephone numbers, fax numbers, and usually a website where eligibility status can be verified (Figure 48-2).

The first element of the process is often to verify **eligibility** status—that is, determine whether the patient has health insurance coverage and will be able to receive health insurance benefits during the proposed time period (Procedure 48-2). The second element is to verify insurance benefits—that is, determine whether the patient's insurance covers the proposed service. The insurance carrier may provide written or electronic verification, or the medical assistant may complete a form when verifying eligibility and/or benefits using the telephone.

The third element is to fulfill the insurance carrier's requirements for notifying the insurance carrier and obtaining authorization to provide the service. **Preauthorization** (or prior authorization) and **precertification** are two terms used to indicate that the patient's health insurance carrier has verified that the service is covered by the patient's insurance policy and/or that the insurance carrier has reviewed the medical necessity for a service and agreed that a procedure is medically appropriate (utilization review). Different companies may use these terms in slightly different ways. In addition, some companies require formal notification of the intent to provide or receive service, either by the provider or the patient. The requirement may be for a telephone call or submission of an electronic or written form depending on the insurance carrier (Procedure 48-3).

Preauthorization (precertification) is usually required for certain medical procedures, therapy (e.g., physical therapy, occupational therapy, speech therapy), certain diagnostic procedures, consultations with a specialist physician, surgery, and hospitalization. Most insurance carriers prefer that requests for preauthorization (precertification) be submitted electronically using the insurance carrier's own website or an affiliate. The response is usually also provided electronically, usually with a form that can be printed and filed in a paper medical record or downloaded to an

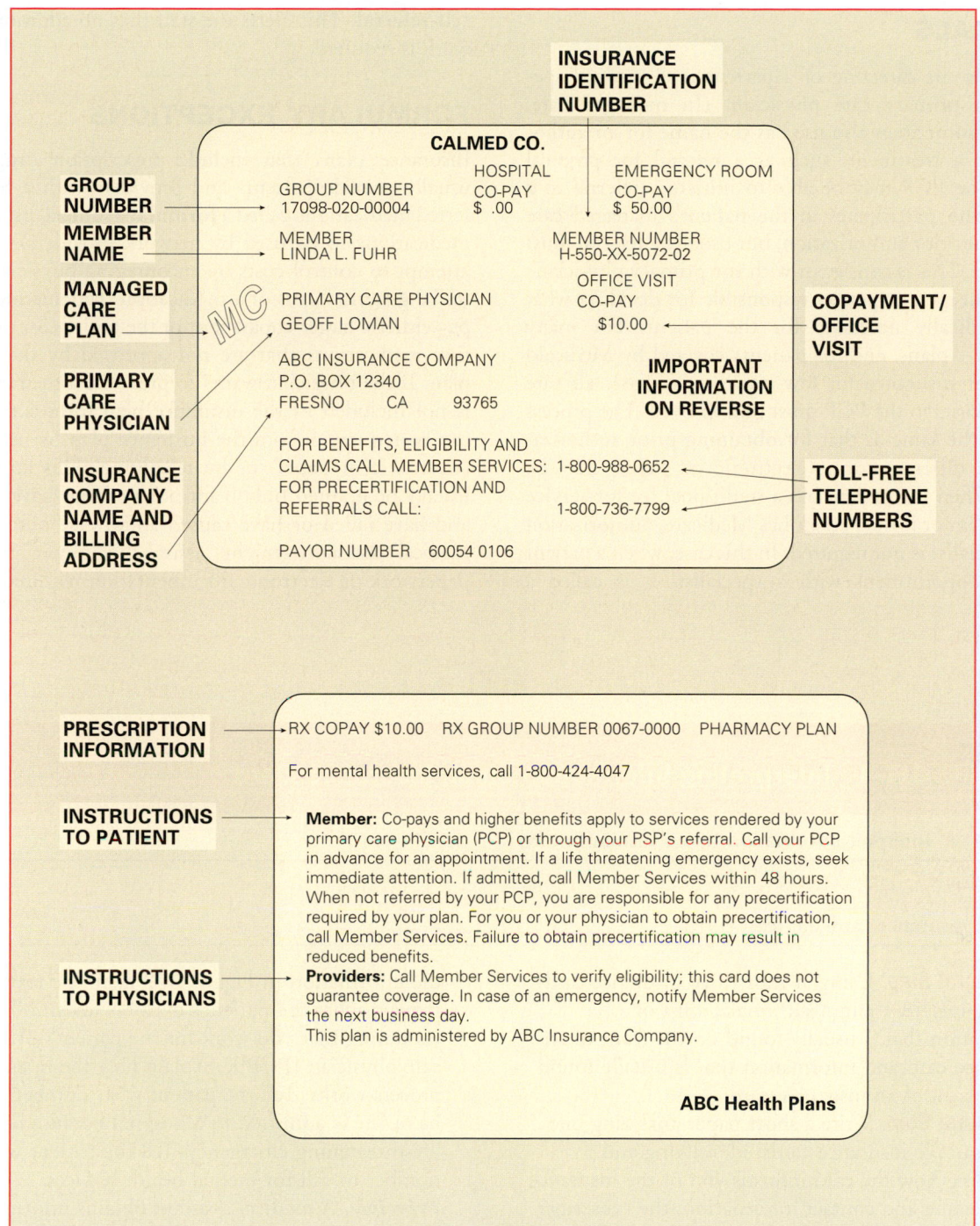

Figure 48-2 The patient's insurance card summarizes important information about the insurance plan. (From Fordney M: *Insurance handbook for the medical office,* ed 13, St Louis, 2014, Saunders.)

electronic medical record. Paper forms can be obtained for fax or mail submission. Electronic requests can be approved more quickly.

The medical assistant should obtain the following information from the physician before initiating the request for preauthorization (precertification): a description of the service (e.g., number of visits to a specialist, type of therapy, surgery), the patient's diagnosis, any relevant information

to justify the need for the service, and the proposed date of service (such as surgery or hospitalization). In addition, the medical assistant will need to provide the patient's demographic and insurance information as well as the National Provider Identifier (NPI) numbers and contact information of the primary care physician, the physician who will perform the service, and the hospital or other health care facility where the patient will receive treatment.

REFERRALS

A **referral** is the directing of a patient to a medical specialist by a primary care physician. (In managed care, a referral is sometimes also used as the name for an authorization for a treatment, such as a referral for physical therapy). The PCP may be able to initiate a referral to a physician who participates in the patient's managed care plan without prior authorization, but usually a referral must be approved. This is consistent with the primary physician's role as gatekeeper, or person responsible for deciding what care is medically necessary for the patient. For many managed care plans, and for patients covered by Medicaid (government insurance for low-income patients), all care other than visits to the PCP must be approved. The process is basically the same as that for obtaining prior authorization, but a different form (electronic or paper) may be required. When the patient has a traditional fee-for-service insurance plan or if the patient has Medicare, authorization to see a specialist is not required. In this case, when a patient makes an appointment with a specialist, it is called a **self-referral.** This alerts the staff that no additional paperwork is required.

FORMULARY EXCEPTIONS

Insurance plans that include prescription drug benefits usually provide patients and providers with a list of preferred medications called a **formulary** (official list of covered medications to be used by network providers). This is an attempt to control costs by encouraging physicians to prescribe generic forms of a medication. Patients may have to pay either a larger copayment or the entire cost of prescription medications that are not approved by the insurance plan. If the physician wants to prescribe a medication that is not included in the insurance plan formulary, approval can be requested from the insurance plan by using a form (electronic or paper) or by telephone. This approval will usually be granted only if formulary drugs have been tried and have failed or have caused an adverse outcome. The medical assistant might assist the physician with the paperwork or electronic documentation required.

PROCEDURE 48-1   Interpreting Information on an Insurance Card

Outcome Interpret information on an insurance card

Equipment/Supplies

• Sample insurance cards (at least three

1. **Procedural Step.** Using at least three insurance cards (see Figures 48-1 and 48-2), make a list of information that is usually found on the front of an insurance card and information that is usually found on the back of an insurance card.
2. **Procedural Step.** Write a short paper analyzing one of the sample insurance cards, identifying and explaining how the card informs you of the insurance carrier name and contact information, the subscriber name and identifying information, the patient payment responsibility for various services, and the type of insurance plan.
3. **Procedural Step.** Role-play the part of a medical assistant with a classmate playing the part of the patient whose insurance card you are viewing using

the information in Figure 48-2 from the textbook. Explain what the patient's copay is for an office visit (assuming that you work for the patient's primary care physician [PCP]). Explain how the referral process works. Tell the patient what number to call if he or she is admitted to a hospital because of a life-threatening emergency. Tell the patient what number to call for mental health services.
Principle. A medical assistant obtains information about a patient's insurance plan from the insurance card and may be required to coach the patient about his or her insurance plan.

4. **Procedural Step.** Hand in your list of information on an insurance card and analysis of an insurance card to your instructor.

PROCEDURE 48-2   Verifying Insurance Eligibility and Benefits

Outcome Verify insurance or managed care eligibility

Equipment/Supplies

- Patient insurance information
- Telephone
- Computer with Internet access
- Pen and paper

1. **Procedural Step.** Assemble information about the patient's insurance plan including name of insurance or managed care company, telephone number or Web address, patient name, patient date of birth, subscriber number, and group number. If possible, obtain this information from a photocopy of the patient's insurance card.
   Principle: The insurance card contains all information to contact a patient's insurance plan.

2. **Procedural Step.** If using the telephone, call the appropriate number and speak to a representative to verify that the patient is eligible for benefits. Record the effective date and the termination date (if any).
   Principle: An individual's insurance coverage can change for many reasons. A patient must have current coverage to obtain insurance reimbursement.

3. **Procedural Step.** Ask the representative for information about the patient's deductible and copayment or coinsurance. If a service other than a routine office visit is planned, determine if it is a covered service and if precertification or preauthorization is required.
   Principle: Knowledge of deductible and copayment or coinsurance helps determine the amount the patient should pay at the time of the visit.

4. **Procedural Step.** If using a plan website to verify eligibility, log in to the website and find the patient using name, date of birth, and subscriber number.

5. **Procedural Step.** Verify that you have found the correct patient on the plan website, and view the eligibility information as described previously for a telephone contact.

6. **Procedural Step.** Note the information according to office policy. There may be a form to fill out or a notation may be required in the patient's medical record. If the insurance carrier provides an electronic verification of eligibility, attach it to the patient's electronic medical record (EMR), or print it and file it in a paper-based medical record.

PROCEDURE 48-3   Obtaining Insurance Preauthorization (Precertification)

Outcome Obtain insurance preauthorization (precertification)

Equipment/Supplies

- Patient's medical record and insurance information
- Physician's directions about the service to be provided
- Computer or paper preauthorization (precertification) request form
- Computer with Internet access
- Pen
- Telephone

1. **Procedural Step.** Assemble information to complete a preauthorization (precertification) request:
   - Patient demographic information
   - Patient insurance information
   - Information about service to be provided, including diagnosis code(s) and procedure code(s), and the patient's name, address, telephone number, and insurance information
   - Forms as needed
     It may be helpful to print and complete a Prior Authorization Request form from SimChart® for the Medical Office (Forms Repository).

2. **Procedural Step.** From the patient's medical record or the physician, determine the service for which preauthorization or precertification is requested. Assemble all information needed to complete the request.
   Principle. Most requests require at a minimum the patient's name, ID number, diagnosis and diagnosis code, proposed procedure and procedure code, physician's National Provider Identifier (NPI) number, and NPI number of other physician or service provider. Assembling information ahead of time facilitates completing the request.

Continued

PROCEDURE **48-3**   Obtaining Insurance Preauthorization (Precertification)—cont'd

3. Procedural Step. Obtain preauthorization or precertification from the patient's insurance carrier or health maintenance organization (HMO). The preferred method is usually by completing a form on the carrier's website. Telephone, fax, or a paper form may also be used. Supply all information requested. If using the telephone, it is helpful to complete the form manually before placing the call to be sure you have all necessary information.

Principle. The patient's medical condition must justify the service requested. Failure to obtain preauthorization or precertification required by the insurance carrier will result in denial of the patient's insurance claim.

For a telephone request, it is helpful to fill out the required form before calling the insurance carrier.

4. Procedural Step. When the form is complete, submit the form for approval using the appropriate method.

5. Procedural Step. Inform the patient that he or she will not be able to obtain service until preauthorization or precertification is received from the insurance carrier.

6. Procedural Step. When approval is received, notify the patient. An electronic form should be accessible to any other health care provider using the Internet. A paper copy must be sent or faxed to a specialty physician or other provider of service.

7. Procedural Step. Instruct the patient how to make the appointment (or assist the patient in making the first appointment).

8. Procedural Step. File the approval form in the patient's medical record or attach an electronic form (scan a paper form) to the electronic medical record (EMR).

INSURANCE CLAIM FORMS

The most commonly used insurance form in the medical office is the CMS-1500. This form began as the Health Insurance Claim Form, which was approved for use by the American Medical Association in 1975. It was gradually accepted by various insurance plans for payment of claims by those plans. In 1990 this form was revised and printed in red. It became the required form for Medicare claims in 1992. It is discussed in greater detail in the next section.

Another commonly used form is the UB-04 form, which is used by hospitals and other institutions to submit paper insurance claims.

THE CMS-1500 CLAIM FORM

Since the 1950s the Health Insurance Association of America has sought to have all medical insurance claims filed on a common form. After considerable work to develop a universal claim form, most insurance companies will accept the CMS-1500 form, either alone or as an attachment to the company's own form. This form was updated in 2005 to accept the NPI, a 10-digit identifier required for all health care providers that replaces all previous identification (ID) numbers. A claim form with minor revisions to accept International Classification of Diseases, 10th Revision, Clinical Modification (ICD-10-CM) diagnosis codes was accepted in 2012 and is required for claim submission effective April 1, 2014 (Figure 48-3).

HEALTH INSURANCE CLAIM FORM

APPROVED BY NATIONAL UNIFORM CLAIM COMMITTEE (NUCC) 02/12

Figure 48-3 The CMS-1500 claim form (2/12 revision).

GUIDELINES FOR PROCESSING INSURANCE CLAIMS

Because payment of a significant part of the bill for most patients is made by a third-party payor, it is important for the office to prepare and track insurance claims so that claims are processed in a timely manner without mistakes that will prevent or delay payment. This improves the cash flow for the office and avoids the need for the medical assistant to take extra time to correct errors. There are several general guidelines to facilitate the claim submission process.

1. Enter all patient and insurance information correctly into the computer, and be sure that insurance information is updated at each visit with an updated photocopy of the patient's insurance card.
2. Be sure there is a signature on file for each patient for whom an insurance claim is submitted.
3. Be aware of and follow requirements of all insurance companies related to verifying patient coverage, notifying before procedures, obtaining prior authorization, and using facilities such as laboratories, hospitals, and surgery centers as required by the insurance carrier.
4. Follow the correct procedure to transmit electronic information (which will be discussed later) or complete paper claims (when they are accepted) so that they can be read by automated equipment.
5. Proofread all claims for accuracy before submitting them. Numbers that are incorrect by one digit, missing information, and/or incorrect information can result in an automatic claim rejection. Be sure to submit additional information with a claim if it is required.
6. Submit claims or claim information promptly, and follow up to make sure that claims have been processed by the insurance carrier.
7. Follow up to correct and resubmit claims rejected for errors in a timely manner.

COMPLETING THE INSURANCE CLAIM FORM

In the medical office, the medical assistant usually prepares insurance claims using a computer billing program or submits claim information to an insurance billing clearinghouse. Since 2004, federal programs such as Medicare require electronic claim submission unless the office has been granted a waiver that allows submission of paper claims. Nevertheless, the medical assistant must know what information should be included so that each claim form can be reviewed before submission (Procedure 48-4).

CARRIER INFORMATION

The name and address of the insurance carrier to which the claim will be sent is printed in the top section of the

insurance claim form. For paper claims this address should be entered in uppercase letters without punctuation (except for the hyphen in the ZIP+4 code.)

PATIENT AND INSURED INFORMATION

Patient Information

The patient section contains the patient's basic demographic information. This includes the patient's name, address, date of birth, and sex. It also identifies whether the physician accepts assignment of benefits, which is authorized by the patient's signature. Instead of asking patients to sign every insurance claim, the phrase **signature on file** or the abbreviation **SOF** is often used to indicate that the office maintains a copy of the patient's signature authorizing submission of the claim and assignment of benefits.

What Would You Do? What Would You *Not* Do?

Case Study 2

Daniel Litton is a 14-year-old new patient who has an appointment with one of the dermatologists in the office. He is brought to the office by his mother, who helps him fill out the new patient information form. In the section for insurance information, his mother indicates that he is covered by family insurance plans through both his father and his mother. His mother says, "I hope you will bill my insurance for him because I have better coverage for things like this." ■

Subscriber and Insurance Information

The insurance information part of the insurance claim form includes the following information about the insured (sometimes called the *subscriber* or the *guarantor*): the name of the insured, address, and relationship to the patient. It is important to be sure that the information about the **guarantor,** the individual with financial responsibility and/or insurance, has been entered into the computer (if he or she is not a patient). In addition, for employer-sponsored plans, the employer's name is listed. The insured has an ID number. In a family plan, other family members may use the same number as the insured, or each may be assigned a different number. For a group plan there is also a group number that is common to all members who obtain insurance from that employer or through that group.

If there is insurance in the name of a second party, this is also included on the claim form with the appropriate information about the insurance policy and ID (policy) and group numbers. On every claim form, information must be included to identify whether the claim relates to a work injury, auto accident, or other accident. This helps the insurance carrier identify which insurance is responsible for covering the claim.

PHYSICIAN INFORMATION

The information about the medical service provided is entered in the lower half of the insurance claim form. In addition to information about the medical problem, the ICD code for each diagnosis must be listed. An ICD indicator must be entered (9 or 10) that corresponds to the type of diagnosis codes being used (ICD-9 or ICD-10). Only ICD-9 codes will be accepted until October 1, 2015. Each procedure must be linked to a primary diagnosis code to justify the procedure. On the lower lines, information about each procedure is given, including the date of service, place of service, pointer to the procedure code, charge for the service, number of units being billed, and NPI number of the provider of each service. See Table 48-1 for a list of codes commonly used for place of service when billing from the medical office.

Table 48-1 Place of Service Codes Used for Billing in the Medical Office

Code	Place of Service
11	Office
12	Home
20	Urgent care facility
21	Inpatient hospital
22	Outpatient hospital
23	Emergency room—hospital
24	Ambulatory surgical center
25	Birthing center
26	Military treatment facility
31	Skilled nursing facility
32	Nursing facility
33	Custodial care facility
49	Independent clinic

PROCEDURE 48-4

PROCEDURE 48-4   Completing and Reviewing an Insurance Claim Form

Outcome Complete or review an insurance claim form

Equipment/Supplies

- Patient information
- Patient account or ledger
- Copy of the patient's insurance card or computer patient information screen
- Insurance claim form
- Computer with medical billing program or SimChart® for the Medical Office
- Pen
- Printer

1. **Procedural Step.** Assemble information needed to prepare an insurance claim, including a claim form, information about the patient, the patient account or ledger, and a copy of the patient's insurance card or insurance information. Review the claim form guidelines for the specific insurance carrier.

2. **Procedural Step.** Enter (or review) information as required on the paper CMS-1500 form according to the following information. If a paper claim will be submitted to be scanned by optical character recognition (OCR) or intelligent character recognition (ICR), do not use commas, dollar signs, or other punctuation unless instructed to do so.
   Principle. Most insurance companies use ICR scanning to digitize information on paper claims, and the equipment works best when the guidelines outlined earlier have been followed. It is usually no longer necessary to use only capital letters.

3. **Procedural Step.** In the carrier section, enter or validate the name and address of the insurance carrier to which the claim will be sent using the following format:
   Line 1: Name of carrier
   Line 2: First line of address
   Line 3: Second line of address (if needed)
   Line 4: City [space] State [space] ZIP
   Example:
   Three-line address:
   Standard Health Care
   1500 Summit Avenue
   Western XY 45000
   Four-line address:
   Standard Health Care
   Suite 620
   1500 Summit Avenue
   Western XY 45000

Continued

PROCEDURE 48-4   Completing and Reviewing an Insurance Claim Form—cont'd

4. Procedural Step. Complete or review the patient and insured information on the claim form.

Box 1—The type of insurance is indicated with an **X**. Only one box can be marked. Insurance obtained through employment is a Group Health Plan.

Box 1a—The ID number of the individual who is insured as shown on the insurance card.

Box 2—The patient's last name, first name, and middle initial (separated by commas).

Box 3—The patient's date of birth in the format MM DD YYYY and the patient's sex (M or F) marked with an **X**.

Box 4—The name of the insured using the format last name, first name, middle initial (separated by commas). If the patient and the insured are the same, this box does not have to be completed.

Box 5—The patient's mailing address beginning with the street. Use the two-letter state code. Do not use commas, periods, or other punctuation in the address with the exception of the hyphen in a nine-digit ZIP code. Do not use a hyphen or space as a separator in the telephone number.

Box 6—An **X** in the box that defines the patient's relationship to the insured (i.e., person whose name is on the insurance policy). The choices include self, spouse, child, and other.

Box 7—The insured's mailing address beginning with the street. Use the two-letter state code. Do not use commas, periods, or other punctuation in the address with the exception of the hyphen in a nine-digit ZIP code. Do not use a hyphen or space as a separator in the seven-digit telephone number. Complete this box if Box 4 is completed.

Box 8—The boxes that best describe the patient's marital status and employment status are checked. If the patient has insurance through the employer, assume that he or she is employed. If the patient is a college student (older than 18), it may be important to determine if he or she is a full-time student. The choices include single, married, and other, and employed, full-time student, and part-time student.

Box 9—If there is secondary insurance, the insured's name using the format described for Box 4.

Box 9a—If there is secondary insurance, the subscriber policy (ID) or group number

Box 9d—If there is secondary insurance, the other insured's insurance plan or program name.

Boxes 9b and 9c have been deleted from ANSI 5010A1, the current data format for electronic claim submission, so these boxes should be left blank.

Box 10a-c—Information related to the cause of the patient's condition(s). The correct boxes are checked (yes or no) to answer the questions. If the patient's condition was caused by an automobile accident, the state where the accident occurred is identified using the correct two-letter code.

Patient and insurance information section.

PROCEDURE 48-4   Completing and Reviewing an Insurance Claim Form—cont'd

Box 10d—Used to report claim codes that identify additional information about the patient's condition when required by public or private payers.

Box 11—The insured's policy group or Federal Employees' Compensation Act (FECA) number. If item number 4 is completed, this field should be completed

Box 11a-d—If the patient is the insured, only box 11d must be completed. The insured's date of birth in the format MM DD YYYY and the insured's sex (M or F) marked with an **X**. The insured's employer and insurance plan name. An **X** is used in the correct box to indicate if there is additional insurance (yes or no). If *yes* is selected, Boxes 9a-d are filled out.

Box 12—If the office has on file the patient's signature on a similar permission form, the initials *SOF* or the words *Signature on File* are placed in this box. Otherwise, the patient must sign and date the form.

Box 13—If the office has on file the patient's signature on a similar permission form, the initials *SOF* or the words *Signature on File* are placed in this box. Otherwise, the patient must sign and date the form.

5. **Procedural Step.** Complete the physician or supplier information using information from the patient charge slip.

   Principle. If incomplete or incorrect information about primary and secondary insurance plans is given, the claim will be denied.

   Boxes 14-16—Not usually required for Medicare, Medicaid, TRICARE, CHAMPVA, and most private insurance. If these boxes must be filled in, the dates are obtained from the patient's medical record and/or the physician. A qualifier code must be entered in box 15 using the following:

   454   Initial treatment
   304   Latest visit or consultation
   453   Acute manifestation of a chronic condition
   455   Last x-ray
   471   Prescription
   090   Report start (Assumed care date)
   091   Report end (Relinquished care date)
   444   First visit or consultation

   Box 17—Name of the physician who ordered the service or referred the patient (first, middle initial, last) or other source followed by the credentials of the professional. If multiple providers are involved and for Medicare claims, use the

following order and enter a qualifier to the left of the dotted line:
   1. DN   Referring provider
   2. DK   Ordering provider
   3. DQ   Supervising provider

   Box 17a—Usually blank. If the provider does not have a national provider identifier (NPI) number, other identifying numbers can be used.

   Box 17b—The 10-digit NPI number of the referring physician.

   Box 18—If the patient's claim is for a hospitalization, either a visit or surgery performed when the patient was hospitalized, and the dates of hospitalization. Otherwise, the box is left blank.

   Box 19—Left blank unless instructed by a specific insurance carrier to use this box for information specific to that carrier.

   Box 20—*No* is usually checked. If the office paid for outside laboratory services that are not itemized on one of the lines in Box 24, *yes* is checked. If *yes* is checked, enter the charges with a space between the dollars and cents. Only one outside service can be billed per claim form.

   Box 21—Enter the International Classification of Diseases (ICD) indicator to identify which version of ICD codes is being reported.
   9   ICD-9-CM
   10   ICD-10-CM
   Enter up to 12 ICD codes with alphanumeric characters and periods. Relate lines A to L to the lines of service in 24E by the letter of the line.

   Box 22—Left blank unless the claim is a Medicaid resubmission, when the code and original reference number are entered.

   Box 23—Left blank unless a referral, preauthorization, or precertification number was assigned by the insurance carrier.

6. **Procedural Step.** Enter information in Box 24 on lines 1 to 6 for each procedure that is being billed to the insurance carrier. For more than six procedures, complete an additional CMS-1500 form.

   Box 24A—The date service began under the "From" section in the format MM DD YYYY in the unshaded area. If the service occurred on 1 day only, the "To" section is left blank or the "From" date may be entered again; otherwise, the date service ended.

   Box 24B—The code for the place of service from Table 48-1.

   Box 24C—This box is usually left blank. For some carriers, a *Y* is placed in this box if the service is an emergency service.

Continued

PROCEDURE 48-4   Completing and Reviewing an Insurance Claim Form—cont'd

Box 24D—The Current Procedural Terminology (CPT) or Healthcare Common Procedure Coding System (HCPCS) Level II code and modifier(s) (if any) in the unshaded area.

Box 24E—The letters(s) (from A to L) that point to ICD code(s) in Box 21 that justify the procedure. Only one letter can be used in this box for Medicare claims.

Box 24F—The charges in the unshaded area, leaving a space between the number of dollars and the number of cents instead of using a decimal point.

Box 24G—If charging for more than one of the same procedure (e.g., visits to a hospitalized patient on 3 consecutive days), the number of units of the procedure charged in the unshaded area. Otherwise, the number 1.

Box 24H—Left blank unless the patient is enrolled in the Medicaid program for Early and Periodic Screening, Diagnosis, and Treatment (EPSDT).

Box 24I—If the provider does not have an NPI number, a qualifier is entered in the shaded part of Box 24I, and the appropriate identification number is entered in the shaded part of Box 24J.

Box 24J—The 10-digit NPI number of the individual who provided service in the lower (unshaded) portion.

7. **Procedural Step.** Complete the remaining boxes on the CMS-1500 form.

Box 25—The tax ID number. If the Social Security number of an individual physician is used, box "SSN" is checked. If the employer ID number of a group practice is used, box "EIN" is checked.

Box 26—The patient account number. The box is left blank if there is no patient account number. Hyphens should not be used in this box.

Box 27—If the physician accepts assignment of benefits, an X is placed in the "yes" box. If assignment of benefits is not accepted, an X is placed in the "no" box.

Box 28—The total charges with a space between the number of dollars and the number of cents.

Box 29—The amount paid toward the covered charges, including any copayment. If the amount is zero, the box is left blank.

Provider and supplier section.

PROCEDURE 48-4 Completing and Reviewing an Insurance Claim Form—cont'd

Box 30—The box should be left blank because information in it is no longer transmitted with electronic submission.

Box 31—SOF, Signature on File, or the physician's legal signature including credentials and the date.

Box 32—The name, address, city, state, and ZIP code of the facility where the services were provided, without punctuation. If services were provided at the same address as the billing address, this box, as well as 32a and 32b, can be left blank.

Box 32a—The 10-digit NPI number of the service facility location.

Box 32b—For purchased diagnostic services (box 20) insert the supplier's PIN.

Box 33—The name, address, and telephone number of the physician group or supplier of services without punctuation. The telephone number is entered to the right of the title of the field without a hyphen. A hyphen is used in a nine-digit ZIP code after the fifth digit.

Box 33a—The 10-digit NPI number of the physician group or supplier of services.

Box 33b—Blank.

8. **Procedural Step.** Submit claim according to office policy. Copy a paper form before mailing, and keep the copy in an insurance claims file.

Completing the Insurance Claim Form in SimChart® for the Medical Office

1. **Procedural Step.** After the superbill and ledger have been created for a patient, select *Claim* from the *Info Panel* of the *Coding and Billing* screen and search for the patient.

2. **Procedural Step.** Select the correct encounter and confirm the autopopulated details on all tabs. On the *Encounter Notes* tab, select the *Yes* radio button to validate that the HIPAA form is on file for the patient, and document today's date in the date field. Then click the *Save* button before proceeding to the *Claim Info* tab. Enter the information requested on this screen. Proceed to the *Charge Capture* screen and enter the information from the superbill as outlined for Box 24 above.

3. **Procedural Step.** Click on the printer icon to print the claim so that you can manually double-check all information before submitting the claim.

4. **Procedural Step.** When you are sure that all information is correct, click on the *Submission* tab, and then click on the "I am ready to submit the Claim" box. Then click the *Yes* radio button and enter the date of service in the date field. Click the *Save* button, then the *Submit Claim* button.

PROCEDURE 48-4

SUBMITTING INSURANCE CLAIMS

ELECTRONIC CLAIMS

Electronic submission speeds things up enormously. Submission is instantaneous, instead of taking a few days to move through the mail. The office may submit insurance claims directly to the insurance carrier or may submit them to a clearinghouse that processes the data and submits the claim to the appropriate carrier. The medical office may also submit information to a billing service that processes and submits claims to the various insurance companies. The procedure for submission depends on the computer software used by the office, clearinghouse, or billing service. Insurance company personnel cannot make errors inputting the information into the company's computer system because the transmission is computer to computer.

Faster delivery and faster and more accurate processing means faster reimbursement. If electronic claim submission is coupled with electronic payment from the company to the practice's operating account, the entire turnaround time from submission to money in the bank can be days instead of weeks.

All parts of the Health Insurance Portability and Accountability Act of 1996 (HIPAA) affect insurance billing, but an important provision is the Transactions and Code Set Rule. This rule requires all health care providers to use American National Standards Institute (ANSI) technical content and format specifications for electronic transmissions. The electronic data interchange (EDI) Health Care Claim Transaction set 837P defines the format that must be used to submit health care claim billing information electronically by medical offices or to transmit this information among and within agencies involved in the reimbursement process. Because of the change from ICD-9 to ICD-10 diagnosis codes, the version of 837P has changed from ANSI version 4010A1 to ANSI version 5010 effective January 2012. This change as well as the change to ICD-10 codes affects the computer systems of almost all medical offices. Usually a new version of the office's electronic billing software incorporates the required changes.

PAPER CLAIMS

The CMS-1500 form is printed in red to facilitate optical scanning when paper forms are submitted. Although rarely used, paper claim forms can be purchased from medical office supply companies. For efficient processing, it is recommended to use all capital letters and no punctuation, to be sure that all information is within the required box, and to proofread for typographical errors that might cause the claim to be rejected. The medical assistant must be sure that the insurance carrier accepts paper claims. (Although there are some exceptions, in general, Medicare and Medicaid now require that all claims be submitted electronically.)

If the office submits claims by mail, the frequency of submission depends on the size of the office, the number of personnel devoted to processing claims, and the number of patients seen who are covered by any particular insurance plan. Submission is usually done daily or weekly.

Memories *from* Practicum

Sandra O'Keefe: My practicum was done in the office of a single gynecologist in a medium-size city. Although the office had a computer billing program, we submitted most of the insurance claims on paper. After I had been at the office for several weeks, the office manager started having me fill out some insurance claim forms by hand. Then she would have me print the forms on the computer and compare my form with the computer-generated form. She said I needed to understand how to fill out the form myself, even if I didn't usually do it, so that I would know what kind of information should be in each box. At first I found it very confusing, but after a while I began to know what to look for. For example, an insurance carrier will deny a claim for a Pap test if the sex of the patient is given as male. I was always glad that I had some experience with insurance, although I don't think I realized how complex it really is until I actually began to work as a medical assistant. ∎

What Would You Do? | What Would You *Not* Do?

Case Study 3

Maria Santos, a 33-year-old woman, has been seen in the office for a physical examination. When reviewing insurance claims in the computer before submission, Sandra notices that the name of the insured on the claim for Maria Santos is Jose Santos, and his date of birth is the same as her date of birth. Sandra also notices that in box 8 there is an X beside the word *Employed.* ∎

TRACKING INSURANCE REIMBURSEMENT

Reimbursement is the payment received by the medical practice from the insurance carrier for the services performed.

USING A CLAIMS REGISTER

A record of every insurance claim filed should be kept using an insurance claims register. An insurance claims register can be kept either manually or on the computer (Figure 48-4).

INSURANCE CLAIM REGISTER

BLACKBURN PRIMARY CARE ASSOCIATES, PC

1990 Turquoise Drive
Blackburn, WI 54937
608-459-8857

Claim number	Service	Insurance and ID and group no.	Date and amount of claim	Date and amount paid	Difference	Follow-up action

Figure 48-4 Insurance claims register.

The claims register includes the claim number (the number given to the claim as part of the office's tracking system); the patient's name and insurance group or policy number; the insurance carrier's name; the date and amount of the claim; a column for any follow-up actions taken (by mail or telephone); the date and amount of the paid claim; and any difference between the amount submitted and the amount paid. If a claim is delayed, the medical assistant should submit an insurance claim tracer to the insurance carrier. A form may be available on the insurance website, or there is a sample form that can be printed from Sim-Chart® for the Medical Office (see the Forms Repository).

The medical assistant should review the claims register on a regular basis to be sure that all claims have been paid and that the insurance carrier has not denied services that should be covered or paid less than it should for those services. If a pattern of rejected claims is seen, the medical assistant should work together with other office staff to improve systems so that claims are not denied.

REMITTANCE ADVICE (EXPLANATION OF BENEFITS) FORMS

After payment has been made by the insurance carrier to the physician, or if a claim is being denied, both the physician and the patient receive a notification explaining payment for the claim. The provider receives a **remittance advice (RA)** or **explanation of benefits (EOB)** form. The form sent to the patient is the EOB form. The provider may elect to receive an electronic remittance advice (ERA) from Medicare or other insurance carrier. Although each insurance carrier has its own form, the type of information contained on any RA or EOB is similar, as shown in Figure 48-5. If the insurance carrier is denying the claim, the physician will receive a remittance advice form showing why the claim was disallowed.

Claims are usually denied for one of the following reasons: transposed names or numbers, incomplete information, incorrect or incomplete codes, or information that does not match codes or other information (Table 48-2). Claims may also be denied for late submission or late resubmission of a denied claim.

FOLLOW-UP AND RESUBMISSION OF CLAIMS

If a claim is denied, it should be resubmitted immediately, following any advice given by the company on the remittance advice form. Any questions about a denial should be discussed with a provider relations representative at the company.

If claims are not being paid or denied in a timely fashion, follow-up is in order. Follow-up can be made via letter or over the telephone. The claims log can be used to find all claims to any company that are becoming delinquent and to follow up with a tracer or telephone call.

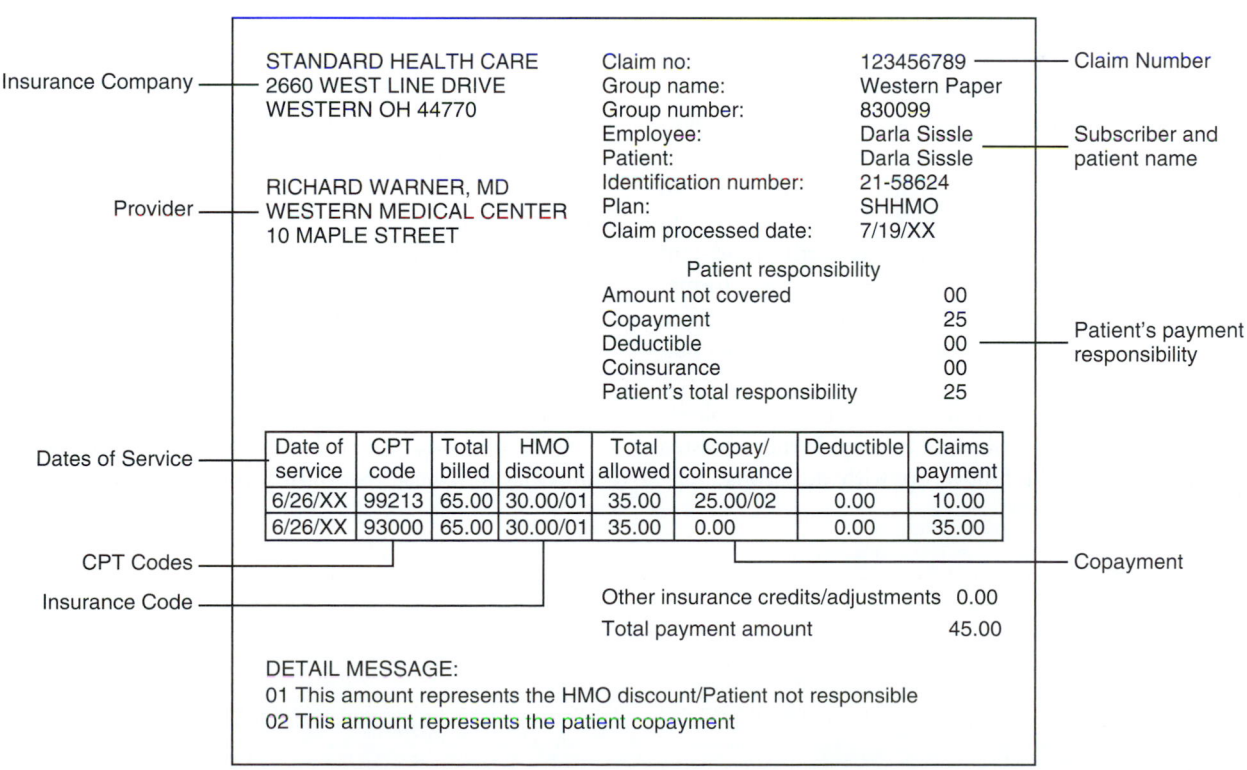

Figure 48-5 Sample explanation of benefits (EOB) form.

Table 48-2 Common Errors on Insurance Claim Forms

Type of Error	Example
Transposing names or numbers	Reversing the name of the patient with the subscriber (guarantor)
	Reversing the primary insurance with the secondary insurance
	Transposing numbers in one of the identification numbers
Missing information	Missing signatures or signature stamps
	Missing or inaccurate physician national provider identifier number for each service, or not a physician registered with plan
	Required attachments missing (e.g., pathology report)
	Incomplete boxes
	Too little information to prove medical necessity
	No preapproval or preauthorization number
Inaccurate or incomplete codes	Inaccurate procedure or service codes (Current Procedural Terminology [CPT] or Healthcare Common Procedure Coding System [HCPCS] Level II codes)
	Missing modifier
Information does not match codes or other information	Diagnosis inconsistent with patient gender
	Diagnosis does not justify procedures performed
	Total amount of billing does not agree with services provided
	Place of service inconsistent with procedure code

EFFECTIVE COMMUNICATION REGARDING MANAGED CARE AND/OR INSURANCE

COMMUNICATION WITH MANAGED CARE AND/OR INSURANCE PROVIDERS

When communicating with managed care and/or insurance providers, it is important for the medical assistant to be polite and tactful, but also to demonstrate assertive communication techniques to maximize reimbursement. Familiarity with a specific plan's requirements and attention to detail when submitting claims helps to minimize claim denials, but when a claim is denied, the medical assistant should telephone the provider and request specific information about the reason for the denial. It may be necessary to ask several questions to determine the type of documentation that will be necessary for the claim to be paid if resubmitted. If necessary, the medical assistant must ask politely for the name of an individual who can provide the requested information and should follow up with additional telephone calls.

COMMUNICATION WITH PATIENTS REGARDING MANAGED CARE AND/OR INSURANCE

The medical assistant must demonstrate different communication skills when discussing insurance benefits with patients. Although the patient has usually signed a form promising to pay for services if they are not covered by insurance, the medical assistant must be willing to explain tactfully that a patient's insurance does not cover a service or that a provider has denied a claim, and the patient is now responsible for the bill. Patients often become upset about gaps in their insurance coverage. By imagining how they would feel in the patient's situation, the medical assistant can empathize with a patient who may be acting angry or hostile. It is important to stay calm, express understanding for the patient's feelings, and if necessary, suggest that the discussion be postponed to give everyone a chance to consider the situation. If a claim has been denied, the medical assistant should offer to resubmit the claim if there is any chance that additional documentation might induce the provider to reverse its decision (Procedure 48-5).

PROCEDURE 48-5 Communicating Effectively Regarding Insurance and/or Managed Care

Outcomes

1. Interact professionally with third-party representatives
2. Display tactful behavior when communicating with medical providers regarding third-party requirements
3. Show sensitivity when communicating with patients regarding third-party requirements

Equipment/Supplies

- Pen
- Paper
- Computer with printer

1. **Procedural Step.** Review the principles of effective communication in the textbook (Chapter 4) including listening skills, measures to facilitate communication, and barriers to effective communication.
2. **Procedural Step.** Working with a group of at least two other students, assign one student to create a role-play situation for each of the following:
   a. A situation in which a medical assistant must demonstrate professional communication with a managed care provider relating to a denied insurance claim.
   b. A situation in which a medical assistant must explain to a physician that a request for a diagnostic test was not approved for a patient by the patient's insurance carrier.
   c. A situation in which a medical assistant must explain to a patient that the insurance carrier has denied an insurance claim and the patient will have to pay for the service.

Principle: A medical assistant must demonstrate effective communication when communicating with managed care and/or insurance representatives as well as with physicians and patients about insurance reimbursement.

3. **Procedural Step.** Review the situations of the other students in your group to be sure that they are specific and realistic. Revise your situation as needed.
4. **Procedural Step.** Role-play each situation with your group members, demonstrating sensitivity, tact, professionalism, and/or other appropriate communication techniques.
5. **Procedural Step.** Add a short summary of the role-play experience to the situation you have created, and explain how you demonstrated professional communication with a third-party representative, tact with a physician, and sensitivity to a patient when discussing a denied insurance claim.
6. **Procedural Step.** Print your paper and hand it in to your instructor.

PROCEDURE 48-5

What Would You Do? What Would You *Not* Do? RESPONSES

Case Study 1
Page 1194

What Did Sandra Do?

☐ Explained to the patient that the original referral authorized treatment of only the lesion on the patient's neck, and the insurance carrier would not pay for other treatment without authorizing it.

☐ Explained that Sandra would contact the insurance carrier and primary care physician and take care of any required paperwork.

☐ Promised to minimize delay as much as possible.

☐ Told the patient that she would be responsible for the cost of removal if proper authorization was not obtained from her insurance carrier.

What Did Sandra *Not* Do?

☐ Did not assume that the referral covered additional lesions not specifically mentioned on the referral form.

☐ Did not assure the patient that her insurance would automatically cover the cost of removing the additional lesions.

☐ Did not schedule the removal of the additional lesions before she received insurance authorization or the patient promised to pay for the procedure.

Case Study 2
Page 1204

What Did Sandra Do?

☐ Explained to Daniel's mother that there are rules governing coverage of children when both parents have insurance plans that cover their children.

☐ Asked Daniel's mother for her birth date and her husband's birth date.

☐ Explained to Daniel and his mother that usually children are covered by the insurance of the parent whose birth date comes first in the year.

Continued

❑ Asked Daniel's mother which insurance plan covers her children for their ordinary medical care.

What Did Sandra _Not_ Do?
❑ Did not promise to send the insurance claim to the carrier the mother prefers unless it was the primary insurance carrier.
❑ Did not tell the mother not to worry because she would take care of it.
❑ Did not tell Daniel's mother that it was her responsibility to find out which insurance was the primary insurance.

Case Study 3
Page 1210

What Did Sandra Do?
❑ Checked the new patient information form to be sure that the insured's name and date of birth had been entered correctly because incorrect information could lead to denial of the insurance claim.
❑ Checked the new patient information form to be sure that the patient had listed an employer.

What Did Sandra _Not_ Do?
❑ Did not assume that it was just a coincidence that the husband and wife had the same date of birth.
❑ Did not assume that a few errors on the insurance claim form would not matter.
❑ Did not assume that the information in the computer was always correct.

TERMINOLOGY REVIEW

Key Term	Definition
Advanced Beneficiary Notice of Noncoverage (ABN)	A written notification to a patient with Original Medicare that a covered service must be paid for by the patient if Medicare denies the claim as medically unnecessary.
Assignment of benefits	Authorization for insurance reimbursement to be made to the provider of a health service rather than the insured individual.
Beneficiary	A person who can receive benefits under an insurance plan.
Benefit	Payment for a covered service under a health insurance plan.
Birthday rule	If both parents of a child have a family health plan, the insurance plan of the parent whose birthday comes earlier in the year is defined as the primary insurance plan covering the child. The insurance of the other parent becomes secondary insurance.
Capitation	A method of paying for insurance in which a fixed amount is paid to the provider per member for a specific time period regardless of the amount of care provided.
Carrier	An insurance company.
CHAMPVA	A government health insurance program that covers dependents of military veterans with service-connected disabilities.
Coinsurance	A percentage of the allowed charge for health services, which the patient is responsible for paying.
Coordination of benefits	Rules followed by insurance companies so that no claim is reimbursed at more than 100% of the charges.
Copayment	A fixed amount of money that the patient must pay for any health care service.
Deductible	An amount of money that an insured person must pay annually before health services are covered by the insurance plan.
Diagnosis-related groups (DRG)	A system to determine Medicare reimbursement for a hospital stay on the basis of the patient's diagnosis.
Eligibility	Enrollment status related to a health insurance plan.
Explanation of benefits (EOB)	A statement issued by the insurance carrier explaining reimbursement for specific procedures.
Fee-for-service insurance	Insurance reimbursement that is directly related to the services provided and the amount charged by the provider.
Formulary	An insurance carrier's official list of covered medications to be used by network providers.
Group plan	One insurance policy that covers a group of people.
Guarantor	A person with financial responsibility for a bill who may or may not also be a patient.
Indemnity	An obligation to provide compensation for loss or damage.
Insured	The individual who has a specific insurance plan.

↻ TERMINOLOGY REVIEW—cont'd

Key Term	Definition
Managed care	A movement in health care based on reducing health care costs while providing high-quality care. The term may be used for the techniques used to reduce costs or for the companies that pay for the care provided.
Medicaid	The government insurance program for low-income individuals and families that is funded both by the federal government and by each individual state.
Medicare	The federal health insurance program that provides insurance coverage for the elderly, permanently disabled, and individuals with end-stage kidney disease.
Medicare Administrative Contractor (MAC)	A multistate, regional independent business that administers both Medicare Part A and Medicare Part B claims under a contract with the Centers for Medicare and Medicaid Services (CMS).
Nonparticipating provider (nonPAR)	A physician who does not have any contract with a third-party payor.
Participating provider (PAR)	A physician who has a contractual agreement with a third-party payor.
Preauthorization	Verification from a patient's insurance carrier that a procedure is covered by the patient's insurance and/or agreement, after review, that the test or procedure is medically appropriate.
Precertification	Verification from a patient's insurance carrier that a procedure is covered by the patient's insurance and/or agreement, after review, that the test or procedure is medically appropriate.
Premium	An amount of money paid in a given period to purchase health insurance.
Primary care provider (PCP)	The health care practitioner chosen by a patient to provide general medical care and also to determine and authorize additional medical services the patient may require.
Primary insurance	The insurance company that must be billed first for any individual.
Referral	The directing of a patient to a specialist physician by the primary care provider. Most managed care plans and some other insurance plans require the primary care provider to obtain prior authorization.
Reimbursement	The amount paid for a procedure by insurance.
Remittance advice (RA)	A statement issued by Medicare or another third-party payer to the provider explaining reimbursement for specific procedures or denial of an insurance claim.
Resource-based relative value scale (RBRVS)	A system to establish the Medicare fee schedule for Medicare Part B based on the service provided and the geographic location of the provider.
Secondary insurance	Insurance that an individual has in addition to primary insurance.
Self-referral	The process by which a patient makes an appointment with a specialist physician without requesting prior authorization from his or her primary care physician, usually because the patient's insurance plan does not require it.
Signature on file (SOF)	An indication on the insurance claim form that the signature of the patient is maintained by the medical office to authorize submission of insurance claims.
Third-party payor	Insurance carrier or managed care organization that pays health insurance claims.
TRICARE	A government insurance plan that provides medical care to spouses and dependents of individuals on active duty in the military. Formerly this program was called *CHAMPUS.*
Usual, customary, and reasonable (UCR)	A system for establishing the amount an insurance carrier will pay for a procedure. The reasonable charge is set by the insurance carrier on the basis of a physician's usual (most frequent) charge for the procedure and the customary charge of other physicians in the same geographic area.
Utilization review	Reviewing proposed or current care to determine medical necessity.
Workers' compensation	An insurance program that covers lost wages and health care costs of workers injured on the job or having work-related illnesses.

ON THE WEB

For information on the Centers for Medicare and Medicaid Services (Medicare, Medicaid, and CHIP):

Centers for Medicare and Medicaid Services: www.cms.gov

Medicare coverage: www.cms.gov/center/PeopleWithMedicareCenter.asp

Advanced Beneficiary Notice of Noncoverage form: http://www.cms.gov/Medicare/Medicare-General-Information/BNI/ABN.html

For information on CHAMPVA:

U.S. Department of Veterans Affairs: www.va.gov/PURCHASEDCARE/programs/dependents/champva/index.asp

For information on CMS-1500 form—National Uniform Claim Committee:

National Uniform Claim Committee: www.nucc.org

For information on health care options and health care law:

U.S. Department of Health and Human Services: www.healthcare.gov

For information on TRICARE:

TRICARE Management Activity: www.tricare.mil

For information on U.S. Department of Labor—Office of Workers' Compensation Programs:

Office of Workers' Compensation Programs: www.dol.gov/owcp/owcpcomp.htm

Billing and Collections

49

e Check out the Evolve site at http://evolve.elsevier.com/Bonewit/today/ to access additional interactive activities and exercises to help you study and prepare for success.

LEARNING OBJECTIVES

1. Describe the process of billing and collections.
2. Describe problems that can occur when patients pay by check.
3. Explain how to adjust patient accounts for an overpayment and process a refund.
4. Develop a collection system.
5. Identify past due accounts and the actions needed.

6. Describe the information to include in a collection letter.
7. Identify legal requirements that affect collections for the medical office.
8. Describe special circumstances affecting collections in the medical office.

PROCEDURES

Process patient statements.
Post a "non-sufficient funds" check.
Process a credit balance and refund.

Create and examine an accounts receivable aging record.
Write a collection letter.

CHAPTER OUTLINE

INTRODUCTION TO BILLING
BILLING CYCLE
BILLING PROCESS
BILLING PROBLEMS
Problems with Checks
Insufficient Funds in the Office Account
Stopping Payment
Insufficient Funds in a Patient Account
Overpayments and Refunds
ACCOUNT AGING
Accounts Receivable Aging Records and Reports
Examining Accounts for Those Overdue
COLLECTION ACTIVITIES
Past Due Accounts
Collection Letters
Credit Agreements

Truth in Lending Agreements
Policy for Patients with Outstanding Balances
Other Collection Techniques and Special Circumstances
Tracing "Skips"
Sending Accounts to a Collection Agency
Small Claims Court
Billing an Estate
Bankruptcy
Laws Affecting Credit and Collection Activities
Equal Credit Opportunity Act
Fair Debt Collection Practices Act
Federal Truth in Lending Act
Fair Credit Reporting Act
Bankruptcy Abuse Prevention and Consumer Protection
    Act of 2005

KEY TERMS

account aging
balance due
bankruptcy
claim message

collection agency
credit balance
overdraft
patient statement

skip
truth in lending

INTRODUCTION TO BILLING

If patients have insurance, a bill is not usually sent to the patient until after the insurance company has paid its portion of the bill. If the patient is covered by a managed care policy, the copayment is usually collected at the time of the visit, and a bill may not be necessary. Often, however, the patient has a deductible and/or coinsurance, and a bill must be sent to the patient after insurance has paid its portion of the patient charges.

If a patient visit will not be covered by insurance, most physicians' offices request that payment be made at the time a medical service is provided. Medical offices usually also accept payment by credit card, which makes payment at the time of service possible and convenient for many patients. However, a number of patients still need to make arrangements to pay for their medical services over a period of time. In this case, the office must establish an account for the patient and send periodic bills. These bills are usually generated by computer software. Each bill is then placed in a window envelope and sent to the patient. Even if the patient's account is being paid by capitation, a billing record is usually kept for that patient, showing the amount of charges and payments.

The billing for physician offices that are affiliated with a hospital or large health group is usually done from a central location, and office employees are responsible only for posting charges. Patients and insurance companies make payments to the central office. Other physician offices may contract with an outside billing service. The medical assistant should understand the billing process, however, because efficient billing maximizes revenue for the medical practice.

BILLING CYCLE

The bills sent to patients are called **patient statements** because they contain not only patient charges but also payments and adjustments that affect the balance that the patient must pay. Patient statements can be sent every 2 weeks, monthly, or at any regular period, such as once every 3 months (quarterly). The time between bills is called the *billing cycle.* A bill sent out at the end of a cycle will show the balance owed at the beginning of the cycle, any payments made during the billing cycle, any new charges for new services that occurred during the billing cycle, and the **balance due** (total amount owed) at the end of the cycle.

Patient accounts are often divided into equal parts, usually alphabetically. Each week a different section of the

accounts receivable is billed. For instance, on the first week of the month, patients with a last name beginning with the letters *A* to *E* may be billed; the second week, *F* to *L*; the third week, *M* to *S*; and the fourth week, *T* to *Z*. The same cycle is followed each month. Dividing the bills in this way makes more efficient use of staff time because billing is spread out over the month instead of being performed only at the end of the month.

BILLING PROCESS

Patient statements can be produced manually using a word processing program and billing template, but in almost all medical offices that do their own billing, they are produced using the medical office practice management program or the administrative part of the electronic medical record (Figure 49-1). If an outside billing service is used, the service can either send a paper record of all of the bills sent out at the end of each cycle or can transfer billing information from its computer to the office's computer, linking the information into the patient's financial record and the office's bookkeeping software.

At regular intervals, patient financial accounts should be examined and the accounts that must be billed should be processed. Sending claims to insurance companies and billing patients are both straightforward transactions. However, the medical assistant should be aware of some special situations. A patient may have been treated for a final illness just before dying. In this case, any charges will have to be billed to the patient's estate. (Billing an estate is discussed in more detail at the end of this chapter.)

A patient may be a minor who sought treatment without his or her parent's knowledge. When minors are brought to a physician by a parent or guardian for treatment, the parent or guardian acknowledges that he or she is the responsible party for financial purposes. However, if a minor is treated without the parent's knowledge, the minor may want be responsible to pay for services in order to avoid parental questions. Minors older than age 12 may give consent for certain kinds of treatment including treatment for sexually transmitted diseases (STDs), human immunodeficiency virus (HIV) testing, and treatment for drug or alcohol abuse. Because of confidentiality, the physician may not release information to the parent or guardian about the reason for the visit.

A patient may have a credit agreement with the practice, which allows the patient to pay bills off over time, sometimes with interest on the balance due. This is important because in such situations, even though an outstanding balance may become old, it should not be considered delinquent and sent out of the office for collection (Procedure 49-1).

WALDEN-MARTIN
FAMILY MEDICAL CLINIC
1234 ANYSTREET ANYTOWN, ANYSTATE 1234
PHONE 123-123-1234   FAX 123-123-5678

Patient Statement

Patient Name:	Sissle, Darla A	**Address:**	10 Maple St. Anytown AL 12345
Account #:	98866	**Insurance Name:**	Aetna
Policy #:	12345		

This statement reflects charges, payments and adjustments for Walden-Martin Family Medical Practice. Payment due upon receipt.

Date of Service	Description	Amount	Patient's Responsibility
6/26/XX	Prob Focused OV, ECG	$121.00	--
7/15/XX	INSPYMT & ADJ	$96.00	$25.00

Total Amount Due: $25.00

Please Pay in Full By: 7/26/XX

Please mail your check or money order to the above address. You can also pay by phone using your credit or debit card.

Figure 49-1 A sample patient statement using SimChart® for the Medical Office.

Putting It All Into Practice

My name is Christa Wilson, and I have been working in the office of three physicians for the past 5 years. There are three medical assistants, and we all assist the physicians during office hours, but I am responsible for most of the billing. We use cycle billing in our office. The first week of the month we send out statements for patients whose last names begin with the letters A-F, the second week G-L, and so on. By the end of the month, every patient with an outstanding balance has received a statement, and we begin again. I am also responsible for posting payments received in the mail. Every month, we run an aging report, and I analyze it to see which accounts are overdue. Our computer program lets us add written messages to the statements, but I add colored stickers for accounts that are older than 60 days because I think they are more likely to get the patient's attention. If there is a balance due from a patient after 90 days, I always follow up with a telephone call. When I first started making these calls, I used to get very nervous, but I have gotten accustomed to it now. I always try to stay calm and keep my cool. I have found that in most cases, there is a financial problem that makes it difficult for the individual or family to keep up with its debts. I try to work with our patients if they have an outstanding balance so that they pay something each month. Eventually we do collect most of the money that is owed to us, and we feel that part of the reason is that we stay on top of our billing. ■

PROCEDURE 49-1   Processing Patient Statements

Outcome Prepare patient statements

Equipment/Supplies

- Computer
- Patient accounts
- Computer program to prepare patient statements or SimChart® for the Medical Office
- Window envelopes or letterhead envelopes and labels
- Word processing program
- Paper or statement forms

1. **Procedural Step.** Locate patient accounts in the computer database.
2. **Procedural Step.** Identify patient accounts with an outstanding balance for which insurance payments have been made.
   Principle. Patients are usually not billed until insurance payments have been received.
3. **Procedural Step.** Create one or more patient bills manually using a word processing program or SimChart® for the Medical Office (see specific steps at the end of the procedure). If using medical billing software, compile outstanding bills using the computer program and view using *Print Preview*. Check all statements for completeness and accuracy.
   Principle. All bills must have the patient's name and address, previous activity for the account, and the amount due from the patient.
4. **Procedural Step.** Print patient statements using the office patient statement form or paper (if statement form prints with the statement). The statement form may be printed with the bills from the computer program, or statement forms may be loaded in the printer.
5. **Procedural Step.** Make sure that statements have printed correctly.
6. **Procedural Step.** Fold statements suitable for window envelopes so that the practice and the patient names and addresses will be visible through the windows in the envelopes. If statements are not suitable for window envelopes (such as those produced by SimChart®), prepare a patient label for each statement.

7. **Procedural Step.** Insert statements in envelopes. Be sure that the names and addresses are visible if window envelopes are used. If labels are used, affix the correct mailing label to a letterhead envelope for each statement.
8. **Procedural Step.** Place postage on envelopes and mail statements.

Preparing a Patient Statement Using SimChart® for the Medical Office

1. **Procedural Step.** From the *Form Repository* click on *Patient Statement* on the *Info Panel* at the left.
2. **Procedural Step.** Click on the *Patient Search* button at the bottom of the *Patient Statement* screen. Search for and select the correct patient.
3. **Procedural Step.** Check to be sure that the information that has populated the top part of the Patient Statement form is correct. Then enter charges and payments that have taken place since the last statement, including the date of service, the description of the service, the amount, and the patient responsibility. All services from a single day can usually be entered on one line. The insurance payment and insurance write-off usually occur on different dates; payment is entered on a separate line (see Figure 49-1).
4. **Procedural Step.** Click the *Save to Patient Record* button. To print the statement, find and select the patient, then open the saved statement and click the *Print* button.

BILLING PROBLEMS

PROBLEMS WITH CHECKS

From time to time the office may encounter a problem either with a check it has written or with one that has been written to the office by a patient.

Insufficient Funds in the Office Account

It is illegal to write a check for more than the amount of money in a bank account. However, this occasionally happens because of an arithmetic error in calculating the balance while writing checks or because of failure to recon-

cile a bank statement. If the office's account accidentally becomes overdrawn, the bank may refuse to honor any check written after the account is overdrawn. In this case the check will be returned to the person or company that deposited it marked NSF ("non-sufficient funds" in the payer's account to cover the check). A check written on an account without adequate funds to cover it is called an **overdraft.**

It is a good practice to have overdraft protection for any office checking account. Although this protection may never be needed, it will prevent a check from bouncing or a problem with a scheduled online payment in the event that the balance in the office checking account becomes too low. In that case, funds will automatically be transferred from another office account, such as a savings account to cover an outstanding check or make an online payment, and the bank will charge a fee for this service every time it is used.

Stopping Payment

From time to time it may become necessary to ask the bank to stop payment on a check. A check might have been lost and a new check issued, or there may be a dispute between the practice and a vendor about a purchase or a previous payment. Banks charge a fee for stopping payment, so this practice should be used sparingly.

Insufficient Funds in a Patient Account

The bank may not honor a check deposited by the practice because a patient's account has insufficient funds. If a check is returned marked NSF, do not hesitate to call the patient and tell him or her of the problem. This may be the first of many checks that are being returned, and it is important for the person to find out why he or she is writing checks against insufficient funds. The bank usually charges fees both to the individual who wrote the check and to the medical office that tried to deposit the check. The amount of the NSF check must be added back to the balance owed by the patient as a positive adjustment that increases the amount owed. The fee charged by the bank is also added to the patient's balance, usually as a separate positive adjustment. As an example, assume that the patient paid a copayment of $20.00 at the time of the visit. The bank returned the check for insufficient funds and charged the medical office checking account a $15.00 fee. The medical assistant would increase the patient's account balance by $35.00 to cover both the amount of the returned check and the additional fee charged by the bank. Most offices have a sign posted in the waiting room notifying patients of the additional charge for each returned check (Procedure 49-2). When a check has been returned, the patient is often asked to make the payment using cash, a bank check, or a money

order instead of another personal check. This should be done tactfully with a professional explanation of the necessity for this step.

OVERPAYMENTS AND REFUNDS

If the total of patient payments and insurance payments exceeds the allowed charge, it is called an *overpayment*. This might happen, for example, if a patient thought that he had not yet paid his annual deductible, when in fact he had. An insurance carrier might overpay if an incorrect code was used on the insurance claim. After all the payments have been posted, the balance on the account will be a negative number, or **credit balance,** indicating that the medical office owes money to the patient or the insurance carrier. Sometimes a small credit balance is left in place when a patient has a visit scheduled in the near future because new charges will be applied. Usually, however, the medical assistant will process a refund. The amount of the refund is posted to the patient's account, bringing the account balance to zero. The medical assistant sends a letter and a check to the patient (or insurance) with a brief explanation about the overpayment (Procedure 49-3).

What Would You Do? What Would You *Not* Do?

Case Study 1

The bank returns a check from a patient for non-sufficient funds (NSF). The amount on the check is $25.00, and the bank includes a notice that the practice will be charged $15.00. Christa makes a telephone call to the patient, and she asks the patient to send the office a bank check or money order in the amount of $40.00 The patient becomes very upset. She says, "The bank will charge me the fee for the returned check, not you. All you have to do is send the check through again. There is money in the account now because I deposited my paycheck yesterday. You can't charge me a fee for this. You are just trying to make money out of this situation." ∎

PROCEDURE 49-2 Posting a Check Returned for Non-sufficient Funds (NSF)

Outcome Post an NSF check

Equipment/Supplies

- Computer
- Patient accounts
- Returned check
- Patient ledger
- SimChart® for the Medical Office or other practice management program
- Pen
- Calculator

1. **Procedural Step.** When the NSF check has been received, locate the patient's old balance in the computer database. In SimChart® for the Medical Office, select *Ledger* on the *Info Panel* of the

Coding and Billing tab, then select the correct patient.

2. **Procedural Step.** Add a new row, and use today's date. Enter "NSF check and fee" in the *Service* field.

Continued

PROCEDURE 49-2   Posting a Check Returned for Non-sufficient Funds (NSF)—cont'd

3. **Procedural Step.** In SimChart® for the Medical Office, enter the total of the returned check and the amount charged by the bank in the *Charges* field. Note that the amount of the returned check is actually a positive adjustment, but in this program all adjustments to the ledger are considered negative adjustments (i.e., they are subtracted from the patient balance) so a positive adjustment must be entered as a charge. If using a practice management program such as Medisoft, the amount of the returned check and the bank fee are added as two separate adjustments. Using the correct code in the *Service* field will prompt the program to add any positive adjustment to the balance appropriately.
   Principle. The amount of the returned check must be added to the patient balance because it did not clear the bank. Any fee charged by the bank is also added to the patient balance as a positive adjustment.

4. **Procedural Step.** Enter zero in the *Payment* and *Adjmt* fields, and the program will calculate the balance for the transaction and the new balance.

5. **Procedural Step.** To post on a day sheet in SimChart® for the Medical Office, select *Day Sheet* from the *Coding and Billing* information panel.

6. **Procedural Step.** Enter the date and patient name, then enter "NSF check and fee" in the *Service* field. The total of the returned check and bank fee is entered in the *Adjmt* field using a minus sign to indicate that it is a positive adjustment. In some practices the bank fee may be added as a charge that is not billed to insurance.
   Principle. The amount of the returned check must be added to return the patient balance to the amount before the check was deducted. Any fee charged by the bank is also added to the patient balance. Normally adjustments are subtracted from the balance, so the minus sign indicates to perform the opposite mathematical operation. When posting manually, parentheses are used.

7. **Procedural Step.** Find the patient's old balance from their ledger and enter in the *Old Balance* field. Then add the total of the bank fee and returned check in the *New Balance* field.

8. **Procedural Step.** Notify the patient by telephone or letter that the check was returned and a fee has been charged. If sending a letter, enclose a patient statement with the letter showing the total amount of the returned check and the fee. Demonstrate professionalism and sensitivity when discussing the returned check and informing the patient of payment conditions (such as a bank check or money order).
   Example. Darla Sissle's previous balance was $40.00. Her check for $15.00 was returned by the bank marked *NSF.* The bank also charged a fee of $15.00.

8

DATE	PATIENT NAME	SERVICE	Column A CHARGES	Column B PAYMENT	Column C ADJMT	Column D NEW BALANCE	Column E OLD BALANCE
6/03/XX	Darla Sissle	NSF check & fee	$ 15.00	$ 0.00	$ 15.00	$ 70.00	$ 40.00

The NSF check and bank fee are posted on the day sheet and to the patient's account.

PROCEDURE 49-3   Processing a Credit Balance and Refund

Outcome Process a credit balance and issue a refund

Equipment/Supplies

- Computer
- Patient accounts
- Payment check(s)
- SimChart® for the Medical Office or other practice management program
- Pen
- Calculator

PROCEDURE 49-3 Processing a Credit Balance and Refund—cont'd

1. **Procedural Step.** When a payment has been made, locate the patient account in the computer. In SimChart® for the Medical Office, select *Ledger* on the *Info Panel* of the *Coding and Billing* tab, then select the correct patient.
   Principle. Both insurance payments and patient payments must be entered in the correct patient account.

2. **Procedural Step.** Add a new row, and use today's date. Enter *Payment* and the check number (if any) in the *Service* field.

3. **Procedural Step.** Compare the amount of the payment against the total amount owed.
   Principle. The total amount owed will be the balance due and charges for new services.

4. **Procedural Step.** Even if the payment is greater than the charges, in a computer billing program post the payment to the computer system using the correct code (i.e., patient payment, check, insurance payment) and link to the visit for which the payment is made. In SimChart® for the Medical Office, post the payment in the *Payment* field. If using a paper day sheet, post the payment in the *Payment* column.

5. **Procedural Step.** If an overpayment has occurred, note that the account balance *(Total)* is a negative number. This means that the medical office owes the patient money.

6. **Procedural Step.** Take steps to clear the balance from the system according to your office policy. If the patient has another appointment scheduled, the negative balance may be carried for a short time. In most cases, a refund should be issued promptly.
   Principle. Office policy guidelines indicate the proper management of a credit balance in a patient account.

7. **Procedural Step.** Calculate the amount to be refunded (usually the amount of the negative balance) and the recipient of the refund. If the patient overpaid because it was not known how much insurance would pay, the refund goes to the patient. If insurance overpaid (e.g., because an incorrect code was used on the claim), the refund goes to the insurance carrier.

8. **Procedural Step.** Add a new row, select the date and enter the patient name. Enter *Refund to [recipient]* in the *Service* field. In SimChart® for the Medical Office, enter the adjustment in the adjustment field with a minus number. In a practice management program, all adjustments are entered as positive numbers with the correct code, and the program performs the correct operation (addition or subtraction). Enter zeros in the other fields. The program will calculate the balance for the transaction.

9. **Procedural Step.** Verify that the *Total* (account balance) is zero.

10. **Procedural Step.** Write a check for the refund amount to the correct recipient including the date, amount in numbers, and amount in words on the line below. Leave the signature line blank.
    Principle. The medical assistant is usually not authorized to sign checks for the medical office.

11. **Procedural Step.** Record the check number, date, payee, and reason for the check on the check stub in the checkbook or in the check register.

12. **Procedural Step.** Subtract the amount of the check from the balance in the check register.

13. **Procedural Step.** Write a letter informing the recipient of the reason for the refund, and prepare an envelope.

14. **Procedural Step.** Sign the letter and your title, and leave the check, letter. and envelope in the correct place to obtain an authorized signature on the check.

ACCOUNT AGING

Account aging is the process of determining how long specific account balances have been outstanding.

ACCOUNTS RECEIVABLE AGING RECORDS AND REPORTS

An accounts receivable aging record should be created to identify accounts that are overdue. Accounts are aged in 30-day intervals. Figure 49-2 shows a sample accounts receivable aging record).

EXAMINING ACCOUNTS FOR THOSE OVERDUE

An account is considered overdue if it is not paid within 30 days of the date billed unless there is an outstanding credit agreement. Accounts for which all the charges are from the previous billing period are considered current (0 to 30

Enter credits in parentheses ( ) and subtract when totaling columns and P

ACCOUNTS RECEIVABLE AGING RECORD

Name			As of Date		Prepared by						Page of Page

NO.	ACCOUNT NAME	Insurance Information Date Claim Filed	Amount of Claim	Date of Last Payment	Current 1 to 30 days	31 to 60 days	61 to 90 days	91 to 120 days	121 days and over	TOTAL
	Amounts brought forward									
1	Mary Smith			8/8/XX	120					120 -
2	John Payne			7/6/XX		250 -				250 -
3	Jack Desmonde			5/25/XX			500			500 -
4	Jill Jayne			4/2/XX		80 -				180 -
5										

A

Blackburn Primary Care Associates
Patient Aging

NAME	CURRENT 0 - 30	PAST 31 - 60	PAST 61 - 90	PAST 91 - 120	PAST over 120	Total Balance
Mary Smith Last Payment on 08/08/XX	$120.00					$120.00
John Payne Last Payment on 07/06/XX		$250.00				$250.00
Jack Desmonde Last Payment on 05/25/XX			$500.00			$500.00
Jill Jayne Last Payment on 04/02/XX		$80.00		$100.00		$180.00
Report Aging Totals Percent of Total Aging	$120.00 11.4%	$330.00 31.4%	$330.00 47.6%	$100.00 9.5%		$1,050.00 100.0%

B

Figure 49-2 Sample accounts receivable aging record: **A,** prepared by hand; **B,** prepared by computer.

days). Overdue accounts are categorized as 30 to 60 days, 60 to 90 days, and longer than 120 days.

An account with an outstanding balance after 120 days requires additional collection activity, such as sending the account out to a collection agency or writing a demand letter informing the account holder that a lawsuit will be brought if the account is not brought up to date (Procedure 49-4). Most of the time, the balance of medical office accounts is small enough to permit legal action in small claims court. (Small claims court is discussed in more detail at the end of the chapter.)

What Would You Do? | What Would You *Not* Do?

Case Study 2

A patient calls the office to say that she has received her bill, and it does not show a payment of $10.00 that she made in cash at the time of the visit. The patient is upset, and she says, "I knew I shouldn't pay cash, because now I can't prove that I made that payment. I don't see why you can't keep accurate records." Christa asks the patient if she received a receipt for the cash payment. The patient says, "How do you expect me to remember that? This happened over a month ago." ■

PROCEDURE 49-4 Creating and Examining an Accounts Receivable Aging Record

Outcome Create and examine an accounts receivable aging record

Equipment/Supplies

- Computer with medical billing software
- Patient accounts
- Accounts receivable aging record analysis form (optional)
- Pen

1. **Procedural Step.** Using the reports function of a computer billing program, create an aging report for patients and for insurance companies. It is also possible to create such a report manually using individual patient ledgers.
   Principle. In a computerized billing system, the computer program can generate the report of all overdue accounts.

2. **Procedural Step.** Review the accounts on the report and mark the proposed action for each account according to your office policy.
   Principle. Efforts to collect outstanding accounts should become increasingly more active as the account ages. Office policy may vary with regard to specific actions.

3. **Procedural Step.** Mark all accounts that are less than 31 days old "No action needed."
   Principle. Accounts that are less than 31 days old are considered current.

4. **Procedural Step.** Mark bills with unpaid insurance claims that are older than 31 days "Follow up with insurance."
   Principle. Patients usually do not pay bills with outstanding insurance claims until they find out how much the insurance will pay. These bills, if overdue, need to be followed up on with the insurance company.

5. **Procedural Step.** Mark accounts that are 31 to 60 days old according to office policy. For example, a note may be attached to the statement indicating "Payment is now due." It may be possible to include payment notices in the computer billing program so that they print on the statement automatically if the account is overdue.

6. **Procedural Step.** Mark accounts that are 61 to 90 days old according to office policy. For example, a note may be attached to the statement indicating "Payment of this bill is now overdue. Please pay the balance or contact the office."

7. **Procedural Step.** Mark accounts that are 91 to 120 days old according to office policy. It may be office

policy to place a telephone call to the patient at this point to discuss the account. Follow up with a letter confirming any agreement made.

8. **Procedural Step.** Role-play a collection telephone call with a classmate to demonstrate a professional manner for interacting with a patient who has a balance that is over 91 days old. Tell the patient a specific amount that is owed, and ask for a commitment for payment by a specific date. Remain calm, and do not threaten the patient. Inform the patient that it is office policy to turn accounts older than 120 days over to a collection agency.
   Principle: Professionalism during collection activities and sensitivity to patients help maximize collections without creating excess negativity that offends and shames patients.

9. **Procedural Step.** For accounts older than 120 days, review previous collection attempts. Unless there are known circumstances that warrant a delay in collection activity, send a collection letter stating that if payment is not received by a certain date the account will be given to a collection agency or payment will be pursued in small claims court (depending on the procedure used by the office to collect on delinquent accounts).
   Principle. After 120 days without activity, especially if the person owing money has been contacted by telephone and letter, it is unlikely that the bill will be paid without more aggressive collection measures.

10. **Procedural Step.** Record all action taken beside each account on the report.
    Principle. This provides a written record of actions taken and results of telephone conversations.

11. **Procedural Step.** Write follow-up letters to document in writing any agreements made during telephone conversations. Attach a copy to the patient's medical record.
    Principle. A written record of verbal communications regarding bills and payments provides evidence in case further legal action is necessary.

PROCEDURE 49-4

COLLECTION ACTIVITIES

Many people who owe money have every intention of paying their bill but are unable to do so in the short term because of some emergency. As accounts age, it is appropriate to increase the forcefulness of any message to the patient that the account is overdue. Patients should always be invited to call the office and make arrangements to pay over time if they have had a true emergency. Sometimes it is medical bills themselves that are piling up, especially in the case of a patient with a chronic illness who does not have adequate insurance or has a large deductible.

Patients are also encouraged to discuss accounts for which insurance payment is expected but delayed. By working with the insurance company, the patient can more easily determine whose responsibility the bill is.

PAST DUE ACCOUNTS

Messages encouraging payment of the bill (often called **claim messages**) can be attached to bills or included in the billing envelope. Some computer programs will print a message on the bill itself.

A bill that is 60 days overdue should be accompanied by a claim message reminding the patient that the bill is overdue. Many offices use a series of messages that become more forceful as time passes without payment.

Bills that are 90 days overdue should be followed up with a telephone call. By contacting patients directly, the medical assistant can determine why there has been no activity related to the account. The medical assistant must be careful to follow legal guidelines when discussing accounts with patients. The Fair Debt Collection Practices Act of 1966 identifies activities that are permitted and not permitted when contacting individuals who owe money. Most states also have debt collection laws with which the medical assistant should be familiar.

COLLECTION LETTERS

Bills that are aged 120 days should either be accompanied by or followed up with a collection letter, such as the one shown in Figure 49-3. When writing a collection letter, the medical assistant should gather information related to the account before composing the letter. The recipient should be clearly informed about what action is expected, as well as the deadline for action. The letter should not threaten legal action or transfer to a collection agency unless the office is prepared to follow through.

Each medical office has its own policy about who should sign a collection letter. In many offices, the medical assistant signs the letters. In other offices there may be an office manager or billing specialist, or each physician may prefer to sign letters to his or her own patients (Procedure 49-5).

If the collection letter does not receive a response, another letter should be sent stating either that the account is now being turned over to a **collection agency** (a company that collects overdue bills for other companies) or that a lawsuit will be filed in small claims court if the account is not paid by a certain date. Some offices will continue to see patients with accounts in collection, but they usually require the

---

Western Medical Center
107 River Street
Western, OH 44770

4/10/20XX

[Patient Address]

Dear [Patient Name],

Your account in this office is now more than 120 days overdue. We have made several previous attempts to set up a mutually agreeable payment schedule with you, but you have not followed through on your commitment. This will be your final notice. If you do not contact our office within 7 days of receipt of this letter, we will have no choice but to turn over this account to our collection agency. Please call us at (490) 220-1156 or send a check to pay the balance of your account if you wish to avoid collection activity.

Yours truly,

Richard Warner, MD

Richard Warner, MD

RW/mt

Figure 49-3 Sample collection letter.

patient to pay any current charges before the patient can be seen.

As in any case where it is important to have documentation that a letter was received, the letter should be sent Certified Mail, with a Return Receipt requested. If the patient is being asked to find a new provider, the letter should allow the patient at least 2 weeks to arrange alternate care.

CREDIT AGREEMENTS

Credit agreements are documents that allow patients to set up a schedule to pay off their bills as long as they make the specified monthly payments. If a patient decides independently to pay his or her bill in installments (i.e., without discussing it with the medical office), no credit agreement is necessary. If the office and patient make an agreement regarding installment payments, even if no interest is charged, the agreement must be in writing. An interest charge may be added to the balance due at the end of each billing cycle when a written agreement exists.

A credit agreement with a medical office is a type of revolving credit, like a department store or gasoline company charge card. As long as the monthly minimum is paid, the account is considered in good standing.

TRUTH IN LENDING AGREEMENTS

Because a credit agreement is a type of revolving credit, it falls under federal and state government fair lending practices. Therefore a truth in lending statement must be supplied to the patient when the agreement is made. **Truth in lending** refers to the legal requirement to disclose the terms of a loan to borrowers so that they can understand them.

This truth in lending statement includes facts about such things as the maximum amount the patient may charge to the account, the interest rate, how the interest is computed (e.g., average daily balance, or balance at the end of the billing period), and how the minimum monthly payment is computed (e.g., percentage of outstanding balance). Figure 49-4 shows a sample credit agreement.

POLICY FOR PATIENTS WITH OUTSTANDING BALANCES

Most medical offices insist that a patient close out any current balance due before a credit agreement is written with that patient. If the practice has had trouble collecting bills from a patient in the past, it may write the credit agreement for a lower maximum balance. But the practice cannot charge a different interest rate or compute the minimum

---

HIGHLIGHT on Guidelines for Telephone Collections

Things to Do

1. A creditor (person or company who is owed money) may contact the person who owes money by telephone during reasonable hours. The medical assistant should gather accurate information before placing the telephone call about an overdue account:
   a. Who owes the money?
   b. How much money is owed?
   c. How long has the money been owed?
   d. Is there any insurance claim pending?
   e. Has the insurance company processed the claim and/or made any payment?
2. A creditor may take measures to locate a person but may not divulge that he or she is trying to collect a bill to anyone other than the person who owes money. The medical assistant should ask to speak with the patient or the person responsible for the account when placing the call.
3. A creditor may not misrepresent himself or herself to trick the person who owes money into taking the call. After asking for the person responsible for the account, the medical assistant should identify himself or herself and the office or physician.
4. A creditor may not harass or intimidate a person who owes money. The medical assistant should speak calmly and professionally. The conversation should include a discussion of the different options for payment, including full payment,

partial payment, and monthly installments. If possible, the medical assistant should obtain a verbal commitment for a date and amount of at least a first payment and/or a payment plan.
5. Although a verbal agreement is legally binding, a written agreement is easier to enforce if legal action becomes necessary. It is important to follow up any verbal agreement with a letter referring to the conversation and the agreement. If an arrangement was established for more than four monthly payments, a truth-in-lending statement must be included, even if the patient will not pay interest.
6. Although it is not permitted to harass patients, the medical assistant may contact them again if payments are not made as agreed. Often, the knowledge that attention is being paid to the account will encourage a patient to adhere to the repayment schedule.

Things *Not* to Do

1. A creditor should not call too early in the day or too late at night.
2. A creditor should not divulge to employers, neighbors, or other third parties that he or she is trying to collect a bill from the patient.
3. A creditor should not threaten.
4. A creditor should not end the conversation on vague terms.
5. A creditor should not call repeatedly. ■

Blackburn Primary Care Associates, PC
1990 Turquoise Drive
Blackburn, WI 54937
608-459-8857

Federal Truth in Lending Statement

Patient _____

Address _____

1. Fee for service of   _____

2. Amount down   _____

3. Amount financed   _____

4. finance charge   _____

5. total of payments 3 + 4   _____

6. number of payments   _____

7. amount of each payment _____

Total no. of payments _____ payable over _____ monthly installments

In the amount of $_____. The first payment is due _____.

Date _____   Signed _____

Figure 49-4 Sample credit agreement.

payment in a different way for different patients depending on past payment history.

OTHER COLLECTION TECHNIQUES AND SPECIAL CIRCUMSTANCES

Tracing "Skips"

Occasionally a bill is returned to the medical office from the post office with the notation "address unknown." This may be an innocent mistake—the result, perhaps, of an incorrect address on file or the patient's failure to notify the office after moving. On the other hand, it may be a deliberate attempt to "skip out" on the medical office's bill and the bills of other professionals and/or merchants.

A potential **skip** (account for which no billing information is available) should be followed up on immediately. The first step is to call the patient's phone number: It is very common to keep the same telephone number even if a person moves, or a person may have had the phone company use a "new number" message to forward calls. Because caller ID is a feature on many land lines and cell phones, a telephone call from a creditor may be ignored or the person answering the call may say that it is a wrong number.

If the patient cannot be contacted using the telephone number given at the office visit and if there is no new number listed, the next step is to call the patient's place

of employment and ask to speak with the individual. The medical assistant can try to get in touch with the person by contacting professional associations, unions, or other organizations with which the person is associated.

The medical assistant should never tell a third party that an individual owes money to the medical office and should not identify the employer; the medical assistant should say only that he or she wishes to speak with the person. Also, it is illegal to call a third party more than once in an attempt to trace a skip unless that person asks the medical assistant to call back. For example, the medical assistant may speak with a third party where the individual with an overdue account works, and that third party might ask the medical assistant to call back at the end of the day when he or she is not so busy.

Another way to attempt collection is to send a letter by Registered or Certified Mail, with a Return Receipt requested, to the individual at the old address. Even if the person did not ask the post office to forward all mail, he or she may have asked for certain types of mail to be forwarded. In this case, the letter should be placed in a plain envelope, with just the return street address and no office name. This minimizes the chances that the individual will refuse to accept the mail.

The medical office may also use one of several Internet resources to trace skips. These services usually charge a fee.

The more information the office has about the individual, the more likely it is that the individual can be located.

If all of these efforts fail, the bill should be turned over to a collection agency used by the office as soon as possible. Most collection agencies handle far more "skips" than individual medical offices do and sometimes use other, more aggressive techniques. The sooner the collection agency receives the account, the better chance it has to collect the amount owed on the bill.

Sending Accounts to a Collection Agency

Collection agencies are in business specifically to collect accounts that have "aged out." This means that by the time a collection agency receives a delinquent account, the business such as a medical office has given the person who owes the money fair warning that the bill is overdue and that a professional collector is going to become involved.

Each state has specific laws under which collection agencies must work. These laws define when collection agency personnel can call, what they can say, and what other tactics they can use to collect the bill.

In general, collection agencies charge 20% to 40% of the amount they collect. They are not allowed to "cut a deal" with a patient and accept less than full payment unless the medical office has agreed to the arrangement for payment.

If a patient's account is in collection, usually the office has a policy not to see the patient unless any new charges are paid in full before the patient is seen by the physician. Other offices notify patients in writing that they will not be seen by any physician in the office until their outstanding balance has been collected.

When an account is turned over to a collection agency, the patient balance in the computer system is often adjusted to zero. The amount owed by the patient can still be seen clearly in the patient ledger, but the current balance is zero. This prevents bills to the patient from being generated, and the account no longer appears as overdue on account aging reports. The medical assistant should become familiar with the exact procedure used in his or her medical office. The medical office makes no further attempts at collection, and any payments received from the patient are sent directly to the collection agency. When a payment for the patient's account is received from a collection agency, it should be recorded on the daily ledger. In addition, it should be posted to the account for which it was collected. The patient's account balance, which is usually zero, is first increased (as a positive adjustment) by the amount of the payment. Then the payment is posted as a payment, bringing the current account balance back to zero.

Small Claims Court

Small claims courts exist in each state. They are special sessions of the local district court that deal only with civil lawsuits involving small amounts of money. Most small claims lawsuits involve disputes over payments. Each state has its own rules for the maximum claim that can be brought in small claims court. This maximum amount runs from about $1500 in some states to as much as $15,000 in others.

The question for a medical practice when choosing to use the court system is always whether it will sacrifice more in "good will" than it will gain in money if the collection is successful. Many offices bring suits in court only after a patient has left the practice without paying a bill in full. Furthermore, winning a judgment in small claims court is only the first step. The office must still collect the judgment.

Small claims courts are set up to reduce the legal fees for those seeking to collect relatively small amounts of money. Because there is no lawyer, the plaintiff (an individual or business) must represent himself or itself. The office manager or medical assistant might have to assume this duty if the office uses small claims court to try to collect on patient accounts. A collection agency cannot represent the office.

The clerk of the court has all of the documents necessary to file a small claim and can usually walk a first-time claimant through the process, explaining how to fill out the forms and which documentation to submit to back up the claim. Only the defendant can appeal a small claims court judgment; for the plaintiff, a negative judgment is final.

Billing an Estate

Patients sometimes die without having paid their medical bills in full. In this instance the office will have to collect the balance due from the estate. Estates fall into an area of the law known as *probate,* and probate law is administered by a special section of the court system in each state.

It is not appropriate to send a bill to a deceased patient's estate immediately after the death while the family is grieving; however, the bill should be sent within 30 days. The bill should be sent to "The Estate of" the patient at the patient's address rather than to a family member or other individual unless that person has made a written promise to cover the deceased's medical costs.

If the deceased patient had a will, it usually has a provision that the costs of the patient's final illness be paid by the estate outside of the probate process. In such a case the bill will probably be paid promptly. The will should be filed within 30 days, and the clerk of the probate court should then be able to furnish you with the name of the executor or administrator (the person responsible for handling the estate's business dealings). An itemized final bill should then be sent to this individual by Certified Mail with a Return Receipt requested.

If the patient did not have a will, the medical practice's bill will be put in with other creditors' bills and paid only when payment is approved by the probate court and the administrator appointed by the court.

Bankruptcy

Bankruptcy laws are federal laws, meaning that they apply equally regardless of the state in which the bankrupt person lives. **Bankruptcy** is a means for an individual or business to "get out from under" a crushing load of debt, either by reorganizing the debt or by liquidating assets and dividing the funds among all of the creditors.

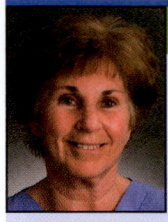

Memories *from* Practicum

Christa Wilson: During my practicum, I observed billing activities and I was allowed to assist in some ways. For example, I got a lot of practice at making sure that all statements printed correctly, checking each statement to make sure that there was an outstanding balance and that the insurance had already paid, and folding the statements to place them in window envelopes. The computer system used by the office where I did my practicum printed the statements with all activity on the account. The patient was expected to pay the balance on the bottom line of the statement. Sometimes patients called the office because they didn't understand what amount to pay. They usually spoke to the medical assistant at the office. I noticed that she was always polite and professional when she spoke to patients. The office also taught me how to post patient payments that were sent by check. I have to say I did not realize how important good billing practices are until my practicum. I was grateful that I had experience at an office with a smooth-running system. ∎

Individuals file for personal bankruptcy under either Chapter 7 or Chapter 13 of the bankruptcy code.

A Chapter 7 bankruptcy is a liquidation of assets. Under such a bankruptcy, only secured creditors will be paid from the proceeds from the sale of any assets. If the bankrupt patient had a credit agreement, the medical office is a secured creditor. But if the office is merely trying to collect a bill, the office is an unsecured creditor and will not receive payment.

A Chapter 13 bankruptcy is an "Adjustment of Debts" bankruptcy. In such a bankruptcy, the debtor (patient) pays a particular amount determined by the bankruptcy court to the court-appointed trustee, who then distributes the money to creditors. The debtor, if he or she has a regular income, can be required to make payments from that income into the trustee account for 3 years, and the trustee makes payments to creditors under payment plans he or she works out.

During the period the debtor is under the jurisdiction of the bankruptcy court, no creditor may try to collect a debt outside the bankruptcy process. However, a medical office can demand payment in full for any additional service it provides to a patient from whom it is collecting old debts under a bankruptcy agreement.

What Would You Do? What Would You *Not* Do?

Case Study 3

On the day that Judith Mason is scheduled for an appointment, Christa notices that she has an outstanding balance of $58.00 from charges that were incurred 4 months ago. It is office policy that patients with a balance over 120 days are not seen until the balance has been paid. ∎

LAWS AFFECTING CREDIT AND COLLECTION ACTIVITIES

Several laws affect credit and collection activities.

Equal Credit Opportunity Act

The Equal Credit Opportunity Act is a federal law that prevents discrimination based on the following when offering credit:

- Sex, marital status, race, national origin, religion, age
- The fact that the applicant receives public assistance income
- The fact that the applicant has exercised rights under consumer credit laws

An applicant must be informed if credit is denied and has 60 days to request, in writing, the reason for denial of credit.

Fair Debt Collection Practices Act

The Fair Debt Collection Practices Act is a federal law that requires the fair treatment of debtors and prevents unfair debt collection measures, including harassment, false statements, and threats.

- The debt collector may not make frightening, verbally abusive, or threatening calls.
- The debt collector may not call before 8 AM or after 9 PM.
- The debt collector may not threaten action that cannot legally be taken or is not intended to be taken.

Federal Truth in Lending Act

Installment agreements must be in writing if more than four payments will be made (or fewer if interest is charged). The Federal Truth in Lending Act is administered by the Federal Trade Commission. It requires creditors to provide applicants with a form disclosing in a clear and obvious way all finance charges and terms.

Fair Credit Reporting Act

The Fair Credit Reporting Act requires credit bureaus to supply correct and complete information to businesses to use in evaluating a person's application for credit, insurance, or employment.

Bankruptcy Abuse Prevention and Consumer Protection Act of 2005

The Bankruptcy Abuse Prevention and Consumer Protection Act of 2005 is a revision of federal bankruptcy laws that attempts to make it more difficult for individuals to file for bankruptcy under Chapter 7, by which most of the debts are forgiven by establishing a means test to determine if individuals are able to pay some of their debts. It also makes the process of filing for bankruptcy more difficult and expensive. Debtors are still able to file for bankruptcy under Chapter 13.

PROCEDURE 49-5   Writing a Collection Letter

Outcome Write a collection letter

Equipment/Supplies

- Accounts aging report
- Computer
- Patient accounts
- Letterhead stationery
- Envelope
- Printer

1. **Procedural Step.** After the accounts receivable aging record has been created, determine which accounts need a letter. In general, this will be the accounts that are 90 to 120 days old.
   Principle. A letter is usually sent after reminders have been sent and a telephone call has been made to collect an outstanding account balance.

2. **Procedural Step.** Review each account for the amount due, how long it has been due, any previous activity, and special situations. If the account is due from the estate of a deceased patient or insurance, or if there is a known reason why delayed payment is acceptable, do not take action on the account.
   Principle. There may be circumstances that justify the delay in payment.

3. **Procedural Step.** Otherwise, prepare a letter for each outstanding account. If using SimChart® for the Medical Office, select *Collection Letter* from the *Correspondence* information panel.

4. **Procedural Step.** Identify the patient's address by selecting the correct patient in the computer billing program.

5. **Procedural Step.** Enter the information in the collection letter template including the amount of the outstanding balance, the date that the charges were incurred, the service provided, and the date by which payment is expected. The tone should be professional without threats or efforts to shame the patient.
   Principle. Even though the bill is overdue, the recipient of the letter is given a reasonable amount of time to respond to this letter. Professionalism during collection activities and sensitivity to patients help maximize collections without creating excess negativity that offends and shames patients.

6. **Procedural Step.** Enter the provider name and medical assistant signature.

7. **Procedural Step.** Print the letter and save the letter to the patient record.

8. **Procedural Step.** If office policy, copy the letter and file it in a collection follow-up file.
   Principle. Future activity to collect on the account should be based on a review of your current activity.

9. **Procedural Step.** Place the letter in the envelope, address the envelope, and mail the letter.

PROCEDURE 49-5

What Would You Do? What Would You *Not* Do? RESPONSES

Case Study 1
Page 1221

What Did Christa Do?
- ❑ Reassured the patient that the situation is upsetting, but it can happen sometimes.
- ❑ Explained that most banks charge both the account of the individual who writes a check against an account with insufficient funds, as well as the account where the check was deposited.
- ❑ Explained that the office has a policy of not sending a check through the bank a second time or accepting a personal check for payment after one check was returned.
- ❑ Suggested that the patient might want to consider overdraft protection.
- ❑ Explained politely that the office is only recovering its out-of-pocket expenses and was not, in fact, charging an additional fee.

What Did Christa Not Do?
- ❑ Did not get angry or raise her voice.
- ❑ Did not imply that the patient was trying to avoid payment or was a bad money manager.
- ❑ Did not make statements such as "This better not happen again!" or "How do you expect us to pay our bills if our patients' checks bounce?"

Case Study 2
Page 1224

What Did Christa Do?
- ❑ Told the patient that she would check the receipt book, then went through the duplicate receipts of the day of the patient's visit.
- ❑ If a copy of the receipt for a cash payment was found, told the patient and entered the payment into the patient's account.
- ❑ If no copy of the receipt was found, explained to the patient that it was office policy to issue a receipt for any cash payment from a book where a duplicate was made automatically.

Continued

What Would You Do? What Would You *Not* Do? RESPONSES—cont'd

❏ If no copy of the receipt was found, suggested tactfully that the patient may not remember this specific visit, and perhaps she was unable to pay her copayment that day or forgot to pay it.

❏ If the patient continued to insist that she paid cash, offered to discuss the matter with the office manager or physician.

What Did Christa *Not* Do?

❏ Did not get angry at the patient or raise her voice.

❏ Did not say that unless the patient can show her a receipt, the office will automatically assume that she had not paid.

❏ Did not accuse the patient of trying to get out of paying the copayment.

Case Study 3
Page 1230

What Did Christa Do?

❏ Attempted to contact Ms. Mason by telephone to inform her of the office policy so that the patient would be prepared to settle her outstanding bill.

❏ If the patient could not be contacted before the appointment, took her to a private room when she arrived at the office to discuss her account.

❏ Strongly encouraged Ms. Mason to settle the account by check or credit card before being seen by the physician.

❏ If Ms. Mason stated that she could not pay the balance on that day, left the final decision about whether she would be seen to the physician because the patient had not been informed of the office policy before coming to the office.

What Did Christa *Not* Do?

❏ Did not take sole responsibility to tell the patient that if she did not pay, under no circumstances would she be seen by the physician.

❏ Did not raise her voice or get angry with Ms. Mason.

❏ Did not discuss Ms. Mason's financial matters where others could overhear the conversation.

↻ TERMINOLOGY REVIEW

Key Term	Definition
Account aging	The process of finding out how long specific account balances have been outstanding.
Balance due	Total amount owed.
Bankruptcy	Legal process by which the debts of an individual or business are resolved if they cannot be paid.
Claim message	Messages encouraging payment of a bill, usually attached to or printed on the monthly statement.
Collection agency	A firm that is in the business of collecting overdue accounts.
Credit balance	A negative balance on a patient account (i.e., money is owed by the medical office), usually a result of an overpayment.
Overdraft	A check (or draft) that exceeds the amount of funds in a bank account.
Patient statement	A bill sent to a patient that contains not only charges but also payments and adjustments that affect the balance that the patient must pay.
Skip	Account for which no billing information is available.
Truth in lending	Legal requirement to disclose the terms of a loan in terms that the borrower can understand.

ON THE WEB

For information on the Federal Trade Commission:

Federal Trade Commission: www.ftc.gov

The Medical Assistant as Office Manager

50

Check out the Evolve site at http://evolve.elsevier.com/Bonewit/today/ to access additional interactive activities and exercises to help you study and prepare for success.

LEARNING OBJECTIVES

1. Describe routine maintenance activities in the medical office.
2. Identify methods to maintain a safe environment and prevent injury to patients and employees.
3. Explain how safety signs, instructions, and labels contribute to a safe office environment.
4. Describe an efficient system of maintaining equipment inventory lists and operator manuals.
5. Maintain administrative and clinical equipment.
6. Describe the process of obtaining new equipment.
7. Explain procedures for taking inventory.
8. Describe an effective method for ordering, receiving, and storing supplies.
9. Explain how to manage office payroll.
10. Describe ways to enhance teamwork in the medical office.
11. Describe the medical assistant's role in orienting and training new employees.
12. Manage the physician's professional schedule.
13. Differentiate between medical office policies and procedures.
14. Create and/or revise medical office policies and procedures as needed to promote smooth office functioning.
15. Locate community resources to assist patients and medical office staff.
16. List types of liability, professional (malpractice), and personal injury insurance for physicians, the medical office, and medical assistants.
17. Describe the process of compliance reporting for unsafe activities, errors in patient care, and conflicts of interest.
18. Describe how incident reports should be used to protect the medical office.

PROCEDURES

Create an environmental checklist and perform a safety inspection.
Comply with safety signs, symbols, and labels.

Perform routine maintenance of equipment.

Take a supply or equipment inventory.

Locate and facilitate referrals to community resources.

Complete an incident report.

CHAPTER OUTLINE

INTRODUCTION TO MEDICAL OFFICE MANAGEMENT
MAINTAINING THE OFFICE
Administrative Area
Examination and Treatment Rooms
Waiting Room
Security Systems
ROUTINE MAINTENANCE
Temperature and Ventilation
General Cleaning
Cleaning Cabinets and Drawers
Miscellaneous Tasks
PATIENT AND EMPLOYEE SAFETY
Safe Work Practices

Monitoring Environmental Safety
Signs and Instructions
MAINTAINING EQUIPMENT
Inventory
Monitoring Equipment Function and Readiness for Use
Service Contracts
Service Calls
New Equipment Purchases
SUPPLIES
Supply Inventory
Restocking
Ordering Supplies
Receiving Supplies

CREATING AN ENVIRONMENT FOR TEAMWORK
Staff Meetings
Orienting and Training Employees
Working With New Employees or Medical Assisting Students
PREPARING PAYROLL
Deductions
Income Taxes
Social Security and Medicare
State Taxes
Employer Obligations
Unemployment Tax
Preparing Payroll Checks

MANAGING PHYSICIAN AND EMPLOYEE SCHEDULES
Physician Schedules
Employee Schedules
PROVIDING RESOURCES FOR STAFF AND PATIENTS
Office Policy and Procedure Manuals
Medical Office Policies
Written Procedures
Locating Community Resources
RISK MANAGEMENT
Minimizing Risk of Injury or Illness
Liability Insurance
Compliance Reporting
Incident Reports

KEY TERMS

back order	*per diem*	service contract
depreciation	policy	Social Security tax
gross pay	procedure	vendor
inventory	purchase order (PO) number	warranty
invoice	reorder point	W-4 form
minutes	risk management	
net pay	salary	

INTRODUCTION TO MEDICAL OFFICE MANAGEMENT

The medical assistant performs many tasks that promote the smooth running of the medical office. These tasks include maintaining the physical space, taking inventory, ordering supplies, monitoring programs such as risk management and employee safety programs, orienting new employees, and processing employee payroll. The responsibility for these management functions may be primarily that of the medical assistant in a small office or primarily that of an office manager in a larger setting. Office management always provides the basis for effective patient care, and its importance cannot be overestimated.

MAINTAINING THE OFFICE

In many medical practices, a medical assistant assumes responsibility for maintaining the physical space of the medical office and performing general maintenance. Heavy cleaning and equipment repair are usually not performed by office staff, but rather by contractors. Thus the medical assistant may also be responsible for managing the relationship between the office and contractors, as well as medical, pharmaceutical, and office supply companies.

ADMINISTRATIVE AREA

When sitting at the front desk, the medical assistant must be able to effectively and efficiently answer two or three incoming calls, greet patients, and handle paperwork.

Depending on the size of the administrative area, supplies and equipment for correspondence and billing may be stored in this area, including stationery, envelopes, billing forms, and coding reference books. In addition to the telephone (discussed in detail in Chapter 41), the reception area usually contains one or more personal computers, which are linked to the office's computer network. Materials for creating new patient folders should also be at hand if a paper medical record system is used.

The administrative area needs to have enough room to perform the required activities without the patient files and other papers becoming mixed up, and it must also allow the medical assistant to maintain patient confidentiality (Figure 50-1).

Again, depending on the size of the office, business operations will take place either in the front office close to the reception area or in a separate area in the office. In the business office are the rest of the pieces of equipment necessary for administering the office, including the photocopy machine, fax machine, and postage meter or electronic mailing system. In small offices, an all-in-one printer-copier-fax may be used.

Figure 50-1 Well organized front office.

Patient billing records are available either in hard-copy files in the business office or on the computer. Charge slips, patient statements, and other documents are usually printed using a laser printer or inkjet printer.

The medical assistant should be familiar not only with the office equipment's operation, but also with the maintenance responsibilities, such as reloading paper and adding toner or printer cartridges. In addition, the medical assistant may need to follow the terms of any maintenance agreements when scheduling maintenance or repairs.

Offices should also have a paper shredder for disposing of confidential documents. Although medical records must be maintained indefinitely, old telephone logs, old payroll records, canceled checks more than 7 years old, and minutes of practice management meetings should all be shredded rather than simply thrown away in the wastebasket or in a wastepaper-recycling bin. Any documents with patient information that have been scanned into the electronic medical record (EMR) should be shredded if they are not retained. Shredded paper can still be recycled, and there is no danger that sensitive personal or business information will be seen by anyone who should not have access to it.

EXAMINATION AND TREATMENT ROOMS

Each examination or treatment room also needs approximately 100 square feet of floor space to hold an examination or treatment table, cabinets and countertop, patient chair and physician stool, and a small surface for the physician to write on. The room should be laid out so that a physician and medical assistant can move freely about the room. Equipment and supplies should be within easy reach or stored in drawers or cabinets that are easy to reach.

Each examination or treatment room needs to have a sink, as well as soap and paper towel dispensers. Hand sanitizer may be in a wall-mounted or freestanding dispenser. The examination room must also contain a wall-mounted

rigid container for the disposal of sharps, such as needles, scalpel blades, or other objects that might puncture a plastic bag. Biohazard wastebaskets with a biohazard plastic liner for materials that contain body fluids, such as blood, mucus, or pus, are located either in each examination room or in the hall. Containers for hazardous waste must be covered, except when adding waste. A foot pedal to open the cover facilitates use. The examination room usually contains an ordinary wastebasket for used paper towels and table paper.

For safety reasons, examination rooms should not contain syringes, needles, or medication samples. Cleaning materials and chemical solutions should never be stored under the counter in an examination room, especially if it is used for children.

WAITING ROOM

The waiting room makes a first impression on a new patient. It must be neat and welcoming. The waiting room needs two to four chairs for each physician in the office at one time, current magazines, and a table or magazine stand to hold them. If the practice sees children, some toys should be available in a separate play area. One person should be assigned to tidy up the waiting room a couple of times during the day.

A waiting room should have signs that inform patients about office policies. The signs depend on the policies of the individual office. Common signs include the following:

- No smoking
- Copayments are expected at the time of service (or some other language regarding the expectation of payment)
- The following credit cards are accepted (followed by names of credit cards)
- No eating or drinking
- A charge will be added for returned checks to cover any bank fees
- Patients will be charged for cancelled appointments unless at least 24-hour notice is given

Some offices have a display rack with health information brochures. Brochures are available from government agencies, public agencies, and many companies. With the approval of the physician(s), these brochures are often provided to help educate patients about health promotion and disease prevention.

Sometimes there is a television or DVD player in the waiting room. In some practices, health information videos are playing. Other practices have a radio tuned to an easy-listening station or a CD player with quiet pop or light classical music. The medical assistant may need to turn on this equipment at the beginning of the day.

SECURITY SYSTEMS

A medical office maintains a number of different security systems.

First, if the office is entered from a corridor in an office building, the building owner or office condominium association most likely has an electronic security system for the building itself.

Second, regardless of whether the office is entered from a corridor or directly from the outside, the practice should maintain an electronic security system against break-ins to the office itself.

The office's security and safety alarm system is monitored by an alarm company and may or may not also be tied to the local police and fire departments. Whether or not the system is tied into the police and fire departments, the alarm company will call the practice's liaison to the company whenever the alarm goes off.

This designated person is often the practice administrator or managing partner. However, two or three people are always listed as backups in case the liaison is not available.

Third, various places within the office require another layer of security. Medication cabinets—with all medications and prescription pads inside—should be locked, and a limited number of people should have keys to the medication cabinet lock. The laboratory, physicians' private offices, medical records cabinet or room, and business office are other areas that often have a lock and limited access.

If controlled substances are stored in the office, they should be double-locked (e.g., in a locked drawer within a locked cabinet). Two separate keys should open the two different locks.

ROUTINE MAINTENANCE

It is important to maintain the physical space of the medical office. Depending on the size of the office, many if not most routine maintenance activities are undertaken by staff. These include controlling the temperature, cleaning cabinets and drawers, changing lightbulbs, replacing batteries in battery-powered equipment, turning the security system on and off, making sure fire protection equipment is in working order, and performing some daily cleaning. In all activities, medical assistants and other staff must be sure to protect themselves and patients from hazards and injury. Good body mechanics should be used to move supplies and equipment and when cleaning, as well as when working with patients. The workplace should be arranged to minimize strain during all routine and maintenance activities.

TEMPERATURE AND VENTILATION

The reception area and examination rooms should be kept at a comfortable temperature. People who are ill are sensitive to cold and drafts. The reception and patient waiting areas and examination rooms should be about 70° to 72° F. The temperature in treatment rooms, the laboratory, and physicians' offices should be about 68° to 70° F. A room used for procedures or minor surgery can be kept a little cooler because the physician and medical assistant may be wearing gowns or lab coats, gloves, and masks.

Ventilation is also important. Keeping air circulating is important both to dissipate odors and to allow germs to escape from the office atmosphere.

Putting It All Into Practice

My name is Kelsey Whitman, and I am a Registered Medical Assistant. I usually work in one of the satellite offices of a large medical group that includes primary care providers and medical specialists. The office where I usually work was formerly a house. They are planning to close it next spring, tear it down, and build a modern office building. Even though there are some disadvantages to the current setting, it has a lot of charm. The waiting room and three small examination rooms are on the first floor with the physicians' office, and we use the rooms upstairs for storage, a break room, and meeting rooms. I have a small office upstairs, but I never have time to sit in it. Usually we have only one physician in the office. I work with one other medical assistant, but since I have been in the practice longer, I am responsible for making sure that everything runs smoothly. I have to go to the main office once a month for a staff meeting. The meetings are held once a month late on Wednesday afternoon. We discuss issues affecting all work areas. We have also been reviewing some of the procedures done by medical assistants to be sure that every medical assistant in every office does things the same way. The other medical assistant will be going out for maternity leave in a few weeks, and we have been interviewing for a replacement. After an initial screening interview, I have been asked to talk to three applicants, to give them a tour of our office, and to give my feedback about how they might fit into this setting. One of the applicants seemed like a real team player, and I hope they hire her. It is so important for everyone to be able to work well together. ■

GENERAL CLEANING

Larger offices may contract for cleaning services, or office cleaning may be included in the monthly rent, especially in buildings that are dedicated to medical offices. Contracted cleaning is usually done one or two times a week, so even if the major cleaning is contracted out, daily cleaning tasks still must be performed.

Daily cleaning includes tidying up all areas of the office—reception and waiting rooms, administrative space, physicians' offices, examination and treatment rooms, and the laboratory.

Sinks should all be toweled dry, and rest rooms should be checked to make sure ample toilet and facial tissue, soap, and paper towels are available. Any spills or puddles on the floor of the rest room should be mopped up using gloves as needed.

Waste containers and recycling containers should be checked daily and emptied as needed. Biohazard sharps containers should be checked daily and replaced when they are three-quarters full. The plastic liners of biohazard waste containers should be changed as needed. Contracted cleaning services will usually not empty biohazard waste containers because they contain regulated medical waste. The medical assistant must handle biohazard waste containers carefully to prevent an exposure incident. The Occupational Safety and Health Administration (OSHA) Bloodborne Pathogens Standard outlines specific actions to take when handling regulated medical waste. These are outlined in Chapter 17.

If the office staff must do more intense cleaning, this should be done at least weekly. These tasks include mopping linoleum floors and vacuuming carpets, cleaning the glass at the reception area, polishing furniture and accessories, dusting, and thoroughly cleaning the rest rooms.

It is important to try to avoid a "medical smell" in the office. This is done by maintaining proper ventilation, as well as by cleaning up spills and accidents immediately, using light or unscented air fresheners in rest rooms and examination rooms, and keeping disinfectants and cleaning materials closed tightly when not in use and out of patients' reach.

CLEANING CABINETS AND DRAWERS

Storage cabinets, drawers, and bookcases are cleaned less frequently, often on a day when the physician or some of the physicians in the practice are absent so that the room is not in use. After cleaning, the medical assistant should check labels on all items before putting them back on shelves. This is a good time to check the expiration date on supplies and make a list of any items that need to be ordered or restocked from the general supply area to the cabinet. Outdated supplies must be disposed of properly (Figure 50-2).

Figure 50-2 Well organized supply cabinet.

MISCELLANEOUS TASKS

Among the miscellaneous tasks that have to be performed daily are rearranging the waiting room chairs and replacing magazines in their racks (as well as toys if toys are available); cleaning mirrors in the rest rooms and examination rooms; and cleaning the tops, fronts, and undersides of cabinets and paper towel dispensers. Toys must be cleaned and disinfected on a regular basis, because they can harbor microorganisms.

The medical assistant may be responsible for replacing light bulbs in gooseneck lamps and other special lighting. Ceiling lighting is usually a responsibility of the maintenance staff employed by the building owner. If the space is owned by the practice, this may be a staff responsibility or may be covered by the cleaning or maintenance contract with an outside service.

PATIENT AND EMPLOYEE SAFETY

In addition to maintaining the physical environment of the medical office, it is also vital for all medical facilities to maintain a safe environment both for patients and for employees. This involves several measures.

1. Manage the environment to reduce hazards.
2. Train employees in general safety and to use correct methods and processes to prevent accident or injury.
3. Maintain equipment and perform regular safety inspections.
4. Create open lines of communication so that mistakes and accidents can be reported without fear of severe consequences.

What Would You Do? What Would You *Not* Do?

Case Study 1

Jean Highsmith has brought her 1-year-old twins, Scott and Lucy, to the medical office because they have been fussy and tugging at their ears. In the waiting room, she puts the twins on the floor to play with the toys while they are waiting. When Kelsey is able to take them to an examination room, she notices that the twins, who also have runny noses, have been chewing on some of the plastic toys in the waiting room. She notices that Mrs. Highsmith has left used tissues on one of the waiting room tables. After a few minutes in the examination room, Mrs. Highsmith comes to the door holding a child under each arm and tells Kelsey that Scott has thrown up a little on the examination room table. ∎

PROCEDURE 50-5 Locating and Facilitating Referrals to Community Resources—cont'd

1. **Procedural Step.** Research local sources to identify community agencies with resources to assist patients. Potential sources of information include the library, local newspapers, local cable television stations, local telephone books, local hospital newsletters, and the Internet.

   Principle. Familiarity with local agencies improves the medical assistant's ability to provide useful information about community resources to patients.

2. **Procedural Step.** As resources are identified, create a list including pertinent information about the resource: name, services available, address, telephone number, website address, contact name or information, and other useful information. The list may be created using pen and paper, but it should be transferred to a word processing file for ease of duplication.

3. **Procedural Step.** Include resources for organizations and support groups that can assist patients and family members of patients experiencing terminal illness.

4. **Procedural Step.** Include resources for complementary and alternative medicine (CAM) practices.

5. **Procedural Step.** Once the document file has been substantially completed, group resources by subject and/or age group served. Alphabetize resources within each group.

   Principle. Arranging lists in alphabetic order facilitates finding specific information and avoids any impression of favoritism or recommending one agency more frequently than another.

6. **Procedural Step.** When the list is complete, save and print copies as needed.

7. **Procedural Step.** Ask the office physicians to review and approve the list.

   Principle. Any referral made by a medical office should have the approval of the practice physicians.

8. **Procedural Step.** Update the list when information changes, when a new resource is identified, and on a periodic basis to be sure information is accurate.

9. **Procedural Step.** Use the list to make appropriate recommendations to patients either in response to patient questions or when instructed to by one of the office physicians.

10. **Procedural Step.** Write a two-page report identifying the specific steps a medical assistant should take to facilitate referrals for a patient who needs a handicap placard for his or her automobile and a patient not taking his or her prescribed brand name medication because the patient cannot afford it.

    Principle: A medical assistant can act as a patient navigator for patients by helping them to identify resources to obtain services such as a handicap placard, or to find out how to apply for the free drug program from the manufacturer of a brand name drug.

RISK MANAGEMENT

Risk management is the process of assessing risk and putting in place policies and procedures that minimize it. Often, the focus of risk management activities is on avoiding lawsuits. Risk in a medical office comes in a number of forms.

MINIMIZING RISK OF INJURY OR ILLNESS

Physical risk involves the risk of injury or illness to employees, patients, and visitors. Business risk also exists: the risk of reduced patient visits because of poor customer relations.

The medical office seeks to minimize these risks and prevent lawsuits that may result from injuries related to patient care or an accident in the office.

The medical assistant or office manager is often responsible for maintaining the risk management program, in close consultation with the physician or the managing partner among the physicians. In larger clinics or hospitals there may be a full-time risk manager, or risk management may be a part of the duties of one of the clinic's top administrators. Policies and procedures are designed by the physicians and the office's top administrator, who work closely with an attorney, an insurance professional, and a risk management professional. When a new policy is adopted, a copy is given to each employee covered by the policy. Policy and procedure manuals, once developed, should be accessible to all employees when questions arise.

LIABILITY INSURANCE

Every office should have adequate insurance protection against liability, both professional liability (commonly called *malpractice*) and liability for any accident that might occur in the office.

Professional liability insurance covers a medical professional against patient claims that diagnostic procedures, tests, or treatments either caused an injury or failed to detect an existing medical condition that should have been detected using good medical practice.

Some physicians purchase insurance in their own name only and have professional staff members purchase their own professional liability policies. If this is the case, the medical assistant can purchase a professional liability policy through an organization that provides insurance to health professionals. In other cases a practice purchases professional liability insurance for the entire staff. If this is the case, every professional staff member should be named on the policy.

The office should also have adequate insurance to cover property damage to the office because of fire, storm, or flooding (similar to homeowner's insurance). In addition, the practice should have adequate coverage against personal injury sustained on the office's property by a patient or employee. Many patients are ill and/or fragile, and a fall can occur at any time. The policy should cover any injury sustained on the property controlled by the practice. If the practice is in an office building, the public hallways are the responsibility of the landlord or medical office condominium association. If the office is in a freestanding building, the practice is responsible for any occurrences that happen on walkways, in the parking lot, or in other outdoor areas up to the public road or sidewalk.

COMPLIANCE REPORTING

Each state board of health requires specific compliance reports for infectious diseases, other diseases, abuse, and injuries resulting from possible criminal behavior as discussed in Chapter 3. In addition, hospitals, nursing homes, and other types of facilities must report specific serious medical incidents. Physicians must also make a report to the state if a patient demonstrates failing eyesight that would interfere with the ability to maintain a driver's license. Depending on the state, reports of unsafe activities and errors in patient care (especially medication errors) must be reported, especially when they occur in relation to individuals with disabilities. Workplace disease and injury reporting is also required in most states.

The "Sunshine" provision of the Patient Protection and Affordable Care Act (PPACA) requires manufacturers of drugs, devices, and biologic and medical supplies covered by Medicare, Medicaid, or the Children's Health Insurance Program to disclose to CMS any payments or other valuable transfers made to physicians and teaching hospitals. It has long been felt that gifts and payments to physicians by the pharmaceutical industry have created a potential conflict of interest, influencing physicians to prescribe the medications of those companies who support them. Some states have placed limits on such gifts. Physicians are also required to disclose any financial interest in laboratories or other health care facilities to which they refer patients.

INCIDENT REPORTS

Whenever something happens in the office for which the office could be considered liable, an incident report should be filled out. An incident can be as simple as a staff member or patient tripping over a chair, or it could be as serious as a staff member sticking himself or herself with a needle that has just been used to give an injection.

The incident report should be initiated by the staff member who is injured or who is closest to the patient or visitor when he or she is injured. A supervisor should review the report before giving it to the individual who manages the risk management program.

Incident report forms vary widely but usually ask for the following information:
- Date and time that the incident occurred
- Name and identifying information of the individual(s) involved
- Address, building, and room number where the incident occurred
- Description of how the incident occurred and exactly what occurred
- Complete description of any injury or potential injury
- Name(s) and identifying information for any witnesses
- Name and contact information for the person in the organization to whom the incident was reported
- Date of receipt and follow-up by supervisor

Incident reports should always be filled out if a patient, employee, or visitor slips or falls, if a medication error is made, if blood is drawn from the wrong patient, if the number of surgical instruments counted after a procedure does not match the number counted before the procedure, or if an employee is stuck with a needle. Any witnesses to the incident should be asked for their name, address, and phone number so that the office's insurance provider can call and investigate the incident further if necessary.

An incident report can usually be created for a patient through the EMR and filed as part of the patient's record. Paper reports are used for visitors and/or employees. A paper report should be dated and signed by the person filling it out. A physician and/or supervisor's signature also goes on the form, according to the office's policy for incident reports (Procedure 50-6). If the incident relates to a reportable occurrence, the information must be forwarded to the correct government agency.

PROCEDURE 50-6 Completing an Incident Report

Outcome Complete an incident report

Equipment/Supplies

- Incident report form (from SimChart® for the Medical Office or OSHA Form 301)
- Index card from instructor describing an incident involving an error in patient care
- Pen
- Notes from witnesses to the incident

1. **Procedural Step.** Interview all witnesses to the incident, and make notes as needed to complete the incident report.
   Principle. The incident report is based on factual information, but individuals involved in the incident may not be available when the report is actually written.
2. **Procedural Step.** Obtain an incident report form and fill in information about the person (or persons) who are the main subject of the incident including name, date of birth, and address. If using SimChart® for the Medical Office, select the Incident Report form in the Office Forms section of the Form Repository.
3. **Procedural Step.** Complete any information about health care provided, including the names and identifying information for physicians or health care professionals who provided treatment.
   Principle. Risk management includes taking all possible steps to minimize an adverse result from an incident.
4. **Procedural Step.** Complete all information to describe the incident in detail including time, location (address, building, room number), what happened, and any injury or illness that resulted from the incident. Include the names and identifying information of any witnesses.

Principle. Documentation of this information as soon as possible after the incident makes it easier to establish the facts about the incident at a later time.
5. **Procedural Step.** Depending on the form used, it may be necessary to include the name and contact information of the individual within the office to whom the incident was reported. The supervisor should add information about any follow-up that occurs at a later date. The supervisor should initiate any additional required reports to appropriate government agencies.
   Principle. Follow-up for an incident is a crucial step in effective risk management.
6. **Procedural Step.** Review the report with the subject of the incident if possible before signing the report and obtaining his or her signature on a paper form, also if possible. Obtain a supervisor's signature as well on a paper form.
   Principle. Signatures on an incident report indicate that parties involved have been informed of the contents of the report.
7. **Procedural Step.** If using SimChart® for the medical office, save the report when it is complete. Create a signed paper report as well if it is office policy.

What Would You Do? What Would You *Not* Do? RESPONSES

Case Study 1
Page 1237

What Did Kelsey Do?
- ❑ Put the twins in an examination room as soon as possible.
- ❑ Asked Mrs. Highsmith to place the used tissues in the wastebasket before taking the twins to the examination room. Then provided hand sanitizer for Mrs. Highsmith.
- ❑ As soon as possible, put on disposable gloves and removed the plastic toys that the twins had had in their mouths so that the toys could be cleaned before other children played with them.
- ❑ When told that Scott Highsmith had thrown up a little, put on disposable gloves, used paper towels to absorb as much liquid as possible, and then promptly cleaned and disinfected the surrounding area.

- ❑ Reassured Mrs. Highsmith that children are ill sometimes and that cleaning up is all in a day's work.
- ❑ Noted the color and amount of vomit so that she could inform the physician.

What Did Kelsey Not Do?
- ❑ Did not ask Mrs. Highsmith to prevent the twins from playing with any toys because they had colds.
- ❑ Did not tell other mothers in the waiting room that they might not want to let their children play with the toys until they could be disinfected.
- ❑ Did not wait to perform routine cleaning until the lunch break or after office hours.
- ❑ Did not tell another staff member or Mrs. Highsmith to clean up when Scott vomited.

What Would You Do? What Would You *Not* Do? RESPONSES—cont'd

Case Study 2
Page 1244

What Did Kelsey Do?
❏ Checked the number of each type of item against the packing slip to be sure the order was complete. Made a notation if any items were missing.
❏ Placed all the items in their assigned storage area, either that night or the next day. Placed newer items behind older items.
❏ When placing items into storage, checked items on the shelves to be sure that none of them had expired.
❏ If any items were missing or backordered, made a notation on the packing slip. Then placed the packing slip in the accounts payable folder to indicate that the order had been received.
❏ Removed the shipping box to the designated area for trash.

What Did Kelsey Not *Do*?
❏ After opening the large box, did not leave the office before checking the packing slip. Another staff member might assume that the individual who opened the box had also checked the contents.
❏ Did not stack the items on shelves in the storage room randomly because she was in a hurry.
❏ Did not discard the packing slip after checking the order.

❏ Did not keep the shipping box because it might be dirty or harbor pests.

Case Study 3
Page 1249

What Did Kelsey Do?
❏ Encouraged Ellen to reach out and find out if there were services that could help her mother.
❏ While Mrs. Brown was present, included her in the conversation.
❏ If speaking to Ellen privately was an option, offered understanding of how difficult it is to know what to do when a parent begins to be less able to function independently.
❏ Offered to help Ellen find resources for delivered meals or homemaking services in the community.
❏ Referred Ellen to local agencies that provide elder services.
❏ Offered to ask the physician if a referral to a visiting nurse would be appropriate.

What Did Kelsey Not *Do*?
❏ Did not exclude Mrs. Brown from the conversation or treat her like a child.
❏ Did not push Mrs. Brown or Ellen to accept her suggestions, but rather just offered information.
❏ Did not promise that the physician would make specific referrals.

↻ TERMINOLOGY REVIEW

Key Term	Definition
Back order	A term used for items ordered that cannot be shipped immediately, usually because they are out of stock.
Depreciation	Accounting methods to respond to the loss of value of a property or piece of equipment over time.
Gross pay	The total amount earned in a time period by an employee before any deductions.
Inventory	A detailed list of items in stock or in possession of an individual or business.
Invoice	An itemized bill for items whose cost has not been prepaid.
Minutes	A written record of the proceedings of a meeting.
Net pay	The actual amount of money paid directly to an employee after taxes and other deductions have been taken out.
Per diem	A term used for employees who do not have a fixed schedule but are scheduled by the day according to office needs.
Policy	A guiding principle for the management of a medical office or business.
Procedure	A list of the steps to handle a certain situation or perform a certain task.
Purchase order (PO) number	A number assigned by a business to authorize and keep track of a purchase request and order.
Reorder point	A number on a supply inventory that indicates when a specific item should be reordered to be sure that the supply will not run out before the new order is received.
Risk management	The process of assessing risk and putting policies and procedures in place to minimize it.
Salary	A fixed amount of money paid on a regular basis that does not depend on the number of hours worked.
Service contract	An agreement that provides for service for a piece of equipment after the warranty expires.

Continued

TERMINOLOGY REVIEW—cont'd

Key Term	Definition
Social Security tax	A tax collected from employers and employees to fund the Social Security program, which provides benefits to retired workers.
Vendor	A company from whom supplies or equipment is purchased.
Warranty	A promise by the manufacturer to repair or replace defective parts in an item during a specific time period.
W-4 form	The form used to claim allowances for federal income tax reporting.

ON THE WEB

For information on U.S. government forms related to payroll and employment:

I-9 form (United States Citizen and Immigration Services): www.uscis.gov/sites/default/files/files/form/i-9.pdf

Internal Revenue Service: www.irs.gov

- W-2 (Wage and Tax Statement)
- W-4 form (for employee withholding)
- Withholding tax tables
- Form 941 (employer's quarterly tax return)
- Form 940 (employer's annual federal unemployment [FUTA] tax return)

Social Security Administration: www.ssa.gov

- Obtain a Social Security number
- Apply for a replacement Social Security card

For information on worker safety:

OSHA Guide to Compliance for Medical and Dental Offices: www.osha.gov/Publications/OSHA3187/osha3187.html

OSHA Small Business Handbook: www.osha.gov/Publications/smallbusiness/small-business.html

Obtaining Employment

51

Check out the Evolve site at http://evolve.elsevier.com/Bonewit/today/ to access additional interactive activities and exercises to help you study and prepare for success.

LEARNING OBJECTIVES

1. Describe the process for locating potential employers when looking for a job.
2. Discuss the steps in preparing a résumé.
3. Describe how to write a cover letter.
4. Differentiate between information placed on a résumé and information required on an employment application.
5. Explain how to provide potential employers with a résumé by mail, using a fax, or using Internet resources.
6. Prepare to answer questions commonly asked in a job interview.
7. Describe measures to prevent job burnout.
8. Identify two professional organizations to which a medical assistant may belong.
9. Identify benefits of joining a professional organization.
10. Discuss why lifelong learning is vital for a medical assistant after graduation.

CHAPTER OUTLINE

INTRODUCTION TO OBTAINING EMPLOYMENT
SUCCESSFUL JOB SEARCH
Setting Goals
Identifying Potential Employers
TOOLS FOR A JOB SEARCH
Preparing a Résumé
Résumé Styles
Information to Include
Formatting the Résumé
Writing a Cover Letter
Sending the Résumé
Filling out an Employment Application
Applying for Employment Using the Internet
GETTING THE JOB
Interview Techniques
Preparing for the Interview
Appearance and Behavior
Questions That the Interviewer Should Not Ask

Discussing Salary and Benefits
Asking Questions
Determining the Timeline for Filling the Position
Follow-up After an Interview
LIFELONG LEARNING
Staying Current
Administrative Skills
Clinical Skills
Preparing for Increased Responsibility
Avoiding Burnout
Professional Organizations and Peer Support
Legislation Affecting Medical Assistants
Continuing Education Units
PLANNING FOR JOB ADVANCEMENT OR CAREER CHANGE
Advancing to Management
Upgrading Technical and Clinical Skills
Transferring Skills

KEY TERMS

burnout
continuing education unit (CEU)

cover letter
networking

résumé

INTRODUCTION TO OBTAINING EMPLOYMENT

After graduating from a medical assisting program, most medical assistants must begin the search for their first job. Sometimes the medical office where the graduate did a practicum asks the student to stay on as an employee. When this happens, it eases the transition from student to employed medical assistant. Because a student cannot count on this, it is important for the new graduate to see the process of learning how to seek employment as just another skill that must be mastered.

Finding a job involves more than simply answering a few newspaper advertisements or responding to one or two help-wanted notices on the school's career bulletin board. To find the right job, a medical assisting graduate needs to put time and effort into the job-hunting process.

SUCCESSFUL JOB SEARCH

Successful job hunting has two parts. The first is setting appropriate goals; the second is identifying potential employers where those goals might be met.

SETTING GOALS

Setting goals means identifying the ideal job for a medical assistant's current circumstances. The medical assistant should ask herself or himself the following questions:

- Do I want to work full-time or part-time?
- In what area of the country or region do I want to work?
- Do I want to work in a city? In the suburbs? In the country?
- What are my particular strengths and weaknesses?
- Am I interested in working in a particular medical specialty?
- Do I have a preference about the size of the organization where I would be happy?
- Do I want to specialize in either clinical or administrative duties, or do I want to do both?

IDENTIFYING POTENTIAL EMPLOYERS

After a graduate has set goals, it is time to begin identifying potential employers. This is done by viewing online want ads and scanning newspaper ads to see what kinds of positions are being advertised and searching online to see what kinds of practices are in the community where the graduate wants to work. It is important to read carefully, because a graduate may be eligible for positions with different job titles. Many large organizations post job openings internally first. The graduate should ask family or friends who work in such institutions to keep an eye on the internal posting boards.

Larger institutions also often have personnel or human resource departments that keep files of potential employees to give to physicians or department administrators who need to fill a position. When an applicant fills out an application for such a facility, the application will stay on file for a period of time—usually 6 months or 1 year. After that, a new, updated application must be submitted.

During the job-hunting period, it is important to set aside some time each day to look for a job. The more opportunities a graduate explores, the better the possibility of not only finding a job but also finding the right job.

When looking for a job, it is important not to underestimate the importance of **networking**—contacting friends and acquaintances who may know of potential jobs. A personal network may include former instructors, contacts made during the medical assisting practicum, classmates, and even physicians the medical assistant knows or has worked with. It is important to develop a habit of maintaining professional contacts. Staying in touch, either through occasional telephone calls, e-mails, or meeting for coffee or lunch, provides opportunities to gain both support and information. A contact may call in the future when there is an opening at work or when someone has asked for names of potential employees.

Potential employers may use the Internet to do research about job applicants, so when the job search begins, a graduate should use a Web browser and enter his or her own name, looking for both websites and images. Potential employers may look at public information on Facebook, Twitter, other social media sites, and blogs. The graduate should be sure that nothing appears that would prevent an employer from granting an interview. For example, a picture showing the graduate at a party, a comment criticizing the school the graduate attended, or even family photographs can create a negative impression. In addition, employers sometimes do credit checks, so it is recommended to review a personal credit history early in the job-hunting process and take steps to correct any errors.

TOOLS FOR A JOB SEARCH
PREPARING A RÉSUMÉ

The primary purpose of a résumé is to obtain an interview for an open position. A **résumé** is a summary of information about a person that describes education, work experience, and other information that employers may find pertinent in deciding whether or not to hire an individual.

A résumé is often important in making a first impression on a potential employer. It must be neat, professional, and informative. A paper résumé looks better if it is printed on high-quality paper. Employers, who often receive several résumés for one position, use the résumé to create a list of people with the desired training and/or experience to call in for personal interviews.

A résumé should describe a medical assistant's education, experience, and skills completely, but not in an exaggerated way. If possible, the résumé should be limited to one type-written sheet. If the résumé is more than one page, which typically should only occur when a person has multiple degrees, the information that is especially pertinent to the job for which the medical assistant is applying should appear on the first page. If a medical assistant is applying for many different types of positions, it may be desirable to have many variations of a résumé available, each one slanted toward the requirements of certain positions.

Personal information should not be included on a résumé. Information such as marital status, children, and hobbies does not relate to a medical assistant's credentials for a position. If personal information is included, the effect is most likely to be neutral or possibly negative, providing a reason not to grant an interview. For example, the employer may be afraid that a medical assistant with two or more children may need to be absent if the children become ill.

Résumé Styles

In general, there are three styles of résumés: chronologic, functional, and targeted.

A chronologic résumé contains a list of formal education, with degrees and certificates earned, followed by work experience (although work experience can come before education in this style). This is the most common type of résumé for applicants with limited work experience, or those who are seeking work similar to their present work.

A functional résumé categorizes experience according to skills or abilities, some of which may be a result of activities other than paid employment (e.g., volunteer work, unpaid work). A functional résumé is useful for an individual who wants to change from one type of work to a different type of work and wants to highlight how particular skills attained in one line of work can be helpful in the new position for which he or she is applying.

A targeted résumé organizes information about an individual who has targeted a particular job opportunity in such a way as to highlight the skills and work experiences being called for in the new employment. This type of résumé often begins with an employment objective that identifies the type of position the individual is seeking.

Information to Include

The basic pieces of information needed for a résumé are personal demographics, objective, education, experience, skills, credentials, and references. A number of computer programs are available for preparing résumés. If a computer program is used, the medical assistant should be sure to personalize the résumé. It is also helpful to use some sample résumés as guides (Figures 51-1, 51-2, and 51-3). Other samples may be available from the placement office of the graduate's college or medical assisting program, as well as résumé-writing books and websites.

Personal Demographics

Personal demographics include the name, address, telephone number, and e-mail address. This information is usually placed at the top of the résumé. The e-mail address should sound professional. If a graduate has been using an e-mail address such as "partyanimal@server.com" or if his or her personal e-mail has a link to Twitter or Facebook, he or she should think about creating a new e-mail account for the job search. The message on the cell phone and home phone should sound professional, without a child's voice or pet name. All identifying information should be large enough and in bold enough type to stand out.

Objective

The objective is a statement of the type of position the medical assistant is looking for. A medical assistant just graduating may be—even *should* be—flexible about the type of position being sought. If the objective is to obtain an entry-level position as a medical assistant, there may be better ways to use the limited space on a single-sheet résumé than stating this as an objective. This becomes a matter of personal preference.

A medical assistant with a more focused goal may wish to use a statement such as "To obtain a clinical medical assisting position in an office specializing in family practice or internal medicine." A specific objective reassures the potential employer that the candidate is interested in the position he or she is trying to fill, but it can limit the positions for which the candidate will be considered.

Education

The education section includes the institutions attended and degrees or certificates received. These should be arranged in chronological order with the most recent first. At least one program should be listed with a degree, certificate, or diploma and the year it was received. Usually the high school diploma is included only if the candidate has no higher credential.

When identifying a school or program, the anticipated graduation date can be included if the résumé is prepared before the medical assistant graduates (e.g., A.S. in Medical Assisting, anticipated June 20XX). After graduation, the résumé should be revised before it is sent to other potential employers.

It is also appropriate to include the grade-point average (GPA) if it is above 3.0 and any honors or awards received from the educational institution, such as Dean's List.

Previous Experience

In the section on previous experience the following are included:
- The job title
- Years of employment
- Employer's name
- The town and state in which the work was performed

A new graduate may wish to present information about previous experience in two sections, titled *Related Experience* and *Other Experience*. The medical assisting practicum (externship) can be included under the heading *Related Experience,* but if the section is titled *Work Experience,* only

Anderson
2314 May Avenue
Western, OH 44770
(490)111-1555
S.Anderson@anyserver.com

OBJECTIVE
To obtain an entry level position as a clinical medical assistant.

EDUCATION/CERTIFICATION
Associate of Science, Western Community College, Western, OH   June 2014
Major: Medical Assisting
GPA: 3.5

RELATED EXPERIENCE
Medical Assisting Externship (160 hours), Western Medical Associates,   2014
Western, OH
- Prepared patients for examination, took vital signs, patient history and chief complaint
- Performed diagnostic tests including throat cultures, rapid strep test, ECG's, dipstick urinalysis
- Answered telephones, filed, scheduled appointments and validated insurance coverage
- Entered patient information, patient charges and payments and insurance payments in the computer

Home Health Aide, Medical Home Care, Newtown, OH   2011-2014

OTHER EXPERIENCE
Cashier, Western Supermarket, Western, OH   2011

SPECIAL SKILLS
- Fluent in Spanish
- Keyboarding 45 wpm
- Microsoft Office, MediSoft, Practice Partner EMR

CERTIFICATIONS
Certified Medical Assistant (AAMA): August 2014
BLS Healthcare Provider Level and First Aid

Figure 51-1 Chronologic résumé of a recent graduate.

paid employment should be included. Most employers do not like to see gaps in a work history, which might reflect jobs that the applicant does not wish to acknowledge. If the applicant has been a homemaker, it is recommended to include the years devoted to this under *Other Experience*. Any volunteer work can also be included.

For each position or type of experience, a short summary of responsibilities should be included. If the experience was in health care or medical assisting, more details should be included than for other jobs or experience. For example, more details should be included about specific responsibilities as a home health aide than as a cashier. Action verbs should be used in the description of previous experience (Figure 51-4). Any special achievements or projects should

be included (e.g., setting up an electronic tickler file in a previous job as a secretary).

When preparing the descriptions of previous experience, the medical assistant should use one of two styles consistently. Either can be written in sentence form or as a list with bullets.

Describing Responsibilities Using Verbs in the Past Tense

Example in sentence form:

Measured vital signs, prepared patients for examination, posted charges and payments, sent monthly bills, etc.

Patricia A. Saychelles

26 Gillian Street
Western OH 44770
(490) 111-2728
saychelles@anyserver.com

OBJECTIVE

To obtain a challenging position as a medical assistant that will utilize my skills and training

EDUCATION

Certificate in Medical Assisting, Shamrock Institute, Western, OH   May 2014

SKILLS

- Developed clinical and medical assisting skills during classes and medical assisting externship at Western Medical Associates.
- Able to use computer programs including Microsoft Word, Microsoft Excel, MediSoft v. 16, Practice Partner EMR
- Managed, implemented and coordinated multiple activities and schedules for family members
- Able to plan events for large and small groups

COMMUNITY ACTIVITIES

- Chairperson of public library committee responsible for obtaining feedback from local community
- Volunteer for the DARE program at Western Middle School
- Secretary of the Western Women's League 2011-2013 responsible for secretarial duties, keeping the financial records and fund raising

CERTIFICATIONS

Registered Medical Assistant: August 2014
BLS Healthcare Provider Level and First Aid

EMPLOYMENT

Package Sorter United Parcel Service, Western, OH   2008-2009

Figure 51-2 Functional résumé of a woman who stayed home with children for several years before training as a medical assistant.

Example in bullet form:
- Measured vital signs
- Prepared patients for examination
- Posted charges and payments
- Sent monthly bills

Describing Responsibilities Using Participle Form of the Verb

Example in sentence form:

Responsible for measuring vital signs, preparing patients for examination, posting charges and payments, sending monthly bills.

Example in bullet form:
Duties included:
- Measuring vital signs
- Preparing patients for examination
- Posting charges and payments
- Sending monthly bills

Special Skills

The special skills section describes skills learned in an education program that may not be reflected in any direct experience, or that are usually not included in a medical assisting program. These may include computer skills with particular programs, ability to perform specific diagnostic

---

John Davidson
16 Carriage Way
Western, OH 44770
(490) 111-3235
airman@anyserver.com

OBJECTIVE

To obtain a position as a medical assistant or administrator in an emergency care setting with both clinical and management responsibilities.

SUMMARY

More than ten years of providing professional military and civilian health care, specializing in emergency treatment, supervision of personnel, physical examination, and health awareness training.

- Received qualifications from the U. S. Navy as Medical Assistant (MA), Nursing Assistant (NA), Emergency Medical Technician (EMT), Emergency Vehicle Operator (EVO) and Emergency Medical Dispatcher (EMD)
- Able to assist with and supervise personnel assisting with occupational, preventative, and emergent medical examinations, ECG's, and emergency procedures
- Able to facilitate hospital admission and maintain medical records
- Provided instruction in personal hygiene, preventative care and sanitary conditions

EMPLOYMENT

United States Navy

- *Hospital Corpsman First Class*, Naval Air Station, Harbor Bay, OH   2004-2014
- *Hospital Corpsman Second Class*, Naval Air Station, Seal Beach, CA   1999-2004

OTHER CREDENTIALS

Instructor: Emergency Medical Technician (EMT-B)

Instructor: American Heart Association BLS

Advanced Life Support (ACLS) provider

EDUCATION

Attended Western Community College from 1998-1999 taking general education courses and introductory health courses.

Figure 51-3 Targeted résumé of a man who received health care training in the Armed Services.

administer	distribute	process
analyze	document	proofread
arrange	establish	propose
assist	file	purchase
authorize	instruct	reconcile
balance	list	run
calculate	log	schedule
classify	mail	send
code	measure	set up
collect	monitor	sort
compose	order	stock
contact	organize	teach
coordinate	perform	write
copy	post	
develop	prepare	

Figure 51-4 Action verbs to use on a résumé.

tests, or knowledge of or fluency in a language other than English.

Activities and Other Credentials

In the section on activities and other credentials, the medical assistant may include certification (as a CMA [AAMA], RMA, or CCMA), memberships in professional organizations such as the American Association of Medical Assistants (AAMA) or the American Medical Technologists (AMT), and any other certifications or credentials including cardiopulmonary resuscitation (CPR) and/or first aid. Membership in community service organizations or disaster relief efforts may be included as well. Lists of unrelated activities, hobbies, and interests should not be included on a professional résumé.

References

Traditional résumés always included the following statement: *References will be furnished on request.* This statement is considered optional on a modern résumé because it is assumed to be the case. Actual references are not listed on the résumé because the goal is to be interviewed before the potential employer checks any references. After the interview, the medical assistant provides a list of references with contact information. Before using someone's name as a reference, the medical assistant should be sure to get that person's permission. It is also polite to call individuals whose names have been used so that they can be ready to receive a phone call or written request for a reference.

For references, a medical assistant who has recently graduated should choose a balance of instructors, practicum supervisor, other job supervisors, or co-workers from volunteer activities. It is not recommended to use friends or family for references. Sometimes the individual who will be used as a reference gives the medical assistant a letter that can be shown to a potential employer. More often, the potential employer contacts the individual given as a reference after interviewing the candidate.

Formatting the Résumé

The résumé should be formatted with at least 1-inch margins. It is important to lay out the résumé so that it looks balanced on the page with clear sections of information. After the résumé has been created, it should be proofread carefully. Spelling and grammar errors are unacceptable. A single spelling or grammar error may prevent a potential employer from offering an interview.

Often, the résumé is sent as an e-mail attachment or is attached to an online job application. If the résumé will be sent through the mail, it should be a printed original, not a photocopy. It makes a good impression if a stationery-weight paper is used, which is slightly heavier than ordinary printer paper. Because medical assistants work in a fairly conservative segment of the job market, it is important to avoid using colored paper, unusual type fonts, or flashy formatting for the résumé.

WRITING A COVER LETTER

A **cover letter** is a letter sent with a résumé that explains briefly why the résumé is being sent. The cover letter clarifies whether the medical assistant is responding to an advertisement, has been referred by another individual, or is simply inquiring about possible job opportunities.

If sent through the mail, the cover letter should use the format for a business letter and should be printed on the same color paper as the résumé. If possible, the medical assistant should call the office to find out the name of the office manager or other individual responsible for hiring medical assistants. If sent online with a résumé, the letter should be addressed to the human resources department.

The letter should begin with the reason for writing the letter and sending the résumé. This should be followed by a brief summary of the position being sought and the candidate's qualifications for filling that position. The final paragraph should be a request for an interview.

Each cover letter should be personalized because this is the first thing the potential employer will see. Of course, it should not contain any grammar or spelling errors. The reader should be referred to the résumé for details (Figure 51-5).

The medical assistant should keep a copy of all cover letters. The results (interview, second interview, job offer) can be written on the copy or on a separate log that keeps track of responses to all letters sent out.

Putting It All Into Practice

My name is Deanna Taylor, and I took the CMA (AAMA) examination in June of the last year that they gave a pen-and-paper examination. During the time that I was waiting for my examination results, I went on six job interviews. I was hired in my present position 3 weeks before I found out that I passed the examination. The combination of searching for my first medical assisting job and hoping that I had passed the certification examination was very stressful. Current graduates are really lucky to take a computerized examination and get a preliminary report the same day, even if potential employers sometimes wait for the official results to hire new grads.

I was looking for a position in obstetrics and gynecology, but I sent a résumé for every medical assisting job that I saw. That turned out to be good because I had a much better idea of what different offices were like, and I became more comfortable in the interview itself. When I first walked through the door of the office that hired me, I felt comfortable. I knew that if I were a patient, I would trust the staff because they were friendly but professional. This office does specialize in obstetrics and gynecology, so I was lucky enough to find exactly the position I had hoped for.

I was interviewed by the practice manager, a woman who works with several medical practices affiliated with a local hospital. We discussed my experience and the position. Later she called me back for a second interview to meet with the physicians and office staff. After that, she offered me the position. I was very excited, and I have to say that it has turned out very well. Even though I have been here for several years, I am always learning new things because there are so many changes. It seems that there is always a new challenge and something new to learn. ■

SENDING THE RÉSUMÉ

It is recommended to send résumés in 9- × 11-inch manila envelopes so that they do not need to be folded. If using a standard No. 10 business envelope, its color and weight should match the paper used for the résumé and cover letter if possible.

2314 May Avenue
Western, OH 44770
September 5, 20XX

Diane Wells, Practice Manager
Medical Practice Associates
525 Main Street
Western, OH 44770

Dear Ms. Wells:

I am sending you a copy of my resumé in response to your advertisement for a medical assistant in the Western Daily Item. As you will be able to see, I have recently completed an Associate's degree in Medical Assisting at Western Community College.

As part of our training, I was placed in an externship for 160 hours, and I was able to practice the skills that I learned in my training program. I have also passed the national certification exam in medical assisting given by the American Association of Medical Assistants.

I hope you will contact me at (490) 111-1555 to schedule an interview for this position. I am looking forward to hearing from you.

Sincerely,

Susan Anderson, CMA (AAMA)

Figure 51-5 Sample cover letter.

Increasingly, it is possible to respond to job openings using the Internet or to fax a résumé to an office. A cover letter is still recommended.

The advantage of a faxed or e-mailed résumé and cover letter is that the material arrives quickly, often within minutes of making a telephone inquiry. The disadvantage is that a fax or a printout of an e-mail does not look as crisp or professional as a mailed résumé and cover letter.

A few days after a mailed résumé should have arrived, a job applicant may call to see if the material did, indeed, arrive. At this time it is appropriate to ask if the person doing the hiring has an idea about the time frame in which a hiring decision will be made. However, a job applicant should not call again after that, to avoid appearing too aggressive.

FILLING OUT AN EMPLOYMENT APPLICATION

Most medical facilities require a completed job application in addition to a résumé. In large facilities, it may be necessary to complete the application before an interview is scheduled. In smaller offices, the application may be filled out at the time of the interview.

It is important to keep a list of information needed to fill out the job application. This includes the name and address of previous employers, dates of employment, names and telephone numbers of supervisors, as well as the names, addresses, and telephone numbers of references. Any letters of reference should be brought to the interview so that the facility can make copies to attach them to the job application.

The medical assistant should answer all questions fully and truthfully on the application. If filling the application out by hand, the medical assistant should print legibly. All questions should be answered. It is not appropriate to refer the reader to the résumé. If a question does not apply, the medical assistant should write *N/A* or *Not Applicable.*

If the application asks for the reason for leaving a previous position, the medical assistant should avoid making any negative statements about the employer or supervisor. Common reasons for leaving are returning to school, relocation for a spouse's job, end of a temporary position, or exploration of new career options.

Some health care facilities may require applicants for medical assisting positions to take a keyboarding test or other skills test before an interview is granted.

APPLYING FOR EMPLOYMENT USING THE INTERNET

The medical assistant may use an online employment website (e.g., Monster.com) to create a résumé, use that résumé to apply for open positions, and also post the résumé on the Web for potential employers to view it. The résumé that is created can be saved as a document file and used to post on various websites or to apply for other positions. Many employers also advertise for medical assistants and accept applications using their own websites. When looking for employment, the medical assistant should visit the websites of potential employers, review job postings, and submit an application online if a suitable position is open. By networking with other students, instructors, and friends, the medical assistant can identify online resources that others have used successfully.

GETTING THE JOB

INTERVIEW TECHNIQUES

An employment interview provides a potential employer with an opportunity to assess a candidate's interpersonal and communication skills and preparation for a position in the medical setting. The interview also provides the medical assistant with a chance to assess the potential employer. The questions asked, the flow of the discussion, and the tour of the facility help the medical assistant decide whether the position fits appropriately with his or her work style and personality.

For a job to be offered, the medical assistant must do well in the interview. Often a candidate whose skills appear excellent on paper does not create a positive impression during the interview. The key for the employer is to find the person who seems to be the best fit for the position.

It is important for a medical assistant to accept any job interview offered, even if the position does not seem ideal. The more interviews a new graduate goes on, the more comfortable the job interview process becomes. It is not appropriate, however, to accept more job interviews after a position has been accepted.

Preparing for the Interview

Before the interview, the medical assistant should try to find out as much as possible about the practice or facility. Information can be obtained by talking to someone who works there or a patient of the office, if possible. The medical assistant should ask friends and other contacts if they know anyone with information about the potential employer.

Many medical offices have a website that describes the practice. The medical assistant should enter the name of the practice and/or physician(s) into a search engine. If the practice has a website, it will probably include the names of the physicians and other practitioners, the philosophy of the practice, and other background information. If the office is small, it may only be possible to locate telephone and address information. This may indicate that the office is not using as much modern technology as some other offices.

When the interview is arranged, the medical assistant should find out whether one person or a committee will conduct the interview, and if one person, the name and position of the individual.

The medical assistant should ask if there are any particular things that the interviewer(s) would like to know and if any background materials should be brought to the interview.

Appearance and Behavior

As always, a professional appearance is important. A female medical assistant should wear tailored, professional-looking clothing, such as a suit or blouse and skirt or dress slacks. Denim skirts, denim jeans, shorts, and mid-calf pants are not appropriate for an interview. Long hair should be worn pulled back and off the collar, as it would be when working as a medical assistant. It is recommended to avoid bulky jewelry, avoid false nails and visible piercings, and present a tailored appearance (Figure 51-6). Visible tattoos should be covered, if possible. For an interview the medical assistant should avoid sandals or athletic shoes and never wear flip-flops. A male medical assistant should wear a suit or dress slacks and sports coat or blazer, with a dress shirt and tie. Hair, including any facial hair, should be clean and neatly trimmed.

It is important to maintain good posture and look alert during the interview. The medical assistant should sit comfortably without slouching and avoid fidgeting or displaying nervous habits. At the same time, the medical assistant presents a better impression if he or she is relaxed and natural instead of reserved and stiff. The interviewer is looking for an individual who interacts well with patients and can make them feel at ease. If a job applicant smiles and makes conversation easily during an interview, it is likely that he or she will be comfortable with patients. A job applicant should never chew gum during an interview. Before the interview, the applicant should turn off his or her cell phone. It is useful to have a pen and notepad handy to make notes. It is also helpful to write down questions

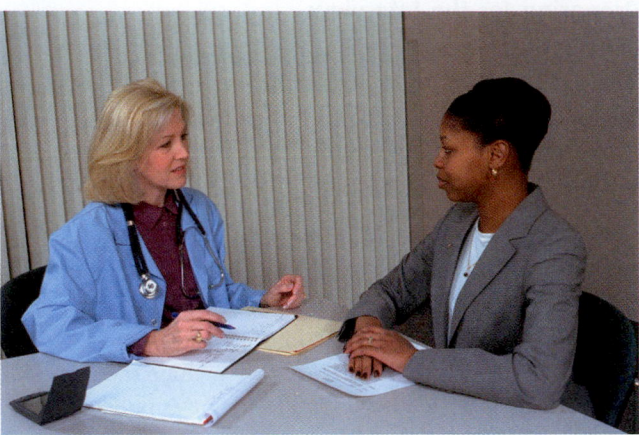

Figure 51-6 At a job interview, the medical assistant should look and act in a professional manner.

that might be encountered in future interviews, to practice answers before the next interview.

Questions That the Interviewer Should Not Ask

Interviewers are not supposed to ask questions that do not relate to the position, including marital status, number of children, and age (unless there is a legal age requirement as part of the job). Various federal and state laws regulate these questions. The 1964 Civil Rights Act prohibits discrimination based on race, sex, color, national origin, and religion. The Age Discrimination in Employment Act prohibits questions about a person's age. The Americans with Disabilities Act of 1990 protects qualified individuals with disabilities from discrimination in employment. If the interviewer asks an illegal question, the medical assistant should try to identify or respond to the underlying concern without directly refusing to answer the question.

Interviewer: "Are you a United States citizen?"
Applicant: "Are you asking whether I am authorized to work in the United States?"

What Would You Do? What Would You *Not* Do?

Case Study 2

When she was looking for a job, Deanna got lost on the way to an interview. The office was located about 30 minutes from her home. Deanna had allowed plenty of travel time, but she took the wrong turn off the highway and didn't realize it until she had gone almost 10 miles in the wrong direction. When she realized she was lost, she knew that backtracking would make her at least 15 minutes late. ∎

Discussing Salary and Benefits

Specific salary is usually not discussed until a job is offered. But it is common for a salary range to be discussed. If the interviewer does not state the salary range, it is acceptable

to ask about it as the interview is winding down. Asking about the salary range early in the interview may give the impression that money is the most important thing about the job. Failing to ask about a salary range may be interpreted as lack of interest.

It is also appropriate to ask a general question about benefits, such as how long an employee must work before becoming eligible for the benefits package and if health insurance is a benefit. It is customary not to ask specifically about vacation, sick days, and personal days until a job offer has been made.

When a position is offered, a discussion of salary and benefits helps the medical assistant make a decision about whether or not to accept the position. If the salary seems low or is less than the medical assistant currently earns, it is appropriate to ask about the specific time frame when performance will be reviewed and a raise will be possible.

Often, especially in larger facilities with rigid salary structures, a position is limited to a particular salary range. It is important to be sure that the salary is adequate to meet expenses before accepting the position. Usually an applicant can ask for 24 to 48 hours to consider a job offer.

Asking Questions

A good interviewer will ask a candidate at the end of the interview if he or she has any questions. The medical assistant may ask about who supervises the position, may ask the interviewer to clarify the job responsibilities, and/or may ask about the availability of training programs in-house or financial support for outside training or college courses. It is helpful to come to the interview with three or four written questions. If these were answered during the interview, the medical assistant can look over the list and say that it seems as though all his or her questions have been answered.

Determining the Timeline for Filling the Position

If the interviewer or lead interviewer on a committee does not state the employer's time frame for making a decision about filling the position, this is an important question to ask. Employers know that people must seek employment at many facilities, and most are willing to get back to applicants who have been interviewed within a few days.

FOLLOW-UP AFTER AN INTERVIEW

Although it may seem old-fashioned to write a written thank-you note after a job interview, most potential employers will be favorably impressed by this courtesy. It also provides an opportunity to include any additional information requested at the interview. See Figure 51-7 for a sample follow-up letter.

If the interviewer has not responded by the date expected, the medical assistant may telephone to ask if the position has been filled.

HIGHLIGHT on Responding to Questions

Based on previous experience at interviews and suggestions from friends about their experiences, the medical assistant should try to prepare for questions the interviewer(s) will ask. Although it may seem awkward, it is helpful to practice answering sample interview questions out loud with friends, family, or a roommate. Several common interview questions and potential answers are presented in the following discussion.

1. *What can I tell you about my organization?*
   It is always important to have questions prepared. The medical assistant might ask about the history of the office or clinic and/or how long it has been in its present location. He or she should have found out how many physicians work there and what specialties are represented, but could ask how many medical assistants are employed.

2. *What was your favorite subject in school?*
   The answer is more powerful if it demonstrates enthusiasm and has some relation to the position being applied for. Math, English, science, computer courses, and medical assisting courses are good answers. If a job applicant says that poetry was her favorite subject, the interviewer may wonder if medical assisting is the applicant's real interest.

3. *Why did you choose to study medical assisting?*
   People who choose this field are usually interested in health, like people, like a job where they can be active, and believe that preventive care and early diagnosis are important components of health. This question also gives the medical assistant an opportunity to demonstrate enthusiasm and caring.

4. *What courses did you like least in school?*
   It is better for the medical assistant to name one course and describe it as "difficult" or "challenging" (even if that does not directly respond to the question) instead of giving a long list of subjects that were boring. It is important to avoid looking like an individual who is uninterested in subjects that may relate to the job and also to avoid complaining or speaking negatively.

5. *What campus activities did you participate in? What did you learn from them?*
   The medical assistant can prepare by thinking of an interesting extracurricular activity he or she has participated in, even if there was not time to be a member of any club or organized activity in school. If the medical assistant worked for several hours while going to school, he or she might say so while identifying a hobby: "I worked as a cashier several hours a week to help pay for school, so I had to leave school right after class. But I'm working with a classmate to arrange for some of our graduates to get together monthly because I think that it would be too bad to lose contact with the friends I made in school."

6. *Describe your responsibilities when you worked for XYZ Company.*
   The medical assistant should identify his or her responsibilities, being sure to emphasize any special projects, promotions, or leadership roles. A medical assistant often has a part-time job while going to school, with some extra responsibility, such as opening or closing, training new employees, or rotating to different departments. If handling money was a job responsibility, it should be mentioned because it indicates reliability.

7. *What types of problems have you encountered in your jobs? How did you handle them?*
   The medical assistant should describe a problem that he or she experienced that might occur in any office setting, such as an angry or unsatisfied customer, telephones ringing off the hook, work backing up, and being overwhelmed at first. When discussing the problem, it is important explain how the problem-solving process was applied to resolve the problem.

8. *What would your instructors or previous supervisors tell me about you if I were to call them?*
   The medical assistant should identify his or her positive attributes and practice saying them calmly, even if it seems like bragging. "They would say that I work hard," "I am organized," "I catch on quickly," "I'm good with people," and "I try hard to be accurate" are some examples. In an effective interview, the job applicant puts his or her best foot forward without exaggerating or distorting the truth.

9. *What are some of your weaknesses or areas you need to work on?*
   The medical assistant should think carefully about weaknesses that may be seen in some lights as positive, or weaknesses that everyone is subject to. Being a perfectionist, not liking to miss work for illness, and double-checking all work to be sure it is correct are examples of weaknesses that employers usually like. Being nervous in a new situation, becoming frustrated when there isn't enough time, and hating to see others sitting around when there is much work to do are traits common to many people. If a medical assistant is shy and reserved, this is a good opportunity to state that he or she is not always outgoing in new situations, but that it doesn't take very long to feel comfortable and open up more.

10. *What are your long-term goals?* or *Where do you plan to be in 5 years?*
    The prospective employer is trying to get a sense of how long the applicant plans to stay in the position if hired. In many areas, turnover of medical assistants is rapid, but an employer would like to be able to count on at least 2 years. If the medical assistant will be returning to school within 6 months, he or she should say so and identify whether part-time work would be possible at that time. ∎

2314 May Avenue
Western, OH 44770
September 18, 20XX

Diane Wells, Practice Manager
Medical Practice Associates
525 Main Street
Western, OH 44770

Dear Ms. Wells:

Thank you for the opportunity to interview with you last week for the position of medical assistant. It is clear that your practice provides high quality care to patients. After meeting with you, I know that I would be glad for the opportunity to join your team.

I look forward to hearing from you about this opportunity. Please feel free to contact me at (490) 111-1555 or by email (S.Anderson@anyserver.com) if you have any questions. Thank you again for your time and consideration.

Sincerely,

Susan Anderson, CMA (AAMA)

Figure 51-7 Sample letter after an interview.

LIFELONG LEARNING

The field of health care is becoming more complex all the time. It is important for every member of the health care team to constantly improve his or her skills and stay up to date on new techniques in his or her field. To provide high-quality patient care, every member of the health care team must engage in lifelong learning.

STAYING CURRENT

Medical assistants must keep their skills current. This means keeping abreast of new techniques, as well as learning how to use the latest technology.

Administrative Skills

On the administrative side, computer software is constantly being updated. This includes operating systems and all programs used routinely in the medical office. Training to use updated versions of operating systems, word processing programs, or other general programs is often available online or through classes. If the office switches to an updated version of office management programs or an electronic medical record, the software company often provides training for office personnel.

Another area that requires constant updating relates to changes in coding and insurance claim submission. The medical assistant should read updates and attend classes as needed to keep skills current.

Clinical Skills

On the clinical side, it is important to learn to use new diagnostic or laboratory equipment. When a new piece of equipment is purchased, training should be arranged for all staff who will use it. The medical assistant must also stay current on new medications. Pharmaceutical representatives leave informational materials for the physician, and the medical assistant should make a point of reading this information.

Preparing for Increased Responsibility

The medical assistant may be trained to assist with special procedures. The medical assistant may be sent to an outside training program at office expense, or the physician or other staff member may provide the training. It is important to pay close attention during the training and take notes to be sure that all information is retained.

The medical assistant may also be given some responsibility to supervise other staff members. Classes or workshops in supervision, appraisal, conflict management, or other subjects may be helpful to ease this transition.

AVOIDING BURNOUT

Burnout is a constant worry, especially for those in repetitive, high-stress jobs. **Burnout** is a term that has come to mean disillusionment with work and physical or emotional exhaustion. It is characterized by a loss of interest or enthusiasm and energy about work.

A person experiencing burnout may exhibit behavioral changes as well, including increased irritability, inability to empathize with patients, chronic fatigue, and poor relations with co-workers. Job burnout can be a precipitator for clinical depression and must be dealt with as a medical issue rather than a disciplinary problem.

Loss of enthusiasm at work may also result from factors outside the job. If an individual's life is out of balance, or if the individual is having problems with relationships within the family, he or she may not have the necessary energy to expend at work. This may appear as depression or burnout.

If a medical assistant arrives at the point where job burnout is a concern, it is important to take action. If possible, the medical assistant should reduce the hours of work, even if only for a 3- or 6-month period. Increased social activities, increased exercise, and focusing on physical and mental health can foster a more positive physical and emotional state. The medical assistant should try to find a hobby to help "decompress" from work.

Sometimes burnout is not recognized until the problems have progressed to such a degree that professional intervention is necessary. The individual with severe burnout may need counseling, therapy, or a job change; and if the individual has developed a substance abuse problem, he or she may even need inpatient rehabilitation. Many large facilities have in-house employee counseling.

For an annual membership fee, many benefits are available, including the following:

- Peer support
- Continuing education programs
- Legislative advocacy on issues important to medical assistants
- Publications and/or newsletters with information related to the profession of medical assisting

Legislation Affecting Medical Assistants

Professional organizations are able to advocate for pending state and federal legislation that may affect the medical assisting profession. Changes in legislation require actions by many people. In some states, issues for medical assistants arise from actions taken by other professionals to define legally who may perform certain procedures. As a result of such actions, medical assistants may not take radiographs in most states, and they may not be permitted to administer injections or draw blood, depending on the state.

A future task for the medical assisting profession will be to organize and help draft legislation giving medical assistants the right to perform in the workplace all skills for which they have been trained. This can best be accomplished by working with the national professional organizations and their state chapters.

What Would You Do? What Would You Not Do?

Case Study 3

After 6 months at the obstetrics and gynecology office where she was first hired, Deanna began to wish that she had more contact with other medical assistants to discuss job-related issues. The other medical assistants in her office seemed to be busy with their families, and they didn't socialize at all after work. Deanna wished that she knew more about new trends, new medications, and new technology. She had joined the American Association of Medical Assistants (AAMA) when she graduated, but there didn't seem to be an active chapter in her area. ■

PROFESSIONAL ORGANIZATIONS AND PEER SUPPORT

The AAMA and the AMT are professional organizations for medical assistants. Even if a medical assistant has not obtained certification, he or she can become a member of an active chapter of one of these organizations. Through local and national meetings and workshops, medical assistants are able to enter a network of peers with whom they can share and from whom they can learn. They can also obtain insurance at reasonable cost, professional journals, and other sources of information important to the profession.

Memories *from* Practicum

Deanna Taylor: The biggest difference between a practicum and employment is that it takes more effort to stay enthusiastic about showing up every day. When I was doing my practicum, everything was new. I was always excited to go because it seemed like there was a new experience every day. Now that I have been working for several years, there are many days that seem very routine. There are new experiences, but I have to remind myself to notice them. One way that I have found to stay fresh and focused is to volunteer to be on committees to gather information or to plan the implementation of new equipment or new software. For example, I took a course and attended seminars to prepare for the transition to the ICD-10, and I have been working with a committee to facilitate the changeover. I also have been taking a general business course at night for the past month. I notice things at work that I never would have before, and I am now planning to take more courses in health administration or business administration. When I was in school, all I could think of was graduating and getting a job, but now that I am a medical assistant, I realize that my career is just beginning. I realize that I am personally responsible to find a way to keep my career rewarding and satisfying. ■

CONTINUING EDUCATION UNITS

A **continuing education unit (CEU)** is a standard measure of qualified instruction as defined by a specific profession.

Most health professions require a certain amount of continuing education for licensure or certification renewal. CEUs or contact hours of instruction are required for recertification as a CMA (AAMA) or RMA. The medical assistant should keep a file with the paperwork acknowledging attendance at classes or workshops, together with the CEU credits or contact hours approved for them. With the constant change in the medical field, it is not merely important but necessary to keep skills up to date, attain new skills, and obtain new information about professional practices.

Medical assisting contact hours and CEUs can be obtained from education programs that have been approved by the particular certifying agency. These education programs may be given through the state and national organization, through other educational institutions, or through home or online study programs.

PLANNING FOR JOB ADVANCEMENT OR CAREER CHANGE

One of the best ways to avoid job burnout is to chart a course of career advancement.

ADVANCING TO MANAGEMENT

If a medical assistant enjoys the administrative part of medical assisting, there are many opportunities to find a management position within the health care industry.

The larger the facility, the more the administrative and management tasks are broken into discrete parts, and the more management and administrative staff are in demand.

If a medical assistant is currently working in such a facility and would like to move up the management ladder, he or she should ask about the possibility of rotating through the various departments to gain experience in finance, billing, marketing, public relations, or any other department. If the medical assistant is working at a small facility or private practice, he or she should take the opportunity to learn about every job within the practice. This makes the medical assistant more versatile and more valuable as an employee. After gaining supervisory experience in a smaller facility, the medical assistant may wish to move to a larger facility.

Business courses or formal education in health administration is invaluable. A number of colleges have both bachelor's and master's degree programs in health care administration. A degree in public administration or business management would also be appropriate.

UPGRADING TECHNICAL AND CLINICAL SKILLS

To advance to a position of greater responsibility on the clinical side, it will probably be necessary to obtain more formal education. After a few years of experience, a medical assistant who wishes to remain in an outpatient setting might consider enrolling in a formal education program to become a physician's assistant, a registered nurse, a medical technologist, or an x-ray technologist.

The opportunities become broader if a medical assistant wishes to work in a hospital or rehabilitation center. The medical assistant should talk to various health professionals and explore several potential career options. Obtaining financial support for additional education may be a concern. The medical assistant must decide if financial support is available to pursue further education full-time. For most candidates, it will be necessary to continue working either part-time or full-time at their present positions. Many employers encourage education and pay all or part of an employee's education costs.

TRANSFERRING SKILLS

Over time, the medical assistant may have built up skills that would make it possible to find a position in a field such as computers, insurance, the pharmaceutical industry, or medical equipment sales. If a medical assistant develops a strong interest in one of these areas, he or she should develop contacts, gather information, and develop a strategy for making a lateral career move.

This discussion would also not be complete without a word about the enormous rewards that can come from teaching—transferring knowledge and abilities to others who would like to become medical assistants.

With a medical assisting degree or certificate, a certified medical assistant may be able to get some work teaching a specific class related to medical assisting skills. A medical assistant who is interested in teaching should speak to the director of the program where he or she trained about teaching opportunities.

To teach full-time, in addition to maintaining certification, the medical assistant should obtain a bachelor's degree and master's degree in a health care field, or in education. Depending on the financial resources available from a spouse or partner's income, family assistance, or scholarships and loans available, this may be as a part-time or full-time student.

What Would You Do? What Would You *Not* Do? RESPONSES

Case Study 1
Page 1263

What Did Deanna Do?
- ❏ Reminded Andrea that employers usually consider work experience to include only paid positions.
- ❏ Pointed out tactfully that putting the practicum in the category of work experience might indicate unreliability or lack of knowledge to a potential employer.
- ❏ Advised Andrea to include the practicum in a section on the résumé called *Related Experience.*
- ❏ Offered to look over Andrea's résumé to see if she could make other helpful suggestions.

What Did Deanna Not *Do?*
- ❏ Did not tell Andrea that she was being dishonest when she listed the practicum as work experience.
- ❏ Did not make a discouraging remark such as, "That won't help you get hired."

Case Study 2
Page 1264

What Did Deanna Do?
- ❏ Made sure to take the name and telephone number of the person with whom she was going to interview.
- ❏ When Deanna realized that she was lost, she called the individual with whom she was scheduled to interview, explained the situation, apologized, and asked if it would be better to come late or reschedule.
- ❏ At the same time, Deanna asked for directions.
- ❏ Resolved always to get very clear directions before any other interview.

What Did Deanna Not *Do?*
- ❏ Did not show up 15 minutes late without making every effort to contact the individual with whom she was supposed to interview.
- ❏ Did not blame any individual for giving bad directions or failing to give directions.
- ❏ Did not act like being 15 minutes late was really not important.

Case Study 3
Page 1267

What Did Deanna Do?
- ❏ Found out where there were chapters of the AAMA in her state and made a point of attending a meeting. Also, she looked into attending the national meeting of the organization.
- ❏ Asked the practice manager if there were any continuing education programs at the local hospital that she could attend.
- ❏ Contacted graduates from her medical assisting program and arranged to get together with graduates with whom she had been friends when she was in school.
- ❏ Looked into the possibility of establishing a local chapter of the AAMA and tried to find one or two other medical assistants who might be interested in helping her.
- ❏ Looked at course offerings at the local community college to see if there were any courses or continuing education programs that she might be interested in attending.

What Did Deanna Not *Do?*
- ❏ Did not avoid taking responsibility to meet her own needs.
- ❏ Did not make excuses for putting off the process of seeking helpful contacts.
- ❏ Did not avoid reaching out to other medical assistants.

↻ TERMINOLOGY REVIEW

Key Term	Definition
Burnout	Disillusionment with work and physical or emotional exhaustion.
Continuing education unit (CEU)	A standard measure of qualified instruction or contact hours as defined by a specific profession.
Cover letter	A letter sent with one or more documents (such as a résumé) to provide an explanation.
Networking	Contacting acquaintances and their contacts who may know of potential jobs.
Résumé	A summary of information about a person that describes education, work experience, and other information related to an individual's suitability for employment.

ON THE WEB

For information about job discrimination:

U.S. Equal Employment Opportunity Commission (EEOC): www.eeoc.gov

For information on professional organizations:

American Association of Medical Assistants: www.aama-ntl.org

American Health Information Management Association: www.ahima.org

American Medical Technologists: http://www.americanmedtech.org/

American Society of Phlebotomy Technicians: www.aspt.org

For information on writing résumés and cover letters:

The OWL at Purdue University: owl.english.purdue.edu/owl/resource/564/01/

Résumé Templates—Microsoft Office Online: https://templates.office.com/en-us/Resumes-and-Cover-Letters

Glossary

ABA routing number A nine-digit number that identifies a bank; the number is printed at the beginning of the magnetic ink character recognition line at the bottom of a check. It also appears in fractional form at the top right of the check under the check number.

Abandonment Failure to continue to provide medical care to a patient without proper notification.

Abortion The termination of the pregnancy before the fetus reaches the age of viability (20 weeks).

Abrasion A wound in which the outer layers of the skin are damaged; a scrape.

Abscess A collection of pus in a cavity surrounded by inflamed tissue.

Absorbable suture Suture material that is gradually digested and absorbed by the body.

Absorption The passage of digestive end products from the gastrointestinal tract into the blood or lymph.

Accommodation Mechanism that allows the eye to focus at various distances, primarily achieved by changing the curvature of the lens.

Account aging The process of finding out how long specific account balances have been outstanding.

Accounting Systematic recording and reporting of financial transactions.

Accounts payable The outstanding bills of a business, such as a medical office.

Accounts receivable Total amount owed to a business for goods and services.

Accreditation Credit or recognition from a regional or national organization for maintaining certain standards.

Accrual basis of accounting Accounting method in which income is entered at the time of sale or provision of service.

Acetylcholine A neurotransmitter at the neuromuscular junction.

Acetylcholinesterase An enzyme that inactivates acetylcholine.

Acronym A word formed from the first letters in a name.

Act A bill or measure that has become law. Often refers to legislation with several parts.

Action potential A nerve impulse; a rapid change in membrane potential that involves depolarization and repolarization.

Active listening Paying close attention to a speaker without thinking of anything else.

Active record The medical record of a patient who has been seen within a time frame specified by the office (usually 2 to 3 years).

Active transport Process that moves substances across or through a membrane and requires cellular energy.

Adenohypophysis Anterior portion of the pituitary gland; the gland that grows below the brain.

Adjustment A change to a patient account that is neither a charge nor a payment.

Adnexal Adjacent.

Adolescent An individual 12 to 18 years old.

Advanced Beneficiary Notice of Noncoverage (ABN) A written notification to a patient with original Medicare that a covered service must be paid for by the patient if Medicare denies the claim as medically unnecessary.

Adventitious sounds Abnormal breath sounds.

Adverse reaction An unintended and undesirable effect produced by a drug.

Advocate A person who intercedes on another person's behalf.

Aerobe A microorganism that needs oxygen to live and grow.

Afebrile Without fever; the body temperature is normal.

Agglutination (as it pertains to blood) Clumping of blood cells.

Agranulocytes White blood cells that lack granules in the cytoplasm.

Allergen A substance that is capable of causing an allergic reaction.

Allergy An abnormal hypersensitivity of the body to substances that are ordinarily harmless.

Alveoli Microscopic dilations of terminal bronchioles in the lungs, where diffusion of gases occurs; air sacs in the lungs.

Alveolus A thin-walled air sac of the lungs in which the exchange of oxygen and carbon dioxide takes place.

Ambulation Walking or moving from one place to another.

Ambulatory Able to walk as opposed to being confined to bed or a wheelchair.

Ambulatory care Medical care that is provided on an outpatient basis. The patient is able to come to the facility providing care and return home after receiving services.

Amenorrhea The absence or cessation of the menstrual period. Amenorrhea occurs normally before puberty, during pregnancy, and after menopause.

Amphiarthrosis A slightly movable joint; plural, amphiarthroses.

Amplitude Refers to amount, extent, size, abundance, or fullness.

Ampule A small sealed glass container that holds a single dose of medication.

Anaerobe A microorganism that grows best in the absence of oxygen.

Analyte A substance that is being identified or measured in a laboratory test.

Anaphylactic reaction A serious allergic reaction that requires immediate treatment.

Anatomic position Standard reference position for the body.

Androgens Steroid hormones that promote male characteristics.

Anemia A condition in which there is a decrease in the erythrocytes or amount of hemoglobin in the blood.

Annotate To underline or highlight important words and phrases in correspondence.

Antagonist A muscle that has an action opposite to that of the prime mover.

Antecubital space The surface of the arm in front of the elbow.

Antibodies Substances produced by the body that inactivate or destroy other substances that are introduced into the body; immunoglobulins. Substances capable of combining with an antigen, resulting in an antigen-antibody reaction.

Antibody-mediated immunity Immunity that is the result of B-cell action and the production of antibodies; also called humoral immunity.

Anticoagulant A substance that inhibits blood clotting.

Antigens Substances that trigger an immune response when they are introduced into the body resulting in the formation of antibodies.

Antioxidant An antioxidant is a molecule that inhibits the oxidation of other molecules.

Antipyretic An agent that reduces fever.

Antiseptic A substance that kills disease-producing microorganisms but not their spores. An antiseptic is usually applied to living tissue.

Anuria Failure of the kidneys to produce urine.

Anxiety A vague, unpleasant emotion of fear or dread often accompanied by restlessness or nervousness.

Aorta The major trunk of the arterial system of the body. The aorta arises from the upper surface of the left ventricle.

Apnea The temporary cessation of breathing.

Aponeurosis A broad flat sheet of connective tissue that connects one muscle to another.

App A specialized program, often small enough to run on a mobile device.

Appendicular skeleton Bones that are attached to the body; upper and lower extremities.

Application software Software designed to accomplish a specific task (e.g., word processing); also called *application program* and *software program*.

Appointment matrix Basic pattern of available appointment times.

Appositional growth Growth resulting from material being deposited on the surface, such as the growth in diamaeter of long bones.

Approximation The process of bringing two parts, such as tissue, together through the use of sutures or other means.

Arbitration A formal process whereby the parties to a dispute agree to submit to the decision of a neutral party.

Arrector pili Muscle associated with hair follicles.

Articular cartilage Thin layer of hyaline cartilage that covers the ends of long bones in joints.

Articulation A joint; area of contact between two bones.

Artifact Additional electrical activity picked up by the electrocardiograph that interferes with the normal appearance of the ECG cycles.

Asepsis Free from infection.

Assets In accounting, a combination of property owned and money owed to a business.

Assignment of benefits Authorization given by the patient to allow the insurance company to make payments directly to the health care provider instead of to the patient.

Assumption of risk A defense to a lawsuit that establishes that the plaintiff assumed the risk of whatever caused the injury.

Astigmatism A refractive error that causes distorted and blurred vision for both near and far objects due to a cornea that is oval shaped.

Atherosclerosis Buildup of fibrous plaques of fatty deposits and cholesterol on the inner walls of an artery that causes narrowing, obstruction, and hardening of the artery.

Atria (singular atrium) Thin walled chambers of the heart that receive blood from veins.

Atrioventricular valve Valve between an atrium and a ventricle in the heart.

Attending physician The physician responsible for the care of a hospitalized patient.

Atypical Deviation from the normal.

Audiometer An instrument used to measure hearing acuity quantitatively for the various frequencies of sound waves.

Auscultation The process of listening to the sounds produced within the body to detect signs of disease.

Autoclave An apparatus for the sterilization of materials, using steam under pressure.

Autonomy Ability to make independent decisions without constraint or coercion by others.

Axial skeleton Bones of the head, neck, and trunk.

Axilla The armpit.

Axon The single efferent process of a neuron that carries impulses away from the cell body.

B

Bacilli (sing. *bacillus*) Bacteria that have a rod shape.

Back order A term used for items ordered that cannot be shipped immediately, usually because they are out of stock.

Backup A duplicate copy of a program or data kept for reference in case the original is damaged, lost, or destroyed.

Balance due Total amount owed.

Bandage A strip of woven material used to wrap or cover a part of the body.

Bankruptcy Legal process by which the debts of an individual or business are resolved if they cannot be paid.

Barcode clear zone The area on the lower right-hand corner of a card or letter that is left clear for the postal bar code to be printed.

Bariatrics The branch of medicine that deals with the treatment and control of obesity and diseases associated with obesity.

Basal ganglia Paired regions of gray matter located within the white matter of the cerebrum.

Baseline The flat horizontal line that separates the various waves of the ECG cycle.

Beneficence Acting in the best possible way; performing good deeds.

Beneficiary A person who can receive benefits under an insurance plan.

Benefit Payment for a covered service under a health insurance plan.

Bilirubinuria The presence of bilirubin in the urine.

Bill A law proposed by a legislative body.

Biopsy The surgical removal and examination of tissue from the living body. Biopsies are generally performed to determine whether a tumor is benign or malignant.

Birthday rule If both parents of a child have a family health plan, the insurance plan of the parent whose birthday comes earlier in the year is defined as the primary insurance plan covering the child. The insurance of the other parent becomes secondary insurance.

Bit The smallest unit of computer storage capacity.

Bladder catheterization The passing of a sterile catheter through the urethra and into the bladder to remove urine.

Blocked Times in the appointment schedule when physicians are not available to see patients.

Blood antigen A protein present on the surface of red blood cells that determines a person's blood type.

Body language Communication that is expressed through facial expressions, body position, muscle activity, and other nonverbal means.

Body mechanics Utilization of the correct muscles to maintain proper balance, posture, and body alignment to accomplish a task safely and efficiently without undue strain on any muscle or joint.

Bookkeeping The process of keeping detailed records of financial transactions.

Bounding pulse A pulse with an increased volume that feels very strong and full.

Bradycardia An abnormally slow heart rate (less than 60 beats per minute).

Bradypnea An abnormal decrease in the respiratory rate of less than 10 respirations per minute.

Brain stem The portion of the brain, between the diencephalon and spinal cord, that contains the midbrain, pons, and medulla oblongata.

Braxton Hicks contractions Intermittent and irregular painless uterine contractions that occur throughout pregnancy. They occur more frequently toward the end of pregnancy and are sometimes mistaken for true labor pains.

Broadband A method of transmitting electronic data that handles a wide range of frequencies.

Bronchi The airways that are formed when the trachea branches.

Bronchial tree The bronchi and all their branches that function as passageways between the trachea and the alveoli.

Buffy coat A thin, light-colored layer of white blood cells and platelets that lies between a top layer of plasma and a bottom layer of red blood cells when an anticoagulant has been added to a blood specimen.

Bulbus oculi The eyeball.

Burn An injury to the tissues caused by exposure to thermal, chemical, electrical, or radioactive agents.

Burnout Disillusionment with work and physical or emotional exhaustion.

Byte A unit of computer storage capacity, usually eight bits. One byte is approximately equal to one character.

C

Calibration A mechanism to check the precision and accuracy of a test system, such as an automated analyzer, to determine if the system is providing accurate results. Calibration is typically performed using a calibration device, often called a *standard*.

Call-in times Blocks of time when a physician accepts telephone calls from patients.

Canthus The junction of the eyelids at either corner of the eye.

Capillary action The action that causes liquid to rise along a wick, a tube, or a gauze dressing.

Capitation A method of paying for insurance in which a fixed amount is paid to the provider per member for a specific time period regardless of the amount of care provided.

Cardiac cycle A complete heartbeat consisting of contraction and relaxation of both atria and both ventricles.

Carrier An insurance company.

Case law Law established by decisions of previous court cases.

Cash basis of accounting Accounting method in which income is entered when payment is received.

Cashier's check A check drawn on a bank instead of an individual account.

Cell-mediated immunity Immunity that is the result of T-cell action.

Celsius scale A temperature scale on which the freezing point of water is 0° and the boiling point of water is 100°; also called the centigrade scale.

Central sulcus The groove or furrow between the frontal and parietal lobes of the cerebrum; also called the fissure of Rolando.

Cerebellum Second largest part of the human brain, located posterior to the pons and medulla oblongata and involved in the coordination of muscular movements.

Cerebrospinal fluid A fluid, similar to plasma, that fills the subarchnoid space around the brain and spinal cord and is in the ventricles of the brain.

Cerebrum The largest and uppermost part of the human brain; concerned with consciousness, learning, memory, sensations, and voluntary movements.

Certified check A check on an individual account that a bank assumes responsibility for, usually by withdrawing funds to cover the check from the checking account at the time the check is certified.

Cerumen Earwax.

Ceruminous gland A gland in the ear canal that produces cerumen or ear wax.

Cervix The lower narrow end of the uterus that opens into the vagina.

CHAMPVA A government health insurance program that covers dependents of military veterans with service-connected disabilities.

Charge slip A form used to keep track of charges and payments at the time of a patient visit.

Chemoreceptor A sensory receptor that detects the presence of chemicals; responsible for taste, smell, and monitoring of the concentration of certain chemicals in body fluids.

Chemotherapy The use of chemicals to treat disease. Chemotherapy is most often used to refer to the treatment of cancer using antineoplastic medications.

Chief complaint A statement of the most important symptom or symptoms for which a patient is seeking care.

Cholesterol A white waxy, fatlike substance that is essential for normal functioning of the body.

Chondrocyte Cartilage cell.

Chronic Existing over a long period of time.

Chyme The semifluid mixture of food and gastric juice that leaves the stomach through the pyloric sphincter.

Cilia Slender, hairlike projections that constantly beat toward the outside to remove microorganisms from the body.

Circadian rhythms Biological clock or a person's 24-hour rhythm such as a natural sleep-wake cycle.

Civil law Law that regulates relationships and interactions between individuals and groups.

Claim message Messages encouraging payment of a bill, usually attached to or printed on the monthly statement.

Clinical age Method of timing in development that begins with the last menstrual period; two weeks more than developmental age.

Clinical diagnosis A tentative diagnosis of a patient's condition obtained through evaluation of the health history and the physical examination, without the benefit of laboratory or diagnostic tests.

Cloning Producing genetically identical cells or individuals artificially.

Closed questions Questions that anticipate a yes or no or a short answer.

Cloud computing A model where the Internet is used to store and access data and programs, and servers are not physically located at the same site as the computer.

Clustering Scheduling similar types of patients or examinations on the same day or part of the day.

Coagulation The process of blood clotting.

Cocci (sing. *coccus*) Bacteria that have a round shape.

Cochlea Spiral or snail-shaped portion of the inner ear.

Coinsurance A percentage of the allowed charge for health services, which the patient is responsible for paying.

Collagenous fibers Strong and flexible connective tissue fibers that contain the protein collagen.

Collate To assemble the pages of a document in numeric order.

Collection agency A firm that is in the business of collecting overdue accounts.

Colonoscope An endoscope that is specially designed for passage through the anus to permit visualization of the rectum and the entire length of the colon.

Colonoscopy The visualization of the rectum and the entire colon using a colonoscope.

Colposcope A lighted instrument with a binocular magnifying lens used to examine the vagina and cervix.

Colposcopy Visual examination of the cervix using a colposcope (a lighted instrument with a magnifying lens).

Common law Unwritten body of law based on general custom.

Comparative negligence A defense to a lawsuit that establishes a percentage of responsibility for injury on the part of the plaintiff.

Complete protein A protein that contains all of the essential amino acids needed by the body.

Complimentary closing Words used as a polite ending to a letter just before the writer's signature.

Compress A soft, moist, absorbent cloth that is folded in several layers and applied to a part of the body in the local application of heat or cold.

Computer An electronic machine that has the ability to process data according to a program in order to produce a desired result.

Computer system All of the hardware and software components making up the computer.

Conduction The transfer of energy, such as heat, from one object to another by direct contact.

Conduction myofibers Cardiac muscle cells specialized for conducting action potentials to the myocardium; part of the conduction system of the heart; also called *Purkinje fibers*.

Consultation report A narrative report of an opinion about a patient's condition by a practitioner other than the attending physician.

Contagious Capable of being transmitted directly or indirectly from one person to another.

Contaminate To soil, stain, or pollute; to make impure. An aseptic object is contaminated when it touches something that is not clean. As it relates to sterile technique, to cause a sterile object or surface to become unsterile.

Contingency A condition that must be met before a contract is binding.

Continuing Education Unit (CEU) A standard unit of measure of continuing education for professionals, defined as 1 contact hour by the AAMA, but also commonly 10 contact hours of participation.

Contractility The ability of muscle cells to shorten to produce movement.

Contrast medium A substance used to make a particular structure visible on a radiograph.

Contributory negligence A defense to a lawsuit that establishes any responsibility for injury on the part of the plaintiff.

Control A solution that is used to monitor a test system to ensure the reliability and accuracy of test results.

Controlled drug A drug that has restrictions placed on it by the federal government because of its potential for abuse.

Controlled substance A drug that has the potential for addiction or abuse.

Contusion An injury to the tissues under the skin that causes blood vessels to rupture, allowing blood to seep into the tissues; a bruise.

Convection The transfer of energy, such as heat, through air currents.

Conversion Changing from one system of measurement to another.

Coordination of benefits Rules followed by insurance companies so that no claim is reimbursed at more than 100% of the charges.

Copayment A fixed amount of money that the patient must pay for any health care service.

Corpora cavernosa Two dorsal columns of erectile tissue found in the penis.

Corpus albicans Scar tissue in the ovary that forms when the corpus luteum degenerates.

Corpus luteum The yellow structure that develops from the mature follicle after ovulation.

Corpus spongiosum Ventral column of erectile tissue found in the penis.

Cover letter A letter sent with one or more documents (such as a résumé) to provide an explanation.

Crash cart A specially equipped cart for holding and transporting medications, equipment, and supplies needed for lifesaving procedures in an emergency.

Credit A posting that is subtracted from an account balance.

Credit balance A negative balance on a patient account (i.e., money is owed by the medical office), usually a result of an overpayment.

Crepitus A grating sensation caused by fractured bone fragments rubbing against each other.

Crime An offense in violation of a law that prohibits or requires certain behavior.

Criminal law Law that regulates offenses against the public welfare.

Crisis A sudden falling of an elevated body temperature to normal.

Crista ampullaris Receptor organ located within the ampulla of the semicircular canals; functions in dynamic equilibrium.

Critical item An item that comes in contact with sterile tissue or the vascular system.

Cross-index To file under one unit and use a guide or card filed under another unit that refers to the primary filing location.

Cryosurgery The therapeutic use of freezing temperatures to destroy abnormal tissue.

Cubic centimeter The amount of space occupied by 1 milliliter (1 mL = 1 cc).

Culture The growth of microorganisms in a culture medium.

Culture medium A mixture of nutrients on which microorganisms are grown in the laboratory.

Curative treatment Treatment that cures disease.

Cutaneous membrane A type of epithelial membrane; skin.

Cyanosis A bluish discoloration of the skin and mucous membranes.

Cytokinesis Division of the cell at the end of mitosis to form two separate daughter cells.

Cytology The science that deals with the study of cells, including their origin, structure, function, and pathology.

D

Data Raw, unorganized facts about subject matter presented to the computer for processing.

Data processing The changing of raw facts or data into usable information following a three-part sequence: input, processing, output.

Day sheet The record of daily transactions in the pegboard or "write-it-once system" and also in computer medical billing programs.

DEA Number A registration number assigned to physicians by the Drug Enforcement Administration for prescribing or dispensing controlled drugs.

Debit A posting that is added to an account balance.

Decontamination The use of physical or chemical means to remove, inactivate, or destroy pathogens on a surface or item to the point where they are no longer capable of transmitting infectious particles or disease; the surface or item is rendered safe for handling, use, or disposal.

Decussation A crossing over; usually refers to motor fibers that cross over to the opposite side in the medulla oblongata.

Deductible An amount of money that an insured person must pay annually before health services are covered by the insurance plan.

Defecation The expulsion of indigestible wastes, or feces, through the anus.

Defendant The person or group against which an action is brought in a court of law.

Deglutition The process of swallowing.

Dendrites The branching (tree-like) afferent processes of a neuron that receive impulses from other neurons and transmit them to the cell body.

Denial Failure to acknowledge the reality of a situation.

Depreciation Accounting methods to respond to the loss of value of a property or piece of equipment over time.

Dermis Inner layer of the skin that contains the blood vessels, nerves, glands, and hair follicles.

Detergent An agent that cleanses by emulsifying dirt and oil.

Detruser muscle The smooth muscle in the wall of the urinary bladder.

Developmenal age Method of timing in development that begins with fertilization; two weeks less than clinical age.

Diagnosis The scientific method of determining and identifying a patient's condition.

Diagnostic procedure A procedure performed to assist in the diagnosis, management, or treatment of a patient's condition.

Diagnosis-related group (DRG) A system to determine Medicare reimbursement for a hospital stay on the basis of the patient's diagnosis.

Diapedesis The process by which white blood cells squeeze between the cells in a vessel wall to enter the tissue spaces outside the blood vessel.

Diaphysis The long straight shaft of a long bone.

Diarthrosis Freely movable joint characterized by a joint cavity; also called a synovial joint; plural, diarthroses.

Diastole The phase in the cardiac cycle in which the heart relaxes between contractions; opposite of systole.

Diastolic pressure The point of lesser pressure on the arterial wall, which is recorded during diastole.

Diencephalon Part of the brain between the cerebral hemispheres and the midbrain; includes the thalamus, and hypothalamus.

Differential diagnosis A determination of which of two or more diseases with similar symptoms is producing a patient's symptoms.

Diffusion Movement of substances from a region of high concentration to a region of low concentration.

Digital image A picture that is stored electronically to allow viewing on a computer.

Digital subscriber line (DSL) Technology that allows digital signals to be transmitted over telephone lines at high speed even if the telephone line is also being used for voice transmission.

Dilation (of the cervix) The stretching of the external os from an opening a few millimeters wide to an opening large enough to allow the passage of an infant (approximately 10 cm).

Disaccharide A simple carbohydrate consisting of two sugar units.

Disaster A sudden event that causes damage or loss of life.

Disbursements Money paid out.

Discharge A brief summary of the significant events of a patient's hospitalization.

Disinfectant An agent used to destroy pathogenic microorganisms but not their spores. Disinfectants are usually applied to inanimate objects.

Dislocation An injury in which one end of a bone making up a joint is separated or displaced from its normal anatomic position.

Diuresis Secretion and passage of large amounts of urine.

Do-not-resuscitate (DNR) order A medical order signed by a physician that relieves health care personnel from the obligation to resuscitate a patient who stops breathing or whose heart stops.

Documentation A written set of instructions accompanying an application program, designed to assist the user in understanding how to operate the program. Examples include the user manual, help screens, and reference cards.

Documenting The process of making written or electronic entries about a patient in the medical record.

Dose The quantity of a drug to be administered at one time.

Double booking Scheduling two patients for the same appointment time.

Drug A chemical used for the treatment, prevention, or diagnosis of disease.

Drug Enforcement Administration (DEA) The federal agency that enforces the Controlled Substances Act of 1970.

Ductus deferens Tubular structure that is continuous with the epididymis; it ascends through the inguinal canal and transports sperm to the ejaculatory duct.

Duplex To produce double-sided copies by storing images from both sides of the original in the memory of a photocopier.

Duty Commitment to act in a certain way.

Dysmenorrhea Pain associated with the menstrual period.

Dyspareunia Pain in the vagina or pelvis experienced by a woman during sexual intercourse.

Dysplasia The growth of abnormal cells. Dysplasia is a precancerous condition that may or may not develop into cancer.

Dyspnea Shortness of breath or difficulty in breathing.

Dysrhythmia An irregular heart rate or rhythm; also termed *arrhythmia*.

Dysuria Difficult or painful urination.

E

Echocardiogram An ultrasound examination of the heart.

Ectocervix The part of the cervix that projects into the vagina and is lined with stratified squamous epithelium.

Edema The retention of fluid in the tissues, resulting in swelling.

Effacement The thinning and shortening of the cervical canal from its normal length of 1 to 2 cm to a structure with paper-thin edges in which there is no canal at all. Effacement occurs late in pregnancy, during labor, or both. The purpose of effacement along with dilation is to permit the passage of the infant into the birth canal.

Ego defense mechanism Unconscious mental process that offers psychological protection.

Elastic fibers Yellow connective tissue fibers that are not particularly strong but can be stretched and will return to their normal shape when released.

Elasticity The ability of tissue to return to its original shape after contraction or extension.

Electrocardiogram (ECG) The graphic representation of the electrical activity of the heart.

Electrocardiogram (ECG) cycle The graphic representation of a heartbeat.

Electrocardiograph The instrument used to record the electrical activity of the heart.

Electrode A conductor of electricity, which is used to promote contact between the body and the electrocardiograph.

Electrolyte A chemical substance that promotes conduction of an electrical current.

Electronic health record (EHR) A patient health record that is stored on a computer.

Electronic signature An electronic sound, symbol, or process added to an electronic record that indicates intent to sign.

Eligibility Enrollment status related to a health insurance plan.

Email A method of composing, sending, receiving, and storing messages that are sent over the Internet.

Emancipated minor A person younger than the age of 18 with the rights of an adult including the ability to consent to medical care.

Embezzlement Fraudulent appropriation of funds or property of an employer or client.

Embryo The child in utero from the time of conception through the first 8 weeks of development.

Embryonic period Stage of development that lasts from the beginning of the third week until the end of the eighth week after fertilization; period during which the organ systems develop in the body.

Emergency action plan A written document that describes the actions that employees should take to ensure their safety if a fire or other emergency situation occurs.

Emergency medical services (EMS) system A network of community resources, equipment, and personnel that provides care to victims of injury or sudden illness.

Emergency preparedness The process of making plans to prevent, respond, and recover from an emergency situation.

Empathy Objective awareness and sensitivity to the feelings and emotions of others.

Empirical Learned from observation or experiment.

Encryption A process by which electronic information is changed into an unreadable form that requires the original encryption software to reverse the process.

Endocardium The thin, smooth inner lining of each chamber of the heart.

Endocervix The mucous membrane lining the cervical canal.

Endocrine gland Gland that secretes its product directly into the blood; opposite of exocrine gland.

Endocrinology Study of the endocrine glands.

Endometrium Innermost mucous membrane layer of the uterine wall.

Endoscope An instrument that consists of a tube and an optical system that is used for direct visual inspection of organs or cavities.

Endosteum Membranous lining of a cavity within a bone.

Enema An injection of fluid into the rectum to aid in the elimination of feces from the colon.

Engagement The entrance of the fetal head or the presenting part into the pelvic inlet.

Enteral nutrition The delivery of nutrients through a tube inserted into the gastrointestinal tract.

Enunciation The act of speaking clearly and concisely.

Epicardium The outer layer of the heart wall; the visceral pericardium.

Epidermis Outermost layer of the skin.

Epididymis Tightly coiled tubule along the posterior margin of each testicle; functions in the maturation and storage of sperm.

Epimysium Fibrous connective tissue that surrounds a whole muscle.

Epiphyseal line The remnant of the epiphyseal plate after the cartilage calcifies and growth ceases.

Epiphyseal plate The cartilaginous plate between the epiphysis and diaphysis of a bone; responsible for the lengthwise growth of a long bone.

Epiphysis The end of a long bone.

Erythema Reddening of the skin caused by dilation of superficial blood vessels in the skin.

Erythrocyte Red blood cell.

Erythropoiesis The process of red blood cell formation.

Erythropoietin A hormone released by the kidneys that stimulates red blood cell production.

Essential amino acid An amino acid that is required by the body, but cannot be manufactured by the body and must be obtained from food.

Established patient A patient who has been seen by one of the physicians in the practice within the past 3 years.

Estrogens Group of hormones that stimulate the development of female secondary sex characteristics.

Ethics The branch of knowledge that deals with standards of behavior or beliefs.

Eupnea Normal respiration. The rate is 16 to 20 respirations per minute, the rhythm is even and regular, and the depth is normal.

Evacuated tube A closed glass or plastic tube that contains a premeasured vacuum.

Evacuation A planned systemic retreat of people to safety in an emergency situation.

Evacuation procedures Clear step-by-step procedures for the rapid, efficient, and safe removal of individuals from a building during an emergency.

Excitability The ability of muscle and nerve tissue to receive and respond to stimuli; also called irritability.

Exhalation The act of breathing out.

Exit route A continuous and unobstructed path of travel from any point within a workplace to a place of safety.

Exocrine gland Gland that secrets its product to a surface or cavity through ducts; opposite of endocrine gland.

Expected date of delivery (EDD) Projected birth date of the infant.

Explanation of benefits (EOB) A statement issued by the insurance carrier explaining reimbursement for specific procedures.

Extensibility The ability of muscle tissue to stretch when pulled.

External os The opening of the cervical canal of the uterus into the vagina.

External respiration Exchange of gases between the lungs and the blood.

Exudate A discharge produced by the body's tissues.

F

Fahrenheit scale A temperature scale on which the freezing point of water is 32° and the boiling point of water is 212°.

False-negative result A test result denoting that a condition is absent when it is actually present.

False-positive result A test result denoting that a condition is present when it is actually absent.

Familial Occurring in or affecting members of a family more frequently than would be expected by chance.

Fasting Abstaining from food or fluids (except water) for a specified amount of time before the collection of a specimen.

Fauces Opening from the oral cavity into the oropharynx.

Fax Transmission of scanned, printed material by telephone. A short form of the word *facsimile*.

Febrile Pertaining to fever.

Fee-for-service A means of payment for health care in which the cost for each service provided is reimbursed in full or in part.

Fee-for-service insurance Insurance reimbursement that is directly related to the services provided and the amount charged by the provider.

Fee schedule List of charges (fees) for specific procedures that may be performed in a medical office.

Fee splitting The practice of sharing fees with colleagues, especially for making referrals.

Felony A serious crime punishable by death or imprisonment.

Fetal heart rate The number of times per minute the fetal heart beats.

Fetal heart tones The sounds of the heartbeat of the fetus heard through the mother's abdominal wall.

Fetal period Stage of development that starts at the beginning of the ninth week after fertilization and lasts until birth.

Fetus The child in utero from the third month after conception to birth; during the first 2 months of development, it is called an *embryo*.

Fever A body temperature that is above normal; synonym for pyrexia.

Fibroblast An immature cell from which connective tissue can develop.

Fidelity Faithfulness.

Filing system The way in which records are arranged. Common filing systems in the medical office include alphabetic, numeric, by subject, or chronologic.

Fire extinguisher A portable device that discharges an agent designed to extinguish a fire.

Fire prevention plan A written document that identifies flammable and combustible materials stored in the workplace and ways to control workplace fire hazards.

Fire protection The implementation of safety measures to reduce the unwanted effects of fire.

Firewall A system that protects a computer network from unauthorized access by users on its own network or another network, such as the Internet.

First aid The immediate care administered before complete medical care can be provided to an individual who is injured or suddenly becomes ill.

Fixed appointment scheduling An appointment scheduling method in which each patient is given a different, specific appointment time. Also called *stream scheduling, time-specified scheduling,* or *single booking*.

Flow rate The number of liters of oxygen per minute that come out of an oxygen delivery system.

Flow sheet A paper document or electronic screen that allows similar data to be recorded and viewed chronologically.

Fluoroscope An instrument used to view internal organs and structures directly.

Fluoroscopy Examination of a patient with a fluoroscope.

Forceps A two-pronged instrument for grasping and squeezing.

Formulary An insurance carrier's official list of covered medications to be used by network providers.

Fracture Any break in a bone.

Fraud Intentional deception resulting in injury or loss.

Frenulum linguae The midline fold that connects the undersurface of the tongue with the floor of the mouth.

Frequency The condition of having to urinate often.

Full block style A letter format in which all parts of the letter are left justified.

Fundus The dome-shaped upper portion of the uterus between the fallopian tubes.

Furuncle A localized staphylococcal infection that originates deep within a hair follicle. Also known as a *boil*.

G

Gametes Sex cells: sperm and ova.

Gastric juice The secretions of the exocrine gastric glands.

Gastrin Hormone secreted by the endocrine glands in the stomach.

Gauge The diameter of the lumen of a needle used to administer medication.

Gene therapy Giving patients new genes or parts of genes to treat a disease or condition.

General senses Senses that are located throughout the body; somatic senses.

Genetic engineering Making, altering, or repairing genetic material.

Gestation The period of intrauterine development from conception to birth; the period of pregnancy. The average pregnancy lasts about 280 days, or 40 weeks, from the date of conception to childbirth.

Gestational age The age of the fetus between conception and birth.

Gigabyte (GB) A unit of computer storage capacity. One gigabyte is equal to a little more than 1 billion bytes or 1000 megabytes.

Gingiva Soft tissue that covers the alveolar processes of the mandible and maxillae; also called gums.

Glomerular capsule Double-layered epithelial cup that surrounds the glomerulus in a nephron; also called Bowman capsule.

Glomerular filtration The movement of blood plasma across the filtration membrane in the renal corpuscle.

Glomerulus Cluster of capillaries in the nephron through which blood is filtered.

Glucocorticoids Hormones from the adrenal cortex that raise blood sugar levels.

Gluten A type of protein found in certain grains such as wheat, rye, and barley.

Glycogen The form in which carbohydrate is stored in the body.

Glycosuria The presence of glucose in the urine.

Glycosylation The process of glucose attaching to hemoglobin.

Gonadocorticoids Sex hormones secreted by the adrenal cortex.

Gonads Primary reproductive organs; organs that produce the gametes: testes in the male and ovaries in the female.

Grammar The study of accepted rules used to create meaning in a language.

Granulocytes Cells that develop granules in the cytoplasm; granular leukocytes.

Gross pay The total amount earned in a time period by an employee before any deductions.

Group plan One insurance policy that covers a group of people.

Guarantor A person with financial responsibility for a bill who may or may not also be a patient.

Gustatory sense Sense of taste.

Gynecology The branch of medicine that deals with the diseases of reproductive organs of women.

H

Hand hygiene The process of cleansing or sanitizing the hands.

Hard copy Printed output from a computer.

Hard disk drive A storage device consisting of one or more rigid, nonflexible platters coated with a magnetically sensitive material and encased in a permanently sealed, airtight container.

Hardware The physical devices making up a computer system (e.g., main computer unit, keyboard, monitor, printer).

Hazardous chemical Any chemical which is classified as a health or physical hazard, a simple asphyxiant, a combustible dust, pyrophoric gas or hazard not otherwise classified.

HAZMAT An acronym constructed from the beginnings of the two words "*haz*ardous *mat*erials." It refers to materials that pose a danger to health or the environment and must be handled with protective equipment.

HDL cholesterol A lipoprotein, consisting of protein and cholesterol, that removes excess cholesterol from the cells.

Health care proxy A legal document that names an agent to make decisions about a person's medical care if he or she becomes unable to make wishes known.

Health coaching A process that helps patients identify their values related to health, set health goals, and take steps to meet their personal goals.

Health history A collection of subjective data about a patient.

Health insurance Purchase of protection for covered services related to health care.

Hematology The study of blood and blood-forming tissues.

Hematoma A swelling or mass of coagulated blood caused by a break in a blood vessel.

Hematopoiesis Blood cell production, which occurs in the red bone marrow; also called *hemopoiesis*.

Hematuria Blood present in the urine.

Hemoconcentration An increase in the concentration of the nonfilterable blood components in the blood vessels, such as red blood cells, enzymes, iron, and calcium, as a result of a decrease in the fluid content of the blood.

Hemocytoblast A stem cell in the bone marrow from which the blood cells arise.

Hemoglobin The protein- and iron-containing pigment of erythrocytes that transports oxygen in the body.

Hemoglobin A_{1c} Compound formed when glucose attaches or glycosylates to the protein in hemoglobin.

Hemolysis The breakdown of blood cells.

Hemophilia An inherited bleeding disorder caused by a deficiency of a clotting factor needed for proper coagulation of the blood.

Hemostasis The control or stoppage of bleeding by natural or artificial means.

Hierarchy Classified according to rank or importance.

Histology Branch of microscopic anatomy that studies tissues.

Holistic Considering the whole; in medicine, considering the entire person when providing health care.

Home health care The provision of medical and nonmedical care in a patient's home or place of residence.

Homeostasis The state in which body systems are functioning normally and the internal environment of the body is in equilibrium; the body is in a healthy state.

Hormones A substance secreted by an endocrine gland.

Hospice Palliative service provided for patients whose life expectancy is less than 6 months, including aiding with comfort, pain relief, and personal care. Services may be provided in the patient's home, a nursing home, or a special hospice facility. Manages care for dying patients including comfort, pain relief, and personal care.

Human anatomy Study of human body shape and structure and the relationships of its parts.

Human physiology Study of the functions of humans and their separate parts.

Hydrolysis Chemical breakdown of complex molecules by the addition of water.

Hyperglycemia An abnormally high level of glucose in the blood.

Hyperopia Farsightedness.

Hyperpnea An abnormal increase in the rate and depth of respiration.

Hyperpyrexia An extremely high fever.

Hypertension High blood pressure.

Hyperventilation An abnormally fast and deep type of breathing, usually associated with acute anxiety conditions.

Hypodermis Below the skin; a sheet of areolar connective tissue and adipose beneath the dermis of the skin.

Hypoglycemia An abnormally low level of glucose in the blood.

Hypopnea An abnormal decrease in the rate and depth of respiration.

Hypotension Low blood pressure.

Hypothermia A life-threatening condition in which the temperature of the entire body falls to a dangerously low level, or below normal body temperature.

Hypoxemia A decrease in the oxygen saturation of the blood. Hypoxemia may lead to hypoxia.

Hypoxia A reduction in the oxygen supply to the tissues of the body.

Ileocecal valve The valve between the small intestine and large intestine.

Immune globulin A blood product consisting of pooled human plasma containing antibodies.

Immunity The resistance of the body to the effects of a harmful agent, such as a pathogenic microorganism and its toxins.

Immunization (active, artificial) The process of becoming immune or of rendering an individual immune through the use of a vaccine or toxoid.

Immunoglobulins Substances produced by the body that inactivate or destroy other substances that are introduced into the body; antibodies.

Impacted Wedged firmly together so as to be immovable.

In vivo Occurring in the living body or organism.

Inactive record The medical record of a patient who has not been seen within the past 2 to 3 years, or some other time frame specified by a given medical office.

Incision A clean cut caused by a cutting instrument.

Incomplete protein A protein that lacks one or more of the essential amino acids needed by the body.

Incubate To provide proper conditions for growth and development. In microbiology, the act of placing a culture in a chamber (incubator) that provides optimal growth requirements for the multiplication of the organisms, such as the proper temperature, humidity, and darkness.

Incubation period The interval of time between the invasion by a pathogenic microorganism and the appearance of first symptoms of the disease.

Indemnity An obligation to provide compensation for loss or damage.

Indexing units Pieces of information used to identify a correct filing location.

Induration An abnormally raised, hardened area of the skin with clearly defined margins.

Infant A child from birth to 12 months of age.

Infection The condition in which the body, or part of it, is invaded by a pathogen.

Infectious disease A disease caused by a pathogen that produces harmful effects on its host (also known as a *communicable disease*).

Infiltration The process by which a substance passes into and is deposited within the substance of a cell, tissue, or organ.

Inflammation A protective response of the body to trauma and the entrance of foreign matter. The purpose of inflammation is to destroy invading microorganisms and to remove damaged tissue debris from the area so that proper healing can occur.

Informed consent Agreement to a medical procedure based on understanding of the procedure and its possible consequences and effects.

Infusion The administration of fluids, medications, or nutrients into a vein.

Inhalation The act of breathing in.

Inhalation administration The administration of medication by way of air or other vapor being drawn into the lungs.

Initiative The ability to begin or carry through on a plan of action independently.

Inpatient A patient who has been admitted to a health care facility for at least one overnight stay.

Input 1. (noun) Data that have been entered into the computer. 2. (verb) The transfer of data to the computer for processing.

Input device A device for entering data into the computer (e.g., keyboard, mouse, scanner).

Internet A global system of interconnected computer networks that use the Internet protocol (TCP/IP) to transmit and exchange data.

Inscription The part of a prescription that indicates the name of the drug and the drug dosage.

Insertion The end of a muscle that is attached to a relatively movable part; the end opposite the origin.

Inspection The process of observing a patient to detect signs of disease.

Instillation The dropping of a liquid into a body cavity.

Insufflate To blow a powder, vapor, or gas (e.g., air) into a body cavity.

Insured The individual who has a specific insurance plan.

Intercostal Between the ribs.

Internal respiration Exchange of gases between the blood and tissue cells.

Interstitial cells Cells between the seminiferous tubules in the testes; produce testosterone; also cells of Leydig.

Interval The length of a wave or the length of a wave with a segment.

Intradermal injection Introduction of medication into the dermal layer of the skin.

Intramuscular injection Introduction of medication into the muscular layer of the body.

Intravenous (IV) therapy The administration of a liquid agent directly into a patient's vein, where it is distributed throughout the body by way of the circulatory system.

Inventory A detailed list of items in stock or in possession of an individual or business.

Invoice An itemized bill for items whose cost has not been prepaid.

Irrigation The washing of a body canal with a flowing solution.

Ischemia Deficiency of blood in a body part.

J

Judgmental Critical or negative; making judgments about what is good or bad based on personal opinion.

Juxtaglomerular apparatus Complex of modified cells in the afferent arteriole and the ascending limb and distal tubule in the kidney; helps regulate blood pressure by secreting renin; consists of the macula densa and juxtaglomerular cells.

K

Keratinization Process by which the cells of the epidermis become filled with keratin and move to the surface where they are sloughed off.

Ketonuria The presence of ketone bodies in the urine.

Ketosis An accumulation of large amounts of ketone bodies in the tissues and body fluids.

Kilobyte (KB) A unit of computer storage capacity. One kilobyte is equal to 1024 bytes (characters).

Kilocalorie The amount of heat needed to raise the temperature of 1 kilogram of water 1 degree Celsius. (Often referred to as a calorie).

Korotkoff sounds Sounds heard during the measurement of blood pressure that are used to determine the systolic and diastolic blood pressure readings.

L

Laboratory test The clinical analysis and study of materials, fluids, or tissues obtained from patients to assist in diagnosis and treatment of disease.

Laceration A wound in which the tissues are torn apart, leaving ragged and irregular edges.

Lacrimal apparatus The structures that produce and convey tears.

Lactation Milk production and ejection from the mammary glands.

Lactose A disaccharide which consists of two sugar units and is found in milk and milk products.

Larceny Stealing another person's property or money without violence.

Laryngopharynx Portion of the pharynx that is behind the larynx and extends from the level of the hyoid bone to the lower margin of the larynx.

Larynx Passageway for air between the pharynx and trachea; commonly called the voice box.

LDL cholesterol A lipoprotein, consisting of protein and cholesterol, that picks up cholesterol and delivers it to the cells.

Ledger A book, card, or computer account used to record financial transactions.

Left justified Lines of type that begin at the left margin of a document.

Length (recumbent) The measurement from the vertex of the head to the heel of the foot in a supine position.

Letterhead A sheet of stationery preprinted with information about a business, including name, address, telephone number, and other information.

Leukocyte White blood cell.

Leukocytosis An abnormal increase in the number of white blood cells (greater than 11,000 per cubic millimeter of blood).

Leukopenia An abnormal decrease in the number of white blood cells (less than 4500 per cubic millimeter of blood).

Liabilities Legal responsibilities. In accounting, the amount owed by a business to creditors.

License Official permission to perform an activity or practice a profession.

Licensure The process by which the state examines qualifications and gives permission to an individual or organization to engage in a profession or business.

Ligate To tie off and close a structure such as a severed blood vessel.

Lipoprotein A complex molecule consisting of protein and a lipid fraction such as cholesterol. Lipoproteins function in transporting lipids in the blood.

Litigation The process of taking a lawsuit through the courts.

Living will A legal document that specifies the kind of medical treatment a patient wants or does not want if he or she becomes incapacitated.

Load The articles that are being sterilized.

Local anesthetic A drug that produces a loss of feeling and an inability to perceive pain in only a specific part of the body.

Lower esophageal sphincter Valve between the esophagus and stomach.

Lower respiratory tract Portion of the respiratory tract that is inferior to the larynx; includes the trachea, bronchial tree, and lungs.

M

Macronutrient A nutrient required in relatively large amounts by the body. Includes carbohydrates, fat, and protein.

Macrophage Large phagocytic connective tissue cell that functions in immune responses; name given to a monocyte after it leaves the blood and enters the tissues.

Macula lutea Yellowish depression on the retina.

Main computer memory The part of the CPU that is responsible for temporarily storing information until it is needed for processing by the computer. Main memory in a microcomputer is known as *RAM*.

Malaise A vague sense of body discomfort, weakness, and fatigue that often marks the onset of a disease and continues through the course of the illness.

Malfeasance A crime or wrongdoing that is illegal or contrary to official obligation.

Malpractice Negligence by a professional.

Man-made disaster An event that causes serious damage through intentional or negligent human actions or the failure of a man-made system.

Managed care A movement in health care based on reducing health care costs while providing high-quality care. The term may be used for the techniques used to reduce costs or for the companies that pay for the care provided.

Manometer An instrument for measuring pressure.

Mast cell A connective tissue cell that produces heparin and histamine.

Mastication The process of chewing.

Mayo tray A broad, flat metal tray placed on a stand and used to hold sterile instruments and supplies when it has been covered with a sterile towel.

Mechanoreceptor A sensory receptor that responds to a bending or deformation of the cell; examples include receptors for touch, pressure, hearing, and equilibrium.

Mediation Negotiation by a third party to help two parties resolve a dispute.

Medicaid The government insurance program for low-income individuals and families that is funded both by the federal government and by each individual state. The Medicaid program has a different name in each state.

Medical asepsis Practices that are employed to inhibit the growth and hinder the transmission of pathogenic microorganisms to prevent the spread of infection.

Medical necessity Health care that is reasonable and necessary for a patient based on evidence-based clinical standards of care.

Medical practice A program that provides instructions to the computer for performing medical practice management procedures.

Medical record A written record of important information regarding a patient, including the care of that individual and the progress of the patient's condition.

Medical record format The way a medical record is organized. The two main types of medical record formats are the source-oriented record and the problem-oriented record.

Medical record management Activities related to the creation, management, use, and disposition of patient medical records.

Medicare The federal health insurance program that provides insurance coverage for the elderly, permanently disabled, and individuals with end-stage kidney disease.

Medicare administrative contractor (MAC) A multistate, regional independent business that administers both Medicare Part A and Medicare Part B claims under a contract with CMS.

Megabyte (MB) A unit of computer storage capacity. One megabyte is equal to a little more than 1 million bytes or 1000 kilobytes.

Megakaryocytes A large cell that contributes to the formation of platelets.

Meiosis Type of nuclear division in which the number of chromosomes is reduced to one half the number found in a body cell; results in the formation of egg or sperm.

Melena The darkening of the stool caused by the presence of blood in an amount of 50 mL or greater.

Melanin A dark brown or black pigment found in parts of the body, especially skin and hair.

Melanocyte A cell that produces the dark or black pigment melanin.

Memo (memorandum) A form of communication within a company that is usually short and limited to one subject.

Menarche First period of menstrual bleeding at puberty.

Meninges Connective tissue membranes that cover the brain and spinal cord.

Meniscus The curved surface on a column of liquid in a tube.

Menopause The permanent cessation of menstruation, which usually occurs between the ages of 45 and 55.

Menorrhagia Excessive bleeding during a menstrual period, in the number of days or the amount of blood or both. Also called *dysfunctional uterine bleeding (DUB)*.

Mensuration The process of measuring a patient.

Mesentery Extensions of peritoneum that are associated with the intestine.

Metered mail Mail for which the postage has been applied using a postage meter.

Metrorrhagia Bleeding between menstrual periods.

Microbiology The scientific study of microorganisms and their activities.

Microcomputer A small general-purpose computer that relies on a tiny microprocessor chip to perform its processing functions.

Micronutrient A nutrient required in very small amounts by the body. Includes vitamins and minerals.

Microorganism A microscopic plant or animal.

Microprocessor The "brain" of the computer housed in the main unit that interprets and executes the instructions that operate the computer. The microprocessor is a chip that resides on the mainboard in the main unit of the computer.

Micturition Act of expelling urine from the bladder; also called voiding or urination.

MICR line A line of numbers containing the ABA transit routing number and the account number that appears at the bottom left of a check. These numbers are read by a magnetic ink character recognition (MICR) system.

Mineral A naturally occurring inorganic substance this is essential to the proper functioning of the body.

Mineralocorticoids A group of hormones secreted by the adrenal cortex that regulates electrolyte balance in the body.

Minutes A written record of the proceedings of a meeting.

Misdemeanor A less serious crime, punishable by a fine or imprisonment for less than 1 year.

Misfeasance Performing a legal act in an improper way.

Mitosis Process by which the nucleus of a body cell divides to form two new cells, each identical to the parent cell.

Modified block style A format for business letters in which the date line, complimentary close, and printed signature line are on a tab at the center or right justified and all other parts of the letter are left justified.

Modified wave scheduling An appointment system that has some fixed appointments and some appointment times during which patients are seen in order of arrival.

Modifier An addition to a *Current Procedural Terminology* code that indicates unusual circumstances related to the procedure, such as a more extensive procedure or two procedures performed in the same session.

Monosaccharide A simple carbohydrate consisting of one sugar unit.

Morphology The study of structure and form.

Motor unit A single neuron and all the muscle fibers it stimulates.

Mucous membrane Epithelial membrane that lines body cavities that open directly to the exterior; secretes mucous.

Multigravida A woman who has been pregnant more than once.

Multipara A woman who has completed two or more pregnancies to the age of fetal viability regardless of whether they ended in live infants or stillbirths.

Myelin White, fatty substance that surrounds many nerve fibers.

Myocardium Middle layer of the heart wall and composed of cardiac muscle tissue.

Myometrium Thick middle layer of the uterus; it is composed of smooth muscle.

Myopia Nearsightedness.

N

Nasopharynx Portion of the pharynx that is posterior to the nasal cavities; extends from the base of the skull to the uvula.

Natural disaster A catastrophic event that is caused by nature or the natural process of the earth.

NEC A diagnosis code that is not elsewhere classified. It is used when a more specific code for the condition is not available.

Needle biopsy A type of biopsy in which tissue from deep within the body is obtained by the insertion of a biopsy needle through the skin.

Negative feedback A mechanism of response in which a stimulus initiates reactions that reduce the stimulus.

Negligence Failure to act (or to refrain from acting) as a reasonably prudent person would in similar circumstances.

Neoplasm Abnormal growth or tumor.

Nephron Functional unit of the kidney consisting of a renal corpuscle and a renal tubule.

Nephron loop The hairpin loop of the renal tubule that extends into the renal pyramids.

Net pay The actual amount of money paid directly to an employee after taxes and other deductions have been taken out.

Network A group of computers that share data and resources.

Networking Contacting acquaintances and their contacts who may know of potential jobs.

Neurilemma The layer of cells that surrounds a nerve fiber in the peripheral nervous system and in some cases produces myelin; also called *Schwann sheath*.

Neuroglia Supporting cells of nervous tissue; cells in nervous tissue that do not conduct impulses; nerve glue.

Neurohypophysis Posterior portion of pituitary gland; the gland that grows beneath the brain and contains axons of neurons.

Neuromuscular junction The area of communication between the axon terminal of a motor neuron and the sarcolemma of a muscle fiber; also called a *myoneural junction*.

Neuron Nerve cell, including its processes; conducting cell of nervous tissue.

Neurotransmitter A chemical substance that is released at the axon terminals to stimulate a muscle fiber contraction or an impulse in another neuron.

New patient For billing purposes, a patient who has not received services during the previous 3 years from any physician in a medical practice.

No-show A patient who does not keep a scheduled appointment.

Nociceptor A sensory receptor that responds to tissue damage; pain receptor.

Nocturia Excessive (voluntary) urination during the night.

Nocturnal enuresis Inability of an individual to control urination at night during sleep (bedwetting).

Nodes of Ranvier Short spaces between segments of myelin in a myelinated nerve fiber.

Non-specific defense mechanisms Body's ability to counteract all types of harmful agents.

Nonabsorbable suture Suture material that is not absorbed by the body and either remains permanently in the body tissue and becomes encapsulated by fibrous tissue or is removed.

Noncritical item An item that comes into contact with intact skin, but not with mucous membranes.

Nonessential amino acid An amino acid that is required by the body that can be synthesized by the body in sufficient quantities to meet its needs.

Nonfeasance Failing to perform an act that should have been performed, resulting in injury.

Nonintact skin Skin that has a break in the surface. It includes, but is not limited to, abrasions, cuts, hangnails, paper cuts, and burns.

Nonmalfeasance Ethical concept requiring that an action do no harm, or do less harm than good.

Nonparticipating provider (nonPAR) A physician who does not have any contract with a third-party payor.

Nonpathogen A microorganism that does not normally produce disease.

Nonverbal Communication that occurs without words, such as through body posture or facial expression.

Nonwaived test A complex laboratory test that does not meet the CLIA criteria for waiver and is subject to the CLIA regulations.

Normal flora Harmless, nonpathogenic microorganisms that normally reside in many parts of the body but do not cause disease.

Normal sinus rhythm Refers to an ECG that is within normal limits.

NOS A diagnosis code that is not otherwise specified. It is used when there is not enough information given to select a more specific code.

Nullipara A woman who has not carried a pregnancy to the point of fetal viability (20 weeks of gestation).

Nutrient A chemical substance found in food that is needed by the body for survival and well-being.

Nutrition Nutrition is the study of nutrients in food including how the body uses them and their relationship to health.

Nutrition therapy The application of the science of nutrition to promote optimal heath and treat illness.

O

Obesity A medical condition in which there is an excessive accumulation of body fat to the extent where it may have an adverse effect on the health and well-being of an individual.

Objective symptom A symptom that can be observed by an examiner.

Obstetrics The branch of medicine concerned with the care of the woman during pregnancy, childbirth, and the postpartal period.

Occult blood Blood in such a small amount that it is not detectable by the unaided eye.

Olfaction Sense of smell.

Oliguria Decreased or scanty output of urine.

Oogenesis Process of meiosis in the female in which one ovum and three polar bodies are produced from one primary oocyte.

Oogonia Stem cells that give rise to ova or egg cells.

Open questions Questions that could have a variety of answers and encourage a personal response.

Operating system A type of system software that performs tasks required by the computer to operate itself.

Ophthalmoscope An instrument for examining the interior of the eye.

Opportunistic infection An infection that results from a defective immune system that cannot defend the body from pathogens normally found in the environment.

Optical disc A storage device consisting of a flat, round portable disk that stores data using laser technology.

Optical disc drive A device installed in a drive bay on the main computer unit that uses a laser to read an optical disc or write onto (burn) an optical disc.

Optimum growth temperature The temperature at which an organism grows best.

Oral Spoken; pertaining to the mouth.

Oral administration Administration of medication by mouth.

Origin The end of a muscle that is attached to a relatively immovable part; the end opposite the insertion.

Oropharynx Portion of the pharynx that is posterior to the oral cavity; extends from the uvula to the hyoid bone.

Orthopnea The condition in which breathing is easier when an individual is in a sitting or standing position.

Osmosis Diffusion of water through a selectively permeable membrane.

Osteoblast Bone-forming cell; immature bone cell.

Osteochondritis Inflammation of bone and cartilage.

Osteoclast Cell that destroys, breaks down, or resorbs bone tissue.

Osteocyte Mature bone cell.

Osteogenesis Formation of bone; also called ossification.

Osteomyelitis Inflammation of the bone or bone marrow as a result of bacterial infection.

Osteon Structural unit of bone; haversian system.

Otoliths Little stones of calcium carbonate in the macula of the inner ear.

Otoscope An instrument for examining the external ear canal and tympanic membrane.

Outguide A cardboard or plastic card to insert in a file when a medical record is removed.

Outpatient A patient who has not been admitted to a health care facility.

Output 1. (noun) Information that has been generated by the computer. 2. (verb) The transfer of processed data back to the user.

Output device A device that transfers processed data to the user (e.g., computer monitor, printer).

Ovarian cycle Monthly cycle of events that occur in the ovary from puberty to menopause; occurs concurrently with the uterine cycle.

Ovarian follicle An oocyte surrounded by one or more layers of cells within the ovaries.

Overdraft A check (or draft) that exceeds the amount of funds in a bank account.

Oxygen therapy The administration of supplemental oxygen at concentrations greater than room air to treat or prevent hypoxemia.

P

Pager An electronic device that notifies the recipient to receive a message or return a telephone call.

Palate Roof of the mouth; separates the oral cavity from the nasal cavity.

Palliative treatment Therapy that reduces the effects of a disease or condition but does not remove the disease itself.

Palpation The process of feeling with the hands to detect signs of disease.

Panel A group of diagnostic tests done in one machine at the same time.

Paper-based patient record A medical record in paper form.

Paraphrasing A restatement of the words of another, often to clarify meaning.

Parenteral Taken into the body through piercing of the skin barrier or mucous membranes, such as through needlesticks, human bites, cuts, and abrasions. Also, administration of medication by injection.

Participating provider (PAR) A physician who has a contractual agreement with a third-party payor.

Parturition Act of giving birth to an infant.

Passive transport Process that moves substances across or through a membrane and does not require cellular energy.

Pathogen A disease-producing microorganism.

Patient-centered medical home A model of primary care that emphasizes patient-centered health care based on a personal relationship between a patient, physician, and the patient's care team.

Patient navigator A person whose role is to remove obstacles that patients face in accessing and receiving treatment.

Patient portal An online application that allows patients to interact with and communicate with their healthcare providers.

Patient self-scheduling The practice of allowing patients to have access to the computer scheduling program so that they can schedule their own appointments.

Patient statement A bill sent to a patient that contains not only charges but also payments and adjustments that affect the balance that the patient must pay.

Payee The person to whom a check is made out.

Peak flow rate The maximum volume of air that can be exhaled when the patient blows into a peak flow meter as forcefully and as rapidly as possible.

Pectoral girdle Attachment for the upper extremities in the chest region; clavicle and scapula.

Pediatrician A physician who specializes in the care and development of children and the diagnosis and treatment of children's diseases.

Pediatrics The branch of medicine that deals with the care and development of children and the diagnosis and treatment of children's diseases.

Pelvic girdle Attachment for the lower extremities; bones collectively shaped like a basin; ilium, ischium, pubis.

Per diem A term used for employees who do not have a fixed schedule but are scheduled by the day according to office needs.

Percent daily value The percentage of a nutrient provided by a single serving of a food item compared to how much is required for the entire day.

Percussion The process of tapping the body to detect signs of disease.

Percussion hammer An instrument with a rubber head, used for testing reflexes.

Pericardial cavity Small space around the heart, between the parietal pericardium and visceral pericardium, that contains a small amount of serous fluid for lubrication.

Pericardium Membrane that surrounds the heart; usually refers to the pericardial sac.

Perimenopause Before the onset of menopause, the phase during which the woman with regular periods changes to irregular cycles and increased periods of amenorrhea.

Perineum The external region between the vaginal orifice and the anus in a female and between the scrotum and the anus in a male.

Periosteum Tough white outer membrane that covers a bone.

Peristalsis Rhythmic contractions of the intestine that move food along the digestive tract.

Peritoneum Serous membrane associated with the abdominopelvic cavity.

Peroxidase (As it pertains to the guaiac slide test) A substance that is able to transfer oxygen from hydrogen peroxide to oxidize guaiac, causing the guaiac to turn blue.

Petty cash A cash account kept in a business office to pay for incidentals, such as postage due and other small items.

pH The unit that describes the acidity or alkalinity of a solution.

Phagocytosis Condition of cell eating; a form of endocytosis in which solid particles are taken into the cell.

Pharmacology The study of drugs.

Pharynx Passageway for air and food; extends from the base of the skull to the larynx and esophagus; throat.

Phlebotomist A health care professional trained in the collection of blood specimens.

Phlebotomy Incision of a vein for the removal of blood; the collection of blood.

Photoreceptor A sensory receptor that detects light; located in the retina of the eye.

Physical examination An assessment of each part of the patient's body to obtain objective data about the patient that assists the physician in determining the patient's state of health.

Physiologic Pertaining to body processes.

Pinealocytes Secretory cells of the pineal gland; secrete melatonin.

Pinocytosis Condition of cell drinking; a form of endocytosis in which fluid droplets are taken into the cell.

Plaintiff The person or group that makes the complaint in a lawsuit.

Plasma The liquid part of the blood, consisting of a clear, yellowish fluid that comprises approximately 55% of the total blood volume.

Pleura Serous membrane that lines the ribs (parietal layer) and surrounds the lungs (visceral layer).

Pleural cavity The small space between the parietal and visceral layers of the pleura.

Plicae circulares Circular folds in the mucosa and submucosa of the small intestine.

Poison Any substance that causes illness, injury, or death if it enters the body.

Policy A guiding principle for the management of a medical office or business.

Polycythemia A disorder in which there is an increase in the red blood cell mass.

Polyuria Increased output of urine.

Position The relation of the presenting part of the fetus to the maternal pelvis.

Postage meter A machine that automatically stamps a piece of mail with the correct postage.

Postal bar code A series of vertical bars of two lengths, which represent the delivery address of a piece of mail. The bar code facilitates automated sorting of mail.

Postexposure prophylaxis (PEP) Treatment administered to an individual after exposure to an infectious disease to prevent the disease.

Postnatal development Development that begins with birth and lasts until death.

Postoperative After a surgical operation.

Postpartum Occurring after childbirth.

Practicum A supervised work experience that is required in an educational program and usually unpaid. Formerly called an *externship*.

Preadmission testing (PAT) A series of diagnostic tests done before surgery to establish the patient's health status and identify any potential problems that may occur during surgery.

Preauthorization Verification from a patient's insurance carrier that a procedure is covered by the patient's insurance and/or agreement, after review, that the test or procedure is medically appropriate.

Precertification Verification from a patient's insurance carrier that a procedure is covered by the patient's insurance and/or agreement, after review, that the test or procedure is medically appropriate.

Preeclampsia A major complication of pregnancy, the cause of which is unknown, characterized by increasing hypertension, albuminuria, and edema. If this condition is neglected or is not treated properly, it may develop into eclampsia, which could cause maternal convulsions and coma. Preeclampsia generally occurs between the 20th week of pregnancy and the end of the first week postpartum.

Preembryonic period First two weeks after fertilization; period of cleavage, implantation, and formation of primary germ layers.

Premium An amount of money paid in a given period to purchase health insurance.

Prenatal Before birth.

Prenatal development Development within the uterus.

Preoperative Preceding a surgical operation.

Presbyopia A decrease in the elasticity of the lens that occurs with aging, resulting in a decreased ability to focus on close objects.

Preschool child A child 3 to 6 years old.

Prescription A physician's order authorizing the dispensing of a drug by a pharmacist.

Presentation Indication of the part of the fetus that is closest to the cervix and is delivered first. A cephalic presentation is a delivery in which the fetal head is presenting against the cervix. A breech presentation is a delivery in which the buttocks or feet are presented instead of the head.

Pressure point A site on the body where an artery lies close to the surface of the skin and can be compressed against an underlying bone to control bleeding.

Primary care provider The physician chosen by a patient to provide general medical care and also to determine and authorize additional medical services the patient may require.

Primary insurance The insurance company that must be billed first for any individual.

Prime mover The muscle that is mainly responsible for a particular body movement; also called *agonist*.

Primigravida A woman who is pregnant for the first time.

Primipara A woman who has carried a pregnancy to fetal viability (20 weeks of gestation) for the first time regardless of whether the infant was stillborn or alive at birth.

Printing speed The number of pages per minute (ppm) generated by a printer.

Privilege A special immunity that protects against legal liability.

Problem Any condition that requires further observation, diagnosis, management, or patient education.

Procedure A list of the steps to handle a certain situation or perform a certain task.

Processing The manipulation and reorganization of data according to the instructions in a program.

Product insert A printed document supplied by the manufacturer with a laboratory test product that contains information on the proper storage and use of the product.

Profile An array of laboratory tests for identifying a disease state or evaluating a particular organ or organ system.

Prognosis The probable course and outcome of a patient's condition and the patient's prospects for recovery.

Program A set of instructions organized in a logical step-by-step sequence, which tells the computer how to perform a specific function.

Projection Experiencing one's own emotions as those of another.

Proofread To identify and correct errors in a document.

Proprioception The sense of body position and movements; responds to stimuli originating within an organism or muscle.

Proteinuria The presence of protein in the urine.

Prudent Using care or common sense.

Puerperium The period of time, usually 4 to 6 weeks after delivery, in which the uterus and the body systems are returning to normal.

Pulmonary circulation The pathway that takes blood from the right side of the heart to the lungs, and then returns it to the left side of the heart.

Pulse oximeter A computerized device consisting of a probe and a monitor used to measure the oxygen saturation of arterial blood.

Pulse oximetry The use of a pulse oximeter to measure the oxygen saturation of arterial blood.

Pulse pressure The difference between the systolic and diastolic pressures.

Pulse rhythm The time interval between heartbeats.

Pulse volume The strength of the heartbeat.

Puncture A wound made by a sharp-pointed object piercing the skin.

Purchase order (PO) number A number assigned by a business to authorize and keep track of a purchase request and order.

Pyloric sphincter Valve between the stomach and first part of the small intestine.

Pyuria The presence of pus in the urine.

Q

Qualitative test A test that indicates whether or not a substance is present in the specimen being tested and also provides an approximate indication of the amount of the substance present.

Quality control The application of methods to ensure that test results are reliable and valid and that errors are detected and eliminated.

Quantitative test A test that indicates the exact amount of a chemical substance that is present in the body, with the results being reported in measurable units.

Quickening The first movements of the fetus in utero as felt by the mother, which usually occur between 16 and 20 weeks of gestation and are felt consistently thereafter.

R

Radiation The transfer of energy, such as heat, in the form of waves.

Radiograph A permanent record of a picture of an internal body organ or structure produced on radiographic film.

Radiologist A physician who specializes in the diagnosis and treatment of disease using radiation and other imaging techniques.

Radiology The branch of medicine that deals with the use of radiation and other imaging techniques (such as ultrasound, CT scans, MRIs, and nuclear medicine) in the diagnosis and treatment of disease.

Radiolucent Describing a structure that permits the passage of x-rays.

Radiopaque Describing a structure that obstructs the passage of x-rays.

Random access memory (RAM) The main computer memory of a microcomputer, which is used to temporarily store items until needed by the computer for processing. Also known as *main computer memory*.

Reagant A substance that produces a reaction with a patient specimen that allows detection or measurement of the substance by the test system.

Reciprocity Automatic issuing of a license in one state to the holder of a license in another state.

Reconciling Making sure that two financial records agree, such as a bank statement and bank balance.

Reference range A certain established and acceptable parameter or reference range within which the laboratory test results of a healthy individual are expected to fall. (Also known as reference value and reference interval.)

Referral The directing of a patient to a specialist physician by the primary care physician. Most managed care plans and some other insurance plans require the primary care physician to obtain prior authorization.

Refraction The deflection or bending of light rays by a lens.

Refractory period Time during which an excitable cell cannot respond to a stimulus that is usually adequate to initiate an action potential.

Regulated medical waste (RMW) Medical waste that poses a threat to health and safety.

Reimbursement The amount paid for a procedure by insurance.

Remittance advice (RA) A statement issued by Medicare or other third party payer to the provider explaining reimbursement for specific procedures or denial of an insurance claim.

Renal corpuscle Portion of the nephron where filtration occurs; consists of the glomerulus and glomerular capsule.

Renal cortex Outer portion of the kidney that appears granular.

Renal erythropoietic factor A substance produced by the kidneys that activates erythropoietin to stimulate the production of red blood cells.

Renal medulla Inner portion of the kidney consisting of renal pyramids.

Renal pelvis Large cavity in the central region of the kidney that collects the urine as it is produced.

Renal threshold The concentration at which a substance in the blood that is not normally excreted by the kidneys begins to appear in the urine.

Renal tubule Tubular portion of the nephron that carries the filtrate away from the glomerular capsule; site where tubular reabsorption and secretion occur.

Renin An enzyme secreted by the kidneys that functions in blood pressure regulation by stimulating the formation of angiotensin.

Reorder point A number on a supply inventory that indicates when a specific item should be reordered to be sure that the supply will not run out before the new order is received.

Reservoir host The organism that becomes infected by a pathogen and serves as a source of transfer of the pathogen to others.

Residency A program to provide training in a medical specialty to a physician who has finished medical school.

Resident flora Harmless, nonpathogenic microorganisms that normally reside on the skin and usually do not cause disease. Also known as *normal flora*.

Resistance The natural ability of an organism to remain unaffected by, or to counteract, the effects of pathogens and other harmful agents in its environment.

Resource-based relative value scale (RBRVS) A system to establish the Medicare fee schedule for Medicare Part B based on the service provided and the geographic location of the provider.

Respiration Exchange of oxygen and carbon dioxide between the atmosphere and the body cells.

Respiratory membrane Any surface in the lungs where diffusion occurs; consists of the layers that the gases must pass through to get into or out of the alveoli.

Respondeat superior A legal doctrine making an employer liable for the negligent acts of employees.

Résumé A summary of information about a person that describes education, work experience, and other information related to an individual's suitability for employment.

Retention The inability to empty the bladder. The urine is being produced normally but is not being voided.

Reverse chronological order Arranging documents with the most recent document on top or in the front, which means that the oldest document is on the bottom or at the back of a section or file.

Rhodopsin Photosensitive pigment in the rods; also called visual purple.

Right A claim that is expected to be honored.

Right justified Type that is aligned with the right margin of a document.

Right lymphatic duct The collecting duct of the lymphatic system that collects lymph from the upper right quadrant of the body.

Risk factor Anything that increases an individual's chance of developing a disease. Some risk factors (e.g., smoking) can be avoided, but others cannot (e.g., age and family history).

Risk management The process of assessing risk and putting policies and procedures in place to protect a health care facility from the risk of legal action.

Router A wired or wireless device used to form or connect networks.

Routine test A laboratory test performed routinely on apparently healthy patients to assist in the early detection of disease.

Rugae Longitudinal folds in the mucosa of the stomach.

S

Safety data sheet (SDS) A sheet that provides information regarding a chemical, its hazards, and measures to take to prevent injury and illness when handling the chemical.

Salary A fixed amount of money paid on a regular basis that does not depend on the number of hours worked.

Saltatory conduction Process in which a nerve impulse travels along a myelinated nerve fiber by jumping from one node of Ranvier to the next.

Salutation The greeting that begins a letter.

Sanitization A process to remove organic matter from an article and to reduce the number of microorganisms to a safe level as determined by public health requirements.

SaO$_2$ (saturation of arterial oxygen) Abbreviation for the percentage of hemoglobin that is saturated with oxygen in arterial blood.

Sarcolemma Covering of a muscle cell; the muscle cell membrane.

Saturated fat A type of fat that is solid at room temperature and comes primarily from animal sources.

Scalpel A surgical knife used to divide tissues.

School-age child A child 6 to 12 years old.

Scissors A cutting instrument.

Sebaceous cyst A thin, closed sac or capsule that contains fatty secretions from a sebaceous gland.

Sebaceous gland An oil gland of the skin that produces sebum or body oil.

Sebum Oily secretion from sebaceous glands.

Secondary insurance Insurance that an individual has in addition to primary insurance.

Segment The portion of the ECG between two waves.

Seizure A sudden episode of involuntary muscular contractions and relaxation, often accompanied by changes in sensation, behavior, and level of consciousness.

Self-actualization The fulfillment of each individual's potential.

Self-referral The process by which a patient makes an appointment with a specialist physician without requesting prior authorization from his or her primary care physician, usually because the patient's insurance plan does not require it.

Semiblock style A letter format in which the date line, complimentary close, and printed signature line are on a tab at the center or right justified, all paragraphs are indented five to eight spaces, and the other parts of the letter are left justified.

Semicritical item An item that comes into contact with nonintact skin or intact mucous membranes.

Semilunar valve Valve between a ventricle of the heart and the vessel that carries blood away from the ventricle; also pertains to the valves in veins.

Seminiferous tubules Tightly coiled structures within which sperm are produced in the testes.

Sensory adaptation Phenomenon in which some receptors respond when a stimulus is first applied but decrease their response if the stimulus is maintained; receptor sensitivity decreases with prolonged stimulation.

Sequela (pl. sequelae) Any condition that results from a disease, injury, or treatment for a disease or injury.

Sequential-access memory Computer memory in which all stored data must be searched sequentially from beginning to end to locate the desired information.

Serous membrane Epithelial membrane that lines closed body cavities.

Serum The clear, straw-colored part of the blood (plasma) that remains after the solid elements and the clotting factor fibrinogen have been separated out of it.

Server A large computer that stores data and manages tasks for other computers on a network.

Service contract An agreement that provides for service for a piece of equipment after the warranty expires.

Shock The failure of the cardiovascular system to deliver enough blood to all of the vital organs of the body.

Sigmoidoscope An endoscope that is specially designed for passage through the anus to permit visualization of the rectum and sigmoid colon.

Sigmoidoscopy The visual examination of the rectum and sigmoid colon using a sigmoidoscope.

Signatura The part of a prescription that indicates the information to print on the medication label.

Signature on file (SOF) An indication on the insurance claim form that the signature of the patient is maintained by the medical office to authorize submission of insurance claims.

Simplified letter style A letter format in which all elements are left justified. The greeting is replaced by a subject line in all capital letters. The complimentary close and typed signature are replaced by a typed signature in all capital letters.

Single booking An appointment scheduling method in which each patient is given a different, specific appointment time. Also called *stream scheduling* or *fixed appointment scheduling*.

Skip Account for which no billing information is available.

Smartphone A cell phone with computer capabilities.

Smear Material spread on a slide for microscopic examination.

Soak The direct immersion of a body part in water or a medicated solution.

SOAP A method of organization for recording progress notes. The SOAP note includes the following categories: subjective data, objective data, assessment, and plan.

Social Security tax (FICA) A tax collected from employers and employees to fund the Social Security program, which provides benefits to retired workers.

Software A general term for the programs or instructions that tell a computer what to do.

Solid state drive Uses integrated circuits (flash memory) to store data permanently.

Somatomotor cortex The primary motor area of the brain; located in the precentral gyrus; transmits motor impulses to the body.

Somatosensory cortex The primary sensory area of the brain; located in the postcentral gyrus; receives sensory impulses from the body.

Sonogram The record obtained with ultrasonography.

Sorter A device that facilitates putting papers or records in alphabetic or numeric order.

Sound card A circuit board connected to the mainboard that converts computer audio output into electronic signals. The electronic signals are then sent to speakers that convert them into sound.

Special keys Keys that issue commands to the computer to perform specific functions on the information displayed on the screen.

Special senses Senses with receptors localized in a particular area; taste, smell, vision, hearing, and equilibrium.

Specific defense Activities of the body that counteract only certain types of harmful agents.

Specific gravity The weight of a substance compared with the weight of an equal volume of a substance known as the standard. In urinalysis, the *specific gravity* refers to the measurement of the amount of dissolved substances present in the urine compared with the same amount of distilled water.

Specimen A small sample or part taken from the body to show the nature of the whole.

Speculum An instrument for opening a body orifice or cavity for viewing.

Spermatogenesis Process of meiosis in the male in which four spermatids are produced from one primary spermatocyte.

Spermatogonia Stem cells that give rise to sperm cells.

Spermiogenesis Morphologic changes that transform a spermatid into a mature sperm.

Sphygmomanometer An instrument for measuring arterial blood pressure.

Spirilla (sing. *Spirillum*) Bacteria that have a spiral or curved shape.

Spirometer An instrument for measuring air taken into and expelled from the lungs.

Spirometry Measurement of an individual's breathing capacity by means of a spirometer.

Splint Any device that immobilizes a body part.

SpO₂ (saturation of peripheral oxygen) Abbreviation for the percentage of hemoglobin that is saturated with oxygen in arterial blood as measured by a pulse oximeter.

Spore A hard, thick-walled capsule formed by some bacteria that contains only the essential parts of the protoplasm of the bacterial cell.

Sprain Trauma to a joint that causes tearing of or injury to the ligaments.

Standard of care Level of appropriate care required of a health professional.

Statute of limitations A law limiting the time period for beginning a lawsuit.

Statutory law Law enacted by a legislative body.

Sterile Free of all living microorganisms and bacterial spores.

Sterilization The process of destroying all forms of microbial life, including bacterial spores.

Stethoscope An instrument used for amplifying and hearing sounds produced by the body.

Storage capacity The maximum amount of information that a device can hold, measured in bytes.

Storage device A device that permanently stores information for later retrieval by the computer.

Strain A stretching or tearing of muscles or tendons caused by trauma.

Stratum basale Bottom layer of the endometrium that is responsible for rebuilding the stratum functionale after menstruation.

Stratum corneum Outermost layer of the epidermis; consists of flattened, dead, keratinized cells.

Stratum functionale Portion of the endometrium that is sloughed off during menstruation.

Stream scheduling An appointment scheduling method in which each patient is given a different, specific appointment time. Also called *fixed appointment scheduling, time-specified scheduling,* or *single booking.*

Stress The body's response to threat or change.

Stem cells Cells that have the capacity to develop into various types of body tissue.

Subcutaneous injection Introduction of medication beneath the skin, into the subcutaneous or fatty layer of the body.

Subcutaneous layer Below the skin; a sheet of areolar connective tissue and adipose tissue beneath the dermis of the skin; also called *hypodermis* or *superficial fascia.*

Subjective symptom A symptom that is felt by the patient but is not observable by an examiner.

Sublingual administration Administration of medication by placing it under the tongue, where it dissolves and is absorbed through the mucous membrane.

Subscription The part of the prescription that gives directions to the pharmacist and usually designates the number of doses to be dispensed.

Subpoena A court order for a witness to appear and give testimony.

Subpoena duces tecum A court order to produce documents or records.

Sudoriferous gland A gland in the skin that produces perspiration; also called *sweat gland.*

Summarizing Expressing the most important points of a conversation or written document.

Superbill An itemized charge slip usually also containing diagnosis codes and procedure codes required for insurance billing.

Supernatant The clear liquid that remains at the top after a precipitate settles.

Superscription The part of a prescription consisting of the symbol Rx (from the Latin word recipe, meaning "take").

Suppuration The process of pus formation.

Suprapubic aspiration The passing of a sterile needle through the abdominal wall into the bladder to remove urine.

Surfactant A substance, produced by certain cells in lung tissue, that reduces surface tension between fluid molecules that line the respiratory membrane and helps keep the alveolus from collapsing.

Surgery The branch of medicine that deals with operative and manual procedures for correction of deformities and defects, repair of injuries, and diagnosis and treatment of certain diseases.

Surgical asepsis Practices that keep objects and areas sterile or free from microorganisms.

Surgical packing Surgical services usually covered by a single procedure code that includes a preoperative visit, postoperative care, and local anesthesia (if applicable).

Surname Last name or family name of an individual; used as the first indexing unit in alphabetic filing.

Susceptibility Lack of resistance to disease.

Susceptible Easily affected; lacking resistance.

Sutures Immovable fibrous joints between the flat bones of the skull. Also, Material used to approximate tissues with surgical stitches.

Swaged needle A needle with suturing material permanently attached to its end.

Sweat glands Glands in the skin that produce perspiration; also called *sudoriferous glands.*

Sympathy Feeling the same emotions as another.

Symptom Any change in the body or its functioning that indicates a disease might be present.

Symptomatic treatment Therapy for symptoms of a disease or condition that does not remove the disease itself.

Synapse The region of communication between two neurons.

Synarthrosis An immovable joint; plural, *synarthroses.*

Synergist A muscle that assists a prime mover but is not capable of producing the movement by itself; two or more muscles work together to produce a movement.

Synovial membrane Membrane that lines the cavities of freely movable joints.

System software A group of programs that control or maintain the operations of a computer.

Systemic circulation Pathways that transport blood from the left side of the heart to all parts of the body and return the blood to the right atrium; excludes pulmonary circulation.

Systole The phase in the cardiac cycle in which the ventricles contract, sending blood out of the heart and into the aorta and pulmonary aorta; opposite of diastole.

Systolic pressure The point of maximum pressure on the arterial walls, which is recorded during systole.

T

Tab A projection of a folder that extends beyond the top or side of the folder.

Tachycardia An abnormally fast heart rate (more than 100 beats/min).

Tachypnea An abnormal increase in the respiratory rate of more than 20 breaths/min.

Target tissue A tissue (cells) that responds to a particular hormone because it has receptor sites for that hormone.

Template A standard form to which additional information can be added as needed.

Teniae coli Bands of longitudinal muscle fibers in the large intestine.

Terabyte (TB) A unit of computer storage. One terabyte is equivalent to a little more than a trillion bytes or 1000 gigabytes.

Terminal digit filing A chronologic filing system that uses the last number or number group as the first indexing unit.

Terminal phase The last stage of illness, usually used when death is expected to occur within 6 months.

Test system A setup that includes all of the test components required to perform a laboratory test such as testing devices, controls, and testing reagents.

Thermolabile Easily affected or changed by heat.

Thermoreceptor A sensory receptor that detects changes in temperature.

Third-party payor Insurance carrier or managed care organization that pays health insurance claims.

Thoracic duct The primary collecting duct of the lymphatic system that collects lymph from all regions of the body except the upper right quadrant.

Thready pulse A pulse with a decreased volume that feels weak and thin.

Threshold stimulus Minimum level of stimulation that is required to start a nerve impulse or muscle contraction; also called *liminal stimulus*.

Thrombocyte One of the formed elements of the blood; functions in blood clotting; also called *platelet*.

Tickler file A chronological file containing reminders of things to be done.

Time management Skills and techniques used to manage time in order to accomplish tasks and meet goals.

Time-specified scheduling An appointment scheduling method in which each patient is given a different, specific appointment time. Also called *stream scheduling, fixed appointment scheduling*, or *single booking*.

Tissue Group of similar cells specialized to perform a certain function.

Toddler A child 1 to 3 years old.

Topical administration Application of a drug to a particular spot, usually for a local action.

Tort An injury or wrong against a person or property that does not involve breach of contract.

Toxemia A condition that can occur in pregnant women that includes preeclampsia and eclampsia. If preeclampsia goes undiagnosed or is not satisfactorily controlled, it could develop into eclampsia, characterized by convulsions and coma.

Toxoid A toxin (a poisonous substance produced by a bacterium) that has been treated by heat or chemicals to destroy its harmful properties. It is administered to an individual to prevent an infectious disease by stimulating the production of antibodies in that individual.

Trachea Passageway for air that extends inferiorly to the carina where it branches into the bronchi; commonly called the windpipe.

Transfusion The administration of whole blood or blood products through the intravenous route.

Triage The process of separating patients by the urgency of their need for care.

TRICARE A government insurance plan that provides medical care to spouses and dependents of individuals on active duty in the military. Formerly this program was called CHAMPUS.

Triglycerides The chemical form in which most fat exists in food, as well as in the body.

Trigone Triangular area in the floor of the urinary bladder formed by the openings for the urethra and the two ureters.

Trimester Three months, or one third, of the gestational period of pregnancy.

Truth in lending Legal requirement to disclose the terms of a loan in terms that the borrower can understand.

Tubular reabsorption The movement of filtrate from the renal tubules back into the blood in response to the body's needs during urine formation.

Tubular secretion The movement of substances from the blood into the renal tubules in response to the body's needs during urine formation.

Transient flora Microorganisms that reside on the superficial skin layers and are picked up in the course of daily activities. They are often pathogenic but can be removed easily from the skin by sanitizing the hands.

Tympanic membrane A thin, semitransparent membrane between the external ear canal and the middle ear that receives and transmits sound waves. Also known as the *eardrum*.

U

Ultrasonography The use of high-frequency sound waves to produce an image of an organ or tissue.

Unsaturated fat A type of fat that is liquid at room temperature and comes primarily from plant sources.

Upcoding Using a code to obtain a higher level of reimbursement than is justified by medical procedures performed as documented in the medical record. This can result in serious fines and penalties.

Upper respiratory tract Portion of the respiratory tract that includes the nose, pharynx, and larynx.

Ureter Tubular structure that carries urine from the renal pelvis to the urinary bladder.

Urethra Passageway that conveys urine from the urinary bladder to the exterior.

Urgency The immediate need to urinate.

Urinalysis The physical, chemical, and microscopic analyses of urine.

Urinary bladder Storage reservoir for urine: located in the pelvic cavity.

Urinary incontinence The inability to retain urine.

URL The characters and/or words used to access a specific website or file on the World Wide Web.

User The individual operating a computer.

Usual, customary, and reasonable (UCR) A system for establishing the amount an insurance carrier will pay for a procedure. The reasonable charge is set by the insurance carrier on the basis of a physician's usual (most frequent) charge for the procedure and the customary charge of other physicians in the same geographic area.

Uterine cycle Monthly cycle of events that occur in the uterus from puberty to menopause; also called the menstrual cycle; occurs concurrently with the ovarian cycle.

Uterine tubes The tubes that extend laterally from the upper portion of the uterus to the region of the ovaries; also called fallopian tubes or oviducts.

Utilization Review Assessing medical services to determine whether they are appropriate, necessary, and of high quality.

V

Vaccine A suspension of attenuated (weakened) or killed microorganisms administered to an individual to prevent an infectious disease by stimulating the production of antibodies in that individual.

Vendor A company from whom supplies or equipment is purchased.

Venipuncture Puncturing of a vein.

Venous reflux The backflow of blood (from an evacuated tube) into the patient's vein.

Venous stasis The temporary cessation or slowing of the venous blood flow.

Ventilation Movement of air into and out of the lungs; breathing.

Ventricle Pumping chamber of the heart; right ventricle pumps blood to the lungs and left ventricle pumps blood into systemic circulation.

Veracity Truthfulness.

Verbal Using words to communicate.

Vertex The top of the head.

Vial A closed glass container with a rubber stopper that holds medication.

Vitamin A type of fat that is liquid at room temperature and comes primarily from plant sources.

Voicemail A method for delivery, storage, and retrieval of telephone messages that is built into the telephone system.

Void To empty the bladder.

Vulva Collective term for the external accessory structures of the female reproductive system; also called the pudendum.

W

W-4 form The form used to claim allowances for federal income tax reporting.

Waived test A laboratory test that meets the CLIA criteria for being a simple procedure that is easy to perform and has a low risk of erroneous test results. Waived tests include tests that have been FDA-approved for use by patients at home.

Warranty A promise by the manufacturer to repair or replace defective parts in an item during a specific time period.

Wave scheduling A method of scheduling appointments in which several patients are given the same appointment time and are seen in the order in which they arrive.

Web browser A software program used to access the World Wide Web.

Webcam Small video camera attached to a computer that allows video to be transmitted on the Internet.

Wheal A tense, pale, raised area of the skin.

Wheezing A continuous, high-pitched whistling musical sound heard particularly during exhalation and sometimes during inhalation.

Workers' compensation An insurance program that covers lost wages and health care costs of workers injured on the job or having work-related illnesses.

World Wide Web A series of interlinked websites or files accessed via the Internet.

Wound A break in the continuity of an external or internal surface, caused by physical means.

Z

ZIP code A five-digit code that identifies the post office to which a given piece of mail is to be delivered.

ZIP+4 code A more detailed mailing code consisting of the original five-digit ZIP code followed by a hyphen and four additional digits. These digits identify a specific geographic segment within the delivery area.

Zygote The single diploid cell that is a fertilized ovum.

Index

Note: Page number followed by "*b*" indicate boxes; "*f*" figure; "*t*" tables.

A

Abbreviations and symbols, 1012*t*-1014*t*, 1104
Abdominis, rectus *vs.* transversus, 143
Abduction, 140, 141*f*-142*f*
ABHES. *See* Accrediting Bureau of Health Education Schools (ABHES).
Acceptance, 76. *See also* Grieving process.
Account aging, 1223-1224. *See also* Billing/collections.
  of accounts receivable, 1223, 1224*f*, 1225*b*
  definition of, 1223
  overdue accounts, 1223-1224
Accountable Care Organizations (ACOs), 2
Accounting, 1147. *See also* Finance management.
  accounts payable, 1147
  accounts receivable, 1147
  accrual basis of, 1147
  vs. bookkeeping, 1147
  cash basis of, 1147
  definition of, 1147
  terminology of, 1152*b*
Accounts receivable, 1223, 1224*f*, 1225*b*
Accreditation, 20-21
Accrediting Bureau of Health Education Schools (ABHES), 20-21
Accuracy requirements, 1185-1187. *See also* Medical coding.
Acetylcholine (ACh), 139
Acetylcholinerase, 139
ACh. *See* Acetylcholine (ACh).
Achilles tendon, 147
ACOs. *See* Accountable Care Organizations (ACOs).
Action verbs, 1260*f*
Active listening, 64, 66*t*. *See also* Listening skills.
Active records, 1112
Acupuncture, 16, 16*f*
Acute period, 898
ADA. *See* American with Disabilities Act (ADA).
Additional credentials, 27-28
Addressing standards, 1139-1141
Adduction, 140, 141*f*-142*f*
Adductors
  brevis, 144-147
  longus, 144-147
  magnus, 144-147
Adenosine triphosphate (ATP), 138-140
Adjectives, 1123, 1125*b*
Administrative components
  appointment scheduling, 1078-1093
  billing/collections, 1217-1230
  job-seeking/employment considerations, 1255-1268
  mail/shipping, 1131-1143
  medical coding, 1168-1185
  medical insurance, 1189-1212
  medical office computerization, 1040-1059
  medical records, 991-1021
  medical records management, 1098-1112
  office manager roles, 1233-1251
  patient reception, 1025-1037
  practice finance management, 1146-1166
  telephone techniques, 1063-1075
  written communications, 1115-1128
Advancement, management, 1268
Adverbs, 1123, 1125*b*
Advocacy, 28
Aerobic exercise, 373*b*
Aerobic respiration, 139. *See also* Respiration.
Agencies, collection, 1226-1227, 1229. *See also* Collections/billing.
Aging, accounts, 1223-1224. *See also* Billing/collections.
  of accounts receivable, 1223, 1224*f*, 1225*b*
  definition of, 1223
  overdue accounts, 1223-1224
Agreements
  credit, 1227, 1228*f*

Agreements *(Continued)*
  service, 1059
  truth in lending agreements, 1227
Allergy and immunology, 13*b*-14*b*, 1008
Allied health professionals, 8, 9*t*
Alphabetic filing system, 1104-1105, 1107*b*. *See also* Filing systems.
  abbreviations, 1104
  cross-indexing, 1104
  hyphenation, 1104
  indexing units, 1104
  names
    companies/businesses, 1105
    identical, 1105
    individual, 1104
    married women, 1105
    nicknames, 1104
    surnames, 1104
  prefixes, 1104
  seniority terms, 1105
  titles, 1105
Alternative medicine. *See* Complementary and alternative medicine (CAM).
AMA. *See* American Medical Association (AMA).
Ambulatory care, 6-10
  activity flow in, 6-8, 7*f*
  definition of, 6
American Board of Medical Specialties, 12, 13*b*-14*b*. *See also* Medical specialties.
American Medical Association (AMA)
  American Nomenclature of Disease, 1169
  Current Procedural Terminology (CPT), 1169. *See also* Current Procedural Terminology (CPT).
American Nomenclature of Disease, 1169
American with Disabilities Act (ADA), 10
Amino acids, 922. *See also* Proteins.
  classification of, 922
  definition of, 922
  essential, 922
  nonessential, 922
Amphiarthroses, 131
Anaerobic respiration, 139. *See also* Respiration.
Anatomy and physiology
  body systems
    circulatory, 196-216
    digestive, 235-248
    endocrine, 186-195
    integumentary, 111-115
    muscular, 136-147
    nervous, 151-168
    reproductive, 266-283
    respiratory, 224-230
    skeletal, 118-133
    urinary, 254-264
  fundamentals of, 80-105
  senses, 173-182
Anemia, 855, 860*b*
Anesthesia codes, 1174. *See also* Medical coding.
Anesthesiology, 13*b*-14*b*
Anger responses, 74, 76
Annotations, 1137. *See also* Incoming mail.
Antagonists, 140
Antecubital space, 818
Antioxidant vitamins, 923, 925*f*. *See also* Vitamins.
Antivirus software, 1058
Anuria, 787
Anxiety responses, 73-74
Apical pulse, 371, 372*f*. *See also* Pulse.
Apical-radial pulse, 373. *See also* Pulse.
Aponeurosis, 138
Appearance considerations, 21-23, 21*f*-23*f*, 1263-1264, 1264*f*
Appendicular skeleton, 122*f*, 126. *See also* Skeletal system.
Applications, employment, 1262

Appointment scheduling, 1078-1093
Appositional growth, 121
Articles, 1123
Articular cartilage, 121, 121*f*
Articulations, 131-132. *See also* Skeletal system.
Asepsis, 290-314
Assessments
    ear, 441-458
    eye, 441-458
    gynecologic, 487-521
    pediatric, 529-556
    physical, 405-436
    specialty, 719-748
Assignment of benefits, 1029-1030
ATP. *See* Adenosine triphosphate (ATP).
Attachments, e-mail, 1126
Attending physician reports, 1006
Audit controls, 1058
Aural temperature, 356, 365*b*-367*b*. *See also* Temperature.
Authorization, 1030-1032. *See also* Medical insurance.
Automated mail processing, 1138, 1139*b*
Axial skeleton, 122-127, 122*f*. *See also* Skeletal system.
Axilla, 354-355
Axillary temperature, 356, 362*b*-363*b*. *See also* Temperature.

B

Bacilli, 899
Backorders, 1244
Backup protocols, 1058
Bacteria, 899-900, 899*f*-900*f*
Balance billing, 1033
Balance due, 1218. *See also* Billing/collections.
Banking activities, 1157-1162. *See also* Finance management.
    account types, 1157-1158
        checking, 1157
        money market, 1157-1158
        savings, 1157
    checks, 1158
    introduction to, 1157
Bankruptcy Abuse Prevention and Consumer Protection Act (2005), 1229-1230
Bar code system, postal, 1132, 1133*f*
Bargaining, 76. *See also* Grieving process.
Basilic veins, 821
bcc notation. *See* Blind copy notation (bcc).
Bedwetting, 787
Behavioral skills, 23-24
    initiative, 23-24
    organizational skills, 24
    task lists, 24
    time management, 23-24
Belly, 138
Benefit/salary discussions, 1264
Biceps
    branchii, 144
    femoris, 147
Bilirubin, 795
Billing cycles, 1218, 1219*b*
Billing/collections, 1217-1230
    account aging, 1223-1224
        of accounts receivable, 1223, 1224*f*, 1225*b*
        definition of, 1223
        overdue accounts, 1223-1224
    billing cycles, 1218, 1219*b*
    billing problems, 1220-1221
        checks, 1220-1221
        non-sufficient funds (NSF) designations, 1220-1221, 1221*b*-1222*b*
        overdrafts, 1220
    case studies of, 1221*b*, 1224*b*, 1230*b*-1232*b*
    collections, 1226-1230
        claim messages, 1226
        collection agencies, 1226-1227, 1229
        collection letters, 1226-1227, 1226*f*, 1231*b*
        credit agreements, 1227, 1228*f*
        estate billings, 1229
        outstanding balance policies, 1227-1228
        past due accounts, 1226
        skips tracing, 1228-1229
        small claims court, 1229
        techniques for, 1228-1230
        telephone, 1227*b*
        truth in lending agreements, 1227
    introduction to, 1218
    laws affecting, 1230
        Bankruptcy Abuse Prevention and Consumer Protection Act (2005), 1229-1230
        Equal Credit Opportunity Act, 1230

Billing/collections (*Continued*)
        Fair Credit Reporting Act, 1230
        Fair Debt Collections Practice Act (1966), 1226, 1230
        Federal Truth in Lending Act, 1227, 1230
        probate, 1229
    overpayments, 1221
        credit balances, 1221, 1222*b*-1223*b*
        refunds, 1221, 1222*b*-1223*b*
    patient statements, 1218, 1219*f*, 1225*b*
        balance due, 1218
        processing of, 1220*b*
    procedures for, 1220*b*-1223*b*, 1225*b*, 1231*b*
    processes, 1218
    terminology of, 1217, 1232*b*
    Web resources for, 1232*b*
Bladder catheterization, 788
Blind copy notation (bcc), 1117
Blood chemistry, 870-891
BMI. *See* Body mass index (BMI).
Board certified physicians, 8
Body mass index (BMI), 932-934, 934*t*
Body of letter, 1117, 1118*f*. *See also* Business letters.
Body systems
    circulatory, 196-216
    digestive, 235-248
    endocrine, 186-195
    fundamentals of, 80-105
    integumentary, 111-115
    muscular, 136-147
    nervous, 151-168
    reproductive, 266-283
    respiratory, 224-230
    senses, 173-182
    skeletal, 118-133
    urinary, 254-264
Bone names, 124*t*
Bookkeeping systems, 1148*b*
Bounding pulse, 373. *See also* Pulse.
Brachial pulse, 371-372. *See also* Pulse.
Bradycardia, 373
Break/lunch rooms, 12
Broadband routers, 1055-1056
Buccinator muscle, 140-143
Burnout avoidance, 1266-1267
Business letters, 1116-1120. *See also* Written communications.
    composition of, 1120, 1121*b*-1122*b*
    definition of, 1116
    enclosures (enc.), 1117
    equipment for, 1116
    examples of, 1118*f*-1120*f*
    format of, 1117-1120
    parts of, 1116-1117, 1118*f*
        complimentary closing, 1117, 1118*f*
        date line, 1116, 1118*f*
        end notations, 1117, 1118*f*
        headings, 1116, 1118*f*
        inside address, 1116, 1118*f*
        letter body, 1117, 1118*f*
        return address *vs.* letterhead, 1116, 1118*f*
        salutation/greeting, 1116-1117, 1118*f*
        signature, handwritten, 1117, 1118*f*
        signature, printed, 1117, 1118*f*
        title designations, 1117, 1118*f*
    procedures for, 1121*b*-1122*b*
    set-up of, 1117
    styles of, 1117-1120
        full block, 1117-1120, 1118*f*
        justification, left *vs.* right, 1117-1120
        modified block, 1117, 1119*f*
        modified block with indented paragraphs, 1117, 1119*f*
        semiblock, 1117, 1119*f*
        simplified, 1120, 1120*f*
    supplies for, 1116
    templates of, 1116
Business managers, 8
Business names, 1105. *See also* Names.
Business office areas, 11-12. *See also* Medical offices.
Butterfly method, 835-836. *See also* Phlebotomy.
Bytes, 1047

C

CAAHEP. *See* Commission on Accreditation of Allied Health Education Programs (CAAHEP).
Calcaneal tendon, 147
Call-in times, 1036

Calories, 917
CAM. *See* Complementary and alternative medicine (CAM).
Capillaries, 138
Carbohydrates, 918-919, 918*f*
    classification of, 918
    complex, 918
    counting system, 938
    definition of, 918
    dietary fiber, 918-919, 919*f*, 919*t*
    simple, 918, 946*f*
Cardiopulmonary procedures, 687-716
Cardiopulmonary resuscitation (CPR) training, 27
Care teams, 8-10
    definition of, 8
    effective teamwork, 9-10
    medical assistant roles in, 8
    members of, 8, 9*t*
Carotid pulse, 372. *See also* Pulse.
Carrier information, 1204
Case studies
    of billing/collections, 1221*b*, 1224*b*, 1230*b*-1232*b*
    of blood chemistry, 764*b*, 768*b*, 775*b*
    of clinical laboratories, 764*b*, 768*b*, 770*b*, 775*b*, 784*b*
    of employment/job-seeking considerations, 1261*b*, 1263*b*, 1267*b*,
        1269*b*
    of health care system, 8*b*-9*b*, 12*b*, 16*b*-17*b*
    of hematology, 857*b*, 861*b*, 863*b*, 868*b*
    of immunology, 764*b*, 768*b*, 775*b*
    of mail/shipping, 1134*b*, 1136*b*-1137*b*, 1143*b*, 1145*b*
    of medical assistant profession, 21*b*-22*b*, 25*b*-26*b*, 31*b*-32*b*
    of medical coding, 1177*b*-1178*b*, 1182*b*, 1185*b*, 1187*b*
    of medical insurance, 1194*b*, 1204*b*, 1210*b*, 1213*b*-1214*b*
    of medical microbiology, 899*b*, 906*b*-907*b*, 911*b*-913*b*
    of medical records management, 1100*b*-1101*b*, 1106*b*, 1111*b*-1113*b*
    of office manager roles, 1236*b*-1237*b*, 1244*b*, 1248*b*-1249*b*, 1252*b*-1253*b*
    of patient interactions, 65*b*, 68*b*, 72*b*, 74*b*, 77*b*-78*b*
    of patient reception, 1029*b*, 1034*b*, 1037*b*-1039*b*
    of phlebotomy, 818*f*, 824*b*, 837*b*, 852*b*
    of urinalysis, 788*b*, 793*b*, 800*b*, 808*b*, 811*b*
    of written communications, 1123*b*, 1125*b*-1126*b*, 1128, 1128*b*-1129*b*
Catheterization, bladder, 788
CBCs. *See* Complete blood counts (CBCs).
CC. *See* Chief complaint (CC).
cc notation. *See* Copy notation (cc).
Celiac disease, 940
Celsius-Fahrenheit conversions, 353*t*
Centers for Medicare and Medicaid Services (CMS), 1169
Cephalic veins, 821
Certificates of Mailing, 1133
Certification, 26-28
    additional credentials, 27-28
    American Association of Medical Assistants (AAMA) and, 26-27
    American Heart Association (AHA) and, 27
    American Medical Technologists (AMT), 27
    American Red Cross (ARC) and, 27
    American Society for Clinical Pathology (ASCP) and, 27
    American Society of Phlebotomy Technicians (ASPT) and, 27
    California Certifying Board for Medical Assistants (CCBMA), 27
    cardiopulmonary resuscitation (CPR) training, 27
    Certified Medical Assistant (CMA), 21, 21*b*, 26-27
    National Center for Competency Testing (NCCT), 27
    National Healthcareer Association (NHA) and, 27
    registered medical assistant (RMA), 27
    registered phlebotomy technician (RPT), 27
Certified Mail, 1133-1134, 1134*f*
CEUs. *See* Continuing education units (CEUs).
CHAMPUS, 1191, 1197
CHAMPVA, 1197
Character traits, 21
Chart dividers, 1100-1101
Check-in procedures, 1029-1036
    assignment of benefits, 1029-1030
    confidentiality and, 1029, 1029*f*
    of established patients, 1033-1034
    forms
        managed care referrals, 1033
        Notice of Privacy Practices acknowledgments, 1030, 1033*f*
        patient histories, 1030
        patient information, 1030, 1031*f*-1032*f*
    Health Insurance Portability and Accountability Act (HIPAA) and,
        1030
    insurance verification/authorization, 1030-1032
    of new patients, 1029-1033
    patient waiting notifications, 1036
Checking accounts, 1157. *See also* Banking activities.

Checks, 1158, 1220-1221. *See also* Billing/collections.
    non-sufficient funds (NSF) designations, 1220-1221, 1221*b*-1222*b*
    overdrafts, 1220
Chemical thermometers, 358-359. *See also* Thermometers.
Chemistry, blood, 870-891
Chief complaint (CC), 999*b*, 1007, 1007*f*
Children's Health Insurance Program (CHIP), 1197
CHIP. *See* Children's Health Insurance Program (CHIP).
Chiropractic practice, 15, 15*f*
Cholesterol, 920
Chronological filing systems, 1106. *See also* Filing systems.
Chronological résumés, 1257, 1258*f*. *See also* Résumés.
Circulatory system, 196-216
Circumduction, 140, 141*f*-142*f*
Civilian Health and Medical Program for the Uniformed Services (CHAMPUS), 5,
    1191, 1197
Claim. *See also* Medical insurance.
    forms, 1202-1204, 1203*f*
        carrier information, 1204
        common errors on, 1212*t*
        completion of, 1204-1205, 1205*b*-1209*b*
        physician information, 1205
        place of service codes, 1205*t*
    messages, 1226
    submissions, 1209-1210
        electronic, 1209
        paper, 1210
Clauses
    dependent, 1124
    independent, 1124
Clean catch midstream specimens, 788-789
Cleft, synaptic, 139
Clerks, file, 8
CLIA 1988. *See* Clinical Laboratory Improvement Amendments (CLIA 1988).
Clinical components
    blood chemistry, 870-891
    cardiopulmonary procedures, 687-716
    clinical laboratories, 752-783
    ear assessments/procedures, 441-458
    emergency medical procedures, 967-988
    emergency preparedness, 944-964
    eye assessments/procedures, 441-458
    first aid, 967-988
    gynecologic examinations, 487-521
    hematology, 854-868
    immunology, 870-891
    intravenous (IV) therapy administration, 613-683
    medical asepsis, 290-314
    medical microbiology, 896-912
    medications, 613-683
    minor office surgery, 560-609
    nutrition, 915-942
    Occupational Safety and Health Administration (OSHA) standards, 290-314
    pediatric examinations, 529-556
    phlebotomy, 814-851
    physical examinations, 405-436
    prenatal care, 487-521
    protective practices, 944-964
    specialty examinations/procedures, 719-748
    sterilization/disinfection, 318-345
    tissue healing physical agents, 467-479
    urinalysis, 786-809
    vital signs, 350-396
Clinical laboratories, 752-783
Clinical Laboratory Improvement Amendments (CLIA 1988), 10-11
Clinical skills, 1266
Clinics, 16
Closed questions, 65. *See also* Questions.
Closed-panel health maintenance organizations (HMOs), 15
Closing procedures, 1027, 1028*b*. *See also* Patient reception.
Closings, complimentary, 1117, 1118*f*. *See also* Business letters.
CMS. *See* Centers for Medicare and Medicaid Services (CMS).
Coaching, health, 30-31
Coagulation analyzers, 867, 867*f*
Cocci, 899
COD. *See* Collect on Delivery (COD).
Coding, 1168-1185
    accuracy requirements of, 1185-1187
        downcoding, 1185
        Local Coverage Determinations (LCDs), 1185
        medical necessity, 1185
        National Coverage Determinations (NCDs), 1185
        upcoding, 1185
    American Medical Association (AMA)
        American Nomenclature of Disease, 1169

Coding *(Continued)*
  Current Procedural Terminology (CPT), 1169
  case studies of, 1177*b*-1178*b*, 1182*b*, 1185*b*, 1187*b*
  Current Procedural Terminology (CPT) codes, 1170-1175, 1175*b*-1177*b*
    anesthesia, 1174
    appendices, 1171
    category II, 1171
    category III, 1169
    established patients, 1173
    Evaluation/Management (E/M) section, 1172-1174
    index, 1171-1172
    inpatients, 1173
    manual sections, 1170-1171
    medical decision making, 1173, 1174*f*
    medical histories, 1173
    Medicine section, 1175
    modifiers, 1171
    new patients, 1173
    outpatients, 1173
    Pathology/Laboratory section, 1175
    physical examinations, 1173
    Radiology section, 1175
    secondary factors, 1174
    selection criteria, 1172-1175, 1172*f*
    Surgery section, 1174-1175
    symbols in, 1170-1171, 1170*f*
    unlisted codes, 1171
  diagnosis coding, 1179
    historical reviews of, 1179
    International Classification of Diseases (ICD), 1179. *See also* International
      Classification of Diseases (ICD).
  Healthcare Common Procedure Coding System (HCPCS)
    Level I, 1169
    Level II, 1169, 1177-1178, 1178*b*
    procedure codes, 1169
    selection criteria for, 1178, 1178*b*
  introduction to, 1169
  procedure codes, 1169
    Centers for Medicare and Medicaid Services (CMS) and, 1169
    definition of, 1169
    Health Insurance Portability and Accountability Act (HIPPA) and, 1169
  procedures for, 1175*b*-1177*b*, 1185*b*-1187*b*
  terminology of, 1169, 1188*b*
  Web resources for, 1188*b*
Collation, 1128
Collect on Delivery (COD), 1133, 1135-1136
Collection agencies, 1226-1227, 1229
Collection letters, 1226-1227, 1226*f*, 1231*b*
Collections/billing, 1217-1230
  account aging, 1223-1224
    of accounts receivable, 1223, 1224*f*, 1225*b*
    definition of, 1223
    overdue accounts, 1223-1224
  billing cycles, 1218, 1219*b*
  billing problems, 1220-1221
    checks, 1220-1221
    non-sufficient funds (NSF) designations, 1220-1221, 1221*b*-1222*b*
    overdrafts, 1220
  case studies of, 1221*b*, 1224*b*, 1230*b*-1232*b*
  collections, 1226-1230
    claim messages, 1226
    collection agencies, 1226-1227, 1229
    collection letters, 1226-1227, 1226*f*, 1231*b*
    credit agreements, 1227, 1228*f*
    estate billings, 1229
    outstanding balance policies, 1227-1228
    past due accounts, 1226
    skips tracing, 1228-1229
    small claims court, 1229
    techniques for, 1228-1230
    telephone, 1227*b*
    truth in lending agreements, 1227
  introduction to, 1218
  laws affecting, 1230
    Bankruptcy Abuse Prevention and Consumer Protection Act (2005), 1229-1230
    Equal Credit Opportunity Act, 1230
    Fair Credit Reporting Act, 1230
    Fair Debt Collections Practice Act (1966), 1226, 1230
    Federal Truth in Lending Act, 1227, 1230
    probate, 1229
  overpayments, 1221
    credit balances, 1221, 1222*b*-1223*b*
    refunds, 1221, 1222*b*-1223*b*
  patient statements, 1218, 1219*f*, 1225*b*
    balance due, 1218

Collections/billing *(Continued)*
    processing of, 1220*b*
    procedures for, 1220*b*-1223*b*, 1225*b*, 1231*b*
    processes, 1218
    processes of, 1218
    terminology of, 1217, 1232*b*
    Web resources for, 1232*b*
Colon and rectal surgery, 13*b*-14*b*
Comma. *See also* Punctuation and grammar.
  rules, 1124-1125
  splices, 1124
Commission on Accreditation of Allied Health Education Programs (CAAHEP), 20-21
Common nouns, 1122-1123
Communications
  telephone techniques, 1063-1075
  written, 1115-1128. *See also* Written communications.
    business letters, 1116-1120
    case studies of, 1123*b*, 1125*b*-1126*b*, 1128, 1128*b*-1129*b*
    confidentiality statements, 1127*f*
    electronic data transmission, 1125-1127
    grammar and punctuation, 1122-1125
    Health Insurance Portability and Accountability Act (HIPPA) and, 1116
    introduction to, 1116
    memorandum/memoranda (memo), 1116, 1123*f*
    photocopying, 1128
    procedures for, 1121*b*-1122*b*, 1127*b*-1128*b*
    proofreading, 1125
    spelling, 1125, 1125*b*
    terminology of, 1116, 1129*b*
    Web resources for, 1130*b*
Community health centers, 16
Community resources, 1249, 1249*b*-1250*b*
Company names, 1105. *See also* Names.
Complementary and alternative medicine (CAM), 16
  acupuncture, 16, 16*f*
  National Center for Complementary and Alternative Medicine, 16
  traditional medicine, 16
Complementary proteins, 922. *See also* Proteins.
Complete blood counts (CBCs), 861
Complete proteins, 922. *See also* Proteins.
Complex carbohydrates, 918. *See also* Carbohydrates.
Complex sentences, 1124. *See also* Sentences.
Complex testing rooms, 12
Compliance reporting, 1251
Complimentary closing, 1117, 1118*f*. *See also* Business letters.
Compound sentences, 1124. *See also* Sentences.
Computerization. *See also* Office computerization.
  backup protocols, 1058
  case studies of, 1046*b*, 1053*b*, 1055*b*, 1059*b*-1060*b*
  computer monitors, 1048-1049
  computer network security, 1057-1058
  computer system components, 1043-1046, 1043*f*
  data processing cycles, 1042-1043, 1043*f*
  electronic information transfer, 1055-1057
  electronic medical records (EMRs), 1057
  fundamental computer concepts, 1042
  input devices, 1049-1050
  introduction to, 1042
  medical office, 1053-1055
  printers, 1050-1052
  service agreements, 1059
  storage devices, 1052-1053
    definition of, 1052
    hard disk drives, 1052, 1052*f*
    jump drives, 1053
    optical disc drives, 1053
    optical discs, 1052-1053
    solid state drives, 1052
    thumb drives, 1053
    Universal Bus (USB) flash drives, 1053
  system maintenance protocols, 1058-1059
    disk cleanup, 1059
    disk defragmentation, 1059
    system administration, 1059
  terminology of, 1041, 1060*b*-1062*b*
  Web resources for, 1062*b*
Computerization considerations, 1040-1059
Conduction, 352
Confidentiality
  patient cheek-in and, 1029, 1029*f*
  statements, 1127*f*
Confusing word pairs, 1125*b*
Conjunctions, 1123
Consecutive numeric filing systems, 1106, 1106*t*. *See also* Filing systems.
Consultation reports, 1005

Contagious diseases, 898
Continuing education units (CEUs), 1267-1268
Continuity of care reports, 1005-1006. *See also* Medical records.
  components of, 1005
    attending physician reports, 1006
    consultation reports, 1005
    discharge summary reports, 1006
    emergency department reports, 1006
    home health care reports, 1005-1006
    hospital documents, 1006
    occupational therapy reports, 1006
    physical therapy reports, 1006
    speech therapy reports, 1006
    therapeutic service documents, 1006
  descriptions of, 1005
Contractility, 137
Control loss responses, 73
Convalescent period, 898
Convection, 352
Copayment acceptance, 1034
Copy notation (cc), 1117
Counting system, carbohydrates, 938
Course of fever, 354
Cover letters, 1261, 1262*f*. *See also* Résumés.
CPR training. *See* Cardiopulmonary resuscitation (CPR) training.
CPT. *See* Current Procedural Terminology (CPT).
Creatine phosphate, 139
Credit agreements, 1227, 1228*f*. *See also* Agreements.
Credit balances, 1221, 1222*b*-1223*b*. *See also* Billing/collections.
Cross-indexing, 1104
Cultural influences, 76-77
Curative treatments, 2
Current Procedural Terminology (CPT), 1175*b*-1177*b*. *See also* Medical coding.
  anesthesia, 1174
  appendices, 1171
  category II, 1171
  category III, 1169
  code selection criteria, 1172-1175, 1172*f*
  established patients, 1173
  Evaluation/Management (E/M) section, 1172-1174
  historical reviews of, 1169
  index, 1171-1172
  inpatients, 1173
  manual sections, 1170-1171
  medical decision making, 1173, 1174*f*
  medical histories, 1173
  Medicine section, 1175
  modifiers, 1171
  new patients, 1173
  outpatients, 1173
  Pathology/Laboratory section, 1175
  physical examinations, 1173
  Radiology section, 1175
  secondary factors, 1174
  Surgery section, 1174-1175
  symbols in, 1170-1171, 1170*f*
  unlisted codes, 1171
Cycles, billing, 1218, 1219*b*. *See also* Billing/collections.

D
Daily activities organization, 1026
DASH eating plan. *See* Dietary Approaches to Stop Hypertension (DASH) eating plan.
Data processing cycles, 1042-1043, 1043*f*
Date line, 1116, 1118*f*. *See also* Business letters.
Decision making, medical, 1173, 1174*f*
Defense mechanisms, 74*b*-75*b*
Delivery confirmation services, 1133-1136. *See also* United States Postal Service (USPS).
  Certificates of Mailing, 1133
  Certified Mail, 1133-1134, 1134*f*
  Collect on Delivery (COD), 1133, 1135-1136
  Insured Mail, 1135
  Registered Mail, 1133-1135
  Restricted Delivery, 1134
  Return Receipt, 1133-1134, 1135*f*
  Signature Confirmation, 1134
  Special Handling, 1135
Delivery services, 1136
Deltoid muscle, 144
Denaturation, 942
Denial, 76. *See also* Grieving process.
Dependent clauses, 1124
Depression, 76
Dermatology, 13*b*-14*b*
Developmental stages, 70

DHL delivery service, 1136
Diabetes, 937-939
  type 1, 937-939
  type 2, 939
Diagnosis coding, 1179. *See also* Medical coding.
  historical reviews of, 1179
  International Classification of Diseases (ICD), 1179. *See also* International Classification of Diseases (ICD).
Diagnostic procedure reports, 1005. *See also* Medical records.
  components of, 1005
    electrocardiogram (ECG) reports, 1005
    Holter monitor reports, 1005
    imaging reports, 1005
    radiology reports, 1005
    spirometry reports, 1005
  description of, 1005
Diaphragm, 138*b*, 143
Diaphragm, pelvic, 143
Diaphysis, 121, 121*f*
Diarthroses, 131-132, 132*f*
Dietary Approaches to Stop Hypertension (DASH) eating plan, 936-937, 936*t*
Dietary cholesterol, 920
Dietary fiber, 918-919, 919*f*, 919*t*
Dietary Guidelines for Americans (2010), 928, 929*b*
Dietary supplements, 927-928
Dieticians, 917
Diets, 917
Differential counts, 862-863, 863*b*-865*b*
Digestion, 917
Digestive system, 235-248
Digital image, 1005
Digital signatures, 1111*b*
Digital subscriber line (DSL), 1055-1056
Diploë, 120
Direct muscle attachments, 138
Disaccharides, 918
Disbursements, 1157
Discharge summary reports, 1006
Disinfection/sterilization, 318-345
Disposable single-use thermometers, 358-359. *See also* Thermometers.
Dividers, chart, 1100-1101
DO degrees. *See* Doctor of osteopathy (DO) degrees.
Doctor of osteopathy (DO) degrees, 8
Domestic mail classifications, 1132-1133
  First-Class Mail, 1132-1133
  Media Mail, 1133
  Standard Post, 1133
Dorsalis pedis pulse, 372. *See also* Pulse.
Dorsiflexion, 140, 141*f*-142*f*
Downcoding, 1185. *See also* Medical coding.
Drug testing, 794*b*
DSL. *See* Digital subscriber line (DSL).
Duiuresis, 787
Duplex photocopying, 1128
Dysrhythmia, 373
Dysuria, 787

E
E codes, 1180
E-mail
  attachments, 1126
  uses of, 1125-1126
E-prescribing, 1056-1057
E/M section. *See* Evaluation/Management (E/M) section.
Ear
  assessments, 441-458
  procedures, 441-458
  temperature, 356. *See also* Temperature.
Earlobe temperature, 358. *See also* Temperature.
Eating disorders, 933*b*-934*b*
ECG reports. *See* Electrocardiogram (ECG) reports.
EDTA. *See* Ethylenediaminetetraacetic acid (EDTA).
Educational programs, 20-21
Effective teamwork, 9-10. *See also* Teams.
Effective treatments, 2
Ego defense mechanisms, 74*b*-75*b*
EHRs. *See* Electronic health records (EHRs).
Elasticity, 137
Electrical shock, 138*b*
Electrocardiogram (ECG) reports, 1005
Electronic claim submissions, 1209
Electronic data transmission, 1125-1127. *See also* Written communications.
  e-mail
    attachments, 1126
    uses of, 1125-1126

Electronic data transmission (Continued)
    fax transmissions, 1127, 1127b-1128b, 1127f
    secure messaging in, 1126
Electronic health records (EHRs), 994
Electronic medical records (EMRs), 994, 1057
    introduction to, 994
    management of, 1110-1111
    medical assistants use of, 1057
    physicians use of, 1057
    secure messaging in, 1126
Electronic signatures, 1111b
Electronic thermometers, 356, 359b-361b. See also Thermometers.
Elimination diets, 941
Emergency
    department reports, 1006
    medical procedures, 967-988
    medicine, 13b-14b
    preparedness, 944-964
Emotional responses to illness, 72-74
    anger, 74
    anxiety, 73-74
    ego defense mechanisms, 74b-75b
    grieving process, 75-76. See also Grieving process.
    loss of control, 73
Empirical evidence, 2
Employee schedules, 1248
Employment/job-seeking considerations, 1255-1268
    advancement and career changes, 1268
        clinical skill upgrades, 1268
        management advancement, 1268
        skill transfers, 1268
        technical skill upgrades, 1268
    case studies of, 1261b, 1263b, 1267b, 1269b
    current opportunity trends, 31
    employment applications, 1262
    interviews, 1263-1264
        follow-ups after, 1264, 1266f
        hiring timeline determinations, 1264
        preparation for, 1263
        professional appearance/behavior and, 1263-1264, 1264f
        questions and responses, 1264, 1265b
        salary/benefit discussions, 1264
        techniques for, 1263-1264
    introduction to, 1256
    job searches, 1256
        goal setting, 1256
        networking, 1256
        potential employer identification, 1256
        tools for, 1256-1263
    law/legislation updates, 1267
    lifelong learning, 1266-1268
        administrative skills, 1266
        burnout avoidance, 1266-1267
        clinical skills, 1266
        continuing education units (CEUs), 1267-1268
        increased responsibility preparation, 1266
    peer support, 1267
    professional organizations, 1267
    résumés, 1256-1261
        action verbs in, 1260f
        activity sections in, 1260
        chronological, 1257, 1258f
        cover letters and, 1261, 1262f
        credential sections of, 1260
        definition of, 1255
        education sections in, 1257
        examples of, 1258f-1260f
        formatting of, 1261
        functional, 1257, 1259f
        mailing of, 1261-1262
        objective sections in, 1257
        personal demographic sections in, 1257
        previous experience sections in, 1257-1259
        reference sections of, 1261
        required information in, 1257-1261
        special skills sections of, 1259-1260
        styles of, 1257
        targeted, 1257, 1260f
    terminology of, 1255, 1269b
    Web resources for, 1270b
Empty calorie foods, 917-918
Enc. notations. See Enclosure (enc.) notations.
Enclosure (enc.) notations, 1117. See also Business letters.
End notations, 1117, 1118f. See also Business letters.

Endocrine system, 186-195
    endocrine glands, 187-194, 188f, 189t
    endocrinology, 187
    hormones, 187, 189t
        action mechanisms of, 187, 188f
        characteristics of, 187
        chemical nature of, 187
        definition of, 187
        target tissues of, 187
    introduction to, 187
    vs. nervous system, 187
    pituitary gland (hypophysis), 188-192, 191f
    terminology of, 186, 195b
    Web resources for, 195b
Endocrinology, 187
Endosteum, 121, 121f
Energy sources, 139-140
Enriched foods, 917
Envelope preparation, 1142-1143, 1144b
    no. 10 envelopes, 1142
    no. 6 3/4 envelopes, 1142
    postal addressing standards, 1139-1141
    window envelopes, 1142
Epimysium, 137
Epiphyseal line, 121
Epiphyseal plate, 121, 121f
Epiphysis, 121, 121f
EPOs. See Exclusive provider organizations (EPOs).
Equal Credit Opportunity Act, 1230
Equipment checks, 1026-1027
Equipment maintenance, 1240-1241
Erector spinae group, 143
Ergonomics, 1048-1050, 1050f
Erickson's stages of psychosocial development, 70, 70t
Essential amino acids, 922. See also Amino acids.
Established patients, 1033-1034, 1173
Estate billing, 1229. See also Billing/collections.
Ethics, 34-57
Ethylenediaminetetraacetic acid (EDTA), 818-819
Evaluation/Management (E/M) section, 1172-1174. See also Current Procedural Terminology (CPT).
Eversion, 140, 141f-142f
Evidence, empirical, 2
Examination rooms, 11-12, 11f
Exchange lists system, 937-938, 938f
Excitability, 137
Exclusive provider organizations (EPOs), 1195
Exercise, aerobic, 373b
Exhalation, 374, 374f
Experimental research, 2
Extensibility, 137
Extension, 140, 141f-142f
External intercostals, 143
External oblique, 143
Externships, 21
Eye assessments and procedures, 441-458

F
Fahrenheit-Celsius conversion, 353t
Fainting, 844b, 845
Fair Credit Reporting Act, 1230
Fair Debt Collections Practice Act (1966), 1226, 1230
Family histories, 1008. See also Histories.
Family medicine, 13b-14b
Fat-soluble vitamins, 923, 925t. See also Vitamins.
Fats, 919-921, 920f
    cholesterol, 920
    classification of, 920-921
    definition of, 919
    saturated, 920
    trans, 920
    triglycerides, 921
    unsaturated, 920
Fatty acids, 139
Fax
    checks of, 1026
    transmissions, 1127, 1127b-1128b, 1127f
Federal Express (FedEx), 1136
Federal Truth in Lending Act, 1227, 1230
FedEx. See Federal Express (FedEx).
Fee-for-service plans, 2-3, 1193-1194
Fellowships, 12
Femoral pulse, 372. See also Pulse.
Fever, 354, 355b, 355t
Fiber, dietary, 918-919, 919f, 919t

Fifth digit selection, 1180-1181, 1180*t*-1181*t*
File cabinets, 1099
File clerks, 8
Filing supplies, 1100-1101, 1101*f*
Filing systems, 1104-1106
  alphabetic, 1104-1105, 1107*b*
    abbreviations, 1104
    companies/businesses, 1105
    cross-indexing, 1104
    hyphenation, 1104
    identical names, 1105
    indexing units, 1104
    individual names, 1104
    married women, names of, 1105
    nicknames, 1104
    prefixes, 1104
    seniority terms, 1105
    surnames, 1104
    titles, 1105
  chronological, 1106
  definition of, 1104
  numeric, 1105-1106, 1108*b*
    consecutive, 1106, 1106*t*
    terminal digit, 1106, 1106*t*
  selection criteria for, 1106
  subject, 1106
Finance management, 1146-1166
  accounting, 1147. *See also* Accounting.
  banking activities, 1157-1162. *See* Banking activities.
    account types, 1157-1158
  bookkeeping systems, 1148*b*
  case studies of, 1145*b*, 1148*b*-1149*b*, 1152*b*, 1162*b*, 1166*b*-1167*b*
  introduction to, 1147
  non-patient accounts, 1157
    accounts payable, 1157
    disbursements, 1157
    petty cash, 1157
  patient accounts. *See* Patient accounts.
  procedures for, 1152*b*-1157*b*, 1163*b*-1165*b*
  terminology of, 1147, 1152*b*, 1163*b*-1164*b*
  Web resources for, 1167*b*
Finger puncture guidelines, 850-851, 851*f*
Firewalls, 1058
First aid, 967-988
First-Class Mail, 1132-1133
First-voided morning specimens, 788
Flexion, 140, 141*f*-142*f*
Folding/inserting letters, 1142, 1142*f*
Food allergies, 941-942, 941*f*
Food labels, 929-932
  ingredient lists, 931-932, 931*f*
  Nutrition Facts panels, 930-931, 930*f*
Forehead temperature, 356. *See also* Temperature.
Formulary exceptions, 1200
Fortified foods, 917
Frequency, 787
Frontalis muscle, 140-143
Full block style, 1117-1120. *See also* Business letters.
Function keys, 1049
Functional résumés, 1257, 1259*f*. *See also* Résumés.
Fundamental concepts
  anatomy and physiology, 80-105. *See also* Anatomy and physiology.
  health care system, 1-16
  medical assistant profession, 19-31
  medical ethics and law, 34-57
  patient interactions, 61-77

G
Gap, synaptic, 139
Gaster, 138
Gastrocnemius muscles, 147
GBs. *See* Gigabytes (GBs).
General surgery, 13*b*-14*b*
Genetics, medical, 13*b*-14*b*
GHz. *See* Gigahertz (GHz).
Gigabytes (GBs), 1047
Gigahertz (GHz), 1047
Glands
  endocrine, 187-194, 188*f*, 189*t*
  pituitary (hypophysis), 188-192, 191*f*
Glucose, 139
Gluten intolerance, 940-941
Gluteus
  maximus, 144

Gluteus (*Continued*)
  medius, 144
  minimus, 144
Goal setting, 1256
Government plans, 5, 1196-1198
GPAs. *See* Grade point averages (GPAs).
Gracilis muscles, 144-147
Grade point averages (GPAs), 1257
Gram stain, 911-912
Grammar and punctuation, 1122-1125
  comma rules, 1124-1125
  confusing word pairs, 1125*b*
  definitions of, 1122
  parts of speech, 1122-1123
  sentences, 1124. *See also* Sentences.
Greeting/salutation, 1116-1117, 1118*f*. *See also* Business letters.
Grieving process, 62
  acceptance, 76
  anger, 76
  bargaining, 76
  denial, 76
  depression, 76
  hospice and, 76
  terminal phase, 75
Group practice, 15
Gynecologic examinations, 487-521

H
Hamstrings, 147
Handwritten signatures, 1117, 1118*f*. *See also* Signatures.
HCG. *See* Human chorionic gonadotropin (HCG).
HCPCS. *See* Healthcare Common Procedure Coding System (HCPCS).
Hct. *See* Hematocrit (Hct).
HDL. *See* High-density lipoprotein (HDL).
Headings, 1116, 1118*f*. *See also* Business letters.
Health care reform, 6
Health care system, 1-16
  ambulatory care, 6-10
    activity flow in, 6-8, 7*f*
    definition of, 6
  case studies of, 8*b*-9*b*, 12*b*, 16*b*-17*b*
  complementary and alternative medicine (CAM), 16
    acupuncture, 16, 16*f*
    National Center for Complementary and Alternative Medicine, 16
    traditional medicine, 16
  health care teams, 8-10
    definition of, 8
    effective teamwork, 9-10
    medical assistant roles in, 8
    members of, 8, 9*t*
    United States Medical Licensing Examination (USMLE) and, 8
  health insurance, 2-6. *See also* Health insurance.
    definition of, 3
    fee-for-service plans, 2-3
    government plans, 5
    health care reform and, 6
    health maintenance organizations (HMOs), 5-6
    managed care, 5-6
    Patient Protection and Affordable Care Act (2010), 6
  historical reviews of, 3*b*-5*b*, 3*f*-4*f*
  introduction to, 2
  medical offices, 10-12
    American with Disabilities Act specifications for, 10
    business office areas, 11-12
    Clinical Laboratory Improvement Amendments (CLIA 1988) regulations for, 10-11
    complex testing rooms, 12
    examination rooms, 11, 11*f*
    laboratories, 11
    layouts of, 10-12, 10*f*
    lunch/break rooms, 12
    medical records storage, 11-12
    Occupational Safety and Health Administration (OSHA) standards for, 10
    patient progress through, 7*f*
    pediatric examination/treatment rooms, 12
    physician private offices, 12
    reception areas, 7*f*, 11
    staff rooms, 12
    surgical procedure rooms, 12
    trauma rooms, 12
    waiting rooms, 11
  medical specialties, 12-15, 13*b*-14*b*
    American Board of Medical Specialties recognition of, 12, 13*b*-14*b*
    chiropractic, 15, 15*f*
    comparisons of, 13*b*-14*b*

Health care system (Continued)
  fellowships and, 12
  osteopathy, 14
  patient-centered medical home (PCMH), 12-14
  podiatry, 14-15
  primary care, 12-14
  practice types, 15-16
    clinics, 16
    group practice, 15
    solo practice, 15
  terminology of, 1, 17b
  trends in, 2
  Web resources for, 18b
Health care teams, 8-10
  definition of, 8
  effective teamwork, 9-10
  medical assistant roles in, 8
  members of, 8, 9t
Health coaching, 30-31
Health histories, 1007-1008. See also Histories.
  components of, 1007-1008
    allergies, 1008
    chief complaint (CC), 999b, 1007, 1007f
    family histories, 1008
    identification data, 1007
    immunizations, 1008
    medications, current, 1008
    past histories, 1008
    present illness (PI), 1007-1008
    review of systems (ROS), 1008
    social histories, 1008
  definition of, 1007
  forms for, 1009f-1010f
  procedures for, 999b
Health insurance, 2-6
  definition of, 3
  fee-for-service plans, 2-3
  government plans, 5
  health care reform and, 6
  health maintenance organizations (HMOs), 5-6
  managed care, 5-6
  Patient Protection and Affordable Care Act (2010), 6
Health Insurance Portability and Accountability Act (HIPAA)
  Check-in procedures and, 1030
Health Insurance Portability and Accountability Act (HIPPA), 1116, 1169
Health maintenance organizations (HMOs), 5-6, 1195
Health, definition of, 2
Healthcare Common Procedure Coding System (HCPCS). See also Medical coding.
  Level I, 1169
  Level II, 1169
  Level II codes, 1177-1178, 1178b
  procedures codes, 1169
  selection criteria for, 1178, 1178b
Hearing impairments, 68
Heat
  loss, 352
  production, 352
Hematocrit (Hct), 856f, 857, 858b-860b
Hematology, 854-868
  case studies of, 857b, 861b, 863b, 868b
  complete blood counts (CBCs), 861
  definition of, 855
  hematocrit (Hct), 856f, 857, 858b-860b
  hemoglobin (Hgb), 855-857, 857f
  introduction to, 855
  iron deficiency anemia, 860b
  posthrombin time/International Normalized Ratio (PT/INR) tests, 866-868
    coagulation analyzers, 867, 867f
    home testing, 867-868, 867f-868f
    purpose of, 866
    specimen collection for, 866-867, 867f
  procedures for, 858b-860b, 863b-865b
  red blood cells (RBCs), 862f
    counts, 861
    indices, 861
  terminology of, 854, 869b
  Web resources for, 854, 869b
  white blood cells (WBCs), 862f
    counts, 861
    differential counts, 862-863, 863b-865b
Hematomas, 820, 844
Hematuria, 787
Hemoconcentration, 819-820
Hemoglobin (Hgb), 855-857, 857f
Hemolysis, 844

Hgb. See Hemoglobin (Hgb).
Hierarchy of needs (Maslow), 69, 69f
High-density lipoprotein (HDL), 921
HIPPA. See Health Insurance Portability and Accountability Act (HIPPA).
Hippocrates, 2
Hiring timeline determinations, 1264
Histories
  coding of, 1173
  family, 1008
  forms for, 1009f-1010f, 1030
  health, 1007-1008. See also Health histories.
    components of, 1007-1008
    definition of, 1007
    procedures for, 999b
  past, 1008
  social, 1008
HMOs. See Health maintenance organizations (HMOs).
Holistic medicine, 14
Holter monitor reports, 1005
Home health care reports, 1005-1006
Horseback riding, 138b
Horserider's muscles, 144-147
Hospice, 76
Hospital documents, 1006
Human chorionic gonadotropin (HCG), 807
Hyperextension, 140, 141f-142f
Hyperpyrexia, 353
Hypertension, 936-937
Hyphenation, 1104
Hypophysis, 188-192, 191f
Hypothermia, 353

I
ICD. See International Classification of Diseases (ICD).
Identical names, 1105
Identification data, 1007
Iliopsoas, 144
Imaging reports, 1005
Immunizations, 1008
Immunoassays, 807-808
Immunology, 870-891
Inactive records, 1112
Incident reports, 1251, 1252b
Incoming mail, 1136-1137. See also Mail/shipping.
  annotations on, 1137
  opening guidelines, 1137
  processing of, 1136-1137, 1137b-1138b
  sorting guidelines, 1136, 1136t, 1138f
Incomplete proteins, 922. See also Proteins.
Incontinence, urinary, 787
Incubation period, 898
Indemnity, 1193
Indented paragraphs, 1117, 1119f
Independent clauses, 1124
Independent practice associations (IPAs), 1195
Indexing units, 1104
Indices
  body mass (BMI), 932-934, 934t
  of Current Procedural Terminology (CPT), 1171-1172
  ICD-10-CM, 1182-1183
  ICD-9-CM, 1180
  red blood cells (RBCs), 861
Indirect muscle attachments, 138
Individual names, 1104. See also Names.
Infectious diseases
  stages of, 898
  treatments for, 3b-5b, 3f-4f
Informational materials, 1037
Ingredient lists, 931-932, 931f
Inhalation, 374, 374f
Initiative, 23-24
Inpatients, 1006, 1173
INR. See International Normalized Ratio (INR).
Inserting/folding letters, 1142, 1142f
Insertion, muscle, 138
Inside address, 1116, 1118f. See also Business letters.
Insoluble fiber, 919, 919f
Instructional notes, 1184f
Insurance, 2-6, 1189-1212. See also Medical insurance.
  cards, 1198, 1199f, 1200b
  case studies of, 1194b, 1204b, 1210b, 1213b-1214b
  claim forms, 1202-1204, 1203f
  claim submissions, 1209-1210
  definition of, 3
  effective communication for, 1212, 1213b

Insurance (Continued)
  fee-for-service plans, 2-3
  government plans, 5
  health care reform and, 6
  health maintenance organizations (HMOs), 5-6
  historical reviews of, 1191
  introduction to, 1190-1191
  managed care, 5-6
  obtaining, 1191-1192
  Patient Protection and Affordable Care Act (2010), 6
  paying for, 1192
  policies for, 1198-1200
  procedures for, 1198-1200, 1200b-1202b, 1205b-1209b, 1213b
  reimbursement tracking, 1210-1211
  reimbursements, 1192-1193
  terminology of, 1190, 1214b-1215b
  types of, 1193-1198
  verification/authorization, 1030-1032
  Web resources for, 1216b
Insurance and delivery confirmation services, 1133-1136. See also United States Postal
    Service (USPS).
  Certificates of Mailing, 1133
  Certified Mail, 1133-1134, 1134f
  Collect on Delivery (COD), 1133, 1135-1136
  Insured Mail, 1135
  Registered Mail, 1133-1135
  Restricted Delivery, 1134
  Return Receipt, 1133-1134, 1135f
  Signature Confirmation, 1134
  Special Handling, 1135
Interactions, patient, 61-77. See also Patient interactions.
  case studies of, 65b, 68b, 72b, 74b, 77b-78b
  communication, 62-68
  cultural influences, 76-77
  emotional responses to illness, 72-74
  interviewing techniques, 65-67
  introduction to, 62
  listening skills, 64-65
  patient needs, 69-77
  procedures for, 71b
  self-boundaries, 72, 73b
Intercostals, external vs. internal, 143
Interjections, 1123
Internal intercostals, 143
Internal medicine, 13b-14b
Internal obliques, 143
Internal respiration, 374, 374f
International Classification of Diseases (ICD), 1179. See also Medical coding.
  historical reviews of, 1179
  ICD-10-CM, 1181-1185
    alphabetic index, 1182-1183
    code selection specificity criteria, 1184-1185, 1184t
    contents of, 1181t
    format of, 1181-1182
    instructional notes, 1184f
    tabular list, 1183-1185, 1183f
    V codes, 1182
    Z codes, 1182
  ICD-9-CM, 1179-1181
    E codes, 1180
    fifth digit selection, 1180-1181, 1180t-1181t
    format of, 1179-1180
    index, 1180
    morphology (M) codes, 1180
    not elsewhere classifiable (NEC) codes, 1180
    not otherwise specified (NOS) codes, 1180
    numeric codes (001-999.9), 1179-1180
    tablular list, 1180-1181
    V codes, 1180
  World Health Organization (WHO) and, 1179
International Normalized Ratio (INR), 866-868
Internet service providers (ISPs), 1055-1056
Internships, 8
Interviewing techniques, 65-67
  closed questions, 65
  open questions, 65
Interviews, 1263-1264
  follow-ups after, 1264, 1266f
  hiring timeline determinations, 1264
  interviews, 1263-1264
  preparation for, 1263
  professional appearance/behavior and, 1263-1264, 1264f
  questions and responses, 1264, 1265b
  salary/benefit discussions, 1264
  techniques for, 1263-1264

Intravenous (IV) therapy administration, 613-683
Inversion, 140, 141f-142f
IPAs. See Independent practice associations (IPAs).
Iron deficiency anemia, 860b
ISPs. See Internet service providers (ISPs).

J
Job-seeking considerations, 1255-1268. See also Employment/job-seeking
    considerations.
  advancement and career changes, 1268
  case studies of, 1261b, 1263b, 1267b, 1269b
  current opportunity trends, 31
  employment applications, 1262
  interviews, 1263-1264. See also Interviews.
  introduction to, 1256
  job searches, 1256
  law/legislation updates, 1267
  lifelong learning, 1266-1268. See also Lifelong learning.
  peer support, 1267
  professional organizations, 1267
  résumés, 1256-1261. See also Résumés.
  terminology of, 1255, 1269b
  Web resources for, 1270b
Job-seeking/employment considerations, 1255-1268
Justification, left vs. right, 1117-1120

K
KBs. See Kilobytes (KBs).
Kcal. See Kilocalories (kcal).
Ketones, 795
Kilobytes (KBs), 1047
Kilocalories (kcal), 917
Kova method, 804b-807b

L
Labels, food, 929-932
Laboratories, 11, 752-783
Lactose intolerance, 939-940
Language barriers, 68
Large medical groups, 15
Latissimus dorsi, 144
Laws and legislation, 34-57
  American with Disabilities Act (ADA), 10
  Clinical Laboratory Improvement Amendments (CLIA 1988), 10-11
  for collections, 1230. See also Collections/billing.
    Bankruptcy Abuse Prevention and Consumer Protection act (2005), 1229-1230
    Bankruptcy Abuse Prevention and Consumer Protection Act (2005), 1229-1230
    Equal Credit Opportunity Act, 1230
    Fair Credit Reporting Act, 1230
    Fair Debt Collections Practice Act (1966), 1226, 1230
    Federal Truth in Lending Act, 1227, 1230
    probate, 1229
  ethics and. See Ethics.
  Health Insurance Portability and Accountability Act (HIPPA), 1116, 1169
  Occupational Safety and Health Administration (OSHA) regulations, 10
  Patient Protection and Affordable Care Act (2010), 6
Layouts, 10-12, 10f. See also Medical offices.
LCDs. See Local Coverage Determinations (LCDs).
LDL. See Low-density lipoprotein (LDL).
Left justification, 1117-1120
Legislation. See Laws and legislation.
Letterhead vs. return address, 1116, 1118f. See also Business letters.
Letters
  business, 1116-1120. See also Written communications.
    composition of, 1120, 1121b-1122b
    definition of, 1116
    enclosures (enc.), 1117
    equipment for, 1116
    examples of, 1118f-1120f
    format of, 1117-1120
    parts of, 1116-1117, 1118f
    procedures for, 1121b-1122b
    set-up of, 1117
    styles of, 1117-1120
    supplies for, 1116
    templates of, 1116
  collection, 1226-1227, 1226f, 1231b. See also Collections/billing.
  cover, 1261, 1262f. See also Résumés.
Level of understanding impairments, 67
Licensed practical nurses (LPNs), 8
Lifelong learning, 1266-1268
  administrative skills, 1266
  burnout avoidance, 1266-1267
  clinical skills, 1266
  continuing education units (CEUs), 1267-1268

Linea alba, 143
Lipoproteins, 921
Listening skills, 64-65
    active listening, 64, 66t
    nonverbal facilitation measures, 64-65, 64f
Local Coverage Determinations (LCDs), 1185. See also Medical coding.
Loss of control responses, 73
Low-density lipoprotein (LDL), 921
Low-nutrient density foods, 918
LPNs. See Licensed practical nurses (LPNs).
Lunch/break rooms, 12

M
M codes. See Morphology (M) codes.
Macronutrients, 917, 917t
Mail/shipping, 1131-1143
    case studies for, 1134b, 1136b-1137b, 1143b, 1145b
    e-mail, 1125-1126. See also Electronic data transmission.
    incoming mail, 1136-1137
        annotations on, 1137
        opening guidelines, 1137
        processing of, 1136-1137, 1137b-1138b
        sorting guidelines, 1136, 1136t, 1138f
    introduction to, 1132
    outgoing mail, 1142-1143
        adding postage, 1142-1143
        envelope preparation, 1144b. See also Envelope preparation.
        folding/inserting letters, 1142, 1142f
        metered mail/postage meters, 1142-1143, 1143b
        online postage services, 1143
        safety precautions for, 1143
    private carrier package delivery services, 1136
    procedures for, 1137b-1138b, 1141b
    résumés, mailing of, 1261-1262. See also Résumés.
    terminology of, 1132, 1145b
    United States Postal Service (USPS), 1132-1136. See also United States Postal Service (USPS).
        automated mail processing, 1138, 1139b
        delivery confirmation services, 1133-1136
        insurance, 1133-1136
        postal addressing standards, 1139-1141
        postal bar code system, 1132, 1133f
        postal money orders, 1136
        Zone Improvement Plan (ZIP) code system, 1132, 1141b
    Web resources for, 1145b
Major minerals, 924, 926t
Malaise, 354
Malnutrition, 917
Managed care, 5-6, 1033
Management components
    appointment scheduling, 1078-1093
    billing/collections, 1217-1230
    job-seeking/employment considerations, 1255-1268
    mail/shipping, 1131-1143
    medical coding, 1168-1185
    medical insurance, 1189-1212
    medical office computerization, 1040-1059
    medical records, 991-1021
    medical records management, 1098-1112
    office manager roles, 1233-1251
    patient reception, 1025-1037
    practice finance management, 1146-1166
    telephone techniques, 1063-1075
    written communications, 1115-1128
Manager roles, 1233-1251
Married women, names of, 1105. See also Names.
Maslow's hierarchy of needs, 69, 69f
Masseter muscle, 140-141
Master of Science in Nursing (MSN), 8
MBs. See Megabytes (MBs).
MD degrees. See Medical doctor (MD) degrees.
Meaningful use, 997b
Media Mail, 1133
Median cubital veins, 821
Medicaid, 1191, 1197
Medical asepsis, 290-314
Medical assistant profession, 19-31
    behavioral skills, 23-24
        initiative, 23-24
        organizational skills, 24
        task lists, 24
        teams, 24
        time management, 23-24
    case studies of, 21b-22b, 25b-26b, 31b-32b
    certification, 26-28

Medical assistant profession (Continued)
    additional credentials, 27-28
    American Association of Medical Assistants (AAMA) and, 26-27
    American Heart Association (AHA) and, 27
    American Medical Technologists (AMT), 27
    American Red Cross (ARC) and, 27
    American Society for Clinical Pathology (ASCP) and, 27
    American Society of Phlebotomy Technicians (ASPT) and, 27
    California Certifying Board for Medical Assistants (CCBMA), 27
    cardiopulmonary resuscitation (CPR) training, 27
    Certified Medical Assistant (CMA), 21, 21b, 26-27
    National Center for Competency Testing (NCCT), 27
    National Healthcareer Association (NHA) and, 27
    registered medical assistant (RMA), 27
    registered phlebotomy technician (RPT), 27
    characteristics of, 21-24
        character traits, 21
        personality traits, 22
        professional appearance, 21-23, 21f-23f
    educational programs for, 20-21
        accreditation, 20-21
        Accrediting Bureau of Health Education Schools (ABHES), 20-21
        Commission on Accreditation of Allied Health Education Programs (CAAHEP), 20-21
        practicums/externships, 21
    employment opportunities, 31
    historical reviews of, 20
    introduction to, 20
    legal scope of practice, 24b
    medical assistant roles, 28-31
        administrative responsibilities, 28-29
        clinical responsibilities, 29-30, 29f
        health coaching, 30-31
        office management responsibilities, 30
        patient education, 30-31, 30f
        patient navigation, 31
    procedures for, 24b
    professional organizations, 28
        American Association of Medical Assistants (AAMA), 20, 26-27
        continuing education units (CEUs) and, 28
        legislative advocacy, 28
        peer support and, 28
        publications, 28
    professionalism, 25-26
        American Medical Assistant Association (AAMA), Code of Ethics, 25
        definition of, 25
        for medical assistants, 25-26
        for physicians, 25, 25b-26b
    terminology of, 19, 32b
    Web resources for, 33b
Medical assisting concepts
    administrative components
        appointment scheduling, 1078-1093
        billing/collections, 1217-1230
        job-seeking/employment considerations, 1255-1268
        mail/shipping, 1131-1143
        medical coding, 1168-1185
        medical insurance, 1189-1212
        medical office computerization, 1040-1059
        medical records, 991-1021
        medical records management, 1098-1112
        office manager roles, 1233-1251
        patient reception, 1025-1037
        practice finance management, 1146-1166
        telephone techniques, 1063-1075
        written communications, 1115-1128
    anatomy and physiology
        circulatory system, 196-216
        digestive system, 235-248
        endocrine system, 186-195
        fundamentals of, 80-105
        integumentary system, 111-115
        muscular system, 136-147
        nervous system, 151-168
        reproductive systems, 266-283
        respiratory system, 224-230
        senses, 173-182
        skeletal system, 118-133
        urinary system, 254-264
    clinical components
        blood chemistry, 870-891
        cardiopulmonary procedures, 687-716
        clinical laboratories, 752-783
        ear assessments/procedures, 441-458
        emergency medical procedures, 967-988

Medical assisting concepts (Continued)
   emergency preparedness, 944-964
   eye assessments/procedures, 441-458
   first aid, 967-988
   gynecologic examinations, 487-521
   hematology, 854-868
   immunology, 870-891
   intravenous (IV) therapy administration, 613-683
   medical asepsis, 290-314
   medical microbiology, 896-912
   medications, 613-683
   minor office surgery, 560-609
   nutrition, 915-942
   Occupational Safety and Health Administration (OSHA) standards, 290-314
   pediatric examinations, 529-556
   phlebotomy, 814-851
   physical examinations, 405-436
   prenatal care, 487-521
   protective practices, 944-964
   specialty examinations/procedures, 719-748
   sterilization/disinfection, 318-345
   tissue healing physical agents, 467-479
   urinalysis, 786-809
   vital signs, 350-396
  fundamentals
   health care system, 1-16
   medical assistant profession, 19-31
   medical ethics and law, 34-57
   patient interactions, 61-77
Medical coding, 1168-1185
  accuracy requirements of, 1185-1187
   downcoding, 1185
   Local Coverage Determinations (LCDs), 1185
   medical necessity, 1185
   National Coverage Determinations (NCDs), 1185
   upcoding, 1185
  case studies of, 1177b-1178b, 1182b, 1185b, 1187b
  Current Procedural Terminology (CPT) codes, 1175b-1177b
   anesthesia, 1174
   appendices, 1171
   category II, 1171
   category III, 1169
   established patients, 1173
   Evaluation/Management (E/M) section, 1172-1174
   index, 1171-1172
   inpatients, 1173
   manual sections, 1170-1171
   medical decision making, 1173, 1174f
   medical histories, 1173
   Medicine section, 1175
   modifiers, 1171
   new patients, 1173
   outpatients, 1173
   Pathology/Laboratory section, 1175
   physical examinations, 1173
   Radiology section, 1175
   secondary factors, 1174
   selection criteria, 1172-1175, 1172f
   Surgery section, 1174-1175
   symbols in, 1170-1171, 1170f
   unlisted codes, 1171
  diagnosis coding, 1179
   historical reviews of, 1179
   International Classification of Diseases (ICD), 1179. See also International
     Classification of Diseases (ICD).
  Healthcare Common Procedure Coding System (HCPCS)
   Level I, 1169
   procedures codes, 1169
  Healthcare Common Procedure Coding System (HCPCS) codes
   Level II, 1169, 1177-1178, 1178b
   selection criteria for, 1178, 1178b
  Healthcare Common Procedure Coding System (HCPCS) Level II codes,
    1177-1178, 1178b
  introduction to, 1169
  procedure codes, 1169
   Centers for Medicare and Medicaid Services (CMS) and, 1169
   definition of, 1169
   Health Insurance Portability and Accountability Act (HIPPA) and, 1169
  procedures for, 1175b-1177b, 1185b-1187b
  terminology of, 1169, 1188b
  Web resources for, 1188b
Medical decision making, 1173, 1174f
Medical doctor (MD) degrees, 8
Medical ethics and law, 34-57
Medical genetics, 13b-14b

Medical histories. See Histories.
Medical impressions, 1002
Medical insurance, 1189-1212
  case studies of, 1194b, 1204b, 1210b, 1213b-1214b
  claim forms, 1202-1204, 1203f
   carrier information, 1204
   common errors on, 1212t
   completion of, 1204-1205, 1205b-1209b
   physician information, 1205
   place of service codes, 1205t
  claim submissions, 1209-1210
   electronic, 1209
   paper, 1210
  effective communication for, 1212, 1213b
  historical reviews of, 1191
  introduction to, 1190-1191
  obtaining, 1191-1192
  paying for, 1192
  policies for, 1198-1200
  procedures for, 1198-1200, 1200b-1202b, 1205b-1209b, 1213b
   eligibility verification, 1198-1199, 1201b
   formulary exceptions, 1200
   insurance cards, 1198, 1199f, 1200b
   National Provider Identifier (NPI) numbers, 1199
   preauthorization, 1198-1199, 1201b-1202b
   precertification, 1198-1199, 1201b-1202b
   referrals, 1200
   requirements, 1198
   self-referrals, 1200
  reimbursement tracking, 1210-1211
  reimbursements, 1192-1193
  terminology of, 1190, 1214b-1215b
  types of, 1193-1198
   armed services members/dependents and veterans, 1197
   Children's Health Insurance Program (CHIP), 1197
   exclusive provider organizations (EPOs), 1195
   fee-for-service plans, 1193-1194
   government plans, 1196-1198
   health maintenance organizations (HMOs), 1195
   independent practice associations (IPAs), 1195
   managed care plans, 1194-1195
   Medicaid, 1197
   Medicare, 1196-1198, 1196f
   point-of-service (POS) plans, 1195
   preferred provider organizations (PPOs), 1195
   worker's compensation insurance, 1197-1198
  Web resources for, 1216b
Medical microbiology, 896-912
  case studies of, 899b, 906b-907b, 911b-913b
  definition of, 897
  historical reviews of, 897-898
  infections, 898
   definition of, 898
   infectious disease stages, 898
  introduction to, 897-898
  microorganisms and disease, 899-901
   bacilli, 899
   bacteria, 899-900, 899f-900f
   cocci, 899
   prevention and control, 912
   spirilla, 900
   streptococci, 899
   viruses, 900-901
  microscopes, 901-903, 901f, 903b-905b
   gram stain, 911-912
   microorganism examinations, 909-912
   smears, 911
   wet mount methods, 909-911
  normal flora, 898
  procedures for, 903b-905b, 908b
  sensitivity testing, 909, 910f
  specimen collection, 906-907
   collection guidelines, 907
   handling guidelines, 906-907
   procedures for, 908b
   transport system, 907, 907f
   transporting guidelines, 906-907
  streptococcus testing, 909, 910f, 911b
  terminology of, 897, 913b
  Web resources for, 914b
Medical necessity, 1185
Medical offices, 10-12
  business office areas, 11-12
  Clinical Laboratory Improvement Amendments (CLIA 1988) regulations for,
   10-11

Nutrition *(Continued)*
    definition of, 936
    Dietary Approaches to Stop Hypertension (DASH) eating plan, 936-937, 936*t*
    nutrition therapy for, 936-937
    sodium intake, 937, 937*b*
  introduction to, 916
  kilocalories (kcal), 917
  lactose intolerance and, 939-940
    definition of, 939
    nutrition therapy for, 939-940, 940*f*
  medications and, 942
  minerals, 923-924
    definition of, 923
    major, 924, 926*t*
    trace, 924, 926*t*
  National Academy of Sciences, Food and Nutrition Board, 917
  nutrients, 917
    classification of, 917-918, 917*t*
    definition of, 916-917
    density, 917
    macronutrients, 917, 917*t*
    micronutrients, 917-918
    roles of, 917
  poor, 917
  proteins, 921-922
    amino acids, 922. *See also* Amino acids.
    classification of, 922
    complementary, 922
    complete, 922
    definition of, 921
    incomplete, 922
  supplements and, 942
  terminology of, 916-917, 942*b*-943*b*
  tools for, 928-942
  vegetarianism, 921*b*-922*b*
  vitamins, 922-923
    antioxidant, 923, 925*f*
    classification of, 922-923
    definition of, 922
    fat-soluble, 923, 925*t*
    water-soluble, 923, 923*f*, 924*t*
  water, 925-927
  weight management, 932-935
    body mass index (BMI), 932-934, 934*t*
    eating disorders, 933*b*-934*b*
    obesity, 932-934
Nutrition Facts panels, 930-931, 930*f*

O

Obesity, 932-934
Objective data, 995
Obliques
  external, 143
  internal, 143
Obstetrics and gynecology, 13*b*-14*b*
Occupational Safety and Health Administration (OSHA), 10, 290-314, 1111
Occupational therapy reports, 1006
OCR. *See* Optical character recognition (OCR).
Office checks, 1026
Office computerization, 1040-1059
  backup protocols, 1058
  case studies of, 1046*b*, 1053*b*, 1055*b*, 1059*b*-1060*b*
  computer monitors, 1048-1049
    care/maintenance of, 1048-1049
    ergonomics of, 1048
    types of, 1048, 1048*f*
  computer network security, 1057-1058
    antivirus software, 1058
    audit controls, 1058
    authentication, 1057-1058
    authorization levels, 1058
    firewalls, 1058
  computer system components, 1043-1046, 1043*f*
    application software, 1044-1045
    care/maintenance of, 1047-1048
    central processing units (CPUs), 1047
    data entry, 1045, 1045*f*
    documentation, 1046
    file formats, 1045-1046
    hardware, 1046
    main computer memory, 1047
    main computer units, 1046-1048
    medical practice management programs, 1044
    microprocessors, 1047
    operating systems, 1043-1044, 1044*b*

Office computerization *(Continued)*
    programs, 1042, 1044-1045
    random-access memory (RAM), 1047
    software, 1043-1046
    spreadsheet programs, 1044
    storage capacity, 1047
    system requirements, 1047
    system software, 1043-1044
    telecommunications applications, 1044
    voice recognition software, 1045
    word processing software, 1044
  data processing cycles, 1042-1043, 1043*f*
    data processing, definition of, 1042
    input, 1043, 1043*f*
    input devices, 1043
    output, 1043, 1043*f*
    output devices, 1043
    processing, 1043, 1043*f*
  electronic information transfer, 1055-1057
    of billing information, 1056
    E-mail, 1056
    E-prescribing, 1056-1057
    encryption and, 1056
    of insurance information, 1056
    Internet, 1055-1056
    patient portals, 1056
    World Wide Web, 1056
  electronic medical records (EMRs), 1057
    medical assistants use of, 1057
    physicians use of, 1057
  fundamental computer concepts, 1042
    cloud computing, 1042
    computer types, 1042*b*
    computers, definition of, 1042
    local area networks (LANs), 1042
    microcomputers, 1042
    networks, 1042
    servers, 1042
    wide area networks (WANs), 1042
  input devices, 1049-1050
    care/maintenance of, 1050
    computer keyboards, 1049
    ergonomics of, 1049-1050, 1050*f*
    mouse, 1049
    QWERTY keyboard layouts, 1049
    special keys, 1049
    touchscreens, 1049
  introduction to, 1042
  medical office computerization, 1053-1055
    advantages of, 1054
    care/maintenance of, 1055
    definition of, 1041
    disadvantages of, 1054
    efficient operation of, 1055
    impact of, 1053
    malfunctions of, 1055
    prerequisite computer concepts, 1053
    qualified operators of, 1055
    selection criteria of, 1055
  printers, 1050-1052
    care/maintenance of, 1051-1052
    hard copy, 1050
    inkjet, 1051
    laser, 1051, 1051*f*
    wireless, 1051
Office manager roles, 1233-1251
  case studies of, 1236*b*-1237*b*, 1244*b*, 1248*b*-1249*b*, 1252*b*-1253*b*
  equipment maintenance, 1240-1241
    function monitoring, 1241, 1242*b*
    new equipment purchases, 1241
    readiness for use monitoring, 1241
    service calls, 1241
    service contracts, 1241
  introduction to, 1234
  office maintenance, 1234-1236
    administrative areas, 1234-1235, 1235*f*
    examination/treatment rooms, 1235
    security systems, 1235-1236
  payroll preparation, 1246-1247
    check preparation, 1247
    deductions, 1247
    employer obligations, 1247
    Federal Insurance Contributions Acts (FICA) deductions, 1247
    federal unemployment tax (FUTA), 1247
    income taxes, 1247

Office manager roles *(Continued)*
    Medicare taxes, 1247
    Social Security taxes, 1247
    state taxes, 1247
    W-2 forms, 1247
    W-4 forms, 1247
  procedures for, 1239*b*-1240*b*, 1242*b*, 1245*b*, 1249*b*-1250*b*, 1252*b*-1253*b*
  resources provision, 1248-1249
    community resources, 1249, 1249*b*-1250*b*
    Health Insurance Portability and Accountability Act (HIPAA) and, 1248
    office policy and procedure manuals, 1248
    written procedures, 1249
  risk management, 1250-1251
    compliance reporting, 1251
    definition of, 1250
    incident reports, 1251, 1252*b*
    liability insurance, 1251
    Patient Protection and Affordable Care Act (PPACA) and, 1251
    risk minimization, 1250
  routine maintenance, 1236-1237
    cabinet/drawer cleaning, 1237, 1237*f*
    general cleaning, 1236-1237
    miscellaneous tasks, 1237
    temperature, 1236
    ventilation, 1236
  safety maintenance, 1237-1239
    environmental safety, 1238, 1239*b*-1240*b*
    ergonomics, 1238*b*
    safe work practices, 1238, 1238*b*
    signs and instructions, 1239, 1239*f*, 1240*b*
  schedule management, 1247-1248
    employee schedules, 1248
    per diem employees, 1248
    physician schedules, 1247-1248
  supplies maintenance, 1242-1244
    backorders, 1244
    inventories, 1243, 1243*f*-1245*f*, 1245*b*
    ordering, 1243-1244
    purchase order (PO) numbers, 1243-1244
    receiving supplies, 1244
    restocking, 1243
  teamwork environments, 1245-1246
    employee orientations, 1246
    employee training, 1246
    medical assistant students, 1246, 1246*f*
    staff meetings, 1246
  terminology of, 1234, 1253*b*-1254*b*
  Web resources for, 1254*b*
Office surgery, 560-609
Offices, medical, 10-12
  business office areas, 11-12
  Clinical Laboratory Improvement Amendments (CLIA 1988) regulations for,
    10-11
  complex testing rooms, 12
  examination rooms, 11, 11*f*
  laboratories, 11
  layouts of, 10-12, 10*f*
  lunch/break rooms, 12
  medical records storage, 11-12
  Occupational Safety and Health Administration (OSHA) regulations for, 10
  Occupational Safety and Health Administration (OSHA) standards for, 10
  patient progress through, 7*f*
  pediatric examination/treatment rooms, 12
  physician private offices, 12
  reception areas, 7*f*, 11
  staff rooms, 12
  surgical procedure rooms, 12
  trauma rooms, 12
  waiting rooms, 11
Oliguria, 787
Online postage services, 1143
Open questions, 65
Opening procedures, 1026-1027, 1028*b*. *See also* Patient reception.
  daily activities organization, 1026
  equipment checks, 1026-1027
  fax checks, 1026
  message checks, 1026
  office checks, 1026
  patient charts, 1026
  safety checks, 1026-1027, 1027*f*
  tickler files, 1026
  waiting room checks, 1026
Optical character recognition (OCR), 1138
Oral communication, 62
Oral temperature, 355-356. *See also* Temperature.

Orbicularis
  oculi, 140-143
  oris, 140-143
Organizational skills, 24
Organizations, professional, 28
Orientation procedures, 1036-1037
  call-in times, 1036
  informational materials, 1037
  for new/prospective patients, 1036, 1037*b*-1038*b*
  patient understanding facilitation, 1036-1037
  physician selection, 1036
Origin, muscle, 138
Orthopedic surgery, 13*b*-14*b*
OSHA. *See* Occupational Safety and Health Administration (OSHA).
Ossification, 121
Osteochondritis, 846-847
Osteogenesis, 121
Osteomyelitis, 846-847
Osteopathy, 14
OTC medications. *See* Over-the-counter (OTC) medications.
Otolaryngology, 13*b*-14*b*
Outgoing mail, 1142-1143. *See also* Mail/shipping.
  adding postage, 1142-1143
  envelope preparation, 1144*b*. *See also* Envelope preparation.
  folding/inserting letters, 1142, 1142*f*
  metered mail/postage meters, 1142-1143, 1143*b*
  online postage services, 1143
  safety precautions for, 1143
Outguides, 1101, 1102*f*
Outpatients, 1173
Outstanding balance policies, 1227-1228. *See also* Collections/billing.
Over-the-counter (OTC) medications, 1003
Overdrafts, 1220
Overdue accounts, 1223-1224. *See also* Account aging.
Overpayments, 1221. *See also* Billing/collections.
  credit balances, 1221, 1222*b*-1223*b*
  refunds, 1221, 1222*b*-1223*b*
Oxygen debt, 139-140

P
Package delivery services, 1136
Palliative treatments, 2
Parts of speech, 1122-1123
PAs. *See* Physician assistants (PAs).
Past due accounts, 1226. *See also* Collections/billing.
Past histories, 1008. *See also* Histories.
Pathology, 13*b*-14*b*
Pathology/Laboratory section, 1175. *See also* Current Procedural Terminology (CPT).
Patient accounts. *See also* Finance management.
  components of, 1148-1152
    charge slips/superbills, 1148-1149, 1150*f*, 1152*b*-1155*b*
    day sheets/daily journals, 1151-1152
    fee schedules, 1149
    superbills, 1148-1149
  introduction to, 1147
  maintenance of, 1147
    credits. *vs.* debits, 1151
    insurance write-offs, 1151
    posting adjustments, 1151, 1156*b*-1157*b*
    posting charges, 1155*b*
    posting payments, 1151, 1156*b*-1157*b*
  statements, 1218, 1219*f*, 1225*b*. *See also* Billing/collections.
    balance due, 1218
    processing of, 1220*b*
Patient charts, 1026. *See also* Opening procedures.
Patient check-in, 1029-1036
  assignment of benefits, 1029-1030
  confidentiality and, 1029, 1029*f*
  of established patients, 1033-1034
  forms
    managed care referrals, 1033
    Notice of Privacy Practices (NPP) acknowledgements, 1030, 1033*f*
    patient histories, 1030
    patient information, 1030, 1031*f*-1032*f*
  Health Insurance Portability and Accountability Act (HIPAA) and, 1030
  insurance verification/authorization, 1030-1032
  of new patients, 1029-1033
  patient waiting notifications, 1036
Patient information forms, 1030, 1031*f*-1032*f*
Patient interactions, 61-77
  case studies of, 65*b*, 68*b*, 72*b*, 74*b*, 77*b*-78*b*
  communication, 62-68
    barriers to, 67-68
    body language, 62
    feedback, 62

Patient interactions *(Continued)*
  inhibitors of, 66-67, 67*t*
  interference with, 62-63
  judgmental, 66
  models of, 62, 63*f*
  styles of, 65-66
  verbal *vs.* nonverbal, 62, 63*f*
cultural influences, 76-77
emotional responses to illness, 72-74
  anger, 74
  anxiety, 73-74
  ego defense mechanisms, 74*b*-75*b*
  grieving process, 75-76. *See also* Grieving process.
  guilt, 72-73
  loss of control, 73
interviewing techniques, 65-67
  closed questions, 65
  open questions, 65
introduction to, 62
listening skills, 64-65
  active listening, 64, 66*t*
  nonverbal facilitation measures, 64-65, 64*f*
patient needs, 69-77
  behavioral impact of, 69-70
  care relationship establishment, 70-72
  developmental stages and, 70
  empathy, 70-71
  Erickson's stages of psychosocial development, 70, 70*t*
  health care expectations, 69
  Maslow's hierarchy of needs, 69, 69*f*
procedures for, 71*b*
self-boundaries, 72, 73*b*
terminology of, 62, 78*b*
Web resources for, 79*b*
Patient navigation, 31
Patient orientation, 1036-1037
  call-in times, 1036
  informational materials, 1037
  for new/prospective patients, 1036, 1037*b*-1038*b*
  patient understanding facilitation, 1036-1037
  physician selection, 1036
Patient portals, 1056
Patient Protection and Affordable Care Act (2010), 6
Patient reception, 1025-1037
  case studies of, 1029*b*, 1034*b*, 1037*b*-1039*b*
  closing procedures, 1027, 1028*b*
  copayment acceptance, 1034
  introduction to, 1025
  Notice of Privacy Practices (NPP), 1025
  opening procedures, 1026-1027, 1028*b*
    daily activities organization, 1026
    equipment checks, 1026-1027
    fax checks, 1026
    message checks, 1026
    office checks, 1026
    patient charts, 1026
    safety checks, 1026-1027, 1027*f*
    tickler files, 1026
    waiting room checks, 1026
  patient check-in, 1029-1036
    assignment of benefits, 1029-1030
    confidentiality and, 1029, 1029*f*
    of established patients, 1033-1034
    forms, managed care referrals, 1033
    forms, Notice of Privacy Practices (NPP) acknowledgements, 1030, 1033*f*
    forms, patient histories, 1030
    forms, patient information, 1030, 1031*f*-1032*f*
    Health Insurance Portability and Accountability Act (HIPAA) and, 1030
    insurance verification/authorization, 1030-1032
    of new patients, 1029-1033
    patient waiting notifications, 1036
  patient orientation, 1036-1037
    call-in times, 1036
    informational materials, 1037
    for new/prospective patients, 1036, 1037*b*-1038*b*
    patient understanding facilitation, 1036-1037
    physician selection, 1036
  procedures for, 1027*b*-1028*b*, 1035*b*-1038*b*
  terminology of, 1025, 1039*b*
  Web resources for, 1039*b*
Patient status designations. *See also* Current Procedural Terminology (CPT).
  established, 1173
  inpatients, 1173
  new patients, 1173
  outpatients, 1173

Patient understanding facilitation, 1036-1037
Patient waiting
  notifications, 1036
  rooms, 11
Patient-centered medical home (PCMH), 12-14
Payroll preparation, 1246-1247
PCMH. *See* Patient-centered medical home (PCMH).
Pectoralis major, 144
Pediatric examination/treatment rooms, 12
Pediatrics, 13*b*-14*b*, 529-556
Peer support, 1267
Pelvic diaphragm, 143
Per diem employees, 1248
Periosteum, 121, 121*f*
Peroneus muscles, 147
Personal boundaries, 72
Personal demographic sections, 1257. *See also* Résumés.
Personality traits, 22
Petty cash, 1157
pH, 794-795
Phlebotomy, 814-851
  blood specimens, 822-823
    anticoagulants and, 823, 823*f*
    clotted blood, 822
    plasma, 823
    serum, 823
    whole blood, 823
  butterfly method of, 835-836
    guidelines for, 836, 836*f*-837*f*
    procedures for, 837*b*-842*b*
  case studies of, 818*f*, 824*b*, 837*b*, 852*b*
  definition of, 815
  finger puncture guidelines, 850-851, 851*f*
  introduction to, 815
  microcollecton devices, 850
    capillary tubes, 850
    microcollection tubes, 850
  Occupational Safety and Health Administration (OSHA) standards for, 823-825
  phlobotomists, 815
  problems encountered with, 842-845, 843*f*
    collapsing veins, 844
    failure to obtain blood, 842
    hematomas, 844
    hemolysis, 844
    inappropriate puncture sites, 843
    premature needle withdrawal, 844
    rolling veins, 843
    scarred veins, 843
    sclerosed veins, 843
    vasovagal syncope (fainting), 844*b*, 845
  procedures for, 830*b*-835*b*, 837*b*-842*b*, 848*b*-850*b*
  serum specimens, 845-846
    serum removal, 845, 845*f*
    serum separator tubes (SSTs), 845-846, 846*f*
    serum, definition of, 845
    specimen preparation, 845
    tube selection for, 845
  skin punctures, 846
    devices for, 846-848
    disposable semiautomatic lancets, 847, 847*f*
    procedures for, 848*b*-850*b*
    site of, 846
  terminology of, 815, 852*b*-853*b*
  vacuum tube method, 824-829, 824*f*
    evacuated tubes, 825-827, 826*f*-827*f*
    guidelines for, 828-829, 829*f*
    multiple tubes, order draw for, 827-828, 828*t*
    needles, 824-825, 825*f*
    plastic holders, 825
    procedures for, 830*b*-835*b*
    satiety-engineered devices, 825, 826*f*
  venipuncture, 815-824
    alternative sites for, 822, 823*f*
    collection requirements, 816, 817*f*
    equipment and supplies for, 816, 816*f*, 818*f*
    guidelines for, 816
    handling requirements, 816, 817*f*
    patient identification, 816
    patient positions, 818-819, 819*f*
    patient preparation for, 816
    patient reassurance, 818
    site selection for, 821-822, 821*f*
    tourniquet application, 819-821, 820*f*-821*f*
  Web resources for, 853*b*
Phlobotomists, 815

Phone techniques. *See* Telephone techniques.
Photocopying, 1128
　collation and, 1128
　duplex, 1128
Physical examinations, 405-436
　codes for, 1173. *See also* Medical coding.
　pediatric, 529-556
　specialty, 719-748
Physical medicine and rehabilitation, 13*b*-14*b*
Physical therapy reports, 1006
Physician assistants (PAs), 8
Physician private offices, 12. *See also* Medical offices.
Physician schedules, 1247-1248
Physician selection, 1036
Physicians, 8
Physiology and anatomy
　body systems
　　circulatory, 196-216
　　digestive, 235-248
　　endocrine, 186-195
　　integumentary, 111-115
　　muscular, 136-147
　　nervous, 151-168
　　reproductive, 266-283
　　respiratory, 224-230
　　skeletal, 118-133
　　urinary, 254-264
　fundamentals of, 80-105
　senses, 173-182
PI. *See* Present illness (PI).
Pituitary gland (hypophysis), 188-192, 191*f*
Place of service codes, 1205*t*
Plantar flexion, 140, 141*f*-142*f*
Plastic surgery, 13*b*-14*b*
Podiatry, 14-15
Point-of-service (POS) plans, 1195
Polycythemia, 855
Polyuria, 787
POMRs. *See* Problem-oriented medical records (POMRs).
Poor nutrition, 917. *See also* Nutrition.
Popliteal pulse, 372
PORs. *See* Problem-oriented records (PORs).
Portals, patient, 1056
POS plans. *See* Point-of-service (POS) plans.
Postage meters, 1142-1143, 1143*b*
Postal addressing standards, 1139-1141
　addresses
　　complete, 1139
　　format of, 1139-1141
　　return, 1141
　　specific delivery, 1140*b*
　　two-letter state/territory abbreviations, 1140*t*
　large envelopes, 1139
　letters, 1139
Postal bar code system, 1132, 1133*f*
Postal money orders, 1136
Posterior tibial pulse, 372
Posthrombin time/International Normalized Ratio (PT/INR) tests, 866-868
　coagulation analyzers, 867, 867*f*
　home testing, 867-868, 867*f*-868*f*
　purpose of, 866
　specimen collection for, 866-867, 867*f*
Potential employer identification, 1256
PPOs. *See* Preferred provider organizations (PPOs).
Practice finance management, 1146-1166
Practice types, 15-16
　clinics, 16
　group practice, 15
　solo practice, 15
Practicums/externships, 21
Preauthorization, 1198-1199, 1201*b*-1202*b*
Precertification, 1198-1199, 1201*b*-1202*b*
Preferred provider organizations (PPOs), 1195
Prefixes, 1104
Pregnancy testing, 807-808
　guidelines for, 808
　human chorionic gonadotropin (HCG), 807
　immunoassays, 807-808
　procedures for, 809*b*-811*b*
　quality control logs for, 809*f*
　vs. radioimmunoassay (RIA), 808-809
　serum, 808-809
Preliminary diagnoses, 1002
Prenatal care, 487-521
Preparedness, emergency, 944-964

Prepositions, 1123
Present illness (PI), 1007-1008
Preventive medicine, 13*b*-14*b*
Primary care, 12-14
Prime movers, 140
Printed signatures, 1117, 1118*f*. *See also* Business letters.
Printers, 1050-1052
Private carrier package delivery services, 1136
Private offices, 12. *See also* Medical offices.
Probate laws, 1229
Problem-oriented medical records (POMRs), 994-995
Problem-oriented records (PORs), 994-995. *See also* Medical records.
　database establishment, 995
　organization of, 994-995
　plans, 995
　problem lists, 995, 995*f*
　　development of, 995
　　problem, definition of, 992
　progress notes, 995
　SOAP progress, 995, 996*f*
Procedure codes, 1169. *See also* Medical coding.
　Centers for Medicare and Medicaid Services (CMS) and, 1169
　definition of, 1169
　Health Insurance Portability and Accountability Act (HIPPA) and, 1169
Procedure reports, 1005. *See also* Medical records.
　components of, 1005
　　electrocardiogram (ECG) reports, 1005
　　Holter monitor reports, 1005
　　imaging reports, 1005
　　radiology reports, 1005
　　spirometry reports, 1005
　description of, 1005
Procedure rooms, 12
Procedures
　for billing/collections, 1220*b*-1223*b*, 1225*b*, 1231*b*
　for blood chemistry, 784*b*
　for business letters, 1121*b*-1122*b*
　cardiopulmonary, 687-716
　emergency medical, 967-988
　eye, 441-458
　for hematology, 858*b*-860*b*, 863*b*-865*b*
　for immunology, 784*b*
　for mail/shipping, 1137*b*-1138*b*, 1141*b*
　for medical assistant profession, 24*b*
　for medical coding, 1175*b*-1177*b*, 1185*b*-1187*b*
　for medical insurance, 1200*b*-1202*b*, 1205*b*-1209*b*, 1213*b*
　for medical microbiology, 903*b*-905*b*, 908*b*
　for medical records management, 1102*b*-1103*b*, 1107*b*-1108*b*, 1110*b*
　minor office surgery, 560-609
　for office manager roles, 1239*b*-1240*b*, 1242*b*, 1249*b*-1250*b*, 1252*b*-1253*b*
　for patient interactions, 71*b*
　for patient reception, 1027*b*-1028*b*, 1035*b*-1038*b*
　for phlebotomy, 830*b*-835*b*, 837*b*-842*b*, 848*b*-850*b*
　specialty, 719-748
　for urinalysis, 790*b*-791*b*, 797*b*-799*b*, 804*b*-807*b*, 809*b*-811*b*
　for written communications, 1121*b*-1122*b*, 1127*b*-1128*b*
Prodromal period, 898
Professional appearance, 21-23, 21*f*-23*f*
Professional appearance considerations, 1263-1264, 1264*f*
Professional medical assistant concepts
　administrative components
　　appointment scheduling, 1078-1093
　　billing/collections, 1217-1230
　　job-seeking/employment considerations, 1255-1268
　　mail/shipping, 1131-1143
　　medical coding, 1168-1185
　　medical insurance, 1189-1212
　　medical office computerization, 1040-1059
　　medical records, 991-1021
　　medical records management, 1098-1112
　　office manager roles, 1233-1251
　　patient reception, 1025-1037
　　practice finance management, 1146-1166
　　telephone techniques, 1063-1075
　　written communications, 1115-1128
　anatomy and physiology
　　circulatory system, 196-216
　　digestive system, 235-248
　　endocrine system, 186-195
　　fundamentals of, 80-105
　　integumentary system, 111-115
　　muscular system, 136-147
　　nervous system, 151-168
　　reproductive systems, 266-283
　　respiratory system, 224-230

Professional medical assistant concepts *(Continued)*
  senses, 173-182
  skeletal system, 118-133
  urinary system, 254-264
  clinical components
    blood chemistry, 870-891
    cardiopulmonary procedures, 687-716
    clinical laboratories, 752-783
    ear assessments/procedures, 441-458
    emergency medical procedures, 967-988
    emergency preparedness, 944-964
    eye assessments/procedures, 441-458
    first aid, 967-988
    gynecologic examinations, 487-521
    hematology, 854-868
    immunology, 870-891
    intravenous (IV) therapy administration, 613-683
    medical asepsis, 290-314
    medical microbiology, 896-912
    medications, 613-683
    minor office surgery, 560-609
    nutrition, 915-942
    Occupational Safety and Health Administration (OSHA) standards,
      290-314
    pediatric examinations, 529-556
    phlebotomy, 814-851
    physical examinations, 405-436
    prenatal care, 487-521
    protective practices, 944-964
    specialty examinations/procedures, 719-748
    sterilization/disinfection, 318-345
    tissue healing physical agents, 467-479
    urinalysis, 786-809
    vital signs, 350-396
  fundamentals
    health care system, 1-16
    medical assistant profession, 19-31
    medical ethics and law, 34-57
    patient interactions, 61-77
Professional organizations, 28
  employment considerations and, 1267
Pronation, 140, 141*f*-142*f*
Pronouns, 1123
Proofreading, 1125
Proper nouns, 1122-1123
Prospective patients, 1036, 1037*b*-1038*b*
Protective practices and emergency preparedness, 944-964
Proteins, 921-922
  amino acids, 922. *See also* Amino acids.
  classification of, 922
  complementary, 922
  complete, 922
  definition of, 921
  incomplete, 922
Provisional diagnoses, 1002
Psychiatry, 13*b*-14*b*
PT/INR tests. *See* Posthrombin time/International Normalized Ratio (PT/INR)
    tests.
Pulled hamstrings, 147
Pulse. *See also* Vital signs.
  apical, 371, 372*f*
  apical-radial, 373
  bounding, 373
  brachial, 371-372
  carotid, 372
  dorsalis pedis, 372
  femoral, 372
  radial, 371
  thready, 373
  ulnar, 372
Punctuation and grammar, 1122-1125
  comma rules, 1124-1125
  confusing word pairs, 1125*b*
  definitions of, 1122
  sentences, 1124. *See also* Sentences.
Pyuria, 787

Q
Quadriceps femoris, 147
Quads, 138*b*
Questions
  closed, 65
  open, 65
  and responses, 1264, 1265*b*
QWERTY keyboard layouts, 1049

R
Radial pulse, 371. *See also* Pulse.
Radiation, 352
Radioimmunoassay (RIA), 808-809
Radiology, 13*b*-14*b*
  reports, 1005
  section, 1175. *See also* Current Procedural Terminology (CPT).
Random specimens, 788
Rapid streptococcus tests, 909
RBCs. *See* Red blood cells (RBCs).
Reagent strips, 796-797, 796*f*, 797*b*-799*b*
Reception, 1025-1037
  areas, 7*f*, 11
  case studies of, 1029*b*, 1034*b*, 1037*b*-1039*b*
  closing procedures, 1027, 1028*b*
  copayment acceptance, 1034
  introduction to, 1025
  Notice of Privacy Practices (NPP), 1025
  opening procedures, 1026-1027, 1028*b*
    daily activities organization, 1026
    equipment checks, 1026-1027
    fax checks, 1026
    message checks, 1026
    office checks, 1026
    patient charts, 1026
    safety checks, 1026-1027, 1027*f*
    supplies checks, 1026-1027
    tickler files, 1026
    waiting room checks, 1026
  patient check-in, 1029-1036
    assignment of benefits, 1029-1030
    confidentiality and, 1029, 1029*f*
    of established patients, 1033-1034
    forms, managed care referrals, 1033
    forms, Notice of Privacy Practices acknowledgements, 1030, 1033*f*
    forms, patient histories, 1030
    forms, patient information, 1030, 1031*f*-1032*f*
    Health Insurance Portability and Accountability Act (HIPAA) and, 1030
    insurance verification/authorization, 1030-1032
    of new patients, 1029-1033
    patient waiting notifications, 1036
  patient orientation, 1036-1037
    call-in times, 1036
    informational materials, 1037
    for new/prospective patients, 1036, 1037*b*-1038*b*
    patient understanding facilitation, 1036-1037
    physician selection, 1036
  procedures for, 1027*b*-1028*b*, 1035*b*-1038*b*
  terminology of, 1025, 1039*b*
  Web resources for, 1039*b*
Records, medical, 991-1021. *See also* Medical records.
Rectal temperature, 356, 363*b*-364*b*. *See also* Temperature.
Rectus
  abdominis, 143
  femoris, 147
Red blood cells (RBCs), 862*f*
  counts, 861
  indices, 861
Reform, health care, 6
Refunds, 1221, 1222*b*-1223*b*. *See also* Billing/collections.
Registered Mail, 1133-1135
Registered medical assistant (RMA), 27
Registered nurses (RNs), 8
Registered phlebotomy technician (RPT), 27
Rehabilitation and physical medicine, 13*b*-14*b*
Reimbursements, 1192-1193
Reproductive systems, 266-283
Residencies, 8
Respiration
  aerobic, 139
  anaerobic, 139
Respiratory system, 224-230
Restricted Delivery, 1134
Résumés, 1256-1261
  action verbs in, 1260*f*
  activity sections in, 1260
  chronological, 1257, 1258*f*
  cover letters and, 1261, 1262*f*
  credential sections of, 1260
  definition of, 1255
  education sections in, 1257
  examples of, 1258*f*-1260*f*
  formatting of, 1261
  functional, 1257, 1259*f*
  mailing of, 1261-1262

Résumés (Continued)
  objective sections in, 1257
  personal demographic sections in, 1257
  previous experience sections in, 1257-1259
  reference sections of, 1261
  required information in, 1257-1261
  special skills sections of, 1259-1260
  styles of, 1257
  targeted, 1257, 1260f
Retention requirements, 1112
Return address vs. letterhead, 1116, 1118f. See also Business letters.
Return keys, 1049
Return Receipt, 1133-1134, 1135f
Reverse chronological order, 994
Review of systems (ROS), 1008
RIA. See Radioimmunoassay (RIA).
Right justification, 1117-1120
Rigor mortis, 138b
Risk management, 1250-1251
RMA. See Registered medical assistant (RMA).
RNs. See Registered nurses (RNs).
Rolling veins, 843
ROS. See Review of systems (ROS).
Rotation, 140, 141f-142f
Rotation diets, 941-942
Rotator cuff muscles, 144
Routers, 1055-1056
Routine care, 5-6
RPT. See Registered phlebotomy technician (RPT).
Rubber tourniquets, 820, 820f
Run-on sentences, 1124. See also Sentences.

S
Safety considerations, 1026-1027, 1027f, 1143. See also Opening procedures.
Salary/benefit discussions, 1264
Salutation/greeting, 1116-1117, 1118f. See also Business letters.
Sarcolemma, 137-138
Sarcoplasm, 137-138
Sartorius, 147
Saturated fats, 920. See also Fats.
Savings accounts, 1157. See also Banking activities.
Scarred veins, 843
Schedule management, 1247-1248
  employee schedules, 1248
  patient appointments, 1078-1093
  per diem employees, 1248
  physician schedules, 1247-1248
Sclerosed veins, 843
Secondary factor codes, 1174. See also Medical coding.
Secretaries, medical, 8
Secure messaging, 1126
Self-boundaries, 72, 73b
Semiblock style, 1117, 1119f
Semimembraneous muscle, 147
Semitendinous muscle, 147
Seniority terms, 1105
Senses, 173-182
Sensitivity testing, 909, 910f
Sentences, 1124
  classification of, 1124
    complex sentences, 1124
    compound sentences, 1124
    simple sentences, 1124
  definition of, 1124
  dependent vs. independent clauses, 1124
  errors in, 1124
    comma splices, 1124
    run-on sentences, 1124
    sentence fragments, 1124
Serum, 845
Serum pregnancy testing, 808-809. See also Pregnancy testing.
Serum specimens, 845-846. See also Phlebotomy.
Service agreements, 1059
Setting goals, 1256
Shelf filing units, 1099-1100
Shipping/mail, 1131-1143
  case studies for, 1134b, 1136b-1137b, 1143b, 1145b
  e-mail, 1125-1126. See also Electronic data transmission.
  incoming mail, 1136-1137
    annotations on, 1137
    opening guidelines, 1137
    processing of, 1136-1137, 1137b-1138b
    sorting guidelines, 1136, 1136t, 1138f
  introduction to, 1132
  outgoing mail, 1142-1143

Shipping/mail (Continued)
  adding postage, 1142-1143
  envelope preparation, 1144b. See also Envelope preparation.
  folding/inserting letters, 1142, 1142f
  metered mail/postage meters, 1142-1143, 1143b
  online postage services, 1143
  safety precautions for, 1143
private carrier package delivery services, 1136
procedures for, 1137b-1138b, 1141b
terminology of, 1132, 1145b
United States Postal Service (USPS), 1132-1136. See also United States Postal Service (USPS).
  automated mail processing, 1138, 1139b
  delivery confirmation services, 1133-1136
  insurance, 1133-1136
  postal addressing standards, 1139-1141
  postal bar code system, 1132, 1133f
  postal money orders, 1136
  Zone Improvement Plan (ZIP) code system, 1132, 1141b
Web resources for, 1145b
Shock, electrical, 138b
Sight impairments, 67-68
Signature Confirmation, 1134
Signatures. See also Business letters.
  handwritten, 1117, 1118f
  printed, 1117, 1118f
  witnessing of, 997
Simple carbohydrates, 918, 946f. See also Carbohydrates.
Simple sentences, 1124. See also Sentences.
Simplified block style, 1120, 1120f
Skeletal system, 118-133
  aging of, 133
  appendicular skeleton, 122f, 126
    bone names, 124t
    lower extremities, 130-131, 130f-131f
    pectoral girdle, 127, 128f
    pelvic girdle, 129-130, 129f
    upper extremities, 127-129, 128f
  articulations, 131-132
    amphiarthroses, 131
    definition of, 131
    diarthroses, 131-132, 132f
    synarthroses, 131
  axial skeleton, 122-127, 122f
    bone names, 124t
    hyoid bone, 125
    skull, 122-125, 123f-124f
    thoracic cage, 126-127, 127f
    vertebral column, 125-126, 126f
  bone classification, 120-121
    flat bones, 120
    inner vs. outter tables, 120
    irregular bones, 120-121
    long bones, 120-121, 121f
    short bones, 120
  bone development, 121
  bone growth in length, 121-122
  bone tissue structure, 119-120
    compact bone, 119, 120f
    lacunae, 120
    osteoblasts, 119, 121
    osteoclasts, 119, 121
    osteocytes, 118-119
    osteons, 120
    spongy (cancellous) bone, 120, 120f
    trabeculae, 120
  divisions of, 122, 122f
  functions of, 119
    movement, 119
    protection, 119
    storage, 119
    support, 119
  introduction to, 119
  overviews of, 119-122
  pathology of, 133t-134t
  terminology of, 119, 135b
  Web resources for, 135b
Skin punctures, 846. See also Phlebotomy.
Skips tracing, 1228-1229. See also Collections/billing.
Sliding filament theory, 139
Small claims court, 1229
Smears, 911
SOAP progress, 995, 996f
Social histories, 1008. See also Histories.
Sodium intake, 937, 937b

Soleus muscles, 147
Solo practice, 15
Soluble fiber, 919, 919f
Sorters, 1101
Sorting guidelines, 1136, 1136t, 1138f. See also Mail/shipping.
Special Handling mail, 1135
Specialties, 12-15, 13b-14b
    ambulatory care, 6-10
    American Board of Medical Specialties recognition of, 12, 13b-14b
    chiropractic, 15, 15f
    comparisons of, 13b-14b
    complementary and alternative medicine (CAM), 16
        acupuncture, 16, 16f
            National Center for Complementary and Alternative Medicine, 16
        traditional medicine, 16
    fellowships and, 12
    osteopathy, 14
    patient-centered medical home (PCMH), 12-14
    podiatry, 14-15
    primary care, 12-14
Specialty examinations/procedures, 719-748
Specific gravity, 792-793
Specimen collection, 906-907
Speech therapy reports, 1006
Speech, parts of, 1122-1123
Spelling, 1125, 1125b
Spirilla, 900
Spirometry reports, 1005
Splices, comma, 1124. See also Comma.
Spoken communication, 62
Staff rooms, 12
Stages of psychosocial development (Erickson), 70, 70t
Standard Post, 1133
Stasis, venous, 819-820
Statements, 1218, 1219f, 1225b. See also Billing/collections.
    balance due, 1218
    processing of, 1220b
Statute of limitations, 1112
Sterilization/disinfection, 318-345
Sternocleidomastoid mules, 143
Storage areas, 11-12
Storage equipment, 1099-1101
Streptococci, 899
Streptococcus testing, 909, 910f, 911b
Styles, business letters, 1117-1120. See also Business letters.
Subject filing systems, 1106. See also Filing systems.
Subjective data, 995
Supination, 140, 141f-142f
Supplements, dietary, 927-928
Suprapubic aspiration, 788
Surgery section, 1174-1175. See also Current Procedural Terminology (CPT).
Surgery, general, 13b-14b
Surgical procedure rooms, 12
Surnames, 1104. See also Names.
Symbols and abbreviations, 1012t-1014t, 1170-1171, 1170f
Symptomatic treatments, 2
Synaptic cleft (gap), 139
Synarthroses, 131
Synergists, 140
Systems
    circulatory, 196-216
    digestive, 235-248
    endocrine, 186-195
    fundamentals of, 80-105
    integumentary, 111-115
    muscular, 136-147
    nervous, 151-168
    reproductive, 266-283
    respiratory, 224-230
    senses, 173-182
    skeletal, 118-133
    urinary, 254-264

T
Tabs, 1102
Tabular list, 1180-1181, 1183-1185, 1183f
Tachycardia, 373
Targeted résumés, 1257, 1260f. See also Résumés.
Task lists, 24
TBs. See Terabytes (TBs).
Teams, 8-10
    definition of, 8
    effective teamwork, 9-10
    medical assistant roles in, 8
    members of, 8, 9t

Telecommunications applications, 1044
Telephone collections, 1227b. See also Collections/billing.
Telephone techniques, 1026, 1063-1075. See also Opening procedures.
Temperature. See also Vital signs.
    aural, 356, 365b-367b
    axillary, 356, 362b-363b
    ear, 356
    earlobe, 358
    forehead, 356
    oral, 355-356
    rectal, 356, 363b-364b
Templates, 1116. See also Business letters.
Temporal artery thermometers, 357-358, 358b, 358f, 367b-369b
Temporal pulse, 372
Temporalis muscle, 140-141
Tendons, 138
Tentative diagnoses, 1002
Terabytes (TBs), 1047
Terminal digit filing systems, 1106, 1106t. See also Filing systems.
Terminal phase, 75. See also Grieving process.
Terminology
    of billing/collections, 1217, 1232b
    of blood chemistry, 871
    of clinical laboratories, 753, 784b-785b
    of employment/job-seeking considerations, 1255, 1269b
    of endocrine system, 186, 195b
    of health care system, 1, 17b
    of hematology, 854, 869b
    of immunology, 871
    of mail/shipping, 1132, 1145b
    of medical assistant profession, 19, 32b
    of medical coding, 1169, 1188b
    of medical insurance, 1190, 1214b-1215b
    of medical microbiology, 897, 913b
    of medical records management, 1099, 1113b
    of muscular system, 136, 149b
    of nutrition, 916-917, 942b-943b
    of office manager roles, 1234, 1253b-1254b
    of patient interactions, 62, 78b
    of patient reception, 1025, 1039b
    of phlebotomy, 815, 852b-853b
    of skeletal system, 119, 135b
    of urinalysis, 787, 812b-813b
    of written communications, 1116, 1129b
Testing rooms, complex, 12
Tetanus, 138b
Therapeutic Lifestyle Changes (TLC) plan, 935t, 936
Therapeutic service documents, 1006
Thermometers, 356-359
    chemical, 358-359
    disposable single-use, 358-359
    electronic, 356, 359b-361b
Thoracic surgery, 13b-14b
Thready pulse, 373. See also Pulse.
Tibialis anterior, 147
Tickler files, 1026. See also Opening procedures.
Time management, 23-24
Tissue healing physical agents, 467-479
Title designations, 1117, 1118f. See also Business letters.
Titles, 1105
TLC plan. See Therapeutic Lifestyle Changes (TLC) plan.
Tourniquet application, 819-821, 820f-821f
Trace minerals, 924, 926t
Traditional medicine, 16
Trans fats, 920. See also Fats.
Transversus abdominis, 143
Trapezius muscle, 143-144
Trauma rooms, 12
Treatment/examination rooms, 12
TRICARE, 5, 1191, 1197
Triceps branchii, 144
Triglycerides, 921
Trimpeter's muscle, 140
Truth in lending agreements, 1227
Tympanic membrane thermometers, 356-357, 365b-367b

U
Ulnar pulse, 372. See also Pulse.
Uniform resource locators (URLs), 1056
United Parcel Service (UPS), 1136
United States Postal Service (USPS), 1132-1136
    automated mail processing, 1138, 1139b
    domestic mail classifications, 1132-1133
        First-Class Mail, 1132-1133
        Media Mail, 1133

United States Postal Service (USPS) (Continued)
  Priority Mail Express, 1132-1133
  Standard Post, 1133
  insurance and delivery confirmation services, 1133-1136
    Certificates of Mailing, 1133
    Certified Mail, 1133-1134, 1134f
    Collect on Delivery (COD), 1133, 1135-1136
    Insured Mail, 1135
    Registered Mail, 1133-1135
    Restricted Delivery, 1134
    Return Receipt, 1133-1134, 1135f
    Signature Confirmation, 1134
    Special Handling, 1135
  postal addressing standards, 1139-1141
  postal bar code system, 1132, 1133f
  postal money orders, 1136
  Zone Improvement Plan (ZIP) code system, 1132, 1141b
Universal Serial Bus (USB) ports, 1046
Unlisted codes, 1171. See also Medical coding.
Unsaturated fats, 920. See also Fats.
Upcoding, 1185. See also Medical coding.
UPS. See United Parcel Service (UPS).
Urgency, 787
Urinalysis, 786-809
  analysis parameters, 791-801
    appearance, 792, 792f
    bilirubin, 795
    blood, 795
    casts, 800
    chemical examinations, 793-796
    color, 792, 792f
    crystals, 800
    glucose, 795
    ketones, 795
    microscopic examinations, 800-801, 804b-807b
    nitrite, 795
    odor, 792
    pH, 794-795
    physical examinations, 791-793
    protein levels, 795
    specific gravity, 792-793
    urine sediment structures, 800-801, 801t-804t
    urobilinogen, 795
  case studies of, 788b, 793b, 800b, 808b, 811b
  definition of, 791
  pregnancy testing, 807-808
    guidelines for, 808
    human chorionic gonadotropin (HCG), 807
    immunoassays, 807-808
    procedures for, 809b-811b
    quality control logs for, 809f
    vs. radioimmunoassay (RIA), 808-809
    vs. serum pregnancy tests, 808-809
  procedures for, 790b-791b, 797b-799b, 804b-807b, 809b-811b
  terminology of, 787, 812b-813b
  testing kits, 793-794
    analyzers, 797, 797f
    guidelines for, 796
    quality control testing, 796-797
    reagent strips, 796-797, 796f, 797b-799b
  urinary tract infections (UTIs), 801b
  urine collection, 787-790
    clean-catch midstream specimens, 788-789, 790b-791b
    first-voided morning specimens, 788
    guidelines for, 787-788
    laboratory request forms, 786-787, 789f
    methods of, 788-789
    random specimens, 788
    twenty-four-hour specimens, 789-790
  urine composition, 787
  Web resources for, 813b
  workplace drug testing, 794b
Urinary incontinence, 787
Urinary system, 254-264
Urinary tract infections (UTIs), 801b
URLs. See Uniform resource locators (URLs).
Urology, 13b-14b
USB ports. See Universal Serial Bus (USB) ports.
USPS. See United States Postal Service (USPS).
UTIs. See Urinary tract infections (UTIs).

V
V codes, 1180, 1182
Vacuum tube method, 824-829, 824f. See also Phlebotomy.
Vascular surgery, 13b-14b

Vasovagal syncope (fainting), 844b, 845
Vastus
  intermedius, 147
  lateralis, 147
  medialis, 147
Vegetarianism, 921b-922b
Velcro-closure tourniquets, 820-821, 821f
Venipuncture, 815-824. See also Phlebotomy.
Venous reflux, 818-819
Venous stasis, 819-820
Verbs, 1123, 1125b
Verbs, action, 1260f
Verification, 1030-1032. See also Insurance.
Very-low-denisty lipoprotein (VLDL), 921
Viruses, 900-901
Visual impairments, 67-68
Vital signs, 350-396
  case studies of, 355b, 371b-372b., 375b
  introduction to, 352
  procedures for, 359b-369b
  pulse, 370-373, 371f, 371t
  respiration, 374-377, 374f-375f, 375t
  temperature, 352-359, 352f-354f, 353t-355t
  terminology of, 351, 401b-403b
  Web resources for, 404b
Vitamins, 922-923
  antioxidant, 923, 925f
  classification of, 922-923
  definition of, 922
  fat-soluble, 923, 925t
  water-soluble, 923, 923f, 924t
VLDL. See Very-low-denisty lipoprotein (VLDL).

W
Waiting rooms, 11, 1026
Water, 925-927
Water-soluble vitamins, 923, 923f, 924t. See also Vitamins.
WBCs. See White blood cells (WBCs).
Web browsers, 1056
Web resources
  for billing/collections, 1232b
  for clinical laboratories, 785b
  for employment/job-seeking considerations, 1270b
  for endocrine system, 195b
  for health care system, 18b
  for hematology, 854, 869b
  for mail/shipping, 1145b
  for medical assistant profession, 33b
  for medical coding, 1188b
  for medical insurance, 1216b
  for medical microbiology, 914b
  for medical records management, 1114b
  for muscular system, 150b
  for office manager roles, 1254b
  for patient interactions, 79b
  for patient reception, 1039b
  for phlebotomy, 853b
  for skeletal system, 135b
  for urinalysis, 813b
  for written communications, 1130b
Weight management, 932-935
Wet mount methods, 909-911
White blood cells (WBCs), 862f
  counts, 861
  differential counts, 862-863, 863b-865b
White line (linea alba), 143
WHO. See World Health Organization (WHO).
Witnessing signatures, 997
Word pairs, confusing, 1125b
Workplace drug testing, 794b
World Health Organization (WHO)
  health definitions, 2
  International Classification of Diseases (ICD) and, 1179
Written communications, 1115-1128
  business letters, 1116-1120. See also Business letters.
    composition of, 1120, 1121b-1122b
    definition of, 1116
    enclosures (enc.), 1117
    equipment for, 1116
    examples of, 1118f-1120f
    format of, 1117-1120
    parts of, 1116-1117, 1118f
    set-up of, 1117
    styles of, 1117-1120
  case studies of, 1123b, 1125b-1126b, 1128, 1128b-1129b

Written communications *(Continued)*
  confidentiality statements, 1127*f*
  electronic data transmission, 1125-1127
    e-mail, 1125-1126
    e-mail attachments, 1126
    electronic medical records (EMRs), secure messaging in, 1126
    fax transmissions, 1127, 1127*b*-1128*b*, 1127*f*
  grammar and punctuation, 1122-1125
    comma rules, 1124-1125
    confusing word pairs, 1125*b*
    definitions of, 1122
    parts of speech, 1122-1123
    sentences, 1124. *See also* Sentences.
  Health Insurance Portability and Accountability Act (HIPPA) and, 1116
  introduction to, 62, 1116
  memorandum/memoranda (memo), 1116, 1123*f*

Written communications *(Continued)*
    photocopying, 1128
      collation and, 1128
      duplex, 1128
    procedures for, 1121*b*-1122*b*, 1127*b*-1128*b*
    proofreading, 1125
    spelling, 1125, 1125*b*
    terminology of, 1116, 1129*b*
    Web resources for, 1130*b*
Wryneck, 138*b*

Z
Z codes, 1182
ZIP code system. *See* Zone Improvement Plan (ZIP) code system.
Zone Improvement Plan (ZIP) code system, 1132, 1141*b*
Zygomatic arch, 140-143
Zygomaticus, 140-143